SURGICAL MANAGEMENT

Surgical Management

Edited by

SELWYN TAYLOR DM MCh FRCS Hon FRCSE Hon FCS(SA)
Dean Emeritus, Royal Postgraduate Medical School,
Hammersmith Hospital, London

GEOFFREY D. CHISHOLM ChM FRCS FRCSE
Professor of Surgery, University of Edinburgh
Honorary Consultant Urological Surgeon, Western General Hospital, Edinburgh
Honorary Senior Lecturer, Institute of Urology, London

NIALL O'HIGGINS BSc MCh FRCSI FRCS FRCSE
Professor of Surgery, University College Dublin
Consultant Surgeon, St Vincent's Hospital, Dublin
Honorary Consultant, National Maternity Hospital, Dublin

ROBERT SHIELDS MD FRCS FRCSE
Professor of Surgery and Dean, Faculty of Medicine, University of Liverpool
Consultant Surgeon, Royal Liverpool and Broadgreen Hospitals, Liverpool

WILLIAM HEINEMANN MEDICAL BOOKS LTD
LONDON

First published 1984
Reprinted 1985

© Selwyn Taylor, G.D. Chisholm, N. O'Higgins, R. Shields 1984

First published as a paperback, 1986

ISBN 0 433 32209 8

Typeset by Phoenix Photosetting, Chatham
Printed and bound in Great Britain by
Butler & Tanner Ltd, Frome and London

Contents

Editors' foreword

It is over fifty years since C.C. Choyce of University College Hospital in London edited a comprehensive work for the practising surgeon and there has been little that is comparable published since that time other than Souttar's *British Surgery*. Other broadly based books have been designed primarily to help senior students achieve qualification to higher diplomas and we hope that this volume may do this.

The present work has, however, been undertaken for the benefit of the practising general surgeon, covering advances in diagnosis, principles of treatment, possible major complications and the available modern procedures in patient care. Thus our aim has been to cover the subjects that constitute the daily task of a general surgeon in, for example, a district hospital; including paediatric and urological problems, chemotherapy and radiation in malignancy, head and neck surgery and much else.

Orthopaedics are omitted as being outside the scope of general surgery except for a discussion of the handling of disaster situations. On the other hand, some specialised subjects such as cardiovascular and brain surgery are included because a knowledge of the potential in these fields is necessary for the general surgeon who is so often involved, even if indirectly with such situations. In this respect we are particularly indebted to Professor Bentall for his help with the cardiothoracic section. The management of fluid and electrolyte balance, nutritional support, blood replacement, the control of clotting and the avoidance of pulmonary embolism all have a place in total patient care and receive attention.

It is our wish that this book should prove a real friend to surgeons of all persuasions, including those in training, refreshing knowledge in their own fields and giving access to that in others, so that they can appreciate the scope of surgical practice as a whole; the generality of surgery.

It will be noted that the four editors are recruited from London, Merseyside, Scotland and Ireland; that they thus constitute a Board broadly based in the teaching of British general surgery.

Selwyn Taylor,
London

Niall O'Higgins,
Dublin

Geoffrey Chisholm,
Edinburgh

Robert Shields,
Merseyside

November, 1983

List of contributors

C.A. BARTZOKAS, MD
Senior Lecturer and Hon Consultant in Medical Microbiology, University of Liverpool and Royal Liverpool Hospital.

P.R.F. BELL, MD FRCS
Professor of Surgery, University of Leicester; Hon Consultant Surgeon, Leicestershire Health Authority.

H.H. BENTALL, MB FRCS
Professor of Cardiac Surgery in the University of London at the Royal Postgraduate Medical School; Consultant Thoracic Surgeon, Hammersmith Hospital, London.

C.A.C. CHARLTON MB MS FRCS
Consultant Urologist, Bath Health District; formerly Consultant Urologist, St Bartholomew's Hospital, London.

A.D. CHEESMAN, FRCS
Consultant Otolaryngologist and Head and Neck Surgeon, Charing Cross Hospital, London; Surgeon, Royal National Throat, Nose and Ear Hospital, London.

GEOFFREY D. CHISHOLM, ChM FRCS FRCSE
Professor of Surgery, University of Edinburgh; Hon Consultant Urological Surgeon, Western General Hospital, Edinburgh; Hon Senior Lecturer, Institute of Urology, London.

RONALD G. CLARK MB ChB FRCS FRCSE
Professor of Surgery, University of Sheffield; Hon Consultant Surgeon, Northern General Hospital, Sheffield.

D.L. COPPEL, MB BCh FFARCS
Consultant Anaesthetist, Royal Victoria Hospital, Belfast.

L.T. COTTON, MCh FRCS
Dean, King's College Hospital School of Medicine and Dentistry; Consultant Surgeon; Director, Dept of Biomedical Engineering, King's College Hospital Medical School, London.

ALAN G. COX, MD FRCS
Consultant Surgeon, Northwick Park Hospital, Harrow.

G. CRUPI, MD
Chief Assistant, Ospedali Riuwiti, Bergamo, Italy.

ROBERT A. DICKSON, MA ChM FRCS FRCSE
Professor of Orthopaedic and Traumatic Surgery, University of Leeds.

HAROLD ELLIS, DM MCh FRCS
Professor of Surgery, Westminster Medical School, London.

R.B. GALLAND, MD FRCS
Senior Registrar, Dept of Surgery, Royal Postgraduate Medical School, Hammersmith Hospital, London.

ERIC S. GLEN FRCSG FRCSE
Consultant Urologist and Director, Walton Urological Teaching and Research Centre, Southern General Hospital, Glasgow; Hon Clinical Lecturer, University of Glasgow.

J.G. GOW, MD ChM FRCS
Emeritus Consultant Urologist, Liverpool Area Health Authority (Teaching).

H.H. GUNSON, DSc MD MRCP FRCPath
Director, Northwestern Regional Blood Transfusion Service; Reader in Human Serology, University of Manchester.

T.B. HARGREAVE, MS FRCS FRCSE
Senior Lecturer, University of Edinburgh; Hon Consultant Urological and Transplant Surgeon, Western General Hospital, Edinburgh.

D.F.N. HARRISON, MD MS FRCS HonFRACS HonFRCSE
Professor of Laryngology and Otology, Institute of Laryngology and Otology, University of London.

R.J. HEALD, MChir FRCS
Consultant Surgeon, Basingstoke Hospital, Hampshire.

J. HIBBERT, MA FRCS ChM
Consultant Otolaryngologist, Guy's Hospital, London.

J.R. HINDMARSH, MD FRCS FRCSE
Senior Lecturer, Institute of Urology, London; Hon Consultant Urologist, St Peter's Hospital, London.

C.W. IMRIE, BSc MB ChB FRCS
Consultant Surgeon, Royal Infirmary, Glasgow.

ALAN G. JOHNSON, MChir FRCS
Professor of Surgery, University of Sheffield.

PETER F. JONES, MChir FRCS
Consultant Surgeon, Woodend Hospital and Royal Aberdeen Children's Hospital; Clinical Professor of Surgery, University of Aberdeen; Surgeon to HM The Queen in Scotland.

R.M. KALBAG, BSc MBBS FRCS
Consultant Neurosurgeon, Newcastle General Hospital, Newcastle-upon-Tyne.

ALLAN E. KARK, FACS FRCS
Consultant Surgeon, Division of Clinical Sciences, Clinical Research Centre, Northwick Park Hospital, Harrow.

CHRISTOPHER LINCOLN, FRCS
Consultant Cardiac Surgeon, Brompton Hospital, London.

E. MCATEER, MB BCh FFARCS
Consultant Anaesthetist, Royal Victoria Hospital, Belfast.

K.C. MCKEOWN, CBE DL MCh FRCS FRCSE
Hon Senior Consultant Surgeon, Darlington Memorial Hospital; formerly Senior Consultant Surgeon, Friarage Hospital, Northallerton and Consultant Surgeon, Hospital of St. John of God, Scorton, Richmond, N. Yorks.

A.G.D. MARAN, MD FRCSE FACS
Head, Dept of Otolaryngology, University of Edinburgh; Consultant Otolaryngologist, The Royal Infirmary, Edinburgh.

JOHN MAYNARD, MS FRCS
Consultant Surgeon, Guy's Hospital, London; Chairman, Salivary Gland Tumour Panel.

W. CAMERON MOFFAT, OBE MB FRCS
Major General Late RAMC; Principal Medical Officer, United Kingdom Land Forces.

ANDREW NICOLAIDES MS FRCS FRCSE
Professor of Vascular Surgery; Director, Irvine Laboratory for Cardiovascular Investigation and Research; Hon Consultant Cardiovascular Surgeon, St Mary's Hospital.

C.S. OGG, MD BSC FRCP
Consultant Renal Physician, Guy's Hospital, London.

NIALL O'HIGGINS, BSc MCh FRCSI FRCS FRCSE
Professor of Surgery, University College Dublin; Consultant Surgeon, St Vincent's Hospital, Dublin; Hon Consultant, National Maternity Hospital, Dublin, Ireland.

M. PANETH, BM BCh FRCS
Cardiothoracic Surgeon, Brompton Hospital, London.

DONALD ROSS, DSc FRCS FACS
Consultant Surgeon, National Heart Hospital, London; Director of Surgery, Institute of Cardiology, London.

DOUGLAS ROY, MB ChB FRCS FRCSE FRCSG FRCSI
Professor of Surgery, Queen's University of Belfast; Consultant Surgeon, Royal Victoria Hospital, Belfast; formerly Professor of Surgery, University of Nairobi, Kenya.

ALAN A. SHARP (deceased), MA BSc MD FRCP FRCPath
Late Consultant Haematologist, John Radcliffe Hospital, Oxford; Lecturer in Haematology, University of Oxford; Consulting Haematologist to the RAF.

THOMAS SHERWOOD, MA MB FRCR FRCP
Professor of Radiology, University of Cambridge.

ROBERT SHIELDS, MD FRCS FRCSE
Professor of Surgery and Dean, Faculty of Medicine, University of Liverpool; Consultant Surgeon, Royal Liverpool and Broadgreen Hospitals, Liverpool; Member of Court of Examiners of Royal College of Surgeons of England.

P.M. STELL, ChM FRCS
Professor of Oto-Rhino-Laryngology, University of Liverpool; Consultant, Royal Liverpool Hospital.

SELWYN TAYLOR, DM MCh FRCS HonFRCSE HonFCS(SA)
Dean Emeritus, Royal Postgraduate Medical School, Hammersmith Hospital, London.

DAVID G.T. THOMAS MA MB BChir MRCP FRCSE
Consultant Neurosurgeon, National Hospital for Nervous Diseases, London; Senior Lecturer, Institute of Neurology, Queen's Square, London.

DAVID TOLLEY MB BS FRCS
Consultant Urologist, Royal Infirmary, Edinburgh; Hon Senior Lecturer, Dept of Surgery/Urology, University of Edinburgh.

R.B. WELBOURN, MA MD HonMD(KAROLINSKA) FRCS FWACS HonMRCS (DENMARK)
Emeritus Professor of Surgical Endocrinology, Royal Postgraduate Medical School, University of London; Hon Consultant Surgeon, Hammersmith Hospital, London; Visiting Scholar, Dept of Surgery, University of California, Los Angeles, USA.

A.W. WILKINSON ChM FRCS FRCSE
Emeritus Professor of Paediatric Surgery, University of London; Surgeon, Hospital for Sick Children, Great Ormond Street, London.

R.F.M. WOOD, MA MD FRCS
Clinical Reader in Surgery, Nuffield Dept of Surgery, University of Oxford; Fellow of Green College; Hon Consultant Surgeon, Oxfordshire Area Health Authority.

D.W. YATES, MA MChorth FRCS
Senior Lecturer in Accident and Emergency Medicine, Manchester University; Member of Scientific Staff, Medical Research Council Trauma Unit; Hon Consultant, Hope Hospital, Salford.

Alimentary tract

Introduction

It is appropriate that the opening section, and by far the largest, in this book on *Surgical Management* should be devoted to the alimentary tract. Surgery of the gut has always formed a major part of the general surgeon's practice and has benefitted greatly in recent years from the setting up of joint medical and surgical gastroenterology units such as that pioneered by Avery Jones. For the most part the quality of surgical care depends on the diagnostic and clinical skills of the operator which today are profoundly influenced by the ever increasing number of laboratory tests, imaging techniques, endoscopy and other supporting services upon which we all depend more than ever before.

It is also most appropriate that the opening chapters of this book should be devoted to that essential subject, the diagnosis of the acute abdomen, which is excitingly and attractively presented here by Peter Jones. His two chapters are so packed with information that they are worth reading and re-reading and are so arranged that reference to them is particularly easy.

The other chapters in this part of the book proceed through the traditional subdivisions of the alimentary tract in anatomical order from oesophagus to anus and it is surprising how new knowledge and new skills are found in almost every field. This is in large measure because modern technology has provided us with new techniques. First the introduction of fibreoptics has revolutionised endoscopy and there are very few parts of the alimentary tract indeed which cannot now be inspected under direct vision and photographed. In

what was once called radiology, but is better described as imaging, a whole gamut of new ways of looking at the gut has evolved. Different types of opaque medium can now be introduced into selected areas and radiology, for example, joins forces with endoscopy in ERCP to demonstrate the pancreatic ducts and the lower end of the common bile duct. There has certainly been an enormous increase in biliary tract disease in the last thirty years and the acutely inflamed gallbladder is now one of the commonest emergencies presenting to the abdominal surgeon, having long since challenged the inflamed appendix from that unenviable position.

Excision of the bowel in such conditions as ulcerative colitis has been greatly benefitted by the new techniques of stoma construction and stoma therapy, improvements in which have made it possible for these patients to live virtually normal lives. At the same time more and more effort has been directed to conserving the anal sphincter when parts of the rectum have to be excised for carcinoma. This has revived interest in stapling, which has so improved that it is being found useful once more in many other parts of the gut.

Endocrine surgery has now come of age and the discovery of a whole new series of hormones arising from cells within or associated with the gut and controlling its functions has added a new dimension to the handling of alimentary disease. The hormonal control not only of acid secretion, but also of the pancreas, gallbladder and much of the small bowel has now to be taken into consideration by the surgeon in this field. It will be useful to turn to the section on endocrinology and, in particular, the chapter on gut hormones, when considering some of these problems.

It seemed appropriate to include the excellent resumé of paediatric surgery by Andrew Wilkinson in this part of the book because so much of what the surgeon is called upon to do in the newborn baby and small child is concerned with abnormalities which occur within the abdomen. Naturally, there must be considerable overlap between the opening chapters on the acute abdomen and those concerned with the individual parts of the gut, but there can be no harm in this and it makes the book more valuable as a work of reference.

In these days of universal travel by air anyone of us can be confronted by a patient who was living in a totally different climatic area only hours before and for this reason, since many diseases have a geographical distribution, there is a chapter concerning those surgical conditions which are seen in tropical countries. Professor Roy, who has headed departments of surgery both in Africa and Northern Ireland, is particularly well suited to guide us in this field.

'No man is an island, entire of itself' and no part of this book should be consulted in isolation. Thus the last four chapters on patient care contain essential information for the proper management of the patient with alimentary problems.

S. T.

Alimentary tract

1

Acute abdomen: (i)

PETER F. JONES

Introduction

Abdominal emergencies occupy one of the few areas of medical practice in which the practitioner can still hope, by the exercise of bedside skills and experience, to reach a diagnosis unaided by numerous investigations. This characteristic, combined with the fact that the accuracy of diagnosis is often checked within an hour or two by laparotomy, makes this a continuously interesting field and one of the most important aspects of surgical training (de Dombal, 1974).

The essential steps in the management of the patient with an acute abdomen are:

History. The importance of a good history is quite as great as that of a careful physical examination. Sit down by the bedside – this is more comfortable for patient and surgeon and encourages the patient to talk. Judicious prompting may be needed. Few women, for instance, provide a gynaecological history, but the vital clue to diagnosis may lie in a missed or abnormal period.

Physical examination. This must be complete because many cases of tonsillitis, pneumonia, pyelonephritis, salpingitis, strangulated femoral hernia and torsion of the testicle have abdominal pain as their first symptom. Rectal and vaginal examination can rarely be omitted, unless abdominal examination already provides inescapable evidence of the need for laparotomy.

Perhaps the most important signs to elicit accurately are localised tenderness and muscle guarding and to do this the patient must be relaxed. This can be difficult to achieve, especially in young children (*see* p. 11). Auscultation of the abdomen is often unhelpful, but when the unmistakable splashing and tinkling of obstructive bowel sounds is heard, this can be a vital clue.

Investigations. Those which can give essential help are few – urinalysis, plain abdominal radiography and estimation of the serum amylase. Microscopy of the urine and testing for albumin and sugar must never be omitted. It is unnecessary to x-ray every acute abdomen but whenever there is doubt about perforation of a viscus or intestinal obstruction, then erect and supine abdominal films (including the diaphragm) must be taken. In any doubtful case of acute upper abdominal pain it is wise to estimate the serum amylase.

Proforma. It is always a help to commit the essential features of history and examination to paper and we have found a check list very useful. Fig 1.1 shows the record sheet used in our children's hospital for some years, adapted for use also in adults. It is much quicker to shade in the diagrams than to write down a description of position and use of the form prevents an essential point being overlooked at 3 a.m.

The possible. In reaching a sensible conclusion on diagnosis and management, it is a help to know which

Name:	Unit No.:	M/F Age: yrs mos

HISTORY

PAIN   Duration   hours   days
     Onset: sudden/gradual

Site at onset 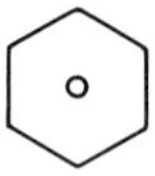   Site now

    Type: steady/colicky/intermittent
        sharp/dull
   Severity:
   Aggravated by
   Relieved by
   Getting better/worse
   Shoulder or back pain
   Loin pain
   Sleep disturbed?

Nausea
Vomiting
Appetite
Constipation   Diarrhoea
Bowels normal

Frequency   Dysuria
Haematuria

Menstruation: LMP
   Normal/abnormal
   Fainting
   Vaginal discharge

Previous illnesses/operations

Drugs

Differential diagnosis

EXAMINATION

General state
Ease of movement
Colour

Temp: °C   Pulse   /min
Rhythm
Respirations   /min   BP   /

Tongue
Fauces
Lungs
Heart

Abdomen
   Movement
   Distension
   Herniae
   Testicles
   Area of tenderness — 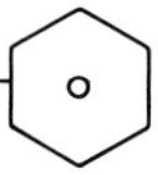
   Scars —
   Guarding
   Rigidity
   Rebound
   Mass — 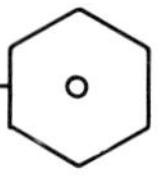
   Bowel sounds
   Rectal
   Vaginal

Urine

X-ray

Final diagnosis

Fig 1.1   Acute abdominal pain record sheet.

conditions are seen in a surgical receiving ward. In children two-thirds of admissions for acute abdominal pain will not require surgery (Table 1), and one-third will have the self-limiting condition known as non-specific acute abdominal pain (NSAP) (Jones, 1969), which is more fully considered on p. 11. In adults NSAP occurs even more frequently (Table 1).

The probable. Having learnt which diseases can present as an acute abdomen and their relative frequency, it is necessary to build up through experience and reading an accurate picture of the various guises in which they can appear. It is useful to know, for instance, that only 50% of patients with acute appendicitis experience a shift of pain and that the tenderness of a high retro-caecal appendicitis is well above and lateral to McBurney's famous point, while pelvic appendicitis may show few abdominal signs until rectal examination is carried out. One-third of children with acute appendicitis have a clean tongue and 10% have a sore head. Most patients with a strangulated femoral hernia are unaware they have a hernia and it is often not tender.

The diagnosis. The vital point of construction of a differential diagnosis and deciding on a course of action has now been reached. It is here that the proforma is so helpful, because all the facts are presented concisely, and odd findings and omissions cannot be overlooked.

Table 1
ADMISSIONS TO SURGICAL WARDS WITH ACUTE ABDOMINAL PAIN

552 patients, adult surgical wards. Leeds, 1972 [1]	% of total	363 patients, up to 13-years-old. Royal Aberdeen Children's Hospital 1974 [2]	% of total
NSAP	50.5	NSAP	30.0
Acute appendicitis	26.3	Acute appendicitis	28.0
Cholecystitis	7.6	Constipation	11.0
Small bowel obstruction	3.6	Upper respiratory tract infection	8.0
Perforated peptic ulcer	3.1	Urinary tract infection	6.9
Pancreatitis	2.9	Gastroenteritis	3.6
Diverticular disease	2.0	Bronchopneumonia	2.2
Miscellaneous	4.0	Small bowel obstruction (incl. intussusception)	2.2
		Mesenteric adenitis (operated)	2.2
		Abdominal injuries	1.0
		Infective hepatitis	1.0
		Torsion of testis	
		Acute pancreatitis	less than 1%
		Otitis media	
		Acute glomerulo-nephritis	
		Diabetic acidosis	

[1] From de Dombal *et al.*, 1974.
[2] From Jones, 1976.

There is a strong temptation for all emergency surgeons to decide simply whether the abdomen needs opening or not. Half the interest, and much valuable experience, of the acute abdomen is lost if this is done, quite apart from the importance of making a positive diagnosis of the many important medical diseases which present as an acute abdomen. The signs of peritonitis and haemoperitoneum can be somewhat similar, but the preoperative preparation of the patient is vitally different.

It is important to recognise that in many patients a firm diagnosis cannot be reached at the first interview. NSAP is a diagnosis which can only be given when the patient leaves hospital, when several examinations over 12–24 h have shown steady improvement. Some children are so restless that they need sedation before they can be usefully examined. The early case of acute appendicitis may only show convincing signs after several hours of observation, and it may be 24 h before the signs of acute catarrhal appendicitis become clear. This process of 'active observation' (Jones, 1976) is just as much a part of surgical management as an operation.

It is equally important to remember that there are very few patients who need to be 'rushed to theatre', and for many this can be dangerous. There are exceptions to this – sudden haemorrhage from a ruptured ectopic pregnancy or the gastroduodenal artery are examples – but the majority of patients with an acute abdomen have been ill for a day or two, have stopped drinking and vomited much of what they have taken. An hour or two in a warm bed with an analgesic injection and an intravenous infusion of Hartmann's solution will greatly improve their readiness for operation. In a child with a ruptured appendix and spreading peritonitis, 3–4 h devoted to giving intravenous Hartmann's followed by some colloid, with a parenteral antibiotic, may make the difference between an easy convalescence and a patient who comes off the table desperately ill. Attention to preoperative preparation is every bit as vital as a high standard of postoperative care.

General peritonitis

Some 60 000 patients are treated each year in England and Wales for acute appendicitis and approximately 1 patient in every 6 will have peritonitis (Office of Population Censuses and Surveys, 1978). In this group 1 patient in every 50 will die, compared with 1 death in 2000 among patients who have appendicitis without peritonitis. Although mortality from peritonitis is now lower than it has ever been, it is still a serious matter if it raises the mortality of appendicitis 40 times, and this is especially true when it occurs in the very young and the elderly. There are many causes of peritonitis, some more lethal than appendicitis, but the principles of management are essentially the same.

Aetiology

Diffuse peritonitis is either primary or secondary.

Primary peritonitis

This is a fairly rare condition almost confined to females, who are usually below the age of 8. It is probably due to retrograde infection via the genital tract. The purulent exudate grows either streptococci or pneumococci (rarely, *E. coli*) and these children are nearly always thought, before operation, to have pelvic appendicitis. At laparotomy, the appendix is found to be normal, but green or yellow inoffensive sticky pus is found in the pelvis and the Fallopian tubes look reddened. A film of the pus should be examined immediately after Gram-staining and if Gram-positive diplococci or streptococci are found, then a full course of intramuscular penicillin should be commenced promptly. Recovery is usually rapid. Primary peritonitis occasionally complicates the ascites of nephrosis.

Secondary peritonitis

In the great majority of patients general peritonitis is secondary to perforation of an abdominal viscus. This may be due to injury – closed or penetrating – or to disease. In Western countries the commonest diseases causing peritonitis are:

acute appendicitis (*see* pp. 11, 200)
perforated peptic ulcer (*see* p. 87)
acute colonic diverticulitis (*see* p. 219)
perforations of intestinal neoplasms, e.g. colonic carcinoma, small bowel lymphomas
fulminant inflammatory bowel disease, i.e. ulcerative colitis or Crohn's disease (*see* p. 223)
gangrene of bowel, e.g. superior mesenteric artery embolism, necrotising enterocolitis of newborn
acute obstructive cholecystitis (*see* p. 121)
stercoral ulceration (Elliott and Jeffrey, 1980).

Perforation of a typhoid ulcer is an important cause of peritonitis wherever this disease is endemic. The final, but unfortunately not the smallest, group are those patients who suffer a leak from gastric or intestinal anastomosis.

Numerous as these causes of peritonitis are, they all produce similar pathological effects or clinical signs.

Pathology

There are four distinct effects:

1 There is an inflammatory reaction throughout the peritoneal cavity and this leads to formation of a copious purulent and fibrinous exudate. This exudate bathes the intestine and causes paralytic ileus (*see below*). Extracellular fluid is lost because intestinal juice is secreted into the dilated loops and is often lost in copious vomiting.
2 Intake of water and food by mouth ceases from the onset of the illness, thus materially contributing to dehydration.
3 Bacterial growth in the exudate may be followed by bacteraemia. Children may become hyperpyrexial.
4 The exudate is rich in fibrin and adhesions form throughout the peritoneal cavity. This is particularly likely to result in encysted collections of pus, either trapped between loops of bowel, or in the subphrenic spaces or the pelvis.

Bacteriology

Although it has been known for a long time that 99% of the faecal bacterial flora are anaerobes (mostly *Bacteroides spp.*), it has only recently been recognised that these organisms play an important part in the development of peritonitis. This is probably due to the fact that anaerobes quickly die when, as is usual, a sample of peritoneal pus is transmitted to the laboratory on a throat swab exposed to air. To obtain a true picture of the bacterial population in pus from peritonitis, it is essential to plunge the pus swab immediately into transport medium (e.g. Cary-Blair). (It is worth remembering that it was in 1938 that Altemeier pointed out that the offensive smell of the pus around a perforated appendix is due to *Bacteroide spp.*, and not to *E. coli* which produces odourless pus.)

Most cases of general peritonitis are due to mixed anaerobic and aerobic infections, *E. coli* being much the commonest aerobe, and *Bacteroides fragilis* the predominant anaerobe. These findings have a major bearing on the choice of antibiotic treatment.

Clinical picture

When the effects of the pathological changes just described are considered, it is not surprising that patients with peritonitis look dehydrated and toxic. Diagnosis is rarely a problem: the history of progressive abdominal pain and vomiting, the ill, often febrile, patient with a rapid thin pulse, the distended diffusely tender and silent abdomen, with tenderness and bulging of the pouch of Douglas on rectal examination, all point to one conclusion.

The clinical picture will vary to some extent with the cause of the peritonitis. The instantaneous board-like rigidity caused by the chemical peritonitis of perforated peptic ulcer is well known. The slow onset of peritonitis in blunt injuries of the small bowel and bladder deserves to be better known, as does the very quiet onset of peritonitis in perforated appendicitis in the elderly; it seems characteristic for them to tolerate abdominal pain for several days until they present with the signs of peritonitis with paralytic ileus and are then thought to have a primary small bowel obstruction. These are the patients who are likely already to have complications in other systems – a developing broncho-pneumonia and a measure of renal failure secondary to dehydration. Blood gases are very likely to show abnormalities in these circumstances. About 20% of patients show air under the diaphragm on x-ray, but most will show the radiographic signs of intestinal ileus.

It is important to distinguish the most serious group of patients – those with faecal peritonitis. This is due either to severe diverticular disease, with disruption of a part of the wall of the sigmoid colon, to gangrene of the colon, to stercoral ulceration, to an anastomotic disruption or to fulminant pan-colitis. All will show the signs of severe generalised peritonitis and, in addition, will rapidly show signs of Gram-negative bacteraemia. Cold hypotensive bacteraemic shock is commoner than the well known warm bacterial shock.

Management

The impulse to rush the patient, who is so obviously gravely ill, to the operating theatre must be resisted: time wisely spent on preoperative treatment may literally be life-saving.

Preoperative treatment

1 The most important task is to achieve a large measure of restoration of water and electrolyte balance. Anyone with diffuse peritonitis is certain to have a considerable deficiency of extracellular fluid. This is partly because the normal intake of water will have stopped for 24–48 h because of the patient's anorexia and nausea, and partly because of vomiting. The extent of vomiting can be estimated from the history and low intake probably means that 500 ml instead of 2500 ml of water will have been taken on each day of the illness. In addition, there will be alimentary secretions sequestrated in the dilated inert loops of intestine.

This lost fluid needs to be replaced by rapid intravenous infusion of Hartmann's solution (BP),

which has the additional advantage that it will help to correct the metabolic acidosis which is very likely to be present. A 70 kg adult with peritonitis is likely to have a water deficit of 5–6 l, so it is safe to give 2.5–3.0 l of Hartmann's solution over 2½–3 h. However, in the elderly, it is important not to err towards giving too much fluid too fast and measurement of central venous pressure (CVP) makes fluid administration easier and safer. A CVP of <10 cm water means that rapid infusion can safely continue. A urinary catheter should be inserted, because the hourly urine volume is a valuable guide to the success of resuscitation. If there is evidence of hypovolaemia (systolic BP of <100 mmHg, peripheral vasoconstriction and sweating, tachycardia, low CVP), it is reasonable to give additionally a colloid solution. Dextran 70 is a reasonable choice and 20% of calculated blood volume can be given over half an hour (the blood volume of children is about 80 ml per kg and of adults about 70 ml per kg). Except in abdominal trauma, whole blood is not likely to be required preoperatively.

The replacement of lost extracellular fluid needs careful control to secure the correct balance between an infusion which is too slow to be effective and so fast that it is harmful: preoperative overtransfusion is probably a factor in the production of shock lung.

2 Antibacterial treatment is almost as important as rehydration because some patients will already be bacteraemic. This is unlikely only a few hours after perforation of a peptic ulcer, but should be assumed to be present in anyone with an established septic peritonitis. It is vital to remove blood for culture before commencing treatment.

Most surgeons and bacteriologists would currently favour using combination therapy. Gentamicin, 5–6 mg per kg per day in 3 divided doses, with ampicillin 500 mg 4–6 times per day. Metronidazole is probably the best choice for treatment of anaerobic infection and 500 mg is infused over 20 min every 8 h.

3 Anyone with peritonitis is uncomfortable and anxious so an analgesic should be given as soon as possible, in consultation with the anaesthetist. The subcutaneous route is useless and a slow intravenous injection is the most effective.

4 Considerable debate still goes on over the value of methyl prednisolone in septic shock. There is evidence to suggest that it is useful (Schumer, 1976), but how far this applies to patients with surgically treatable peritonitis is not clear. If it is decided to use methyl prednisolone the dose is 30 mg/kg which is given in 100 ml of normal saline. This dose can be repeated, once only, in 4–6 h.

5 Abdominal rigidity causes rapid shallow breathing and it is reasonable to give oxygen, inhaled through a mask, at 5 l/min.

6 Before inducing anaesthesia, if not before, a 16F

nasogastric tube should be passed and the stomach kept empty. If this is an Andersen-type tube, with an air inlet, this can usefully be placed on continuous suction.

Operative treatment

This is the most controversial part of the treatment of peritonitis. Everyone would agree that the ruptured appendix should be removed and the perforated peptic ulcer closed, but there is considerable controversy over the place of immediate resection of the ruptured colon, the value of peritoneal lavage, and the routine use of antibiotics for appendicular peritonitis.

In these circumstances it seems best to describe the writer's methods and to show why they have been adopted.

1 Incision. There are strong arguments for using a long vertical incision, either midline or paramedian. When there are signs of diffuse peritonitis, it can be difficult to know where the perforation is situated. Also, there are strong grounds for carrying out a thorough toilet of the whole peritoneal cavity and this can only be done through a generous vertical incision. In pelvic appendicitis access is much easier through a vertical than through a gridiron incision.

2 Dealing with the source of contamination. In the case of acute appendicitis, appendicectomy will almost always be carried out. When acute cholecystitis goes on to perforation, cholecystectomy is the treatment of choice because the wall of the gallbladder is often gangrenous: however, if dissection of the cystic duct proves to be difficult, it is safer to perform cholecystostomy, after the removal of all available gallstones. The perforated peptic ulcer will be oversewn or definitive gastric surgery performed.

The most serious forms of peritonitis are those due to colonic perforation, and of these perforated diverticular disease is the most common cause. These patients are usually elderly and often medically unfit and they require very careful management (Tagart's paper (1974) is well worthy of study). However, even though these patients are seriously ill, their one hope is to have expert and timely surgery. In those who have a faecal peritonitis the breach in the wall of the colon is likely to be large, and one which is virtually unclosable: these are the patients who can benefit from a quick excision of the affected segment of colon by a surgeon who is well used to colonic resection. This operation usually takes the form of a Hartmann's resection, but if the distal sigmoid segment is long enough, it can be brought up to the surface as a Paul-Mickulicz type of double-ended colostomy. There is no justification for advising restorative anastomosis in these circumstances, in spite of some very good reported results (Ryan, 1958).

(These were achieved by expert surgeons who were trying to prove a method, but this does not make them generally applicable.)

The rare case of stercoral ulceration will also need resection because a considerable area of the wall of the colon will have given way and be irreparable (Elliott and Jeffrey, 1980).

When a patient has to be reopened on account of a free leakage of faeces into the peritoneum from an anastomosis, it is essential to take down the anastomosis and exteriorise the two ends of bowel separately or convert the operation into a Hartmann's procedure.

When perforation occurs in fulminant colitis, the whole colon is usually severely ulcerated, and a total colectomy with ileostomy is indicated (*see* p. 224).

In purulent, as opposed to faecal, peritonitis, secondary to diverticular disease, it is important to study the bowel carefully. Sometimes a single diverticulum appears to have perforated (it is sometimes situated in the proximal colon) and it may be quite correct to trim the edges of the perforation and suture it. If the area affected is too large, then it may be possible to exteriorise it as a loop colostomy. Sometimes, resection is again the correct treatment with the proximal end of the colon brought out as an end-draining colostomy.

In injuries of the colon and rectum the hardly-learned lesson of every war is that they must be treated with the greatest respect. Much the safest procedure is to exteriorise the torn segment of colon: if this cannot be done, the injured colon should be resected and the two ends of colon brought out as stomata.

3 Peritoneal lavage. This is an ancillary form of treatment for peritonitis which has been used for a long time by a few surgeons but has only achieved popularity over the last 10 years. Burnett *et al.* (1957) gives an impressive description of his first case, in 1942, when lavage with many pints of sulphanilamide in saline in an advanced and apparently hopeless case of appendiceal peritonitis was followed by an uneventful recovery. Hudspeth (1975) has recently reported very impressive results with 'radical surgical debridement' in advanced peritonitis and the writer is convinced, from considerable personal experience of advanced and faecal peritonitis, that complete and thorough intraoperative peritoneal toilet is an essential part of treatment.

It is this need to enter every part of the abdomen that makes it essential to use a long vertical incision. At the start of the operation all pus is sucked out and faeces scooped and washed away. It is then usually wise to proceed to the appropriate treatment of the cause of the peritonitis. Finally, and most important, the whole of the small bowel is gently drawn out of the abdomen, fibrinous plaques being removed wherever possible. This process, in the case of advanced peritonitis of several days' standing, involves some very careful mobilisation of adherent loops of bowel. Sometimes interloop abscesses are found and drained. When all the small bowel has been drawn out of the abdomen and cleaned and washed, the cleaning process must be extended to the subphrenic and subhepatic spaces – fibrin, debris, food, faeces must be washed and picked out of all those areas and finally the same process carried down the paracolic gutters to the pelvis. Once the whole peritoneum is well cleaned in this way, warm normal saline containing 1 g of tetracycline per litre is poured into the abdominal cavity and the edges of the incision are also thoroughly washed. Care is taken to ensure that this solution is thoroughly washed over the undersurface of the diaphragms and around the pelvis and paracolic gutters. The first washing is sucked out and replaced with a second wash which is allowed to remain in the peritoneal cavity during closure of the incision.

If drains are introduced into the peritoneum, these are clipped until the end of the operation and then the saline with tetracycline is allowed to drain away.

Stewart and Matheson have carried out an extensive investigation into the effects of peritoneal lavage, both in patients and in the rat (Stewart and Matheson, 1978a,b), and their conclusions are that it results in a striking decrease in wound and other septic complications. What is also very clear from their work is that lavage with noxythiolin solution, which is still popular, is nothing like so effective as tetracycline solution, and probably secures most of the effects by mechanical cleansing (Stewart, 1978).

My own experience over the past 10 years of patients with faecal peritonitis treated by thorough lavage leaves me in no doubt that this results in a smooth recovery which is quite strikingly different from that expected before the introduction of antibiotic lavage. So strong is this belief that it would not be possible for me to take part in a controlled trial of lavage because I could not conscientiously withhold this treatment from the control group.

The question arises whether it is wise to leave peritoneal dialysis catheters within the peritoneal cavity for subsequent postoperative lavage and this has recently attracted some attention (Fowler, 1975), and has been reported on favourably. So far there is no trial which compares thorough intraoperative antibiotic lavage with a similar series who also, in addition to intra-operative lavage, receive postoperative irrigation through dialysis catheters. Postoperative peritoneal lavage is harmless if carefully controlled and in a severely contaminated peritoneum is worth considering.

What stands out quite clearly from the various papers is that thorough lavage of the peritoneal cavity using saline containing an antibiotic leads to a highly significant diminution in the number of residual abscesses and wound infections. It appears to be harmless and, in

particular, there is no evidence that it tends to diffuse infection into parts of the abdomen previously unaffected.

4 Intestinal intubation. In the advanced case of peritonitis with paralytic ileus, the small bowel is dilated and oedematous, with considerable fibrin deposition on the inflamed serous surface. Clearly many adhesions are going to form and an adhesive kink causing obstruction during the recovery period would be very unwelcome. In these severe cases we have used intestinal intubation (*see* p. 21) and believe that it has been helpful in securing a smooth convalescence by keeping the bowel free of kinks, and decompressed. This must remain a clinical impression but we believe the method to be useful. It is relevant that Hudspeth (1975) used intubation as a part of his 'radical surgical debridement' in 92 critically ill patients between 3 and 69 years of age, and all recovered.

5 Drainage. This continues to be another controversial subject, but most surgeons would agree with Yates's (1905) conclusion that there is no way of draining the general peritoneal cavity. Provided the source of peritoneal contamination has been removed, and thorough lavage performed, there is nothing to be gained by leaving drains in the peritoneal cavity (this does not, of course, apply if resection has been followed by intestinal anastomosis, or the perforation has been oversewn with difficulty and a localised area, therefore, requires drainage).

6 Wound closure. This is a situation in which postoperative gaseous distension of the intestines is very likely, so the closure of the incision must be secure. Those who favour a midline wound will probably choose to use mass-closure after the manner of Jenkins. The writer more often uses a paramedian incision which is closed with deep retention all-layer sutures of 1 nylon and a 'bunching' suture of 0 prolene for the posterior and anterior rectus sheath. Thorough lavage of the wound with the tetracycline solution has a marked effect in preventing wound sepsis and in very contaminated cases 1 g of ampicillin powder should be sprinkled in the wound, or the skin left unsutured. With these two prophylactic measures, it is very rare for even a heavily contaminated wound to become infected.

Postoperative care

Nasogastric suction. This is always worth practising and an 'Andersen' tube which allows continuous suction is useful, because it is particularly effective in evacuating swallowed air, which is the principal cause of distension in paralytic ileus.

Intravenous fluids. This is so standard a part of the postoperative care of a patient with peritonitis that little need be said. It is important to maintain a good urine output: the hourly urine volume should reach 40–50 ml. In the elderly some care is needed to maintain adequate urine output whilst avoiding fluid overloading, so CVP measurement can be very helpful. In spite of an adequate fluid load, the elderly quite often have a low urine output after operation and then frusemide is a safe and effective diuretic. The patient with peritonitis is likely to be on intravenous fluids for some days, so careful attention to sodium and potassium balance is essential from the start: the volume of nasogastric aspirate, which can be high, is therefore highly relevant.

Antibiotic treatment will be continued. Gentamicin is potentially nephrotoxic and whenever there is reason for concern about renal function – and this must include all elderly patients with diffuse peritonitis – the blood gentamycin level must be measured. The desirable peak serum concentration is 5–12 μg per ml and it is also important that the serum concentration should fall below 3 μg per ml between injections. If it appears that the trough concentration is too high, then the dose of gentamicin should be kept the same, but it should be given less often e.g. 80 mg b.d. instead of 80 mg t.d.s.

Postoperative shock. When this is present after operation for peritonitis the situation needs careful analysis. Hypovolaemia must be corrected appropriately – preoperative losses should have been made good before and during surgery, but the calculations must be checked again. Intraoperative blood loss should have been measured and corrected. If hypovolaemia does not appear to be the cause of shock, bacteraemia may be responsible. If the suggestions made for preoperative treatment have been carried out, there may not be much more to be done. Uncorrected metabolic acidosis, especially in the elderly, can aggravate the situation and blood gases should always be checked in this situation. The use of vasopressors is controversial and in the past these have probably done more harm than good. However, dopamine has the virtue that it increases both cardiac output and renal blood flow and appears to be the drug of choice: the dose is 2–5 μg per kg per minute. The value of methyl prednisolone remains debatable (Schumer, 1976).

Sedation is an important part of the care of the postoperative patient. In peritonitis, the patient is going to be ill for some days and require much attention, so it is essential that some rest is obtained. Constant disturbance of the patient by taking the blood pressure can be avoided by careful observations of the general state of the patient and the pulse and urine output, and when these are satisfactory the sphygmomanometer readings can be left until the patient wakes. A good sedative mixture is methadone 7.5–10.0 mg with promazine 25 mg intramuscularly. Some favour measured administration of omnopon intravenously.

Pulmonary complications are especially likely in ill patients with a distended abdomen and a painful incision. In patients with known respiratory disease, it is wise to leave a fine perforated catheter in the layers of the incision and inject through it, for 48–72 h, via an ultrafilter, a 0.5% solution of bupivacaine postoperatively – this strikingly diminishes wound pain and allows the patient to move and cough more easily. Underventilation of the lung bases due to the high diaphragms means that a very close clinical and radiological check on the lungs is essential, and in the elderly the blood gases will also need to be checked.

It is vital to remember that major sepsis is an important cause of the syndrome known as 'adult respiratory distress' and the earliest signs of this are hyperventilation, hypoxaemia which is not improved by inhaling oxygen, and a clear chest x-ray. These findings are an indication for seeking expert advice from an anaesthetist.

Paralytic ileus. This has, happily, become an unusual condition, presumably due to a better understanding of possible causes and the more effective treatment now offered to patients with peritonitis.

There is no precise time at which it can be said that a slow recovery from the effects of diffuse peritonitis becomes an established paralytic ileus. However, most surgeons would consider ileus to be present if, on the fourth postoperative day the patient still looks unwell, has a distended tympanitic, silent abdomen, there is a large volume of nasogastric aspirate, and flatus has not been passed per rectum. The picture is completed if a plain abdominal film shows gas and fluid distension of the large as well as the small bowel.

The first step in management of paralytic ileus is to consider whether any of the known contributory causes of ileus are operating – any sodium or potassium insufficiency or a residual abdominal abscess. If not, there are, on the fourth day, no special extra steps to be taken. Careful intravenous replacement of fluid and electrolytes, repair of any anaemia, and maintenance of nasogastric decompression continue.

From about the sixth day, if there is no immediate sign of improvement, it is necessary to give more thought to the nutrition of the patient. It is a serious error to allow the patient to become visibly wasted and only then to consider intravenous nutrition. On about the sixth day, the catabolic response to surgery is declining and intravenous nutrients begin to be useful, so this is a logical time at which to start parenteral feeding (for details, *see* p. 845). It is always difficult to know whether to take the decision to commence intravenous feeding, but in this situation it is highly unlikely that the patient is going to take a useful amount of food by mouth for another week, so it is certainly worth while to start intravenous nutrition. If the ileus resolves quickly, then the patient has a speedier convalescence. However, if some complication, such as an adhesive obstruction, further delays recovery the early start to parenteral feeding will be of great value to the patient.

There is a sense in which intravenous feeding is a dangerous treatment in so far as it can keep the patient in good general condition for weeks and possibly mask an overall deterioration in the situation. Perhaps the most important feature of this difficult waiting period in the treatment of paralytic ileus is the twice-daily visit of the surgeon, when all aspects of the patient's progress are reviewed. If there is no apparent progress towards deflation of the abdomen, and passage of flatus and stool per rectum, the two main questions to ask are: 'is there a residual intraperitoneal abscess?', and, 'is the paralytic ileus really due to mechanical adhesive obstruction?' Standard clinical radiographic and ultrasonic investigation should answer the first question. The second must be answered by careful examination of the abdomen (not forgetting the hernial orifices), auscultation, and serial plain abdominal x-rays, but this is always a difficult problem. Generally, the presence of obstructive bowel sounds and increasing small bowel distension, with diminution of the amount of gas in the colon, suggests that an adhesive kink in the small bowel has become the reason for persistent obstruction (*see* p. 19).

If, however, the abdomen remains distended and quiet, and the x-rays show gas distension of large as well as small bowel then ileus continues, and the question must be, how long should the surgeon wait for natural resolution of the ileus? The work of Neely and Catchpole (1971) suggests that the more clear it is that a patient has paralytic ileus, the more logical is it to treat the inhibitory state being mediated through the splanchnic nerves. If there is no evidence of active sepsis, which will in itself perpetuate ileus, and if sodium and potassium balance is correct, there is a good case for initiating pharmacological treatment. Catchpole and Neely advise that blood pressure and pulse rate be recorded on a chart, and then 20 mg of guanethidine is infused in 5% dextrose over 40 min. Auscultation may reveal the gradual appearance of intestinal sounds and when this occurs a dose of prostigmine can be given intravenously, commencing with 0.05 mg: this can be repeated several times at 3–4 min intervals. Occurrence of colicky pain is an indication to stop the prostigmine injections.

We have now used this regime in 15 patients and are convinced of its safety and it has certainly been followed by termination of ileus in most cases – failure has indicated a persisting, but unnoticed, cause for ileus. This pharmacological treatment is a valuable advance in the management of a difficult problem.

Residual abscesses. Any patient who has generalised peritonitis is liable to develop a residual abscess and this must be remembered throughout the recovery period. These are no longer the lethal complications that they used to be, but they cause major delays in recovery. It is, indeed, remarkable to see how large a collection of pus can reside under the diaphragm or in the pelvis whilst the patient looks reasonably well, and only a continued swinging fever points inescapably to an undrained abscess. Standard methods of diagnosis and treatment are used. After excision of the rectum, it can be difficult to diagnose a pelvic abscess and then ultrasound is a most valuable aid to diagnosis.

Much the most difficult residual abscesses to diagnose and treat are inter-loop abscesses. These loculi of pus can occur anywhere in the abdomen, securely sealed off by adherent loops of bowel and by omentum. Thorough peritoneal lavage is a most important preventive measure, but such abscesses will occasionally be seen and it is essential to think of the possibility. Ultrasonic scanning is particularly valuable in picking up these collections. Drainage calls for great delicacy and skill because the bowel which forms the wall of the abscess is necessarily oedematous and friable: if torn the chances of successful suture repair are very slim and the subsequent small bowel fistula has been a major contributor to the high mortality of peritonitis.

Fortunately, the peritoneum is the best ally of both patient and surgeon and in the great majority of patients its reparative powers, with timely surgical help, will lead to the complete resolution of peritonitis.

The acute abdomen in infants and young children

The infant with an acute abdomen presents the surgeon with several problems. There is no history, at least from the patient. These small patients are miserable and in pain and they can see no point in a stranger coming to the bedside and making the pain worse by pressing on the abdomen, so they cry and struggle. This makes useful abdominal examination difficult or impossible, so diagnosis is delayed and it is not surprising that most acutely inflamed appendices in children below school age are perforated when they are removed.

Some conditions such as ileo-caecal intussusception are peculiar to early childhood whilst others, such as the complications of Meckel's diverticulum, are most often seen then.

The problem of the absence of a history is not usually serious because most mothers are fairly expert observers of their children. The tendency of young children to cry when asked to lie flat in bed and allow examination of the sore abdomen is more awkward because no useful signs can be obtained until the child is quiet. Very often patience, talking to the child, a toy to play with, warm hands, and gentle palpation of a non-tender area of the abdomen will reassure the child and the tensing of the abdominal muscles will relax and allow an area of tenderness and guarding to be found, or a mass palpated. If the child is inconsolable, then it is essential to give a sedative: diazepam in a dose of 1 mg/kg administered per rectum, is safe, and will, after an hour or so, allow the child to relax and then a useful abdominal examination can be made.

It is very important to remember that a high proportion of children with acute abdominal pain do not have a surgical cause for it (Jones, 1976). Roughly one-third have a medical condition such as pneumonia, urinary tract infection, constipation, tonsillitis, or gastroenteritis, so a full examination including the chest, throat, ears and microscopy of the urine is essential (*see* Table 1, p. 5). Another one-third will have a surgical condition – mostly appendicitis or intestinal obstruction. The remaining one-third will recover without a precise diagnosis being made. This syndrome of 'non-specific acute abdominal pain' (NSAP; Jones, 1969) is not confined to children, but is certainly important because it can produce a good imitation of acute appendicitis during the first 6–12 h of the illness. Pain often commences in the right iliac fossa, the child feels nauseated and may vomit and there can be localised and definite tenderness in the right iliac fossa. However, guarding is rarely found and although pain may persist, tenderness soon diminishes and usually within 24 h the child is better. There is no convincing explanation so far for this common condition, but it does mean that every child with acute abdominal pain needs careful examination followed by close observation. We have called this 'active observation' (Jones, 1976) to signify that it is a continuing and important part of management: the child is starved, kept on an hourly pulse chart and re-examined by the surgeon who first saw the child every 3–4 h. It soon becomes apparent that cases of early appendicitis are developing more convincing signs and these children are operated upon, but the NSAP children show a lessening of discomfort and tenderness, and it is soon evident that they are recovering. In a few children, it will not be possible to be certain, even after 6–8 h of the diagnosis and with persistent abdominal signs these patients must be operated upon. However, with the careful application of 'active observation', the number of normal appendices removed should not exceed 10%, and most important, cases of acute appendicitis are operated on as soon as the diagnosis can be made.

Acute appendicitis

This is very rare in the first year, but thereafter it is increasingly common and more cases are seen between 12 and 15 years of age than at any other time of life. It is vital to realise that the presentation of acute appendicitis in the young child differs markedly from the classical picture (Williams, 1947). The infant becomes fretful, refuses feeds, vomits, feels hot and holds the abdomen, which may become a little distended. There is often diarrhoea and this is all too likely to suggest gastroenteritis. The child looks ill, there is fever, up to 39°C, and tachycardia. The abdomen may show restricted respiratory movement, with consequent tachypnoea, and there will be tenderness and guarding, the extent of this depending on whether there is already a perforation with peritonitis. If these signs are inconclusive a gentle rectal examination must be done, seeking for a tender fullness in the Pouch of Douglas. The white cell count is not, as a rule, of much help, but in a recent series of 32 infants under 2 years with acute appendicitis (Grosfeld *et al.*, 1973), all of whom had a plain abdominal x-ray, 25 showed signs of paralytic ileus and 9 showed a radio-opaque faecolith: these x-ray findings can be very helpful when diagnosis is in doubt.

In older children, the clinical picture becomes progressively more like acute appendicitis in the adult.

Acute intussusception

This is a specific disease of the first 18 months of life and 60% of cases occur between 4 and 12 months of age (Hutchison *et al.*, 1980). It is almost certain that a viral infection of the alimentary tract causes the Peyer's patches in the terminal ileum to swell up (Bell and Steyn, 1962), and this mass is swept on by peristalsis to initiate the intussusception: this is most often ileo-colic and produces a very well-known clinical syndrome of colicky abdominal pain and vomiting, followed by the passage of altered blood per rectum in about 50% of cases. The diagnosis is established by palpating the sausage-like mass of intussuscepted bowel, usually in the epigastrium, below the liver edge. Occasionally the intussusception advances further down the colon and the apex becomes palpable on rectal examination. In 50–60% of children there will be altered blood on the examining finger. In a small, but important, group of patients there is no clearly felt lump in spite of a suspicious history. These children are often 2–3 years of age and they have a soft subacute form of intussusception which is therefore difficult to feel, and tend to grumble on for a day or two, sometimes well and sometimes miserable and sick. In these children it is essential to perform a barium enema, which will make the diagnosis quite clear.

Ileo-ileal intussusception is fortunately rare (5% of all cases), because it is the most difficult to diagnose and the most dangerous form. The child has severe colicky abdominal pain and vomiting, but it is not always possible to feel a mass and blood is not usually passed per rectum. If it is recognised clinically, and on examination of plain abdominal films, that the child has intestinal obstruction then laparotomy will be advised and the diagnosis will become clear. Owing to the small calibre of ileum ischaemic changes occur quickly and it is often necessary to resect this type of intussusception.

There are considerable national variations in the treatment of intussusception (Pollet, 1980). In North America, Australia and Scandinavia a high proportion of children are treated by hydrostatic reduction with a barium enema under x-ray screen control. This method can work very well when the intussusception is early, but it is only safe if some precautions are faithfully observed.

1 The radiologist must be experienced in the method and be able to assure himself that reduction is complete by seeing barium flowing freely up the ileum.
2 Surgeon and radiologist must work together and the theatre be ready for surgery immediately if the radiologist is not satisfied about reduction.

Even with these precautions occasional perforation of the colon occurs and there is always the possibility that a cause for the intussusception such as a Meckel's diverticulum will be overlooked. In a recent survey in Aberdeen (Pollet, 1980), nearly one-third of the children would not have been properly treated without an operation.

In Great Britain there is a fairly strong tendency to treat intussusception surgically, probably dictated by the fact that most emergency surgery is done in general, not paediatric, surgical units. This trend is clearly safer than practising hydrostatic reduction in unsatisfactory circumstances, and is associated with a very low mortality (Hutchison *et al.*, 1980). Happily, the majority of intussusceptions are readily reduced at operation, though a few require firm pressure over the apex to reduce the last few cm of bowel through the ileo-caecal valve. In the occasional irreducible intussusception, or when gangrene has already occurred, then resection is essential and an emergency right hemicolectomy with immediate ileo-colic anastomosis produces excellent results. There is a surprising difference between different hospitals in the frequency with which resection is needed (Thomas, 1980), and this is related to the fact that considerable delay in diagnosis still occurs (Hutchison *et al.*, 1980). Few general practitioners see more than the occasional case of intussusception, and only

half these infants show blood per rectum: this is another example of the difficulties of diagnosis of the acute abdomen in infancy and underlines how important it is that all trainees in general practice should have experience in a children's surgical ward.

Meckel's diverticulum

This small appendage of the distal ileum is the commonest congenital deformity in the alimentary tract and makes itself known most often during the early years of life (Soderlund, 1959). Most of the emergencies due to this organ occur because about half of these diverticula are lined by ectopic gastric mucous membrane and so can be the site of peptic ulceration. If this ulceration occurs it can *perforate*, causing a peritonitis which is indistinguishable from that due to acute appendicitis, or it can produce rectal *haemorrhage*: this condition is much the commonest cause of severe rectal bleeding in childhood and may occasionally require urgent laparotomy because of the severity of the bleeding. The other main complication is *intussusception* due to a Meckel's diverticulum forming the apex of an ileal intussusception – this usually presents in exactly the same way as other intussusceptions in childhood and the true cause is only revealed when the intussusception is reduced at laparotomy. Sometimes a Meckel's diverticulum which has remained attached to the umbilicus forms the axis of rotation of a small bowel *volvulus*. Another complication which cannot be distinguished preoperatively from acute appendicitis is acute *Meckelian diverticulitis*.

The treatment for all these conditions is diverticulectomy, and the first step must be ligation of the omphalo-mesenteric artery and vein which runs directly from the ileal mesentery over the wall of the ileum to the diverticulum. It is most important to remember that gastric mucosa can extend to the point of attachment to the ileum and the only safe way to remove a pathogenic diverticulum is to excise a small amount of ileum adjacent to the base of the diverticulum: then the defect in the antimesenteric wall of the ileum can be closed, with a Connell suture of 3/0 silk or nurolon. This is a safer technique than placing a Kocher's forceps obliquely across the base, removing the diverticulum and inserting an over-and-over suture over the clamp. This is, however, a reasonable way of removing a diverticulum which is found incidentally in the course of treating some other condition.

Mayo's dictum – 'frequently suspected, often looked for, seldom found' – remains true, but, for the few concerned, the effects of possessing a Meckel's diverticulum can still be serious.

The acute abdomen in pregnancy and the puerperium

This event can present both obstetrician and surgeon with some difficult problems, but these arise fairly infrequently so no clinician can build up a body of experience. Pregnancy can substantially modify abdominal signs and there is always the problem of trying to meet the needs of the mother and also to save the baby.

In early pregnancy there is immediately the difficulty that the patient does not realise that she is pregnant (or has reserves about revealing this fact) and this can only be overcome by taking a very careful menstrual history in any young woman with acute abdominal pain. Later on, there will be no doubt about the existence of a pregnancy, but it can too easily be considered to be the origin of abdominal symptoms which in reality derive from a surgical emergency.

Emergencies arising from the presence of a pregnancy

Ectopic pregnancy

This is still a very dangerous condition and the fact that, in Great Britain, management is shared between gynaecologists (70% of patients) and surgeons (30%) (Hughes, 1979) means that both specialties have their total experience reduced and both need to be constantly on the watch for examples. There are remarkable geographical variations in incidence; in Jamaica there is an ectopic pregnancy for every 28 live births (Douglas, 1963) whereas the ratio in Aberdeen, Scotland, is about 1:200 births.

A history of a missed period is usually obtainable, but some of the most serious bleeds follow rupture of a pregnancy embedded in the isthmus, and this tends to occur early when the period is only a little overdue. However, bleeding is so profuse that no one can overlook this situation.

In the more typical case which presents around 7–8 weeks, there is a history of a missed period, or of an unnaturally scanty loss at the normal period time. Lower abdominal pain starts either sharply (47%) or more slowly (50%) (Hughes, 1979) and there is vaginal bleeding, either constant or (more commonly) intermittent. Fainting is a highly characteristic symptom.

Features of the history which are significant are a previous laparotomy or episode of pelvic sepsis, use of an intrauterine contraceptive device, and established infertility – all these are associated with an increased likelihood of ectopic pregnancy. It is important not to be put off by the fact that a previous laparoscopic sterilisation has been performed. It is now clear that there

is a significant failure rate with this procedure and in 16% the subsequent pregnancy is ectopic in position (Hughes, 1979).

The most important sign is cervical excitation – severe pain on gentle movement of the cervix – and it is a serious error to try to feel a forniceal mass in outpatients or the ward, because at this stage the pregnancy is unruptured and the patient not in immediate danger: if the mass is pressed upon, rupture and brisk haemorrhage are likely to follow. Pregnancy tests are not of great help in this situation.

A pelvic haematocele (i.e. a large pelvic haematoma due to a slowly-leaking tubal abortion) is the most difficult condition to diagnose because it produces mild symptoms, but the tell-tale missed period should give the essential clue.

Units which are used to carrying out diagnostic laparoscopy are increasingly using this in the doubtful ectopic pregnancy, although, of course, it has no place in the management of patients whose ectopic pregnancy has already ruptured, and produced haemoperitoneum. Proof puncture of the posterior fornix has been superseded by laparoscopy.

Once an ectopic pregnancy is diagnosed then salpingectomy must follow, urgently. The most important points to remember are:

1 Resuscitation should *not* precede, but should be *coincidental with operation*. This rather goes against much modern teaching that resuscitation comes first. However, the point is that the loss can be so fast that it will always exceed the speed of replacement transfusion, so the safest course is to get on with laparotomy.

2 Once the abdomen is opened, do not waste time sucking out blood but thrust in a hand, identify the abnormal tube, bring it to the surface and put on two curved artery forceps, one on the proximal end of the tube and the broad ligament and one on the infundibulo-pelvic fold. This will arrest haemorrhage and allow blood to be scooped or sucked out of the abdomen: in suitable circumstances this can be used for autotransfusion. The whole of the tube must be removed. It is usual to preserve the ovary, provided it is normal.

Abortion

It is most unusual for a general surgeon to see a spontaneous abortion because of the free vaginal loss of bright red blood. However, a septic abortion is a different matter, because it tends to follow an illegal and often concealed operation and is likely to present as severe lower abdominal peritonitis. The diagnosis will be readily made once the open cervix and foul vaginal discharge are recognised. Intensive therapy for Gram negative and anaerobic bacteraemia is likely to be needed (*see* p. 7).

Emergencies having no direct connection with pregnancy

Acute appendicitis

Acute appendicitis and pregnancy are both common conditions and will sometimes occur together – about one pregnancy in 2000 will be complicated in this way (Finch and Lee, 1974). It is generally fairly easy to make a timely diagnosis of appendicitis during the early months of a pregnancy, but later on and especially in the puerperium it is appreciably more difficult to do, and it is then that there is a real risk to the fetus and some risk to the mother.

The incidence of appendicitis in the three trimesters is roughly equal. Early in pregnancy there is often some nausea, vomiting and abdominal discomfort, but the progressive pain should demand attention and then a careful history will often elicit a tell-tale history of a shift of pain. A past history suggesting a previous attack of appendicitis is especially common. Generally the signs are clear and it is unusual to have major difficulties in diagnosis during the first three to four months. Thereafter the stretching of the abdominal wall by the growing uterus makes it progressively less likely that muscle guarding will be found over the inflamed appendix: this is so much a feature of appendicitis that it is difficult to make allowances for its relative weakness or absence, but fortunately tenderness continues to be a most valuable localising sign. The other feature to remember is that the enlarging uterus will elevate the appendix until at term it lies close to the right costal margin.

Many reports show that delay in diagnosis becomes progressively more likely the later in pregnancy that appendicitis occurs, and these features are especially noticeable in the puerperium (Munro and Jones, 1975), when guarding is absent even in the presence of peritonitis.

Most of these difficulties can be overcome if the possibility of acute appendicitis is remembered by the obstetrician and allowance made for the changed clinical presentation. The commonest cause of acute right-sided abdominal pain in pregnancy is acute pyelitis and in these circumstances there are few doctors who would not examine the urine. However, this may be misleading because a few pus cells are not infrequently seen in pregnancy when there is no pyelitis. When in real doubt about the possibility of acute pyelitis, it is wise to pass a ureteric catheter under local anaesthesia and obtain a specimen of ureteric urine: occasionally the ureter is

obstructed and there is little or no pus in bladder urine, but if the urine withdrawn from the ureter is clear then pyelitis is excluded. Too many pregnant patients with a surgical abdominal emergency have had the diagnosis delayed by the finding of a few pus cells in a mid-stream urine specimen.

The lesson which comes out most clearly from the many papers on this subject is that if there is a reasonably strong suspicion of acute appendicitis and steps have been taken to exclude pyelitis of pregnancy then the right thing for both mother and the fetus is to go ahead with appendicectomy (Parker, 1954). It is general experience that there is virtually no risk to the pregnancy if the appendix proves to be normal so the surgeon need not be inhibited by this consideration. On the other hand, the surest way of promoting an abortion or premature labour is to delay appendicectomy until perforation has taken place (Babaknia *et al.*, 1977).

It is standard practice to use a muscle-splitting incision centred over the point of maximum tenderness. This provides good exposure of the appendix, and avoids the handling and retraction of the uterus which is almost inevitable if a central vertical incision is used.

Maternal mortality used to be considerable – Parker in 1954 found it to be 20%. Nowadays it is extremely uncommon for the mother to lose her life, but all papers quote cases of late diagnosis in which there is grave risk to the mother before she recovers. The Confidential Report on Maternal Mortality (DHHS, 1979) found no maternal deaths among the 1 939 010 births analysed during 1973–75 and there are a number of other reports in which no mother died. As has been said, the prevention of fetal death hinges almost entirely on early diagnosis. If the appendix perforates during the second half of pregnancy, the uterus will be the immediate medial relation of the appendix and will form part of the wall of an appendix abscess: this is more than likely to induce uterine contractions. There is no reported series without some fetal deaths, but this has now fallen to less than 10% (Finch and Lee, 1974).

There is no doubt that in a few patients acute appendicitis precedes labour by a few hours, but is not diagnosed until after the completion of delivery (Munro and Jones, 1975). This is a situation in which dissemination of infection throughout the peritoneal cavity is especially likely and thorough peritoneal debridement (*see* p. 8) will be of special importance at the time of appendicectomy.

Very rarely, when acute appendicitis occurs near term, the question of performing simultaneous Caesarean Section will arise. There is no doubt that appendicectomy for a perforated appendix with peritonitis is likely to be followed by a stillbirth. I have personal experience of a successful lower segment Caesarean Section performed through a right paramedian incision, followed by appendicectomy and thorough peritoneal lavage. This was done in an elderly primipara carrying a much-wanted child and certainly seemed a right decision. Very careful postoperative care as outlined on pages 7 to 11 is an essential part of this treatment.

Intestinal obstruction

This is a rarity, being seen once in about 6000 pregnancies. It occurs more in the second than the first half of pregnancy, and is particularly likely to complicate the puerperium (Munro and Jones, 1975). In at least half of these patients the obstruction is due to adhesions, and volvulus of the small or large intestine causes a further 25% of cases (Goldthorp, 1966). These conditions are especially likely to produce strangulation so, although obstruction is a rare complication of pregnancy, it offers a very serious threat to the mother's life. This rarity, and the fact that most obstructions occur in the second half of pregnancy or the puerperium, means that diagnosis is especially difficult.

Abdominal discomfort, vomiting and constipation are symptoms which can easily be attributed to the pregnancy, and signs of obstruction can be difficult to obtain beside the large uterus or in the flaccid puerperal abdomen. Auscultation of obstructive bowel sounds may give a vital clue. It is essential to pay close attention to the history of recurrent severe periumbilical central abdominal pain, and so to realise that it is not likely to come from the uterus or cervix. When there is real doubt there should be no hesitation in requesting a plain abdominal x-ray.

An unusual cause of obstruction is carcinoma of the colon, although Goldthorp (1966) reported 3 examples among 12 consecutive patients: treatment will depend very much on the stage which the pregnancy has reached.

Another unusual and difficult condition is known as 'pregnancy ileus' and must be regarded as a special form of colonic pseudo-obstruction (Shaxted and Jukes, 1979). This is particularly likely to complicate the puerperium, and results in very wide distension of the colon which can go on to caecal ischaemia and perforation. A barium enema can be very helpful in showing that there is no organic obstruction, but caecal distension must not be allowed to progress too far and decompression via a caecostomy may be essential.

Peptic ulcer in pregnancy

Although many women find that the symptoms of a peptic ulcer improve during pregnancy, in some there is no remission and both haemorrhage and perforation can occur (Jones *et al.*, 1969). There are several records of successful suture of a perforated duodenal ulcer and of gastrectomy for persistent haematemesis, with a sub-

sequent live birth. These rare problems must be managed on their merits, but it is important to remember Sandweiss's advice that 'pregnancy or the puerperium should not be regarded as contraindications to surgery when this is indicated for peptic ulcer' (Sandweiss *et al.*, 1943).

Acute pancreatitis

There is a slight but definite connection between pregnancy and acute pancreatitis and if an episode of hyperemesis is accompanied by epigastric pain, this diagnosis should be considered and the serum amylase estimated. Among 78 patients seen recently in Glasgow (Imrie and Whyte, 1975) 3 were pregnant, but all had gallstones.

Surgery of the elderly

It is evident to everyone that the hospital population is becoming steadily older, and it is also clear that the inhibitions about operating on the elderly have become progressively less. With improvements in anaesthesia and resuscitation there are now few elderly who cannot be successfully operated upon. The main question to ask is, therefore, whether there is any difference between the abdominal emergencies seen in the elderly and those in younger people.

There is no question that the elderly can tolerate abdominal pain with little complaint. This is well illustrated by acute appendicitis, which often presents to the doctor only after 2 or 3 days of lower abdominal pain. The patient tolerates this, believing that the anorexia and constipation mean a disordered bowel, which only needs a laxative for cure. As the pain continues, the abdomen becomes distended and vomiting becomes more troublesome so the doctor is summoned on the 2nd or 3rd day of the illness. At that time the signs suggest a small bowel obstruction and the patient may be opened with this diagnosis only to find that the obstruction is due to paralytic ileus secondary to acute appendicitis.

Some conditions are seen more often in the elderly than in younger patients, and the complications of diverticular disease and carcinoma of the large bowel are obvious examples of this. Vascular accidents are very much more likely to be seen in the elderly and ruptured aortic aneurysm is increasingly recognised as an important cause of sudden collapse, with loin and abdominal pain, in older patients. Ischaemic colitis and superior mesenteric artery obstruction are much less often seen, but need to be particularly remembered in patients of this age.

There is no question that the prognosis of these serious conditions is worsened when they occur in the elderly because older patients are much more likely to have serious coincidental disease of the cardiovascular or respiratory systems, and their kidneys are more susceptible to the effects of stress. However, providing these problems are recognised, the skills now available in an intensive care unit can often bring a patient through such a crisis, and in general terms the age of the patient does not make very much difference to the urgent treatment required for these serious emergencies. It is very difficult to assess the outcome at the time of admission of an unknown patient and it is a serious mistake to give too much weight to calendar age. Some patients of fifty are already a poor operative risk, while alert and active 80-year-olds can come through a major emergency operation and continue to enjoy their lives and to contribute most positively to the lives of their family and friends.

References

Altemeier W.A. (1938). The cause of the putrid odor of perforated appendicitis peritonitis. *Ann. Surg*; **107**:634–6.

Babaknia A., Parsa H., Woodruff J.D. (1977). Appendicitis during pregnancy. *Obstet. Gynaecol*; **50**:40–4.

Bell T.M., Steyn J. (1962). Virus in lymph nodes of children with mesenteric adenitis and intussusception. *Brit. Med. J*; **2**:700–2.

Burnett W.E., Brown G.R., Rosemond G.P. *et al.* (1957). The treatment of peritonitis using peritoneal lavage. *Ann. Surg*; **145**:675–81.

de Dombal F.T., Leaper D.J., Horrocks J.C. *et al.* (1974). Human and computer-aided diagnosis of abdominal pain. *Brit. Med. J*; **1**:376–80.

Department of Health and Social Security (1979). Report on confidential enquiries into maternal deaths in England and Wales 1973–1975. In *Report on Health and Social Subjects*, 14 (Tomkinson J. *et al.* eds.). London: HMSO.

Douglas C.P. (1963). Tubal ectopic pregnancy. *Brit. Med. J*; **2**:838–41.

Elliott M.S., Jeffrey P.C. (1980). Stercoral perforation of the large bowel. *J. Roy. Coll. Surg. Edin*; **25**:38–40.

Finch D.R.A., Lee E. (1974). Acute appendicitis complicating pregnancy in the Oxford Region. *Brit. J. Surg*; **61**:129–32.

Fowler R. (1975). A controlled trial of intraperitoneal cephaloridine administration in peritonitis. *J. Ped Surg*; **10**:43–50.

Goldthorp W.O. (1966). Intestinal obstruction during pregnancy and the puerperium. *Brit. J. Clin. Prac*; **20**:367–76.

Grosfeld J.L., Weinberger M., Clatworthy H.W. (1973). Acute appendicitis in the first two years of life. *J. Ped. Surg*; **8**:285–93.

Hudspeth A.S. (1975). Radical surgical debridement in the treatment of advanced generalised bacterial peritonitis. *Arch. Surg*; **110**:1233–6.

Hughes G.J. (1979). The early diagnosis of ectopic pregnancy. *Brit. J. Surg*; **66**:789–92.

Hutchison I.F., Olayiwola B., Young D.G. (1980). Intussusception in infancy and childhood. *Brit. J. Surg*; **67**: 209–12.

Imrie C.W., Whyte A.S. (1975). A prospective study of acute pancreatitis. *Brit. J. Surg*; **62**:490–4.

Jones P.F. (1969). Acute abdominal pain in childhood, with special reference to cases not due to acute appendicitis. *Brit. Med. J*; **1**:284–6.

Jones P.F. (1976). Active observation in management of acute abdominal pain in childhood. *Brit. Med. J*; **2**:551–3.

Jones P.F., McEwan A.B., Bernard R.M. (1969). Haemorrhage and perforation complicating peptic ulcer in pregnancy. *Lancet*; **ii**:350–1.

Munro A., Jones P.F. (1975). Abdominal surgical emergencies in the puerperium. *Brit. Med. J*; **4**:691–4.

Neely J., Catchpole B. (1971). Ileus: the restoration of alimentary tract mobility by pharmacological means. *Brit. J. Surg*; **58**:21–6.

Office of Population Censuses and Surveys (1978). *Mortality Statistics, Cause, England and Wales, 1976*, Series DH2 No. 3. London: HMSO.

Parker R.B. (1954). Acute appendicitis in late pregnancy. *Lancet*; **i**:1253–7.

Pollet J.E. (1980). Intussusception: a study of its surgical management. *Brit. J. Surg*; **67**:213–15.

Ryan P. (1958). Emergency resection and anastomosis for perforated sigmoid diverticulitis. *Brit. J. Surg*; **45**:611–16.

Sandweiss D.J. *et al.* (1943). Deaths from perforation and haemorrhage of gastroduodenal ulcer during pregnancy and puerperium. *Amer. J. Obstet. Gynecol*; **45**:131–6.

Schumer W. (1976). Steroids in treatment of clinical septic shock. *Ann. Surg*; **184**:333–41.

Shaxted E.J., Jukes R. (1979). Pseudo-obstruction of the bowel in pregnancy. *Brit. J. Obstet. Gynaecol*; **86**:411–13.

Soderlund S. (1959). Meckel's diverticulum: a clinical and histological study. *Acta Chir. Scand*; Suppl:248.

Stewart D.J. (1978). Antibiotic lavage in the treatment of intraabdominal sepsis. *Ann. Roy. Coll. Surg. Eng*; **60**:240-3.

Stewart D.J., Matheson N.A. (1978a). Peritoneal lavage in appendicular peritonitis. *Brit. J. Surg*; **65**:54–6.

Stewart D.J., Matheson N.A. (1978b). Peritoneal lavage in faecal peritonitis in the rat. *Brit. J. Surg*; **65**:57–9.

Tagart R.E.B. (1974). General peritonitis and haemorrhage complicating colonic diverticular disease. *Ann. Roy. Coll. Surg. Engl*; **55**:175–83.

Thomas D.F.M. (1980). The management of childhood intussusception in a district hospital. *Brit. J. Surg*; **67**:33–5.

Williams H. (1947). Appendicitis in the young child. *Brit. Med. J*; **2**:730–2.

Yates J.L. (1905). Experimental study of the local effects of peritoneal drainage. *Surg. Gynecol. Obstet*; **1**:473–92.

Further reading

de Dombal F.T. (1981). *Diagnosis of Acute Abdominal Pain*. Edinburgh: Churchill Livingstone. (Strongly recommended)

Jones P.F. (1974). *Emergency Abdominal Surgery in Infancy, Childhood, and Adult Life*. Oxford: Blackwell Scientific Publications.

2

Acute abdomen (ii)

PETER F. JONES

Intestinal obstruction

As recently as the 1930s patients with intestinal obstruction admitted to British hospitals had a 1 in 3 chance of succumbing to their disease. Although this high mortality has now been reduced to less than 10%, intestinal obstruction is still a dangerous condition which faces the surgeon with many difficult decisions, both in diagnosis and treatment.

Pathology

All patients with intestinal obstruction show three pathological changes:

1 Loss of alimentary secretions. The normal adult secretes 7–9 l of alimentary juice per day and all but 100 ml of this is reabsorbed. In high intestinal obstruction a large proportion of this fluid is lost by vomiting. In low small bowel obstructions, there is a very substantial volume of fluid (up to 2 l) sequestered from the circulation in distended loops of bowel above the obstruction, and there will be further loss by vomiting. Distended bowel also secretes more juice than normal bowel.

2 Increasing intestinal distension. When drainage from the obstructed bowel is easy – as in the upper jejunum, by vomiting – distension and consequent rise of intraluminal pressure may be slight. If,

however, obstruction occurs in a closed loop – as in the colon – when the lips of the ileocaecal valve close to produce an air and water-tight seal, then pressure above an obstruction can rise very high. Pressures over 25 cm water are common and can cause necrosis of the bowel wall (Saegesser and Sandblom, 1975). It is now generally agreed that the source of the gas trapped in obstructed bowel is swallowed air.

3 Bacterial growth. Although the small bowel is normally more or less sterile, bacterial multiplication quickly occurs above an obstruction, as is clearly seen in 'faecal' vomiting. The main danger from this fluid is if it is spilt, either into the lungs or the peritoneum. Bacterial overgrowth also has an adverse effect in intestinal strangulation (*see below*).

Some patients suffer a further serious change:

4 Intestinal strangulation. This means that blood supply to the bowel is impaired and it necessarily carries the implication of necrosis and perforation. Most strangulations are caused by bowel or mesentery being caught under a band or in the neck of a hernial sac and this usually produces immediate venous obstruction. Much damage can be caused by venous engorgement, with or without arrest of the arterial supply.

The effects of strangulation are very seriously compounded by the bacterial multiplication which occurs in closed loops. Bacteria hasten proteolysis and disruption of ischaemic bowel and produce an exudate with highly lethal qualities which can produce either peritonitis or Gram-negative septicaemia.

In addition to these changes, a long loop caught under a band which only causes venous obstruction will accommodate progressively more of the circulating blood volume. This is an uncommon situation, but can cause severe hypovolaemia.

The causes of intestinal obstruction change with time and place of occurrence. Seventy years ago, when little abdominal surgery was done, most obstructions were due to irreducible hernias or to neoplasms, and only the hernias were effectively treated. Now, postoperative peritoneal adhesions have become one of the major causes of intestinal obstruction in Western countries. In other parts of the world, where natural high-fibre diets are the rule, neoplastic obstruction is almost unknown, but sigmoid volvulus is relatively common. In the newborn, several unique forms of intestinal obstruction are seen – atresia and stenosis, Hirschsprung's disease and meconium ileus *see* Chapter 13.

Diagnosis

As ever in the acute abdomen, it is vital to listen closely to the history. The sudden onset of severe central abdominal pain in band obstruction of the small bowel and the gradual onset of abdominal discomfort, distension and constipation over days or weeks in neoplastic obstruction of the colon are both equally characteristic. While the patient is talking watch the face closely and, if attention wanders and the thread of the history is lost, bare the abdomen, whip out the stethoscope, and watch and listen. This may be the vital moment when a spasm of intestinal colic absorbs all the patient's attention and when it will be possible to see visible peristalsis and to hear a rush of high pitched tinkles and splashes. Once these events have been witnessed, they will always be recognised.

Abdominal distension, though often seen in intestinal (and especially in colonic) obstruction, depends on a sufficient length of intestine being distended to produce this physical sign, so it will be absent in high small bowel obstructions.

The rule that the hernial orifices are examined in every case of acute abdominal pain must be scrupulously observed. It is characteristic of strangulated femoral hernia that the patient complains of intestinal colic and vomiting, but is often unaware that there is a lump in the groin. So, if it is not positively looked for, it will be missed; even when found, the hernial swelling can be surprisingly lacking in tenderness (*see* p. 00).

Whenever possible examine the vomit, and remember that it is in intestinal obstruction that plain abdominal radiography makes one of its major contributions to abdominal diagnosis.

Adhesive intestinal obstruction

Adhesions and bands are now responsible for about one-third of all bowel obstructions in Western countries and the great majority will date from a previous laparotomy (Räf, 1969).

Every surgeon who has to reopen the abdomen for any reason knows that some patients make and retain extensive adhesions, whilst others show little or no evidence of the previous laparotomy. This individual variation seems to be the major determining factor in the formation of adhesions and bands. Closure of raw peritoneal areas after resection (Williams, 1955), seromuscular sutures (Thomas and Rhoads, 1950), hot packs and innoculation of talc powder are all ways of making adhesions which are largely avoidable.

Broadly, adhesions can cause trouble at two distinct times, immediately after operation, or months or years later.

Intestinal obstruction in the days after laparotomy is one of the more worrying situations with which the surgeon has to deal. The time taken for the return of full gastrointestinal activity after major abdominal surgery is highly variable. A patient who, 6 days after anterior resection of the rectum, has still not passed flatus is a worry, but is not necessarily obstructed, and to judge when the limit of normal recovery has been reached is difficult. Nearly all these problems in slow convalescence resolve with 'drip and suck', but modern skills in fluid and electrolyte balance and intravenous nutrition can allow this phase to be prolonged almost indefinitely and some rules are needed for the safe management of the postoperative period.

1 After major intestinal surgery, it is passage of flatus per rectum or colostomy, *not* the return of bowel sounds, which signals recovery of the whole alimentary tract and permits commencement of oral feeding. If this rule is not observed, there is a serious risk that the normal phase of intestinal inactivity which follows major surgery will be unnecessarily prolonged.

2 Although rare, a strangulating band obstruction can occur in the postoperative period. Anyone who has a lot of steady abdominal pain with vomiting and rise of pulse rate must be closely watched. If these complaints continue, with some abdominal tenderness, the only safe course is to reopen the abdomen. Abdominal x-rays are of little help in this situation.

3 If the period of a normal convalescence has passed, then it is important to distinguish between paralytic ileus and mechanical obstruction.

a If the clincial and x-ray picture suggests paralytic ileus look for the cause – a continuing peritonitis or a leaking anastomosis – and treat it. Remember that a persistent 'paralytic ileus', for which there is no obvious cause, is likely to be due to unrecognised mechanical obstruction.

  b If the clinical and x-ray findings suggest a mechanical obstruction, then the likely cause will be fibrinous adhesions causing a kink in the small bowel. These are still at the stage when fibrinolysis can lead to improvement and if the bowel is kept decompressed, resolution can occur. On the other hand, this is by no means guaranteed and the fact that, with intravenous nutrition, the patient can be kept in good condition almost indefinitely, offers a serious temptation to delay making a decision. This must be recognised and resisted.

If 'drip and suck' is going to work, then there should be clear evidence of some improvement when the patient is examined every 8–12 h. Softening of the distended abdomen, appearance of gas in the colon in plain abdominal x-rays, passage of flatus per rectum and a general impression of relaxation in the appearance of the patient are all promising signs. Generally speaking, an absence of any signs of improvement after 48 h of 'drip and suck' means that the adhesions are not resolving and a definite time should be set for reopening the abdomen.

The *operation* for adhesive obstruction within days of laparotomy can be difficult and is emphatically not for the tyro. At this stage some adhesions separate easily, but others are very tacky, the bowel is distended and oedematous and it is all too easy to produce a tear, with disastrous leakage of infected obstructed bowel content. Patience, experience, and a light touch, are the keys to successful separation of adhesions. If a tear occurs, repair it with interrupted non-absorbable sutures and consider the passage of a long intestinal tube, to decompress the small bowel (Munro and Jones, 1978). Tracing the small bowel as far distally as possible and then doing an ileo-transverse side-to-side anastomosis has little to commend it. The best procedure is patiently to unravel all the coils of small bowel, and then splint the whole length of the small bowel with a long intestinal tube (*see* p. 22).

Late adhesive intestinal obstruction

Clinical picture

Every patient with late adhesive obstruction complains of *abdominal pain* and it is characteristic that this has a definite time of onset. Fortunately, the severity of the pain seems to be directly related to the likelihood of strangulation. Sudden onset of severe central abdominal colicky pain, which does not relent and goes on to become almost continuous, is highly suggestive of strangulation of a loop of bowel under a band. *Vomit-*

ing soon follows, at first food, and then green, becoming brown, offensive fluid. *Constipation* is usual.

The general condition is likely to be good for a time, until dehydration from low intake and vomiting takes effect (although remember that if a considerable length of small bowel is caught under a band, it can accommodate a large volume of blood which cannot return through the veins compressed by the band. This leads to increasing hypovolaemia.)

The hernial sites should be carefully examined first, so that they are not forgotten. Abdominal tenderness is highly significant, because it is almost always noticeable, often acute, in strangulating obstructions. Obstructive bowel sounds coinciding with an episode of colicky pain are an invaluable diagnostic sign, but they are not always heard and it is essential to wait for the onset of a spasm of colic. If a considerable length of bowel is strangulated, bowel sounds are likely to be infrequent because this change is usually accompanied by ileus. Occasionally, a mass of strangulated loops caught under a band are palpable as a mass.

In most patients with adhesive obstruction, there will be a history of a laparotomy and an abdominal scar, but these may be absent. Spontaneous adhesions – usually of strands of omentum – are common and certainly cause some cases of adhesive obstruction.

Plain radiography of the abdomen is an invaluable aid to diagnosis of adhesive small bowel obstruction. The classical appearances of the parallel-sided gas distended small bowel loops, with fluid levels in erect films, and absence of colonic gas are well known. However, it is vital to remember that one-third of patients with strangulating small bowel obstruction show *no* radiographic evidence of obstruction (Frimann-Dahl, 1960) and this is true for 15–20% of all adhesive obstructions.

Treatment

If a firm diagnosis of late adhesive obstruction is made then the treatment should be by operation unless:

  1 Symptoms of obstruction are clearly improving when the patient is first seen.
  2 There have been multiple previous laparotomies (*see below*).

All patients with intestinal obstruction need a short period of preparation for operation with nasogastric suction to empty the stomach and intravenous fluids to replace the water and electrolytes lost through cessation of drinking, vomiting and sequestration of gastrointestinal secretions in the obstructed intestine.

If it is decided to reopen the previous incision, it is wise to prolong it either upwards or downwards and to open the peritoneum there, very cautiously. With luck, the peritoneal cavity will be free and any adhesions of bowel to the back of the scar can be felt and carefully separated from it with a scalpel. As soon as the peritoneum is open, it may be obvious that strangulation has occurred because discoloured bowel is seen or blood-stained fluid appears.

The first step is to find the site of the obstruction and it is usually easiest to draw out distended bowel first and to empty it back into the stomach, where it can be aspirated by the anaesthetist (Jones and Matheson, 1968). The withdrawal of this bowel will finally reveal the cause of the obstruction, and if it is a band, the trapped bowel beneath it will be seen. This may be just slightly cyanosed, deeply engorged, or frankly gangrenous. The band should be divided and removed and the bowel gently brought up through the incision and closely observed. It may be immediately obvious that the colour is improving and that the whole loop is viable, but it is always vital to pay very close attention to the constriction ring where the band actually held down the loop. This often looks pale and grey, but if it feels of normal consistence, it is almost certainly viable. A constriction ring which feels thin is suspect and must be carefully watched for change of colour and will at least require oversewing with Lembert sutures.

If the strangulated loop shows no signs of changing colour then *tests of viability* must be applied.

1　The colour of the bowel wall (*not* the subserosal ecchymoses) must be watched over several minutes. It is helpful if good pulsation is seen in the mesentery, but the crucial sign is a return of pink colour to the muscular layer.

2　Peristalsis is not very helpful, because it is often absent from recovering bowel and may be seen in non-viable bowel.

3　A flabby and thinned-out feeling to the bowel wall is a grave sign and almost certainly means loss of viability.

4　When in real doubt place the suspect bowel in a saline towel at 37–40°C and look round the rest of the abdomen for other adhesions and other pathology.

Generally speaking, if there is still serious doubt about viability after 10 min observation, then resection of the doubtful loop is needed. The trainee surgeon should certainly ask for senior advice, because this is a difficult decision to take, even for the experienced. A sound method of small bowel resection and anastomosis, carefully applied, is much safer than leaving bowel of dubious viability in the abdomen (Fig 2.1).

Careful closure of the incision with non-absorbable material is of special importance in intestinal obstruction because a period of abdominal distension is highly probable. Mass closure or the use of deep all layer retention sutures of nylon are essential.

Recurrent adhesive obstruction

It is natural for adhesions to recur after a laparotomy for adhesive obstruction, so further episodes of obstruction can occur. In some patients these are mild and respond quickly to intravenous fluids and nasogastric suction and these are almost certainly due to impaction of a bolus of food at a kink. It is wise to warn patients who have had their first division of adhesions that food must be chewed thoroughly, especially fresh fruit.

When an episode of recurrent intestinal obstruction is accompanied by severe abdominal pain and tenderness, there is no alternative to laparotomy because there may be strangulation. When pain is less severe and tenderness slight, but obstruction does not respond to 'drip and suck', the surgeon is faced with a difficult choice between unprofitable delay and a further laparotomy which, in turn, will produce fresh adhesions.

There is as yet no reliable way of preventing adhesions (Ellis, 1974). There is considerable evidence that peritoneal lavage diminishes adhesion formation, and special claims have been made for noxythiolin and polyvinyl pyrrolidone solutions. (Gilmore and Reid, 1979). However, lavage is not going to prevent further adhesions in everyone. The best available plan at the moment is to operate when it is clear that the obstruction is not resolving, followed by lavage and intubalation of the intestine (Munro and Jones, 1978).

The technique of the operation follows the same pattern as that already described for band obstruction. It is best to work away determinedly to divide all adhesions and free the whole small intestine. When there are numerous adhesions this can be a daunting task, but the only answer is to work steadily with a No. 10 scalpel, first at one point making progress as far as possible, and then at another. With patience and care, the bowel can be freed. When in doubt stop, because it is serious to open the lumen of the bowel. However carefully the cut is closed with interrupted non-absorbable sutures, this incision will be a weak point during any postoperative ileus and may leak. The adhesion causing the obstruction will eventually be reached and identified, because the intestine beyond it will be collapsed.

At this point completely decompress the small bowel by retrograde emptying into the stomach and then wash the peritoneum and the bowel thoroughly. Finally, encourage the adhesions which are bound to re-form to do so in a benign manner. Noble's plication was used for this purpose for a long time (Noble, 1937), but it is not reliable (Wilson, 1964) and operative intubation of the whole small intestine (White, 1956) is safer and more effective. A specially-designed Foley-type catheter, 3.25 m long, 18 F gauge,* is introduced through a

*Manufactured by Searle Medical Products. High Wycombe, Bucks. HP12 3TD. Product order code: 463018.

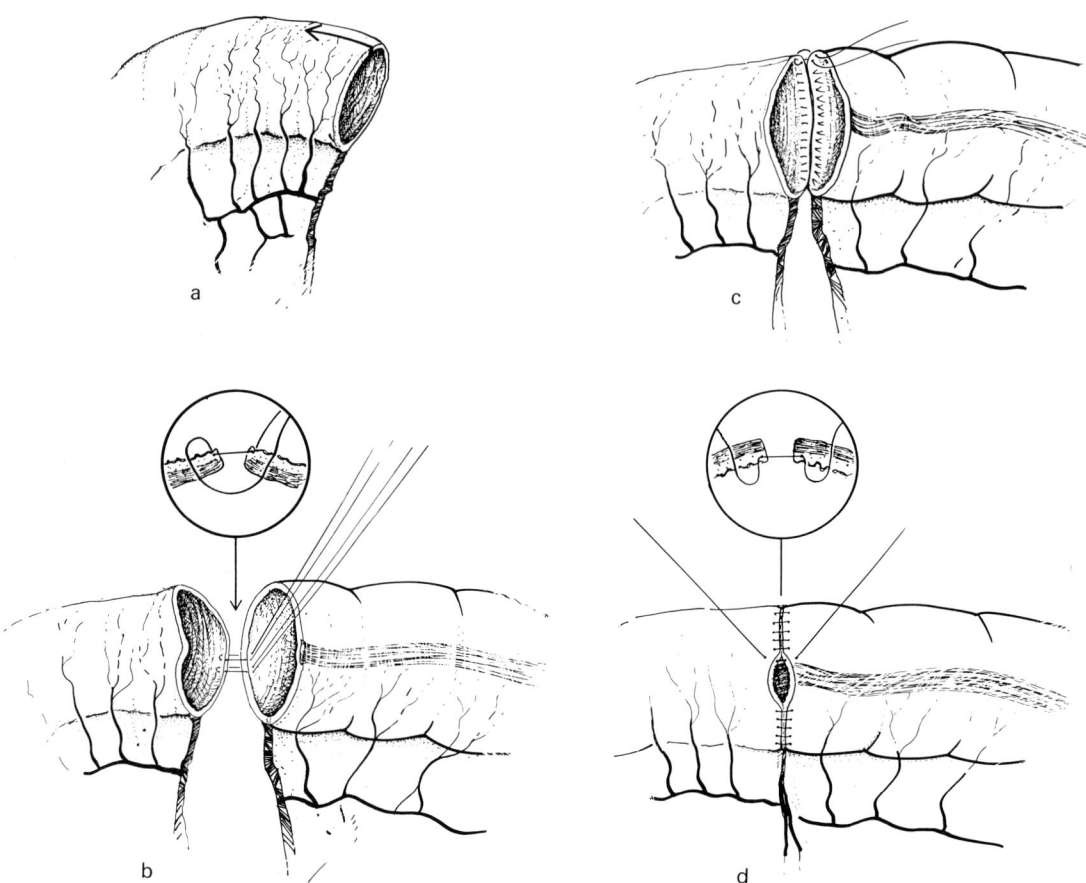

Fig 2.1 Standard method of end-to-end anastomosis of small or large intestine. (a) Back-cut to equalise circumference of two ends of bowel. (b) Interrupted vertical mattress sutures in posterior layer. (c) Posterior layer completed: corners being sutured by continuing interrupted mattress sutures onto anterior layer of anastomosis. (d) Completion of anterior layer with interrupted Gambee sutures.

stab incision in the left flank and then introduced into the upper jejunum, as close as possible to the duodeno-jejunal flexure. The balloon is inflated to about the size of a marble and this allows the tip of the tube to be drawn easily down the small bowel. The assistant advances the tube through the jejunostomy, as the operator manipulates the tip through the loops of intestine. When the tip of the tube reaches the ileocaecal valve, the balloon is deflated, the tube advanced into the caecum and the balloon is then blown up to about 2.5 cm diameter. This prevents the tip of the tube retracting into the ileum. The jejunum is closed snugly around the tube with 2 catgut purse-string sutures and the jejunum sewn to the peritoneum at the point at which the tube passes through the abdominal wall (Fig

2.2). A number of side holes are cut in the tube and this allows gas and fluid to drain, keeping the bowel decompressed. (If any incisions into the bowel have been made this manoeuvre promotes safe healing.) The intestine is laid back in the abdomen in an orderly ladder-pattern and the tube keeps the bowel in smooth open curves at the flexures, while adhesions form in favourable positions. The tube is left on open drainage until flatus passes per rectum and is then spigotted. The tube remains *in situ* for 12–14 days to allow adhesions to form and the balloon is then deflated and the tube withdrawn.

We have now used this tube on over 70 occasions and are convinced of its safety and of its value in preventing further obstructive episodes. A full report is given by Munro and Jones (1978).

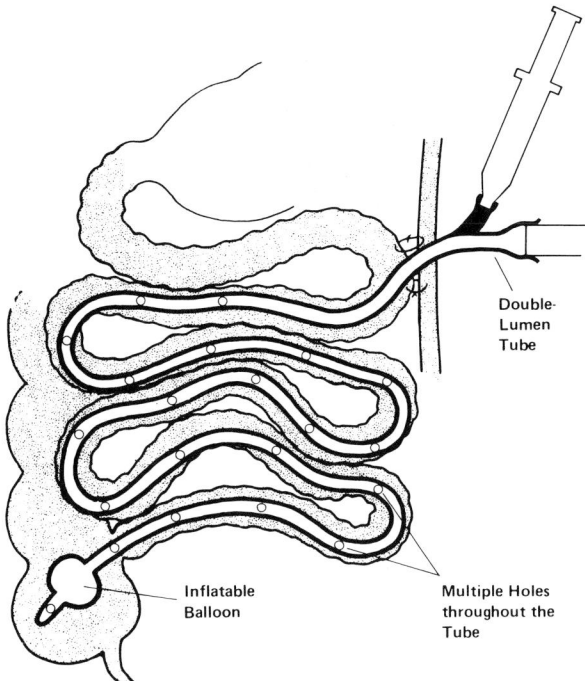

Double-
Lumen
Tube

Inflatable
Balloon

Multiple Holes
throughout the
Tube

Fig 2.2 Long intestinal tube inserted via proximal jejunostomy and threaded through small bowel to caecum. Note the side holes to decompress the small intestine.

Strangulated external hernia

This type of intestinal obstruction has been familiar to surgeons throughout the ages and in pre-Listerian times the occasional patient was successfully relieved by operation. In the early years of this century a strangulated hernia was much the commonest cause of small bowel obstruction, and in developing countries it still is, although in Western countries it now takes second place to postoperative adhesions.

Only 4% of inguinal hernias present with strangulation, but 32% of femoral and 15% of umbilical hernias are strangulated when first seen (McIver, 1933). The male-female ratios for strangulated hernias are inguinal 10:1, femoral 1:3 and umbilical 1:5. Strangulation is rare in the first 25 years of life, except as an occasional complication of the irreducible inguinal hernia often seen during the first year of life.

The point of constriction in a strangulated external hernia is often the neck of the sac, and this is particularly true for femoral hernia. However, at operation on an inguinal hernia, it is often clear that the external abdominal ring is the main point of constriction.

The diagnosis of a **strangulated inguinal hernia** usually presents little difficulty. Typically, a man of 40–70 years of age, who knows he has a rupture, complains of sudden pain and tightness in the hernia, finds it is irreducible and begins to have intestinal colic and vomiting. Only 2% of strangulated inguinal hernias are not painful and tender.

It cannot be too strongly emphasised that this ease of diagnosis does not hold true for **strangulated femoral and umbilical hernias**. Only *one-quarter* of patients with a strangulated femoral hernia complain of pain in the hernia (Dunphy, 1940) and *less than one-half* (42%) know that they have a hernia. Patients are usually well-covered women and it is easy to miss the lump unless it is looked for; hence the golden rule – *make a thorough examination of the hernial sites in any case of acute abdominal pain*. In the minority of patients who complain of pain in the hernia, but not in the abdomen, it will be found to contain strangulated omentum.

The other misleading feature of strangulated femoral hernia is that in nearly 50% the lump is not tender. This is so different to the tenderness of a strangulated inguinal hernia that it tends to put off the inexperienced observer.

Another hazard which characteristically complicates femoral hernia is **Richter's hernia**, in which 'a portion of the circumference of the gut is imprisoned, so reducing, but not obliterating, the lumen of the intestine' (White, 1912). Over half of these hernias occur in femoral hernial sacs, most of the others in umbilical or incisional hernias. The characteristic feature is, interestingly, that the sac is *tender*, although *not* always palpable. Patients complain of abdominal pain and two-thirds of them have signs of intestinal obstruction, but diagnosis is very difficult in those who have only abdominal pain, nausea and some tenderness over the hernia, and these are the patients likely to have ischaemia of the strangulated portion of bowel.

Only 10% of strangulated hernias are **umbilical**, but the mortality is three times greater than in other strangulated external hernias. There are two main reasons for this – the patients are generally elderly, obese and unfit, and the hernia itself presents considerable problems. Nearly all umbilical hernias have been present for some time, many are quite large and patients are used to episodes of tightness and discomfort in the hernia. The signal that strangulation has occurred is likely to be the onset of abdominal colic and vomiting, but the signs in the hernia may be very equivocal. Unfortunately, some patients delay calling for help until there is external evidence of cellulitis in the hernial coverings. The risks to the patient are greatly increased by the fact that colon can be strangulated in an umbilical hernia, making treatment more difficult, with a very high risk of serious infection.

Incisional hernias are becoming less common as more care is exercised by surgeons and gynaecologists over the selection and closure of incisions. Recognition of the weaknesses of catgut has been especially helpful (British Medical Journal, 1977). Strangulation is usually readily diagnosed, unless the size of a hernia masks the signs, as in an umbilical hernia.

Strangulated obturator hernia is a rarity which every surgeon hopes he will recognise before operation. Its features have been well summarised by Desmond and Hutter (1948): 'the combination of intestinal obstruction with pain referred down the front and inner side of the thigh to the knee in an elderly wasted woman suggests strangulation of bowel in an obturator hernia'. This emphasises that nearly all patients are women between 60 and 80 years of age. They are characteristically in poor condition from dehydration and have often had symptoms for 24–48 h. Signs of intestinal obstruction are usually obvious, but it is most unusual to feel a lump, because it lies deep to the femoral vessels and pectineus. However, if the diagnosis is entertained, the sac can often be felt by making forward and lateral pressure through the vaginal wall. The age and poor state of many of these patients make the history difficult to obtain and pain in the distribution of the obturator nerve (Howship's sign) is only described by 50%.

Failure to recognise this condition is disappointing for the surgeon, but not harmful to the patient because laparotomy for intestinal obstruction is clearly indicated, after a few hours spent on rehydration of the patient.

Strangulated internal hernia

This is a rare cause of intestinal obstruction and very unlikely to be diagnosed preoperatively. The patient will present as a case of small bowel obstruction and will almost certainly be thought to have a band obstruction.

About one-half of these hernias are *paraduodenal*. These arise in the embryo, during rotation of the midgut, and a right paraduodenal hernia means that the small bowel lies retroperitoneally behind the ascending and transverse mesocolon. In a left paraduodenal hernia, the small bowel lies behind the descending mesocolon. In both hernias, it is only terminal ileum which becomes intraperitoneal and it is here that the bowel kinks or twists. The right hernia is released by mobilising the proximal colon, as in right hemicolectomy. The left hernial neck contains the inferior mesenteric vein and left colic artery, so considerable care is needed when enlarging the hernial neck. It may help to mobilise the splenic flexure and descending colon.

Bowel may be strangulated in peritoneal pouches around the caecum, the sigmoid mesocolon or the bladder (supravesical). Occasionally strangulation occurs when bowel is caught in a hole in the small bowel mesentery and herniation through the Foramen of Winslow is well known, though fortunately rare. Diaphragmatic hernia is a rare, but dangerous form of internal herniation.

Treatment

It is hardly necessary to say that any patient with a strangulated hernia requires a few hours devoted to intravenous replacement of fluid and aspiration of gastric content through a 16F nasogastric tube. If the hernia is *inguinal*, this time can also very profitably be devoted to *postural treatment*. After a very long experience, Bowesman (1951) noticed that he had never seen gangrene at operation if the duration of strangulation did not exceed 24 h. He found that if 60 cm blocks were placed at the foot of the bed and 30 mg of morphine injected, that 72% of patients with a history of less than 24 h achieved reduction of the strangulated bowel, on average within 4 h. Clearly nothing is lost by this regime, because the patient must in any case be prepared for operation. Postural treatment is well recognised in the treatment of infants with an unreducible inguinal hernia, but it is not so well known among adults.

If posture fails, the hernia should be operated upon, using an incision made in the line of the sac. Often the hernia reduces while this is being made and then the repair is completed in the usual manner. If reduction does not occur, the external oblique is incised in the line of its fibres and the external ring opened up. This may also release a constriction and allow bowel to return to the abdomen. The tense sac needs to be opened very carefully and a hernia director can be helpful. Draw out the discoloured bowel and continue opening the sac until the neck is reached. Viability of the bowel is assessed as already described and action taken accordingly. A repair favoured by the operator is then carried out.

The major technical problem in inguinal hernia is when the caecum or sigmoid colon is strangulated and is of doubtful viability. The 'second-look' procedure may be very valuable here, or a primary resection and anastomosis may be feasible and indicated. This is a situation in which experienced help is likely to be needed.

Reduction *en masse* is well recognised, but very unusual and can be defined as the presence of unreduced gut within a hernial sac after taxis. This occurs when an inguinal hernia is forcibly reduced through the deep abdominal muscular ring, but the bowel is not reduced from the hernial sac. There is usually a history of forceful painful taxis with later onset of colicky abdominal pain and signs of intestinal obstruction. When suspected, this hernia is best approached from above, via a low paramedian incision.

There is no place for posture in the treatment of strangulated femoral hernia. As soon as preoperative preparation is complete, the patient should be operated upon. There can be no hesitation in recommending the extraperitoneal approach developed by McEvedy (1950), because it is both safer and easier to perform than the alternatives, and can be performed easily under local nerve block if the patient is very unfit.

The transverse muscle-splitting incision first described for appendicectomy in 1900 by Fowler is much the best, because it gives good access and yet heals strongly and almost painlessly. The incision follows the skin crease which runs in from the anterior iliac spine. External oblique is split and held open to reveal the lateral edge of the rectus sheath, which is split medially over rectus and the split carried laterally into internal oblique and transversus. This is really a grid-iron incision and is opened up by traction with the fingers. If the lower edge of the incision is now retracted downwards, the extraperitoneal plane easily opens up and leads down, behind the inguinal ligament, to the point where the neck of the femoral hernial sac disappears into the femoral canal. The peritoneum is opened here and the loops of bowel entering and leaving the neck of the sac are secured with Babcock's forceps. The neck of the sac now needs dilatation and a Moynihan's gallbladder forceps firmly opened up does this well. Gentle traction may now allow the loops to slide back into the peritoneal cavity and be closely inspected for viability, and appropriate action taken. If the fundus of the sac cannot be drawn up through the femoral canal, then it can be exposed by raising the lower skin flap, cutting it off at the level of the saphenous opening, the neck of the sac being then drawn out of the femoral canal and the peritoneum repaired. One or two silk or prolene sutures can be passed through the inguinal and Gimbernat's ligament to close the entrance to the femoral canal.

This approach has several virtues. It is easy to understand and at all the important stages, vessels are under direct view so that it is safe. There is early control of intestine, thus a loop of doubtful viability is not lost. There is good access to the peritoneal cavity if resection is needed.

A strangulated umbilical hernia can set even an experienced operator some difficulties. Generally speaking, the contents tend to adhere to the sac at the fundus more than at the neck. However, the neck is a difficult place to open, so it is usually best to open the sac on the side and work gradually to open it up and see what it contains. There is often much adherent omentum, and this is best amputated. As soon as a good view is achieved, incise the neck of the sac by horizontal cuts out into the rectus sheath at 3 and at 9 o'clock. If colon is strangulated there are two possible solutions; resection and formation of separated proximal and distal end or draining colostomies, or primary extended right hemicolectomy and ileocolic anastomosis. Careful judgement is needed to choose the right method. If in doubt, choose the colostomy.

In these circumstances very thorough lavage of the abdomen and abdominal wall with tetracycline solution is important. If possible, carry out a Mayo repair of the hernia. The poor condition of some of these patients may considerably limit what can be done at operation.

Obturation of the intestines

This is an unusual form of intestinal obstruction which is more or less confined to the small intestine.

Gallstone obstruction is a rare but serious cause of obstruction. The patients are nearly always elderly and obese, 85% are women, and the symptoms are often intermittent and confusing. Hence, all too often the diagnosis is not accurately made and patients present late.

It has been estimated that 5% of gallstones migrate into the intestine and 0.5% cause intestinal obstruction. Almost all these stones pass through a cholecyst-duodenal fistula, the formation of which has rarely caused any upset to the patient. Stones which produce obstruction are usually more than 3 cm in diameter and there is considerable speculation on whether stones grow by accretion and so only cause obstruction some time after passing into the lumen of the small bowel. The standard site of arrest is the terminal ileum.

An elderly obese lady complains of vague abdominal pain and vomiting. By the next day she feels better and then the trouble returns. This may be repeated as the stone is sometimes held up and sometimes free to advance down the small intestine. In one reported series, patients took 7 days to reach hospital and another 3 days to reach theatre (Cooperman *et al.*, 1968). The best opportunity to make a diagnosis is when the patient has an episode of colic, when obstructive bowel sounds may be heard. An erect plain abdominal film, apart from showing the signs of small bowel obstruction, should show the diagnostic sign of gas in the biliary tree in about 50% of patients. Only rarely is a radio-opaque gallstone visible in the middle of the abdomen. Often the decision to operate will be taken on the evidence of an unrelieved obstruction, the origin of which is not clear.

These patients are generally poor risks because they have been ill for several days and are dehydrated and immobile. A few hours should be spent over careful rehydration.

A vertical exploratory incision will usually be used and the diagnosis is made as soon as the distended bowel is traced down to the stone. Sometimes the stone can be milked into the caecum but if the stone is stuck, it is usually best to deliver it by enterotomy. Before doing this, empty the distended ileum and jejunum back into the stomach: this makes enterotomy safer and also allows a second stone to be identified, if present. It also gives the opportunity to inspect the cholecyst-duodenal fistula. If another big stone is still present in the gallbladder, this should be removed by cholecysto-tomy and the gallbladder drained, but the fistula should *not* be disturbed. This, when attempted at the time of the obstruction, has carried a high mortality (Anderson and Zederfeldt, 1969). The enterotomy should be made longitudinally over the stone, the stone removed and the incision studied closely. If the edges bleed and the bowel is of reasonable thickness, then it should be closed transversely with interrupted 3/0 nurolon Gam-bee sutures. If viability is seriously in doubt, then this segment must be resected.

Bolus obstruction by food

Not many patients will suffer impaction of a turtle's egg, or grasshoppers eaten whole, which are among the 61 foods which Stephens (1966) listed as causes of bolus obstruction, but dried fruits, peanuts and oranges are often swallowed unchewed and are a regular cause of this type of obstruction, which causes a remarkably severe degree of intestinal colic. Most patients fail to connect their symptoms with the food that is causing them, and direct enquiry is usually needed, which means that the surgeon has to remember this cause of intestinal obstruction. It is more likely to occur in a patient with a partial gastrectomy.

The difficulty in managing these patients is that there is no way of being certain of this diagnosis except by laparotomy, but many patients will cure themselves. Careful observation is needed, and if symptoms and signs continue, it will be necessary to open the abdomen, to treat the impaction and to make certain that another cause of obstruction, such as a band, is not the more important condition to treat.

Obturation of the intestine by worms is almost unknown in the West, but small bowel obstruction by masses of *Ascaris lumbricoides* is well known in Africa and the East (*see* Chapter 14).

Intussusception in the adult

Although this event is not common, most busy surgical units will see one or two examples of this condition each year, the great majority due to a neoplasm, which may be benign or malignant.

In the small bowel the initiating tumour is most often an adenoma, and this is a well-known problem in Peutz-Jeghers syndrome. In the large bowel, the tumour is usually a carcinoma and the intussusception may occur anywhere from the caecum to the rectum. Meckel's diverticulum can cause an intussusception at any age, although the great majority occur before the age of 10. In a small number of patients there is no demonstrable cause. Very rarely intussusception is seen in typhoid fever and dysentery.

Diagnosis is not often suspected before laparotomy, although it should be suspected in patients who show an intermittently palpable abdominal mass. Occasionally, an intussuscepting colonic carcinoma can be felt on rectal examination. Resection is nearly always the correct treatment, because reduction can be difficult and because operation rids the patient of both neoplasm and the source of further trouble.

Retrograde jejunogastric intussusception, although well known, is a very unusual occurrence. It can occur after Polya partial gastrectomy or simple gastro-jejunostomy and it may present at any time from 1 week to 20 years after the operation. In four out of five cases it is the efferent loop which intussuscepts back into the stomach.

In acute postoperative intussusception, the patient is generally making a good recovery when, some 5–7 days after operation, there is a complaint of epigastric pain and vomiting, which continues intermittently. A barium meal shows a characteristic filling defect in the stomach and often the weight of the barium seems to reduce the intussusception, so that no operation is needed.

In the delayed form of acute intussusception, which occurs months or years after operation, the patient is suddenly smitten with severe epigastric pain and vomiting. A mass may be palpable in the epigastrium and the vomitus often contains blood. The diagnosis is readily made if a small barium meal is given, but most of these patients come to operation as high small bowel obstruction and the usual treatment is reduction of the intussusception; occasionally this is irreducible and then resection is required.

Iatrogenic obstruction

After abdomino perineal excision

It used to be the custom to bring out the terminal colostomy across the peritoneum, thus leaving a hiatus lateral to the colostomy in which small bowel could strangulate. This complication has more or less disappeared with the general adoption of extraperitoneal colostomy.

Retroanastomotic hernia

When an antecolic gastrojejunostomy is constructed as the last step of a Polya gastrectomy, a new intra-abdominal hiatus is made between the jejunal loops and transverse colon. Through this a loop of small bowel can pass or become strangulated. This usually causes severe pain and vomiting and sometimes there is a palpable epigastric mass. Surgical relief is essential and may involve a difficult dissection. Stammers (1954) gave an excellent description of this condition.

Potassium-induced stenosis

For a time, in the 1960s, it was common to prescribe potassium chloride with thiazide and it was found that pure potassium chloride tablets caused a severe fibrosis in the wall of the small intestine in a few patients. This could cause a stricture which went on to complete intestinal obstruction. Now that potassium is safely dispensed, this problem has largely disappeared.

Obstruction of the large intestine

Although the colon is a wide bore viscus and capable of great dilatation, it is quite commonly the site of obstruction. In Western communities carcinoma is far and away the commonest cause and volvulus is rare, the exact opposite of the situation in the vegetarian peoples of Asia and Africa.

Whatever the cause, all forms of large bowel obstruction offer problems both in diagnosis and treatment. The correct operative treatment may call for considerable surgical skill, so senior advice and assistance is nearly always needed for the safe and successful treatment of these patients.

Neoplastic obstruction

It might be expected that obstruction would more easily occur in the distal large bowel, where faeces are more solid than in the proximal colon. However, Table 1 (which compares the total incidence of all large bowel neoplasms in N E Scotland with the site of 57 obstructed neoplasms treated consecutively in a surgical unit in Aberdeen) shows that in fact the opposite is true, and 70% of large bowel obstructions occur proximal to the sigmoid colon.

Clinical

The onset of neoplastic obstruction of the large bowel is characteristically insidious. Irregularity of the bowel and recurrent lower abdominal colic gradually

Table 1
57 CONSECUTIVE PATIENTS WITH LARGE BOWEL OBSTRUCTION DUE TO CARCINOMA

	Number of obstructed carcinomas	%	All tumours in Grampian region %
Caecum, A C + Hepatic flexure	21	37	27
Transverse colon	6	10	8
Splenic flexure	7	14	4
Descending colon	5	8	3
Sigmoid	12	20	19
Recto-sigmoid and rectum	6	10	39
Total	57	99	100

become more noticeable and some may observe increasing distension and audible peristaltic sounds. In contrast to small intestinal obstruction, vomiting is unusual and only occurs late, and mainly in caecal tumours.

This slow progress toward obstruction allows time for the colon to distend above the neoplasm and it is usual to see a relatively well patient with enormous tympanitic abdominal distension. In distal obstruction the bowel immediately above the tumour does not distend as much as the proximal colon, because hypertrophy of the muscle in the wall is maximal just above the tumour. The caecum may be hugely distended and can often be both seen and felt. Distinctive obstructive intestinal sounds and splashing are usually audible.

In obstructions of the caecum and ascending colon the distended bowel will be mainly small intestine and the slow progression of the constricting neoplasm will have allowed the muscle in the intestinal wall to have hypertrophied. This can lead to the invaluable sign of intermittent hardening of these loops, which can be both seen and felt. This is diagnostic of a slowly progressive obstruction and is not seen in acute small bowel obstruction.

It is unlikely that rectal examination will reveal an obstructing carcinoma, but occasionally a sigmoid carcinoma in the Pouch of Douglas can be felt, or an intussuscepting carcinoma. Sigmoidoscopy is always worth doing and sometimes reaches an obstructing tumour low in the sigmoid colon.

Plain abdominal x-rays can be very helpful, showing the whole of the obstructed colon outlined in gas, with wide fluid levels, especially in the caecum. The ileocaecal valve remains remarkably competent in many patients, so that the colon between the valve and the carcinoma becomes a closed space, and there is little or no sign of small bowel obstruction. In obstructions of the proximal colon it is likely that the small bowel will be dilated and obstructed. However, it is not unusual for gas distension of the colon to stop short of the actual site of obstruction and there should be no hesitation in asking for an emergency barium enema: this is a harmless and extremely valuable investigation.

The two main differential diagnoses are sigmoid volvulus and pseudo-obstruction. A sigmoid volvulus has a characteristically short history, quite extreme distension of the twisted loop, and a typical x-ray picture. Pseudo-obstruction offers a much more difficult diagnosis. (*see* p. 31)

Treatment

Nearly all these patients are middle-aged or elderly and have been unwell for some time. They often have other medical problems. Their relative well-being may be deceptive and they may be both undernourished, underhydrated and anaemic. A little time spent on simple investigations and treatment may make a great difference to the outcome. On the other hand, the absence of pain and vomiting should not lead to delay because the tightly distended caecum in some of these patients can be dangerously close to rupture (Saegesser and Sandblom, 1975).

There has been considerable change in methods of treatment over the last 20 years and there is still no general agreement. For practical purposes, the colon can be conveniently divided into proximal and distal parts.

Proximal colon obstruction. This is taken as including all neoplasms causing obstruction up to and including the splenic flexure. For these one operation can be applied in nearly all cases, with a high degree of success.

It will be common ground among nearly all surgeons nowadays that carcinoma of the caecum or ascending colon, which has produced intestinal obstruction, should be treated by urgent right hemicolectomy and primary end-to-end anastomosis of the ileum to the right half of the transverse colon. The distended small bowel should be emptied back into the stomach by gentle stripping, which is far and away the safest and most effective way of emptying small bowel. The anaesthetist can aspirate the fluid and gas via a nasogastric tube (Jones and Matheson, 1968). A standard right hemicolectomy is then carried out. The open end of the empty ileum is cleaned with swabs soaked in Savlon or perchloride of mercury, and the same is done to the collapsed transverse colon. An end-to-end anastomosis is then done by the method favoured by the surgeon: we use a single layer of interrupted mattress sutures of 2/0 nurolon (Fig 2.1). In our last 21 patients so treated, 19 made a straightforward recovery; the two who died after operation had a palliative resection.

Most surgeons would tend to extend right hemi-

colectomy to cover obstructing carcinomas in the right half of the transverse colon and we have found this to be a useful operation throughout the transverse colon (Fig 2.3). It may seem that a lot of colon is being removed, but these are often elderly patients who will be more appreciative of a single curative operation than a staged procedure. All the ten patients on whom we have used this operation for obstructed carcinoma of the left transverse colon or splenic flexure have been over 70 years of age and they had a satisfactory recovery.

If the colon is only moderately distended, it can be removed without preliminary decompression. If, however, the degree of distension is severe it is better to decompress it rather than to mobilise tense fragile caecum and colon and the safest way to do this is illustrated in Fig 2.4 (Jones, 1974).

A Foley catheter of 28 or 30 F gauge is attached to a Y-connection, one arm of which goes to the sucker and to the other is attached a 10 cm length of tubing. The catheter tip is introduced into an enterotomy made just proximal to the ileocaecal valve, passed through the valve and the ballon inflated with 15 ml of water. The tubing is then pinched and gas and fluid is aspirated along the wide catheter, decompressing the colon. When this process is complete, the extended right hemicolectomy can be safely carried out, the segment

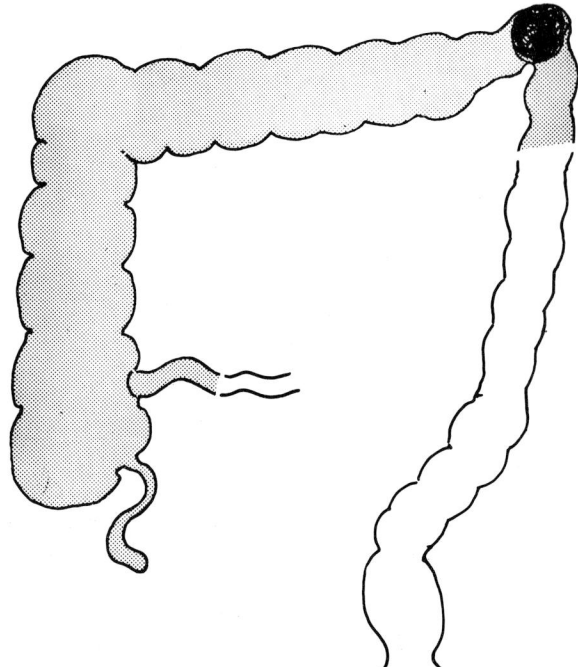

Fig 2.3 Extended right hemicolectomy: the shaded area is resected.

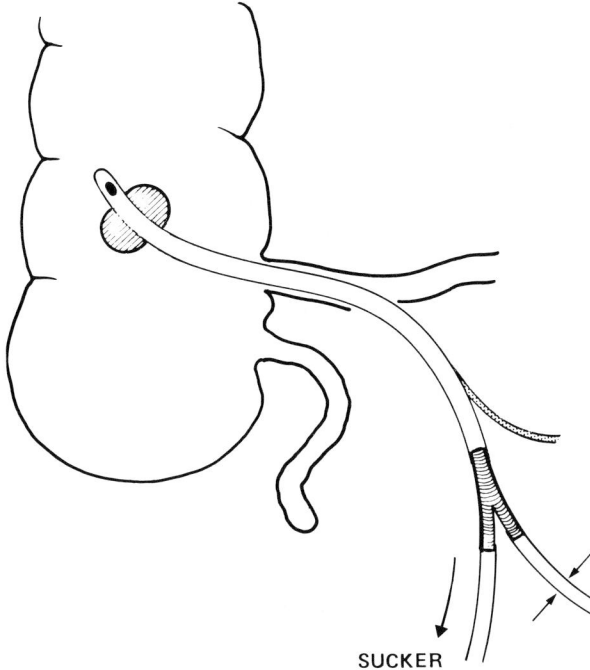

Fig 2.4   Method of decompression of distended colon by large bore Foley catheter. The two opposed arrows show where finger pressure will cause aspiration of the colon.

of ileum containing the catheter is resected, thus completely avoiding any contamination. The two open ends of ileum and colon are cleansed and joined end-to-end.

If a less extensive operation is preferred, then the best alternative is to make a loop colostomy in obstructed transverse colon, as close to the obstructing neoplasm as possible. As soon as the patient has recovered, the patient is re-explored through a left upper paramedian incision, the colostomy and the neoplasm are excised together, the transverse colon is then mobilised and anastomosed end-to-end to the upper descending colon.

It will be noted that nothing has been said about ileo-transverse anastomosis as a method of treatment. This is because it is not a successful treatment – 40% mortality among 61 patients so treated (Samencus, 1962). The only circumstance in which a simple short circuit is useful is when the proximal colon tumour is irremovable, when a palliative side-to-side anastomosis will give a period of relief.

Obstruction beyond the splenic flexure. Until recently, most surgeons treated this situation with a simple loop colostomy in the transverse or sigmoid colon, depending on the site of the carcinoma, and this is still a useful method when no experienced help is available. However, although this may be a simple operation, it carries a high mortality (Fielding *et al.*, 1979) and it suffers from two other serious disadvantages – the resection of the carcinoma is delayed for weeks, sometimes months, and an elderly patient has to face up to two or three staged operations.

When no experienced surgeon is available or when the degree of colonic distension is extreme and the patient is a poor operative risk, a loop colostomy should be established as close to the carcinoma as is reasonable. The aim will then be to return in 2–3 weeks, carry out a radical resection of the carcinoma on decompressed bowel, and to include the colostomy in the resected specimen (Fig 2.5). Proximal and distal colon is then mobilised and an end-to-end anastomosis performed on prepared colon. This method, suggested by Brooke (1955), is a useful one insofar as it cuts the stages from 3 to 2, but it still involves some delay in removing the carcinoma.

On the rare occasion when a low rectal carcinoma causes obstruction, it is wiser to make a sigmoid colostomy only, rather than attempt immediate abdomino-perineal excision.

Whenever the experience of the surgeon and the condition of the patient allow, there is a great deal to be said for performing immediate radical resection of the carcinoma (Fielding *et al.*, 1979). This can be done either as Hartmann's resection or resection with anastomosis.

Hartmann's resection is a sound radical operation for cancer of the sigmoid or upper rectum and avoids an

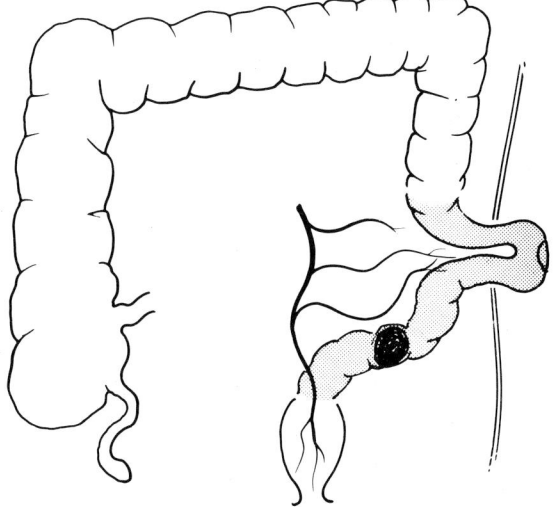

Fig 2.5   The Brooke (1955) operation. The shaded area shows the extent of resection at the second operation.

anastomosis on unprepared distended colon. However, if the colostomy is to be closed, another major operation must be done to mobilise and connect the descending colon to the rectal stump.

Immediate resection and anastomosis appears to break all the rules by using obstructed colon for an anastomosis, but good results can be obtained (Valerio and Jones, 1978). This method can be applied to an obstructing neoplasm at the splenic flexure, in the descending or sigmoid colon, or at the recto-sigmoid junction.

The first, and most important, step is to decompress and cleanse the obstructed proximal bowel, and it is here that the recent suggestion of Dudley and his colleagues (1980) has proved most valuable. The small bowel, if distended, is emptied retrogradely to the stomach whence the air and fluid is aspirated by the anaesthetist through a nasogastric tube. The proximal colon is then intubated with a 16F Foley catheter. Dudley suggests introducing it through an enterotomy in the terminal ileum, but we prefer to perform an appendicectomy and pass the catheter through the appendix stump, a temporary ligature around stump and catheter securing a water-tight seal. The balloon of the catheter is then inflated to prevent accidental withdrawal. The colonic tumour is then mobilised in the standard manner and the mesentery divided above the tumour in the usual way. However, this division is then carried 5 cm proximally and a clamp applied to the colon. In the cleared colon an incision is made and about a metre of corrugated plastic anaesthetic tubing is tied in very securely with tape. The clamp is removed and immediately gas and fluid faeces from the obstructed colon begins to pass down the tubing, the distal end of which discharges into a large plastic bag on the floor beside the operating table. Warm tap water can now be run through tubing into the Foley catheter and used to irrigate and cleanse the proximal colon. This may sound a somewhat crude device, but it is safe and effective and in our hands has now allowed us to carry out a primary resection with immediate end-to-end anastomosis, without protective colostomy, on six patients with a serious degree of colonic obstruction. In every case recovery has been straightforward.

The choice between these two forms of immediate resection must be made by the surgeon in the light of the conditions in the abdomen and the state of the patient. In the course of treating 22 obstructed carcinomas in the distal colon and rectum, 9 were treated by immediate resection (2 Hartmann's operation, 7 resection and anastomosis), and all made a good recovery. The 13 patients treated by initial colostomy had either irremovable tumours, very severe obstruction, or grave general ill-health; 5 of them went on to later resection, so eventually 14 of the 22 had a radical resection of the carcinoma.

Whenever a loop colostomy is made the use of a sub-cutaneous rod or catheter (Valerio and Jones, 1978) is much to be preferred to the classical rod and rubber tubing at skin level. The method is much neater, it allows easy application of the colostomy bag and, most important, it allows immediate mucocutaneous suture of the whole circumference of the stoma (Fig 2.6).

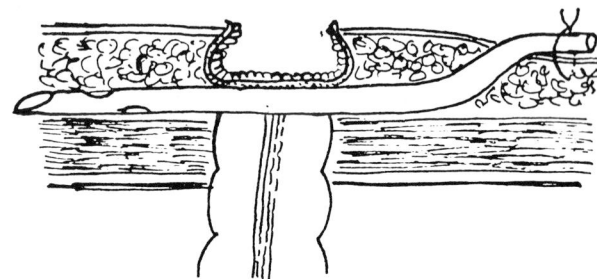

Fig 2.6   Construction of a loop colostomy. This sectional view shows a 22F whistle tip or Jacques catheter supporting the colon and lying subcutaneously. The colon has been opened and sutured to the skin edges. This leaves the skin around the colostomy clear for easy application of the adhesive bag. The catheter is withdrawn after 10 days.

Perforation of a colorectal carcinoma

This is unusual compared to obstruction, although we saw 12 such patients whilst treating 56 obstructed large bowel carcinomas. This appears to be a spontaneous complication and must be clearly distinguished from perforation of the obstructed, overstretched caecum. Immediate resection with thorough peritoneal lavage is certainly the treatment of choice for perforation of a carcinoma and was done on 11 of the 12 patients, with recovery in each case.

Volvulus of the colon

Volvulus of the sigmoid is much commoner than volvulus of the caecum but, even so, only makes up 1–2% of all cases of intestinal obstruction seen in Western Europe and North America. However, reports from Russia, Iran, Africa and India show that volvulus of the colon is one of the commonest causes of intestinal obstruction, and this appears to relate largely to the intake of a bulky vegetable diet (Shepherd, 1968).

Volvulus is the only common cause of ischaemic necrosis of the colon and when perforation occurs the mortality is very high. However, the clinical picture of sigmoid volvulus is generally characteristic, so that diagnosis should be possible before gangrene sets in. Patients who suffer sigmoid volvulus are predisposed to it insofar as they have a long sigmoid loop with a narrow base, but no one knows why rotation occurs. There is an unusually high incidence among patients with mental abnormality.

Sigmoid volvulus has three characteristics: sudden onset of lower abdominal colicky pain, absolute constipation and progressive abdominal distension which can occur very rapidly and produce great tension. A short history, severe pain, an ill patient with abdominal tenderness and guarding, should suggest a strangulating obstruction and lead to urgent laparotomy. The radiological signs of a sigmoid volvulus are quite characteristic – great gaseous distension of the sigmoid loop, with fluid levels in both limbs, and there is usually a dense curved line running down to the pelvis where the two loops are pressed together. The important difference between this picture and the changes in neoplastic obstruction of the distal sigmoid colon is that the proximal colon is not much distended in sigmoid volvulus, because the volvulus forms a closed loop.

The choice of treatment depends on whether gangrene of the loop is suspected (Shepherd, 1968). This possibility, although it is rare, must always be considered and when it cannot be excluded must lead to laparotomy and resection of the sigmoid loop. If gangrene is present, deflate the distended loop by direct puncture before untwisting it, because this manoeuvre is likely to lead to rupture of the friable colon, especially in the area of the twist. Paul-Mickulicz resection is rarely possible because the distal resection line usually runs through upper rectum which cannot be brought up to the surface. The safest operation is a Hartmann's resection.

In the majority of patients gangrene is not likely and then sigmoidoscopy offers a simple way of confirming the diagnosis and deflating the loop. This is one of the occasions when the knee-elbow position is very helpful. The sigmoidoscope will travel a surprisingly long way before meeting the twist (often 20–25 cm). Inspect the mucosa closely for signs of discolouration which would suggest that ischaemic changes are occurring at the twist and indicate prompt laparotomy. If the area of the twist looks healthy, hold the sigmoidoscope steady and pass along it a well-lubricated rectal tube of 1 cm internal bore and in 90% of patients it will slip through the volvulus into the distended loop with an explosive discharge of flatus and liquid faeces. Again, if the fluid is blood-stained, suspect ischaemia of the loop and go straight ahead with laparotomy. The tube can be left *in situ* for 24 h to drain.

Serious consideration must then be given to planned resection of the sigmoid, because recurrence of volvulus is so likely. This will depend on a history of previous episodes of volvulus, and the health and wishes of the patient.

Volvulus of the caecum

This is a rarity and most general surgeons will see only three or four cases during their working lives. The torsion occurs in people who have a mesentery to the caecum and ascending colon and in whom a twist causes the ileum to wrap around the ascending colon. Remarkable distension of the caecum follows as in sigmoid volvulus, and often forms a visible and palpable mass. In 25% of patients gangrene of the caecum occurs. There is an association with pregnancy, especially at the time of delivery.

These patients often have a past history of episodes of abdominal pain. By the time they present they have had abdominal pain for a day or two, with vomiting and constipation. Abdominal distension is usual and the distended caecum may be visible and palpable, somewhere to the left of its usual position 'about the size of a fetal head, resonant on percussion and quite soft on palpation' (Marnoch, 1914). The distended caecum will be seen in a plain abdominal film, but may not be recognised for what it is – in the left upper quadrant it can look like stomach.

Although the precise diagnosis is not always clear, these patients show the signs of intestinal obstruction and need opening. This reveals the tense blue dilated volvulus, at considerable risk of perforation. Aspiration of the volvulus with a trocar and cannula should precede untwisting and if there is the slightest doubt about viability, immediate right hemicolectomy should be done. The risk of recurrence is very high because of the anatomy of the right colon and, if the patient is fit, right hemocolectomy is the best way to prevent recurrence.

Pseudo-obstruction of the colon

In this condition the patient presents with what appears to be a typical large bowel obstruction, but there is no mechanical cause for it, and this condition is probably best called 'ileus of the colon'. The aetiology of this condition is still obscure, but it is clearly associated with:

1 severe systemic infections,
2 abdominal operations, especially caesarean section,
3 focal abdominal sepsis, such as cholecystitis and cystitis, and parturition,
4 antecedent episodes of hypoxia or hypotension.

These are all common events, and it is not clear why

ileus of the colon only rarely complicates them (Caves *et al.*, 1970; Bardsley, 1974).

Typically, a middle-aged or elderly patient complains of lower abdominal pain followed by constipation and abdominal swelling. There is tense gaseous distension of the abdomen and a plain abdominal x-ray shows wide gas distribution of the colon, sometimes with fluid levels, and the appearances are very like those of obstructed carcinoma of the sigmoid colon. A very careful examination of the films usually shows a little gas in the rectum in pseudo-obstruction. However, it must be stressed that these cases are very deceptive. Sigmoidoscopy is rarely helpful, but a gentle barium enema is of great value because in pseudo-obstruction the barium will flow easily into distended colon. This should allow a firm diagnosis to be made.

This does not, however, rule out the possibility that a laparotomy may be needed, because there are reports of the caecum being so tensely distended in pseudo-obstruction that it becomes ischaemic and requires removal. This means that although the correct initial treatment of pseudo-obstruction is to withold fluids by mouth, give intravenous fluids, and treat any coincident sepsis vigorously, there must be a very careful clinical and radiological watch on the colon. Increasing caecal distension, especially if accompanied by tenderness is an indication for laparotomy; caecostomy seems to be particularly useful in this situation.

Neoplastic obstruction of the small intestine

The surgeon will see 50–60 colorectal neoplasms for every small bowel tumour that is encountered, but most will be seen as emergencies, causing obstruction, so it is necessary to be prepared for this situation. A few cases will be due to intussusception of an adenoma or a leiomyoma and can be dealt with readily by a limited resection.

When a patient is opened for small bowel obstruction and the cause is found to be a small hard white lump in the bowel wall it may be a carcinoma, carcinoid, or lymphoma, (and occasionally Crohn's disease and endometriosis can also present in this way). In 168 tumours seen in the Birmingham region over 10 years (Brookes *et al.*, 1968), one-third were carcinomas, one-third lymphomas, 20% were carcinoids and in the remainder there was no histology. Some adenocarcinomas will be metastases from a distant primary which is not always recognisable. Some 45% of carcinoids occur in the appendix and are usually silent, and it is most important, therefore, always to examine the histology of all excised appendices. If the carcinoid tumour arises in the jejunum or ileum and is more than 1 cm in diameter, 50% of patients will have metastases.

Among 50 patients with a small bowel neoplasm

reviewed in Boston (Botsford *et al.*, 1962), two-thirds presented with intestinal obstruction and most of the remainder caused melaena. There is often a history of some weeks before these patients present with acute intestinal obstruction, during which they have suffered from recurrent intestinal colic. Intestinal lymphomas have a strong tendency to perforate and when this occurs the perforation lies at the centre of a penetrating mucosal ulcer (this is not always palpable so whenever non-traumatic perforation of the small bowel is seen, a biopsy must be performed, either by incision or resection) (Green *et al.*, 1979).

Treatment will usually entail a resection. but it is unlikely that these neoplasms will be easily distinguished. A carcinoma will produce a hard white nodule in the wall of the bowel, the lymphomas tend to produce a length of thickened pale intestine with considerable mesenteric thickening and lymphadenopathy and the carcinoids cause a small firm yellowish tumour which may have spread into mesentery and adjacent nodes. Unfortunately, endometriosis can produce an almost identical appearance and Crohn's disease can also affect a very localised area of intestine.

The pathology of small bowel neoplasms suggests that radical excision is well worth while, especially for carcinoid, so it is wise to attempt biopsy. Excision of the primary or of a node and imprinting of the cut surface on to a glass slide, with immediate staining and microscopy is a promising method of examination and may prevent a needlessly extensive resection for endometriosis (Green *et al.*, 1979). If, on the other hand, examination suggests a lymphoma there is a good opportunity to carry out a liver biopsy, and to remove any other suspicious nodes, to assist in the accurate staging of the lymphoma as a guide to subsequent radio- and chemotherapy.

Acute alimentary tract haemorrhage

One of the basic surgical tasks is to arrest haemorrhage. There is no site of bleeding which calls for greater diagnostic ability, sound judgement and surgical skill than acute haemorrhage from the alimentary tract.

The problems presented by acute upper gastrointestinal (UGI) haemorrhage are largely different from those encountered when copious red blood is passed per rectum so these topics are treated separately.

Acute upper gastrointestinal haemorrhage

Each year this emergency accounts for some 30 000 admissions to hospitals in the UK, and about 2500 of these patients die. The district general hospital serving a population of about 200 000 is likely to admit about 150 patients per annum so the relatively high mortality rate of 8–10% is not due to unfamiliarity (Allan and Dykes, 1976). The principal factors accounting for death are:

1   Age. Half the patients are over 60 years of age and one quarter are over 70, and these proportions are increasing.
2   Coincidental serious diseases. These are common, as in any elderly population.
3   Severity of bleeding. Twenty per cent of patients require the transfusion of more than 8 units of blood. Some of the causes of bleeding, e.g. portal hypertension, carry an intrinsically high mortality.

Until ten years ago the exact cause and site of acute UGI bleeding was often uncertain. The wide adoption of fibreoptic endoscopy has brought much greater precision to diagnosis, but has so far not greatly affected mortality rates. There are several comments to be made on this:

1   Thirty years ago the proportion of patients more than 60 years of age admitted with UGI bleeding was about 30%, is now 50% and will go on rising. To hold mortality steady in these circumstances means that the quality of care has improved.

2   The increasing use of emergency surgery has led to many more young patients surviving. Thirty years ago a number of these patients died from exsanguination and this is now a very rare event.

3   The patients who have to be operated on as an emergency, i.e. those who continue to bleed after admission, are the same group as required operation in the days before endoscopy was widely used and they are a high-risk group with a mortality rate around 28%. They are often elderly, unfit, have other serious diseases (such as cirrhosis), and the surgery required can be difficult and liable to carry a high complication rate. These facts have not changed with the coming of endoscopy.

4   One consequence of using surgery freely among acute UGI bleeders is that these patients are generally speaking cured of their ulcer. They are freed of their symptoms and also no longer exposed to subsequent risks of perforation and bleeding. This is a hidden advantage which, to some extent, offsets operative mortality.

The great contribution of endoscopy has been to bring greater certainty to diagnosis and so allow, as will be seen later, more discriminating treatment.

Clinical assessment

A history of peptic ulceration is only of limited help (though it is associated with a lowered mortality) and in 40–50% of patients there is no useful history. Knowledge of the result of a previous barium meal is not a dependable guide to the site of the present haemorrhage. There is a highly significant association between aspirin ingestion and subsequent bleeding, but this is not true for alcohol ingestion alone. However, alcohol and aspirin taken together have a synergistic effect in precipitating bleeding. A history of cirrhosis or portal hypertension is a valuable warning.

Apart from its importance in assessing the circulatory state, and the great diagnostic value of splenomegaly and signs of liver disease, physical examination does not contribute very much to diagnosis.

Although in the hands of experts, emergency barium meal examination of patients with UGI bleeding yielded very useful results, there can be no doubt that in almost all hospitals radiology has yielded to fibreoptic gastroduodenoscopy. Endoscopy can not only show lesions, such as Mallory–Weiss tears and gastric erosions, which are invisible in barium meals, but it can often demonstrate which lesion has actually bled, or is still bleeding.

The source of haemorrhage

Although peptic ulceration is always much the commonest cause of acute UGI haemorrhage, the incidence of the various causes of such bleeding varies from country to country. In Great Britain there have been a number of careful surveys of all admissions for haematemesis and melaena received from a district and these are summarised in Table 2. Four were made before endoscopy became established and two are based largely on endoscopic findings; a large recent series from Melbourne, Australia, is also included. It is interesting that the four pre-endoscopic surveys are remarkably similar, and the three later surveys, with a high percentage of early endoscopies (which might be expected to give greater accuracy of diagnosis) show less consistent findings.

Further haemorrhage

There can be no doubt that the most important feature of acute UGI haemorrhage is whether it continues or recurs after admission to hospital. If there is further haemorrhage (FH) in hospital then mortality is four times higher, and half these patients need emergency surgery (Jones *et al.*, 1974). If there is no FH after admission, then few of the patients die and when they do,

Table 2
SOURCE OF HAEMORRHAGE

	Endoscopy little used				Endoscopy extensively used		
	St James's Hospital, SW London[1] 1940–70	Central Middlesex Hospital, NW London[2] 1941–65	Radcliffe Infirmary, Oxford[3] 1953–67	Aberdeen Hospitals Scotland[4] 1968–9	St Thomas's and Brook Hospitals, SE London[5] 1971–2	St James's Hospital Leeds[6] 1975–7	Prince Henry's Hospital, Melbourne, Australia[7] 1972–8
Total number of patients	3938	3856	2149	817	208	277	894
Duodenal ulcer	36	35	29	48	24	21	31
Gastric ulcer	36	17	15	9	28	16	11
Gastric erosions	8	27	3	7	9	4	18
Mallory-Weiss tear	1			1	1	12	7
Oesophageal varices	3	3	2	3	3	11	11
Gastric carcinoma	3	2	2	3	2	1	–
Source unknown	4			5	15	20	13

The sources of the references are as follows: (1) Desmond and Reynolds, 1972; (2) Jones *et al.*, 1968; (3) Schiller *et al.*, 1970; (4) Johnston *et al.*, 1974; (5) Cotton *et al.*, 1973; (6) Foster *et al.*, 1978; (7) Hunt *et al.*, 1979.

it is from coincident diseases such as heart failure or malignant disease.

It is very clear, therefore, that it is to the FH group that maximum attention must be given. It makes no difference to the risk whether FH is manifested as haematemesis or melaena and FH which appears 48 h after admission carries a higher mortality than bleeding occurring in the first two days (Jones *et al.*, 1974). Any patient with gastric ulceration or oesophageal varices is especially at risk because half these patients have FH, compared with 25% of duodenal ulcers.

Nearly one-third of all patients with acute UGI haemorrhage have FH and two-thirds of these continue to bleed from the time of admission, so there is no difficulty in identifying this group. Some will recommence bleeding between 24 and 48 h and an important 20% will only start bleeding again after 48 h in hospital – and will suffer a higher mortality rate. Can any of these late bleeders be identified before bleeding recommences? Foster *et al.* (1978) have made a very useful contribution by showing that if, at endoscopy, the signs or stigmata of recent bleeding (a bleeding point, adherent clot or a vessel protruding from the base of an ulcer) are seen, then more than half of these patients will experience FH and two-thirds of them will need urgent surgery.

How far do these findings influence the decision to operate? The major influence will be the basic pathology – a non-operative approach may be wise in bleeding from oesophageal varices, carcinoma of the stomach

and erosive gastritis (*see later*). Generally speaking, anyone with a chronic peptic ulcer in the FH group is a strong candidate for emergency ulcer surgery and this is reinforced if the patient was admitted in hypovolaemic shock and has a recent history of severe ulcer symptons. Some emphasise the particular need to operate on those over 50-years-old, but this receives little support from the mortality figures, which are very high for emergency operations in the elderly. It can also be argued that young patients have more to lose from the dangers of recurrent bleeding and by having definitive surgery at the time of bleeding are saved later readmissions.

General principles of treatment

The policy, adopted forty years ago by Avery Jones, of treating all patients with haematemesis and melaena in a combined medical and surgical gastroenterological unit, is gradually being adopted and these units are producing impressive results (Hunt *et al.*, 1979). Early endoscopy, early identification of patients likely to have FH, efficient resuscitation and early surgery in all suitable patients, are the keys to reducing mortality and they can be most easily achieved where physician and surgeon work alongside each other.

1   The management of a patient admitted after UGI bleeding follows the line adopted for any patient after

haemorrhage. Blood is withdrawn for grouping, cross matching and counting, and an infusion is set up. When bleeding is urgent, this takes precedence over all other examinations and volume replacement is the first priority. A central venous pressure line can be very helpful in these circumstances. These patients select themselves for surgery (unless the bleeding comes from oesophageal varices or stress ulcers). They can often be those in whom it is most difficult to obtain a useful view with the endoscope, the stomach being full of blood clot. Our practice (having excluded varices) is not to waste time trying to wash out the stomach and secure a view, but to get on with the operation as soon as vigorous resuscitation through one or two wide intravenous cannulas allows the patient to be anaesthetised.

2   In those in less desperate circumstances, there is then time to take a history, make a full physical examination, hear the blood count result and decide on the level of transfusion required. Endoscopy within 12 h of admission is highly desirable – this greatly increases the chances of seeing signs of recent bleeding (which means that the patient has a 50/50 chance of FH), and of seeing erosions.

3   Collection of evidence of FH is most important, A half-hourly pulse rate and blood pressure record must be made. Aspiration of a nasogastric tube can give helpful evidence of fresh bleeding, but a negative result does not exclude continued bleeding in the duodenum. Serial haemoglobins are helpful – a stationary haemoglobin, in spite of continued adequate blood transfusion, is clear evidence of continued blood loss. Material vomited and the contents of bedpans should always be kept by nursing staff until they have been inspected, or a note made of volume and character.

4   Everyone knows that delay in treating a patient with UGI bleeding is undesirable and yet surgeons are still called to medical wards late at night to see patients who have been bleeding all day. Needham and McConachie in a pioneer paper published in 1950 on FH suggested that 'a reasonable arrangement would be to regard the first recurrence of bleeding in all patients below 50 years as well as above, as an indication for joint medical and surgical consultation on immediate treatment'. Many units do this already, but there are still too many hospitals in which medical and surgical consultation is not coordinated.

Peptic ulcer haemorrhage

In Great Britain between 50 and 60% of all UGI bleeds come from peptic ulcers.

Indications for surgery

1   Further haemorrhage (*see above*).
2   Continued abdominal pain in a patient who con-

tinues to bleed, albeit slowly, is serious, suggests the possibility of perforation, and is generally a strong indication for operation.

3   The occasional combination of bleeding with pyloric stenosis is another strong indication for urgent surgery.

Technique

This is emphatically not an operation to be undertaken by the inexperienced; registrars-in-training must learn how to deal with these patients, but only with experienced help on the opposite side of the operating table.

1   In almost all patients the history and examination will have identified patients with portal hypertension. If there are still doubts about this, oesophagoscopy should be the first step.

2   Study the shape of the epigastrium. A mid-line incision is quick and useful, but many men with bleeding duodenal ulcers are big and deep chested, with horizontally placed costal margins. A right subcostal incision, prolonged as necessary to the left across the mid-line, gives excellent access and heals very well. Coughing after operation is much easier than with a mid-line incision and this is important, because many of these men are smokers.

3   In many patients the site of bleeding is known from endoscopy, but there are still a number of patients who are bleeding fast in whom clot prevents a good view. Chronic duodenal and gastric ulcers are usually easy to see or to feel, but special attention is needed to find:

a   small penetrating ulcers on the posterior wall of the stomach or first part of duodenum;
b   ulcers in the second part of the duodenum (post bulbar). Kocher's manoeuvre can be helpful here;
c   an ulcer in a hiatus hernia within the thorax.

When the site of bleeding is uncertain, even after inspection and palpation, the duodeno-jejunal junction should be found and the small intestine looked at closely. If the bleeding is gastroduodenal and acute, there should be blood in the small bowel. Be particularly careful over this search in patients with melaena only.

4   If the source of bleeding remains uncertain, then the most likely source of UGI haemorrhage is an acute gastric erosion(s) or Mallory-Weiss tears. The latter are usually seen on endoscopy and rarely require surgical treatment. A wide gastrotomy should, therefore, be made, holding up the anterior wall of the stomach and opening it with the diathermy needle. Ligate the largest of the bleeding vessels and then suck or scoop out all clot, of which there can be very large quantities. Insert

Deaver retractors and, with the operating light tilted suitably, carry out a careful inspection of the whole of the stomach mucosa, commencing on the lesser curve and working up to the fundus. Most acute ulcers which bleed are on the lesser curvature, and they can sometimes be felt more easily than seen. These ulcers contain a single projecting artery, which feels like a hair bristle as the pulp of the examining index finger slides over the mucosa.

If this careful search is negative, then the next place to look is in the duodenum, which should be exposed through a longitudinal incision in the anterior wall which can be converted into a pyloroplasty. Beware of a postbulbar ulcer hiding round the corner in the second part of the duodenum. Very occasionally tumours hide in the third or fourth parts of the duodenum and this is where an aorto-duodenal fistula is found.

5   **Gastric ulcer.** An acute gastric erosion may be properly treated by simple oversewing with a Z stitch of 2/0 chromic catgut. These seem most likely to appear (when they are not stress ulcers) in the elderly and this treatment has proved to be effective and quick and seems reasonable, especially when there is some cause, such as aspirin ingestion, which can be stopped. None of our patients re-bled after suture and this experience is general. It is important to remember that these ulcers can be multiple.

Suture of the bleeding chronic gastric ulcer, with vagotomy and pyloroplasty, has been advised by some surgeons (Schiller *et al.*, 1970; Foster *et al.*, 1965), who have suggested that this method carries a lower mortality than gastrectomy and gives good long-term results. It would certainly be the method of choice in the elderly, in whom speed is of some importance, and when the surgeon is not an experienced gastrectomist.

Billroth I partial gastrectomy remains a favourite method among surgeons for treating this situation. This is partly because this operation gives consistently high quality results in elective surgery for chronic gastric ulcer, and partly because a number of bleeding ulcers can be dealt with safely only in this way. This is because many chronic gastric ulcers are large and penetrating and cannot be oversewn. They can erode the splenic artery, when the only safe treatment is to disconnect the stomach from the artery which it has eroded. Some bleeding gastric ulcers are carcinomas and removal provides the opportunity for histological examination.

In the last 30 bleeding gastric ulcers which I have treated, 29 have had a gastrectomy and one very unfit patient had oversewing and vagotomy and pyloroplasty; there was one postoperative death. The wise advice would seem to be to adapt the method to the needs of the patient and the experience of the surgeon. There will then be very little difference between the mortality rates for oversewing and gastrectomy.

6   **Duodenal ulcer.** Over the past ten years there has been a steady change from partial gastrectomy to oversewing of the ulcer, vagotomy and pyloroplasty as the routine method of treating haemorrhage from a duodenal ulcer.

Polya gastrectomy has become an uncommon elective operation for duodenal ulcer, so the majority of surgeons operating on emergencies have a fairly small experience of closing a difficult duodenal stump and so choose the method which, for them, is both easier and safer. Surgeons who were brought up on a diet of numerous gastrectomies will probably continue to deal with the bleeding duodenal ulcer by gastrectomy. I believe that every senior registrar should be able to cope with a difficult duodenum, because there are times when this is essential for safe treatment. Sometimes the ulcer is large and it is impossible to do a safe pyloroplasty and sometimes the ulcer is both perforated and bleeding and cannot safely be sutured. It is, therefore, important that senior registrars are assisted to learn how to perform a gastrectomy.

The essentials of the technique of closure of the duodenal stump beyond a posterior penetrating ulcer are illustrated (Figs 2.7–2.9).

The distal end of the stomach is freed on both the greater and lesser curvatures and divided just proximal to the pylorus. If the cuff of pylorus is now held up (Fig 2.7), the proximal edge of the posterior penetrating ulcer will be seen and is usually easily broken into, using the tip of an artery forceps as a blunt dissector. The duodenum is eased up off the ulcer, leaving the crater in the pancreas – this allows a bleeding point to

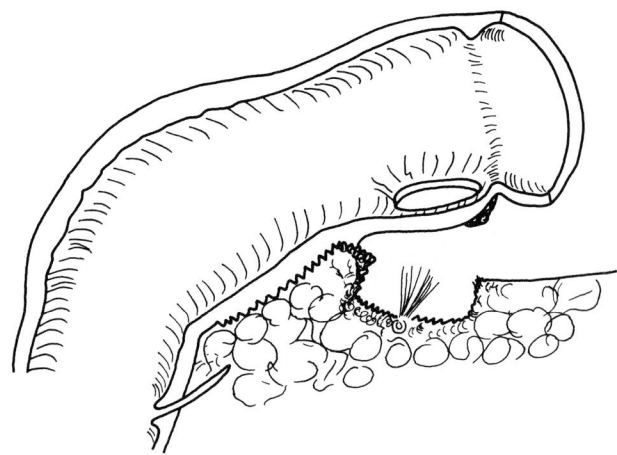

Fig 2.7 Longitudinal section of distal stomach and proximal duodenum. The stomach has been divided close to the pylorus, on the proximal side of the duodenal ulcer. The proximal edge of the penetrating duodenal ulcer has been opened, revealing the bleeding gastroduodenal artery in the base of the ulcer.

be securely under-run (Fig 2.8). A cuff of duodenum must now be obtained distal to the ulcer. The essential point here is that it is possible to find a plane between the wall of the duodenum and the fibrosed inflamed pancreas, which usually dissects up quite readily. The points of Dunhill forceps, opened up to develop this plane, is often the best instrument to use (Fig 2.8). Once 6–7 mm of duodenal wall has been separated off the pancreas in this way, the duodenum is divided, leaving more of the lateral wall (Fig 2.9) and the

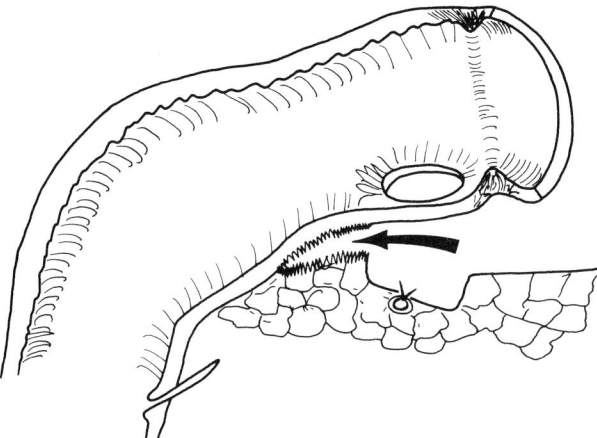

Fig 2.8 Strong non-absorbable sutures have under-run the artery below and above the erosion into the arterial wall. Dissection has been taken into the plane between the duodenal wall and the pancreas.

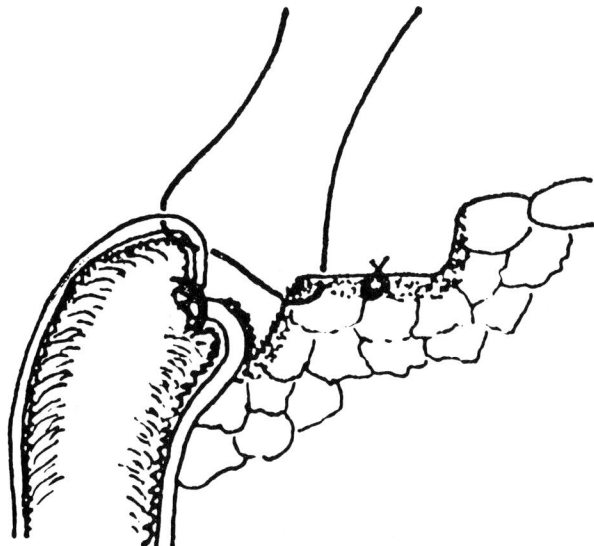

Fig 2.9 The duodenum has been closed by a Connell non-absorbable suture. This layer is being inverted by interrupted sutures which draw the longer lateral wall of the duodenum down into the ulcer base.

duodenal stump can then be closed. If a 2/0 nurolon or silk Connell suture is inserted from each end, the stump will close securely, with inversion of the mucosa. A second layer of interrupted Lembert sutures (Fig 2.9) will then allow the longer lateral wall of the duodenum to fold over the suture line and these sutures can take a good bite of the fibrosed ulcer wall.

As is suggested in the diagrams, the common bile duct usually lies some distance from this dissection. If there is reason for real anxiety about its position, then it is wise to open the duct in the free edge of the lesser omentum and pass an 8F Jacques catheter down it, through the Ampulla of Vater. This usually shows that the duct is further away from the field of dissection than was feared, but is well worth doing when in real doubt. Leave an 8F latex T-Tube in the duct for a few days.

The Polya gastrectomy can now be completed by the technique favoured by the operator. There is one essential step: before completing the suture of the anterior layer of the gastrojejunostomy, clamps (if used) must be removed and all blood and clot sucked out of the gastric stump; a surprising amount of clot can be obtained. If clot should be vomited during recovery, some can be inhaled and produce fatal respiratory obstruction.

It is difficult to decide whether a preference should be expressed for oversewing, vagotomy and pyloroplasty, or for gastrectomy. In the latest published series from Melbourne (Hunt *et al.*, 1979), 266 patients with bleeding duodenal ulcer were treated and 120 (43%) underwent emergency surgery. The two different operations were used equally and produced identical mortality rates of 7%.

I have used these two operations selectively, performing a Polya gastrectomy for preference in 52 patients with 3 deaths and underrunning with vagotomy and pyloroplasty in 13 patients who were old, or who had severe respiratory disease or a postbulbar ulcer, with 2 deaths. The advantage that can be claimed for the gastrectomies is that there was no case of rebleeding from the ulcer bed and this is a complication noted in all reports of the vagotomy/pyloroplasty operation.

This selective approach seems rational especially in elderly patients. The high mortality of operations on the elderly should, contrary to general advice, make us pause before operating, and when we do, the greater safety of vagotomy and pyloroplasty (Schiller *et al.*, 1970) should make this the preferred operation.

Mallory-Weiss tears

In 1929, Mallory and Weiss reported from the Boston City Hospital on 5 patients who, 'after a long alcoholic debauch developed massive gastric haemorrhage with haematemesis'. Haematemesis had been preceded by repeated retching. At postmortem 4 showed 'strikingly identical lesions . . . two to four definite fissure-like lesions of the mucosa . . . arranged around the circumference of the cardiac opening, from 3 to 25 mm in length and from 2 to 3 mm in width. In some of the microscopic sections definite ruptured arterioles were observed'.

In 1963 Lion-Cachet reproduced this lesion by removing the oesophagus and stomach immediately after death, and observing the cardio-oesophageal junction through a cystoscope whilst the stomach was progressively distended with water. The mucosa at the cardia is less elastic than the muscularis and splits longitudinally before the wall of the cardio-oesophageal junction disrupts. However, if distension continues, a typical Boerhaave pressure-rupture of the left wall of the lower oesophagus occurs.

The presumption is, therefore, that something – often alcoholic excess – precipitates vomiting, but the usual relaxation of the cardia and diaphragm fails, pressure rises suddenly within the stomach and the tear occurs. About half the patients with these tears give a clear history of violent retching and vomiting before haematemesis occurs.

Until endoscopy became a standard investigation, most reports of UGI haemorrhage considered Mallory-Weis tears to be rarities, (about 1% of all cases, Table 2) because a barium meal failed to demonstrate them. However, in a recent report from Leeds (Foster *et al.*, 1976) on 277 episodes of acute UGI bleeding 33 (12%) Mallory-Weiss tears were seen on endoscopy (although only 18 (6%) showed signs of recent bleeding).

It is clear from these figures that Mallory and Weiss described an important cause of acute UGI bleeding. There is a strong likelihood that bleeding will stop spontaneously. However, in a minority – about 10% – surprisingly severe and continued bleeding compels operation for these rather insignificant-looking lesions. Gastrotomy, good retraction (Deaver's are best) and simple suture of the tear with chromic catgut is all that is required.

Solitary gastric erosions

Erosions, by their name, should be superficial and therefore relatively minor in their effect. Although they may be small and superficial, they develop speedily in uninflamed mucosa, in which no fibrosis has occurred, as in more chronic ulceration. Erosion into a patent submucous arteriole can, therefore, easily occur so that haemorrhage from a gastric erosion can be fierce and does not always cease with medical treatment.

Solitary gastric erosions are a specific and not clearly understood entity, although their features are well known (Markby, 1965). In only a minority has aspirin been taken, and most patients are over 80 years of age. Opinions vary on whether solitary erosions are more common in men or women.

Before endoscopy was generally used, these erosions could only be diagnosed by laparotomy and gastrotomy, because they were not seen in a barium meal and were impalpable from the outside of the stomach. However, on opening the stomach and retracting widely with Deaver retractors, these ulcers can be seen and the artery projecting from the base can usually be felt as a bristle. Simple oversewing with chromic catgut is quite sufficient treatment.

Acute haemorrhagic gastritis

This condition has been defined as one in which there are 'multiple acute minute gastric erosions distributed throughout the stomach which literally weep blood' (Lulu and Dragstedt, 1970). The body and fundus of the stomach are much more often affected than the antrum.

In its mildest form, this type of gastritis is self-limiting, well illustrated by the temporary after-effects of an alcoholic binge, but once a certain point of severity is reached, acute haemorrhagic gastritis is self-perpetuating, unless vigorously treated, and can cause death by exsanguination. Broadly speaking, there are two causes for this severe type of acute gastritis, drug ingestion and severe injury or illness.

Drug ingestion. One of the features of this type of gastritis which has caused some surprise is that the gastric aspirate contains little acid. It is now clear that gastric acid output represents a balance between acid output and acid absorption across the mucosa, and salicylates have been shown to increase this 'back diffusion' of H ions (Davenport, 1967). This phenomenon is associated with brisk bleeding. It is promoted by gastric acid and inhibited by alkalinisation of the gastric contents.

Aspirin, particularly aspirin taken with alcohol, is the best known drug likely to cause bleeding, especially when taken regularly, but anticoagulants and possibly cortico-steroids can also be responsible. If a careful drug history is taken, it will be found that 40–50% of patients with haemorrhagic gastritis have ingested a known gastric irritant.

'Stress' ulceration in severe illness or injury. This condition has been increasingly recognised over the past ten years, especially among the victims of the fighting in Vietnam where very rapid evacuation resulted in the resuscitation of very gravely wounded men (Kunzman, 1970). The combination of severe injury causing hypovolaemic shock, with the development of surgical sepsis is especially important in aetiology. Severe burns may also cause haemorrhagic gastritis, but Curling's ulcer is a different entity (*see below*). Stress ulceration is also characteristically seen in fulminant liver failure.

The interval between injury and onset of gastric haemorrhage varies between a few days and three weeks, but 7–9 days is the commonest. The grave aspect of these bleeds is that they occur in patients who are already most seriously ill; a typical patient will have peritonitis and loculated pus after a penetrating wound of the colon. Others are in the process of rejecting a kidney transplant or have advanced liver failure.

The amount of blood which can be lost is very great and these patients, already seriously ill, respond to operation poorly and often fail to heal suture-lines. Fortunately, it now appears that this is the one form of gastroduodenal haemorrhage in which cimetidine has an important part to play (La Brooy *et al.*, 1979). Arrest of bleeding comes after only one or two doses and in a controlled trial (Macdougall *et al.*, 1977) in patients with fulminant hepatic failure, there was a highly significant fall in the number of patients showing bleeding in the cimetidine group. A commonly used dose has been 300 mg of cimetidine, six-hourly, but in some patients this is not enough and the gastric juice pH should be checked so that the pH remains above 5. It is to be hoped that this therapeutic advance will obviate the desperate surgery – sometimes total gastrectomy – which used to be employed as a last resort in these patients.

Curling's ulcers

In 1842, Curling described 3 seriously burned children who had bled severely from the duodenum 10–18 days after burning, each had a large posterior penetrating duodenal ulcer which had eroded the gastroduodenal artery. This remarkably specific ulceration has been seen regularly, though not frequently, since then and Sevitt (1967) has given a very clear description of these solitary penetrating ulcers which are seen especially in children. They are totally different from the shallow and usually multiple gastric erosions also seen in burned patients, which appear indistinguishable from the 'stress ulcers' just described (and which should not be referred to as Curling's ulcers even though they follow burns).

However, burns are not the only injuries to cause this specific type of duodenal ulceration. Cushing described a patient who died from a deep perforating duodenal ulcer after craniotomy for a tumour, and Lewis (1973) has recently collected 16 children who, after head injury or craniotomy, had gastroduodenal haemorrhage: 8 required surgery to stop bleeding and 7 of these had a posterior penetrating ulcer with erosion of the gastroduodenal artery.

These ulcers are certainly rare and in burns have an incidence of about 0.2%. However, as can be imagined, when haemorrhage does occur it is likely to cause severe loss in a patient already gravely ill with extensive burns and mortality is very high – only 2 children have survived surgery for this complication, and in adults there is a 60% mortality.

If operation is called for, this seems to be a time when pylorotomy, underrunning of the artery, and pyloroplasty would be the correct treatment. Evidence about hyperacidity as a factor in the causation of these ulcers is conflicting, but certainly in children there seems little justification for adding vagotomy to what is essentially an operation to stop bleeding as simply and swiftly as possible.

Chronic peptic ulceration and stress

Not all UGI haemorrhage in the seriously ill or injured is due to new ulceration. There are circumstances in which a quiescent chronic peptic ulcer may become active and bleed and require appropriate surgical treatment.

Bleeding oesophageal varices

These are dealt with fully in Chapter 8, Portal hypertension.

Rebleeding and negative laparotomy

The great majority of emergency explorations for bleeding are done during or very soon after an episode of brisk haemorrhage so that failure to find a bleeding point at laparotomy should be a very rare event and even in the days before the general use of endoscopy this was most unusual. If the patient has undoubtedly had a haematemesis, then the search can reasonably be concentrated proximal to the duodeno-jejunal flexure (although I have seen a haemangioma of the upper jejunum produce haematemesis), and suggestions have already been made about the important sites to search (p. 35). There is very little to be said in support of doing a blind two-thirds gastrectomy in these circumstances.

If a patient has only had melaena and the duodenum seems entirely normal then the search must extend all down the intestine (*see* the next section).

Copious lower alimentary tract haemorrhage

The passage of bright or dark red blood in quantity from the rectum is not a common occurrence, but it is always alarming, and sometimes dangerous, for the patient and can set the surgeon considerable problems both in diagnosis and treatment (Table 3).

The age at which such haemorrhage occurs is relevant. In infancy and childhood the most likely cause

Table 3
SEVERE RECTAL HAEMORRHAGE

Childhood
Meckel's diverticulum
Juvenile polyps
Haemangioma

Youth and middle age
Inflammatory bowel disease
Endometriosis
Typhoid fever
Small bowel neoplasm
(Peptic ulcer)
(Haemorrhoids)

Older patients
Diverticulosis colon
Vascular malformations (Angiodysplasia)
Aorto-intestinal fistula
Ischaemic colitis
(Carcinoma)
(Coagulation disorder)
(Chemotherapy)

of the rapid loss of dark red blood per rectum is peptic ulceration in **Meckel's diverticulum** (Rutherford and Akers, 1966), associated with the presence of ectopic gastric mucosa. When bleeding is copious and continuous in a child, it is reasonable to assume that this is the source and, as soon as resuscitation is complete, to open the abdomen and look for a Meckel's diverticulum. This course is safer than waiting for further investigations, because these are not always useful and the rate of blood loss can be high. Nearly all are sited in the lower ileum and are readily excised. A single episode of brisk bleeding may be due to spontaneous separation of a juvenile polyp, with continued bleeding from the stalk, but definite diagnosis is difficult unless the polyp is recovered from the stools.

Rarely congenital haemangiomas in the small bowel cause rectal bleeding and fortunately, they are often associated with one or more haemangiomas in the skin, and in addition are visible on the peritoneal surface of the intestine (Shepherd, 1953).

In young and middle-aged people, it is very unusual for gastric or duodenal ulceration to cause red rectal bleeding but if it is rapid enough to do so, the patient will show signs of hypovolaemia. I have seen a reticulum cell sarcoma of the jejunum present in this way and this is an occasional (10%) complication of small bowel neoplasms (Miles *et al.*, 1979). Ulceration in Meckel's diverticulum should not be forgotten in this age group.

Severe rectal bleeding is rare in ileocaecal Crohn's disease, but it is a well-known and serious complication of typhoid fever and, contrary to traditional teaching if bleeding continues, is probably better treated by resection rather than by repeated transfusion, (Wong, 1978). Ulcerative colitis only occasionally results in profuse

and continued rectal haemorrhage, and twice I have had to perform urgent colectomy for this rare complication (Buckell and Lennard-Jones, 1979).

The great majority of patients with severe sudden loss of red blood per rectum are middle-aged or elderly and, until recently, the situation was well summarised by Corry (quoted by Fraenkel, 1954) who said that if, in this age group, there was 'sudden, unexpected and alarmingly profuse rectal haemorrhage of perhaps several pints, full investigation is likely to reveal **diverticulosis** of the colon and the bleeding is unlikely to continue'. This statement, though still largely true, is no longer a complete summary (Boley *et al.*, 1979) (Table 3) **Vascular malformations** in the proximal colon and 'ischaemic colitis' have been increasingly recognised over the last 10 years as causes of severe rectal bleeding and, with the increasing number of aortic aneurysms coming to surgery, **aorto intestinal fistula** must also be remembered. A few patients with colorectal carcinoma present with a continuous flow of altered blood per rectum.

Two distinct clinical situations can be recognised. In the majority there is an episode of brisk rectal haemorrhage which is either single or repeated two or three times and then settles, usually before the patient reaches hospital. The patient is in good condition, although pale, and digital examination of the rectum shows the finger stained with fresh altered blood. In these patients the standard processes of investigation should proceed. Sigmoidoscopy rarely reveals more than a normal rectum full of dark red blood. A barium enema often reveals diverticulosis which often extends throughout most of the colon and in these patients it is generally assumed that the blood has come from a diverticulum. Meyers and his group (1976) have shown how this occurs through rupture of a colonic arteriole (vas rectum) lying in the submucosa of a diverticulum.

If haemorrhage has stopped spontaneously in a patient with diverticulosis, there is nothing to be gained by attempting arteriography and the patient is simply warned to watch for further episodes of rectal bleeding. There is a tendency for diverticular bleeding to recur and we have carried out two elective total colectomies with ileorectal anastomosis in patients with repeated severe bleeding and total involvement of the colon with diverticulosis. These patients have had no further bleeding over 3–4 years.

However, diverticulosis is not the only cause of repeated rectal haemorrhage in older patients and, in particular, the importance of the entity named **angiodysplasia** has been increasingly recognised. These causes of severe bleeding share the very serious disadvantage that the bleeding point is not detectable by external examination of the bowel and it is here that preoperative selective visceral angiography can be such a help (Tarin *et al.*, 1978).

In a minority of these patients bleeding continues and it can be severe; one obese 60-year-old lady was recently taken to theatre after receiving 17 units of blood in 36 h. These patients are usually elderly, often stout and unfit and, if opened, usually present a colon full of blood without evidence of a local lesion. Emergency visceral angiography can demonstrate a bleeding point (Tarin *et al.*, 1978), but the difficulty is that to produce useful pictures an expert radiologist and team are needed and are not necessarily available at all times. We have not found this investigation of much help, so a plan must be made which will enable the bleeding point to be found (Fig 2.10).

If vigorous rectal haemorrhage continues, then the surgeon is left with no alternative but to open the abdomen. It is important that the patient should be in lithotomy-Trendelenburg position and this may allow manual expression of blood per rectum, followed by

intraoperative colonoscopy. This is not easy, because blood often obscures the view, but we have found it helpful, the surgeon performing the colonoscopy and the assistant guiding the instrument round the colon. Alternatively, rigid colonoscopy has also proved its value, using the 2 cm × 30 cm Lloyd-Davies sigmoidoscope. The abdomen is opened through a generous vertical incision and the whole small and large bowel closely inspected. If there is blood in the colon, but not in the small bowel, and there is no obvious cause for the bleeding except scattered diverticula, then the splenic flexure is fully mobilised, held up between stay sutures, a small incision made in it and the sterile lubricated sigmoidoscope manoeuvred, with the obturator still *in situ*, up to the caecum. The obturator is withdrawn and the surgeon goes dirty to perform 'sigmoidoscopy' in the usual way as he withdraws the sigmoidoscope. Much altered blood is seen, but the surgeon is especially watching for bright red blood, because it is this which draws attention to the true site of the bleeding, If this sign is not found between the caecum and the splenic flexure, the sigmoidoscope is cleaned with Savlon swabs, relubricated, the obturator re-inserted and the sigmoidoscope passed, with help from the scrubbed-up assistant, to the sigmoid and the inspection repeated. This method has guided us to the segment of colon needing resection and a local operation is much to be preferred to total colectomy in an elderly and unfit patient. However, if no definite area containing fresh blood can be identified, the only safe operation is total colectomy, otherwise the area of diverticulosis which is bleeding may be left *in situ*. This is well discussed by Drapanas *et al.* (1973) and Eaton (1981). It may be safer to terminate this operation with closure of the rectal stump and terminal ileostomy rather than ileorectal anastomosis.

Vascular malformations are less likely to produce severe exsanguinating haemorrhage, but they can produce sustained losses requiring 2–3 units of blood to be transfused every day and are especially likely to cause repeated intermittent rectal haemorrhage. The dramatic case reported by Rutter in 1956 was undoubtedly an example of what is now called 'angiodysplasia'. The essential lesion is telangiectasia of the mucosal capillaries and veins, and current theory is that these are degenerative changes due to slowly developing obstruction to the submucosal veins. It is not clear why these telangiectases occur mainly in the right colon.

The first patient we saw with this condition illustrates many of its features. A retired teacher aged 67, with known aortic stenosis, passed clots of blood per rectum in 1973, but all investigations were normal. In 1976 she complained of tiredness and the haemoglobin was 6.7g. Barium enema and sigmoidoscopy were again negative. In November she repeatedly passed dark blood and clots per rectum, and after receiving 9 units of blood

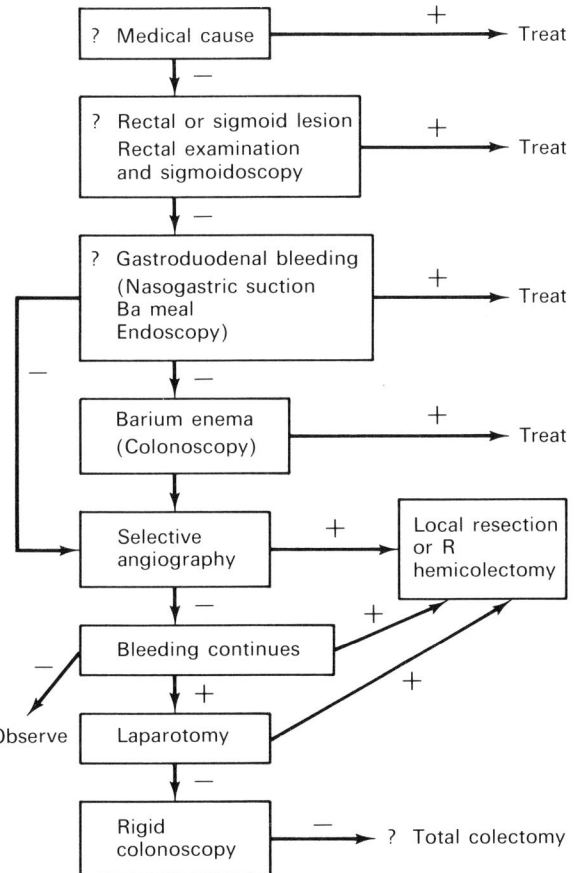

Fig 2.10 Decision tree for management of severe rectal haemorrhage.

the haemoglobin was 11g. Further haemorrhage in the ward led to laparotomy, when blood was seen throughout the colon. Rigid colonoscopy, as already described, showed a polyp in the descending colon which was not bleeding. On passing the sigmoidoscope to the caecum bright red blood was seen so a caecotomy was performed, revealing two bright red plaques 7–8 mm diameter in the mucosa, which bled briskly when touched. These appeared to be haemangiomas and were removed. Bleeding stopped and has not recurred over 3 years. The specimens showed dilated vascular channels just under the mucosa, with a central thrombus at the point of rupture.

Many papers (Baum *et al.*, 1977; Boley *et al.*, 1977) now describe these vascular malformations. Some (Welch *et al.*, 1978) suggest that they are a more frequent cause of serious rectal bleeding than diverticulosis and most reproduce angiograms showing the characteristic capillary vascular tuft with early filling of large veins which distinguishes these malformations. However, although angiography is good at showing extravasation of medium in bleeding diverticulosis, it rarely shows up the bleeding point in angiodysplasia. It is important to recognise the limitations of angiography and when there is no clear lead from it or it cannot be done (our last two patients both had calcified femoral arteries), the surgeon may have to operate because of continued bleeding. In these circumstances, if the general inspection of the alimentary tract gives no definite information, and the haemorrhage appears to be colonic, the rigid colonoscopy described above can be of great help. Right hemicolectomy is usually the correct treatment for angiodysplasia.

In **ischaemic colitis** (Marston, 1977) the patient is nearly always middle-aged or elderly and often has ischaemic heart disease. There is sudden left-sided abdominal pain with nausea and vomiting, followed by the passage of dark red blood and clots per rectum. This bleeding is not sufficient to produce hypovolaemia, but the patient looks pale and unwell and shows fairly acute tenderness over the distal colon. There is altered blood in the rectum, which shows a normal-looking mucosa. Plain x-rays of the abdomen may show some distal colonic distension, with 'thumb printing' in the wall, and this is shown much more clearly in a barium enema, which can clinch the diagnosis. It is most unusual to have to operate on these patients and nearly all settle with rest and a few days of intravenous fluid.

Although these changes are known to occur when the colon suffers sudden diminution in the blood supply, very little is known of the true causes.

Aortointestinal fistula is fortunately rare, because it can cause disastrously rapid rectal bleeding. The patient will either have an abdominal aortic aneurysm (Rekless *et al.*, 1972) or have had an aneurysm treated by insertion of a graft. Anyone who shows a warning melaena and who also has an aneurysm or has had a graft inserted must immediately be suspected of having this grave complication and be operated upon. Once haemorrhage commences from such a fistula, it rapidly becomes torrential and the situation is very difficult to retrieve.

Although colorectal cancers rarely bleed enough to cause rectal haemorrhage, this does occasionally occur and these patients will be the small minority in whom the traditional steps of sigmoidoscopy and barium enema yield a precise localisation of the source of bleeding.

Finally, the small bowel must not be forgotten. Our latest patient with uncontrollable rectal haemorrhage was a 65-year-old woman with rheumatoid arthritis who had multiple bleeding ulcers in the terminal ileum due to vasculitis.

References

Allan R., Dykes P. (1976). Study of the factors influencing mortality rates from gastrointestinal haemorrhage. *Quart. J. Med*; **45**:533–50.

Anderson A., Zederfeldt B. (1969). Gallstone ileus. *Acta Chir. Scand*; **135**:713–17.

Bardsley D. (1974). Pseudo-obstruction of the large bowel. *Brit. J. Surg*; **61**:963–9.

Baum S., Athanasoulis C.A., Waltman A.C. *et al.* (1977). Angiodysplasia of the right colon: a cause of gastrointestinal bleeding. *Amer. J. Roentgenol*; **129**:789–94.

Boley S.J., DiBiase A., Brandt L.J. *et al.* (1979). Lower intestinal bleeding in the elderly. *Amer. J. Surg*; **137**:57–64.

Boley S.J., Sammartano S.R., Adams A. *et al.* (1977). On the nature and aetiology of vascular ectasias of the colon: degenerative lesions of ageing. *Gastroenterology*; **72**:650–60.

Botsford T.W., Crowe P., Crocker D.W. (1962). Tumours of the small intestine. *Amer. J. Surg*; **103**:358–65.

Bowesman C. (1951). Reduction of strangulated inguinal hernia. *Lancet*; **i**:1396–7.

British Medical Journal (1977). Burst abdomen: a preventable condition? (leading article). *Brit. Med. J*; **1**:534.

Brooke B.N. (1955). Simplified operative routine for carcinomatous obstruction of colon. *Lancet*; **i**:945–6.

Brookes V.S., Waterhouse J.A.H., Powell D.J. (1968). Malignant lesions of the small intestine: a 10-year survey. *Brit. J. Surg*; **55**:405–10.

Buckell N.A., Lennard-Jones J.E. (1979). How district hospitals see acute ulcerative colitis. *Lancet*; **i**:1226–9.

Caves P.K., Crockard H.A. (1970). Pseudo-obstruction of the large bowel. *Brit. Med. J*; **2**:583–5.

Cooperman A.M., Dickson E.R., ReMine W.H. (1968). Changing concepts in the surgical treatment of gallstone ileus. *Ann. Surg*; **167**:377–83.

Cotton P.B., Rosenberg M.T., Waldram R.P.L. *et al.* (1973). Early endoscopy of oesophagus, stomach and duodenal bulb in patients with haematemesis and melaena. *Brit. Med. J.*; **2**:505–9.

Curling T.B. (1842). On acute ulceration of the duodenum in cases of burn. *Med. Chir. Trans*; **25**:260–81.

Davenport H.W. (1967). Salicylate damage to the gastric mucosal barrier. *New Engl. J. Med*; **276**:1307–12.

Desmond A.M., Hutter F. (1948). Strangulated obturator hernia. *Brit. J. Surg*; **35**:318–20.

Desmond A.M., Reynolds K.W. (1972). Erosive gastritis: its diagnosis, management, and surgical treatment. *Brit. J. Surg*; **59**:5–13.

Drapanas T., Pennington G., Kappelman M. *et al.* (1973). Emergency subtotal colectomy: preferred approach to massively bleeding diverticular disease. *Ann. Surg*; **177**:519–26.

Dudley H.A.F., Radcliffe A.G., McGeehan D. (1980). Intraoperative irrigation of the colon to permit primary anastomosis. *Brit. J. Surg*; **67**:80–1.

Dunphy J.E. (1940). The diagnosis and surgical management of strangulated femoral hernia. *J. Amer. Med. Ass*; **114**:394–6.

Eaton AC. (1981). Emergency surgery for acute colonic haemorrhage: a retrospective study. *Brit. J. Surg*; **68**:109–12.

Ellis H. (1974). Intraperitoneal adhesions. *Brit. J. Hosp. Med*; **11**:401–8.

Fielding L.P., Stewart-Brown S., Blesovsky L. (1979). Large bowel obstruction caused by cancer: a prospective study. *Brit. Med. J*; **2**:515–17.

Foster D.N., Miloszewski K.J.A., Losowsky M.S. (1976). Diagnosis of Mallory-Weiss lesions. *Lancet*; **ii**:484–5.

Foster D.N., Miloszewski K.J.A., Losowsky M.S. (1978). Stigmata of recent haemorrhage in diagnosis and prognosis of upper gastro-intestinal bleeding. *Brit. Med. J*; **1**:1173–7.

Foster J.H., Hickok D.F., Dunphy J.E. (1965). Changing concepts in the surgical treatment of massive gastroduodenal haemorrhage. *Ann. Surg*; **161**:968–74.

Fowler G.R. (1900). New and improved method of entering the abdominal cavity in the ileo-caecal region. *Med. News*; **76**:321–4.

Fraenkel G.J. (1954 quoting Corry D.C. (1954),). Rectal bleeding and diverticulitis. *Brit. J. Surg*; **41**:643–5.

Frimann-Dahl J. (1960). *Roentgen Examination in Acute Abdominal Diseases*. Oxford: Blackwell.

Gilmore O.J.A., Reid C. (1979). Prevention of intraperitoneal adhesions. *Brit. J. Surg*; **66**:197–9.

Green J.A., Dawson A.A., Jones P.F. *et al.* (1979). The presentation of gastrointestinal lymphoma: study of a population. *Brit. J. Surg*; **66**:798–801.

Hunt P.S., Hansky J., Korman M.G. (1979). Mortality in patients with haematemesis and melaena: a prospective study. *Brit. Med. J*; **1**:1238–40.

Hunt P.S., Korman H.G., Hansky J. *et al.* (1979). Bleeding duodenal ulcer: reduction in mortality with a planned approach. *Brit. J. Surg*; **66**:633–5.

Johnston S.J., Jones P.F., Kyle J. *et al.* (1974). The epidemiology and presentation of major gastro-intestinal haemorrhage in North-East Scotland. *Brit. Med. J*; **3**:655–60.

Jones F.A., Gummer J.W.P., Lennard-Jones J.E. (1968). *Clinical Gastroenterology*, 2nd edn. pp. 423. Oxford: Blackwell Scientific Publications.

Jones P.F. (1974). *Emergency Abdominal Surgery* pp. 343. Oxford: Blackwell Scientific.

Jones P.F., Johnston S.J., McEwan A.B. *et al.* (1974). Further haemorrhage after admission to hospital for gastrointestinal haemorrhage. *Brit. Med. J*; **3**:660–4.

Jones P.F., Matheson N.A. (1968). Operative decompression in intestinal obstruction. *Lancet*; **i**:1197.

Kunzman J. (1970). Management of bleeding stress ulcers. *Amer. J. Surg*; **119**:637–9.

La Brooy S.J., Misiewicz J.J., Edwards J. *et al.* (1979). Controlled trial of cimetidine in upper gastrointestinal haemorrhage. *Gut*; **20**:892–5.

Lewis E.A. (1973). Gastroduodenal ulceration and haemorrhage of neurogenic origin. *Brit. J. Surg*; **60**:279–83.

Lion-Cachet J. (1963). Gastric fundal mucosal tears. *Brit. J. Surg*; **50**:985–6.

Lulu D.J., Dragstedt L.R. II. (1970). Massive bleeding due to acute haemorrhagic gastritis. *Arch. Surg*; **1010**:550–4.

Macdougall B.R.D., Bailey R.J., Williams R. (1977). H_2 receptor antagonists and antacids in the prevention of acute gastrointestinal haemorrhage in fulminant hepatic failure. *Lancet*; **i**:617–19.

Mallory G.K., Weiss S. (1929). Haemorrhages from lacerations of the cardiac orifice of the stomach due to vomiting. *Amer. J. Med. Sci*; **178**:506–15.

Markby C.E.P. (1965). Massive haemorrhage from superficial gastric erosions. *Brit. J. Surg*; **52**:685–91.

Marnoch J. (1914). Cases of acute intestinal obstruction due to rare causes. *Brit. J. Surg*; **1**:644–9.

Marston A. (1977). *Intestinal Ischaemia*. London: Arnold.

McEvedy P.G. (1950). Femoral hernia. *Ann. Roy. Coll. Surg*; **7**:484–96.

McIver M.A. (1933). Acute intestinal obstruction. *Amer. J. Surg*; **20**:171–99.

Meyers M.A., Alonso D.R., Gray G.F. *et al.* (1976). Pathogenesis of bleeding intestinal diverticulitis. *Gastroenterology*; **71**:577–83.

Miles R.M., Crawford D., Duras S. (1979). Small bowel tumour problem assessment based on a 20-year experience with 116 cases. *Ann. Surg*; **189**:732–40.

Munro A., Jones P.F. (1978). Operative intubation in the treatment of complicated small bowel obstruction. *Brit. J. Surg*; **65**:123–7.

Needham C.D., McConachie J.A. (1950). Haematemesis and melaena. *Brit. Med. J*; **2**:133–8.

Noble T.B. (1937). Plication of small intestine as prophylaxis against adhesions. *Amer. J. Surg*; **35**:41–4.

Räf L.E. (1969). Causes of abdominal adhesions in cases of intestinal obstruction. *Acta Chir. Scand*; **135**:73–6.

Rekless J.P.D., McColl I., Taylor G. W. (1972). Aortoenteric fistulae: an uncommon complication of abdominal aortic aneurysms. *Brit. J. Surg*; **59**:458–60.

Rutherford R.B., Akers D.R. (1966). Meckel's diverticulum; a review of 148 patients, with special reference to the pattern of bleeding. *Surgery*; **59**:618–26.

Rutter A.G. (1956). Submucous telangiectasis of the colon. *Lancet*; **ii**:1077–9.

Saegesser F., Sandblom P. (1975). Ischemic lesions of the distended colon. *Amer. J. Surg*; **129**:309–15.

Samencus B. (1962). Treatment of acute obstruction due to carcinoma of right half of colon with special reference to primary hemicolectomy. *Acta Chir. Scand*; **123**:415–21.

Schiller K.F.R., Ttruelove S.C., Williams D.G. (1970). Haematomesis and melaena, with special reference to factors influencing the outcome. *Brit. Med. J*; **2**:7–14.

Sevitt S. (1967). Duodenal and gastric ulceration after burning. *Brit. J. Surg*; **54**:32–41.

Shepherd J.A. (1953). Angiomatous conditions of the gastrointestinal tract. *Brit. J. Surg*; **40**:409–21.

Shepherd J.J. (1968). Treatment of volvulus of the sigmoid colon: a review of 425 cases. *Brit. Med. J*; **1**:280–3.

Stammers F.A.R. (1954). Remarks on fifteen cases of small-bowel obstruction following ante-colic partial gastrectomy and one case following retro-colic partial gastrectomy. *Brit. J. Surg*; **42**:34–8.

Stephens F.O. (1966). Intestinal colic caused by food. *Gut*; **7**:581–2.

Tarin D., Allison D.J., Modlin I.M. *et al.* (1978) *Brit. Med. J*; **2**:751–4.

Thomas J.W., Rhoads J.E. (1950). Adhesions resulting from removal of serosa from an area of bowel. *Arch. Surg*; **61**:565–7.

Valerio D., Jones P.F. (1978). Immediate resection in the treatment of large bowel emergencies. *Brit. J. Surg*; **65**:712–6.

Welch C.E., Athanasoulis C.A., Galdabini J.J. (1978). Haemorrhage from the large bowel with special reference to angiodysplasia. and diverticular disease. *World J. Surg*; **2**:73–83.

White C.S. (1912). Richter's hernia. *Surg. Gynaecol. Obsetet*; **14**:46–8.

White R.R. (1956). Prevention of recurrent small bowel obstruction due to adhesions. *Ann. Surg*; **143**:714–9.

Williams D.C. (1955). The peritoneum: a plea for a change in attitude towards this membrane. *Brit. J. Surg*; **42**:401–5.

Wilson N.D. (1964). Complication sof the Noble procedure. *Amer. J. Surg*; **108**:264–8.

Wong S.H. (1978). The emergency surgical management and persistent intestinal haemorrhage due to typhoid fever: a report of 3 cases. *Brit. J. Surg*; **65**:74–5.

Further reading

Dykes P.W., Keighley M.R.B. (1981). *Gastro-intestinal Haemorrhage*. Bristol: Wright.

Ellis H. (1982). *Intestinal Obstruction*. New York: Appleton Century Crofts.

3

Incisions and drains

NIALL O'HIGGINS

This chapter deals with principles governing the making and closing of incisions and describes specific incisions commonly employed in general surgical operations. Apart from operations on the skin itself, the main purpose of the skin incision is to provide the best means of access to the structure requiring surgical attention. The difficulty or ease by which many operations are carried out depends on the exposure of the area which, in turn, is determined by the incision. Where accurate diagnosis of the diseased organ and the condition affecting it has been made before operation, the surgical procedure is elective and all operative steps can be planned in advance with regard to the anticipated lesion and the nature of the operation to be carried out. The incision to be used in these circumstances is focussed on the target organ or tissue. In general, the incision in this type of operation is placed directly over the organ involved. In anticipation of unplanned difficulties it is important that the incision be capable of being elongated. Where two or more organs need to be approached, or where the site of injury or disease is in doubt, a more versatile incision is required, or one that can be modified either by direct extension or by change in direction. The damage to skin, blood vessels and nerves caused by skin incisions should be kept to a minimum if the ease and safety of the operation is not compromised by so doing. Muscle-splitting incisions, where muscles are divided along the line of their fibres, are associated with minimal trauma or scarring (Fig 3.1).

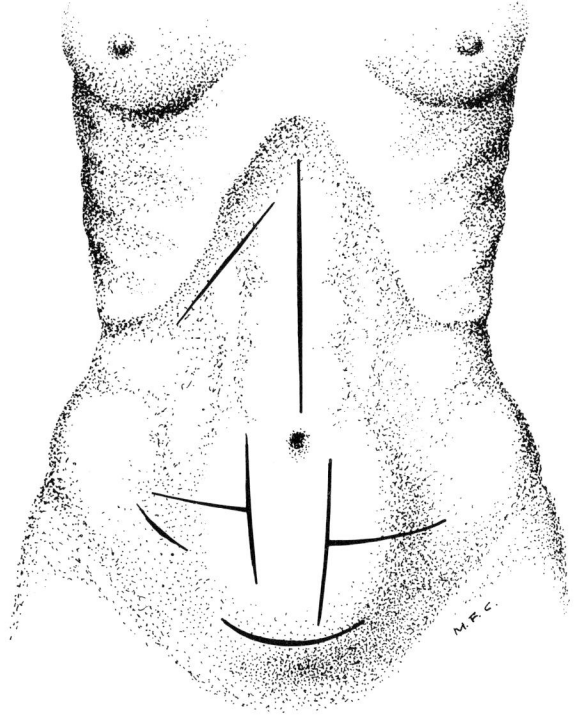

Fig 3.1 Types of abdominal incision.

Subcutaneous bleeding must be arrested before deeper structures are incised. This may be carried out by the use of small haemostats, care being taken to pick up the bleeding vessel only. If fatty or other tissue is caught in the forceps, not only may haemostatis be incomplete, but the damaged adjacent tissue may become a focus for infection. If the forceps are allowed to lie over the edge of the wound for some minutes, bringing about retraction by their own weight, they can be removed without need for ligation of small subcutaneous vessels. Alternatively, coagulating diathermy may be used for small subcutaneous bleeding points which have been picked up by a fine toothed dissecting forceps. Care must be taken not to use diathermy too close to the dermis or a burn in the skin will result. Where more substantial subcutaneous vessels require to be divided, they should be isolated cleanly with artery forceps, divided and ligated with fine chromic catgut. Wound retractors, either self-retaining or hand-held, are useful in exposing the deeper layers, but contact with the skin by instruments should be reduced to a minimum.

Planning the incision

Many considerations, especially surgical experience, apply in the planning of operative incisions and each assumes its own relative importance depending on the circumstances. So many variables arise that what becomes a most important consideration in one patient may be of little consequence in another. It is, therefore, essential in the correct planning of the operative approach that the surgeon understands the relevant background and clinical features of the patient's condition.

Access

Adequate access to the area or organ involved is fundamental to good surgical technique. Simple operations are rendered difficult and dangerous by poor exposure and difficult procedures often become greatly simplified by proper display. A good incision must not only allow the target organ to be exposed, but also facilitate mobilisation during the course of the procedure. Thought must be given to the possibility that the organ may be adherent, displaced, enlarged or otherwise diseased. In this case an incision planned to expose a normal organ may not be appropriate. For example, while a mid-line or left paramedian incision may be perfectly suitable for removal of a normal-sized spleen, it may be quite out of place for excision of a grossly enlarged spleen which is adherent to the diaphragm and lateral abdominal wall. While good exposure depends on adequate lighting, retraction, replacement of sponges and other instruments, the most important factor is an incision suitably placed over the organ and long enough to allow the procedure to be carried out without tension on the edges of the wound or on viscera.

Speed

The urgency of the operation may determine the type of incision used. For patients with life-threatening intra-abdominal haemorrhage or other major catastrophe, a mid-line incision is chosen because it can be carried out quickly and safely and is capable of being extended.

Certainty of diagnosis

When an elective operation on a specific site is being conducted, an incision is made appropriate to the area to be dealt with. Versatility is not required in such an incision and, while full access to the structure concerned is necessary, exposure of other structures is not required. The same point may be made in emergency surgery when the diagnosis is certain. In acute appendicitis, appendicectomy is best carried out through a grid-iron incision, which may be wholly unsuitable for dealing with other conditions in the lower abdomen. When genuine doubt exists, a vertical incision either mid-line or paramedian is preferable.

Local factors

Injury, sepsis or other lesions in the skin or underlying structures may become important in the making of incisions. Incisions through infected areas should be avoided where possible. The infected area should be cleansed and sealed off and the incision placed as far from the areas as is consistent with adequate exposure. Similarly, incisions should not encroach upon skin lesions, which should be excised where possible if they encroach on the line of the planned approach. If it is not feasible to excise them, an alternative incision should be made.

General factors

When a patient requiring operation suffers from some condition associated with debility or poor wound healing, the making of an incision likely to produce the soundest and most secure type of scar becomes of prime importance.

Build of patient

The build or configuration of the patient should be considered, especially in abdominal incisions. A midline incision provides good access to all upper abdominal viscera in a thin patient with a narrow subcostal angle, but may be unsatisfactory in an obese patient with a wide subcostal angle, in whom a transverse or oblique subcostal incision is preferred. Lateral extension at the upper or lower margins, or even at the centre of a vertical incision may provide good access to laterally placed structures, in broadly built patients, particularly if they are fat. These extensions are often useful in operations on the ascending or descending colon.

Safety

The dominant factor in the making of a safe incision is adequate length, so that the entire procedure may be carried out under direct vision. For example, in removing cervical lymph nodes, the incision should be sufficiently long to allow exposure of the important adjacent veins, nerves and arteries.

Soundness of scar

The security of an incision is promoted more by careful surgical technique rather than by the type of incision made, but incisions which divide rather than split or retract muscles tend to be weaker than those where little or no damage to muscle fibres occurs. Vertical incisions in the lower abdomen tend to be weaker than vertical upper abdominal incisions because of the weakness and deficiency of the posterior rectus sheath in the lower abdomen.

Appearance of scar

Cosmetic factors should be considered in all incisions and in some patients and some operations the particular sites are the major concern. In exposed parts of the body, special care should be taken to ensure that the incision is made along the lines of Langer where possible. Where transverse incisions cross the mid-line of the body, they should be placed symmetrically, especially in the neck and lower abdomen.

Making the incision

To ensure symmetry and precision in approximating skin edges during closure of the wound, transverse marks may be made at right angles to the proposed incision. These marks may be made with a sterile skin marker. They serve as a particularly helpful guide when the incision is curved, angled or complicated, particularly in exposed areas of the body. Transverse 'scratch marks' made with the tip of a scalpel should be avoided as they frequently result in an ugly red wheal in the skin. Incisions along Langer's lines or skin creases heal best and should be employed where cosmetic considerations are important. Straight longitudinal incisions over the flexor aspects of joints cause contractures and should be avoided, particularly in the fingers. More acceptable healing occurs where, in crossing the flexor surface of a joint, the incision is curved to follow the joint crease or a line parallel with it. Incisions should be avoided over bony prominences where the movement and friction of the scar overlying the bone may delay healing or lead to keloid formation.

The incision should be made cleanly and decisively, utilising as much of the cutting edge of the scalpel as possible in the circumstances. Tentative and repetitive incisions in the skin give a ragged and unhealthy appearance to the edge of the wound and should be avoided.

Bleeding can be diminished by subcutaneous injection of vasoconstrictor substances such as adrenaline, by identifying and ligating vessels before dividing them and by utilising a median incision where bleeding is less than with paramedian or transverse incisions. Avoidance of cutaneous nerves is achieved by incisions which run parallel to the course of these nerves. Interference with muscle is reduced by the use of midline abdominal incisions or by retraction or displacement rather than transection of muscles.

Closing the incision

In most areas of the body, incisions are closed in layers. A wide variety of suture materials and methods of closure are used depending more on the preference of the surgeon that on proven scientific data. Continuous rather than interrupted sutures are used in the closing of peritoneum lest any intraperitoneal tissue protrude between the sutures. Whether the peritoneum should be closed with chromic catgut or nylon is debatable. Even though it is absorbed in time (minimum of 20 days) chromic catgut evokes more tissue response and this may predispose to the development of adhesions to the suture line. Since the peritoneum heals rapidly and bridges gaps effectively, close apposition of the peritoneal edges may not be necessary. While most surgeons, when closing a transperitoneal incision, suture the peritoneal layer, the value and need for this have been questioned. Experimentally and in clinical trials abdominal incisions have not been found to be weaker in cases where the incision was closed without any peritoneal suture. A practical advantage of closing the peritoneum is that superficial sutures may be placed in layers with more ease and safety.

Layered closure

Traditionally, abdominal and other wounds have been closed in layers, each layer being sutured separately (Fig 3.2). Whether continuous or interrupted sutures are used, it is clear that catgut sutures should not be used for all layers of an abdominal operation. The incidence of wound dehiscence and incisional hernia following the use of catgut alone is as high as 10%. It is customary to close the peritoneum with continuous chromic catgut or monofilament nylon; the same type of material is used for the posterior rectus sheath together with the peritoneum and strong non-absorbable suture material, such as nylon, is used in the anterior rectus sheath. It is important that large bites of tissue are taken, for if the needle is passed less than 1.5 cm from the edge of the divided fascia during suturing, the tissues tend to tear out and predispose to weakening and disruption of the wound. Where muscles have been split, there is seldom need to suture them, although they can be approximated more easily by interrupted catgut sutures to the overlying fascia. If muscles are to be sutured, the sutures should not be

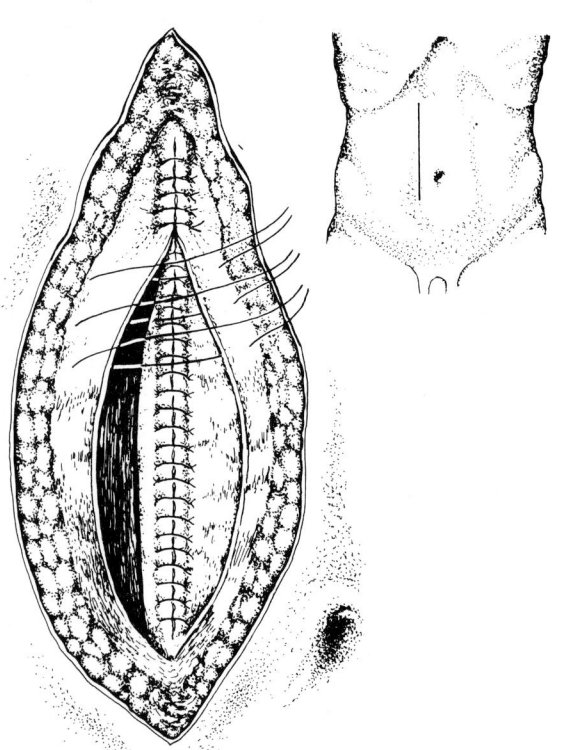

Fig 3.2 Layered closure of paramedian incision.

drawn tight as they will become strangulated and necrotic. All tissues become ischaemic if sutured too tightly and allowances must be made for the reactive oedema and tissue expansion which occurs after the trauma of suture insertion. After the anterior sheath or linea alba has been sutured, the subcutaneous 'dead space' may be closed with interrupted absorbable sutures of chromic catgut or polyglycolic acid (Dexon). Although sutures act as foreign bodies before absorption and, therefore, become potential sites of sepsis, they help prevent infection by obliterating dead space where blood and coagulum, with their tendency to encourage the proliferation of micro-organisms, may collect. Subcutaneous sutures also facilitate the apposition of skin edges and allow easier placement of skin sutures.

Mass ligature technique

The suturing of all layers of the abdominal wall, with the exception of the skin, by interrupted or continuous non-absorbable sutures, has been found to be as effective as a layered closure when the soundness of the wound is considered. Strong monofilament nylon or stainless steel wire sutures are used most commonly in this technique and several clinical trials attest to the integrity of laparotomy incisions closed in this fashion. As with the layered closure, the sutures are placed 2 cm from the edge of the wound and, if interrupted sutures are used, they should be placed 2.5 cm apart. A figure-of-eight interrupted wire suture is suitable for this kind of closure.

Skin closure

When suturing skin, a non-absorbable suture is generally employed, unless the wound is in a particularly sensitive area, such as the scrotum or areolar region, where absorbable sutures are more appropriate. Skin sutures should be tied loosely, their function being to appose the edges of the skin. Nylon, being the least reactive, should be used where cosmetic considerations are important. Sutures should not be placed too closely together and the use of adhesive tapes, coapting the edges of wounds, allows fewer skin sutures to be inserted. Many skin wounds may be closed exclusively with tapes and puncture wounds avoided entirely. Special care must be taken to ensure that the wound is completely dry, otherwise the tapes may become dislodged at an early stage by the seepage of blood from beneath. A subcuticular suture often gives a neat appearance, is especially useful in straight clean incisions and in children avoids the upset of stitch removal. If a non-absorbable subcuticular suture is to be used, strong nylon is recommended, as it slips out readily and does not break. This type of suture should not be used where infection is anticipated, as the entire suture will have to be removed for the drainage of subcutaneous pus.

Laparotomy

In emergency laparotomy for abdominal trauma, or general peritonitis of uncertain origin, where cosmetic considerations are secondary, a mid-line incision is quick and relatively bloodless. The umbilicus should not be crossed however, because of the likelihood of contamination. Even with thorough preoperative cleansing with antiseptic agents, it is almost impossible to sterilise the umbilicus. The incision can be extended upwards or downwards in the mid-line while skirting the umbilicus to the left or right. Incisions through the largely avascular linea alba heal slowly so that, in repairing mid-line incisions, the use of non-absorbable suture material is mandatory. A mid-line incision does not interfere with an intestinal stoma, where this requires to be fashioned. A paramedian incision, if placed too far laterally, may get in the way when the stoma is being made. Mid-line incisions do not affect the blood or nerve supply to muscles and they are easy to make, the point of decussation of fibres in the linea alba being a sure guide to the mid-line. They are also easy to close. Extraperitoneal fat can be pushed aside by gauze and need not be transected. When operating for trauma, it is important to remember that more than one organ may be injured and a long mid-line incision gives good access to most of the peritoneal cavity, particularly when full relaxation of muscles allows the edgess of the wound to be retracted fully. If there is difficulty in exposing the four corners of the peritoneal cavity, the upper or lower end of the incision can be extended to one or other side, either transversely or obliquely. If necessary, such extension can be brought across the costal margin and into the chest to improve exposure of organs such as the liver, diaphragm and oesophagus.

For urgent exploratory surgery where the site of disease is uncertain, a transverse incision is unsuitable, except in paediatric surgery. Although transverse incisions are said to be associated with less pain than vertical abdominal incisions, usually give a better cosmetic result and may be less prone to dehiscence or incisional hernia, these advantages are offset by the lessened access which they provide to the peritoneal cavity.

Specialised abdominal incisions, by definition, lack versatility and, if the diagnosis is incorrect, may be inadequate to deal safely with the involved organ. Many of these incisions can be extended, but in some cases it is better to close the incision and make another more suited to the operative requirements.

Specific incisions

Mid-line incisions

In making a mid-line upper abdominal incision (Weichert and Drapanas, 1972), the linea alba should be cleaned of fat so that its decussating fibres can be defined since this denotes the mid-line, and if this point is chosen to incise the linea alba, there is no risk of opening the rectus sheath inadvertently. In operations on the region of the oesophago-gastric junction, the mid-line incision may be extended to the left or to the right of the xiphisternum or the xiphoid process can be removed. At the lower end of the mid-line incision the umbilicus should be avoided by carrying the incision to the left or to the right. If the incision is brought to the left of the umbilicus, the round ligament (ligamentum teres) can be avoided.

If the incision avoids the umbilicus to the left, an upper mid-line can be extended to a lower mid-line incision; the urachal remnant is found in the mid-line as it passes across between the umbilicus and the bladder. The peritoneal incision is made to one or other side of the urachus. Care is taken to avoid damage to the bladder at the lower end of the mid-line incision. The bladder may be pushed downwards behind the pubis or the peritoneum may be incised to one or other side of the mid-line in order to protect the bladder.

Paramedian incision

A paramedian incision is not as versatile as the midline because the obliquity of the costal margin reduces its extent. However, when the organ to be operated on is known, a suitably placed paramedian incision is strong, safe and appropriate. The anterior rectus sheath is incised along the line of the skin incision about 1.0–1.5 cm lateral to the medial edge. If the sheath is incised nearer to the mid-line, difficulty may be encountered when suturing the wound at the end of the operation. The medial edge of the anterior rectus sheath is elevated and the rectus muscle retracted laterally, while vessels at the site of the tendinous intersections are divided between ligatures. This part of the incision may be difficult if the anterior sheath is divided too far laterally, while an incision too far medially spoils the flap effect by which the incisions in the anterior and posterior rectus sheaths are separated by muscle. Instead of retracting the rectus muscle laterally, it may be split vertically in the line of its fibres 1 cm from its medial border with little loss of blood and without damage to the blood supply of the medial strip.

Rectus splitting incisions

Controversy exists as to the desirability of rectus splitting incisions. They are quicker to carry out than the formal paramedian incision where the rectus muscle is retracted laterally. If the muscle is split through its extent, however, the nerve and blood supply of the medial portion of the muscle suffers interference and muscular atrophy may occur. There being no posterior rectus sheath in the lower abdomen, it is particularly important that vertical lower abdominal incisions be closed with non-absorbable sutures.

Subcostal incison

A right subcostal incision (Kocher or Courvoisier) parallel with and 2 cm below the costal margin is suitable for gallbladder surgery, while the spleen is exposed well by a similar incision on the left, particularly if it is enlarged. Subcostal incisions heal well, are probably less painful than vertical incisions and give adequate access to the common bile duct. They are also less likely to be followed by adhesive small bowel obstruction than are vertical incisions, but take longer to make and involve cutting of muscle. Muscle may be cut with a pointed diathermy needle, but since many of the vessels are too large to be fulgurated while being cut, it is preferable to transect muscles with a scalpel. Vessels, thus exposed, can be coagulated with certainty and precision. Because the transversus muscle is a thin sheet, it is advisable not to use diathermy to cut it as the peritoneal cavity may be entered prematurely with the possible risk of damage to underlying viscera. The 8th and 9th thoracic nerves are at risk of injury when this incision is made. The 9th nerve is usually large and can be seen and protected. The biliary apparatus can also be exposed through a transverse incision or a semilunar one beneath the right costal margin, the convexity being towards the umbilicus.

Transverse abdominal incision

Transverse abdominal incisions are widely used in paediatric surgery where they provide excellent access to all parts of the peritoneal cavity. In adult surgery, they are employed less frequently. Transverse incisions across the whole abdomen are made by transecting the rectus abdominus sheath and muscle on each side in the same line as the skin incision. Bleeding from the cut muscles can be reduced by using two parallel rows of catgut sutures through the anterior rectus sheath and muscle before dividing it. The peritoneum is opened in the same line. If the posterior and anterior sheaths are repaired accurately, little muscular weakness occurs

afterwards and the cosmetic results of transverse incisions are generally better than those of vertical ones.

An alternative method of transverse abdominal incision involves the retraction rather than the transection of the rectus muscles. The skin and anterior rectus sheaths are incised in the same line. The anterior sheaths are then dissected off the muscle upwards and downwards for about 7.5 cm, care being taken to ligate the blood vessels at the tendinous intersections and within the muscle. After the flaps have been developed, the rectus muscle is retracted laterally on each side and the posterior rectus sheath and peritoneum are incised transversely. No damage to the rectus muscle occurs within this incision. It is not a speedy incision and, in the adult, does not give access to the entire peritoneal cavity, but incisional hernia or wound failure are most unusual and the scar is cosmetically satisfactory as it is made along Langer's lines.

Transverse abdominal incisions may be extended upwards in the mid-line by dividing the linea alba vertically after the rectus sheaths and muscles have been transected horizontally.

Lateral extensions of vertical incisions

Various lateral extensions may be made from vertical incisions if these prove to give incomplete exposure in a particular instance. Extensions at right angles to a midline or paramedian incision may be made in the middle or at the upper or lower ends of the vertical incision. Occasionally a T-incision is made where the transverse limb is made across the top of the vertical incision. For better access to laterally placed sites, such as the hepatic and splenic flexures of the colon, such transverse extensions may make a difficult procedure easy. Alternatively, an oblique subcostal extension of a vertical incision may be made but, in a patient with a narrow subcostal angle, the nerve and blood supply to the skin between the limbs of the incision may be put at risk. Useful incisions providing excellent exposure of the left or right colon, are the 'ten-past-six' or 'ten-to-six' incisions (Wyllie, personal communication). In these, an oblique extension is made at the upper end of a paramedian lower abdominal incision. These oblique extensions to the left or to the right are brought as far as the costal margin in the anterior axillary line.

Czerny incision

The Czerny incision provides good exposure of the pelvic organs. It is a predominantly transverse incision, slightly concave upwards, in the suprapubic region. The anterior sheath of the recti and the external and internal oblique aponeurosis are divided in the same line as the skin incision. The lower flap of anterior rectus sheath with the external and internal oblique aponeurosis is elevated off the muscle and developed downwards to the pubic symphysis. The tendinous insertions of the recti at the pubis are divided and the muscles reflected upward. The bladder is then exposed clearly. The peritoneum is incised transversely.

Pfannenstiel incision

This incision is particularly suited for gynaecological surgery and some operations on the bladder and prostate. It is a transverse suprapubic incision some 12 cm in length, slightly concave upwards, with its centre about 3 cm above the pubic symphysis. The aponeurosis anterior to the rectus muscle is incised along the line of the skin incision and may be extended on each side lateral to the rectus muscle. Aponeurotic flaps are developed upwards for 5 or 6 cm and downwards to the pubis. After separation of the rectus muscles in the mid-line, the peritoneum is opened vertically.

Compared with a mid-line lower abdominal incision, the Pfannenstiel incision takes longer, is associated with a higher incidence of haematoma formation and provides less exposure. The scar is, however, inconspicuous and fundamentally stronger.

Reopening the abdomen

If reoperation is required, it is desirable to utilise the previous incision, excising the previous scar. Non-absorbable suture material should be removed in the course of re-exploration but it is unnecessary to trace each suture or to remove all of them. It is usually easy to incise as far as the peritoneum, but entry into the peritoneal cavity may be difficult. The peritoneal layer may not be found and intraperitoneal adhesions may have caused loops of bowel to be attached to the parietal peritoneum. Entry into the peritoneal cavity at a fresh area is then advised and may be achieved by extending the incision slightly. Once safely into the peritoneal cavity the opening can be extended. If a separate, parallel incision is made for reoperation, the abdominal wall is weakened. A separate incision may be advisable, however, when the patient is being reoperated on for small bowel obstruction, a likely cause of which is adhesive obstruction. The obstructed loop of bowel may be related closely to the peritoneal surface of the previous incision and may be endangered by reopening the peritoneum at the previous site. It is not necessary to divide all intra-abdominal adhesions (*see* Chapter 1).

Grid-iron appendicectomy incision

Appendicectomy, particularly when the appendix is perforated, is commonly followed by wound infection. The grid-iron incision is rarely followed by the serious sequelae of wound dehiscence and incisional hernia which can complicate infected vertical incisions.

McBurney's point lies one-third of the distance along a line connecting the right anterior superior iliac spine with the umbilicus. The incision crosses McBurney's point at right angles to the line, one-third of the incision being above, two-thirds of the incision below, the line. In the approach to appendicectomy, slight variations on the skin incision are commoner than the classical incision. A Lanz incision is almost transverse, being slightly oblique, in the line of a skin crease in the right iliac fossa. Being aware of the numerous positions in which the appendix may lie, it is useful to mark the site of maximal tenderness before operation and to place the incision accordingly. The external oblique aponeurosis is divided in the line of the skin incision and the underlying internal oblique and transversus muscles are split along the line of their fibres by separating the blades of haemostat or scissors. The ilio-inguinal nerve is protected. The incision can be extended by cutting the muscles laterally if necessary (Rutherford Morison manoeuvre) or medially by opening into the rectus sheath, or by incising vertically along the lateral border of the rectus muscle.

Thoraco-abdominal incision

This incision converts the abdominal and thoracic compartments into one space and is used for operations on intraperitoneal or retroperitoneal upper abdominal viscera and structures in the lower thorax (Madden, 1980). A right thoraco-abdominal incision provides exposure for hepatic and upper biliary tract surgery, while a left-sided incision is used for removal of grossly enlarged and adherent spleens, large lesions of the tail of pancreas, left adrenal and left-sided retroperitoneal tumours and occasionally for spleno-renal shunts. It is commonly used for operations on the upper stomach and lower oesophagus.

The incision is made over the 7th or 8th interspace, extends across the costal margin, and is carried obliquely to the mid-line of the abdomen. The deepened incision transects the latissimus dorsi, serratus anterior muscle and the anterior rectus sheath and rectus abdominis muscle. The intercostal muscles are then divided, together with the anterior fibres of the diaphragm and the abdominal muscles. The parietal pleura and peritoneum are incised to give full access to the underlying viscera.

When closing the incision, the diaphragm is repaired with interrupted non-absorbable sutures. With the use of a rib approximator and strong non-absorbable pericostal sutures or sutures passed through holes in the ribs made with an awl, or intramedullary rib pegs, the intercostal muscles are apposed and repaired with interrupted silk sutures. Figure-of-eight sutures are used to reunite the transected costal margin and the peritoneum closed with continuous chromic catgut. The latissimus dorsi, serratus anterior and transversus abdominis muscles are repaired with interrupted non-absorbable sutures and continuous monofilament nylon is utilised to repair the internal oblique, the external oblique aponeurosis and the anterior rectus sheath. Subcutaneous interrupted chromic catgut sutures are inserted and the skin closed with interrupted nylon sutures. A drain with underwater seal is placed in the pleural cavity.

Incisions in the neck

Parotid

The parotid gland is approached through a Y-shaped incision, the limbs of the Y enclosing the lower half of the lobe of the ear and the stem of the Y extending downwards behind the angle of the mandible (*see* Chapter 41). This approach allows the facial nerve to be identified at an early stage as it lies below the external auditory meatus (EAM) in the space between the mastoid process and the posterior border of the mandible. An alternative is Patey's incision which starts in front of the EAM, dips below the lobe of the ear and then to the anterior edge of the sternomastoid muscle. It is continued upwards and downwards along the anterior edge of the muscle.

Block dissection

Many types of incision, all giving satisfactory exposure have been devised for this operation since Crile in 1906 described the T-shaped incision, in which the transverse limb was slightly concave upwards and extended from the mastoid process around the borders of the mandible to the symphysis menti. The vertical limb extended downwards as far as the junction of the inner two-thirds and outer third of the clavicle. A double Y incision was described by Martin which, by fashioning Y incisions at the upper and lower ends of the vertical component, avoids tethering of the skin often associated with long vertical incisions (Martin *et al.*, 1951). The ladder incision of MacFee involves two parallel transverse incisions separated by a broad flap of skin in the upper and lower part of the neck, allowing wide exposure when the skin and platysma have been undermined. To avoid vertical wounds over the carotid vessels, other incisions which cross the carotids at right angles are in use. In the Schobinger incision the transverse component is as in the Crile operation, but the vertical limb starts far back on this line just anterior to the upper end of the sternomastoid and describes a curved course taking it in a wide C behind the sternomastoid. A modification has been described where the transverse component is Y-shaped rather than curved. A hockey-stick or Grandons incision has its ascending limb along the posterior border of the sternomastoid muscle and its horizontal part crossing the neck about 2 cm above the clavicle. This incision has the advantage that it lies outside the field of irradiation. In a patient who has had the cervical nodes irradiated previously, this is an important consideration because of the poor healing of irradiated tissue.

Drains

The purpose of a drain is to evacuate fluid or gas which is present or which is likely to accumulate in a localised cavity.

The placement or otherwise of drains has been determined largely by habit, custom and fashion rather than by valid evidence. In recent years there has been a trend to insert drains less frequently than in the past. They should be utilised only for specific reasons, such as drainage of an abscess cavity, underwater negative pressure drainage for pneumothorax or after thoracotomy and in circumstances where complete haemostasis is unattainable. Drains cannot be easy substitutes for careful attention to haemostasis and they provide no security in areas where significant bleeding continues. While they are effective in evacuating fluid from localised areas, they cannot be expected to drain large areas or multiple compartments, such as the general peritoneal cavity.

Advantages and disadvantages of drains

Drains may be harmful and dangerous. Most patients find that a drain is an inconvenient nuisance for it restricts their mobility both in and out of bed, is commonly uncomfortable and sometimes painful. It may allow infection from the outside to pass along the track, particularly if an open rather than a closed system is used, and if the drain is left in position longer than a few days. Drains always induce an inflammatory and fibroblastic response around them and can damage tissue, sometimes with serious consequences. Moreover, they may not function as intended and thus lead to delay in diagnosis of major internal collections of fluid. Perhaps it is not surprising, therefore, that there is a tendency to move away from routine use of drains, even for operations such as cholecystectomy, thyroidectomy and splenectomy, where the traditional practice was to 'always use a drain'.

Drains are, however, effective in promoting the discharge of pus and in removing localised collections of liquid blood or transudates. They also aid the approximation of tissue if negative pressure is applied and they can be used as vehicles for irrigation of cavities.

Types of drainage

Open and closed systems are used widely (Fig 3.3). When open, e.g. corrugated, drains are used, external dressings on the skin around the drains are required. It is difficult to measure the quantity of fluid drained and seepage of fluid may damage the surrounding skin or an adjacent incision.

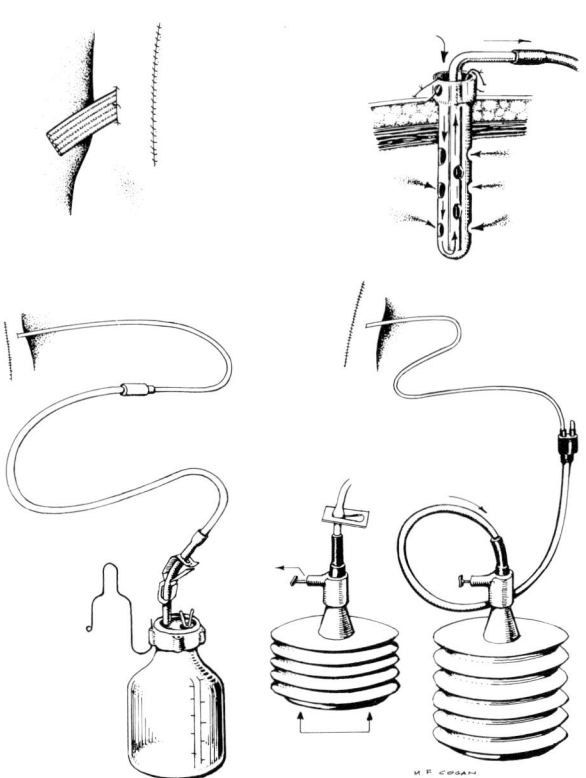

Fig 3.3 Drains. *Top left:* corrugated drain; *top right:* sump drain; *bottom:* vacuum drains.

Tube drains are used as part of a closed system when they are connected to a container. The volume of discharge can be recorded, there is little risk of contamination of skin or incisions in the vicinity and the system is more convenient for patients and nurses.

Sump drains are useful in permitting drainage against gravity. A perforated tube is inserted in the lumen of a larger tube with side holes. The double lumen system prevents plugging by tissue of the side holes of the internal tube. Several effective types, such as the Shirley sump drain, are available commercially. They are of particular use when draining the pelvis or areas where copious fluid loss is to be expected, e.g. pancreatic fistula.

While tissue reaction occurs with all drains, some are more irritant than others. Rubber drains are most irritant and should be avoided if possible. Drains of silicone, silastic or polyethylene material are less damaging to tissue. If a drain is too rigid it may damage viscera, but if it is too soft it may twist, kink and become blocked. Soft latex Penrose drains or Paul's tubing or soft corrugated drains are adaptable and suitable for subcutaneous tissue where vacuum drainage is not needed. They are most unlikely to cause damage to delicate tissue. Smooth drains are superior to rough drains because fibrin and clot do not adhere to them so readily.

Drains are placed in subcutaneous spaces where there has been a major degree of dissection, as in block dissections of lymph nodes or at mastectomy. In these circumstances suction drains are used and are more effective than those which rely on gravity. Subcutaneous vacuum drains may be brought out through the end of a wound, through separate stab incisions or by using a Redon trocar needle to which the drain is attached. Suction drains such as the Redivac, Sterivac or Surgivac apparatus are reliable and effective in subcutaneous tissues.

Intraperitoneal drainage

To be effective intraperitoneal drains should be brought out as far laterally as possible and if dependent drainage cannot be ensured, a sump drain should be considered. Intraperitoneal drains should not be brought out through the laparotomy incision as they predispose to wound infection.

With the exception of oesophageal, pancreatic and extraperitoneal rectal anastomoses, the placement of drains to intestinal anastomoses is probably unnecessary. If drains are applied to an area of bowel anastomosis, they must not press on the bowel wall. Rigid drains have been shown to damage colonic anastomoses and increase the incidence of anastomotic leaks. Vacuum drains, which have negative pressures of 10–25 kPa, can cause intestinal oedema, haematoma and even perforation if placed against the bowel wall.

Where drains are placed in intraperitoneal abscesses, they are usually left in place until the discharge ceases. If drains are placed in the splenic bed after splenectomy they should be removed within 3 days, otherwise they become foci for intra-abdominal sepsis.

References

Madden J. (1980). The thoracoabdominal incision. In *Abdominal Operations*, 7th edn. (Maingot R., ed.) p. 38. New York: Appleton-Century-Crofts.

Martin H., Del Valle B., Ehrlich H., Cohan W.G. (1951). Neck dissection. *Cancer*; **4**:441.

Weichert R.F., Drapanas T. (1972) Abdominal wall and peritoneum. In *Operative Surgery. Principles and Techniques* (Nora P.F., ed.) p. 343. Philadelphia: Lea and Febiger.

4

Oesophagus

K.C. McKEOWN

The oesophagus, a strap-like muscular tube (35 cm in length), is deeply situated in the neck, passes through the posterior mediastinum to traverse the diaphragmatic hiatus, and enters the stomach deep under the dome of the diaphragm. Its muscle coat consists of an outer longitudinal and an inner circular layer. In the upper third of the oesophagus the muscle fibres are striated, giving way to smooth fibres in the lower two thirds. It is lined mainly with squamous epithelium, interspersed with a few mucus-secreting glands. At the lower end it changes to columnar epithelium of the gastric type. This epithelium of the lower oesophagus does not secrete acid or pepsin. The columnar-squamous junction does not lie at the oesophago-gastric junction, but rather in the lower oesophagus.

Arterial supply

The arterial supply to the oesophagus has a segmental arrangement, as shown in Fig 4.1:

1   The cervical portion is supplied mainly from the inferior thyroid arteries, and from the pharyngeal arteries. Another vessel frequently present arises directly from the subclavian artery and is known as the artery of Luschka.

2   The retroaortic and retrobronchial portion is supplied from the bronchial artery arising directly from the under surface of the aortic arch. This large vessel divides into ascending and descending branches which anastomose with vessels from the cervical and the lower thoracic segments.

3   The lower half of the thoracic oesophagus derives its blood supply from segmental branches arising directly from the descending aorta. Usually three in number, the superior is the lesser oesophageal artery, inferior to it is the accessory oesophageal artery, and the most inferior and largest is the greater oesophageal artery. These vessels anastomose with each other and with neighbouring vessels.

4   The intra-abdominal oesophagus is supplied by ascending branches from the left gastric artery, reinforced by branches from the recurrent branch of the left inferior phrenic artery.

The *venous drainage* of the oesophagus starts in an extensive submucous plexus which drains through the muscular coat to a perioesophageal plexus which is particularly marked in the lower third. The cervical segment drains into the inferior thyroid, bronchial, and superior intercostal veins. The mid-segment drains into the azygos and hemi-azygos veins. From the lower third venous drainage is into the portal system by way of the left gastric vein, and the vasa brevia of the splenic vein. A collateral anastomosis, therefore, exists in the lower oesophagus between the systemic and the portal venous systems which is of great importance in portal hypertension.

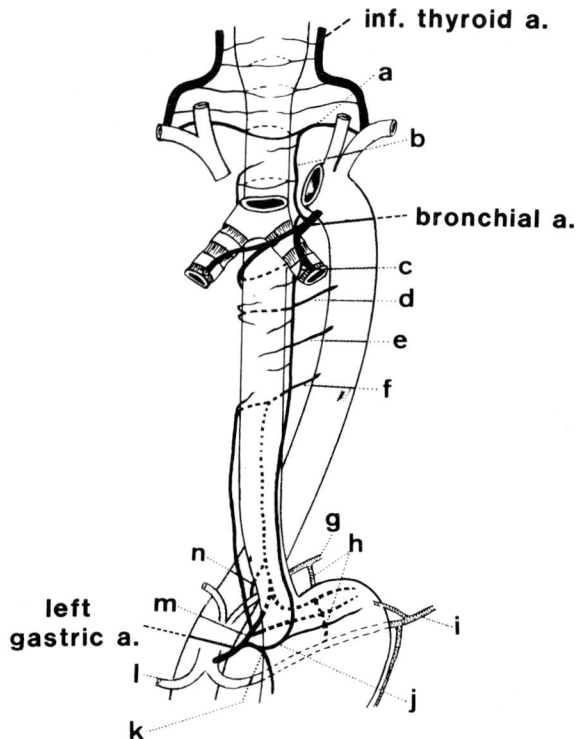

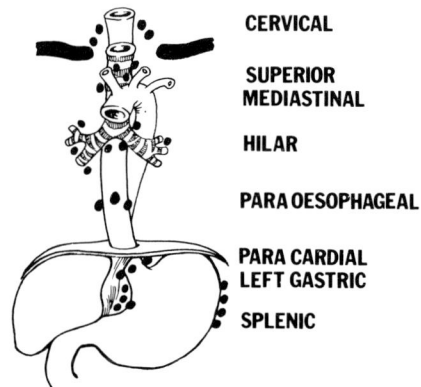

Fig 4.2 Lymphatic drainage of the oesophagus (By courtesy of the editors of *Digestive Cancer*, and the publishers Pergamon Press.)

Fig 4.1 Arterial supply to the oesophagus. 1. *Cervical segment:* inferior thyroid, pharyngeal and subclavian branches; 2. *Mid-oesophagus:* bronchial and (aortic) branches; 3. *Lower thoracic segment:* segmental vessels direct from the aorta; 4. *Intra-abdominal segment:* vessels from the left gastric artery and inferior phrenic.
a = oesophageal artery of Luschka; b = ascending tracheo-oesophageal A; c = ascending oesophageal A; d = lesser oesophageal A; e = accessory oesophageal A; f = greater oesophageal A; g = recurrent br. L. inferior phrenic; h = posterior oesophagofundic A; i = splenic A; j = anterior oesophagofundic A; k = br. of left gastric; l = hepatic A; m = postcardiofundic A; n = abdominal oesophageal A. (Modified from *Diseases of the Oesophagus*, 1958, Terracol J., Sweet R.H., eds., by courtesy of the authors and the publishers W. B. Saunders.)

Lymphatics

Each segment of the oesophagus has a characteristic lymphatic drainage (Fig 4.2). The cervical and supra-aortic segments drain into the cervical and superior mediastinal lymph nodes. The mid-oesophagus drains into the glands at the hilum of the lung. The lower oesophagus drains widely into the paraoesophageal, paracardial, splenic and left gastric lymph nodes. These nodes can be removed en bloc in cancer of the lower third of oesophagus.

Nerve supply

The nerve supply of the oesophagus is both parasympathetic and sympathetic. The parasympathetic supply is by the 9th, 10th, and 11th cranial nerves and by the right and left vagi, while sympathetic fibres arise from the splanchnic trunks and from the periarterial branches from the left gastric artery. The intrinsic plexus has no Meissners network; Auerbachs plexus is confined to the lower third.

The function of the gullet is (a) to transmit food from the mouth into the stomach without allowing gastric contents to enter the lower oesophagus, (b) to allow gastric air to escape upwards and (c) not to interfere with the act of vomiting. The upper end of the oesophagus is kept closed by tonic contractions of the cricopharyngeus muscle so that air is prevented from entering the oesophagus during respiration. This upper oesophageal sphincter actively relaxes when a bolus of food is propelled downwards by the inferior constrictor muscle during the act of swallowing. The lower end of the oesophagus is another high pressure zone which extends for a distance of 3 to 5 cm and which in association with other factors prevents gastro-oesophageal reflux. The thoracic oesophagus is a segment of low pressure which closely follows the negative pressure of the thoracic cavity.

The act of swallowing is a coordinated sequence of neuromuscular contractions involving the voluntary muscles of the pharynx and the smooth muscle of the oesophageal wall. Disease or dysfunction of part of the oesophagus affects the whole organ, so that a lesion at the lower end of the oesophagus may cause symptoms referrable to the oesophageal inlet.

Methods of investigation

Clinical

The presenting symptoms of oesophageal disease are usually dysphagia, heartburn, reflux and pain. An indication of the nature of the disease can often be made by analysis of these symptoms. Complete physical examination includes palpation of the left supraclavicular fossa, examination of the liver, observation of finger clubbing and of the general nutritional state.

Radiology

Straight x-ray of the chest may show air in the gullet, the presence of a foreign body, or a soft tissue shadow. Of equal importance is a search for pulmonary or mediastinal lesions, in particular for aortic aneurysm or vascular abnormalities.

Barium swallow shows that a primary wave of peristalsis begins at the upper end of the oesophagus, followed by secondary waves starting at the level of the aortic constriction. In elderly patients tertiary contractions may occur, which, when marked, produce the appearance of a 'cork screw' oesophagus. Transit time through the upper oesophagus, where the muscle is striated, is very rapid and lesions may be overlooked unless techniques using rapid photography or cine radiography are used. Passage through the thoracic oesophagus is much more leisurely and, above the level of the oesophageal hiatus, there may be a delay in the area known as the phrenic ampulla. The gastro-oesophageal junction requires careful examination and reflux should be looked for both in the vertical and more especially in the head down position (Figs 4.3, 4.4).

Oesophagoscopy

This examination must always be preceded by barium swallow to avoid entering an oesophageal diverticulum, or to prevent damage to an aneurysm of the thoracic aorta. Oesophagoscopy is used chiefly in diagnosis, so that the mucosa can be inspected, the level of the lesion noted, and tissue biopsied. Therapeutically, it is used for the removal of foreign bodies, the dilatation of strictures and for the insertion of tubes.

Instruments may be either rigid of the Chevalier Jackson or Negus type, or flexible as in the fibreoptic oesophagogastro-duodenoscopes. The rigid instrument is more difficult to pass, especially if the patient has a

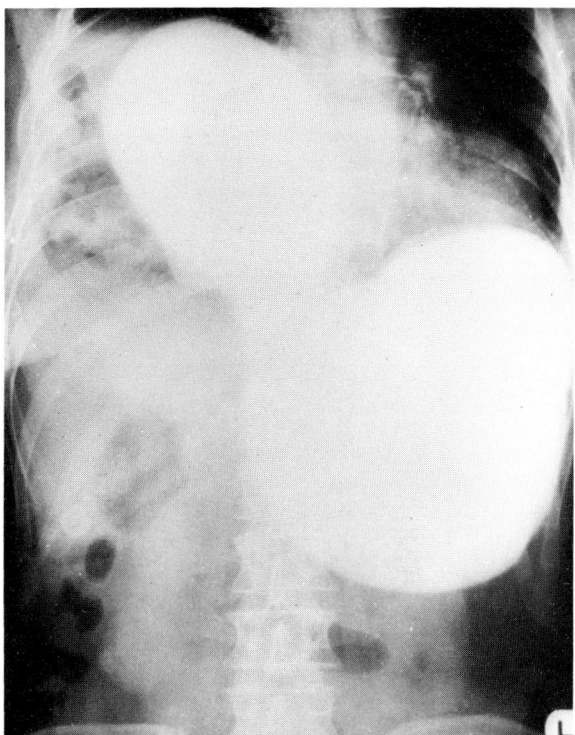

Fig 4.3 Paraoesophageal hernia. Barium meal showing a large paraoesophageal hernia extending upwards into the right side of the chest. The patient also has multiple gallstones.

small mouth, prominent incisor teeth, or spinal arthritis. However, an adequate biopsy can be obtained and the degree of fixity of a growth may be assessed by manipulation of the oesophagoscope. The fibreoptic instrument is more suitable for difficult subjects, especially those with severe spinal kyphosis, but the biopsy specimens tend to be small.

Technique

The fibreoptic instrument may be passed under sedation usually with intravenous diazepam. It is preferable to pass the rigid instrument under general anaesthesia with the use of a short acting relaxant. Positioning of the patient at each phase of the instrumentation is of great importance. With the patient in a supine position and the shoulders slightly raised, the instrument is introduced over the dorsum of the tongue while the neck is flexed. The instrument is advanced under direct vision as the neck is slightly extended. The instrument passes behind the endotracheal tube and its tip is brought gently forward. If difficulty is encountered at this stage, the anaesthetist should grasp the larynx and

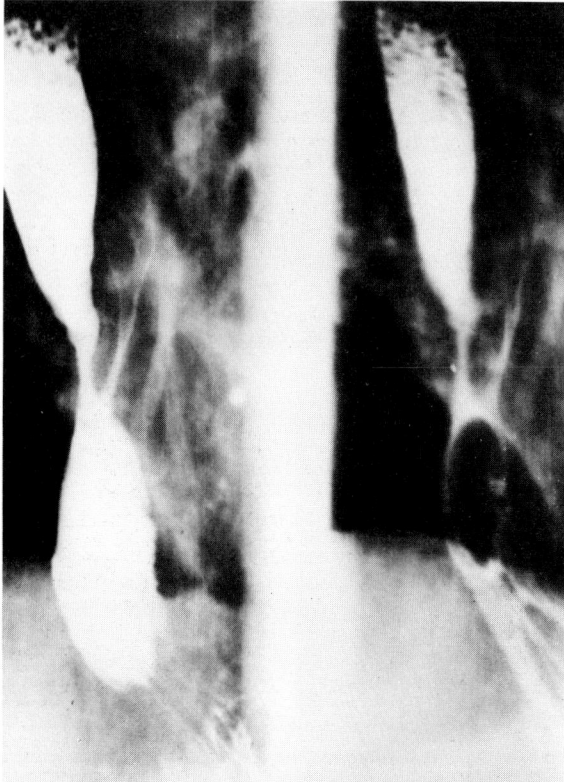

Fig 4.4 Brachy-oesophagus or congenital short oeso-phagus showing the oesophago-gastric junction in mid-chest.

pull it forward so that the upper oesophageal sphincter is drawn open. The instrument is advanced into the cervical oesophagus 16 cm from the incisors. As the head and neck are further extended, the oesophagoscope is advanced, reaching the aortic indentation at 25 cm and the lower end of the oesophagus at 40 cm (Fig 4.5). At this point the mucosa shows a puckered rosette appearance and as the head is further extended the instrument is advanced to the gastro-oesophageal junction.

Bronchoscopy

This examination is of special importance in growths of the mid-oesophagus. Increased vascularity, invasion of the bronchus by the growth, or presence of a fistula may be noted. Widening of the carina usually indicates extensive mediastinal involvement by the tumour.

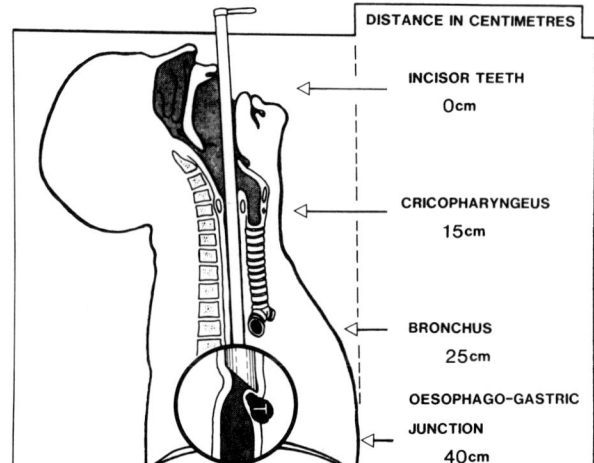

Fig 4.5 Oesophagoscopy showing the positioning of the head and the distances of adjacent structures from the incisor teeth.

Cytology

Balloon or brush biopsies are used widely in countries with a high incidence of cancer of oesophagus in screening programmes to detect the disease at an early stage.

Manometry and motility studies

For oesophageal manometry a multilumen tube is inserted with radiomarkers to enable the position of the tube to be identified. Pressures are recorded using transducers connected to a multichannel recorder. These investigations are of great value in the diagnosis of disorders of motility.

pH probe

This instrument measures the acidity within the lumen of the oesophagus and stomach. It is used in tests for oesophageal reflux. By positioning the probe in the lower oesophagus, acid reflux is noted (standard acid reflux test), and 24 h monitoring can be carried out. Similarly, the clearance rate of acid from the lower oesophagus is measured (acid clearance test).

Congenital abnormalities

Developmental abnormalities in the gullet, in the great vessels of the neck, or in the diaphragm can all cause symptoms of oesophageal disease, and are dealt with in the chapter on paediatric surgery.

Neuromuscular disorders

The act of swallowing, a coordinated sequence of muscular contractions and relaxations, may be impaired by a wide variety of diseases of nerve and muscle, such as myasthenia gravis or multiple sclerosis. As a result of disorders in the swallowing mechanisms *structural changes* may take place in the oesophagus. Dysfunction may occur at various levels:

1   The pharynx
2   The upper oesophageal sphincter
3   The body of the oesophagus (thoracic oesophagus)
4   The lower oesophageal sphincter (LES)

The pharynx

The inferior constrictor muscle acts as an impellor into the upper oesophagus. Nerve palsy, as in bulbar poliomyelitis and muscular dystrophy may affect this function.

The upper sphincter

There are three well recognised conditions associated with dysfunction of the upper oesophageal sphincter.

Cricopharyngeal spasm

This condition occurs in elderly patients who complain of food sticking in the throat and of episodes of regurgitation. These symptoms may cause embarrassment especially if they occur in public and the patient becomes apprehensive. It is perhaps because of this functional overlay that the condition is sometimes known as 'globus hystericus'. With persistence of spasm, or as the result of fibrosis in the muscle, the patient may develop a diverticulum of the pharynx. Barium swallow shows distension of the hypopharynx and folds of mucosa produce the appearance of an oesophageal web. Pharyngoscopy confirms the presence of mucosal folds and of spasm at the oesophageal inlet. Periodic dilatations may produce some improvement in symptoms, but myotomy of the fibres of the cricopharyngeus may be required.

Pharyngeal pouch (Zenker's diverticulum)

This type of diverticulum accounts for 90% of cases of pulsion diverticula, and is caused by neuromuscular

incoordination, spasm, or fibrosis in the pharyngo-oesophageal musculature.

Pathogenesis. At the pharyngo-oesophageal junction an area of potential weakness is situated posteriorly between the lower fibres of the inferior constrictor muscle and the upper fibres of the cricopharyngeal sphincter. This area of weakness is known as the dehiscence of Killian (Fig 4.6). In swallowing, contraction of the

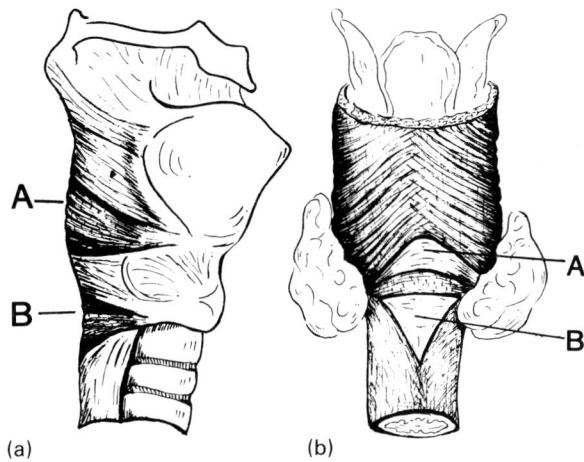

(a)   (b)

Fig 4.6 Sites of origin of pharyngo-oesophageal diverticula in (a) lateral and (b) posterior aspect. A = upper triangular weak spot between the lower margin of the inferior constrictor muscle and the upper margin of the cricopharyngeus. (Dehiscence of Killian). B = lower diamond shaped weak spot below the cricopharyngeus between the diverging muscle fibres of the oesophagus.

inferior constrictor is accompanied, or preceded, by active relaxation of the cricopharyngeus muscle. Should relaxation of the upper sphincter fail to occur or should there be spasm of the cricopharyngeus, mucosa may herniate through the area between the two muscles. The mucosal sac protrudes posteriorly and passes downwards and slightly to the left side of the neck and may reach the superior mediastinum. The sac comes to lie in line with the oesophagus, which is itself pushed forward and constricted (Fig 4.7).

Clinical features. The condition affects patients in later life and is twice as common in men. After a long history of intermittent spasmodic discomfort in the neck, the patient begins to suffer from progressive dysphagia, with regurgitation of unaltered food. The subject may notice swelling and gurgling in the left side of

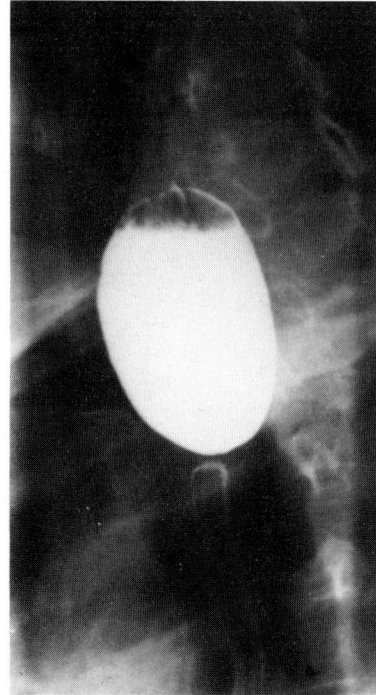

(a)

(b)

Fig 4.7 X-ray appearance of pharyngo-oesophageal diverticulum. (a) Anteroposterior view; (b) Lateral view showing that the diverticulum comes to lie in the line of the oesophagus and presses on it from behind.

the neck and pressure on this area or bending the head forward may help swallowing. Inflammatory changes may occur in the diverticulum and cough and chest complications due to aspiration are common. Malignant changes occur in 10% of untreated pharyngeal pouches.

Diagnosis. Barium swallow shows the typical features of a globular sac with an air bubble, and compression and displacement of the oesophagus may be demonstrated. Oesophagoscopy is unwise, since there is danger of rupturing the thin walled sac which lies in the anus of the normally positioned oesophagus.

Treatment. Formerly the sac was excised and the muscular defect repaired. Alternatively, the sac was dissected free and its fundus suspended by attachment to the prevertebral fascia. Because spasm of the cricopharyngeus muscle is an essential element of the condition, myotomy of the sphincter is desirable. If the diverticulum is small, myotomy alone may suffice, but larger sacs should be excised or diverticulopexy performed.

The cervical oesophagus is approached through a left oblique cervical incision, in the plane between the lateral lobe of the thyroid and the carotid sheath. The middle thyroid vein and the omohyoid muscle should be divided. The cervical oesophagus is rotated to expose the neck of the sac which is situated posteriorly, and great care is taken not to damage the left recurrent laryngeal nerve. If the sac is difficult to locate, a tube may be passed by mouth into its lumen. The sac should be excised and its margins sewn with inverting sutures, without narrowing the pharynx. The muscle defect should be repaired or, alternatively, a myotomy of the cricopharyngeal sphincter extending for a distance of 3 cm may be performed. If reflux oesophagitis is a coexisting condition, this must be dealt with before the pharyngeal pouch is treated.

Complications of operation. Failure to invert the neck of the sac or to deal with the spastic condition of the cricopharyngeus muscle may result in rupture with mediastinitis or fistula formation (4%). Excessive excision of mucosa at the neck of the sac may produce a stricture and inadequate excision may lead to recurrence. Recurrent laryngeal nerve injury occurs in 3% of cases.

Patterson-Kelly (Plummer-Vinson) syndrome

This syndrome, first described by Blakenstein in 1893, has now become known as the Patterson-Kelly or

Plummer-Vinson syndrome because of the various clinical features emphasised by these four observers over the decade 1912 until 1922.

Clinical features. The condition occurs predominantly in edentulous women between 30 and 50 years of age. There is a slow onset of difficulty in swallowing interspersed with acute episodes of spasm in the throat, often described as 'globus hystericus'. Solids are difficult to swallow and symptoms are worse if the patient is fatigued. All features of the syndrome are not present in every case.

1 *Mucosal changes.* The tongue is smooth and devoid of papillae, and the mucosa of the mouth thin, red and atrophic. These changes extend into the pharynx and loss of sensitivity in the mucosa impairs the neuromuscular reflex of swallowing. Thin crescentic webs of mucosa are present at the oesophageal inlet (Fig 4.8). Leucoplakia is sometimes present.

2 *Soft tissue changes.* There is atrophy of the lips which are thin and melanotic, and the angles of the mouth show chronic fissures. The hair is dry and the finger nails are thin, brittle and spoon shaped.

3 *Haematological changes.* There is hypochromic anaemia and the serum iron is low. The spleen is enlarged and there may be gastric achlorhydria. The cause of the condition is iron deficiency often associated with avitaminosis, especially riboflavin.

Diagnosis. The association of the clinical features should make the diagnosis clear. Barium swallow shows a pseudo-web at the oesophageal inlet (Fig 4.8); pharyngoscopy confirms the mucosal changes and the presence of cricopharyngeal spasm.

Thoracic oesophagus

Oesophageal dyskinesia of childhood

This condition usually starts at the age of two weeks and is often mistaken for pyloric stenosis. Regurgitation rather than vomiting occurs. On investigation, peristalsis is absent in the oesophagus and the lower oesophageal sphincter is incompetent allowing gastric reflux.

Treatment. Provided that organic disease can be excluded, this condition is treated conservatively. Regulation of the feeds and keeping the infant in the head-up position diminish the risk of aspiration and of pulmonary complications. The symptoms usually disappear within the first year.

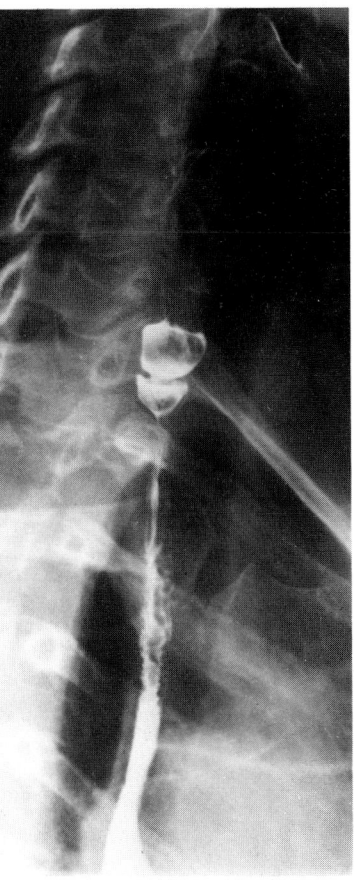

Fig 4.8 Patterson-Kelly syndrome. Barium swallow showing an oesophageal (sideropaenic) web.

Diffuse oesophageal spasm

This condition is one of disordered oesophageal peristalsis, characterised by oesophageal hypermotility and by chest pain and dysphagia. The lower two-thirds of the oesophagus are affected and may present either diffuse or segmental muscle spasm. Diverticula are found in the oesophagus, especially at its lower end. In some cases the lower oesophageal muscle is grossly thickened. The cause of the condition is unknown.

Clinical features. The patients, usually in late middle life, complain of intermittent attacks of retrosternal pain and dysphagia. Occasionally the pain is very severe and radiates to the back and up into the neck, so that a diagnosis of anginal pain is sometimes considered. Attacks which may occur spontaneously are often precipitated by rapid eating or by anxiety.

Investigations. Barium swallow demonstrates the presence of muscle spasm, which may be diffuse and constant, or segmental and transitory, affecting the lower two-thirds of the oesophagus. In the case of segmental contractions, the appearance may be quite striking, the so-called cork screw oesophagus or if the spasm is more marked, there may be a 'pearl necklace' appearance. In extreme cases, multiple pseudo-diverticula may be present (Fig 4.9).

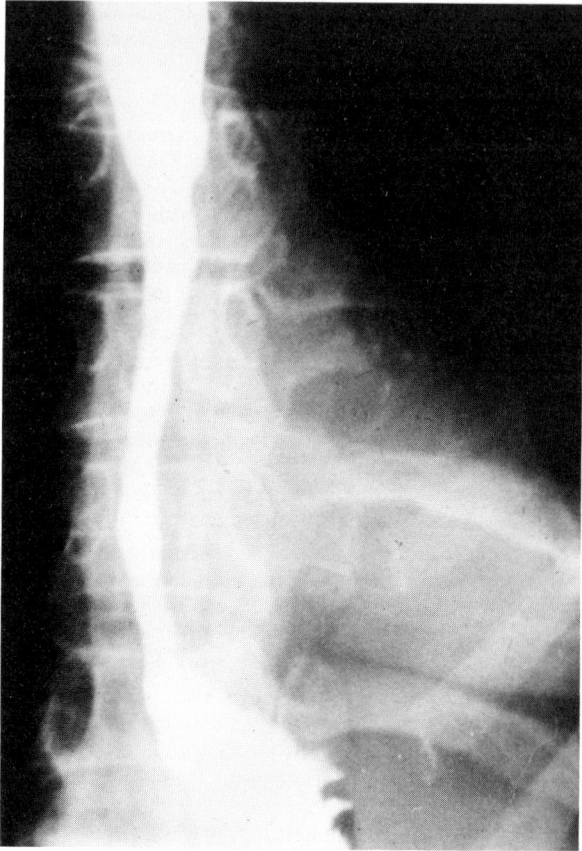

Fig 4.10 Diffuse muscular hypertrophy. The oesophagus shows a long narrow segment, but hold-up of barium is minimal.

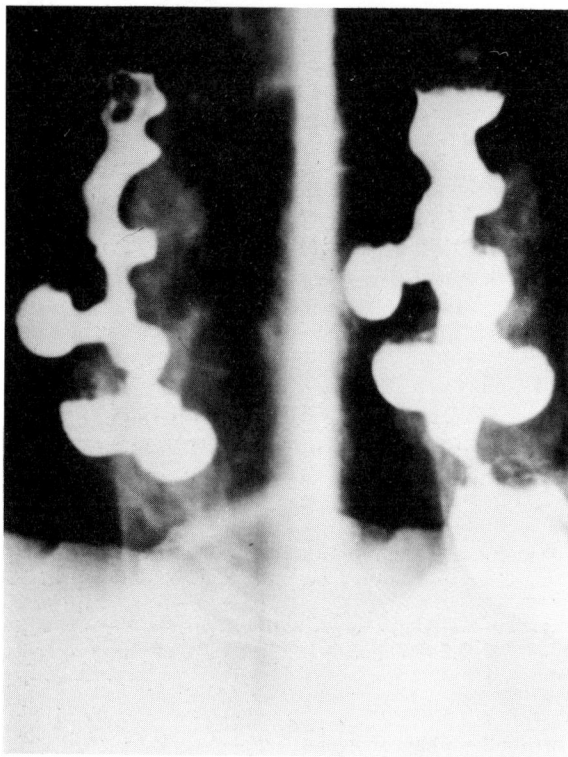

Fig 4.9 Corkscrew oesophagus. An extreme case of oesophageal spasm, showing the formation of pseudo-diverticula. (Dr T.L.C. Pratt's case).

Occasionally diffuse muscular hypertrophy produces a long narrow segment, but the narrowing is not constant as in fibrous or malignant stricture. In spite of the presence of spasm, there is no serious delay in the passage of food (Fig 4.10).

Oesophageal manometry shows contraction waves of high amplitude with pressures up to 140 mmHg. Increased frequency and duration of the peristaltic waves are noted and these are frequently repetitive. Increased pressure in the lower oesophageal sphincter is not a feature of this condition.

Treatment is not often required, but may be indicated if the patient has severe pain, persistent dysphagia or if a large diverticulum with a narrow neck has developed. Through a left thoracotomy, a long oesophagomyotomy extending the entire length of the affected oesophagus is performed. Pseudodiverticula do not require treatment, but a large diverticulum with a narrow neck should be excised.

Diverticula of the thoracic oesophagus

Traction diverticula occur in the mid-oesophagus and are caused by fibrous contracture in old tuberculous glands at the bifurcation of the trachea. All layers of the oesophagus are involved, but the diverticulum is pulled upwards so that symptoms rarely occur.

Pulsion diverticula are of greater clinical significance. They occur in the lower thoracic oesophagus and are true hernial protrusions of the mucosa. Like pharyng-eal pouches they are associated with disorders of peristalsis (Fig 4.11). Achalasia or oesophageal spasm may be present, and other lower oesophageal disease must be looked for.

The lower oesophageal sphincter (LES)

Achalasia

Achalasia of the cardia has two essential features: obstruction at the cardiac inlet and absence of peristal-

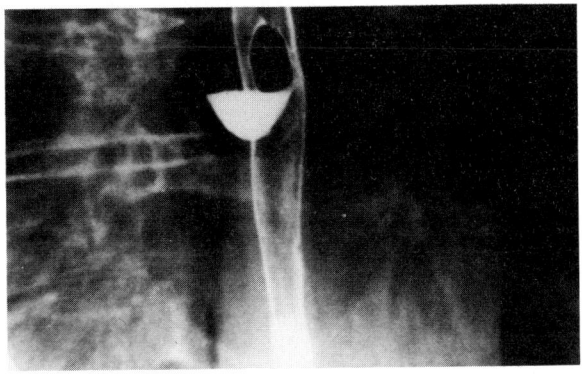

(a)

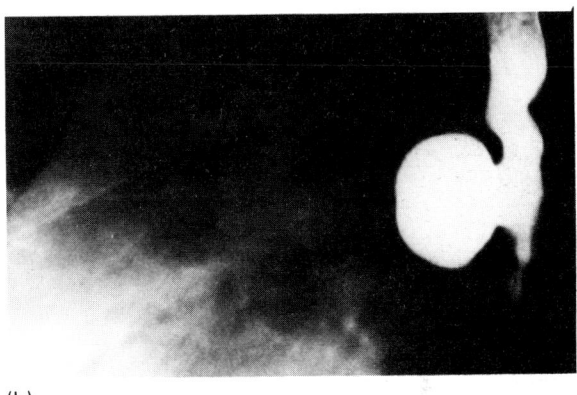

(b)

Fig 4.11 Epiphrenic diverticulum. (a) AP view showing the opening outlined with barium. (b) Lateral view.

Spontaneous rupture of the oesophagus

This condition is caused by muscular incoordination. If during vomiting the cricopharyngeus fails to relax and the pylorus is closed, an area of high pressure develops in the oesophagus which ruptures at its weakest point near the lower end. The tear is longitu-dinal and is situated posteriorly on the left side about 5 cm above the diaphragm (*see below*).

Scleroderma and oesophageal fibrosis

Infiltration of connective tissue into the smooth muscle of the oesophagus can produce dysphagia.

In scleroderma, a systemic disease of adult life in which there is diffuse fragmentation and homogenisa-tion of the connective tissues, the oesophageal wall is infiltrated and becomes thickened and oedematous. Peristalsis is impaired and the patient suffers from dys-phagia and regurgitation. The oesophagus becomes narrowed, and shortened; a hiatal hernia is often pre-sent. Oesophageal dilatation is occasionally required. Resection is hazardous and should be avoided, since in this condition, healing is poor, Reflux oesophagitis due to the failure of the lower oesophageal sphincter also leads to infiltration of the oesophageal wall with fibrous tissue, and may produce somewhat similar clinical features.

sis with dilatation of the oesophagus. Depending on the theories of origin, the obstruction may be referred to as cardiospasm, phrenospasm, or more accurately, as achalasia.

Pathogenesis. Manometric studies show an increase in tone in the lower oesophageal sphincter (LES) usually above 30 mmHg, and a failure of relaxation of the sphincter on swallowing. Primary waves of peristal-sis fade out in the upper oesophagus, while in the lower portion feeble repetitive contractions and occasional churning movements are observed. There is no proper coordinated peristalsis. Histological studies show abs-ence, or a marked decrease in the number, of ganglion cells in Auerbachs plexus with degeneration of pre-ganglionic fibres. The cause of the degeneration is unknown although infection, vitamin deficiency or vagal abnormality have all been incriminated. In accordance with Cannon's Law of denervation sensitiv-ity, there is a marked response of the oesophageal wall to cholinergic agents such as methacholine chloride (Mecholyl) which causes considerable pain. This observation forms the basis of a diagnostic test. In addi-tion, the lower oesophageal sphincter (LES) is hyper-responsive to the hormone gastrin which is thought to act on preganglionic nerve fibres.

Changes in the oesophagus. Because of the absence of peristalsis, food accumulates in the oesophagus which becomes dilated and atonic; it may be fusiform in shape, but sometimes assumes a sigmoid curve. The intra-abdominal segment becomes elongated. The muscle wall hypertrophies and inflammatory changes occur in the mucosa which may show leucoplakia or ulceration. After several years, malignant change may supervene in the dilated segment in 12% of patients.

Clinical features. Achalasia usually presents in adults of either sex between the ages of 30 and 50. It may occur in children and occasionally even in infancy. Of slow onset, the patient usually feels food sticking at the level of the lower sternum and difficulty is more marked with solids than with fluids. At first dysphagia may be intermittent and is aggravated by swallowing cold food. Unaltered food may be regurgitated and choking may be experienced at night. Pulmonary complications result from the aspiration of oesophageal contents and sometimes chest trouble may be the presenting symptom. Nutrition is impaired and the patient may develop arthritis of rheumatoid type.

Diagnosis. This depends on the clinical history, x-ray examination and manometric studies.

X-ray. Straight x-ray of the chest may show a mediastinal shadow with air or fluid levels in the dilated oesophagus. Barium swallow demonstrates a fusiform dilatation of the oesophagus with a tapering lower end or on occasions a sigmoid oesophagus with gross dilatation and haustrations (Fig 4.12). Octyl nitrite or Busco-

pan relaxes the sphincter while mecholyl causes contraction of the gullet associated with pain.

Treatment. The aim of treatment is to relieve the obstruction at the lower oesophageal sphincter and prevent oesophageal reflux.

Drug treatment with the use of nitrites and cholinergic agents has proved disappointing.

Dilatation has been used either alone under general anaesthesia or in combination with various hydrostatic dilators. Good results with pneumatic dilatation have been claimed in 65% of patients, but improvement is usually short-lived and there is danger of oesophageal rupture.

Operation. Lower oesophageal myotomy, first described by Heller in 1913, consisted of the division of the muscle in the front and back wall of the oesophagus. In 1923 Zaaiger advocated the single anterior myotomy which is now common practice.

TECHNIQUE. The lower oesophagus is approached either through the upper abdomen, especially in a thin asthenic patient, or preferably, by thoracotomy through the 8th left interspace. The lower 10 cm of the oesophagus are mobilised and the vagi carefully preserved. The circular fibres of the lower oesophagus are divided, with care not to damage the mucosa. The extent of the division is controversial because of the opposing needs to relieve obstruction and to prevent reflux. Some surgeons advise that the lower circular fibres should be preserved to prevent reflux,

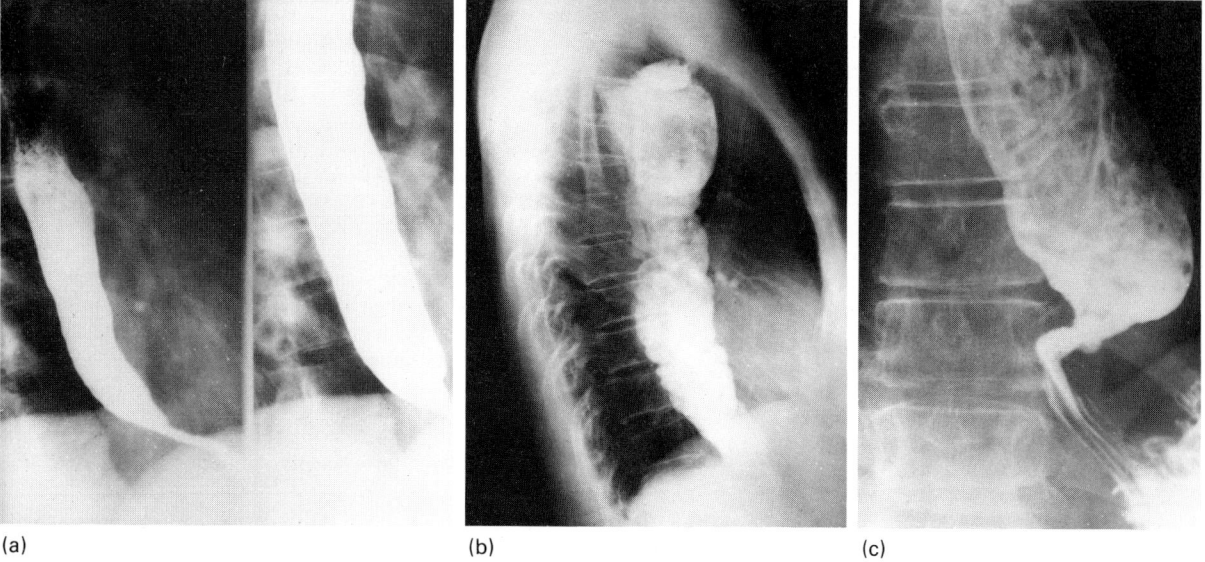

(a)   (b)   (c)

Fig 4.12 Achalasia of the cardia x-ray appearances of (a) a mild case with a smooth tapered lower end of oesophagus (Dr Michael Allen's case); (b) grossly dilated oesophagus with haustrations; (c) megaoesophagus with a sigmoid curve at the lower end.

while others advocate that section should extend over 7 cm and pass through the oesophagogastric junction into the stomach wall. This latter procedure must, however, be combined with an operation to prevent reflux. Failure of the operation is related either to inadequate relief of obstruction, because too small a segment of muscle has been divided, or to reflux after operation, leading to oesophagitis and stenosis. Because of the high risk of carcinoma developing in the oesophagus careful postoperative review and yearly oesophagoscopic examinations are essential. Malignant change does not necessarily occur in the narrow segment, but often at a much higher level in the dilatated oesophagus, where its presence may well be overlooked.

Rupture of the oesophagus

Rupture of the oesophagus is caused by instrumentation or by over-distension of its lumen.

Instrumentation

In the upper oesophagus there is an area of weakness on the posterior wall. While introducing the rigid oesophagoscope this weak area may be torn if the head is over-extended, if prominent teeth prevent proper alignment of the instrument, or if there are osteophytes in the cervical spine. A pharyngeal diverticulum may present an additional hazard. In the mid-oesophagus rupture results from dilating a stricture or intubating a malignant growth. Biopsy of a thin-walled oesophagus may cause perforation.

Over-distension of the lumen

Over-distension may occur in a variety of situations: during childbirth, defaecation, weight lifting, crush injuries, but more particularly after vomiting. Oesophageal damage is especially dangerous in the unconscious patient as in head injury or after general anaesthesia. Postconcussional vomiting may cause bleeding due to a tear in the lower end of the oesophagus or rupture of the oesophagus.

Spontaneous rupture of the oesophagus (Boerhaave's syndrome) and oesophago-gastric mucosal lacerations (Mallory-Weiss syndrome) are both thought to be due to severe vomiting or retching, especially in those suffering from alcoholism. The lower oesophagus and upper cardia are the sites usually involved, and the Mallory-Weiss syndrome presents with painless haematemesis or melaena.

Clinical features

The patient experiences excruciating pain in the back between the shoulder blades, retrosternally and in the upper abdomen. Even pethidine in full doses may not relieve the pain. The patient becomes breathless, shocked and cyanosed. Examination shows board-like rigidity in the epigastrium as in duodenal perforation, and surgical emphysema appears in the left supraclavicular fossa, spreading into the neck. Signs of left sided hydropneumothorax develop after about 6 h. In the early stages x-rays show minimal changes, but later on mediastinal emphysema and left-sided hydropneumothorax can be seen. The condition may resemble myocardial infarction, pulmonary embolus, acute pancreatitis or perforated peptic ulcer.

Treatment

Early operation is required to suture the perforated oesophagus and to establish drainage. Obstruction below the perforation must be relieved because simple suture would be doomed to failure. In the case of perforation of an oesophageal growth, immediate oesophagectomy holds out the best prospect of survival. In perforation of the lower oesophagus the left thoracic approach is appropriate, but in the middle oesophagus a right thoracotomy is preferable.

Oesophagitis

There are many causes of oesophagitis which may be acute or chronic in type, but two conditions are of special surgical interest; acute oesophagitis due to swallowing corrosive chemicals such as acids, alkalies, lye, phenol, or organic solvents, and chronic oesophagitis due to reflux of intestinal fluids such as acid pepsin, bile, and alkaline intestinal juices.

Chemical burns

Chemical burns are usually the result of accident or an attempt at suicide. The degree of damage depends on the type, concentration and volume of the ingested substance. In the Orient, attempted suicide accounts for most of the cases, but in the West, accident is the main cause. In both cases the substances swallowed are those easily accessible in the home or in the factory. Lysol or caustic soda are the commonest used, but in Malaysia acetic acid is often swallowed because it is readily available. Hydrochloric acid and carbolic acid also are causes of oesophageal burns.

Pathological changes

The type of tissue damage depends on the chemical agent. Acid tends to cause coagulation necrosis and the damage is more superficial; alkalis cause liquefaction of the tissues and the changes penetrate more deeply into the oesophageal wall, often causing vascular thrombosis. Burning may affect the lips, mouth, pharynx, oesphagus and stomach in varying degrees. Usually the upper oesophagus suffers least because of the rapid transit of the swallowed fluid. Slower transit in the lower oesophagus and spasm of the lower sphincter results in more severe damage in that area. Extensive sloughing and perforation may occur.

Clinical features

The patient usually presents with retrosternal pain and is severely shocked. The lips may not obviously be burned, but there is usually oedema of the mouth and glottis. Dysphagia is severe and there may be dyspnoea due to tracheal and bronchial damage. Acute symptoms last for one or two weeks during which period the patient may bleed, vomit slough, or perforate the oesophagus leading to mediastinitis.

A barium swallow shows flattening of the mucosa and loss of oesophageal motility. Muscle spasm is present and stenosis may appear especially at the lower end. A long thread-like lumen may be demonstrated. Oesophagoscopy when acute symptoms have subsided is required to show the extent of mucosal damage and to identify zones of stenosis.

Treatment

This is directed initially to the relief of pain and the treatment of shock. Blood is transfused followed by intravenous glucose and saline to maintain fluid and electrolytic balance. If the nature of the chemical agent is known, antidotes may be given, but these are probably of limited value. If possible the patient should be given sips of bland fluid, but if dysphagia is severe a fine nasogastric tube may be passed for drip feeding. In very severe cases gastrostomy is required. Antibiotics are given and after two or three weeks, cortisone may be administered in the hope of avoiding stricture formation.

Treatment of stricture. Dilatation of stricture should be carried out under direct vision through an oesophagoscope. Great gentleness is required to avoid haemorrhage and perforation. The Eder Puestow dilator has proved a safe and satisfactory instrument (*see* Fig 4.17). With an apparently impassable stricture, a thread may be swallowed to act as a guide for a dilator passed from above, or the thread may be identified at

gastrostomy and used to draw a dilator through the stricture.

Operative treatment is reserved for those patients in whom (a) the stricture is impassable, (b) dilatation is difficult, (c) there is frequent haemorrhage or (d), recurrence takes place rapidly. In short localised strictures, oesophagoplasty or local excision and end-to-end anastomosis may suffice. In the longer and more massive strictures bypass or excision with oesophageal replacement using stomach, colon or jejunum may be required.

Gastro-oesophageal reflux

Pathogenesis

The ability of the lower oesophageal mechanism to prevent gastro-oesophageal reflux depends on a complex mechanism involving the gastro-oesophageal junction, the 'physiological' lower oesophageal sphincter, and the anatomical arrangements of the diaphragmatic hiatus. These factors are depicted in Fig 4.13.

The oesophago-gastric junction

The oesophagus enters the stomach obliquely at a point about 7 cm below the dome of the fundus, forming with the fundus an angle known as the angle of His. Gastric distension approximates the fundus to the lateral wall of the oesophagus, and makes reflux less likely by narrowing the angle.

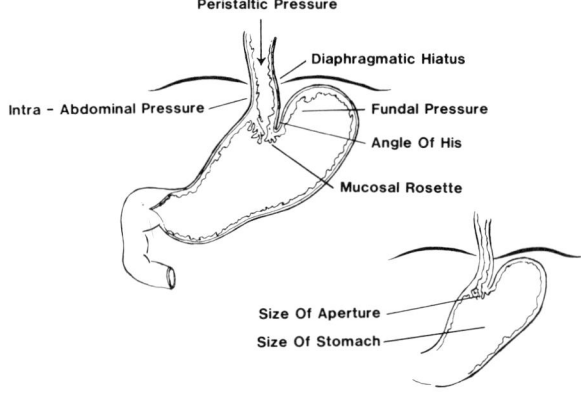

Fig 4.13 Mechanisms which prevent gastro-oeso-phageal reflux. The size and obliquity of the gastro-oesophageal junction contribute to gastro-oesophageal continence, while the mucosal rosette acts as a plug at the opening. Fundal and intra-abdominal pressure squeeze the lower oesophagus and tend to prevent reflux.

The oesophago-gastric opening is protected by folds of mucosa containing muscle fibres which form a 'mucosal rosette' which acts as a mucosal plug and makes the competence of the opening complete. The physical size of the fundus compared with the small size of the opening into the oesophagus makes distension of the fundus easy and that of the oesophageal opening more difficult.

Lower oesophageal sphincter (LES)

Though an anatomical sphincter has never been demonstrated in the lower oesophagus, manometric studies demonstrate a high pressure zone with pressures reaching 15–25 mmHg in the lower 3–4 cm of the gullet. Sphincteric tone is increased by cholinergic drugs such as metaclopramide (Maxolon), by gastrin and a high protein diet. The pressure in the sphincter is reduced by cholecystokinin, secretin and glucagon as well as by fatty meals, alcohol and nicotine. The presence of a portion of the oesophagus within the abdomen will allow the intra-abdominal pressure to act as a squeeze in the region of the lower oesophageal sphincter and tend to prevent reflux.

The anatomical arrangement

The anatomical arrangement of the hiatus probably acts by preventing reflux, particularly during such actions as coughing, lifting or straining at stool.

Reflux occurs in many subjects who experience no symptoms whatever. Whether symptoms are experienced may be explained on the basis of oesophageal sensitivity, the nature of the reflux (whether it be acid-pepsin or bile-trypsin), or on the duration of the reflux. This latter factor may be determined by measuring the rate at which the lower oesophagus clears acid (acid clearance tests).

Aetiology

Oesophageal reflux may be idiopathic, but is more frequently associated with abnormality at the hiatus, or as a consequence of some surgical procedure.

Sliding hernia

The association of gastro-oesophageal reflux with a sliding hernia is now a well recognised clinical entity. The oesophago-gastric junction and a portion of the stomach protrude upwards through the diaphragmatic hiatus into the chest cavity. The term 'sliding hernia' is used to denote that the stomach wall forms part of the hernial sac. The condition is comparable to the 'hernia en glissade' in the inguinal canal. The condition is said to occur in 5 patients per 1000, but all cases of sliding hernia do not have reflux and those who do, do not always complain of symptoms.

Postoperative

Operative procedures such as cardiomyotomy for achalasia, or oesophagogastrectomy for carcinoma of the fundus or lower end of the oesophagus inevitably result in gastro-oesophageal reflux. Even vagotomy in the treatment of peptic ulcer may affect lower oesophageal competence. A special type of reflux may follow Polya gastrectomy resulting in oesophagitis and stenosis.

Pathological changes

The lower oesophagus may be exposed to reflux of acid-pepsin, in the case of sliding hernia, or the action of bile and jejunal juices after partial gastrectomy. The first changes in the mucosa are the loss of the surface cells and elongation of the vascular papillae. Round-cells infiltrate into mucosa and the inflammatory changes lead to linear erosions along the crests of the oesophageal folds. In severe cases chronic peptic ulcer develops. The mucosa regenerates, but is of columnar rather than squamous type. Muscle spasm is present and true fibrous stricture may occur. Carcinomatous changes are apparently more common in cases of oesophageal reflux (Fig 4.14).

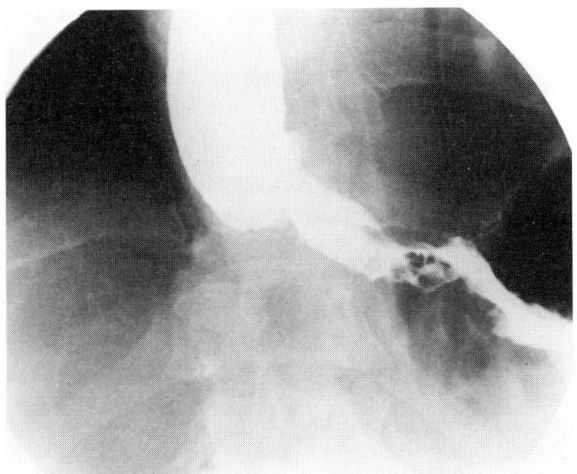

Fig 4.14 Malignant change occurring in a case of long-standing oesophagogastric reflux.

Symptoms

Though this condition may occur in young people, it is typically a disease of obese women in middle life.

Heartburn

This is present in 90% of cases, and epigastric or retrosternal pain after meals may lead to suspicion of peptic ulcer or cardiac disease.

Regurgitation

Regurgitation of bitter tasting fluid may occur after food, on straining, bending or when lying flat in bed at night. Belching of wind is common and occasionally vomiting occurs.

Dysphagia

This may occur, and hot fluids or alcohol cause burning pain in the epigastrium and sometimes in the back between the shoulder blades.

Bleeding

This may occur and the patient may present with haematemesis, melaena, or unexplained anaemia.

Diagnosis

This is made on clinical symptoms and confirmed by radiology, oesophagoscopy, and the special tests already mentioned.

1 **Barium swallow** shows gastro-oesophageal reflux especially when the patient is in the head-down position or lying on the side. The presence of a sliding hernia may be demonstrated and ulceration or stenosis may be noted.

2 **Oesophagoscopy** shows the inflamed mucosa often with linear ulceration along the crests of the mucosal folds. Contact bleeding is common. If an ulcer is seen, a biopsy should be taken to exclude malignant change.

3 **Special tests.** The use of the pH probe enables oesophageal reflux to be detected. As the probe is withdrawn from the stomach a change in the pH occurs as the instrument enters the lower oesophagus (Tuttles test). By positioning the probe above the gastro-oesophageal junction, changes in pH indicate reflux (standard acid reflux test); 24-hour monitoring with the probe in the lower oesophagus may be carried out. In Bernstein's test the lower oesophagus is perfused with 300 ml of 0,1N HCL to produce oesophageal pain, which can be relieved by replacement of the acid solution with bi-carbonate of soda. This test acts as a measure of oesophageal sensitivity and is used to differentiate oesophageal from coronary pain. The rate of clearance of acid from the lower oesophagus may also be measured (acid clearance test). Ambulatory monitoring of oesophageal pH can be employed using a portable radiotelemetry system.

Medical treatment

Medical treatment is directed to the prevention of reflux, the protection of the lower oesophagus, and the lowering of gastric acidity.

Prevention of reflux

This may be achieved by alterations of diet, slimming, maintaining an upright posture and by the use of drugs.

Diet. Meals should be small, and of low fat and high protein content.

Posture. The patient should avoid bending, and should sleep with the head of the bed raised on 10″ blocks. Slimming and the avoidance of tight corsets may ameliorate the symptoms.

Drugs. Metoclopramide (Maxolon) increases the tone of the lower oesophageal sphincter, increases oesophageal peristalsis and encourages gastric emptying so that reflux is diminished or prevented.

Protection of the lower oesophagus

Sucking alkaline tablets is often effective; alkalis combined with alginates (Gaviscon) form a protective layer on the surface of the lower oesophagus and may give greater relief. Alkalis with defoaming agents such as polymethyl siloxane (Asilone) or local anaesthetics (Mucaine) are also of value. Cases of biliary reflux after polyagastrectomy or pyloroplasty are better treated by altacite which has an affinity for bile salts.

Lowering gastric acidity

This may now be more easily achieved by the use of histamine receptor antagonists, such as cimetidine, which decrease both basal and food-stimulated secretion of acid.

Surgical treatment

This is reserved for those patients who have failed to respond to intensive medical treatment, to those with a sliding oesophageal hernia and to those who have developed stricture.

Treatment of sliding oesophageal hernia

Repair of the oesophageal hernia and fixation of the stomach in the abdominal cavity are the essential aims. There are three main techniques used in the treatment of sliding hernia.

Allison (1951). Through a left thoracotomy, the diaphragm is incised to expose the gastro-oesophageal junction. The perioesophageal fascia is exposed as the sliding hernia is reduced. The crura are defined and the hiatus narrowed by approximating the margins of the crura behind the oesophagus. The perioesophageal fascia is reefed and sutured around the margins of the diaphragmatic hiatus (Fig 4.15a).

Hill (1967). Through an abdominal incision the diaphragmatic hiatus is defined and the crura approximated posteriorly. The upper part of the lesser curve is fixed to the preaortic fascia and to the arcuate ligaments on the posterior abdominal wall. Finally the fundus is approximated to the left lateral wall of the oesophagus to accentuate the angle of His (Fig 4.15b).

Belsey (Mark IV) (1966). The lower oesophagus and cardia are extensively mobilised from above through a left thoracotomy. The peritoneal folds are dissected and the vagi displaced. The crura are narrowed as in the previous operations and finally the oesophagus is fixed to the edge of the crura by two rows of interrupted mattress sutures. These produce a buttress of plicated stomach round the oesophageal hiatus (Fig 4.15c).

In addition to these three procedures, designed to narrow the oesophageal hiatus and to reduce the sliding hernia, a further procedure has gained much prominence in recent years.

Nissen fundo-plication. This operation is somewhat different in principle, in that it is designed primarily to prevent gastro-oesophageal reflux. The operation may be performed through the abdomen or left chest. The lower oesophagus is freed, and after mobilising the fundus by dividing the upper vasa brevia, the fundus is wrapped round the lower oesophagus (Fig 4.16).

To prevent narrowing of the lumen of the oesophagus the suturing is performed over an indwelling 40F gauge oesophageal tube. This procedure prevents reflux by maintaining a segment of intra-abdominal oesophagus, by exerting pressure at the gastro-oesophageal junction, and probably by producing an ink-well effect.

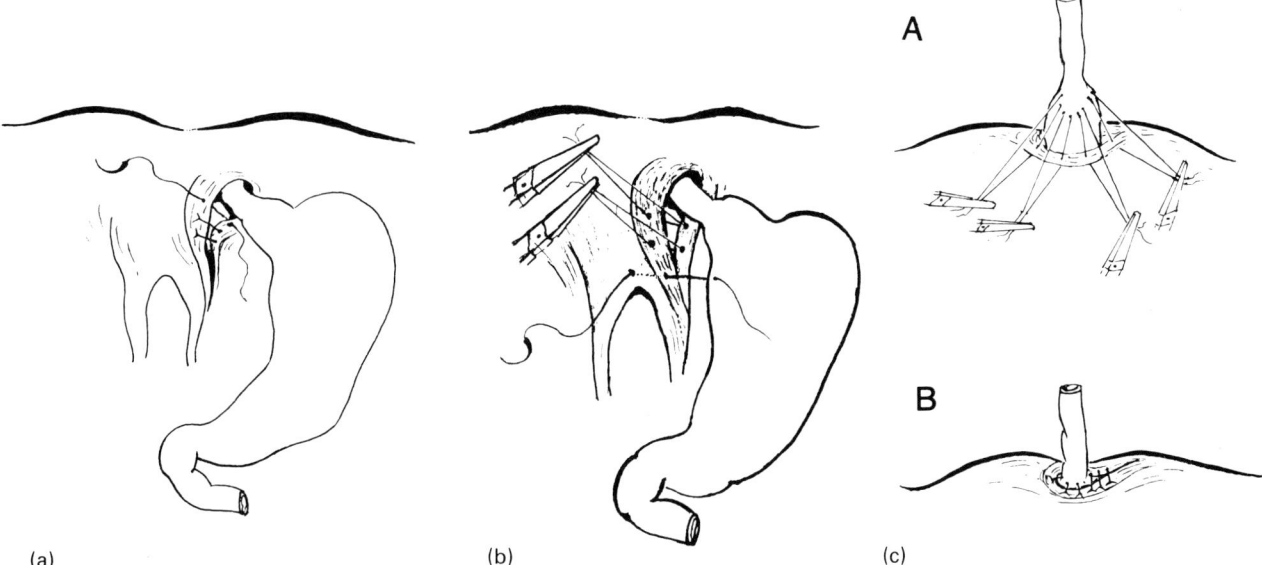

(a) (b) (c)

Fig 4.15 Repair of sliding oesophageal hernia. (a) *Allison.* Approximation of the crura behind the oesophagus. (b) *Hill.* Narrowing of the crura and fixation of the lesser curvature of the stomach to the arcuate ligament. (c) *Belsey.* Buttressing the stomach to the narrowed oesophageal hiatus.

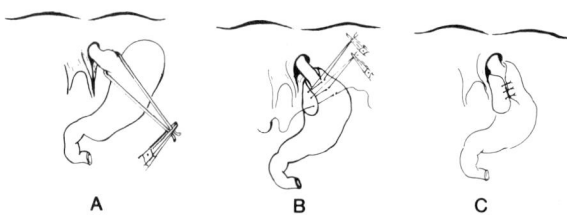

A   B   C

Fig 4.16 Nissen fundo-plication. After mobilisation of the lower oesophagus the fundus is wrapped around with interrupted sutures to produce a high pressure zone.

Results of operations. The Allison procedure produces good clinical results, though in 45% of cases there is evidence of oesophageal reflux on x-ray examination. The Hill procedure is said to produce somewhat better results and 97% of patients are symptom free. The Belsey operation relieves symptoms in 85% of cases, and the recurrence rate is between 10 and 15%. The Nissen procedure is highly effective as an antireflux measure and review of the literature shows a success rate of 95%. Criticism of the procedure centres round a small proportion who have some dysphagia (perhaps due to too tight suturing of the wrap around), or to inability to eructate wind or vomit. This latter problem may result in upper abdominal distension and is referred to as the 'gas-bloat' syndrome.

Treatment of stricture

When stricture complicates gastro-oesophageal reflux, attention must be directed not only to the treatment of the hiatal defect, but also to the narrow oesophageal segment.

Dilatation. Most patients respond to repair of the hernia and simple dilatation of the stricture. The use of the Eder Puestow dilator is a major advance in the treatment of strictures (Fig 4.17). A guide wire with an articulated tip is threaded through the stricture under direct vision using an oesophagoscope. The position of the tip of the guide wire in the stomach is confirmed on an x-ray television monitor. A graduated series of olivary dilators on a flexible wand are threaded over the guide wire and holding the guide wire firmly in position the wand and dilators are passed through the stricture under direct x-ray vision.

Oesophagoplasty. For narrow but not extensive strictures, a simple plastic operation is all that is required. The stricture is cut longitudinally and the mucosa allowed to bulge into the incision somewhat in the manner of Ramstedt's operation. The incised area may be reinforced by suture of the adjacent fundus (Thal procedure) or the fundus of the stomach may be wrapped

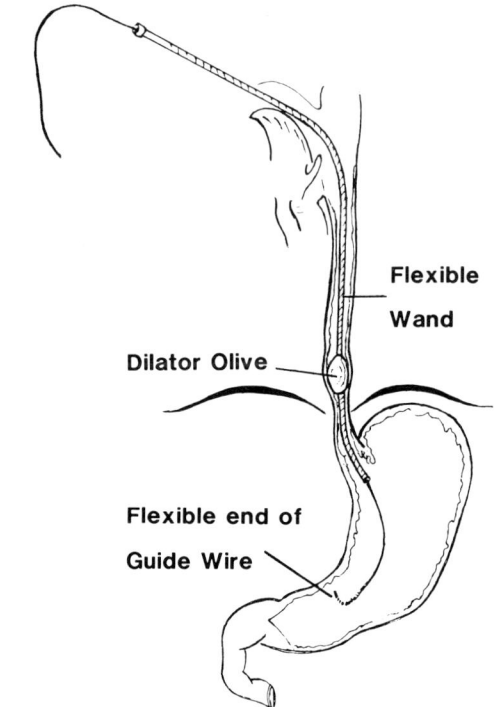

Flexible

Wand

Dilator Olive

Flexible end of

Guide Wire

Fig 4.17 Showing the mechanism of dilatation with the Eder Puestow dilator.

around to cover the denuded area (Woodward procedure).

Where oesophageal shortening is associated with fibrosis, the oesophagus can be lengthened by the procedure described by Leigh Collis. The portion of the sliding hernia above the level of the diaphragm is incised in the line of the oesophagus down to the level of the diaphragm. The sectioned fundal pouch is reflected downwards and the wound sewn up longitudinally (Fig 4.18a,b). The operation is combined with restoration of the angle of His, narrowing of the hiatus in front of the oesophagus and fixing the oesophagus to the edges of the hiatus. In patients with ulceration and extensive fibrosis involving the perioesophageal tissues, a more extensive procedure is recommended by Milstein (1975). Through an eighth left interspace incision, the oesophagus is mobilised to the level of the aortic arch with, if possible, preservation of the vagi. The stomach is freed through the diaphragmatic hiatus and the vasa brevia divided. The stricture is divided longitudinally through the floor of the ulcer, if necessary, and the defect repaired transversely over a full-sized oesophageal tube. This procedure brings the fundus up into the chest cavity. To prevent reflux a Nissen fundoplication is added. Various modifications of this procedure have been described.

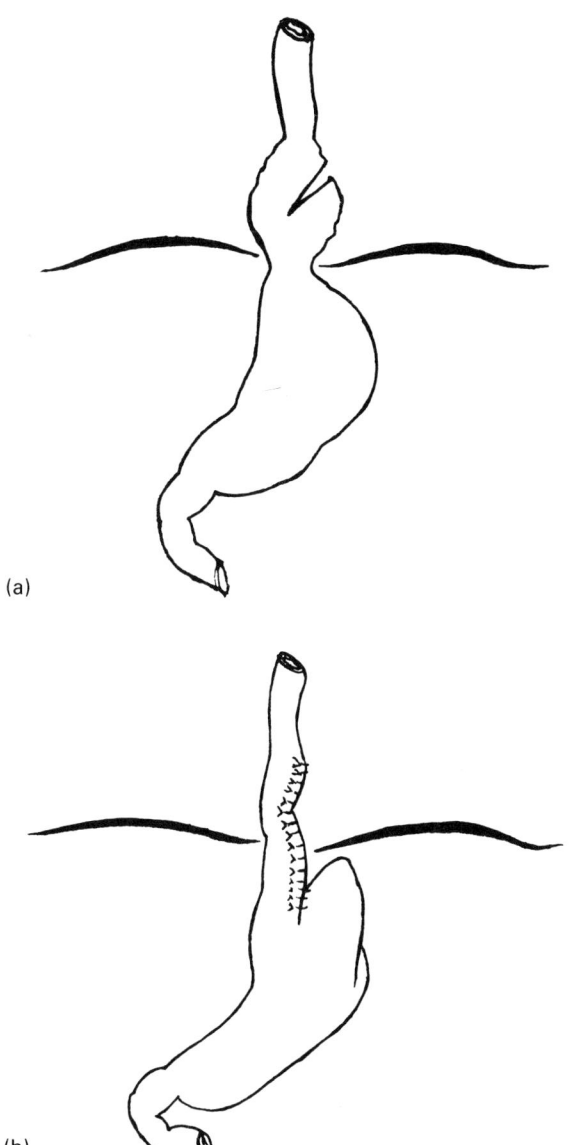

(a)

(b)

Fig 4.18 (a) and (b) Oesophagoplasty (Leigh Collis) for oesophageal stenosis with shortening.

Resection. In cases where there is very marked shortening of the oesophagus, resection and oesophageal replacement may be required. Colonic replacement may be used. With gastric replacement there is less likelihood of further peptic oesophagitis, since the stomach is vagally denervated and reflux seldom occurs if the oesophagogastric anastomosis is above the aortic arch.

Oesophageal webs and rings

In the upper oesophagus a fibrous eccentric web is present just below the cricopharyngeus in cases of Patterson Kelly syndrome (Fig 4.8) and also in certain cases of ulcerative colitis. In mid-oesophagus fibrous rings usually present a congenital malformation and much attention has been directed to the lower oesophageal ring described by Schatzki and Gary (1953). The characteristic features of Schatzki's ring are that it occurs in the lower gullet, it is circumferential and symmetrical and consists of a mucosal fold with little or no inflammatory changes (Fig 4.19). The condition occurs between the ages of 30 and 71, and is frequently associated with a sliding hernia and only gives rise to symptoms of dysphagia if the lumen of the ring is reduced to less than 10 mm.

The ring is situated at the squamo-columnar junction, and it is thought to be due to a hypertonic inferior sphincter, to fibrosis following reflux, or as the result of shortening of the oesophagus associated with hiatal hernia (concertina effect). With severe symptoms, dilatation or removal of the ring may be required and the sliding hernia will require repair.

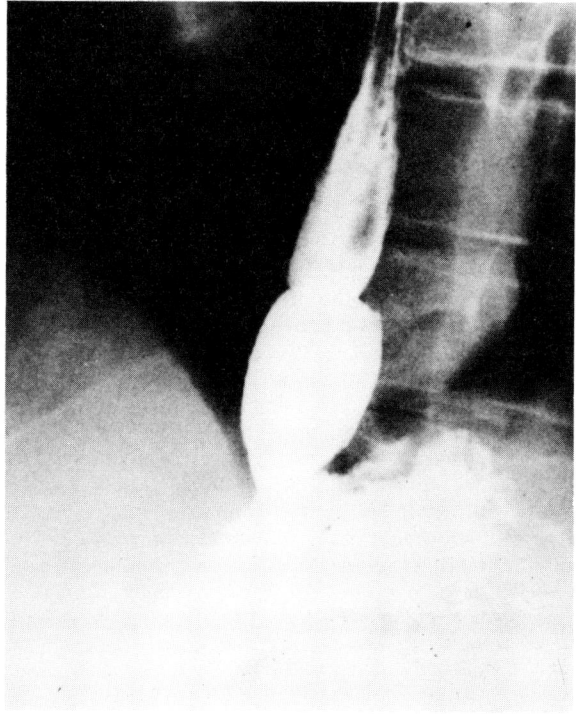

Fig. 4.19 Schatzki's ring. Oesophageal hernia with a circumferential and symmetrical constriction in the lower oesophagus.

Tumours of the oesophagus

Tumours of the oesophagus (Nakayama, 1961) may be innocent or malignant. Simple tumours are exceptionally rare and account for less than 1% of all cases, but they have an importance disproportionate to their frequency, since surgical treatment can be curative, and death from oesophageal obstruction and starvation can thereby be avoided.

Simple tumours. These may arise from the epithelium, (papillomas or adenomas), from mesenchymal tissue (as fibromyomas or leiomyomas, or more rarely lipomas, haemangiomas and lymphangiomas). Fibromas develop in the submucosa and present as intramural swellings, but with increase in size may become pedunculated. Myomas usually occur in the lower end of the oesophagus and are said to be associated with muscular dyskinesia and occasionally with oesophageal diverticula.

Malignant tumours. These usually arise from the squamous epithelium of the oesophagus and account for 90% of cancers. Adenocarcinoma account for about 9% while, more rarely, tumours may possess both glandular and squamous features (adenoacanthoma). Malignant tumours arising from mesodemal structures are very rare, and present as various types of sarcoma. Mixed tumours showing both sarcomatous and carcinomatous features are also rare as are malignant melanomas.

Cancer of the oesophagus

In its modern context oesophageal cancer is of special interest on account of its unusual global distribution, its aetiology and the problems of treatment.

Aetiology

Environmental factors appear to play an important part in the aetiology. There are certain specific regions where the condition is quite common. In the Transkei province of South Africa the condition is common in the Bantu tribesmen, but is not especially prevalent in the other inhabitants. Another region of high incidence is the Bulawayo district of Zimbabwe. Perhaps the region of highest incidence is in the north east of Iran where along the south east border of the Caspian Sea 200 cases occur in every 100 000 of population. A similar region of very high incidence is in the Honan province of China. A belt of high incidence seems to extend from Turkey through northern Iran, Afghanistan, part of Russia, and through Mongolia to northern

China. The condition is, however, rare in Europe and in countries of the West. In the British Isles it accounts for 3600 deaths per year, which represents only 5% of all cases of malignant disease.

Another characteristic feature of the disease is the wide variation of incidence in certain areas and over very short distances. The only genetic association that has been demonstrated is with tylosis.

Social factors

Carcinoma of the oesophagus tends to occur in the lower socio-economic group. It is commoner in peasant farmers on poor land where the soil is deficient in molybdenum, iron, zinc, and copper and where the grain is frequently affected by moulds.

Environmental studies suggest a strong association with the type of diet. The food of those affected is often poor in protein and deficient in vitamins C and riboflavin. In China a close association has been noted between the incidence of cancer of the oesophagus in humans and cancer of the gullet in chickens. When the population of the town of Lin Xian was transposed to another area, the chickens in the new area began to show an increased incidence of cancer of the gullet, presumably due to eating scraps of discarded human food.

Alcohol

Alcohol appears to be an aetiological factor. The condition is commoner in hoteliers, barmen, commercial travellers and in those associated with the catering trade.

Tobacco

The condition is commoner in pipe smokers. In Iran the chewing of 'nass' which is a mixture of tobacco, wood ash and vegetable oil is a possible factor. The combination of alcohol and tobacco is especially harmful.

Physical factors

Hot fluids and the trauma of food roughage is thought to be important. In Russia the drinking of hot tea laced with vodka may be a factor.

Chemical factors

Recently nitrosamines have been incriminated as a cause. Nitrites in the food or those used in the preparation of food as in the canning industry, may combine with amides to make the N-nitrosamines which are carcinogenic. Contamination of foods such as nuts, beans, and cereals by a mould (*Aspergillus flavus*) produces aflatoxin which is also carcinogenic.

Age and sex

In Great Britain the disease is one of late middle life and old age. Among those affected is a preponderance of males to females, in the ratio 1.7:1. In France, males predominate over females in the ratio of 12:1 but in the high incidence areas in Iran and in the Transkei women are more commonly affected.

Clinical associations

An association is thought to exist between carcinoma of the oesophagus and three clinical conditions.

Patterson-Kelly syndrome. While this association appears to be strong in Sweden, in Great Britain few patients admit to symptoms of this before the development of malignant disease of the oesophagus.

Achalasia of the cardia. About 7% of patients with achalasia develop cancer of the oesophagus. The growth develops in the upper dilated oesophagus where irritation and oesophagitis may initiate malignant changes in the epithelium.

Hiatus hernia. Much confusion and contradiction exists regarding the association of hiatal hernia and oesophagogastric cancer. Recent investigations appear to confirm an association between reflux oesophagitis and cancer of the lower end of the gullet.

Pathology

Cancer of the oesophagus is usually a growth of high malignancy often pursuing an aggressive course and spreading locally, regionally and generally.

Macroscopic features

The growth may present in various forms of which three are characteristic:

Fungating. This type of growth is bulky and polypoidal and distends the lumen of the oesophagus (Fig 4.20a).

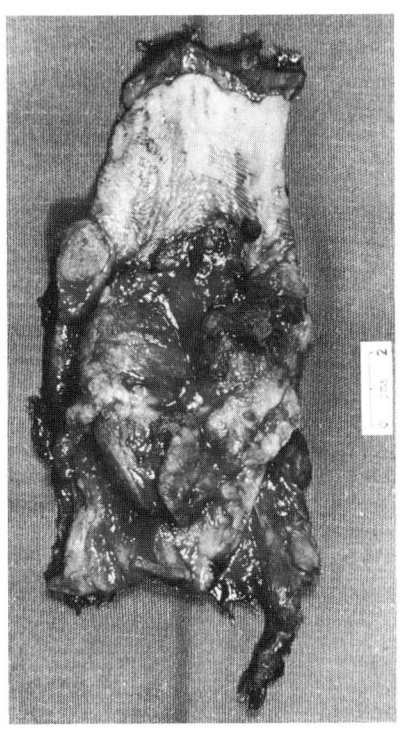 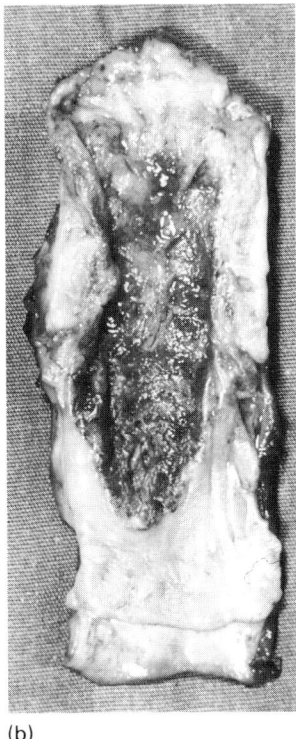 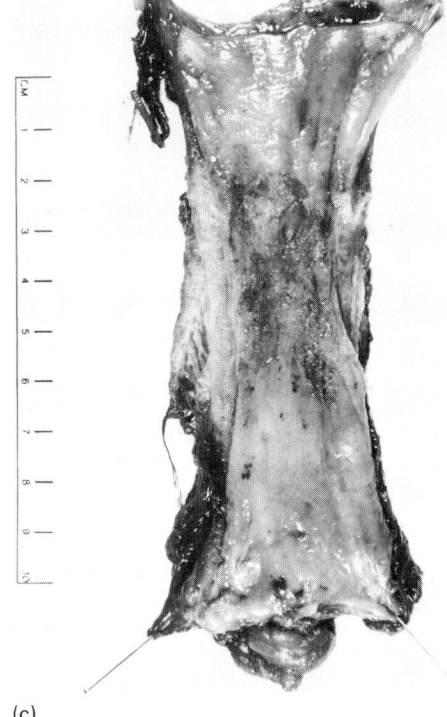

(a)   (b)   (c)

Fig 4.20 Carcinoma of the oesophagus. (a) A large polypoidal growth at the lower end. (b) Ulcerative growth with heaped-up margins. (c) Desmoplastic stenosing growth in the middle third.

Ulcerative. The characteristic feature is that of a deep ulcer with rolled everted edges, but occasionally the margins of the ulcer are clear cut (Fig 4.20b).

Desmoplastic-stenosing. In this condition there is widespread invasion of the oesophagus, comparable to the condition of linitis plastica of the stomach (Fig 4.20c).

Microscopic appearances

Ninety per cent of oesophageal growths are squamous in type and show prickle cell formation and keratinisation. On occasions there may be little differentiation. Ten per cent of cancers are adenocarcinoma, usually but not always, situated at the lower end of the oesophagus. In this region the growth arises from the cardiac glands, or from the gastric mucosa of the lower oesophagus. Adenocarcinoma, at a higher level, may arise in islets of ectopic gastric mucosa, or from the mucus secreting glands of the oesophagus.

Modes of spread

Knowledge of the modes of spread of carcinoma of the oesophagus is important to the clinician for assessment, to the surgeon in planning operation, and to the radiotherapist in the technique of irradiation.

Submucous spread. The tumour spreads readily in the loose connective tissues underlying the epithelium. The tendency to burrow under the mucosa leads to submucous spread well beyond the apparent margins of the growth.

Direct spread. Longitudinal and circumferential spread leads to a long tortuous stricture, often eccentric in position and with rolled upper and lower margins. Spread through the muscular coat takes place fairly readily, and in the lower third the diaphragm and the crura are often involved. In the middle oesophagus the mediastinum is invaded and the air passages are soon involved leading to the possibility of broncho-oesophageal fistula.

Regional spread. Each segment of the oesophagus has its regional lymph node drainage area (*see* Fig 4.2). In the lower third spread is to the paracardial, splenic, left gastric and coeliac lymph nodes. Since these nodes are amenable to excision radical surgery is possible so that the spleen, crura, pancreas and even the left lobe of the liver may be removed 'en bloc' (an ideal type of operation for cancer). In the middle third, lymphatic drainage is to the bronchial, broncho-pulmonary and hilar glands, so that surgery for growths in this situation is essentially palliative. For growths in the upper third, drainage to the extensive cervical lymph nodes makes radical operation even more difficult.

Distant spread. With increasing survival rates after operation, more cases of osseous and subcutaneous secondary deposits are being encountered, a feature which emphasises the high malignancy and aggressive nature of oesophageal carcinoma.

Site of tumour

It is usual to consider the oesophagus as being divided into three segments: an upper third above the aortic arch, a middle third behind the hilum of the lung, and a lower third extending from below the inferior pulmonary vein down to and including the oesophago-gastric junction. In Great Britain 19% of tumours occur in the upper third, 50% in the middle segments, and 31% in the lower third (Fig 4.21).

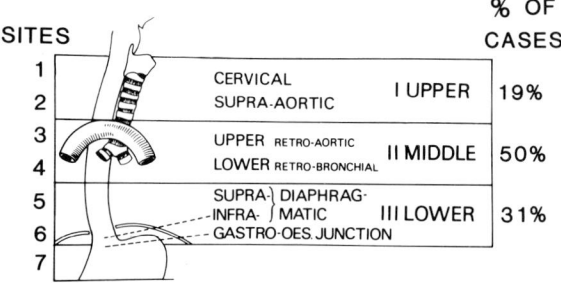

Fig 4.21 Division of the oesophagus into an upper, middle and lower third can be modified with advantage by subdivision. The upper third above the aortic arch consists of a cervical and a supra-aortic segment; the mid-third a retroaortic and retrobronchial segment; and lower third a supradiaphragmatic and an infradiaphragmatic segment. The frequency with which various sites are affected is shown in percentages excluding those arising from the oesophagus junction.

From the point of view of therapy there is advantage in subdividing the three segments so that the upper third consists of a cervical and supra-aortic segment (Sites 1 and 2), the middle third of a retro-aortic and retro-bronchial segment (Sites 3 and 4), while the lower third consists of a supradiaphragmatic portion (Site 5) and an infradiaphragmatic portion (Site 6). The gastro-oesophageal junction is referred to as Site 7.

Symptoms

Symptoms are often delayed until the disease is well advanced because the oesophagus may be almost completely encircled before the patient complains of difficulty in swallowing.

Dysphagia

The presenting symptom is difficulty in swallowing, first noticed with solid food which tends to stick and the patient indicates the site of obstruction, sometimes with fair accuracy. Growths at the lower end of the gullet usually give a sensation of obstruction at the xiphisternum, but occasionally discomfort may be located at the level of the jugular notch. Growths in the mid-oesophagus give a sensation of discomfort behind the sternum and the level of the obstruction in this segment is often accurately located. In the upper third, the sensation of obstruction is felt in the lower neck, and in the region of the jugular notch. At first, fluids may pass easily, but the symptoms are always progressive and in time fluids and even saliva cannot be swallowed. Occasionally a piece of meat may cause sudden and complete obstruction.

Regurgitation

If the patient attempts to overcome the obstruction by taking more food, regurgitation of completely undigested food debris may occur. More often the patient brings up saliva mixed with offensive discharge from the growth surface.

Pain

Retrosternal discomfort and occasional pain through to the back between the shoulder blades may occur, but pain on swallowing is not a marked feature.

Cough

Excessive salivation is common and in the presence of oesophageal obstruction fluid may over-spill into the larynx, causing troublesome cough especially at night. Rarely spasmodic coughing may occur after taking food or fluid, indicating the presence of a tracheal or broncho-oesophageal fistula. Aspiration of infected oesophageal contents causes chronic pulmonary infection, and on occasions acute pulmonary oedema with bronchospasm causes great respiratory distress.

Nutritional state

Weight loss is progressive and is usually associated with anaemia, though on blood examination the anaemia is frequently masked by dehydration.

Voice changes

Hoarseness is usually due to involvement of the recurrent laryngeal nerves and often indicates inoperability.

Diagnosis

The diagnosis is usually clear from the clinical features of the case. Confirmation is, however, required by barium swallow, endoscopic examination and by biopsy.

Barium swallow

This is the first investigation in all cases of suspected oesophageal carcinoma. In the upper oesophagus the tumour is difficult to visualise, because of the rapid transit time through this section of the gullet. With cineradiography or with modern equipment capable of taking two photographs per second, satisfactory x-ray films can be obtained. With growths in the cervical oesophagus there is a tendency for overspill into the trachea (Fig 4.22).

In the mid-oesophagus the x-ray appearances may be characteristic. Barium swallow demonstrates a long irregular stricture (Fig 4.23). In the lower thoracic segment a long filling defect due to carcinoma (Fig 4.24) may somewhat resemble the appearance produced by oesophageal displacement due to a mediastinal tumour or as the result of cardiac enlargement. Rupture of the oesophagus with resultant cellulitis produces a rather bizarre filling defect while on occasion the presence of a fistula may allow barium to enter the trachea.

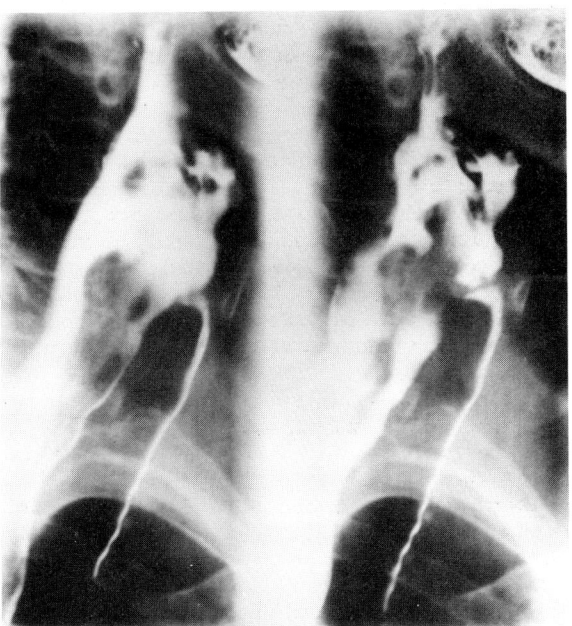

Fig 4.22 Carcinoma of the upper oesophagus showing an overspill of barium into the air passages.

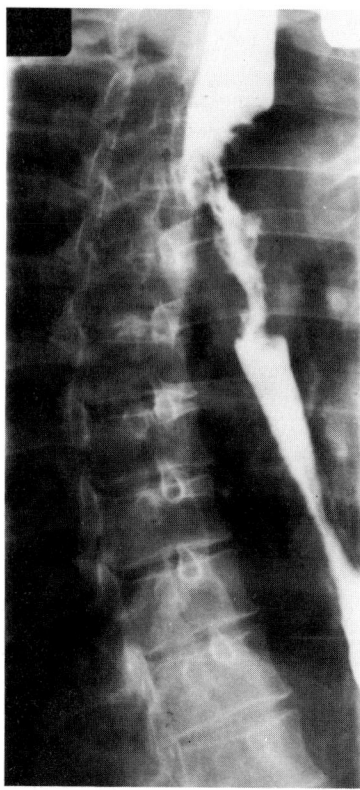

Fig 4.23 Carcinoma of mid-oesophagus showing characteristic radiological appearance of growth (lateral view).

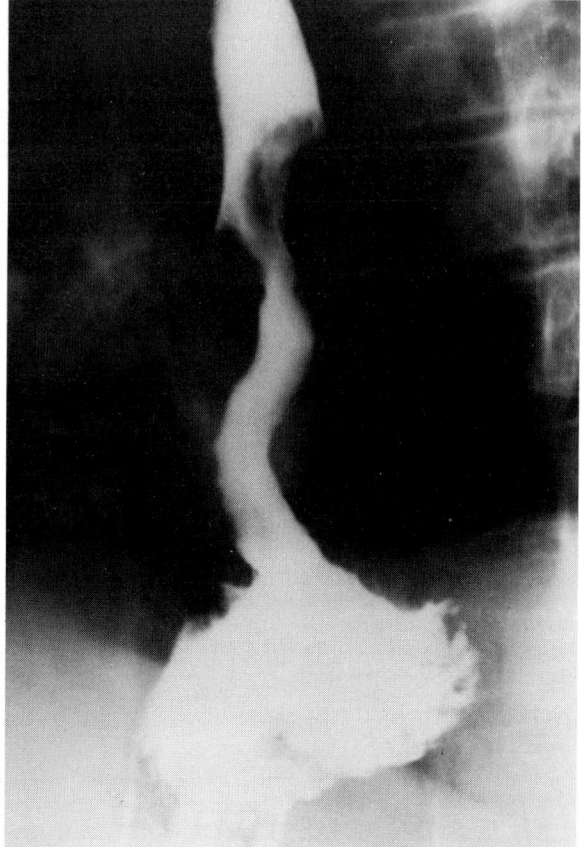

Fig 4.24 Carcinoma of the lower thoracic oesophagus.

At the lower end of the oesophagus, an early carcinoma may easily be overlooked. Achalasia presents with a smooth appearance at the narrowed segment and there is greater oesophageal dilatation. Reflux oesophagitis with shortening of the gullet is more likely to cause confusion than the stenosis that occurs in some cases of sliding hernia.

Rarely, cancer may involve the entire oesophagus and produce on barium swallow an irregular distorted appearance with multiple filling defects and oesophageal deviation (Fig 4.25).

Endoscopy

Oesophagoscopy is essential in all cases of stricture. The lesion is inspected, biopsy is taken, and the distance from the incisor teeth is recorded. The use of the rigid Negus or Chevalier Jackson oesophagoscope allows the operator to assess the degree of fixity of the growth and to obtain a large biopsy specimen. The fibreoptic instrument is easier to pass and is particularly appropriate in patients with small mouths or prominent

incisor teeth, and in those subjects with cervical spondylosis or with a marked thoracic kyphosis; the biopsy specimen is, however, less adequate than that obtained by the rigid instrument. In cases of mid-thoracic growths bronchoscopy is also required. Widening of the carina suggests mediastinal involvement while direct invasion of the bronchus may be observed.

Biopsy

Normal epithelium may overlie a growth that has burrowed under the mucosa, and care must be taken to obtain the biopsy specimen from the centre of the lesion, so that a false negative result is avoided.

Early diagnosis

In western countries where the incidence of carcinoma of the oesophagus is low, most cases present late in the disease. In regions of high incidence such as Iran,

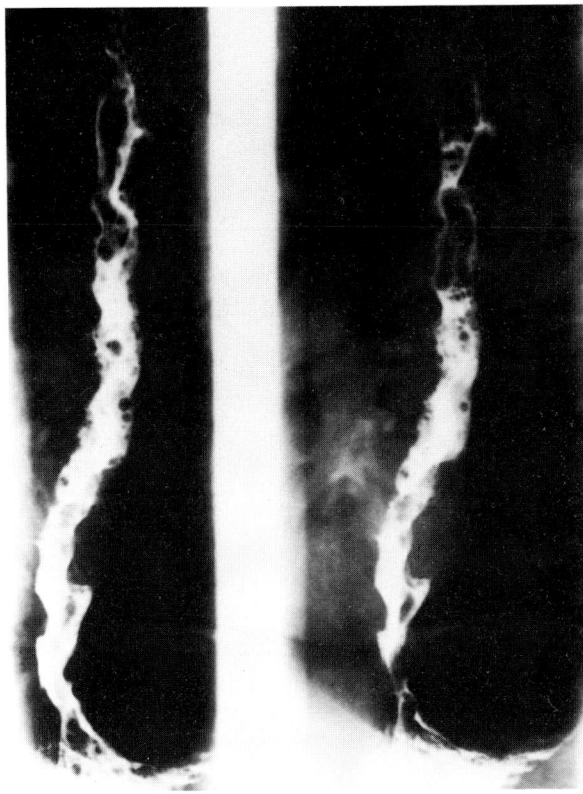

Fig 4.25 Diffuse carcinoma affecting the entire oesophagus in a woman aged 54. There are multiple filling defects with oesophagus irregular and distorted.

China and Japan, population screening has been introduced in an attempt to obtain early diagnosis. Mass examinations of patients by balloon or brush biopsy are now used to detect early precancerous changes in the mucosa. In consequence a diagnosis of carcinoma *in situ* is more frequent.

Treatment of oesophageal cancer

Because of the age groups involved, the frequency of concomitant disease and the aggressive nature of the growth, the results of treatment of whatever type are frequently disappointing. Though the primary aim is to restore the ability to swallow, in some cases treatment also tries to attain a worthwhile survival period. In this limited sense, treatment may be described as palliative or radical. In patients where the disease is very advanced or the physical condition of the patient poor, the simplest palliative measures should be chosen.

The measures avilable are surgical excision, radiotherapy, surgical bypass, intubation and chemotherapy. Gastrostomy should not be performed since it does not relieve dysphagia and merely prolongs the act of dying. In broad principle, radiotherapy alone is most appropriate to growths in the cervical oesophagus, and surgical excision alone for those growths situated at the lower end. In the middle segments both surgical excision or radiotherapy may be used individually or in combination, while chemotherapy is beginning to claim a role as a supplement to other measures.

Surgical management

This is considered in three phases, preoperative, operative, and postoperative, each phase having its own importance.

Preoperative

The most important advance of recent years is an appreciation of preoperative preparation. This should be directed to correction of haematological abnormalities, improvement in the nutritional state, assessment of the pulmonary and cardiac status and measures to diminish sepsis.

Haematological abnormalities. Dehydration is frequently present and often masks severe anaemia. Intravenous glucose and saline should be given to correct dehydration and when anaemia is present, blood is transfused well before operation, so that the patient is in a stable haemodynamic state at the time of operation.

The nutritional state should be improved since it has a significant influence on wound healing and on tumour immunology. After diagnostic oesophagoscopy and removal of food debris from above the stricture, the patient can often take a fluid or semifluid, minced diet. An intake of 3000 calories per day should be aimed at and supplementary vitamins should be given. Food supplements such as Hycal, Complan, or an elemental diet help. If oral feeding is not possible enteral or intravenous feeding are preferable to gastrostomy or jejunostomy, since the latter often interferes with surgical treatment.

The pulmonary condition is frequently unsatisfactory in patients in the affected age group and emphysema and bronchitis are major problems. Physiotherapy with deep breathing exercises help to diminish postoperative chest complications. The patient should be treated by postural drainage before operation, so that the procedures are well rehearsed and can be employed should pulmonary collapse occur after operation. In cases of chronic bronchitis, the sputum should be cultured and an appropriate antibiotic given the day before and for 5 days after operation.

Cardiac irregularities are frequent. Thoracotomy often precipitates or exacerbates these disorders of rhythm. If necessary Lanoxin should be given before operation and its dose regulated appropriately for a week postoperatively.

Measures to diminish sepsis include dental treatment and oesophageal lavage. In patients where jejunal or colonic replacement may be required full bowel sterilisation with sulphonamides, metronidazole or neomycin should be carried out.

In addition to these specific measures, all the problems likely to occur following surgery in aged patients should be considered, e.g. urinary retention due to enlarged prostate.

Operative

Good access to the growth is essential so that excision may be adequate and anastomosis made without undue difficulty. The organ and the route of oesophageal replacement as well as the operative procedure depend on the site of the growth, and for this purpose the subdivisions of the oesophagus shown in Fig 4.21 (p. 74) are helpful in relating the most appropriate operation to the site of the growth.

Carcinoma of the lower end (Sites 6 and 7). Because of the position of the growth at the lower end of the oesophagus and its related lymphatic drainage, it is possible to carry out a radical 'en bloc' excision of the growth and the surrounding structures. The left thoracoabdominal approach along the line of the 7th rib, with the patient in the right lateral position provides ease of access. After exploring the abdomen to confirm operability, the thoracic segment of the incision is opened up. The spleen is mobilised together with the tail and body of the pancreas, so that the growth with its related lymph nodes can be removed 'en bloc'. If the growth is at the oesophago-gastric junction, the entire stomach may be removed and reconstruction by Roux-en-Y anastomosis performed. If the growth is in the lower oesophagus the pyloric end of the stomach may be retained and oesophagogastrostomy carried out (Fig 4.26).

Carcinoma of the lower thoracic oesophagus (Sites 4 and 5). A two-stage operation is most suitable for tumours in this situation (Nakayama, 1961). It consists of an abdominal stage to mobilise the stomach and a thoracic stage to excise the oesophagus.

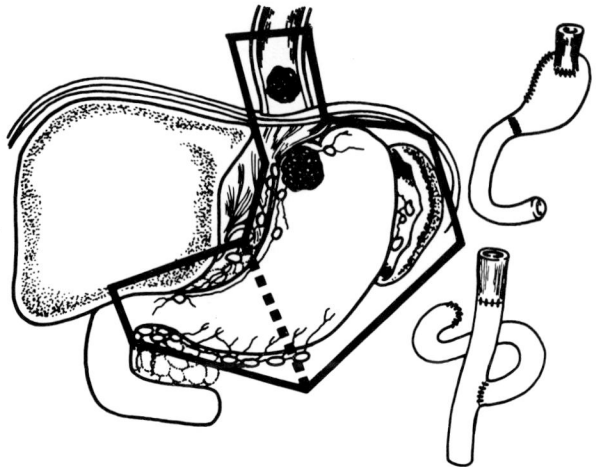

Fig 4.26 Excision of growths at the lower end of the oesophagus. The extent of the excisions and the methods of reconstruction are shown. (By courtesy of the Editors of *Surgery Annual* and the publishers, Appleton Century Crofts.)

Carcinoma of the mid and upper thoracic oesophagus (Sites 4, 3 and sometimes 2). Growths in the mid and upper thoracic oesophagus require total thoracic oesophagectomy in order to avoid the dangers of inadequate excision, or the performance of an anastomosis high up in the superior mediastinum. After total thoracic oesophagectomy the organ and its route of replacement must be chosen.

The organ of replacement should be of adequate length, have a blood supply amenable to surgical manipulation, and a mucosa which joins readily to the mucosa of the cervical oesophagus.

The route for replacement may be presternal, retrosternal or posterior mediastinal. Each route has advantages and drawbacks in regard to its safety, distance, and the effect on swallowing. The posterior mediastinal is the shortest and easiest route, but should leakage occur is the most dangerous. The presternal is the safest, but the least direct and swallowing is always somewhat impaired.

Various techniques may be employed for total thoracic oesophagectomy.

1   *Total three-phase oesophagectomy.* Perhaps the simplest and best way of dealing with a high or mid thoracic growth is by the total three-phase operation (McKeown, 1972), in which a cervical phase is added to the Lewis Tanner procedure (Fig 4.27).

The advantages of this technique are that it requires only a single anastomosis which can be performed easily in the neck and should leakage occur in this situation, it is seldom fatal. There is less risk of infection,

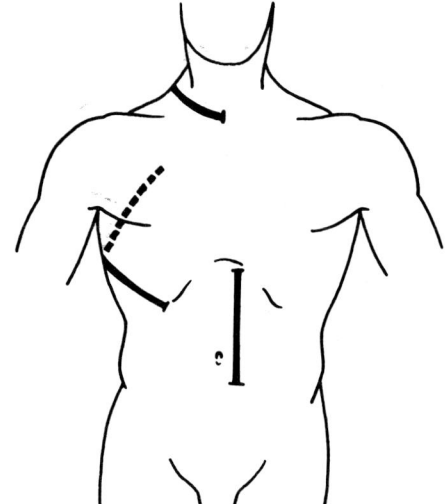

Fig 4.27 Incisions for three-phase oesophagectomy. It is easier and safer to perform anastomosis in the right side of the neck.

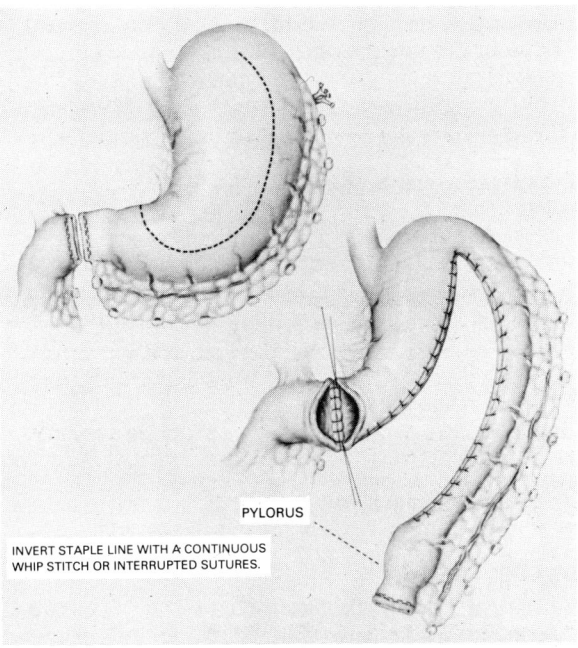

PYLORUS

INVERT STAPLE LINE WITH A CONTINUOUS
WHIP STITCH OR INTERRUPTED SUTURES.

Fig 4.28 The extended Heimlich-Gavriliu gastric tube showing the method of formation. (*Left*) the line of incision and (*right*) formation of gastric tube.

since the gut is not opened until the final stage of the procedure, and stomach contents are seldom highly infected. The patient is able to take a full meal and reflux is rare. If areas of suspected infiltration in the mediastinum are marked at operation by the insertion of Michel's clips, postoperative irradiation can be directed to the areas involved without damage to the anastomosis in the neck.

2   *Reversed gastric tube (Gavriliu-Heimlich) replacement.* In this procedure (Gavriliu, 1975) a long tube is formed from the greater curvature as far as, or sometimes including the pyloric antrum, with its vascular supply based on the left gastroepiploic vessels (Fig 4.28). After reconstructing the main stomach, the tube is passed up in a retrosternal tunnel to be anastomosed with the cervical oesophagus, after total thoracic oesophagectomy.

3   *Presternal gastric replacement* is recommended by various surgeons, but has the disadvantage of the indirectness of the presternal route.

4   *Colonic replacements.* Colonic replacement (Stephens, 1971) presents an alternative to gastric replacement and is, of course, of particular value in cases who have previously had gastric resection. The ascending, transverse or descending and pelvic colon may be utilised (Fig 4.29). The advantages of colonic replacement are an amenable blood supply and adequate reach. Multiple anastomoses are however required and rates of leakage and infective complications appear to be higher than in gastric replacement.

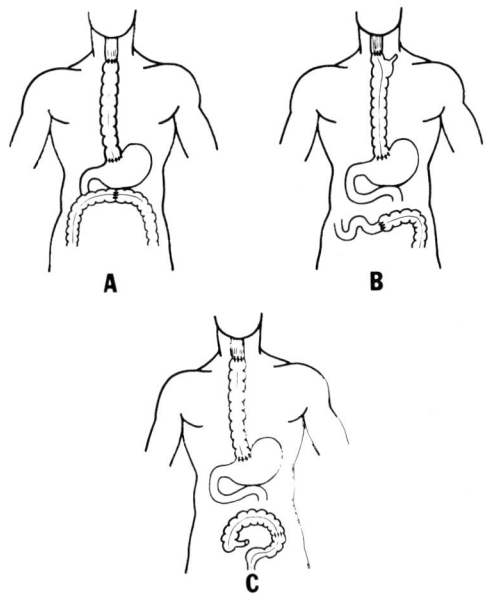

Fig 4.29 Colonic replacement in total thoracic oesophagectomy. (A) transverse colon; (B) right colon; (C) left colon. (By courtesy of the editors of *Surgery Annual* and the publishers, Appleton Century Crofts.)

Growths in the supra-aortic segment (Sites 2 and 1). Carcinoma in the uppermost part of the thoracic cavity may be dealt with by total three-phase oesophagectomy or by the presternal splitting technique described in 1971 by Ong.

Postoperative management

Postoperative care should anticipate and prevent postoperative complications. As after all major procedures, blood replacement and the maintenance of fluid and electrolyte balance require constant attention, but special care must be directed to the lungs, the heart and the prevention of aspiration of oesophagogastric contents.

The lungs. At the end of operation, respiratory movements and pulmonary ventilation must be confirmed as adequate. Blood gas analysis is a helpful guide, but it must be realised that the arterial P_{AO_2} is lowered for many days after operation. The venti-mask is useful and the mask also acts as a humidifier. Should the patient's colour be unsatisfactory and respiratory movements inadequate, assisted respiration may be required for an hour or two postoperatively. Fully controlled positive pressure ventilation should be reserved only for those whose pulmonary ventilation remains inadequate. If prolonged controlled respiration becomes necessary, it is better to perform tracheostomy.

Chest physiotherapy started before operation should be resumed immediately in the postoperative period. Daily x-rays of the chest are taken to confirm pulmonary expansion. Should segmental collapse occur, postural drainage is required. If this measure is not successful and if the collapsed segment is large, bronchoscopy under local anaesthesia should be carried out in the ward.

Underwater drainage systems require constant supervision to prevent blocking of the tube and the accumulation of fluid or blood in the chest cavity. Should tension pneumothorax develop for any reason, continuous thoracic suction is required.

The heart. Continuous cardiac monitoring is required so that changes in rhythm are observed immediately. The blood pressure is recorded at intervals of 30 min.

Prevention of aspiration. Hourly aspiration of the nasogastric tube prevents the accumulation of oesophagointestinal contents and the instillation of 30 ml of water down the tube after aspiration prevents its blockage. The use of the Salem sump tube provides continuous aspiration and these tubes seldom block. On the second day after operation 60 ml water can be instilled into the tube after aspiration, and by progres-

sively increasing the amount, intake may be maintained. Fluid additives such as Hycal may be used to provide additional caloric intake.

The patient should be nursed in the upright position as an additional precaution against reflux. Heavy sedation, especially at night, should be avoided to prevent inhibition of the pharyngeal reflexes. After the nasogastric tube is removed on the sixth day, oral feeding of semifluids should start, but the danger of aspiration is not yet over, large meals in the evening should be avoided and the patient should be encouraged to sleep well propped up.

Should aspiration occur, the ensuing pulmonary pneumonitis may be severe. The use of intravenous cortisone in high dosage combined with aminophylline diminishes bronchial spasm, while potential infection is dealt with by the use of broad spectrum antibiotics. Tracheostomy may be required.

In addition to these special problems, oesophagectomy presents all the difficulties of surgery in old age. The prevention of bed sores, urinary problems and thromboembolism all require routine attention. Mental symptoms and disorientation in aged patients can be a serious problem and are often drug induced. Sedation, especially at night, should be kept to a minimum.

Mortality rate

The definition of operative mortality and the criteria of case selection vary and make comparison of figures somewhat misleading. Most patients are old and are, therefore, high risk subjects, but age alone is of less importance than the presence of serious cardiac or pulmonary disease.

The mortality rate is closely related to the experience of the operator and the efficiency of the surgical team. The overall mortality rate for all cases of oesophagectomy in expert hands is about 12%, but the rate is specially related to the site at which the growth occurs, and the complexity of the procedures required. For growths at the oesophago-gastric junction, the operative mortality is about 6%, but for growths in the thoracic segment the rate varies between 12 and 38%.

Survival time

In the age groups concerned and in the presence of severe concomitant disease, it is unrealistic to talk in terms of 5 and 10 year 'cures'. The primary objective of treatment is to enable the patient to swallow and prolonged survival must be regarded as a fortunate outcome. Many patients die in the first postoperative year, and to a lesser extent in the second year. If, however, the patient survives this period, the outlook is more hopeful and individual survivals for as long as 25 years are occasionally observed. Generally, however, the results are poor.

Ability to eat

Assessment of the results of surgery are measured not only by the operative mortality and survival time, but largely by the restoration of the patient's ability to eat. Ease of swallowing, the ability to take a reasonable meal, and the absence of reflux and postprandial symptoms all have to be taken into consideration. The ability to eat depends largely on the type of anastomosis and the organ and route of replacement.

Total three-phase oesophagectomy with oesophago-fundic anastomosis produces the best results, both in ease of swallowing, the size of the meal and, paradoxically, the absence of reflux even in the head-down position. The reverse gastric tube (Gavriliu Heimlich) (Gavriliu, 1975) provides an alternative to total gastric replacement. In cases of oesophagoantrostomy, reflux can be troublesome and the size of the meal somewhat limited. In colonic replacement, swallowing is slow, though gastric capacity is not reduced. In retro-peristaltic replacements using the left colon, reflux may occur. In the Roux-en-Y jejunal replacements the size of the meal is reduced but biliary reflux is rare.

Palliative procedures

When there are extensive metastases, when the growth is unresectable, or when the general condition of the patient precludes major operation, palliation may be obtained by a variety of procedures.

Bypass operations

Resection is the best form of palliation, but fixity of the growth, or the presence of oesophagobronchial fistula may make resection dangerous or impossible. In these circumstances, various bypass procedures are used. A segment of colon, jejunum or stomach may be brought up for anastomosis with the side of the oesophagus above the level of the tumour. In the case of inoperability due to the presence of tracheo-oesophageal fistula the procedure of Kirschner (Ong, 1971) is of value. In this operation the cervical oesophagus is divided and its distal end closed. After division of the oesophago-gastric junction, the stomach is mobilised and brought up in front of the sternum for anastomosis with the cervical oesophagus. The lower oesophagus is anastomosed by a Roux-en-Y loop to the jejunum to provide drainage for the isolated oesophagus.

Intubation

Intubation (Das and John, 1973) of malignant strictures of the oesophagus using the tube introduced by Souttar (1924), consisting of coiled German silver wire with an expanded upper end has the great advantage of being self-retaining and can be introduced through the oesophagoscope. In modified form it is still in use today. More recently, tubes made of reinforced latex have been used, in which the upper end has a large flange, while the lower end tapers to the size of a naso-gastric tube, e.g. the Mousseau-Barbin and the Celestin tubes.

To prevent upward displacement of the tube, the Livingstone-Proctor tube has a flange at both upper and lower ends. The various types of tubes are shown in Fig 4.30.

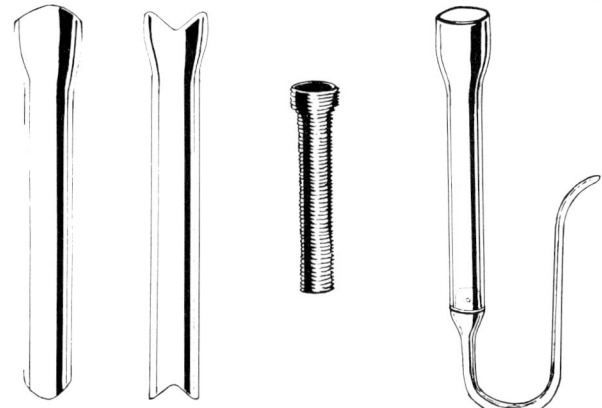

Fig 4.30 Oesophageal intubation. The Proctor Livingstone tubes (*left*) with fish-mouth openings; the Souttar tube of spiral metal wire (*centre*) and the Celestin modification of the Mousseau Barbin tube, (*right*).

Introduction of the tube is either by an 'endoscopic push' (Collis and Kahloor, 1976) or by 'pull through' involving laparotomy and gastrotomy. In the push-through technique the stricture is dilated under direct vision at oesophagoscopy. A modified Souttars tube or a Proctor Livingstone tube is passed over the dilator and pressed down into position either by the rigid oesophagoscope or by a rammer. The alternative procedure is to pass the dilator through the stricture under direct vision as before, and to perform laparotomy so that the tip of the dilator is identified against the stomach wall. Gastrotomy is performed and a strong suture attached to the dilator, which is then withdrawn upwards through the stricture into the mouth. The tip of a Mousseau Barbin or Celestin tube is attached to the suture which is then pulled on from the gastrotomy wound, so that the tube is lead through the growth until the upper flange rests securely above the upper margin of the growth. The lower end of the tube is cut off at an appropriate length and the gastrotomy closed.

Intubation is particularly appropriate to growths in the mid-thoracic oesophagus. In growths of the upper oesophagus the flange may cause respiratory obstruction, while in growths at the gastro-oesophageal junction, reflux of gastric contents may be a problem.

Results of intubation. Intubation is a procedure not without risk, and cannot always be accomplished. There is a risk of tearing the growth or rupturing the oesophagus as well as the dangers of aspiration leading to pulmonary complications.

The recorded mortality rates vary from 6.6 to 46%. The 'push through' procedures in very skilled and experienced hands are less hazardous than the 'pull through' method where laparotomy and gastrotomy are required. Complications are many and bronchopneumonia, perforation or haemorrhage from the growth are frequent, while blocking or displacement of the tubes often occur. In cases of longer survival, disintegration of the tube leading to intestinal complications such as obstruction, ulceration and bowel perforation are recorded. Stay in hospital is short after the 'push through' method (average 3-4 days) while in the 'pull through' procedure the average stay is about 19 days. The degree of palliation is reasonable but not always complete, and diet has to be fluid or semifluid to prevent blockage of the tube. The survival period is usually short and on average is about 4½ months.

Radiotherapy

Radiotherapy is used in the treatment of cancer of the oesophagus as a form of radical treatment, as a palliative, or as a supplement to surgery or chemotherapy.

Radical treatment is reserved for the early case, and is contraindicated in patients with severe cachexia and in the presence of secondary deposits. The use of the cobalt unit, megavoltage and linear accelerator has made it possible to deliver to the affected tumour area the recommended dose of 5000 rads with precision. Radiotherapy is the treatment of choice for growths in the cervical oesophagus. Squamous or undifferentiated tumours in the thoracic oesophagus of 4 cm or under are suitable for radiotherapy. A course of therapy extends over a period of 3 weeks, but tumour shrinkage is not always rapid, so that healing of the irradiated area may not be complete for 2 or 3 months.

The advantages of radiotherapy are the low initial mortality and the preservation of the larynx, oesophagus and stomach. The irradiated area can be wider than that dealt with during surgical excision, and the long-term survivals are comparable to those of surgery. The disadvantages are that in only 50% of patients are all

the tumour cells destroyed and either local recurrence or fibrous stricture formation results in failure to relieve dysphagia. Pulmonary fibrosis may also be a serious complication in elderly subjects in whom the cardiopulmonary reserve is low.

In patients with large and inoperable growths, irradiation in lower dosage of 2000 rads may produce palliation comparable to that attained by intubation.

Combination of surgery and radiotherapy

As with all preoperative radiotherapy, the advantages of obtaining shrinkage of the tumour and the reduction of the liability to local recurrence, must be set against the risk of producing operative difficulties, ischaemic changes or the failure of epithelial union and leakage at the site of anastomosis. A dosage of 2000 rads is given over a period of 10 days and operation is performed about one week later. With larger doses, a longer interval is required before surgery is undertaken.

Routine irradiation after successful operation is of doubtful value and may contribute to postoperative complications. If, however, at operation, areas of possible or known tumour infiltration are marked by the insertion of Michel clips, irradiation can be focused without the risk of damage to the anastomosis.

Chemotherapy

The value of this form of treatment is still debatable for these turnovers but further developments may well transform the position. Chemotherapy may be employed alone or in combination with surgery or radiotherapy, all three being frequently employed. The drugs commonly used are methotrexate and bleomycin. Methotrexate is usually administered intravenously over a period of 4 h in doses of 140–180 mg depending on the patient. Three injections are given at weekly intervals for a total of three doses. Leukopaenia and thrombocytopaenia may occur and blood examinations are required during treatment. Bleomycin may be used as an alternative to or in combination with, methotrexate. The usual dose is 10 mg given intramuscularly daily for one week. Pulmonary complications with fibrosis of the lung may occur.

References and further reading

Akiyama H., Hiyama M., Hashimoto C. (1978). Resection and reconstruction for carcinoma of the thoracic oesophagus. *Brit. J. Surg*; **63**:206.
Allison P.R. (1951). Reflux oesophagitis, sliding hiatal hernia and the anatomy of repair. *Surg. Gynecol. Obstet*; **92**:419.

Belsey R. (1966). Functional diseases of the oesophagus. *J. Thorac. Cardiovasc. Surg*; **52**:169.

Collis J. Leigh. (1971). An appraisal of the methods of treating hiatal hernia and its complications. *Brit. J. Surg*; **58**:801.

Collis J. Leigh, Kahloor G.J. (1976). Palliative push-through intubation for malignant obstruction of the gastro-oesophageal junction. *J. Thorac Cardiovasc. Surg*; **72**:796.

Das S.K., John H.T. (1973). Oesophageal intubation in obstructive lesions of the oesophagus. *Brit. J. Surg*; **66**:403.

Franklin R.H. (1971). Milestones in oesophageal surgery. *Proc. R. Soc. Med*; **64**:257.

Gavriliu D. (1975). Aspects of oesophageal surgery. In *Current Problems in Surgery*. Chicago: Year Book Medical.

Hill L.D. (1967). An effective operation for hiatal hernia. An eight-year appraisal. *Ann. Surg*; **166**:681.

Jackson J.W., Cooper D.K.C., Guvendik L., Reece Smith H. (1979). The surgical management of malignant tumours of the oesophagus and cardia: a review of the results in 292 patients treated over a 15-year period (1961–75). *Brit. J. Surg*; **66**:98.

McKeown K.C. (1972). Trends in oesophageal resection for carcinoma. Hunterian lecture. *Ann. Roy. Coll. Surg*; **51**: 213–38.

McKeown K.C. (1979). Cacinoma of the oesophagus. *J. Roy. Coll. Surg. Ed.*; **24**: 253–74.

Mannell A. (1982). Carcinoma of the oesophagus. In *Current Problems in Surgery*. (Ravitch M.M., ed). Chicago: Year Book Medical.

Milstein B.B. (1975). An operation for the treatment of intractable peptic stricture of the oesophagus. *Isr. J. Med. Soc*; **2**: 281–6.

Nakayama K. (1961). *Tumours of the Oesophagus* (Tanner N.C., Smithers D.W., eds). Edinburgh: Livingstone.

Ong G.B. (1971). Resection and reconstruction of the oesophagus. In *Current Problems in Surgery*. Chicago: Year Book Medical.

Ong G.B., ed. (1981). Progress in the treatment of cancer of the oesophagus. *Wrld. J. Surg*; **5**:487–552.

Royston C.N.S., Dowling B.L., Spencer J. (1975). A modification of the McKeown three phase oesophagectomy. *Brit. J. Surg*; **53**:112.

Saunders N.R. (1979). The Celestin tube in the palliation of carcinoma of the oesophagus and cardia. *Brit. J. Surg*; **66**:419–21.

Schatzki R., Gary J.E. (1953). Dysphagia due to a diaphragm-like localized narrowing in the lower oesophagus. ('lower oesophageal ring'). *Amer. J. Roenty*; **70**:911.

Stephens H.B. (1971). Colon by-pass of the oesophagus. *Amer. J. Surg*; **122**:27.

Thomas H.F., Clarke J.M., Rayl J.E., Woodward E.R. (1972). Results of the combined patch fundoplication operation in the treatment of reflux oesophagitis with stricture. *Surg. Gynecol. Obstet.*; **135**:241.

5

Stomach and duodenum

ALAN G. COX and ALLAN E. KARK

Two subjects dominate the surgery of the stomach and duodenum – benign peptic ulcer and gastric cancer. This chapter is devoted to these important topics almost exclusively since the surgeon must have an easy familiarity with both.

Benign peptic ulcer

ALAN G. COX

In this section, duodenal ulcer and benign gastric ulcer will be discussed both electively and in an emergency. Descriptions of the operations are followed by a consideration of recurrent ulcer and other long-term complications.

Duodenal ulcer

Duodenal ulcer is a very common disease, but surgeons see only a small minority because most patients either do not seek medical advice or are managed reasonably well by conservative measures. Thus the surgeon is most often presented with a neatly packaged patient with the appropriate history and a confirmed duodenal ulcer. His problem is then to decide whether to advise operation and which operation to choose. Other patients present either urgently or as a true emergency with perforation, haemorrhage or stenosis.

Pathophysiology

Almost all chronic duodenal ulcers – excluding those in the Zollinger-Ellison syndrome (see Chapter 37) – occur in the first part of the duodenum where a small area of the mucosa breaks down with inflammatory change in the underlying submucosa and eventually, replacement of the muscle layers by fibrous tissue. Most ulcers do not go beyond this but, occasionally, they ulcerate into a large artery causing a major haemorrhage, or penetrate through the wall into the peritoneal cavity, or are associated with so much fibrosis that the gastric outlet is obstructed.

Fibreoptic duodenoscopy has now revealed a more diffuse erosive duodenitis in patients with typical symptoms, but it is not known if this condition is a forerunner of classical ulcer disease or if it is a different condition. Nothing of any significance is known about the cause of duodenal ulcer despite intensive investigation. Most effort has been devoted to the measurement of gastric acid secretion. It has certainly been established that patients with duodenal ulcer secrete more acid *as a group* than does a group of normal subjects, and that some patients with duodenal ulcer secrete more acid than any normals (Fig 5.1). These observations do not explain the cause, particularly since many patients secrete amounts of acid well within the range of normal.

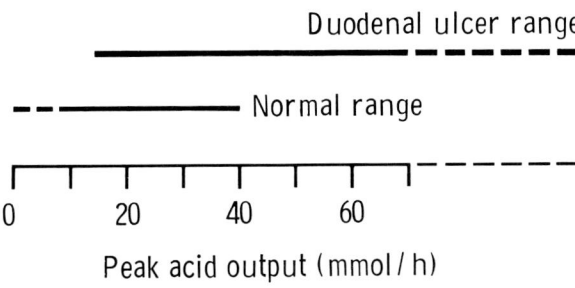

Fig 5.1 The range of peak acid outputs in mmol/h in different groups, showing the overlap between normals and duodenal ulcer patients.

Clearly there is at least one other factor, the most commonly cited being the mucosal defences. Very little indeed is known about these although, recently, prostaglandins have been found to confer some protection in an experimental situation. It would be all too easy to write at length discussing and speculating about the cause of duodenal ulcer. In the end the conclusion would be that the cause is not known, but the practising surgeon need not be concerned, although he must clearly base his treatment on facts that are known.

Clinical features

The patient's history is often virtually diagnostic. Typically, he complains of episodes of a gnawing epigastric pain which is relieved by food, milk and antacids and which characteristically wakes him at 1 or 2 a.m. Other alimentary symptoms, except those of specific complications, are not characteristic and may even be pointers to a different diagnosis. In the uncomplicated case, there may be some epigastric tenderness, but no other physical sign. The natural history is of discrete episodes between which the patient feels perfectly well. The duration, frequency and severity of these episodes vary widely from patient to patient and from time to time in the individual. In some, there are mild attacks lasting a few days every few months or even less frequently. In others, the attacks may be so severe as to prevent the patient working and occur so frequently that one almost merges into the next. It has been observed that the disease tends to burn itself out in 10 to 15 years, but serious complications may occur at any time and, often without warning, change the course of even the mildest of duodenal ulcers.

Treatment of the uncomplicated ulcer

By the time he sees a surgeon, the patient with duodenal ulcer will undoubtedly have tried a whole series of antacids, antispasmodics, liquorice derivatives,

sedatives and other miscellaneous drugs backed up by advice on diet, smoking, alcohol and other aspects of life's pleasures. Recently, there has been a significant development in the conservative treatment of duodenal ulcer with the introduction of H_2- receptor antagonists, in particular cimetidine. This agent specifically inhibits the secretion of gastric acid and almost invariably gives dramatic relief of duodenal ulcer symptoms. However, its place in the treatment of duodenal ulcer has yet to be established. There is reluctance to use it for permanent treatment, because earlier generations of the same family of agents have caused neutropenia. It is possible that cimetidine, or its successors, may become the regular and only treatment required in the majority of duodenal ulcers. If that prediction becomes true, then the surgeon's role in the treatment of duodenal ulcer will be reduced to the occasional failures and the complications in untreated patients. Meanwhile, there are some who argue that the response to cimetidine is a good indicator of the likely outcome of surgery, i.e. if cimetidine relieves the symptoms of duodenal ulcer, the patient is likely to benefit from operation, and *vice versa*. Logic backs this viewpoint, since the aim of surgery is to reduce gastric acid secretion which is also the principal effect of cimetidine.

Indications for surgery

It is frankly difficult, if not impossible, to lay down criteria for advising operation in the uncomplicated case. Somehow, the surgeon has to balance the unpleasantness and risks of surgery against the likelihood of continued disability. Since it is impossible to predict the future behaviour of a duodenal ulcer, it is only possible to judge from past experience. If the ulcer has relapsed repeatedly over two or three years and caused a great deal of discomfort each time, perhaps with loss of time at work, then there is a great deal to be said for operation. In advising operation, it is best to be totally frank with the patient and to point out the possibility of failure, either due to a recurrent ulcer or with the development of new gastrointestinal symptoms. This not only helps in the management of the failures that do occur, it also is an indirect method of assessing the severity of the patient's symptoms. If they are relatively severe, he is more likely to choose surgery, despite the risk of disappointment. It is wise to be wary of the patient with typical symptoms in whom the ulcer may not be the cause of much real trouble, but has become the scapegoat for other problems.

Choice of operation

This is so controversial that it would be impossible to rehearse all the arguments for and against every operation that is available without occupying much of this book. Some surgeons are totally convinced that there is one operation, and one only, that can be justified, others are less confident, and the individual has to make his own choice based upon his experience and what he reads of the experience of others. There are four broad criteria by which operations on duodenal ulcer are judged. These are:

1 Early mortality and complications
2 Recurrence of the ulcer
3 Persistent new gastrointestinal syndromes
4 Malnutrition.

Briefly the operations available and the arguments about each are:

1   Gastrojejunostomy. In this a simple side-to-side anastomosis is made between the antrum and the upper jejunum. This diverts gastric acid away from the duodenum and undoubtedly allows the ulcer to heal in the majority of patients. Unfortunately, this leads to a high incidence of ulceration at the anastomosis – in as many as 50% of patients. Except in the aged very few surgeons would now use it for this reason, even though its performance in terms of the other criteria is very good indeed.

2   Partial gastrectomy. The distal two-thirds of the stomach are removed, the duodenal stump is closed and the gastric remnant anastomosed end-to-side with the upper jejunum. Often a 'valve' is made at the anastomosis, which simply means that part of the opening in the gastric stump is closed, the rest being used for the actual anastomosis. This operation – the Polya gastrectomy – was favoured for many years and is, indeed, still used successfully by a number of surgeons. In its favour is a relatively low recurrence rate – 5% or less. However, it has gained an evil reputation on the other counts – a relatively high mortality and complication rate, a distressing array of new gastrointestinal symptoms which led to the term 'postgastrectomy syndromes' which will be discussed later and the development of malnutrition, principally anaemia and loss of weight. The widespread condemnation of the Polya gastrectomy is probably misplaced, since some surgeons get very good results with it, and the worst results may be due to bad technique and too extensive a resection.

3   The vagotomies. The rationale of dividing the vagus nerves is that this eliminates the nervous drive to gastric acid secretion and reduces peak secretion by an average of about 60%, although there is an unexplained wide range. The earliest vagotomy was *truncal* vagotomy in which all the vagus nerves passing through the oesophageal hiatus were divided; since this leads also to gastric stasis, a gastric drainage procedure is routinely added, either a pyloroplasty or a gastrojejunostomy. The mortality of this operation is relatively low, less than 1%; the recurrence rate is debatable, but certainly higher than that of partial gastrectomy – a figure of about 10% is probably not an exaggeration and is due to failure to divide all the nerve trunks. This operation was popular for many years and was even described by some as 'physiological'. However, it provoked the disapproval of some surgeons who detected an appreciable incidence of distressing diarrhoea, rather like repeated attacks of gastroenteritis. Because this was thought to be due to the division of the vagal nerve supply to extragastric structures such as the biliary tree, pancreas and small intestine, *selective vagotomy* was introduced. In this, only the vagus nerve trunks going to the stomach are divided leaving the other branches of the vagus nerve intact; again a drainage procedure is added. This operation won a number of converts, but it remained controversial and has now largely disappeared from the scene with the introduction of yet a third type of vagotomy which has had many names, the two commonest being *highly selective vagotomy* and *proximal gastric vagotomy*. The principle of this operation is to divide the vagus nerve supply only to the acid-secreting part of the stomach. This is achieved by dividing the tissue between the lesser curvature of the stomach and the nerve of Latarjet from the upper border of the antrum up to the oesophagus, the lower 4 to 5cm of which are also cleared. The object of this meticulous operation is to preserve the vagal nerve supply to the antrum and pylorus, the motor function of which is largely to control gastric emptying; as a consequence, a drainage procedure is not required and this can be expected to have considerable advantages. Indeed, very few of the patients have serious side effects after this operation and the mortality rate is also very low although a few patients have died of ischaemic necrosis of the lesser curvature of the stomach. The question mark that still hangs over this operation is the risk of recurrence. It is already as high as that of truncal vagotomy and there is a fear that it may increase further with longer follow-up.

4   Vagotomy with antrectomy. Both hormonal and nervous phases of gastric secretion are abolished by this operation which has gained particular favour in the United States because of the exceptionally low recurrence rate. It is not popular in the United Kingdom because of the fear that it combines the disadvantages of both gastrectomy and vagotomy. It has not been studied so intensively as the other operations in terms of side effects and malnutrition, but most reports are favourable and it is surprising that it has been largely ignored in the United Kingdom.

Benign gastric ulcer

Surgeons see fewer benign gastric ulcers than duodenal ulcers and yet, paradoxically, they are likely to see a much higher proportion of those that are diagnosed. This is because of the fear that a gastric ulcer is malignant which is a powerful influence on its management.

Almost all gastric ulcers occur on the lesser curvature, the majority at about the middle, but with some in the prepyloric region and others just below the gastro-oesophageal junction. The histopathology is identical to that of chronic duodenal ulcers. Their aetiology remains as much a mystery as does that of duodenal ulcer. The most popular theory at present is that abnormal reflux of bile and pancreatic juice into the stomach leads to inflammation in the lower stomach, thus weakening mucosal resistance to ulcerogenic forces. The reason for the excess reflux is unknown, but it is of interest that a gastric ulcer is almost always at the junction of non-acid secreting mucosa with the parietal cell bearing area. Gastric ulcers are not associated with hyperacidity, except for those in the prepyloric region which have many of the clinical characteristics of a duodenal ulcer, including a tendency to high gastric acid secretion. Some gastric ulcers are apparently caused by drugs such as indomethacin and steroids, and these are often large and slightly more likely to be on the greater curvature of the stomach.

The symptoms of gastric ulcer are not as characteristic as those of duodenal ulcer. The usual pattern is of a gnawing epigastric pain which may be aggravated by eating and which is far less likely to be relieved by antacids. The symptoms may be episodic, but the patient often finds that they wax and wane without ever really disappearing. The patient is often a rather depressed and gloomy individual, but this may well be a result of the pain rather than a basic characteristic of patients who develop gastric ulceration. In a small proportion it is possible to elicit a preceding history of symptoms characteristic of duodenal ulcer, for there seems to be a definite progression from duodenal ulceration to combined gastric and duodenal ulcer in some patients. The diagnosis is most often made on a barium meal and the decision must then be made whether to advise immediate surgery or conservative treatment.

If operation is decided upon because of the duration or severity of the symptoms, then no further specific investigations are needed, although gastroscopy is often employed to obtain biopsies in an attempt to exclude malignancy. It is, however, impossible to *exclude* malignancy by biopsy, but the combination of the opinion of an experienced endoscopist with examination of multiple biopsies can reduce the chances of missing a malignancy to a low level. If conservative treatment is decided, then it is mandatory to enlist endoscopic and histopathological services to substantiate as far as possible the benign nature of the ulcer, for it is a particular tragedy to miss an early cancer of the stomach. By the same token, it is essential to have review endoscopies at intervals of a few weeks to ensure that the ulcer is healing and remains healed under conservative treatment. Many benign gastric ulcers respond well to carbenoxolone sodium and other similar preparations; it is best if this management is under the supervision of a medical gastroenterologist who is likely to be more alive to the dangers of salt and water retention and hypertension which these preparations can cause.

The choice of operation is relatively simple in the majority of cases – partial gastrectomy, including the ulcer, with gastroduodenal anastomosis (Billroth I gastrectomy). Some surgeons employ a vagotomy operation combined with biopsy or excision of the ulcer, but they are in the minority. However, a good case can be made for vagotomy for prepyloric gastric ulcer, but the fear of a missed early cancer must be allayed by excision or generous biopsy of the ulcer. For different reasons, vagotomy and excision biopsy may be used in the high ulcers in which a gastrectomy to remove the ulcer would leave an unacceptably small gastric remnant with a risk of developing the postoperative symptomatic disorders described later in this chapter. Segmental resection of a gastric ulcer is no longer practised because of the high incidence of recurrence.

Emergencies

The three common ways in which a benign peptic ulcer can present as a clinical problem requiring either immediate or urgent clinical attention are: perforation, severe vomiting due to pyloric stenosis and haemorrhage.

Perforation

This occurs almost always in ulcers on the anterior wall of the first part of the duodenum. It is usually a sudden process when the floor of the ulcer gives way and gastric and duodenal contents flood into the peritoneal cavity causing a chemical peritonitis. The patient experiences an almost instantaneous agonising abdominal pain with the rapid development of a rigid silent abdomen. So severe is the pain that the patient seeks immediate medical advice and is soon admitted to hospital, usually with the correct diagnosis already made on clinical grounds. Further confirmation can be obtained by a plain x-ray of the abdomen which shows air free in the peritoneal cavity under the diaphragms.

The description in the previous paragraph applies to almost all patients, but some comment is needed on the differential diagnosis and alternative modes of presentation. Air under the diaphragm is diagnostic of perforation of a hollow viscus (except after a recent laparotomy) and a perforated peptic ulcer is almost always the cause; however, a perforation elsewhere in the alimentary tract, especially of a diverticulum of the sigmoid colon, must be considered. Often the patient can give a clue by indicating where the initial pain was. The absence of a previous history of dyspepsia does not exclude a peptic ulcer, for it is not uncommon for the perforation to be the first sign. Similarly the absence of air under the diaphragm does not exclude a perforation. For example, a gastric ulcer may perforate into the lesser sac where air is more difficult to see. Again, the leakage of air may be minimal due to spontaneous sealing of the perforation by the great omentum and, although radiologists claim to be able to detect just a few millilitres of free air under ideal conditions, less than perfect x-rays taken in the middle of the night may fail to show the air. There is also the 'silent' perforation in which the patient experiences severe pain, but not severe enough to require immediate attention. This is particularly common in the old in whom the dangers of a delayed diagnosis are high. The principal alternative diagnoses are myocardial infarction and any of the causes of sudden severe abdominal pain such as pancreatitis, ruptured aortic aneurysm and mesenteric infarction.

There are three approaches to the treatment of perforation. Whichever is used, treatment must be undertaken immediately. A very few surgeons treat the condition conservatively by nasogastric aspiration to keep the stomach empty, thereby preventing further contamination of the peritoneal cavity and allowing the hole to seal off the omentum. However, most surgeons are apprehensive about this approach which demands continuous observation so that operation can be undertaken if there are signs of deterioration, e.g. failing circulation or toxaemia. All are agreed that gastric aspiration (with intravenous infusions) should be limited only to those seen within a very short time of onset of the symptoms.

The policy of most surgeons is to proceed to an immediate operation, but there is some controversy about its nature. Some believe that the right operation is always the simplest, i.e. suture of the perforation with two or three sutures placed across the hole to close it with onlay of a patch of omentum for added security. Other surgeons take the view there are many circumstances in which closure of the perforation should be accompanied by a definitive ulcer-curing operation such as a vagotomy. This latter policy seems to be reasonable and demonstrably successful – but only under ideal circumstances. The appropriate criteria for definitive surgery are: a patient with an ulcer history which merits definitive surgery irrespective of the perforation, a relatively clean peritoneal cavity, a surgeon who is experienced in vagotomy, and a theatre team which is not exhausted by a long list of emergencies in the middle of the night. In the absence of such conditions, it is better to perform simple suture which is by itself a life-saving procedure.

Pyloric stenosis

This is the condition in which intensive scarring has occurred in response to a duodenal ulcer with narrowing of the gastric outlet sufficient to cause persistent vomiting of food and gastric secretions, characteristically stained only slightly or not at all with bile. The vomiting may be projectile and contain food eaten the day before. It is often associated with gross belching of gas which is said to be explosive. The patient may complain relatively early when there will be little metabolic disturbance. Alternatively, he may have fought shy of medical advice for weeks and present in an advanced state of malnutrition with a severe metabolic alkalosis in need of urgent correction before operation can be safely undertaken. It is these patients particularly in whom the outline of a distended stomach can be seen on inspection of the abdomen, and peristaltic waves are seen crossing from left to right.

The diagnosis is usually clear on the history and examination, but a barium meal is done for confirmation of gastric out-flow obstruction. It is rare for any detail to be visible because of the accumulated secretions and food in the grossly dilated stomach. For this reason and because of the imminence of the operation, gastroscopy is a waste of time.

There are a few other causes of the same syndrome such as adult hypertrophic pyloric stenosis, annular pancreas and a low gastric cancer. A duodenal ulcer can also cause the same clinical features by inducing persisting, but reversible, spasm at the pylorus. This is usually diagnosed as pyloric stenosis (which is by definition irreversible) and is therefore treated in the same way.

Correction of any metabolic disorder is an important preliminary to operation which is essential to successful treatment. The object is to secure a functioning outlet to the stomach which will usually be a pyloroplasty or gastrojejunostomy, accompanied by vagotomy of the surgeon's choice. Some surgeons do a Polya gastrectomy and others do a proximal gastric vagotomy with dilatation of the pylorus. Most patients recover rapidly after operation, but a small minority experience a prolonged period of gastric atony. This is best treated conservatively by a fine naso-enteric feeding tube. Re-exploration to search for an organic obstruction at the anastomosis should be deferred as long as possible because rarely is any cause found.

Haemorrhage (*see also* Chap. 2)

Severe bleeding from a peptic ulcer occurs when the ulcer erodes through the wall of an artery in its base, for example a branch of the gastroduodenal artery or, in the case of a gastric ulcer, a branch of the left gastric artery. Sometimes the bleeding is torrential and may be lethal if a laparotomy is not *immediately* performed with no preliminaries such as the anaesthetic premedication.

Typically the patient with haemorrhage from a peptic ulcer is admitted to hospital with haematemesis or melaena sufficient to cause alarm but not an immediate crisis. There are then several problems to be solved. How much blood has been lost, is the bleeding still active, and how should the blood loss be corrected? Where is the bleeding coming from? Does it require surgery? In most hospitals, the management of such problems is undertaken jointly by surgeons and physicians, at least one of whom must have endoscopic expertise.

The first stage in the management is an immediate assessment of the patient's haemodynamic state, as judged by the history, blood pressure, pulse rate, haemoglobin and packed cell volume. In some patients, especially the relatively young with a resilient cardiovascular system, the need may be for a relatively leisurely blood transfusion or even none at all. At the other extreme are those who have lost a great deal of blood and may still be bleeding. In these, it is often necessary to start an immediate infusion of plasma or electrolyte solutions while urgent cross-matching of blood is being carried out – as well as preparation of the operating theatre for operation forthwith. In such patients, a central venous pressure line is mandatory to maintain control of the situation. It is a matter of considerable clinical judgement to decide the timing of an operation, excluding those with continuing major blood loss in whom no time is to be lost. Several factors have to be considered. Does it appear that the bleeding is continuing? Is the patient otherwise fit or does he have other conditions, e.g. myocardial insufficiency, which would impair his chances of surviving a recurrent bleed? Is the patient over 45? It is well known that the mortality rate incurred in delaying surgery is known to rise in this age group.

Provided instant surgery is not indicated, a major factor in deciding for or against operation is knowledge of the origin of the bleeding. The best way of determining this is undoubtedly fibreoptic gastroduodenoscopy which must be done by a skilled endoscopist who can usually discriminate between lesions that may bleed and those that are actively bleeding or have done so recently. Endoscopy should be regarded as an urgent investigation to be done once the patient is in a reasonably stable haemodynamic state. Armed with a definite diagnosis, the surgeon is in a stronger position to decide when to proceed with operation. He may decide to let the patient escape without operation if the bleeding has stopped, but will certainly wish to keep the patient in hospital for a few days in case there is a recurrence. Alternatively, he may decide that the risks of rebleeding are so high that an operation should be done as soon as convenient. On the whole, it is probably better to err on the side of early surgery when a peptic ulcer has been identified as the source of bleeding.

For a duodenal ulcer, there is now widespread agreement that the operation of choice is exposure of the ulcer via a pyloro-duodenotomy, underrunning the bleeding vessel and ulcer with non-absorbable sutures, followed by closure of the incision as a pyloroplasty, and vagotomy. For a gastric ulcer, the choice is likely to be a partial gastrectomy including removal of the ulcer; for a high lesser curve ulcer, however, the surgeon may opt for an operation similar to that used for a duodenal ulcer. Although these operations can be relatively simple, they may be technically demanding, partly because of a large inflammatory mass associated with an ulcer active enough to erode into an artery of appreciable size and partly because these patients are all too often obese.

There is an appreciable mortality from operations for bleeding peptic ulcer for which several reasons may be adduced. One, which should be less and less common, is failure to operate early enough – a failing often attributed to physicians calling in the surgeon only when the patient has reached a desperate state. Another factor is co-existent disease which limits the patient's ability to withstand the extra strain of blood loss and a major operation. Re-bleeding from the ulcer also occurs in some patients, more often after a vagotomy operation than after gastrectomy, and may require further surgery which is clearly more hazardous than the first operation.

Occasionally, a surgeon may be forced to operate on a patient for haematemesis without foreknowledge of the site of bleeding. Although he will most often find an obvious ulcer at laparotomy, this may not be the case. In these circumstances, it is essential to undertake a gastroduodenotomy and make a detailed inspection of all mucosal surfaces and crevices. With adequate exposure, good assistance and illumination he will usually find a cause, which is most often a small ulcer high in the fundus or a bleeding mucosal tear at the gastroesophageal junction. Failure to find the cause of bleeding is a disheartening and perplexing problem for which there is no satisfactory solution. The author prefers to close the incision and treat the patient conservatively rather than perform a 'blind gastrectomy', which is rarely successful.

Gastric operations

Detailed operative techniques are best learnt by study of one of the excellent illustrated texts and particularly by assisting and being assisted by experienced surgeons. What follows is, therefore, no more than a brief outline of the commonest operations.

Partial gastrectomy (Fig 5.2)

This consists of removal of approximately the distal two-thirds of the stomach, with anastomosis of the gastric remnant to the duodenum (Billroth I gastrectomy) or to the proximal jejunum (Polya or Billroth II gastrectomy).

The excision may be simple or difficult depending partly on the build of the patient and partly on the extent and nature of the disease process. The usual practice is to start by mobilising the greater curvature by division of the gastrocolic omentum between clips from just beyond the pylorus to above the planned line of proximal excision; this dissection starts half-way along the greater curvature and proceeds upwards and downwards. It is wise to mobilise upwards far enough to ensure that the gastric remnant can be brought down without tension and this may involve a careful dissection at the level of the short gastric vessel to the spleen. Distally, it is important to separate the transverse mesocolon to avoid damage to the middle colic artery and to free the proximal duodenum of multiple vessels, principally venous, which are easily torn and can cause irritating bleeding. A finger is then passed behind the duodenum and breaks through the lesser omentum, leaving the right gastric artery running upwards immediately adjacent to the lesser curvature; this artery is divided between ligatures. The duodenum is then transected against a crushing clamp just distal to

the pylorus with a non-crushing clamp about 2cm more distally, leaving the duodenal stump open either for closure or anastomosis. The lesser omentum is then divided upwards to reach the left gastric vessels just above the proximal line of dissection. These are carefully isolated and divided. Particular care is needed to secure these vessels safely; if the ligature slips, it is better to deal with the vascular pedicle with a transfixion suture than attempt to tie these vessels individually. The operation is then continued differently for the two main types of anastomosis.

In a *Billroth I gastrectomy* a crushing clamp is placed across the stomach just distal to the line of transection and a non-crushing clamp more proximally, and the stomach transected just above the crushing clamp. This leaves a gastric remnant with an opening far wider than the duodenum to which it is to be anastomosed. A continuous haemostatic, all-layers suture is used to close the lesser curvature side sufficient to leave an opening about the same size as or a little larger than that of the duodenum. The opening in the gastric remnant is then anastomosed end-to-end to the duodenum with two layers of suture – one haemostatic and one seromuscular. Finally, a continuous seromuscular suture is used to close the lesser curve end of the gastric remnant. The author uses 2/0 chromic catgut throughout this anastomosis. Many different materials are available. It cannot be emphasised too strongly that each surgeon will have his own detailed way of accomplishing the same end result, and some use complicated clamps. The surgeon-in-training is best advised to follow in detail the techniques used by his chief, and only experiment with modifications when he has gained confidence.

In a *Polya gastrectomy* it is convenient to use Lanes Twin Clamps which hold the gastric remnant and a loop of jejunum in position during three-quarters of the anastomosis. Thus one of the clamps is placed across the stomach proximal to the line of excision and the other along the loop of jejunum, and the two clamps are then fixed together. The gastric remnant is retracted over the left costal margin, exposing the posterior surface which is sutured with a seromuscular continuous stitch to the side of the loop of jejunum. A crushing clamp is placed across the stomach distal to the line of section and the stomach is divided. This leaves the opened gastric remnant and the still unopened loop of jejunum adjacent to each other. Some surgeons then complete the anastomosis by opening a length of jejunum equal to the length of the gastric remnant, and performing an all-coats, haemostatic suture to create a wide anastomosis, completed by an anterior seromuscular layer. Others close one end of the gastric remnant and open a smaller length of jejunum for completion of a narrower anastomosis. The closed part of the gastric remnant in this case is often called a 'valve' which has the theoretical benefits

Billroth I gastrectomy   Polya gastrectomy

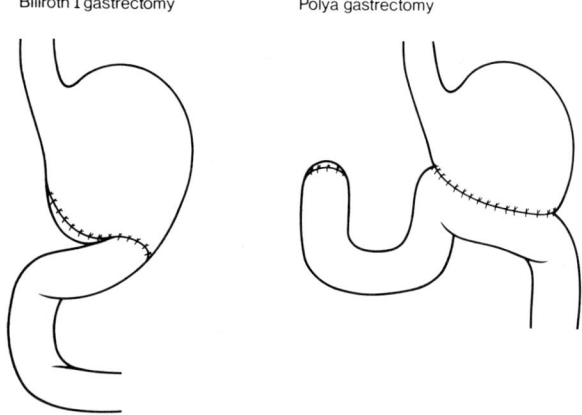

Fig 5.2 The two principal partial gastrectomies.

of delaying gastric emptying and of preventing reflux of duodenal contents into the stomach. Once again, there are probably as many different ways of doing this anastomosis as there are gastric surgeons. Two aspects are, however, desirable. First, the jejunum selected should be as close as possible to the duodeno-jejunal flexure. Second, the anastomosis is best made in the retrocolic position, i.e. a hole is made in the transverse mesocolon and the jejunum is taken up through this for anastomosis to the gastric remnant; when completed the anastomosis is brought below the mesocolon and the gastric remnant is sutured to the defect. However, it is conventional to make the anastomosis in front of the colon if the resection is for carcinoma. There is still controversy over which way the jejunum should lie along the gastric remnant, i.e. afferent limb to lesser curvature or *vice versa*.

Gastrojejunostomy

This anastomosis is done in a manner quite similar to that in a Polya gastrectomy. In an elective operation, it is common to start by making a hole in the mesocolon to expose the posterior surface of the stomach. The latter is then cleared towards the pylorus, because the anastomosis should be in the middle or lower part of the antrum. Lanes Twin Clamps are then applied to a segment of the posterior wall of the stomach and to the selected loop of jejunum and a two-layer anastomosis done. In this case the stomach is only opened for the planned length of the anastomosis, usually about 5cm. It is important to tack the stomach to the edges of the defect in the mesocolon, so that the anastomosis lies below this level. Some surgeons make the anastomosis antecolic which is slightly easier unless there is a bulky, obtrusive greater omentum. Again, it is conventional for an emergency gastrojejunostomy to be antecolic, but there is no particular reason for this.

Pyloroplasty

Stay sutures are placed across the pylorus above and below the planned incision which is made longitudinally from the stomach across the pylorus into duodenum. A very long incision is not necessary, about 2cm on either side of the pylorus being quite adequate. The incision is closed *transversely* using a single layer of a continuous inverting suture, with some reinforcing sutures if the closure is felt to be inadequate. A second, invaginating layer is unnecessary and probably inadvisable for fear of narrowing the lumen.

Vagotomy (Fig 5.3)

Truncal vagotomy by the abdominal approach is aided by preliminary mobilisation of the left lobe of the

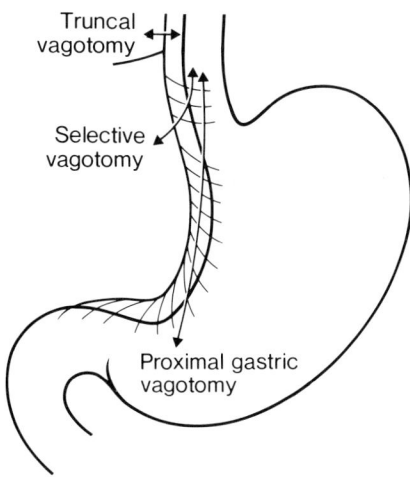

Fig 5.3 Three different vagotomies. Gastrojejunostomy or pyloroplasty is done with truncal and selective vagotomy.

liver so that it can be tucked away and give clearer access to the hiatus. The peritoneum is divided at the hiatus and finger dissection is used to mobilise the lower oesophagus. During this process, it is helpful to feel deliberately for the posterior trunk of the vagus which can often be brought out with the right index finger as it goes round behind the oesophagus from left to right and then breaks through on the right side. The posterior trunk is almost always a very stout, cord-like structure with a glistening white surface. Some surgeons just divide it and others excise short segments, using ligatures or diathermy to deal with the cut ends. With the oesophagus mobilised, a further search should be made for a second posterior trunk, but there rarely is one. Vagal trunks are searched for on the anterior surface and dealt with in the same way. These are smaller than the posterior vagus and there are almost always two (and often more) especially if the lower most part of the oesophagus is being examined, because the vagus at this level is dividing into smaller and smaller fibres as it approaches the stomach. Indeed, it is vital to be obsessional in the search for large and small vagal fibres, if the aim of a complete vagotomy is to be achieved.

It is a useful training exercise to send excised specimens for histology so that the surgeon can discover if he is identifying vagal fibres or excising other tissue unnecessarily. However, histology reports will rarely help in deciding whether the vagotomy is complete. In the case of excision of a single piece of tissue posteriorly which proves to be other than nerve, the vagotomy is clearly incomplete. Anteriorly, no surgeon can realistically fail to find some nerve fibres so that the histologist will always report some nerve tissue; he cannot say if any has been left behind.

Selective vagotomy

Having enjoyed considerable popularity, this has now been virtually superseded by proximal gastric vagotomy. It is performed by a careful dissection around the hiatus and division only of branches of the vagus going to the stomach.

Proximal gastric vagotomy

This is a meticulous operation which is started at what is judged to be the junction of the body and antrum on the lesser curvature of the stomach. It can be identified fairly reliably by recognising the nerve of Latarjet appearing to end in several fibres branching claw-like to the lesser curvature of the stomach. The nerve of Latarjet runs down in the lesser omentum parallel to and within a few mm of the lesser curvature. The dissection proceeds proximally dividing the lesser omentum in this gap and thus dividing the tiny branches of the nerve. Care has to be taken to avoid damage to the nerve of Latarjet and the wall of the stomach respectively, while at the same time ensuring haemostasis, venous bleeding being particularly likely. When the gastro-oesophageal junction is reached, the dissection proceeds close to the circumference of the oesophagus to clear the lower 4 to 5cm.

Recurrent ulcer

Recurrent ulcer is a general term used when a peptic ulcer develops after an operation for gastric or duodenal ulcer. It may be regarded as truly recurrent if it is at essentially the same site, for example on the lesser curvature after operation for gastric ulcer or in the duodenum after vagotomy and pyloroplasty for duodenal ulcer. If the original operation involved a gastrojejunostomy, the 'recurrence' is mostly commonly at or very close to the anastomosis and more properly called a stomal ulcer. Whatever the site, the pathology is the same as that of a peptic ulcer.

There are clearly identifiable causes of most recurrent ulcers. Because vagotomy is so popular as the primary operation, at least for duodenal ulcer, recurrences are most commonly seen after vagotomy operations and failure to achieve a complete vagotomy is almost always the reason. This is a reproach to the surgeon and an indication of how important it is to be obsessional in the search for vagal trunks and small branches, whichever vagotomy operation is employed. After partial gastrectomy, the most likely cause is removal of an insufficient part of the stomach, but there

is one more specific cause for recurrence after gastrectomy with gastrojejunostomy. This is when part of the antrum has been left behind – either inadvertently, or deliberately when a large inflammatory mass associated with a duodenal ulcer prevented the surgeon from making his lower resection line below the pylorus. The so-called retained antrum is then excluded from the flow of gastric acid and is bathed in alkaline secretions. This stimulates the constant liberation of gastrin into the circulation and hence hyperacidity which leads to ulceration of the stoma. A third cause of recurrence is the existence of an actively secreting gastrinoma which again causes hyperacidity. Although rare, it is always worth considering the possibility and measuring the gastrin activity in the blood of patients with recurrent ulcer.

The clinical presentation of a recurrent ulcer may be identical to that of the original ulcer. This is particularly likely to be the case after vagotomy with pyloroplasty. In other cases the patient may present with atypical epigastric pain or an unheralded gastrointestinal bleed from a gastrojejunal ulcer which had previously been completely symptom free.

The investigation of a patient suspected of having a recurrent ulcer should be more extensive than that of the primary peptic ulcer. This is because it is necessary both to confirm the diagnosis and, if possible, to identify the cause. Barium meal studies may be sufficient to confirm the presence of a recurrence, but all too often they fail because of the radiologist's difficulty in distinguishing between an ulcer crater and the distortions caused by the previous operation. Fibreoptic gastroscopy is of particular value and is undoubtedly the method of choice in making the diagnosis. Since recurrences are now seen most often after a vagotomy operation, it is important to try to establish whether or not the vagotomy was complete. This is done by the Hollander insulin test. This is the only measurement of gastric acid secretion which has real clinical value. The principle underlying the insulin test is simple. It is that hypoglycaemia stimulates vagal activity which, in turn, stimulates increased gastric acid secretion; if the vagal nerve supply to the stomach has been efficiently disrupted, then hypoglycaemia will no longer evoke a rise in gastric acid secretion. The criteria by which a genuine rise in acidity is judged to have occurred are controversial. However, it is commonly accepted that provided adequate hypoglycaemia (3.0 mmol/l) has been secured by insulin, then incomplete vagotomy can be assumed if the stimulated secretions show a rise in concentration of 22 mmol/l above the basal level (or of 10 mmol/l if the basal secretions contained no acid). As already stated, it is important to measure fasting blood gastrin levels to see if there is any suspicion of a gastrinoma, which is discussed in Chap 37 and also Chap 35 for parathyroid involvement.

By tradition, the treatment of a recurrent ulcer is surgical, although there is really no good reason why this should be the case in every patient. For example, unless a patient with recurrence after vagotomy and pyloroplasty is in exactly the same situation as he was before the operation, it is legitimate to apply the same criteria for deciding on an operation – with the additional consideration that a second abdominal operation will be more hazardous. Recurrences at a gastrojejunostomy are almost always treated by operation because of the risk of haemorrhage and the occasional, but potentially disastrous, development of a gastrocolic fistula. However, there is no evidence that recurrent ulcers are a greater risk to life than primary peptic ulcers.

The choice of operation for recurrent peptic ulcer is not so wide as that for primary peptic ulcer, but must be carefully considered. For a recurrent gastric ulcer after gastrectomy, the natural choice might seem to be a more extensive gastrectomy, but some surgeons prefer to try vagotomy with the aim of sparing the patient a very small gastric remnant. For recurrent ulcer after partial gastrectomy for duodenal ulcer, the most common choice is a vagotomy unless there is a retained antrum, in which case excision of the antral remnant – usually a simple operation – is carried out. If the recurrence is after a vagotomy operation for duodenal ulcer, the choice lies between an attempt to complete the vagotomy, a partial gastrectomy or antrectomy, possibly combined with re-vagotomy. Completion of a transabdominal vagotomy via the abdomen is often technically difficult and, therefore, relatively hazardous. For this reason, it is best to complete the vagotomy by a trans-thoracic approach. This is a relatively easy operation but it must not be regarded as giving a guarantee of completeness of vagotomy; just as much care is needed to find and divide all vagal nerve trunks as at a primary vagotomy below the diaphragm. A disadvantage of transthoracic vagotomy is that it does not allow examination of the abdominal organs, but this is usually no more than theoretical. If gastrectomy or antrectomy are chosen, it is important to recognise in advance the difficulties likely to be encountered in dissection around a duodenum when a pyloroplasty has been done in the past. Operations for recurrent ulcer are generally successful, but further recurrences can occur when it is necessary to investigate with even more care to exclude a gastrinoma and a parathyroid adenoma.

Symptomatic disorders after gastric operation

One of the important reasons for taking great care in selecting patients for elective operation for benign peptic ulcer is the possible occurrence of one or more of those symptomatic problems which are still popularly grouped together as 'postgastrectomy syndromes'. Unfortunately, this phrase gives the false impression that the same problems do not occur after vagotomy operations. Although the incidence may vary, depending on the operation employed, it is best to assume that each operation may give rise to any of these syndromes. In the absence of a better term, they can be called the 'symptomatic disorders of gastric surgery'. They are often badly understood by doctors, surgeons and others, and therefore the patients who are their victims are often also badly handled. One of the reasons why doctors find difficulty in getting to grips with these problems is that there is no agreed nomenclature, so that different terms are used for the same problem. The following is a list of the common symptomatic disorders:

Dysphagia
Small stomach syndrome
Dumping
Hypoglycaemia
Bilious vomiting
Diarrhoea

Dysphagia

This is a rare postoperative symptom, but occurs particularly after vagotomy. Typically it is noticed early after operation, sometimes with the first solid food. Usually it is mild in nature and can be confidently expected to resolve spontaneously within a few weeks. Occasionally it is persistent and relatively severe when oesophagoscopy and dilatation are required. Usually one dilatation is sufficient. The cause of the dysphagia remains a matter of debate. It may be due to oesophageal trauma or extrinsic pressure from a postoperative haematoma. It has been suggested that it is a denervation phenomenon, but this has not been substantiated.

Small stomach syndrome

The small stomach syndrome is a good descriptive term, but not strictly accurate because it can occur after vagotomy operations when the stomach is, anatomically at least, unchanged in size. The patient complains that he is prevented from taking a normal sized meal because he feels a fullness in the epigastrium at some stage during the meal. It is so common that it is almost normal after gastric surgery in mild degree. However, it constitutes a severe disability in a small proportion to the extent that it is a cause of malnutrition. The treatment of severe examples is extremely difficult and is best undertaken by a dietitian with an understanding of the specific problems. With luck and persistence, she may be able to devise a diet of adequate variety and amount. In the worse cases, it may be necessary to consider revisional gastric surgery (q.v.), but this is often disappointing.

The cause of the small stomach syndrome is uncertain. The likely explanation in most patients is that loss of control of normal gastric emptying, e.g. by excision of the antrum and pylorus in gastrectomy, leads to rapid gastric emptying and rapid filling of the small bowel from which the symptoms probably come. Indeed, it seems likely that many of the symptomatic disorders are initiated by this abnormality of gastric emptying. After vagotomy the complaint may have a dual origin – rapid gastric emptying and failure of 'receptive relaxation', which is absent in the vagotomised stomach.

Dumping

This is the most commonly mis-used term in this context. The usual mistake is to use it for any alimentary symptom after gastric surgery. It is also often described as 'early' or 'late', meaning the time relation of the relevant symptoms of the last meal. 'Early dumping' is dumping in the correct sense of the word and 'late dumping' refers to the hypoglycaemic syndrome. Another term used is the 'efferent loop syndrome'.

There are two essential components to the symptoms of dumping – alimentary and systemic – and the condition can only be diagnosed if this feature is recognised. The alimentary symptoms consist of a feeling of epigastric fullness often associated with nausea and excessive borborygmi, and occasionally with vomiting or diarrhoea or even both. The systemic symptoms are characteristically lethargy, even to the point of falling asleep, and sweating. All these symptoms start either during or soon after a meal, and may last for up to one hour. The reader will surely recognise these symptoms in himself as occurring after a large meal and they can also be induced in any normal subject by fairly rapid instillation of a hypertonic glucose solution (say 50%) directly into the jejunum via a nasojejunal tube. This fact gives the clue to their pathogenesis. Rapid gastric emptying leads to overfilling of the small bowel with hypertonic food causing jejunal distension and hyperperistalsis, partly contributed to by osmotic drag or circulating fluid into the lumen. This, in turn, may reduce the circulating blood volume and cause systemic symptoms. However, it seems likely that some of the latter are also due to the release of an unidentified polypeptide hormone from the small bowel mucosa into the general circulation.

Dumping symptoms are quite common in the first weeks or months after a gastric operation and there seems a distinct tendency to improvement over the months, whether by small bowel adaptation or unconscious modification of the diet. Therefore, it is proper to give genuine reassurance to patients soon after their operation. The symptoms persist and can be very severe in a small percentage of patients. Once persistence of symptoms is recognised, it is important to attempt to give patients a simple explanation of what is happening, so that they can understand the dietary advice they should follow. This is to eat small meals often, to avoid too much fluid and to restrict the carbohydrate intake. This will help an appreciable proportion of sufferers who may also discover for themselves that certain goods are particularly likely to cause the symptoms. If this fails, it is reasonable to try the effect of one or more of the alimentary 'panaceas' in the pharmacopeia, but they are unlikely to help except perhaps in placebo-responders. Ultimately, it may be necessary to consider revisional gastric surgery, but without any great optimism.

Hypoglycaemia

Hypoglycaemia is probably not so rare as is thought, because the diagnosis is so easily missed if the right question is not asked. The symptoms consist of sweating, dizziness and extreme hunger at about 1½ hours after a meal. The crucial feature is the hunger which attains almost pathological proportions in some. If, after questioning, the hunger symptom is established, the diagnosis can be made in a matter of moments and the treatment prescribed i.e. always carry, say, some barley sugar sweets and take them when the symptoms begin. The pathogenesis of hypoglycaemia is almost certainly attributable to rapid gastric emptying and hence a rapid and high rise in the blood sugar with a relatively profound rebound fall to low levels when the symptoms occur. This is the so-called 'steeple' oral glucose tolerance curve.

Bilious vomiting

A good descriptive term for a most unpleasant symptom, bilious vomiting can follow an entirely predictable or very variable pattern in the individual patient. The essential symptom is of vomiting of bile-stained fluid which occurs after a period of 15 to 30 min of epigastric discomfort after a meal; the vomitus is characteristically free of any food. In some patients, the symptom starts almost immediately after the operation and continues without remission; in a few, it is of late onset starting months or even years after the operation. Again, some experience the symptom daily and in others its occurrence is quite erratic. Finally, although the vomit in most patients is free of food, some report seeing food, but rarely is there much; indeed a significant amount of food suggests poor gastric emptying which is most likely to be due to stenosis at an anastomosis.

There are two main theories about the cause. The older is that some abnormality at the anastomosis, particularly gastrojejunostomy, prevents bile and pancreatic juice secreted in response to a meal leaving the afferent loop normally. This leads to accumulation of the secretions which are then expelled explosively, some going into efferent loop and some entering the stomach and being vomited. The evidence for this theory is largely anecdotal, but there are certainly some patients in whom re-exploration reveals a hugely dilated afferent loop. Hence the synonym 'afferent loop syndrome' for this condition. The newer theory – and the two are not necessarily mutually exclusive – is that bile and pancreatic juice enter or reflux continuously into the stomach and cause an alkaline gastritis which causes the vomiting.

There is no effective medical treatment for bilious vomiting, although an occasional patient may respond to one agent or another, such as metoclopramide or propantheline. In the patient with severe and persistent symptoms, the advice can be given fairly confidently that revisional surgery will help. The aim of such an operations, described elsewhere, is to divert the duodenal secretions away from the anastomosis and to a lower level of the jejunum.

Diarrhoea

Most commonly regarded as a complication of truncal vagotomy, diarrhoea can occur after any gastric operation. It may be mild and even welcomed as an unexpected relief from the constipation which so many patients believe they 'suffer'. At the other extreme, it can be disabling although such patients are unusual.

Apart from the rather frequent bowel motions which affect quite a large number of patients in the first few weeks after operation, there are two main varieties of diarrhoea. One is when the patient has more frequent motions every day after operation, and the other is when a usually normal bowel habit is punctuated at more or less regular intervals by a bout of severe diarrhoea lasting a few hours to one or two days during which he is afraid to venture too far from a lavatory because of the associated urgency. It is this second variety which can be particularly distressing. Very occasionally a patient may become constipated after operation and be equally reproachful of the surgeon who caused the affliction!

Despite intensive study, the cause of these changes in bowel habit has not been discovered. Rapid gastric emptying, and hence rapid intestinal transit, seems to be a real factor in some patients, but there is no convincing explanation for the episodic diarrhoea which has all the characteristics of recurrent enteritis of infective origin. Neither type is associated with steatorrhoea.

The treatment of persistent diarrhoea is difficult. Codeine phosphate is often effective in those with a daily problem, but is difficult to prescribe rationally when the problem is periodic. Some patients are able to recognise the onset of an attack and can be helped by *immediately* taking a large dose of codeine phosphate. Revisional surgery can be tried, either to eliminate a gastrojejunostomy or to restore a pylorus after pyloroplasty, and some success has been reported. Reversal of a short loop of jejunum to delay intestinal transit has been used with benefit in a few patients.

Malnutrition after gastric surgery

A great deal of research has been done into aspects of malnutrition after gastric surgery, but it is not really a very complicated problem for the surgeon, provided he recognises its existence and is prepared to refer the patient to an interested gastroenterologist if he finds himself unable to master the situation. Without doubt, the commonest evidence of malnutrition is loss of weight or inability to gain weight. In almost all patients, this can be attributed to inability to eat adequately, due to abdominal discomfort after a normal meal. In many patients, the problem consists of a drop in weight in the first few months after operation to a new level which then stays steady. Unless this new level is particularly low, there is no need to take special measures except to ensure that the patient's diet is adequate in variety. If the weight loss continues and it appears that the main contributory factor is reduced intake due to, say, dumping, then help should be sought from a dietitican who understands the specific problem. If dietary intake is normal, it is likely that the patient has malabsorption. In these circumstances, faecal fat excretion must be measured and, if significant steatorrhoea is confirmed, a full gastro-intestinal investigation is required. Two aspects of this must be emphasised. First, it is important to recognise that a mild degree of steatorrhoea is extremely common after gastric surgery and usually of no clinical importance. Next, significant steatorrhoea is usually due to a combination of the effect of the operation and some pre-existing, previously unrecognised condition such as coeliac disease. However, it must be remembered that severe steatorrhoea can be a direct result of the operation in two different ways. One is the formation of a very poorly emptying afferent loop leading to a 'blind-loop' syndrome. The other is the inadvertent anastomosis of the stomach or gastric remnant to a low level in the jejunum or even to the ileum.

The most common problem is of iron deficiency. This is sufficiently frequent, especially in premenopausal women, to cause some to advocate regular medication with oral iron. Various programmes have been suggested, but patients lose interest after the first few months or year. Studies of patients many years after gastric surgery have often uncovered a considerable reservoir of iron-deficiency anaemia. Too few doctors and surgeons seem to be aware of this problem. There is much to be said for measuring the haemoglobin level in any patient seen for any reason if he had a gastric operation many years ago.

Other specific deficiencies are rare. They include vitamin B12, folic acid, calcium and vitamin D disorders. Undoubtedly megaloblastic anaemias and metabolic disorders occur in a small minority of patients and must be remembered. However, they appear to be decreasing in frequency, possibly due to the diminishing use of partial gastrectomy (especially very extensive resections) and possibly due to improved diet in the community as a whole. It is also likely that the 'clean air policy' has contributed in allowing more ultra-violet rays to reach the body.

Revisional gastric surgery

This term is used for operations done in an attempt to alleviate or cure symptomatic disorders or malabsorption after gastric surgery; it does not apply to operations for recurrent ulcer. There is an almost infinite variety of such operations and only the main ones will be mentioned here.

It is hard to lay down clear cut criteria for undertaking such operations. However, the indications are in some measure similar to, but more stringent than, those for elective surgery for benign peptic ulcer. The symptoms should have failed to respond to conservative management and they should be clearly persistent and severe enough to warrant the risk which is greater than for primary operations. Since the chances of success are not particularly great, it is important that the patient should understand completely the purpose of the operation and accept the possibility of failure. For all these reasons, these operations are best undertaken by a surgeon who is familiar with both the techniques and the general management of patients with symptomatic disorders. Too frequent resort to revisional surgery is likely to lead to disappointment.

Restoration of gastrointestinal continuity

This is a common aim of revisional operations, since many of the postsurgical problems can be blamed at least in part on by-pass of the duodenum. Thus a Polya gastrectomy can be converted to a Billroth I gastrectomy, and a gastrojejunostomy can be replaced by a pyloroplasty. This operation can be quite successful for bilious vomiting and occasionally for diarrhoea.

Jejunal interposition

Loss of gastric capacity can sometimes be corrected by interposing a segment of jejunum between the gastric remnant and the duodenum. The segment is usually some 4″ to 6″ long and may be placed in an isoperistaltic or antiperistaltic fashion – the aim of the latter being to slow down gastric emptying. A particular hazard of this operation is peptic ulceration at the new gastrojejunal junction, so vagotomy must always be added. This operation should only be used in those with severe degrees of dumping or small stomach syndrome.

Biliary diversion

This variety of operation is used most often for severe bilious vomiting and is often successful. A simple version is jejuno-jejunostomy between the afferent and efferent limbs of a gastrojejunostomy where the former is quite long. An alternative common variety is the Roux-en-Y in which the afferent loop is disconnected from the gastrojejunostomy and reanastomosed to the efferent loop some 10″ distal to the stoma. Again, vagotomy should be added to reduce the risk of gastrojejunal ulceration.

Reversal procedures

In addition to the reversed jejunal loop between stomach and duodenum, there are two reversal procedures which have been used occasionally for diarrhoea after vagotomy. One is to 'reverse' a pyloroplasty – literally to open the transverse suture line (as nearly as possible) and close the opening longitudinally. The other is to reverse a short segment of jejunum. There is relatively little experience of both, but the former seems to have been more successful.

Correction procedures

Occasionally a gross anatomical error was made at the primary operation. An example of this is when the stomach was anastomosed to a low point in the small intestine – even to the ileum in a few patients. Such errors can be disastrous and clearly need correction.

Carcinoma of the stomach

ALLAN E KARK

Much that is new and fascinating for the surgeon has been uncovered about this disease in the past decade. Although there has been little of comfort for most patients, there have been significant advances which offer striking improvement in treatment for some. Only one patient in ten survives 5 years after the only treatment of proven value, namely gastrectomy. However, we know considerably more about who that one patient is likely to be and how modern techniques may increase this number; why the disease has occurred in some of these patients; and the pitfalls which arise in the course of surgical treatment. The value of this new information will be assessed and emphasis will be placed on the importance of early diagnosis, the principles of surgical reconstruction, the pre- and postoperative care and the long-term risks.

Incidence and epidemiology

It is surprising that cancer of the stomach is not more common considering its daily confrontation with an endless variety of solid and liquid material with their extremes of temperature, ice cold to near boiling, and sheer volume of toxic additions to the human diet ranging from alcohol to artificial preservatives. In the UK, it is third to lung and breast in frequency and numbers around 16 000 new cases a year. The incidence ranges from 27 to 40 per 100 000 in different areas, lowest in Scotland and highest in the West Midlands and N Wales. Canada and India have low incidences (13 and 15) and the black population of South Africa even less. Only in the USA has there been a significant reduction in the incidence which has fallen from 31 to 13 per 100 000 in the decades 1950-1970. A small reduction has occurred in the UK and Finland, and even in high risk countries like Japan and Chile, which have an incidence of over 110 per 100 000.

These differences strongly suggest that environmental and biological factors play a major role in pathogenesis. It is generally recognised that exogenous carcinogenic agents, especially chemical but also viral, are involved in human cancer development, either by promoting malignant transformation or enhancing host susceptibility. This view is strengthened in gastric cancer by the lack of hereditary or racial factors, the evidence of specific risk factors in gastric cancer and the experimental production of gastric cancer by chemical carcinogens. Of special interest is the role of N-nitrosamine compounds, well established as carcinogens in animals. The human stomach forms these substances when nitrates and amines are present in an acid environment. Their constant contact with gastric mucosa over many years may well be a potent factor in carcinogenesis.

From recent epidemiological studies, it is likely that gastric cancer may be initiated by more than one carcinogen. Chemical agents either swallowed or formed *in vivo* appear to be inducing agents and the development of the tumour is very slow. The role of exogenous factors is supported by the observations that different races resident in low risk zones (such as the USA) or in high risk zones (Japan) have similar rates, while migration from one area to another results in an incidence approaching that of the host country. The influences of common dietary products has been demonstrated: high milk diets tend to be protective (Chile), while low fat diets tend to be associated with a high incidence.

Genetic factors in the incidence of the disease are not impressive. There does appear to be a familial factor – a fourfold increase in incidence among relatives, but this may also be related to environmental similarities such as equivalent socio-economic group and life style of family members. It has been shown, however, that there is a significant excess of gastric cancer in patients with blood group A.

Predisposing gastric factors

A number of local gastric changes are associated with an increased risk of malignant change. These include atrophic gastritis, intestinal metaplasia and gastric polyps. Evidence from a number of sources in Japan, USA, Sweden, Finland and Colombia demonstrates a clear correlation between the incidence of both atrophic and chronic gastritis, and cancer. Although the evidence is largely statistical, it is very likely that the inflammatory change permits the action of carcinogens possibly through a stage of intestinal metaplasia of the gastric epithelium. Pernicious anaemia is associated with a threefold incidence of cancer which usually occurs in the upper half of the stomach, is polypoid and often of low grade malignancy. There is no good evidence that benign gastric ulcers develop into cancers except in a small minority (5-7%) of cases.

Of great interest to the surgeon is the recent evidence that cancer in the gastric stump is an increasing risk following gastrectomy or gastroenterostomy for benign ulcer disease. The risk is proportionate to the length of time after resection; few occur in the first 10 years, but by 20 years the incidence in one series had risen to 9% and by 25 years to 21%. Thus the risk of cancer 25 or more years after gastrectomy is six times the normal. The tumours are sited near the suture line, and they have a poor prognosis, probably because of delay in diagnosis.

The implications of these observations are considerable. The heyday of gastrectomy for duodenal and gastric ulcer was in the period 1950-1965, and the 25-year follow-up period of patients thus treated is now beginning and will peak in the coming decade. The surgeon must be aware of this likely bulge in numbers in a specifically predisposed group, and any symptoms in previously asymptomatic gastrectomy patients must be regarded as especially sinister. Not only is it essential to endoscope any such symptomatic patients, but there is a strong argument for annual endoscopy in patients 20 years or more after operation and especially in those who show dysplasia on biopsy.

Thus some tentative conclusions about pathogenesis have emerged. Gastric tumours have a prolonged latency period, in most cases exceeding 30 years. During this period the predominant mucosal changes in those at high risk are progressive chronic atrophy and intestinal metaplasia. There is evidence that there are two types of gastric cancer. One is usually preceded by a long period of gastric mucosal change and subsequent atrophy and associated with a number of risk-associated factors in both environment and diet; socio-economic factors, chemical carcinogens, food conservation (pickling or smoking), food preparation (frying), concentration of trace elements and nitrates are all significant factors in determining the development of cancer in predisposed individuals. The other type appears to be largely independent of these exogenous factors, and closely linked to factors of heredity.

Pathology

The very wide range of histological types, growth rates, pattern of spread and prognosis has led to a good deal of confusion and differing classifications. Perhaps the most commonly used, that of McNeer and Pack (1967), divides the lesion into (1) fungating (polypoid), (2) ulcerating and (3) diffuse infiltrating. The fungating polypoid type, about 10% is usually slow growing, is of low grade malignancy and metastasises late. Thus the prognosis is usually good. The ulcerating tumour may resemble a benign ulcer and be quite small, but there is often submucous infiltration and the base is usually shaggy and necrotic. The diffuse group may be in the form of a superficial spreading lesion or an infiltrating cancer. The former is slowly progressive with a tendency to involve the mucosa and submucosa while sparing deeper or muscular layers. It also has a good prognosis, a 75% 10-year survival being reported from the Mayo Clinic and it is similar to early gastric cancer discussed below. The commonest variety of the diffuse type is the infiltrating cancer which involves all layers and extends well beyond all palpable or visible tumour growth. It varies from a well-differentiated to anaplastic tumour with the serosa studded with nodules and rapid invasion of adjacent structures with early lymphatic spread. Linitis plastica is a variant of this type with marked mural thickening and contraction – the 'leather bottle' stomach.

The classification of Lauren (1965) emphasises a new aspect. This author has proposed, on the basis of differences in histological types in low and high risk areas, a distinction between:

a   *An intestinal type* which is well-differentiated, with a glandular pattern and much inflammatory cell infiltration. It occurs predominantely in high risk areas and in the aged.

b   *A diffuse type* which is an undifferentiated tumour with scattered cells or clusters and poorly formed lumina. It occurs mostly in younger patients and is commoner in women and has a relatively constant incidence in all areas.

There is much value in staging stomach tumours. Survival has been well shown to be proportional to the degree of spread through the stomach wall and the extent of lymph node involvement. Follicular hyperplasia in lymph nodes has been shown to have a favourable prognosis as has lymphocyte infiltration within the tumour, a feature comparable to the better outlook when present in breast and colon tumour.

It is important that the pathological report should include a number of features of gastric tumours, not only type and degree of differentiation, but with special attention being paid to the following:

a   Grading based on the most poorly differentiated cell types in the specimen.

b   Presence and extent of intracellular and extra-cellular mucus.

c   Stomal reaction and lymphocyte accumulation around the tumour cells.

d   Depth of spread through the stomach wall.

e   Involvement of lymph nodes and the number of nodes involved.

f   Where possible, grouping according to Lauren (1965) as intestinal or diffuse.

g   Degree of intestinal metaplasia and gastritis.

Finally the special types of tumours with a good prognosis should be recognised and noted (Table 1).

Table 1
HISTOLOGIC DESCRIPTIONS OF STOMACH CANCERS WHICH HAVE A MORE FAVOURABLE PROGNOSIS

	% Frequency	% 5-yr survival
1 Early gastric cancer (Murakami, 1971)	5–30	95
2 Superficial spreading carcinoma (Stout, 1945) (? same as e.g.c.)	8	90
3 Polypoidal carcinoma (McNeer and Pack, 1967)	10	50
4 Medullary carcinoma with lymphoid infiltration (Steiner *et al.*, 1948)	4	'good'
5 Mucoid carcinoma (Brander *et al.*, 1947)	1	'good'

Early gastric cancer

A major step forward has been the recognition of a clearly defined category – 'early' gastric cancer (e.g.c.) which is limited to the mucosa and submucosa and distinguished from carcinoma-*in-situ* and more deeply infiltrating growths. It is not meant to describe a stage in the development of a cancer. This concept of early gastric cancer has been especially developed in Japan, where it is now being diagnosed by endoscopy in asymptomatic individuals.

Japanese workers define early cancer as one which can be cured and in which infiltration does not extend beyond the submucosa. This entity has been subdivided into three groups: polypoid, superficial and excavated. The latter accounts for more than half the cases, but combinations are more common than simple types. Most tumours are under 2 cm in diameter, although larger ones are found, and they occur most commonly in the antrum and along the lesser curvature. Involvement of lymph nodes varies with the depth of penetration into the wall; it is very unusual in intra-mucosal cancer, but occurs in 10% or more of submucosal lesions.

The most notable feature of this form of stomach cancer is a 5-year survival rate of over 95% following resection. Furthermore, recurrence is very rare and then usually only in those with submucosal lesions. Although this entity presently accounts for one-third of all gastric cancers in Japan, far higher than appears to be the case in Western countries, its importance lies in the fact that it is becoming increasingly diagnosed elsewhere where sophisticated techniques are available, and with correspondingly excellent results.

Symptoms

Much of the pessimism surrounding the picture of stomach cancer is because almost half the patients have incurable disease when they first present themselves. There is no doubt that this picture is changing and the increasing number of cases of early gastric cancer, notably in Japan, and now being identified in Europe, is a product of public education, doctor awareness and the availability of sophisticated techniques.

The catalogue of symptoms includes mild degrees of discomfort in the epigastrium, fullness, ulcer type pains after meals or periodic discomfort unrelieved by alkalies, vomiting after meals and mild degrees of dysphagia. However vague, any of these must be investigated in all patients of middle age when they persist for more than a few days. The importance of this has been repeatedly confirmed and it is no longer acceptable medical practice for dyspepsia to be treated without investigation and the use of x-ray and or endoscopy.

Diagnostic techniques have developed greatly. Radiological accuracy has been considerably improved by the double contrast barium meal technique using a thin layer of barium in a gas distended stomach; minor mucosal alterations are thus detected more easily. A negative standard barium meal is not acceptable any longer in the presence of symptomatic dyspepsia. Endoscopy should follow any such negative x-ray and any ulcer biopsied, remembering that a negative report is not proof that malignancy is not present. An additional weapon is brush cytology, which should be added to biopsy. This technique, in the hands of experienced cytologists increases the diagnostic yield.

Finally there is a place for diagnostic laparotomy. When all other techniques have been used and clinical suspicion still exists despite a negative biopsy, recourse may be had to direct examination, manually, visually, and if necessary by opening the stomach and direct excision biopsy. Unfortunately, there are no reliable diagnostic laboratory methods available at present.

The logical extension of the search for early disease is the use of mass screening techniques. The cost effectiveness of this is unknown; one Japanese analysis demonstrated that of 3 000 000 patients examined endoscopically a little over 3000 stomach tumours were found of which half were early tumours. The evidence is not strong yet that the effort and expense is justifiable for the level of yield so far reported.

Treatment

At present the only curative method is surgical excision. The tendency towards pessimism over the results of surgery is, in a sense, borne out by the overall statistics. On the other hand, the wide variation in pathological types, differential growth rates and extent of lymph node involvement make it imperative that the fullest potential of surgical treatment should be applied whenever possible. Like breast cancer, gastric cancer presents a spectrum of diseases from a most benign form with slow growth to the rapidly advancing tumour. In the past decade there has been a widespread tendency to reduce or modify the extent of operative excision in many areas e.g. breast and rectum, but in stomach cancer increasing survival rates after surgery have repeatedly confirmed that there is every indication for taking the opposite view. A radical approach refers not only to total or subtotal removal of the stomach itself, but means the addition of *en bloc* resection of omentum, assessment and removal of the involved lymph nodes around the coeliac and hepatic arteries, removal of the spleen, and, if they are involved, the distal pancreas and colon (Fig 5.4). This view is not new, but needs to be emphasised to offset the oft-expressed advice of a minimal approach and palliative techniques because of overall poor salvage rates.

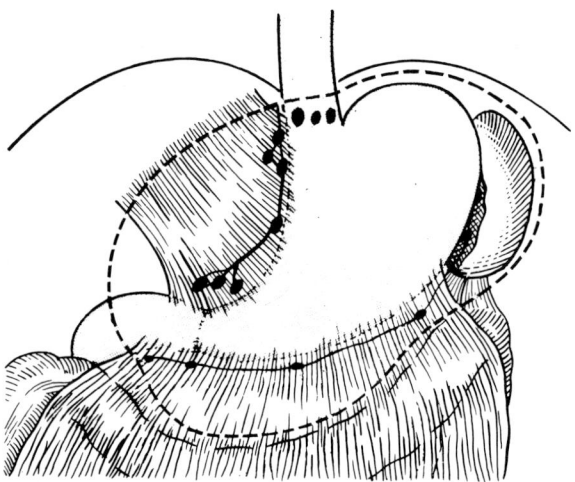

Fig 5.4 Radical total gastrectomy means removal of the whole stomach, first 3 cm of duodenum, associated lymph nodes, spleen and, if necessary, distal pancreas or colon.

Therefore, once a stomach tumour has been diagnosed, laparotomy should be carried out in all but those in the terminal stages of the disease. Age certainly is not a contra-indication and palliative excision may bring great relief even if only for a matter of months. Fortunately, operability rates have increased in recent years from around 65 to 90% and this is a reflection of readier referral to surgery of such patients, as well as of the increased interest in early diagnosis and treatment. Resectability rates, however, although showing the same upward trend, presently account for only half of all patients so diagnosed, and radical surgery is still only possible in about one-quarter of all patients.

Preoperative preparation must be meticulously carried out including restitution to near normal levels of haemoglobin, protein and electrolytes. It is particularly important to look for signs of obvious and occult weight loss reflecting poor nutrition. The major metabolic disturbance even in malnourished underweight patients is the energy deficit. Unless this is corrected, no amount of protein given by whatever route is of proven value. Thus the prime needs are firstly to estimate whether in the days before operation the patient's self-selected oral diet is sufficient, or if it should be supplemented by an easily assimilated energy source via a fine nasogastric feeding tube. In those with difficulty in swallowing or with marked anorexia, the help of a trained dietitian is valuable to establish exactly the quantity and quality of the patient's intake and secondly to restore water and electrolyte balance together with vitamin supplements and trace metals in the 48 h preceding the operation. Energy for basal needs may be given in this

period in the form of 2 l of 20% glucose solution and a third litre consisting of 9 g of protein-containing fluid. There is no clear evidence of the value of intravenous 'long-line' protein feeding using some of the present expensive preparations and the provision of 1500-2000 calories (1 cal = 4.2 J) a day for the immediate pre-operation period appear to be as satisfactory.

Pulmonary function studies are necessary in the elderly, and pre-operative breathing exercises should be taught. A significant number of gastric tumours become involved with omentum, transverse meso-colon and colon itself, so that at least the colon should be thoroughly cleansed to prepare it for possible *en bloc* resection. Barium enema may be helpful, but this depends on facilities and time available.

There is undoubtedly a significant wound infection rate following stomach cancer operations where the tumour is often heavily infected in the presence of low or absent acid values; therefore, it is wise to use peroperative antibiotics. A combination of one of the new cephalosporins such as cefotaxime 1 g i.v. 8-hourly for 3 doses together with metronidazole 500 mg i.v. 8-hourly for 3 doses, both starting at the time of induction, has proved of value.

As a general principle, the operation of choice is a radical gastrectomy, either subtotal or total. The extent of stomach removed is in part determined by the pattern of spread within the organ which is different to that occurring in the colon. In the stomach, creeping submucous extension is characteristic – often impalpable and microscopic – whereas, in the colon, distal spread is seldom more than 2-3 cm beyond the palpable limit of the lesion. Therefore, distal resection of the stomach must include not less than 3-4 cm of duodenum as at least a third of antral tumours invade across the pylorus. Proximal resection must be wide enough to include at least 6 cm of free margin. Frozen section of the resected edge is mandatory if less than this is removed, but should be regarded as good surgical practice in all cases. Inadequate local resection will result in a high proportion, 50% or more, of patients having recurrence in the gastric remnant.

A salutary lesson of the value of wide clearance and radical surgery was demonstrated by Desmond (1976) who showed that the 5-year survival in patients who were re-explored after an initial mistaken diagnosis of benign gastric tumour was more than twice as good as those in whom nothing further was done (56% and 23%).

The pattern of lymphatic spread has been emphasised by Kajitani (1968) and his extensive experience is worth reviewing. The lymph nodes are designated as first, second and third tiers of nodes (N1, N2 and N3) which is simply a modification of the system used for breast or colon. Correspondingly, gastrectomies are therefore R1, R2 or R3 resections according to the extent of lymph node removal. The results demonstrate that where N2 node involvement is found, radical surgery is more than justifiable with a 55% 5-year survival rate, whereas where N3 nodes are present the case is less compelling for radical surgery, because of markedly increased morbidity, and only a 22% 5-year survival rate.

Early tumours of the middle and distal stomach with limited lymph node involvement (N2) and no gross attachment to adjacent organs should be treated by radical subtotal removal of the stomach. Tumours at the cardia (about 15%) have a worse prognosis and are better treated by the radical total gastrectomy and oesophagojejunal anastomosis. The reason for this is the large number of these growths which spread in the submucosal space; a distal resection line in the antrum is not often free of disease, even though appearing so to touch and naked eye. Wide submucous spread occurs less often in a proximal direction in the case of distal growths.

Subtotal gastrectomy

The technique follows accepted gastric operative principles with special attention to avoidance of spillage. The method of reconstruction may be either by a direct gastroduodenal anastomosis which is less commonly performed, but which has the advantage of lessening the incidence of bilious vomiting, or by a standard Polya gastrojejunostomy. This should be placed in an antecolic position which makes involvement of the anastomosis by subsequent recurrence less likely. The anastomosis is usually made with two suture layers, either an outer silk and an inner catgut or both layers of catgut, both continuous. When a gastroduodenal anastomosis is made, it is often easier to place the outer silk layer with interrupted sutures along the posterior wall. A nasogastric tube is usual for the first 24 h. Suction drainage of the splenic bed is a wise precaution. Postoperative feeding should be delayed for 3-4 days and it is most helpful to have a preliminary gastrografin swallow to ensure that no leak is present. Postoperative mortality from this operation performed for cure, ranges worldwide from 10-25%. The five-year survival figures depend on the extent of infiltration and lymph node involvement; these average about 30%, but figures as high as 41 and 46% have been recorded (Tables 2 and 3).

Radical total gastrectomy

This is undertaken in perhaps 1 in 4 of putative curative operations. The cumulative evidence from many sources is persuasive that the method of reconstruction after total gastrectomy should consist of an end-to-side

Table 2
RESULTS OF SURGICAL TREATMENT OF CANCER OF THE STOMACH

	% Frequency	% 5-yr survival	% Op. mortality
1 Early gastric cancer	10	95	1–2
2 Good prognostic variations (*see* Table 1)	15	50–70	3–8
3 Infiltrating adenocarcinoma	60–70	25–40	10–25

Table 3
RESULTS OF GASTRECTOMY FOR CANCER OF THE STOMACH

	% 5-yr survival	% Op. mortality
Curative gastrectomy – in 25% of patients		
(a) curative radical subtotal (in 2/3)		
without nodes	40	10–18
with nodes	15–20	20–40
(b) curative radical (in 1/3)	15–20	15–40
Palliative surgery	0–2	20–25
Overall	10	33

oesophago-jejunostomy with or without an entero-enterostomy or a Roux-en-Y arrangement with at least an 18″ (40 cm) vertical limb; and a feeding jejunostomy or duodenostomy. These precautions may well provide an increase in proximal capacity and improved nutritional status, even with the simplest end-to-side arrangement with a small 3-5 cm closed off jejunal stump. The miserable complications of bile regurgitation and oesophagitis are largely avoided by a Roux-en-Y loop, and jejunal tube feeding helps reduce the heavy penalty associated with leaks at the oesophagojejunal junction which are the main cause of high early mortality.

The problems and risk following total gastrectomy are clearly defined and the surgeon undertaking this operation is obliged to take every precaution to minimise them.

Anastomotic failure is the most serious complication following total gastrectomy or oesophago-gastrectomy (7-29%), and its shadow is ever-present. Mortality following this complication is reported at least 50%. A recent 5-year study from Cardiff (Leinster and Hughes, 1980) showed 10 of 38 patients with radical resections died and 6 of these were due to anastomotic leaks at the oesophago-jejunostomy site. Many factors have been examined or implicated, including sepsis, malnutrition, hypotensive periods during operation, age and surgical technique. A recent instructive survey undertaken by Fortner produced a number of valuable observations.

In a series of 350 patients, there was an overall mortality of 21% and anastomotic dehiscence occurred in 11%, two-thirds of whom died. The incidence of anastomotic failure was as high in early as in advanced disease and, very significantly, was no higher when tumour was detectable at the proximal (oesophageal) margin of the resected specimen than in those (276) with a tumour-free edge. Technique did not appear to be statistically significant although jejunal pouch methods seems to be less prone to dehiscence. End-to-side oesophago-gastrectomy, however, definitely gave poorer results and appears to be a less safe method.

Many factors play a role but one, in particular, deserves to be stressed – the reduction in blood supply of the lower oesophagus following radical resection. No matter how masterly the technique, or free from sepsis or hypotension throughout the operation, the healing of the anastomosis, on which hangs the patient's life, depends on the remaining arterial twigs left by the surgeon. The main arterial supply of the lower oesophageal segment is primarily from the left gastric artery and the left inferior phrenic artery arising from the coeliac artery. These main sources of supply anastomose with twigs coming from the segmental oesophageal arteries which arise directly from the aorta. The left gastric artery is divided completely at its origin as an integral part of a radical gastrectomy so as to achieve as complete a removal of lymph nodes as possible. The inferior phrenic is then the only remaining major source from below and this is frequently divided during mobilisation of the lower oesophagus especially in a thoraco-abdominal approach with division of the diaphragm and wide opening of the hiatus. Thus the blood supply is invariably reduced, and often remains marginal after a total gastrectomy, and anastomotic survival then depends on the 3-4 small segmental vessels supplying the lower thoracic oesophagus (Fig 5.5).

Every surgeon has seen at autopsy a whole anterior or posterior wall of the oesophagus replaced completely by slough for 1-2 cm, or even a slough of the total circumference of the lower oesophagus after an operation where the surgeon was satisfied with the naked eye appearance of the anastomosis – 'the cut edge seemed to bleed well'. No matter how careful, meticulous or experienced the surgeon is, the viability of the oesophageal component of the anastomosis must in some degree be a matter of chance.

The only way a surgeon can attempt to reduce this lethal complication is (a) to preserve, when possible, the upper branches of the left gastric or the inferior phrenic branches, (b) avoid the use of any clamp, however non-traumatic, across the oesophagus and (c) so to buttress the anastomosis with a peritoneal surface that small dehiscences may be localised and protected in the hope of eventual closure.

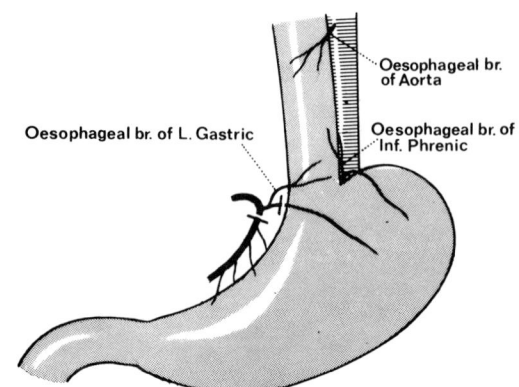

Fig 5.5 Arterial supply of the lower oesophagus (last 3 cm). *Note:* division of left gastric artery and the origin of the oesophageal branch.

It is not always possible to combine a radical resection with preservation of infradiaphragmatic arterial supply, especially with tumours high on the lesser curvature. However, whenever possible, and this applies particularly to fundic and body cancers on the greater curvature or anterior and posterior walls, the left gastric artery should be isolated, cleaned of its associated lymphatic nodes and its gastric branches ligated close to the gastric wall, so preserving the branch or branches that run up to the oesophagus (Fig 5.5). Sometimes this is not possible, but additional dissection should be attempted to test the feasibility of preserving as much blood supply as possible.

One of the pioneers of oesophageal surgery with unrivalled experience in this field, John Garlock, insisted that any clamp, however soft, applied across the oesophagus damaged the wall. He divided the oesophagus after inserting holding stay sutures and handled the cut edge with the utmost gentleness. The margin for error in this area is indeed small. Many technical modifications of reconstruction have been described. Lesley brought an anterior flap of peritoneum over the junction; Roscoe Graham's technique, first described in 1946, has largely fallen into disuse as enthusiasm for radical total gastrectomy has waned. However, the application of Graham's principle of serosal covering has been developed by a number of European surgeons, especially in Germany. The end of the oesophagus is anastomosed to the side of the jejunal loop about 3″ from its closed-off distal end. The junction is made nearer the mesenteric border so that the jejunal circumference may lie behind and above the anastomosis, so buttressing it posteriorly. Two layers of interrupted sutures usually silk and catgut or both non-absorbable are placed, taking care not to narrow the oesophageal opening. Then the free distal end of the jejunal loop is brought over the anastomosis and joined anteriorly to the ascending limb similarly rolled over the anterior surface, so covering the anastomosis with a serosal layer (Figs 5.6a, b). Some surgeons have added an entero-anastomosis to the two jejunal loops. The operation is completed by a Roux-en-Y junction (Fig 5.7).

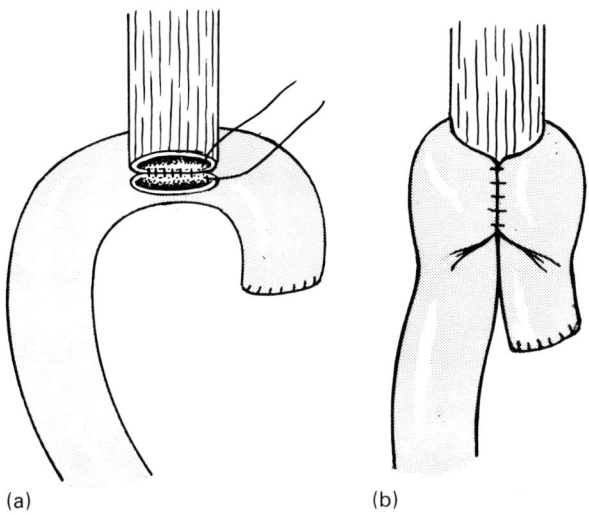

(a)   (b)

Fig 5.6 (a) Oesophagojejunal anastomosis: jejunal opening made near mesenteric border. (b) Oesophago-jejunal anastomosis: proximal and distal jejunal limbs wrapped around anastomotic site so producing a serosal covering.

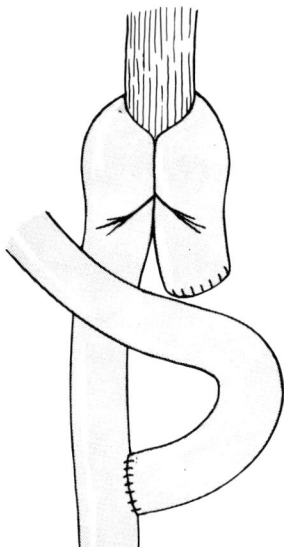

Fig 5.7 Intestinal continuity restored by a Roux-en-Y junction making a 40 cm (16″) ascending limb to minimise biliary reflux.

Using this technique, there has been a significant reduction in mortality from anastomotic leaks, with a dehiscence rate nearly halved to 6-12% and the mortality correspondingly reduced. Such results reflect the value of a peritoneal protection for a very vulnerable suture line, but they are equally a function of precise technique and expertise. There is an increasingly good case to be made for this type of radical resection, which has a mortality often higher than oesophageal resections in the chest, to be undertaken in units which have a special interest in gastric surgery or where the procedures are performed frequently. Surgeons doing occasional radical resections will inevitably have unacceptable death rates.

The correlation between prognosis and lymph node involvement has been well established. However, the observations of Cantrell (1971) are of special importance as he showed that the survival rates were related to the proportion of nodes involved. When less than half the nodes were involved the figures were 35% 5-year survival compared to 46% when no nodes were involved; but when the majority of nodes were involved the figure was 8% 5-year survival.

Palliative surgery

Careful attention should be paid to this aspect of treatment both in terms of surgical judgement and technique, as it will apply to at least 50% of all patients coming to surgery. As survival is measured in a matter of 4-8 months, radical surgery is clearly not indicated. However, the best palliation that can be offered is removal of the tumour. In some patients this produces a gratifying response for many months with relief from chronic anaemia due to bleeding and from the ill-defined toxicity of a fungating tumour. Thus palliative resection is advisable in middle and distal gastric tumours where a subtotal excision of the primary tumour can be done and a recent study from Cardiff (Leinstar and Hughes, 1980) demonstrated the same survival rates from palliative radical surgery as from curative radical surgery. Reconstruction should be by a Polya antecolic anastomosis. An alternative in distal tumours is a highly placed gastroenterostomy. In proximal third tumours, removal is justified although the mortality is high. Proximal tumours causing obstruction which are not resectable may be managed by a Roux-en-Y jejunal loop brought up behind the pancreas and anastomosed to the side of the lower oesophagus, the anastomosis thus being placed away from the tumour, or by insertion of a Celestin tube as used in oesophageal tumour obstruction. A newly described alternative is to insert a plastic prosthesis by direct vision using a small calibre endoscope after dilatation of the stricture with Eder-Puestow metal olives. If, at laparotomy there are widespread peritoneal metastases, nothing further should be done, If, however, there are a few small liver metastases, it is well worth resecting the primary tumour if possible.

Mortality from all palliative procedures is high, being in the region of 15-30% and, of note, no less following the insertion of a Celestin tube. In the absence of obstruction, palliation in terminal stages should be actively pursued. This includes adequate and regular pain relief, the use of antacids for dyspepsia, chlorpromazine and a liquid diet for nausea and vomiting. Local recurrence following gastric resection occurs in a significant number of cases. Others have reported selected groups in which recurrent gastric cancer has been resected with good palliation so that a further small group of patients may be significantly helped in the later stages of this disease.

Radiotherapy

This method has so far had little role to play. Radical treatment with 6000r has been disappointing. However, the development of radiosensitisers and their effects on hypoxic cells has led to increased interest in this method as the presence of hypoxic cells are believed to be the main foci of resistance to radiation therapy. Another method which has had encouraging reports is neutron irradiation (Catterall *et al.*, 1975); 16 or 19 palpable epigastric masses resolved, but the radiation damage to the stomach required gastrectomy in many of these. Nevertheless, these two new approaches offer interesting and exciting lines for further treatment either primary or adjunctive.

Chemotherapy

Stomach cancer has been generally considered to be resistant to chemotherapy. Recent work has shown that it is, in fact, the most sensitive and responsive area in the gastrointestinal tract. Several drugs have shown some degree of effectiveness in the presence of advanced cancer. These include fluorouracil, doxorubicin, and 1-3-bix (2-chlorbethyl)-1-nitrosourea. However, survival is hardly prolonged and complete remission is still uncommon, but enough evidence has accrued of the value of chemotherapy in some cases, and in a small group of patients unresectable lesions have become resectable, perhaps as many as 10% (Levi *et al.*, 1979).

A combined chemotherapeutic regimen has been described which consists of 5-fluorouracil (fluorouracil), mitomycin, the nitrosoureas 1,3-bis (2-chloroethyl)-1-nitrosourea (BCNU) and 1-(2-choroethyl)-3-4 methyl-cyc lohexyl-1-nitrosourea (methyl CCNU), and doxorubicin (adriamycin). This has produced an overall partial response rate of 52% with complete remission in 2 of 35 patients with advanced disease. In addition, those patients responding

to treatment have a longer time until relapse (median 48 weeks compared to median 16 weeks), during which period the disease does not progress. Thus combination chemotherapy would seem to be superior to one or two drug regimens. Myelosuppression is the main side-effect and this was significant in 30% of patients; in few did it require any treatment. Patients who do not respond after two courses of treatment should have the drug stopped, while those who show response should continue until no response is forthcoming.

It appears, therefore, that stomach tumours are more susceptible to chemotherapy than was previously thought and the evidence points to chemotherapy now beginning to establish for itself a place in the treatment of advanced disease, especially after the bulk of tumour has been resected. Two important potential roles for chemotherapy are the possibility of resection of large or irremovable tumours after response to chemotherapy and the use of these drugs as an adjuvant treatment following resection aimed at cure.

Gastric polyps

Gastric polyps have not been easy to assess in the past. The picture is clearer now with the recognition of three groups. The commonest group are regenerative polyps, usually about 1 cm, smooth surfaced and often multiple, occuring at the junction of the body and antral mucosa. These rarely undergo malignant change. The second group comprise hamartomatous polyps and heterotopias, especially aberrant pancreatic tissue. Neoplastic polyps constitute 21% of all gastric polyps. These are lobulated, single and sessile occurring in the antrum and are usually large, averaging 4 cm. They are adenomas and are liable to undergo malignant change in nearly 50%, particularly in larger lesions. It is, therefore, important that multiple sections of the adenoma should be examined for signs of tumour. Polyps which are single should be biopsied and if smooth and less than 2 cm may be left if biopsy is negative. If ulcerative, the polyp should be removed by wedge resection if shown to be benign by microscopy, or partial gastrectomy if malignant. Widespread polyposis should, if symptomatic, be treated by gastrectomy.

Other gastric tumours

Lymphoma

These represent about 5-8% of malignant tumours of the stomach. Primary gastric lymphomas predominate especially lymphosarcoma. The stomach is the most commonly involved part of the gastrointestinal tract, 30-50% in generalised lymphomatosis. A feature of these tumours is the invasion of adjacent organs and metastases to surrounding lymph nodes. Lateral spread of the tumour along the stomach wall is also more common and extensive than vertical penetration through the wall. Multiple foci are demonstrated histologically in two-thirds of cases.

Symptomatically there are a number of distinguishing features dependent upon the fact that orifices are seldom involved and, therefore, vomiting and dysphagia are not common. Weight loss, however, is often disproportionate and ulcer-type pain is frequent. The importance of biopsy as a diagnostic tool is apparent with the increasing pre-operative diagnosis of the disease.

The principles of treatment are similar to those of cancer of the stomach and all resectable cases should be so treated. The particular feature of this tumour is its radiosensitivity, although this is not uniformly so in all gastric lymphomas. Nevertheless, every case should have postoperative radiotherapy. The overall survival rate is in the region of 50% 5-year survival and 30% 10-year survival, being somewhat better, therefore, than cancer of the stomach.

Non-lymphomatous tumours include leiomyosarcomas and, more rarely, apudomas arising from endocrine cells scattered throughout the gastrointestinal tract some of which are in the stomach (*see* chapter 37). The leiomyosarcomas are distinctively slow growing, well differentiated tumours with a relatively better prognosis after resection. The apudomas arise in the stomach from the G cells and are gastrinomas. These are similar in their behaviour to the gastrin producing tumours of the pancreatic islets.

Volvulus of the stomach

The stomach can undergo volvulus around two axes – either the long axis (organoaxial) or the transverse axis (mesenteroaxial). In some examples, there is a specific predisposing factor such as adhesions, but in the majority the only abnormality is considerable laxity of the mesenteric attachments of the stomach, and of the duodenal attachments in the mesenteroaxial variety. In the organoaxial variety, the transverse colon is often included in the volvulus, with the colon and stomach rotating upwards and entering a large hiatal hernial sac which is frequently present.

Most patients present with a history of attacks of profuse vomiting and upper abdominal cramping pains which may start and stop abruptly. The correct diagnosis can be difficult to make unless the radiologist is alive to the possibility when he does the barium meal and moves the patient in different ways to assess the mobility of the stomach. Very rarely, volvulus presents as an acute abdominal emergency requiring urgent operation to avert the risk of gastric necrosis.

The treatment of recurrent attacks is by operation at which the surgeon sutures the stomach to the abdominal wall to prevent further twisting or performs either a partial gastrectomy or gastrojejunostomy. Disappointment with the results of these operations has led to the development of an operation in which the surgeon divides the gastrocolic omentum and fixes the transverse colon in the left subphrenic space to prevent the stomach rotating upwards.

Adult hypertrophic pyloric stenosis

This is a rare condition usually seen in the geriatric age group. There is considerable thickening of the wall around the pylorus and a barium meal shows a dilated stomach emptying slowly through the relatively long, thin and featureless channel. The nature of the condition is unknown. The clinical features are those of pyloric stenosis, but without the preceding history of intermittent dyspepsia. Treatment is surgical – either gastrojejunostomy or Polya partial gastrectomy.

Gastric and duodenal diverticula

Gastric diverticula are uncommon and are usually found by chance at a barium meal for epigastric symptoms. They are rarely the cause of the patient's complaints. Other conditions must be sought before contemplating excision of the diverticulum which can be hazardous.

There are two types of duodenal diverticulum (excluding those associated with the deformity of chronic duodenal ulcer). Small whole thickness diverticula are quite often seen at the ampulla of Vater in cholangiography. They are of no significance except that failure to recognise them may lead to misinterpretation of the x-rays. Similarly, diverticula arising from the concavity of the second and third parts of the duodenum are quite often found on a barium study in the middle-aged or elderly. Even though they can be quite large and occasionally multiple, it is unsafe to attribute clinical problems to them until all other possibilities have been ruled out. There are some well documented causes in which they have been found to be a cause of quite severe bleeding.

References and further reading

Baron J.H. (1978). *Clinical Tests of Gastric Secretion*. London: Macmillan

Brander W.L., Needham P.R.G., Morgan A.D. (1947). Indolent mucoid carcinoma of the stomach. *J. Clin Pathol*; **27**:536–41.

Bushkin F.L., Woodward E.R. (1977). *Post Gastrectomy Syndromes*. Philadelphia: W.B. Saunders.

Cantrell E.G. (1971). The importance of lymph nodes in the assessment of gastric carcinoma at operation. *Brit. J. Surg*; **58**:384–6.

Catterall M., Kingsley D., Lawrence G., Grainger J., Spencer J. (1975). The effects of fast neutrons on inoperable carcinoma of the stomach. *Gut*; **16**:150–6.

Cox A.G., Alexander-Williams J., eds (1973). *Vagotomy on Trial*. London: Heinemann Medical.

Desmond A.M. (1976). Radical surgery in treatment of carcinoma of stomach. *Proc. Roy. Soc. Med*; **69**:867–9.

Fromm D. (1977). *Complications of Gastric Surgery*. Chichester: J. Wiley.

Johnson A.G., Reynolds K.W. (1979). *Techniques of Vagotomy*. London: Edward Arnold.

Kajitani T. (1968). Results of surgical treatment of gastric carcinoma. Gann Monograph Ser; **3**:245–51.

Lauren P. (1965). The two histological main types of gastric carcinoma: diffuse and so-called intestinal type carcinoma. An attempt at a histo-chemical classification. *Acta Pathol. Microbiol. Scand*; **64**:31–49.

Leinster S.J., Hughes L.E. (1980). The role of resection in advanced gastric cancer. *Clin. Oncol*; **6**:55–61.

Levi J.A., Dalley D.N., Aroney R.S. (1979). Improved combination chemotherapy in advanced gastric cancer. *Brit. Med. J*; **2**:1471–3.

McNeer G., Pack G.T. (1967). *Neoplasms of the Stomach*. Philadelphia: J.B. Lippincott.

Morson B.C., Dawson T.M.P. (1979). Benign epithelial tumours and 'polyps'. In *Gastrointestinal Pathology*. pp. 140–7. Oxford: Blackwell Scientific Publications.

Murakami T. (1971). Pathomorphologic diagnosis: definition and gross classification of early gastric cancer. In *Early Gastric Cancer* (Marakami T., ed.) pp. 53–5. Gann Monograph on Cancer Research 11. Tokyo: University of Tokyo Press.

Nyhus L.M., Wastell C., eds (1976). *Surgery of the Stomach and Duodenum*, 3rd edn. Boston: Little, Brown.

Papachristou D.N., Fortner J.G. (1979). Anastomotic failure complicating total gastrectomy and oesophagogastrectomy for cancer of the stomach. *Amer. J. Surg*; **138**:399–402.

Stammers F.A.R., Williams J.A. (1963). *Partial Gastrectomy*. London: Butterworths.

Steiner P.D., Maimon S.N., Palmer W.L., Kirsner J.B. (1948). Gastric cancer: morphologic factors in five-year survival after gastrectomy. *Amer. J. Pathol*; **24**:947–69.

Stout A.P. (1945). Superficial spreading types of carcinoma of the stomach. *J. Nat. Cancer Instit*; **5**:363.

Wastell C. (1974). *Chronic Duodenal Ulcer*. London: Butterworths.

Williams J. Alexander, Cox A.G., eds (1969). *After Vagotomy*. London: Butterworths.

6

Liver and biliary system

ALAN G. JOHNSON

There are two important areas of surgical anatomy that must be understood by any surgeon working in this field. The first is the basic 'lobe' structure of the liver and the second is the marked variability of the extrahepatic bile ducts and vessels which is discussed on p. 122 (Balasegaram, 1970; Rob and Smith, 1977).

The liver is a paired organ with right and left halves, or lobes, having their own main branches of hepatic artery, bile duct and portal vein. The plane between left and right lobes passes through the gallbladder anteriorly, and inferior vena cava posteriorly, and lies to the right of the falciform ligament (Fig 6.1). Each

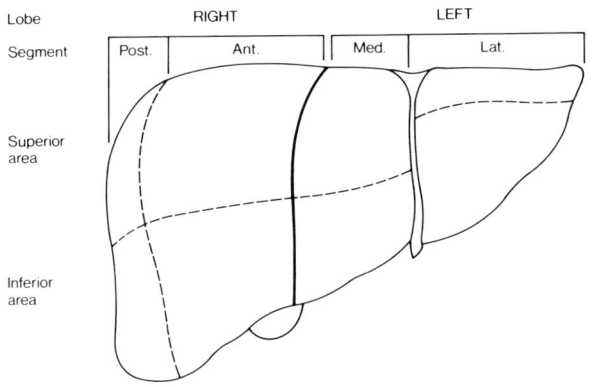

Fig 6.1 Diagram of the basic lobe structure of the liver.

half is divided into segments, but they are not so clearly defined as in the lung and resection is usually limited to either a local wedge resection without ligating major vessels or a right or left hepatic lobectomy; sometimes that part of the left lobe lateral to the falciform ligament is removed preserving the medial part of the left lobe (left lateral segmentectomy). The liver surrounding the porta hepatis is peripheral in anatomical terms and, therefore, can be divided or removed for better access without encountering large vessels (*see* p. 116). The intrahepatic *arteries* are not entirely end arteries, as there are some translobar and subcapsular collaterals. The hepatic arteries contribute 25% of the hepatic blood supply and the portal veins 75% (30–35% of oxygen requirement). The hepatic *veins* occupy an interlobar position and drain into the inferior vena cava (IVC). There is usually a large right hepatic vein and a smaller left hepatic vein which may be joined by a middle vein, or this may enter the IVC separately. These main veins have a very short extrahepatic course if any. In addition, there are several small veins draining into the IVC throughout its course. The anatomy of the portal veins is discussed in the next chapter.

Liver injuries

Damage to the liver must always be suspected with any abdominal or right chest injuries, whether due to blunt trauma, penetration by a knife or bullet, or deceleration (Watt, 1978). Any penetrating injury of the abdominal wall or chest must be thoroughly explored under general anaesthesia. Closed trauma is more difficult to diagnose and intraperitoneal bleeding may be delayed, although not as often as with splenic injuries (Mays, 1976).

Spreading peritonism and right shoulder-tip pain are classical signs and symptoms, but may be difficult to elicit when there is multiple trauma and associated head injury. Often increasing shock, otherwise unexplained, alerts the surgeon. Peritoneal lavage, if positive for blood, will confirm the diagnosis of intraperitoneal bleeding and a liver scan or ultrasonography may occasionally help when the diagnosis is in doubt.

Treatment

Resuscitation

Rapid replacement of the blood loss is the first priority, but liver bleeding can be so rapid that it may be unwise to delay operation until the blood pressure has recovered.

Operation

It is important to be prepared with the correct instruments (*see below*) as well as with sufficient surgical expertise for liver surgery, before exploring an abdomen for trauma. With the increasing use of high velocity bullets, a small entry wound into the liver may conceal extensive intrahepatic damage. In the same way, the size of a stellate tear on the surface due to blunt trauma may be misleading.

The two principles in evaluating a liver injury at operation are:

1 Obtain sufficient exposure, by a lateral extension of a mid-line or paramedian incision, and by dividing the peritoneal reflections, so that the superior and inferior surfaces of the liver can be palpated and inspected. A right thoracotomy is required to visualise the posterior surface and hepatic veins.
2 Palpate the liver carefully to assess the internal damage. The index finger must not be inserted into a tear without great care, otherwise bleeding may restart. If there is an extensive gelatinous mass, rather than firm liver tissue, a major resection may be required. To close the superficial wound in these circumstances, even if bleeding is controlled, will lead to abscess formation and perhaps secondary haemorrhage. Packing a deep liver wound with absorbable sponge is not satisfactory and can also lead to abscess and secondary haemorrhage. However, occasionally effective packing may be life-saving when it is used to control bleeding

temporarily while a patient is transported to a larger hospital or when there is injury to both lobes of the liver precluding resection. The packs are cautiously removed several days later at a *second* laparotomy.

Procedures

There are three possible procedures: simple suture; some form of resection; hepatic artery ligation (Blumgart *et al.*, 1979).

Small tears, particularly of the peripheral parts of the liver, may be treated by simple suture over liver buffers (Fig 6.8) (Wood *et al.*, 1976). If there is pulped liver substance or the tissue lateral to a larger tear is nonviable, a resection is required. It is when most of a lobe is involved that a decision has to be made whether to risk a hemihepatectomy or rely on hepatic artery ligation. Whatever the procedure, good postoperative drainage is essential. Techniques of liver resection are given below (*see* p. 115), but most cases of trauma can be dealt with by resectional debridement rather than formal hemihepatectomy.

Some surgeons recommend right or left hepatic artery ligation as the treatment of choice to stop bleeding from one or other lobe. They argue that the risks are less than the high mortality of major emergency resection, except in the most experienced hands under ideal conditions. Selective ligation should always be considered as an alternative to resection by surgeons with less experience and in hospitals without full intensive care facilities. Once the bleeding is controlled, the patient can be transferred to a larger centre. However, often the bleeding is from portal veins or hepatic veins and hepatic artery ligation will not stop the haemorrhage. A resection may be required for later complications, but it can then be done electively in a non-shocked patient. When selective hepatic artery ligation is done, the two main branches must be carefully isolated and distinguished from each other and the gall-bladder removed (with right-sided ligation) to prevent ischaemic necrosis.

Postoperative complications

Can the hepatic artery or portal vein be ligated with safety to stop bleeding?

There has been much discussion on these subjects, but certain conclusions are generally agreed:

1 Ligation of both the main hepatic artery and main portal vein is fatal.
2 The main portal vein can be ligated without liver necrosis but with (temporary) portal hypertension.
3 Hepatic artery ligation in the presence of normal

portal flow does not necessarily lead to hepatic necrosis unless the patient is shocked or there is significant pre-existing cirrhosis.

Injury to bile ducts and major vessels

These must always be suspected and searched for, especially with penetrating injuries, and pancreatic tears are not uncommon (*see* Ch. 44). Damage to the vena cava and hepatic veins is the most serious problem and may be uncontrollable unless the liver is quickly and adequately mobilised as described above. Temporary control may be obtained by inserting a large Foley catheter into the vena cava through a purse string in the wall above the renal veins and below the liver. The balloon is inflated at the level of the diaphragm and flow from below is controlled by a tape encircling the IVC. Alternatively, a large silicone rubber catheter can be inserted and held with tapes above and below the injury; this, unlike the Foley catheter, will allow venous return to the heart, but usually such procedures are academic as the patient is already exsanguinated. The structures in the porta hepatis and free border of the lesser omentum must be carefully inspected and tears of the common bile duct closed over a T-tube. More extensive damage of the bile ducts requires reconstruction by one of the methods described below (p. 132).

Hepato-cellular failure

Liver failure may result from fulminating hepatitis or advanced cirrhosis, but the surgeon meets the problem most acutely in the first few days after massive hepatic resection for injury or tumour. Fig 6.2 shows the post-operative biochemical changes. Functional recovery takes about 3 weeks, so intensive support must be given during this time. In fully established failure, the patient is hypoglycaemic, comatose, jaundiced with ascites and has a bleeding tendency. The surgeon's aim is to prevent these problems by anticipating four main changes:

1   *Hypoglycaemia*, because much of the stored glycogen has been removed. Glucose 10% should be given i.v. during the first few days.

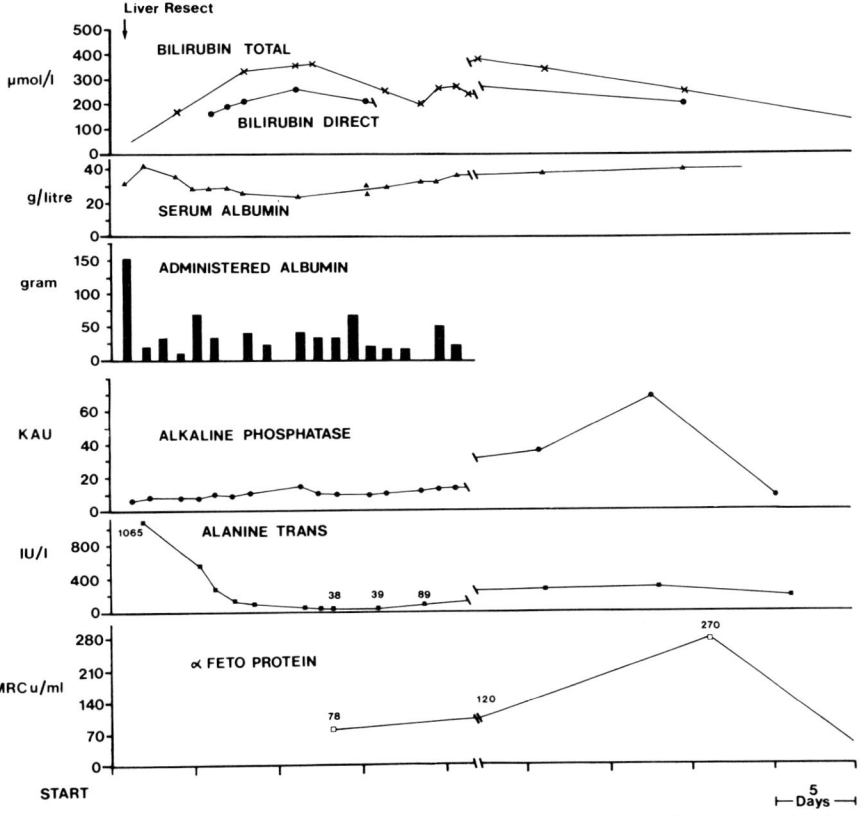

Fig 6.2 Diagram of the biochemical changes following right hepatic lobectomy for trauma.

2 *Hypoalbuminaemia*, because of failure to synthesise albumin. This will have to be given i.v. during the first week to maintain the intravascular osmotic pressure (*see* Fig 6.2 for an example of the albumin requirements).

3 *Jaundice*, because the residual liver cannot cope with the bilirubin load particularly after massive transfusion. Often there is also a raised alkaline phosphatase that does not parallel the bilirubin levels. The jaundice itself is not very important provided it resolves as the liver regenerates, but failure to do so suggests some biliary obstruction.

4 *Disorders of clotting factors*. Vit K synthesis will be reduced giving a prolonged prothrombin time and fibrinogen synthesis is defective. These changes can be improved by administration of Vit K and fresh frozen plasma (FFP). Platelets may also be required.

In patients with liver failure from any cause, intravenous normal (physiological) saline should be avoided as it merely increases the oedema and ascites; and drugs metabolised in the liver, particularly the opiates and other sedatives, must be given with great caution. An H_2 antagonist is important in preventing so-called gastric 'stress' ulceration.

Artificial liver support

Unfortunately extracorporeal liver support systems, whether dialysis, charcoal column, or perfusion through pig liver have not yet provided an effective answer to liver failure.

Hepatic regeneration following major resection

The liver has remarkable powers of regeneration and in man this is probably complete in 3–4 months. The regenerated part is round and bulbous and its progress can be followed on scintiscan. It is not clear yet whether portal blood flow, gastrointestinal hormones or other humoral factors are most important in stimulating regeneration and present knowledge comes mainly from animal work rather than man. The alpha feto protein level in the serum gives an indication of liver cell turnover and it is very high in the first few days of regeneration and returns to normal when regeneration ceases (Fig 6.2).

Classification of investigations used in diagnosis of liver and biliary disease

Over the last few years, an increasing number of investigations has been developed, with a welcome trend towards non-invasive methods (*Lancet*, 1979), but there has been a tendency to add the new to the existing tests rather than substitute them (Smith, 1974). This is because the new must be evaluated against the old and no two tests show the same thing: some just show anatomical abnormalities while others depend on hepatic and biliary function. The list given here is to show the benefits and limitations of each and, in subsequent sections, a guide will be given to the most appropriate investigations for each clinical problem (Triger, 1981).

Radiology

Plain film

This shows calcified gallstones in about 15% of cases or calcification in the liver as with an old hydatid cyst.

Oral cholecystogram

This depends on intestinal absorption, liver secretion and gallbladder concentration of the contrast medium and is, therefore, of no use in jaundiced patients and in some patients with liver disease without jaundice. A number of 'accidents' can occur to give an apparently non-filling gallbladder, such as the patient not taking or vomiting the capsules, or eating afterwards, and so emptying the gallbladder. Before assuming that non-opacification means a stone impacted in Hartmann's pouch or chronic cholecystitis, it is wise to repeat the examination with a double dose of contrast medium. An oral cholecystogram does not show the bile ducts reliably and giving a fatty meal merely confirms that the gallbladder contracts and that any apparent stones remain within the gallbladder outline.

Intravenous cholangiogram (IVC)

IVC depends on liver secretion, but not on gallbladder concentration of the medium and is, again, of no use in moderately or heavily jaundiced patients; but if the jaundice is fading, satisfactory radiographs can be obtained. However, the opacification of the bile ducts is not usually very good and tomograms are needed to produce adequate pictures of stones in the ducts. Although it is relatively non-invasive, a significant number of patients have anaphylactic reactions to the intravenous injection and it is an investigation being used less in many centres, giving way to the following two methods of introducing contrast medium directly into the ducts.

Percutaneous transhepatic cholangiogram (PTC)

This is the direct puncture of a bile duct within the liver via the skin and injection of contrast medium into the duct. This gives a far greater concentration in the ducts than IVC. If the ducts are dilated, the investigation is technically successful in 99% of cases, but with non-dilated ducts the figure is 50–60%. With the larger needle the incidence of bleeding and bile leak from the puncture meant that a surgeon had to be available to operate afterwards should the need arise. With the newer Chiba ('skinny') needle this risk is not so great, but patients should still be kept in hospital for at least 24 h afterwards. Broad spectrum antibiotics are given before the x-ray to prevent septicaemia.

Endoscopic retrograde cholangiopancreatography (ERCP)

The bile duct is cannulated through the ampulla via the flexible duodenoscope. This has the advantage that the ampulla itself can be inspected to exclude a carcinoma, but has the disadvantage that the state of the proximal ducts above an obstructing stone or stricture cannot be seen, and it demands greater technical expertise than PTC.

Operative cholangiography

This is normally performed by passing a cannula through the cystic duct into the CBD and not only shows up suspected or unsuspected stones in the CBD, but also identifies anatomical anomalies before the main dissection is started (*see* p. 124). However, x-rays must be technically of very good quality or they may give the surgeon a false sense of security.

Arteriography

Selective hepatic arteriograms can show up abnormal tumour circulation in the liver, displacement of vessels by a cyst or vascular anomalies. It is an essential investigation if major liver surgery is being considered, but is not used initially.

Isotope scanning

The use of isotopes taken up by various liver cells is an attractive investigation because it is non-invasive, involves minimal radiation to the patient and is relatively cheap in terms of the expendable items once the equipment is installed. There are four substances in common use:

1 Technetium 99^m labelled sulphur colloid which is taken up by the Kupffer cells of the reticuloendothelial system and shows the structure of the liver. Areas that contain no Kupffer cells, such as secondary carcinomatous deposits, show as 'cold' areas.

2 More recently, Technetium labelled millimicrospheres of aggregated albumin in colloid solution have been used in place of sulphur colloid.

3 HIDA (2:6 dimethyl phenyl carbamyl methyl amino diacetic acid) labelled with ^{99m}Tc is secreted in the bile and therefore shows up the bile ducts. However, it shows up delay in flow down the ducts but is not as clear as PTC in showing filling defects or strictures. It is not widely used routinely, although some claim it is more effective than either oral cholecystography or ultrasound in diagnosing acute cholecystitis by the absence of a gallbladder image. Delay in imaging the common bile duct suggests a stone in the duct or other form of obstruction. A newer, alternative isotope is ^{99m}Tc-pyridoxylidene glutamate.

4 Rose Bengal labelled with ^{131}I or ^{123}I is taken up by the bile-secreting cells and, therefore, shows the architecture of the liver in a similar way to (1) and (2).

Figure 6.3 shows the information given by three different investigations in a case of a cyst of the liver.

Ultrasound

As techniques and experience improve, this reliably can show dilated bile ducts inside and outside the liver, gallstones in ducts or gallbladder, filling defects in the liver and whether they are solid or cystic. Imaging is made difficult by overlying gas shadows, but it does not depend on liver function. The prefix 'B mode, grey scale', refers to the method of imaging.

Computerised axial tomography (CAT scan)

This newest technique of all shows structure not function; like ultrasound, it is entirely non-invasive, but it does employ ionising radiation. Structural abnormalities of the liver such as cysts, abscesses and primary and secondary tumours are well shown. Its expense is likely to limit its general availability and it remains to be seen whether it is really superior to high quality ultrasound. Figure 6.4 (p. 114) shows a CAT scan of a large, benign liver tumour.

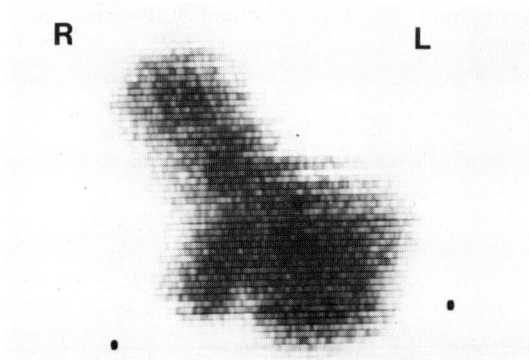

(a)

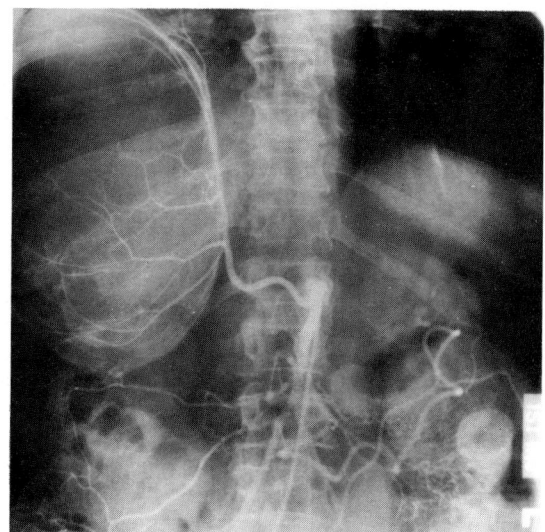

(b)

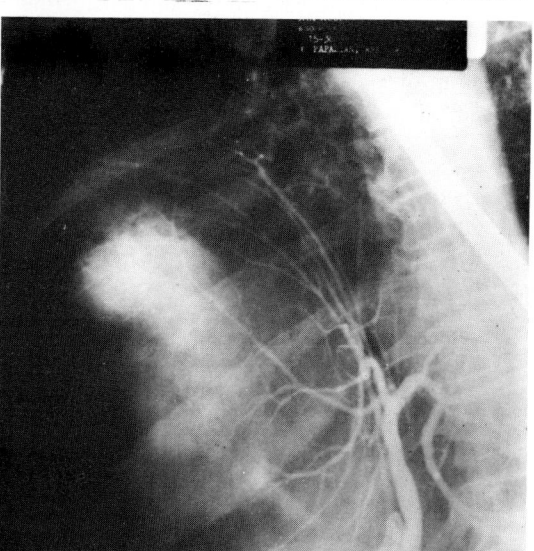

(c)

Biochemical tests

The traditional 'liver function tests' have their place in diagnosis, but it is *not* true that obstructive jaundice can always be distinguished from hepatitis by a raised alkaline phosphatase and low levels of liver enzymes. Drug induced cholestasis can produce a mixed picture and in severe liver failure, the enzyme levels may drop as the patient's condition worsens. In general, the *changes* in liver function tests during the course of an illness are more significant than the absolute levels on one occasion.

Those most commonly used are:

Bilirubin (not now normally divided into direct and indirect Van den Bergh).

Alkaline phosphatase (normally secreted in the bile). This can now be distinguished from bone alkaline phosphatase by estimation of 5-nucleotidase. It is often raised with liver secondaries from a distant primary.

Aspartate aminotransferase (SGOT) released by liver cell damage

Alanine aminotransferase (SGPT) released by liver cell damage

γ-glutamyl transferase, an index of microsomal enzyme activity is elevated in intra- or extrahepatic obstruction and by substances such as phenobarbitone and ethanol.

Total serum protein and albumin (indicates liver cell synthesis).

Haematological tests

The most useful and important is the prothrombin time as an indication of defective Vit K synthesis and risk of haemorrhage during operation. The hepatitis B antigen should be measured in all jaundiced patients and those with liver disease. Before the result is known, disposable gloves should be used for venesection and other reasonable precautions taken. If the surgeon does prick his finger while operating on a patient who is

---

Fig 6.3 (a) Technetium scan of liver showing large filling defect in right lobe. (b) Hepatic arteriogram of same patient showing filling defect to be an avascular cyst displacing the arteries. (c) ERCP showing displacement of the intrahepatic bile ducts but contrast filling the cyst indicating a communication with a duct.

hepatitis B antigen positive, hyperimmune globulin can be given.

Electroencephalogram (EEG)

In hepatic encephalopathy the EEG initially shows slowing of the rhythm, progressing to theta activity. These are non-specific, but progress later, as coma deepens, to the characteristic triphasic waves. While not being essential for diagnosis, the EEG may have a prognostic value, gross changes being associated with a poor chance of recovery.

Liver tumours

The general picture of malignant liver tumours has been depressing (Smith 1979b). Most are multiple secondary tumours, when resection is not possible and primary hepatomas, if resectable, may require very extensive surgery (Ong and Chan, 1976). However, the better understanding of liver physiology and the effects of resection have made it possible to remove 80% of the liver substance (Bismuth and Malt, 1979). Newer methods of palliating unresectable tumours are being developed and there is hope for the future.

Liver tumours may be classified (Anthony, 1978) as shown in Table 1

Of the benign tumours, haemangioma and adenoma are the most important. Haemangiomata in children may cause heart-failure through arterio-venous shunting, or may give severe pain due to spontaneous thrombosis or intrahepatic bleeding. They also may cross the anatomical lobes of the liver making operation very difficult. To biopsy a haemangioma can be disastrous and highlights the place of arteriograms in assessing liver tumours before biopsy. At operation the ability to empty them by pressure gives the clue. Benign adenomas may present with intraperitoneal bleeding, as a palpable lump, or as an incidental finding at operation. The smaller tumours can be removed by local excision without the need for ligating major vessels.

Hepatocellular carcinoma (loosely termed 'hepatoma') is the most common malignant liver tumour and is very common in parts of Africa and South-East Asia where it coexists with macronodular cirrhosis and occurs at a relatively young age (about 40 years). In the West it is rare, but it may become more common possibly due to the large increase in the use of steroid contraceptives (*see below*) in non-cirrhotic patients and to prolonged survival of alcoholic and hepatitis B associated cirrhotic patients, owing to better treatment. The high incidence in Africa (Terblanche, 1977) is associated with chronic hepatitis B infection in 70% and the ingestion of aflatoxin produced by the moulds, *Aspergillus flavus* and *parasiticus*, which contaminate foods such as maize and groundnuts. Neither bilharzia nor malnutrition is associated with the development of hepatocellular carcinoma. Men are more commonly affected than women and the hepatitis infection may be acquired in early childhood and macronodular cirrhosis may be more prone to malignant change than the micronodular cirrhosis that is commonly associated with alcoholic liver disease.

Macroscopically, the tumour may be a single expanding mass, multinodular or diffuse; the latter two forms metastasise early and are usually inoperable. Indeed, any tumour in the presence of significant cirrhosis is usually inoperable, because the cirrhosis precludes major resection. It is the younger patient with a single expanding tumour who may well be helped by early diagnosis and surgical treatment. Presentation may be with non-specific symptoms such as intermittent pain, worse after food, anorexia, malaise and fever or, occasionally, by sudden haemorrhage. Weight loss is usual. An enlarged liver may be felt or a mass in an already enlarged liver, with or without ascites, but pre-existing cirrhosis is apt to confuse the physical signs. The presence of jaundice is a poor prognostic sign. In view of the frequency with which liver tumours give non-specific symptoms, especially in the early stages, the surgeon must always bear such a diagnosis in mind.

Angiosarcoma is rare, but has a well documented association with exposure to vinyl chloride or thorotrast and there may be a very long latent period. Cholangiocarcinoma of the extrahepatic bile ducts is discussed on p. 131. Intrahepatic cholangiocarcinomas present in the same way as other primary malignant tumours and may be multifocal.

Table 1

	Benign	Malignant
Epithelial tumours	Liver cell adenoma	Liver cell (hepatocellular) carcinoma
	Bile duct adenoma	Bile duct (cholangio) carcinoma
	Bile duct cystadenoma	Bile duct cystadenocarcinoma
		Hepatoblastoma
Non-epithelial tumours	Haemangioma	Haemangiosarcoma
	Infantile haemangioendothelioma	Embryonal sarcoma leiomyo- and other sarcomas
Miscellaneous	Mesenchymal haemartoma	
	Teratoma	

Investigation of liver tumours

Liver function tests

These may not be abnormal in primary liver tumours unless there is associated cirrhosis or obstruction of a main bile duct. However, a high level of α-fetoprotein is present in 80% of liver cell carcinoma in Africa and in 40% in Europe and the USA and elevated alkaline phosphatase is a common abnormality. The patient should always be screened for hepatitis B antigen.

Isotope scanning

One of the first investigations of a suspected liver mass, isotope scanning can show whether the tumour is single or multiple, but it cannot determine the nature of the mass. It may be difficult to interpret in the presence of severe cirrhosis because the uptake is so patchy.

Ultrasound or CAT scan (Fig 6.4)

These can distinguish between a cyst and a solid filling defect, and ultrasound is now taking over from isotope scanning as the first investigation.

Other investigations

Selective coeliac arteriogram. If a tumour is suspected, a selective coeliac arteriogram should be the next investigation to show an avascular area or a tumour (Figs 6.3 and 6.5). This is essential, if operation is contemplated in order to establish the blood supply

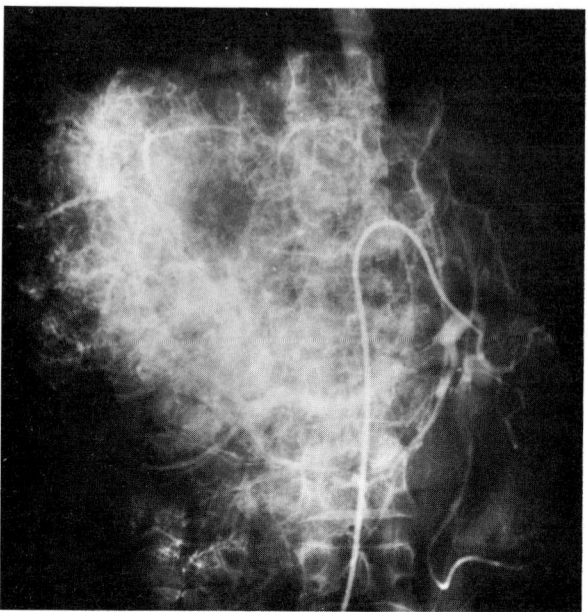

Fig 6.5 Selective hepatic arteriogram of massive malignant liver tumour showing abnormal tumour circulation.

of the tumour and any anomalies of the main vessels passing to the liver. Before resection, the involvement of the vena cava, hepatic veins and portal veins can be checked by *venography* and the diagnosis must be confirmed by histology. *Percutaneous needle biopsy* or *laparoscopic biopsy* under direct vision will make the histological diagnosis, but they should be done with caution when the tumour is very vascular.

Tumours causing bile duct obstruction are investigated initially as described under obstructive jaundice (*see below*). The surgeon should always remember that a primary malignant liver tumour can give secondaries elsewhere – in lungs and bone – and so the appropriate x-rays or scans should be done before attempting a radical resection.

This seems a formidable series of investigations and is only justified if there is a real chance of resection with cure or prolonged palliation.

Is the tumour operable?

The resectability of primary malignant liver tumours varies in different parts of the world from 2 to 17%. A tumour is considered inoperable if the inferior vena cava, or both main branches of the portal vein are invaded; if there is tumour in both lobes of the liver; or if there are metastases outside the liver. However, if

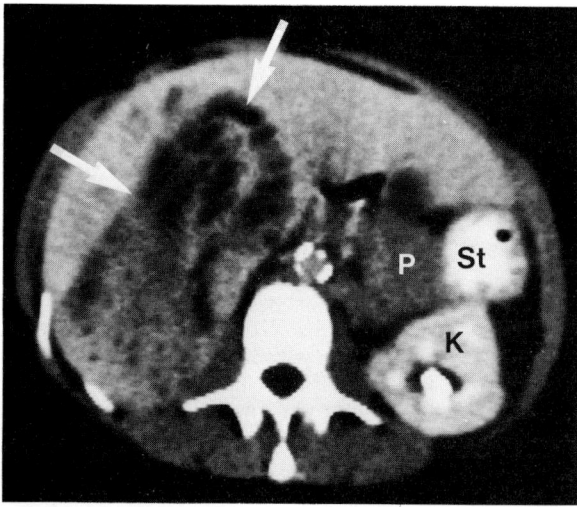

Fig 6.4 CAT scan of large, benign liver tumour with cystic changes (arrowed). St = stomach; P = pancreas; K = right kidney.

both portal vein and hepatic artery are invaded on the same side, but not on the other side, the tumour is still operable. Hepatocellular carcinoma complicating cirrhosis is nearly always inoperable on presentation as, even if it is confined to one lobe, the remaining diseased liver cannot support life and does not regenerate. Palliative measures such as infusion of cytotoxic drugs (eg. split dose adriamycin or 5-fluorouracil) may be used for unresectable tumours.

Hepatic disease and steroids

A number of hepatic lesions are associated with the taking of contraceptive and anabolic steroids. Liver cell adenomas are being reported in increasing numbers in women on 'the pill' and there is evidence to suggest that a woman of 27 or older who has taken a high-dose oral contraceptive for longer than 7 years has a 500-fold increased risk compared with the normal population. The evidence for liver cell carcinoma and hepatoblastoma is not so definite, but gives cause for anxiety when there may be a latent period of many years. Focal nodular hyperplasia, although not a liver tumour, is also associated with 'the pill'. Peliosis hepatis is a rare complication of anabolic steroids, but is more commonly seen in the proximity of liver tumours. It consists of varying sized blood-filled cysts in otherwise normal liver tissue. They may communicate with a central vein and occasionally rupture into the peritoneal cavity.

Major liver resection

It must be stressed that an inexperienced surgeon must beware of doing a laparotomy for suspected liver trauma or tumour without experienced help at hand.

Incision

A right paramedian or bilateral subcostal ('roof top') incision (Fig 6.6) is adequate for the initial exploration, but a right thoracic extension with division of the diaphragm may be required to expose the vena cava. Some surgeons recommend a median sternotomy extension to avoid opening either pleural cavity.

Special equipment

For any liver resection, a specialised liver clamp is important (Fig 6.7). Due to the cross-sectional shape, ordinary intestinal clamps will only compress one edge or the other. The other very useful recent invention is the absorbable liver buffer to hold sutures at the edge and compress the liver tissues tight enough to stop bleeding (Fig 6.8).

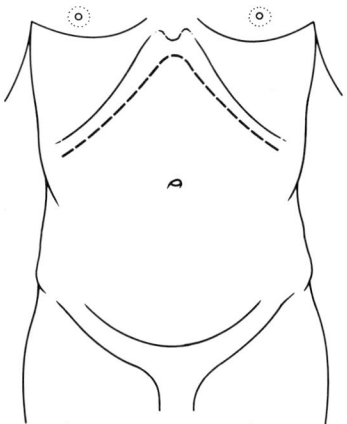

Fig 6.6 'Roof top' incision for access to liver.

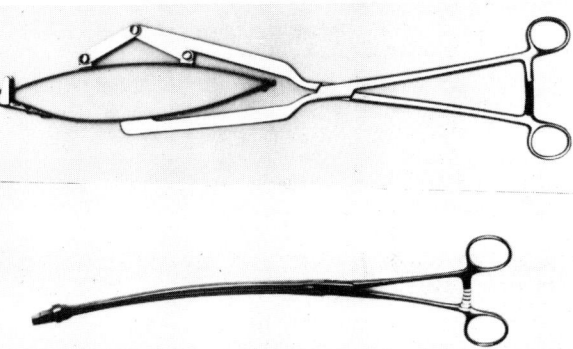

Fig 6.7 Specialised liver clamps: Longmire (*above*); Balasegaram (*below*).

Resections for trauma

The really difficult decision is whether or not a major resection is required and this has to be made on many criteria such as the position of the injury, the patient's condition, the theatre and intensive care facilities and the surgeon's experience. The mortality of major resection is very high in severely shocked patients and it must only be done when any other procedure is more dangerous. The place of selective hepatic artery ligation has been discussed above.

The following procedure is suitable for limited peripheral trauma:

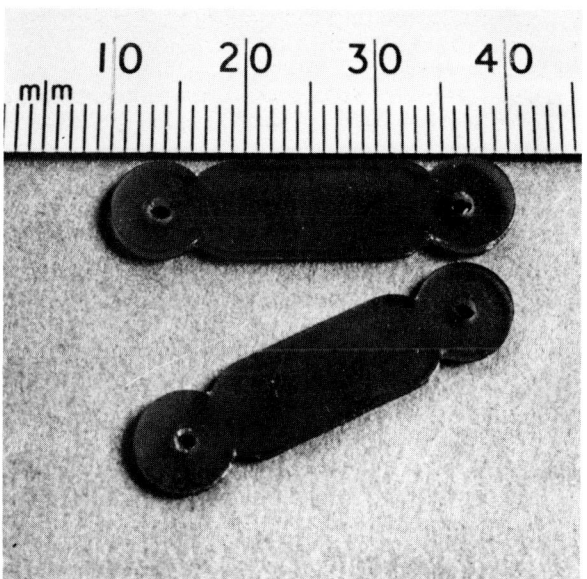

Fig 6.8 Absorbable liver buffers. (Illustration by courtesy of Ethicon Ltd.).

Resectional debridement for injuries of peripheral parts of the right or left lobe merely means removing the already pulped liver edge by *blunt* dissection and securing haemostasis with a combination of ligatures, clips and sutures over liver buffers.

Resections for trauma or tumour

Segmental resection is the removal of part of a lobe without securing the major vessels, but is a more formal procedure than resectional debridement. Neither is appropriate for central stellate ruptures. Left lateral segmentectomy means resecting the liver to the left of the falciform ligament.

Right or left lobectomy is resection through the central anatomical plane to the right of the falciform ligament (*see* Fig 6.1).

Extended right lobectomy (trisegmentectomy) is right lobectomy plus the medial segment of the left lobe (*see* Fig 6.1).

Technique of right hepatic lobectomy

There are five main stages:

1 Mobilisation of the lobe by division of its ligaments (peritoneal folds).
2 Cholecystectomy, dissection and identification of structures in the porta hepatis.

3 Ligation of the right branches of the main structures in the porta hepatis. A probe up the CBD may aid identification and prevent the wrong duct being ligated. It is not now normal practice always to drain the duct with a T-tube postoperatively.
4 Isolation of hepatic veins at the back and ligation of the right. This can be done from below or above by careful dissection to avoid tearing veins or obstructing the vena cava.
5 Division of liver substance after clamping. This may be done by blunt dissection with finger and thumb, isolating the larger bile ducts and vessels, and ligating and clamping them before they are divided. Some surgeons divide the liver before identifying the hepatic veins and then ligate the right vein from within the liver substance.

Lasers. It has been claimed that a laser can cut across the liver without causing bleeding by sealing the vessels as it cuts. For this to happen the blood flow must be temporarily stopped and lasers have not been generally accepted as a major advance in liver surgery.

Ultrasound probes have been claimed to cut liver substance, but not ducts or vessels and it remains to be seen whether they are a significant improvement on standard techniques.

Complications

The mortality of operations for resectable liver tumours is over 20% even in experienced hands.

A special complication of hepatic lobectomy is liver emboli, when pieces of pulped liver reach the circulation via the larger veins. In addition, bile leak, sepsis and reactionary or secondary haemorrhage, disseminated intravascular coagulation and haemobilia all need to be remembered. When the posterior peritoneum has been penetrated, bleeding and leaking bile can lead to a spreading cellulitis in the flank.

Secondary liver tumours

When liver secondaries are present, they can be felt at laparotomy in 95% of cases. Occasionally, a solitary secondary may be deep in the liver substance. However, there are often good reasons to investigate the liver preoperatively. In some patients when the primary is giving little trouble, discovery of the presence of liver metastases by ultrasound or isotope scan would avoid a laparotomy or modify the operative approach and procedure. Both isotopic scan and ultrasound in experienced hands are equally good at showing liver secondaries, and there is not much difference in the cost of the expendable items once the machines are installed. However, unless the alkaline phosphatase is raised, secondaries are unlikely to be shown up by these procedures, but CAT scan can now pick up very small liver secondaries.

Differential diagnoses of liver secondaries

Isotopic scans and ultrasound show multiple cold areas in the liver. The same picture can be given by multiple abcesses, but then the patient is usually febrile with a high white cell count. Sometimes at laparotomy, through a lower abdominal incision, nodules may be felt, but not seen, on the liver surface. These may be simple bile cysts, not secondaries, and may lead the surgeon to abandon a curative for a palliative operation on the primary. Whenever possible, liver nodules should be seen and biopsied. When a decision is being made about whether to operate to remove a carcinoma in an elderly patient, laparoscopy and liver biopsy is a less traumatic alternative to a full laparotomy, as biopsy of the secondary can be done under direct vision. Unguided (blind) percutaneous liver biopsy often misses the secondary nodule.

Treatment of liver secondaries

Should secondaries be removed? If the secondary is truly solitary, removal can prolong life significantly and 5-year survivals have been reported. In the carcinoid syndrome, removal of as much tumour bulk as possible may relieve the symptoms and because of the strange behaviour of these tumours, prolong life significantly.

Infusion of cytotoxics into hepatic artery or portal vein. The choice of drug will depend on the nature of the secondaries, e.g., 5-fluorouracil for gastrointestinal adenocarcinoma, and there is some evidence that both portal vein and hepatic artery should be perfused. So far results have not been dramatic, but the procedures are worth continuing in a few selected patients provided there is a means of monitoring the response. There is no place for giving these expensive and powerful drugs 'in case they may help', without carefully following the patient's progress and assessing that the side effects are not worse than the initial symptoms.

Embolisation of liver tumour

This is a palliative technique for symptomatic liver secondaries or an unresectable primary (Allison, 1978). Particles of polystyrene, dura or foam, are infused through an arterial catheter, via the right or left hepatic artery. It is important to outline the arterial tree first and to ensure that the catheter tip is beyond the origin of the cystic artery, otherwise the gallbladder will become necrotic and perforate. There is often acute pain and fever after the procedure for 24 h and a broad spectrum antibiotic is advisable. However, even though these tumours appear to have a selective arterial supply, they tend to recover and grow again after weeks or months.

Liver abscesses

About half are multiple and half solitary (Rubin *et al.*, 1974).

Multiple abscesses

Multiple abscesses from portal pyaemia or cholangitis, or occasionally, a generalised septicaemia, are very serious as they cannot be drained individually. The presentation is with swinging temperature, and rigors and blood cultures are often positive. The multiple filling defects can be detected by liver isotope scan or ultrasound and the clinical features differentiate them from multiple secondaries. The treatment is with long-term antibiotics and draining the bile duct if appropriate. Common infecting organisms are *E.coli, Klebsiella* species, streptococcus and staphylococcus. As the organisms are often gut bacteria, metronidazole should be added to a broad spectrum antibiotic active against Gram negative organisms, to deal with the bacteroides.

Solitary abscesses

These may be due to *E.histolytica* or *Actinomyces*, or bacteria, and can sometimes be due to secondary infection in a necrotic tumour. They may present as chronic cryptogenic abscesses with an insidious onset, when the patient may complain of anorexia, malaise and loss of weight and have a persistently raised ESR (and raised diaphragm), but may have no local signs or symptoms and the liver need not feel abnormal if the abscess is deep within its substance. It is a diagnosis always to be borne in mind, as it can be diagnosed by ultrasound liver scan and distinguished from a tumour by arteriogram. Under antibiotic cover, these abscesses can be drained transperitoneally and if there is bile duct obstruction, the duct is drained as well. Needle aspiration may be used for diagnosis and bacterial culture and uncomplicated abscesses in the right lobe may sometimes be drained by a needle under ultrasound control. However most abscesses contain thick pus and debris and are best treated by open operation. The mortality of patients whose abscesses are drained is about 15% but rises to 100% if they are not drained.

Amoebic abscesses

These are due to *Entamoeba histolytica* which is becoming more common in Britain due to immigration and rapid air travel from the tropics (British Medical Journal, 1980). It is spread by contamination of the water supply by sewage and the infection may remain dormant for long periods, so there need not be a recent history of bowel symptoms. Although the primary hepatic infection is derived from the colon via the inferior mesenteric and portal veins, there is commonly secondary bacterial infection. The diagnosis is made on finding the parasites in the fresh stool, seeing on sigmoidoscopy large amoebic ulcers with relatively normal mucosa between, or by a positive amoebic fluorescent antibody test.

Treatment

This has been improved by the introduction of metronidazole which is now the treatment of choice. Formerly emetine and chloroquine were used. If the abscess fails to resolve (its size can be monitored on ultrasound), it must be drained, otherwise it will rupture into the peritoneal cavity or through the diaphragm into the pleural cavity. (It is not uncommon to find a pleural effusion on the right side above an hepatic abscess.) An indwelling drain should not be employed as the skin can easily be infected. Therefore, percutaneous needle aspiration is preferred under x-ray control.

Actinomycosis

Although rare, this condition must be thought of when draining a liver abscess and a suitable culture arranged because the textbook 'sulphur granules' are not often noticed. The infection spreads to the liver mainly from the gut via the portal vein and the surgeon should bear in mind the possibility of doing a laparotomy to make this diagnosis in a patient with longstanding undiagnosed pyrexia following an operation on the appendix or colon. High dose penicillin is given intramuscularly for at least 6 weeks.

Hydatid disease of the liver

Hydatid disease of the liver is due to infection with the cyst stage of the dog tapeworm *Echinococcus granulosus*. The sheep is normally the secondary host, but cattle and man can be infected. It is common in the sheep rearing districts of Australia and New Zealand, South America, Greece, Turkey and the Middle East. In Britain it occurs sporadically in the sheep rearing districts. It can affect many organs of the body, but the liver is the most common.

It may lie dormant for years and then give symptoms due to its size or a complication such as jaundice, from pressure on ducts or rupture of a cyst into a bile duct or the peritoneal or pleural cavity. It may also become secondarily infected. Intraperitoneal rupture is a very serious complication leading to shock and dissemination of scolices throughout the peritoneal cavity. The prognosis is poor despite careful cleaning of the peritoneal cavity.

It is important to exclude hydatid disease in susceptible patients before doing a liver biopsy as puncturing the cyst can give an anaphylactic reaction.

Pathology

The cyst consists of two layers:

1 The adventitia, or pseudocyst, which is the liver's reaction to the cyst.
2 The laminated membrane with its internal germinal layer which buds off scolices and secretes the fluid.

There is a natural plane of cleavage between these two layers allowing the cyst proper to be removed intact. Sometimes, however, the second layer disintegrates producing multiple daughter cysts which have to be removed with care from inside the cavity.

Diagnosis

Some cysts die, the wall calcifies and shows on straight x-ray. However, although the calcified cyst needs no treatment, there may well be other non-calcified living cysts in the same liver.

Ultrasound will show a fluid-filled cyst with daughter cysts (Fig 6.9); arteriography will confirm that it is not a tumour, and ERCP may show the separation of the intrahepatic bile ducts and, occasionally, a leak of contrast into the cyst showing communication with the duct system (Fig 6.3). However, ultrasound alone usually gives sufficient information. *Percutaneous transhepatic cholangiogram* should not be attempted if hydatid disease is suspected for fear of puncturing the cyst. Formerly, confirmation of hydatid disease was by the Casoni skin test, but the complement fixation test is now more accurate. Once a cyst has died and calcified, the test may remain positive for many years.

Treatment

A symptomless, calcified cyst can be left alone. Otherwise, the treatment is surgical, the main principle

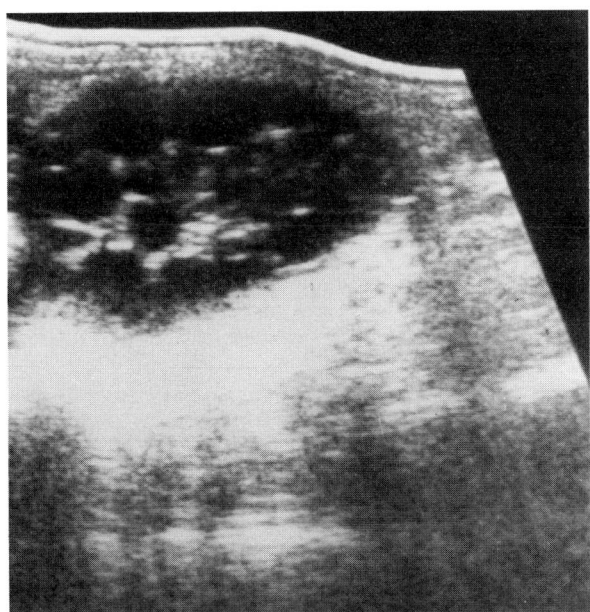

Fig 6.9 Ultrasound of liver showing hydatid cyst full of daughter cysts.

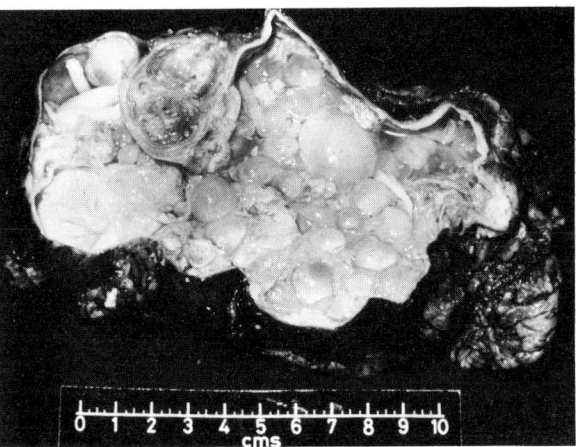

Fig 6.10 Opened hydatid cyst showing daughter cysts (same patient as Fig 6.9).

being to avoid spilling the contents into the peritoneal cavity. Dark coloured towels are used to detect any spilled daughter cysts more easily. Once the cyst is exposed, the fluid is carefully aspirated with a needle and hypertonic (20%) saline or formalin 10% injected into it and left for 10 min to kill the parasites. Care must be taken not to spill formalin which can damage surrounding structures. The adventitia is then incised and the laminated membrane removed intact if possible. The cavity in the liver is either obliterated by sutures, packed with omentum or drained – especially if there is secondary infection or a bile leak. No attempt is made to *excise* the adventitia, as it will induce bleeding from the liver. If the cyst is peripheral, especially in the left lobe of the liver, a segmental resection is the best treatment (*see* p. 116) (Fig 6.10). The prognosis if the primary cyst is completely removed is good. If there is generalised disease due to rupture into the peritoneal cavity, or cysts are inaccessible, the outlook is poor and claims for the new drug merbendazole have not yet been proved.

Other parasitic diseases of the liver are discussed under the section on bile ducts (p. 135).

Simple liver cysts

There is a whole spectrum of non-parasitic liver cysts, from the small dark bile cysts not infrequently seen on the surface of the liver, to large solitary cysts of unknown cause. The danger of mistaking small bile cysts for secondaries has already been mentioned (p. 117). Large cysts, if causing symptoms, should be drained and the cyst cavity marsupialised or obliterated with omentum.

Congenital polycystic disease

This may be associated with polycystic disease of the kidney and presents in adult life with slow, irregular enlargement of the liver, but surgery has little place.

Trauma may leave a cyst which is really a liquified haematoma, sometimes with bile contamination.

Gallstones

Distribution

Over one million operations are performed for gallstones in the world each year. Apart from some tribes of North American Indians who seem to have an hereditary defect in bile salt metabolism, cholesterol gallstones are acquired and we must look to environmental factors. The worldwide distribution varies considerably, being rare in many developing countries, but very common in Western 'affluent' societies. The incidence in Canada after one generation is eight times that in Britain and France, from whence the immigrants came. There is a statistically valid increase in Britain over the last few years with a decrease in the age of onset. It is no longer true that gallstones occur mainly in 'fat, fair, fertile females of forty'.

Composition and causes

In the West, stones mainly consist of cholesterol, although they may also contain some calcium and many other ions and incorporate some bile pigment in the centre. These are the so-called mixed stones. Cholesterol, being insoluble, needs molecules with hydrophylic radicles to form micelles; these are the primary bile acids chenodesoxycholic acid and cholic acid, plus the phospholipids lecithin and cephalin. When the cholesterol concentration is high in proportion to the solubilising agent, a 'supersaturated' solution is formed ('lithogenic bile') leading to a suspension of microcrystals which may then combine to form gallstones. The basic defect in the formation of cholesterol stones is a failure of the liver to synthesise sufficient bile salts to keep the cholesterol in solution. There has been an interesting trend in Japan, where predominantly calcium bilirubinate stones (rare in the West, *see* p. 119) have given way to predominantly cholesterol stones since the Second World War.

Pure pigment (bilirubin) stones have a quite different aetiology and are seen specially in chronic haemolytic anaemia. In congenital spherocytosis or sickle cell disease, pigment stones may be present in children and this should be remembered if the patient is having a splenectomy, as the gallbladder can be removed at the same operation.

Factors leading to gallstone formation

Anything that increases the faecal loss of bile salts, or reduces the reabsorption, such as in ileal disease or resection, will increase the tendency to gallstones (Bouchier, 1973). However, there are a number of other not so precise causes:

Sex. The female:male ratio is about 3:1 before the menopause, but the increasing incidence in young women is partly related to the wider use of the contraceptive pill. In the Boston study, a similar relationship was found with oestrogens given to postmenopausal women.

Obesity. The incidence of gallstones is greater in obese than non-obese people, but a causal relationship is difficult to establish.

Diet. There is epidemiological evidence that a diet rich in refined carbohydrate and deficient in fibre is related to gallstones and to a change in bile composition which favours gallstone formation, but, again, the evidence is circumstantial rather than direct. A high cholesterol diet would, at first sight, be an obvious cause of gallstones, but it has been difficult to produce clear evidence of this.

Stasis. There is a slightly increased incidence of gallstones following polya gastrectomy and truncal vagotomy, and in about 50% of postvagotomy patients, gallbladder emptying is sluggish. These side effects have not been established after more selective vagotomies.

Clinical presentation of gallstones and diagnosis

Gallstones may present in a variety of ways, from an incidental finding on x-ray or at operation, to life-threatening cholangitis or Gram negative septicaemia.

The problem of silent gallstones

Sometimes gallstones are found incidentally at an operation for another condition and sometimes they are found on an abdominal x-ray. The decision to proceed to cholecystectomy depends on many factors. The few studies of long-term follow-up of unoperated gallstones suggest that about 50% will get significant complications within 10 years, but it is difficult to predict for the individual. At operation, if the main procedure is a bowel operation, it is unwise to add a cholecystectomy, particularly if the facilities for operative cholangiogram have not been arranged beforehand. During peptic ulcer surgery, where the gallstones could be contributing to the symptoms, if the main procedure has gone smoothly, cholecystectomy may be added, but there is a suggestion that the combination of cholecystectomy and a gastric drainage procedure can give severe diarrhoea. Ideally, gallstones should have been excluded preoperatively. At no time, however, should cholecystectomy be considered 'a minor procedure'. When stones are discovered incidentally on plain x-ray, the patient's general health and social situation must be considered. It might be better, for example, to defer operation on a housewife with young children for a year or two. Before deferring operation, a cholecystogram to check gallbladder function is advisable, because stones in a non-functioning gallbladder, indicating obstruction of Hartmann's pouch, are more likely to produce cholecystitis, a mucocoele or an empyema. In the elderly, there is a risk of leaving a carcinoma if the gallbladder cannot be visualised on cholecystography.

Gallstones and flatulent dyspepsia

Middle-aged female patients commonly present at the outpatient clinic with symptoms of belching, bloating, reflux, nausea and fatty food intolerance – the syndrome of flatulent dyspepsia (Johnson, 1975). It is entirely reasonable to do a cholecystogram in these patients and gallstones will be found in approximately

50%. Others may have duodenal scarring or evidence of gastric ulcer on subsequent barium meal, but many will have no structural abnormality. However, if the 50% with gallstones have a cholecystectomy, only about half of these will be completely free of symptoms afterwards and a quarter will be no better. The symptoms are related to motility abnormalities of the pylorus, stomach and lower oesophageal sphincter and the connection with gallstones is indirect. This is important, for it is unwise to do a cholecystectomy *solely* for symptoms of flatulent dyspepsia, while implying to the patient that these symptoms will disappear. The patient must be told that the reason for operating is to prevent a number of serious complications and that there is a fair chance of their indigestion being improved (the chances are better if there are stones in a functioning gallbladder) (Lund, 1960). There is no need to give a fat-restricted diet postoperatively – it is better to see first how the patient manages.

Complications of gallstones

1   Acute cholecystitis
2   Chronic cholecystitis
3   Empyema and mucocoele
4   Biliary colic
5   Obstructive jaundice
6   Suppurative cholangitis leading to septicaemia and liver abscesses
7   Carcinoma of gallbladder
8   Acute pancreatitis
9   Choledocho-enteric fistula and gallstone 'ileus'

Although gallstones are popularly regarded as a condition merely causing unpleasant symptoms, the surgeon must still consider them as a potentially lethal disease.

Acute cholecystitis

Initially this is probably a chemical inflammation which later becomes infected and is nearly always associated with gallstones; it is characterised by pain, fever, vomiting and right upper quadrant tenderness with sometimes a palpable, tender mass or positive Murphy's sign. Usually the diagnosis is not difficult, but there are some important pitfalls. The appendix tip may be up under the liver and an inflamed carcinoma or diverticular disease of the hepatic flexure of the colon can mimic acute cholecystitis. Acute pancreatitis may be a differential diagnosis or be present at the same time, so a serum amylase estimation is an important screening test. If right shoulder-tip pain is present, it implies that the inflammation has involved the diaphragm. Slight jaundice or a trace of bilirubin in the urine can be caused by oedema around the common

bile duct as well as a stone in the duct. A perforation of a duodenal ulcer must also be borne in mind and it may be sealed by the gallbladder (*see* choledocho-enteric fistula).

In empyema of the gallbladder there is persistent tenderness and both an empyema and mucocoele may give a palpable gallbladder (Courvoisier's Law does not apply in the absence of obstructive jaundice).

Emergency or elective cholecystectomy for acute cholecystitis? It has been the tradition in Britain not to operate on acute cholecystitis unless there are signs of (1) spreading peritonitis suggesting that the gallbladder has ruptured or the infection is not contained, (2) inability to control pain, and (3) empyema. The reason behind this policy is that most cases settle with conservative treatment, and it has not always been possible to be sure of the diagnosis because a cholecystogram is of little help in the acute stage. The operation is sometimes more difficult and dangerous in the presence of acute infection, leading to an increased chance of damage to the common bile duct and hepatic arteries. Septic complications are said to be more common, but prophylactic antibiotics have reduced these. In the USA, on the other hand, emergency cholecystectomy has been the rule. Apart from financial factors, acute cholecystitis does seem to be a more dangerous condition in North America, leading more often to septicaemia and shock, especially in the elderly. The diagnostic problem has been partly overcome by the ability of grey scale ultrasound to detect gallstones even in an acutely inflamed gallbladder (Fig 6.11), or by a HIDA scan failing to show the gallbladder.

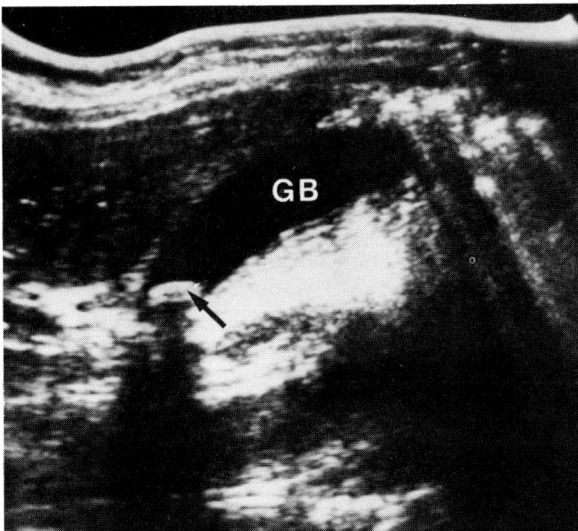

Fig 6.11 Ultrasound in acute cholecystitis showing gallbladder containing stones (arrow) and a thickened oedematous wall.

The policy in Britain is being rethought in the light of the pressure on surgical beds. Operating in the acute stage probably halves the total hospital stay. On the other hand, it is usually impossible to add one or two extra operations to an already planned list. The incidence of duct damage and retained stones will increase if it becomes the practice for inexperienced assistants to do emergency cholecystectomies without adequate help in the middle of the night. The worst time to operate is 5–7 days after the acute attack. It may, however, be possible in some hospitals to operate within a day or two of admission and still observe the precautions for biliary surgery: (a) facilities for operative cholangiography are available, (b) the surgeon is experienced and there is able assistance at the operation. More general practitioners are now treating acute cholecystitis at home and then later referring the patient for confirmation of the disease and elective surgery.

Conservative management of acute cholecystitis. The principles are to refrain from stimulating the gallbladder with food, to use nasogastric suction if there is vomiting, replace oral fluid by intravenous infusion and give antibiotics if there are systemic signs and symptoms. The antibiotic should be given to yield a high blood level, not high bile level and be active against the organisms which are likely to be *E. Coli*, *Klebsiella sp.*, *Streptococcus faecalis* and *Bacteroides*. The patient should be examined frequently to detect complications.

Is there a place for cholecystostomy?

The introduction of cholecystostomy preceded cholecystectomy by several years. There is still a place for it in an elderly, frail patient with an empyema or mucocoele in whom dissection around the ducts would be difficult or time-consuming in the acute stage. It may also be a useful way of biliary tract decompression if acute pancreatitis is discovered at laparotomy. All stones should be removed from the gallbladder and a connection between the gallbladder and common bile duct confirmed by passing a fine catheter or by a cholangiogram if available. A large Foley balloon catheter is fixed into the gallbladder with a purse-string. The fundus of the gallbladder is sutured to the parietal peritoneum where the catheter passes through the abdominal wall. A cholangiogram is performed at 7 days and the catheter removed at 10 days. If no stones are left, once the catheter is removed, the gallbladder may fibrose and give no further trouble.

Anatomy of gallbladder and bile ducts

The key to the anatomy of this region is its variability. The so-called 'normal' arrangements of ducts and arteries occurs in less than half the patients. It is of no practical use to the surgeon to know the percentage of patients having a particular variation as he does not know to which group his particular patient belongs. Guesswork has no place in biliary surgery, the only safe rule being to identify the anatomy accurately before dividing any important structures. A knowledge of the variations, therefore, is essential and the operative cholangiogram, as well as identifying stones, is of great help in confirming the anatomy. The sessile gallbladder is particularly dangerous when a thin common duct can be mistaken for the absent cystic duct. On the other hand, the long cystic duct that crosses the CBD and descends on its left-hand side to join low down can be equally misleading. An anterior right hepatic artery lying in front of the cystic duct can be mistaken for the cystic duct, but the mistake is realised as soon as an attempt is made to cannulate it to do the operative cholangiogram. Hopefully, if this is done, the vessel will only be incised, not divided, and can be repaired with fine silk sutures.

Figure 6.12 shows the common variation of the ducts and Fig 6.13 the common variations of the arteries. After previous operations and sepsis, there may be distortion of any of the patterns. In this case, it may help to do a cholangiogram by direct puncture with a fine needle into the first part of the common bile duct to be exposed, if preoperative percutaneous transhepatic cholangiography has not made the arrangement clear.

Technique of cholecystectomy

Only the techniques for dealing with particular problems will be highlighted here. Instruments for exploring the CBD should always be readily available, including stone forceps, malleable scoops, Fogarty balloon catheters, together with catheters and syringes for flushing the ducts.

A Kocher or right paramedian incision may be used. The former has the advantage that it gives a better cosmetic result and heals well, but the latter gives better access to the pelvis should an ovarian cyst or other pelvic pathology be found on routine laparotomy. Whichever is chosen, really good access is vital, especially to the upper part of the bile ducts. Packs are used to displace the hepatic flexure caudally and the assistant uses a pack to pull the duodenum to the left and keep the common bile duct on the stretch. A good assistant is particularly important in these operations; unfortunately the least experienced surgeon often has to operate with the least experienced assistant! The gallbladder is freed from adhesions and the ducts dissected by carefully dividing the overlying peritoneum so that they can be identified clearly. It is at this stage that familiarity with the anatomical variations is important, but the

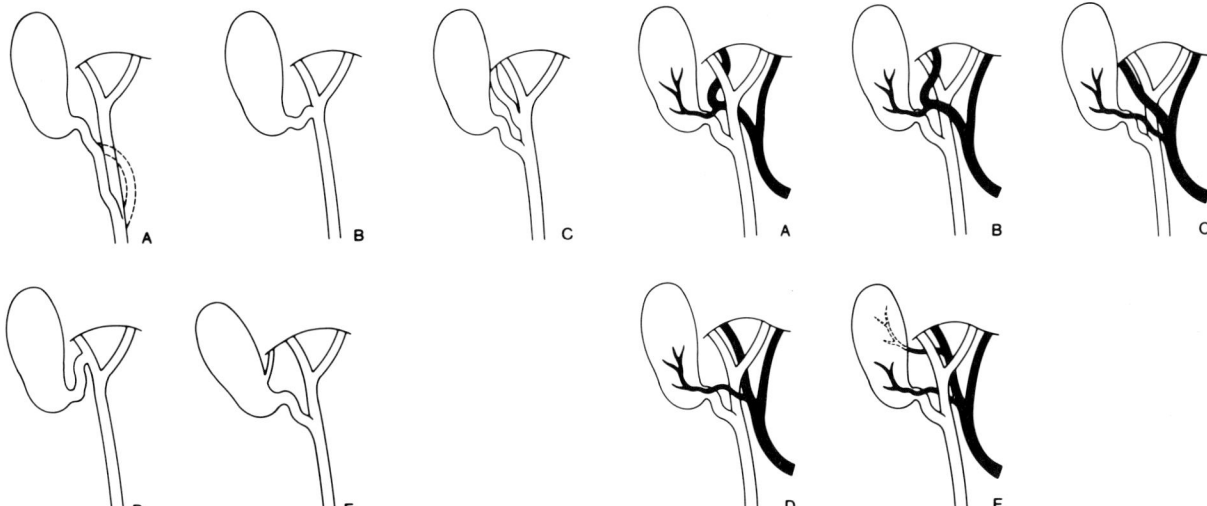

Fig 6.12 Common anatomical variations of bile ducts. (Modified after Benson E.A. and Page R.E., 1976. *Brit. J. Surg*; **63**:853–60.)

Fig 6.13 Common anatomical variations of hepatic and cystic arteries. (Modified after Benson E.A. and Page R.E., 1976. *Brit. J. Surg*; **63**:853–60.)

anatomy must be defined before any important structures are divided. Two 'T's' must be identified, i.e. the junction of the cystic duct with the common hepatic and common bile ducts should be seen and the cystic artery with its main feeding artery palpated. The peroperative cholangiogram is performed through the cystic duct at this stage – the technique and problems are discussed below. The cystic duct will be ligated close to its junction and the cystic artery close to the gallbladder. The cystic artery can be ligated and divided either before or after the cystic duct. It usually arises from the right hepatic artery at a right angle. If there is an anterior ('caterpillar') right hepatic artery, it may have to be dissected carefully off the gallbladder wall. Apart from anatomical variations, the particular danger to the common bile duct comes from 'tenting' it by pulling on the gallbladder when the assistant is not keeping the common bile duct on the stretch. Late stricture of the common bile duct can result from interruption to its blood supply (Fig 6.14) as well as direct damage. It is dangerous to dissect the CBD on both sides for most of its length and, although a flush ligation is ideal, it is safer to leave a small length of cystic duct rather than risk damage to the common bile duct. A residual length of cystic duct probably does no harm unless it has a stone left in it. Some surgeons suture the gallbladder bed, others rely on diathermy haemostasis to the liver. Both are acceptable and the choice can depend on how much gallbladder mesentery can be left. At the end of the operation, a final check is made of the integrity of the common bile duct.

To divide the common bile duct is unfortunate, but not to recognise it is disastrous. Ironically, the duct is usually divided during apparently simple and straightforward operations. If there appears to be an extra cystic duct at the end of the operation, check again that this is not the proximal end of a divided common bile duct.

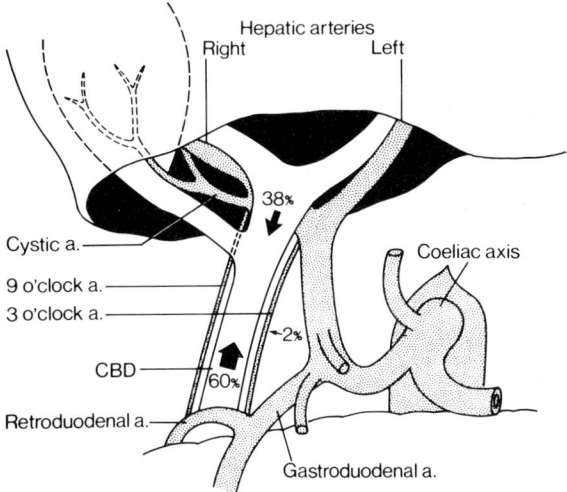

Fig 6.14 Diagram of arterial supply to common bile duct by two 'radial' arteries. The percentages indicate the proportion of blood flow from proximal and distal ends. (Modified after Northover J.M.A. and Terblanche J., 1979. *Brit. J. Surg*; **63**:379–84.)

If the common bile duct is, by chance, divided during cholecystectomy, immediate repair should be done, if necessary calling in a more experienced surgeon. Usually a segment of common bile duct has been removed, making end-to-end suture over a T-tube impossible without tension. A choledochoduodenostomy end-to-side is sometimes possible, but the safest technique is a choledocho-jejunostomy en Roux over a long T-tube which emerges from the jejunum through the abdominal wall (*see* Fig 6.20, p. 133) or over a transhepatic tube. This is a difficult operation because the duct is thin-walled and not dilated. The T-tube should be retained for 3 months to reduce the chance of stricture during healing.

Wound infection

Use of antibiotic prophylaxis is indicated when there is fever, recent inflammation, stones in the CBD, obstructive jaundice, or the patient is elderly, as there is high incidence of wound infection in these patients, usually due to the same organism as is recovered from the bile.

Operative cholangiography

Although careful palpation of the duct for stones should still be done, the routine use of operative cholangiography has helped in three ways:

1 Identification of anatomical variations.
2 Diagnosis of unexpected stones in the CBD.
3 Avoiding exploring the CBD which would otherwise have been explored on the standard clinical criteria, viz. a history of biliary colic or jaundice, a dilated duct and multiple small stones in the gallbladder.

Having said that, the technique must be meticulous and the quality of the film very good, otherwise the surgeon has a false sense of security. For the busy surgeon with a long operating list the procedure must be quick. Operative cholangiography is not a good way of assessing duct size, because of varying film distance from the patient. The justification for doing cholangiography in every case is that a routine can be established, the nursing staff and radiographers know exactly what to do; and the very case the surgeon decides *not* to x-ray may have silent CBD stones! The technique used will depend on the facilities. A TV monitor for screening with video playback does give useful information about the flow down the duct, hold-up at the sphincter and may show the initial injection of contrast flowing round a stone that is later obscured by the greater volume of contrast; but rarely is the quality of the picture good enough to exclude stones. 'Still films' are required as well, for accuracy of detail and for a permanent record, but the screening shows the surgeon the best time to take the film. Without screening facilities, it is best to take two or three films after injecting progressive amounts of contrast, starting with 2–4 ml, according to duct size. Though expensive, the ideal is to have a split beam so that a series of x-ray pictures can be taken during fluoroscopy without having to change film by hand. Stones in the CBD can be differentiated from gas shadow outside the duct on screening, by rotating the patient to either side and seeing that the shadow remains within the duct outline.

Exploration of common bile duct

Once it is decided to explore the common bile duct, the peritoneum is carefully dissected from the anterior surface for a distance of about 2 cm. There is no need to dissect along the medial side or behind the duct. Two catgut stay sutures are inserted and the duct wall incised longitudinally, the bile being carefully sucked away. If a stone can be palpated, it can be milked up the duct into the incision and removed. Otherwise a variety of instruments should be available for extracting stones, i.e. Desjardin's stone forceps, a malleable lead spoon, Fogarty biliary balloon catheters and irrigation catheters. Care must be taken not to push stones further up into the intrahepatic ducts (Orloff, 1973).

Choledochoscopy

Once the common bile duct has been opened, it is difficult to be sure that all stones and debris have been removed and at least 10% of patients are left with retained stones after exploration. Passing Bakes dilators through the sphincter 'just to make sure' is unreliable, because they can easily pass a stone in the duct, and is sometimes dangerous, because they can make a false passage or damage the sphincter, starting acute pancreatitis. A postexploratory cholangiogram is important, but not as easy as a preoperative x-ray, as it is difficult to exclude all the air bubbles and, if there has been a stone at the lower end, oedema may prevent flow through the sphincter.

Choledochoscopy offers an alternative way of excluding stones. It does not take the place of cholangiography as it is only useful when the decision has been taken to explore the common bile duct. There are two types: the flexible fibreoptic choledochoscope and the rigid angled choledochoscope. The rigid instrument is cheaper and is less likely to be damaged and to be able to move the tip is not as necessary as with gastroscopy or colonoscopy, as the bile duct itself can be moved. Stones and gravel can be removed with forceps passed down the choledochoscope and biopsies can be taken of any suspicious lesion in the duct. With the meticulous use of operative cholangiography and choledochoscopy, the incidence of retained stones should be less than 1%.

Manometry of the CBD

For years there has been a vogue on the continent of Europe for measuring the duct pressure at operation to determine narrowing or 'spasm' in the sphincter of Oddi. The whole matter has been studied by a few surgeons in Britain and America. Measurement of pressure may be made at constant flow or measurement of flow at constant pressure, and the variation and flow problems of the apparatus itself and effects of anaesthetics and drugs must all be taken into account. Once the lumen of the duct is filled and any elasticity taken up, the flow or pressure will reflect the ability of the sphincter to transmit the fluid load into the duodenum. In most cases, a significant narrowing of the lower end is obvious from the operative cholangiogram, particularly if screening is used, but in the hands of an enthusiast, the technique may help to decide in a few patients whether to do a sphincteroplasty or choledochoduodenostomy (*see* p. 126). There is no indication for vagotomy or splanchnicectomy for biliary dyskinesia.

T-tube or no T-tube?

It has always been traditional to close the common bile duct around a T-tube to allow any distal duct oedema to subside and prevent leakage from the duct incision. T-tubes should be of latex. Attempts to introduce various plastics were dangerous because (a) some plastics hardened in bile and were, therefore, very difficult to take out and, (b) they caused no irritation and produced no 'track' around them as they crossed the peritoneal cavity, so when they were removed bile leaked. However, some surgeons do not use a T-tube provided there has been no instrumentation at the lower end of the duct and choledochoscopy or post-exploration cholangiogram shows a normal sphincter with free flow into the duodenum. If a T-tube is not used, a drain should be placed near the duct. Avoiding a T-tube certainly reduces the time of convalescence and the loss of electrolytes in the immediate postoperative period.

Postcholecystectomy 'syndrome'

This is an unfortunate name for a group of symptoms that persist or recur after cholecystectomy. They are hardly ever due to the operation, as the name would imply. Reference has already been made to the post-operative persistence of flatulent dyspepsia.

The other main symptom is a biliary type of pain. Occasionally this is due to a retained or recurrent CBD stone, but usually the IVC or ERCP is normal. A long cystic duct stump is not responsible unless it happens to contain a stone. Spasm of the sphincter of Oddi and 'dyskinesia' of the CBD have not been proven. Sometimes, a chronic pancreatitis or other lesion of the upper GI tract has been overlooked at laparotomy and the frequency of these symptoms highlights the need to exclude any other possible cause of the patient's pain at the first operation.

If investigations such as ERCP are negative, re-exploration of the patient is usually unrewarding and has significant risks. If the symptoms recur some time after operation, the surgeon should think of a *new* cause and not assume that the symptoms are linked with the previous operation.

Treatment of residual stones

Over the whole of Europe and North America, the incidence of retained stones after exploration of the CBD is more than 10% (Orloff, 1978). If a T-tube cholangiogram at 7 days shows a retained stone, what should be done? There are three alternatives:

1. Try to flush it through or dissolve it.
2. Remove it by non-surgical methods.
3. Reoperate, remove it and possibly do a choledochoduodenostomy.

1. If a T-tube cholangiogram at 7 days shows a small filling defect at the lower end of the common bile duct, the first course is continuous irrigation with N-saline in conjunction with an antispasmodic in the hope of washing it through the sphincter of Oddi. It may be an air bubble, small stone or blood clot. The cholangiogram is repeated after 3 days. Figure 6.15 shows a blood clot at the lower end of the bile duct washed out by heparin/saline infusion. Many other solutions have been in vogue over the years such as chloroform and ether, but have no advantage over mechanical irrigation and may be dangerous. The only infusable substances likely to dissolve non-calcified stones are cholic acid, or more recently, mono-octanoin. An oral alternative is long-term chenodeoxycholic acid and this has helped in 50% of these patients.

2. If the stone persists, there are at least two other approaches that avoid a second operation. The first is endoscopic papillotomy and removal of the stone from below; Fig 6.16 shows the ERCP findings. This, in experienced hands, has had a 93% success rate if the stone is 1 cm in diameter or less, but it is not entirely without risk of acute pancreatitis and bleeding and it remains to be seen how many patients later develop

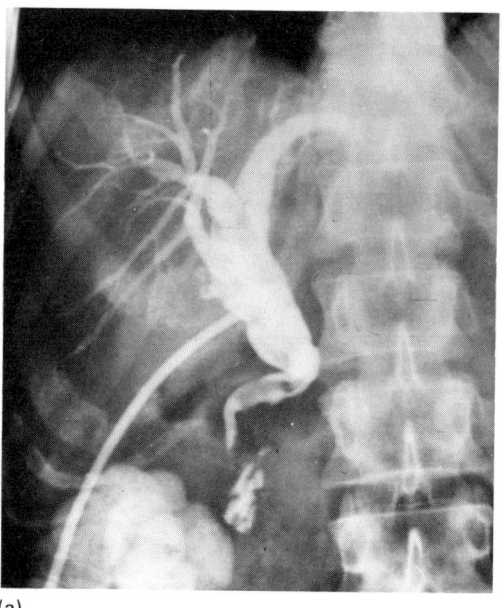
(a)

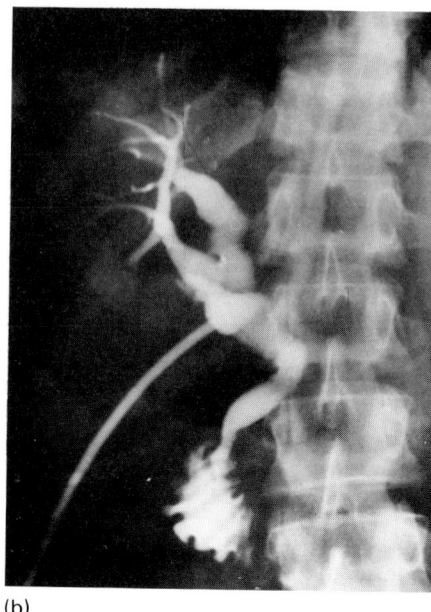
(b)

Fig 6.15   (a) T tube cholangiogram at 7 days showing blood clot at the lower end of the duct. (b) Repeat x-ray 3 days later after irrigation with heparin saline showing a clear duct.

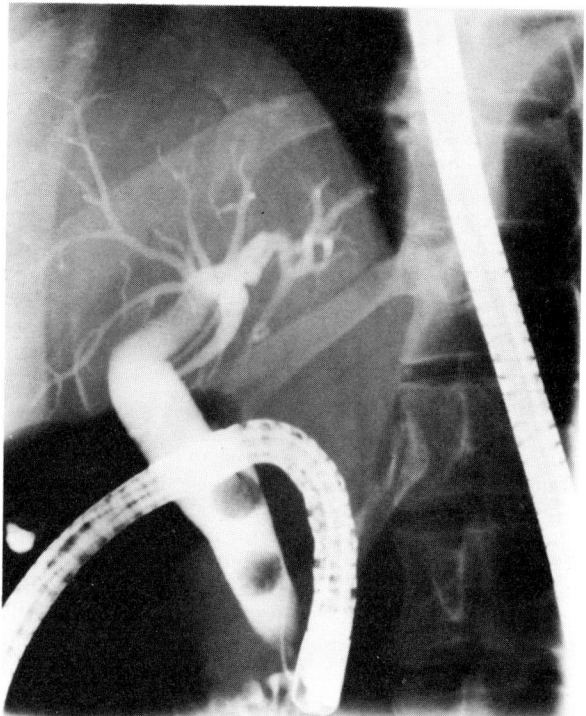

Fig 6.16 ERCP after cholecystectomy showing residual stones in the common bile duct.

stenosis of the sphincter. The second approach is extraction by a Dormia basket through the T-tube sinus track under x-ray control, provided a moderately large diameter T-tube has been used. This is done at least 4 weeks after operation so that a firm T-tube track has been established and it has a success rate of 95% in experienced hands. The basket is passed through a catheter with a manoeuvreable tip. Antibiotics should be given before such manipulations.

3   Reoperation must not always be considered as a last resort and may be the quickest and best treatment for the young, fit patient. However, there is a 25% chance of leaving stones behind at a second exploration. Operation should be preferred to non-operative methods if the stone is large, multiple, or if there is evidence of stenosis or hold-up at the lower end of the duct. At a second exploration it may well be wise to consider a sphincteroplasty or choledochoduodenostomy.

The role of sphincteroplasty and choledochoduodenostomy

These procedures for establishing internal biliary drainage are options that can be used at a first or second operation on the bile duct. The general indications are:

1 when it is impossible to extract all the duct stones through the choledochotomy or stones are impacted at the ampulla;
2 when the biliary tree is packed with stones and it is difficult to be sure that all were removed;
3 when there are primary duct stones (usually soft, muddy stones) without stones in the gallbladder. These can reform if there is any stasis in the duct;
4 when bile duct stones are associated with stenosis of the sphincter of Oddi.

Sphincteroplasty is, perhaps, preferable in the younger, fit patient, but is more difficult to perform and carries a small risk of pancreatitis. Choledochoduodenostomy is ideal for the elderly, less fit patient and is easy to do, but the bile ducts must be dilated and the stoma size at least 2.5cm (Fig 6.17).

There is no place for the surgeon to do a mere sphincterotomy; it must be a long incision up the duct with multiple mucosal to mucosal sutures so that the diameter of the opening is equal to the diameter of the CBD. Care must be taken to identify and avoid the opening of the pancreatic duct (Fig 6.18). Postoperatively, it is advisable to avoid skins and pips in the diet as these occasionally reflux into the duct. In assessing the anastomosis postoperatively an IVC is of no value, but barium taken orally can be seen to reflux into the duct if the stoma is patent and should quickly empty again. Air will normally be seen in the ducts on plain abdominal x-ray.

Dissolution of gallstones

Following the early success in dissolving gallstones with chenodesoxycholic acid or ursodesoxycholic acid, the popular press has given the impression that operation is no longer required for the treatment of gallstones. This is very misleading. There is no doubt that

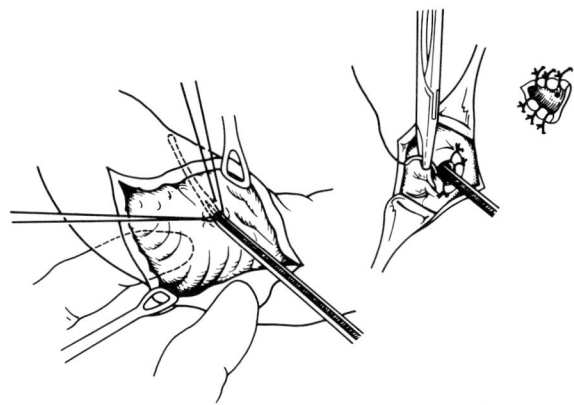

Fig 6.18 Technique of sphincteroplasty. A grooved director is placed in the sphincter. Catgut sutures are placed on either side and the tissue between them cut; this is continued up the duct until the opening is as wide as the CBD. Note that the pancreatic duct must be identified at the end to ensure that it is not narrowed by a suture.

there are now a number of well-documented cases of dissolution of gallstones and this experience validates the theory of gallstone formation (*see* p. 120), but dissolution is only possible if three criteria are present:

1 The gallbladder is functioning and the cystic duct is not obstructed.
2 The stones are not calcified.
3 The stones are relatively small.

The treatment takes many months and may be accompanied by diarrhoea. When treatment stops, stones may reform as the bile again becomes lithogenic.

The practical clinical use is mainly for frail patients who are experiencing symptoms or those with other medical conditions in whom operation carries a high risk. There is no indication to try to dissolve symptomless gallstones.

Cholesterosis

The mucosal surface of the gallbladder has yellow subserosal cholesterol specks in it, resembling a strawberry. The cholecystogram usually shows very good concentration of the contrast medium with a fine irregularity of the outline. Although the mucosal changes are inflammatory, there is still discussion whether without associated gallstones, this condition produces symptoms. If biliary symptoms persist, cholecystectomy is justified and, not infrequently, small cholesterol stones are found at operation.

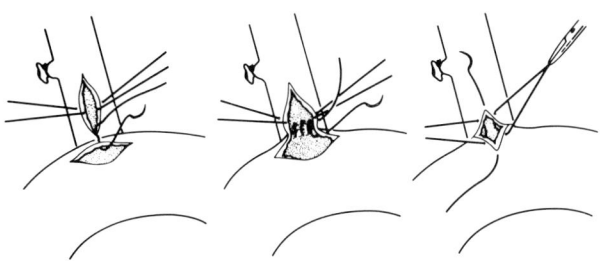

Fig 6.17 Technique of side-to-side choledochoduodenostomy. The CBD is opened longitudinally between stay sutures and the duodenum is also opened in its longitudinal axis. Interrupted catgut sutures are inserted alternately in each side as the duodenum is rolled up over the duct. The last three sutures are all inserted and then tied, to ensure good apposition at the corner.

Cholecystoenteric fistulae

A spontaneous connection between the gallbladder and intestine is uncommon, but the most common site is between the gallbladder and duodenum. It may result from acute cholecystitis and gallstones when the inflamed gallbladder become adherent to the duodenum and eventually erodes through, allowing a stone to pass into the intestine. Sometimes a large stone then impacts in the terminal ileum giving gallstone obstruction (badly named gallstone 'ileus'). Alternatively, the fistula may result from a large superior or anterior duodenal ulcer that perforates and becomes 'plugged' by the gallbladder, but a penetrating ulcer usually causes the rarer choledochoduodenal fistula.

The symptoms are those of the underlying ulcer or gallbladder disease, but sometimes cholangitis may complicate the fistula. The diagnosis is confirmed by a plain abdominal x-ray showing air in the biliary tree as is seen after an operative choledochoduodenostomy or sphincteroplasty. A barium meal will show reflux into the gallbladder and biliary tree, but an i.v. cholangiogram is of little use.

The ideal treatment is to disconnect the fistula and treat the gallbladder disease or duodenal ulcer in the appropriate way. An operative cholangiogram is advisable to ensure that the common bile duct is not obstructed at its lower end and this is especially important in a choledochoduodenal fistula. However, when the patient is ill from gallstones without obstruction and there is an inflammatory mass around the gallbladder, it may be safer to leave the gallbladder alone and merely remove the stone from the terminal ileum. If it is round, all is well, but if it is faceted there is probably another stone somewhere proximal that could also obstruct if not removed!

Carcinoma of the gallbladder

Carcinoma of the gallbladder is more common than is generally realised, but it does not always involve the surgeon. It ranks fifth or sixth in frequency of gastrointestinal malignancies and accounts for 500 deaths annually in Britain and 6500 in the USA. Ninety per cent of cases are in patients over 50 years of age. The prognosis is very poor, because there is usually spread directly into the liver as well as the lymph nodes before there are symptoms and 75% are inoperable. However, in about 1 in 300 gallbladders removed for stones, a small carcinoma is found incidentally and when this is confined to the mucosa or submucosa there is a good prognosis – 64% surviving 5 years. The disease may present with biliary tract pain, jaundice, metastases or be asymptomatic. Up to 80% of patients also have gallstones, which is the main known associated condition. The risk of eventually developing cancer (estimated at around 8% after the age of 50) is one more indication for the removal of a gallbladder containing stones, but must be weighed against the increased risk of operation in the more elderly patient.

Treatment

If the symptoms are due to invasion of the CBD, then a bypass or intubation procedure is indicated. If, on the other hand, the lesion is found as a histological 'surprise' and it is confined to the mucosa or submucosa, nothing more need be done. However, if rarely, the carcinoma has invaded through the wall, but there are no obvious secondaries, or if an operable carcinoma is discovered at laparotomy, a radical excision is justified as the only hope of cure. This involves a limited excision of the neighbouring liver tissue and dissection of the lymph drainage around the porta hepatis and down the CBD to the posterior pancreaticoduodenal and para-aortic nodes (after Kocher's mobilisation of the duodenum).

Benign 'tumours' of the gallbladder

There are a number of benign 'tumours' of the gallbladder which probably do not progress to carcinoma, at least in the absence of gallstones.

Adenomyosis

Adenomyosis consists of an overgrowth of smooth muscle and/or cystic glands in the gallbladder wall and is not a neoplasm but a chronic inflammatory condition. It has a variety of other names such as cholecystitis glandularis proliferans', 'cholecystitis cystica' and 'gallbladder dysplasia' and may be diffuse or localised. The localised form typically presents at cholecystography as a filling defect in the fundus of the gallbladder and other appearances resemble a polyp, septum, or occasionally, a diverticulum with or without stones. The difficult question is whether the condition is responsible for symptoms. Most surgeons would perform a cholecystectomy having carefully excluded other obvious causes for the pain.

Polyps

Polyps are relatively common, but are not necessarily neoplastic. They may be a particular form of adenomyosis, be inflammatory or be cholesterol deposits. Other things being equal, they are best removed.

Investigation of obstructive jaundice

One of the most important clinical problems the surgeon meets is the differential diagnosis of the patient presenting with jaundice (Blumgart, 1978). It is tempting to think that with all the new diagnostic aids, a clinical diagnosis is no longer necessary. This is not so, as the surgeon must not only decide which series of investigations are required, but also must be able to interpret the findings in the light of the clinical picture; for example, the finding of non-dilated bile ducts does not exclude extrahepatic obstruction if the history of jaundice is short, but makes it very unlikely if the jaundice has been present for 5 or 6 weeks. He must first distinguish surgical jaundice from cirrhosis, hepatitis or drug-induced jaundice. A history of malaise or influenza-like illness before the jaundice develops suggests viral hepatitis, and it is extremely important to take a detailed drug history bearing in mind that cholestasis may be produced by a very small dose of such drugs as chlorpromazine. Pain of the biliary colic type preceding the jaundice supports a diagnosis of common bile duct stone and persistent pain radiating into the back suggests pancreatic carcinoma or chronic pancreatitis, but both can be painless. Viral hepatitis or cholestatic jaundice may produce a dull ache over the liver from stretching of the capsule. Pale stools and dark urine indicate obstructive jaundice, but the real problem is that there may be some intrahepatic bile duct obstruction with 'medical jaundice' and, conversely, secondary hepatocellular change from extrahepatic obstruction. This is why the routine liver function tests, at any one time, may be misleading. Screening for hepatitis B antigen is advisable at the patient's first visit.

The presence of constitutional disturbance, such as a fever, is important and points to a primary infection such as hepatitis, malaria, amoebiasis or secondary infection such as cholangitis with stones in the common bile duct. A history of a previous operation makes the surgeon consider residual stones, CBD stricture or metastases from a previously resected primary carcinoma elsewhere in the gastrointestinal tract.

Examination

The associated clinical sign of liver failure – flapping tremor, clubbing, spider naevi, gynaecomastia, testicular atrophy, ascites and encephalopathy – point to cirrhosis or the later stage of hepatitis.

A palpable gallbladder in the presence of obstructive jaundice makes gallstones unlikely and, by inference, carcinoma of the pancreas likely (Courvoisier's Law), but the exception to the rule is when there is a stone impacted in Hartmann's pouch as well as in the lower end of the common bile duct.

A palpable spleen in the presence of jaundice suggests haemolysis or portal hypertension, but it can be enlarged by viral infection or splenic vein thrombosis from carcinoma of the pancreas.

The liver itself may be large, hard and nodular, suggesting malignancy, or firm and finely irregular, suggesting cirrhosis, but in the later stages of cirrhosis it may be small. In viral hepatitis it may be large, smooth and tender.

The presence of ascites indicates widespread malignancy or cirrhosis. Rectal examination will confirm pale stools as well as reveal other unsuspected pathology.

Investigation

Urine

The urine may appear 'dark' merely due to concentration and it must be tested for bilirubin. An excess of bilirubin and absence of urobilinogen confirms obstructive jaundice while absence of bilirubin confirms haemolytic (prehepatic) jaundice.

Liver function tests

These may be pointers to the diagnosis, but are often not diagnostic. Serial measurements are more valuable by indicating the progress of the illness, although it is quite unnecessary to do daily liver function tests when the jaundice is obviously clearing clinically. Prothrombin time is important not only as an indication of abnormal liver function but also to allow correction with Vit. K. before surgery.

Blood urea and creatinine levels

These are a useful indication of renal function which can deteriorate rapidly at operation in the presence of jaundice.

Special diagnostic aids

Once obstructive jaundice is suspected on clinical grounds and with the help of simple laboratory tests, the diagnosis must be confirmed and the cause found without delay. There is no place now for 'steroid white washes' in a modern gastroenterological surgical unit and the delay of 'expectant treatment' is not justified unless the jaundice is obviously fading rapidly, not just fluctuating, as it can in carcinoma of the ampulla or common bile duct stones. A suggested order of investigations is:

Grey-scale ultrasound

This is used to detect dilated intrahepatic ducts, gallstones (Fig 6.11), carcinoma of head of pancreas, or multiple secondaries in the liver. The success rate in distinguishing surgical from medical jaundice varies from 80–97%, but it is very unlikely to give a false positive, i.e. show dilated ducts when they are not present except when the CBD is confused with the portal vein.

Percutaneous transhepatic cholangiography (PTC).

The use of the fine needle has greatly improved the value of this test (Fig 6.19). There is a lower risk of bile leak or bleeding and the needle will enter ducts that are only slightly dilated. ERCP is an alternative investigation and has an advantage in examining the ampulla directly for an ampullary carcinoma and investigating pancreatic disease. The choice of these will depend on the expertise available. PTC is overall more likely to get good pictures of the upper bile ducts and gallbladder, and it is usually more important to know the upper rather than the lower extent of a lesion.

Laparotomy

This is the final arbiter, but nowadays there is no excuse for the surgeon to operate without a knowledge of what he is likely to find. The more information he can have about the bile duct anatomy and pathology the better, especially if there have been previous operations.

Cholangitis

Inflammation of the bile ducts can be of two sorts, acute suppurative or primary sclerosing.

Acute suppurative cholangitis

Acute suppurative cholangitis is secondary to obstruction (partial or complete) due to stones, carcinoma or stricture. It presents as the classic triad of Charcot: recurrent pain, fever with rigors and fluctuating jaundice. Its importance, particularly in the elderly,

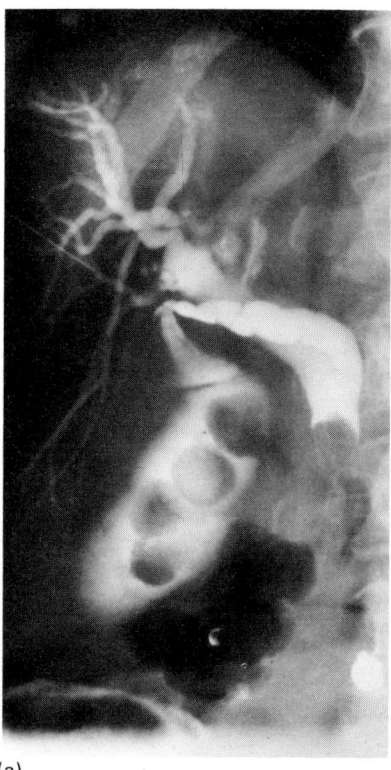
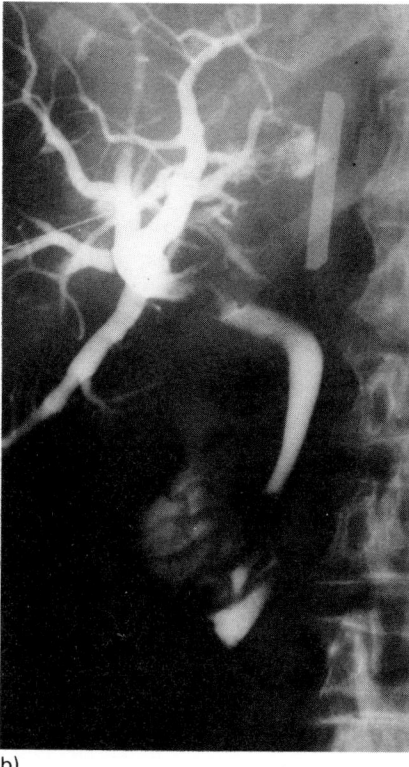
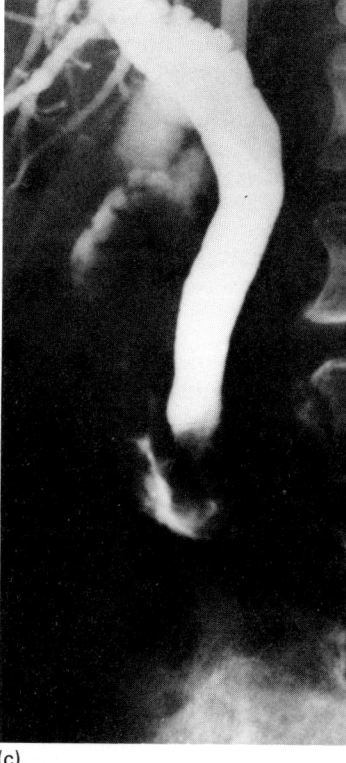

(a)   (b)   (c)

Fig 6.19 PTC in differential diagnosis of obstructive jaundice showing (a) gallstone impacted at lower end of duct, (b) malignant stricture of CBD at junction with cystic duct, (c) carcinoma of ampulla.

lies in the complication of Gram negative septicaemia, sometimes leading to multiple liver abscesses. The question whether it is an 'ascending' or 'descending' infection is of no value in treatment and the patient should be given antibiotics, e.g. gentamicin and metronidazole, but if there is not a rapid response the duct must be drained. The mucosa of the duct is found to be acutely inflamed ('red-hot duct') and there may be frank pus. The immediate aim is to decompress the duct; when stones are present they are removed and a T-tube inserted; in the case of a stricture, the duct alone may merely be drained and a definitive operation performed later when the infection has subsided, or if the stricture is low, a wide stoma choledochoduodenostomy is used to drain the distended duct. This is not the time to do complicated reconstructions of the biliary tree.

Primary sclerosing cholangitis

This is an uncommon and difficult condition characterised by fibrosing inflammation of the bile ducts. It was first described in 1924 and has also been called 'stenosing cholangitis', 'obliterative cholangitis' and 'fibrosing cholangitis'. Since the introduction of endoscopic retrograde cholangiography, the diagnosis is being made more frequently. It particularly affects males under the age of 50 years and presents with jaundice, pruritus and hepatomegaly, but there is disagreement about the criteria for diagnosis. The initial criteria were 'diffuse inflammatory thickening of the extrahepatic bile ducts in patients without previous biliary surgery, in the absence of gallstones, and after cholangiocarcinoma had been excluded'. Some would also add 'in the *absence* of primary biliary cirrhosis'. An association with ulcerative colitis (but not Crohn's disease) is well recognised but it does not necessarily improve after colectomy or remission of the colitis. (Some purists argue that this group should not be called primary: this merely seems a matter of semantics as the disease can still be a *primary* disease of the bile ducts and be associated with an inflammatory process elsewhere.) The aetiology is unknown but an autoimmune process is suggested (*see* chapter 34). Recent work has shown an hepatic copper overload as in primary biliary cirrhosis. The duct walls may be eight times their normal thickness and the lumen reduced to a diameter of 3 mm. Characteristically, the whole duct system is involved, but sometimes the intrahepatic ducts are spared making an operative bypass possible. *Histologically* the main ducts show fibrosis in the submucosa and subserosal portions with oedema between, but liver biopsy is only diagnostic in about one third of patients. The diagnosis is suggested by a disproportionate elevation of serum alkaline phosphatase compared with bilirubin. Transhepatic percutaneous cholangiogram or ERCP show uniformly narrow ducts with a characteristic beaded appearance and no obstruction at the ampulla of Vater. Confirmation of the diagnosis can be made at operation by feeling a thickened cord-like duct and it is sometimes necessary to exclude a diffuse bile duct carcinoma by biopsy and frozen section.

Treatment has been with steroids and immunosuppressive drugs, but they seem to give only temporary relief. Because of the similarities to primary biliary cirrhosis, a trial of D-penicillamine has been suggested. The role of surgery is limited but can be used (a) to confirm the diagnosis and exclude carcinoma, (b) to insert a T-tube to drain the duct while steroids are started, (c) occasionally to do a hepaticojejunostomy if the hepatic ducts are spared or, (d) rarely, to insert a plastic tube through the narrowed segments if there are normal ducts above and below. The advantage of a T-tube is that the effect of drugs can be monitored by serial cholangiograms.

Haemobilia

Haemobilia is a rare cause of acute or chronic blood loss from the gastrointestinal tract, but must be thought of when other common causes have been excluded. It occurs as a complication of hepatic injury, due to an arterial-biliary communication, or may follow a difficult exploration of the CBD. A carcinoma of the bile duct or an hepatic tumour communicating with a duct are possibilities while in the Orient, parasitic infestation is the commonest cause. The associated symptoms are biliary colic and obstructive jaundice.

The diagnosis can easily be made if a T-tube is already in place but, in the unoperated patient, blood may be seen emerging from the sphincter of Oddi on ERCP. An arteriogram can locate the site of the bleeding within the liver and the treatment is to ligate the feeding vessel as close as possible to the leak. Occasionally a partial hepatectomy is needed for heavy post-traumatic haemobilia arising deep in the liver substance.

Strictures of the common bile duct

Malignant strictures

Primary carcinoma can occur in any part of the biliary tree, but the junction of the right and left hepatic duct and the lower end of the common bile duct are the most frequent sites (Fig 6.19). They may be associated with gallstones or parasitic infestation (*see* p. 135). Although the primary may be small, there are commonly secondaries in lymph nodes or liver or direct spread into the surrounding structures. Bile duct cancers also tend to spread up and down the duct in the submucosal plane, but they may be slow-growing making palliative operation worthwhile.

They may be classified *macroscopically* as nodular, diffuse, infiltrating, scirrhous, constricting and polypoid, or *microscopically* as undifferentiated, moderately well differentiated or papillary adenocarcinoma. However, it is a combination of presenting symptoms, position along the duct and degree of spread outside the wall that determine the choice of treatment. The presentation in 90% of patients is progressive painless jaundice while about one-fifth also have dyspepsia, anorexia, weight loss or non-dyspeptic pain. Fever is rare.

The differential diagnosis is from a gallstone and sclerosing cholangitis. If there is doubt, a frozen section biopsy should be taken at operation, either by incising the wall of the duct or opening it from below and taking a biopsy with the choledochoscope.

Resection is sometimes possible with a Roux-en-Y jejunal anastomosis to the hepatic duct and this gives a 5-year survival of about 30%. The prognosis of the polypoid type is significantly better than the others. Occasionally, a low duct primary in a younger patient justifies a Whipple's operation and offers the only hope of cure. However, usually the surgeon has to consider the different forms of palliation similar to those used for bypassing benign strictures, but he must always remember that the simplest and least traumatic method should be chosen for palliating malignant disease.

Benign tumours of CBD

Occasionally benign papillomas occur, particularly at the lower end of the duct. They may show as a filling defect on cholangiogram and need to be distinguished from gallstones and carcinoma by biopsy if necessary.

Secondary nodes from a distant gastrointestinal primary in the porta hepatis may obstruct the bile ducts by external pressure. As there are usually multiple secondaries, direct operation on the ducts is not justified and various forms of intubation are the simplest way of relieving the jaundice (*see below*).

Benign strictures

These, unfortunately, are usually due to operative trauma during cholecystectomy, either narrowing part of the duct or interrupting the blood supply to the duct by a carelessly applied artery forceps. The precautions necessary to avoid duct damage during cholecystectomy have been outlined above, but the duct can also

be damaged during over-enthusiastic underrunning of a bleeding duodenal ulcer or in other forms of duodenal surgery. We are concerned here with strictures that occur postoperatively or damage that is not recognised at operation.

Presentation

Postoperatively, the patient either becomes progressively jaundiced or develops a biliary fistula which may cease spontaneously only to be replaced by jaundice as the duct heals by stenosis. Sometimes there may be an intraperitoneal bile collection which becomes infected and can be confused with cholangitis. Occasionally a stricture presents long after operation with progressive jaundice due to interruption to the blood supply rather than direct trauma to the duct.

Management

Electrolyte loss must be quickly replaced and infection brought under control by antibiotics or drainage of a subphrenic abscess if necessary. The prothrombin time must be checked and the haemoglobin brought to a satisfactory level before operation.

Investigation

In this situation a percutaneous, transhepatic cholangiogram is definitely preferable to an ERCP as it is the duct *proximal* to the stricture that needs to be outlined.

Operations for malignant and benign bile duct strictures

There are a number of different techniques of bypassing strictures, one of which is not necessarily superior to the others, but better in a particular situation (Whelton *et al.*, 1969). The surgeon operating on bile duct strictures must be familiar with all the options and choose the right one for each patient. Each option will be described with its advantages and disadvantages, indications and contraindications. Each, however, requires a really good exposure and thorough mobilisation of the hepatic flexure of the colon. Identification of the bile duct may be helped by aspirating likely structures with a fine needle and syringe.

Choledochoduodenostomy

Choledochoduodenostomy either end-to-end or side-to-side is simple and safe for a low bile duct stricture and should be made as high up in the duct as possible.

For higher strictures it should only be done if the duodenum can easily be mobilised and there is no tension.

Cholecystojejunostomy

Cholecystojejunostomy is suitable for low malignant strictures, *provided* it is confirmed by operative cholangiography (through the gallbladder) that the cystic duct joins the common duct well above the lesion.

Hepaticojejunostomy

This is the treatment of choice for high strictures with some extrahepatic duct remaining. It is best performed with a Roux loop end-to-side with a mucosa-to-mucosa anastomosis on to an opening in the front of the dilated portion of the bile duct. Alternatively, the duct may be divided and the proximal portion anastomosed end-to-side to the Roux loop. A tube may be placed across the anastomosis to prevent late stenosis and brought out either further down the jejunum (Fig 6.20), through the liver (Fig 6.21) or in both directions as a modified U tube. If the hepatic duct is very dilated and the wall thickened, a tube may be unnecessary. When there is much fibrosis, the front of the duct may be cut away and the Roux limb attached end-to-side to the wall of the duct widely around it, rather than doing a mucosa-to-mucosa suture.

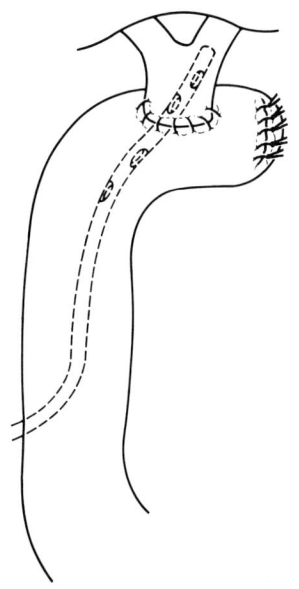

Fig 6.20 Diagram of hepaticojejunostomy.

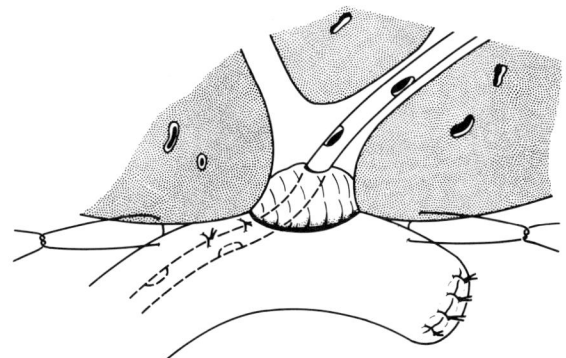

Fig 6.21 Diagram of 'mucosal graft' hepaticojejunostomy. (After Knight M. and Smith R., 1977. *Operative Surgery: Abdomen*, 3rd edn, p. 376. London and Boston: Butterworth.)

Mucosal jejunal graft (Smith)

In order to get the mucosa of the jejunum into contact with the epithelial lining of a duct high in the liver, a tube with transhepatic extension is used to pull a cuff of mucosa protruding from the jejunal wall against the open intrahepatic duct, avoiding the need for any mucosal sutures (Fig 6.21). The jejunum is sutured to the liver capsule to hold it in place. Six hundred of such operations have now been performed with a very low mortality, but it is always difficult to assess long-term results in patients of this kind (Smith, 1979a).

Longmire's procedure

When the porta hepatis is grossly scarred from previous operations or trauma, it is very difficult to find a suitable bile duct for anastomosis. Longmire *et al.* (1974) devised a technique for avoiding the porta hepatis and anastomosing the jejunum to a dilated intrahepatic duct by resecting part of the right or left lobe or the quadrate lobe until a dilated duct was found. Dilated ducts do not always reach to the surface of the liver, but the position of such ducts can be shown before resection by percutaneous or operative transhepatic cholangiography. An end-to-side or side-to-side hepaticojejunostomy is performed with fine interrupted catgut sutures (Fig 6.22).

Liver split

In a high, benign or malignant stricture, the liver substance can be split or excised at the junctions of the functional right and left lobes to obtain access to an

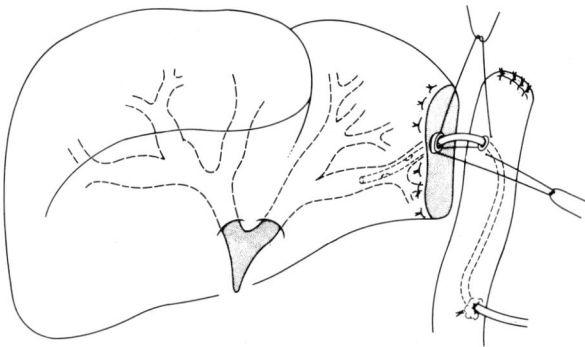

Fig 6.22 Diagram of Longmire procedure. (In this case both main ducts are blocked so only the left lobe will be decompressed.)

intrahepatic portion of the right and left hepatic ducts. Because of the anatomy, it is easier to expose a significant length of the left duct by this approach.

Bypass using artificial materials

For years a search has been made for a bile duct substitute. Vein has been used but receives no oxygenation as it may when used for arterial bypass. Dacron has been used with limited success and newer, non-porous, tubes may be more effective but more expensive. Such substances should be considered as a last resort when other procedures are not possible, or in malignant disease when the overall prognosis is short. For patients with a benign stricture, one of the other procedures using the patient's own tissues is far preferable.

Operative intubation

Internal tube

When a malignant obstruction is found to be inoperable, effective palliation can be obtained by opening the duct and inserting a stiff plastic tube through the stricture from the bile duct below. A number of side holes should be cut in the tube above and below the part that will be in the stricture and the length of the tube should enable it to reach the sphincter of Oddi, but not pass through it; this helps to keep it in position. The stricture may have to be dilated with Bake's dilators to enable a reasonable sized tube to be introduced (George *et al.*, 1981).

U tube

Because the straight tube tends to block after a time with tumour or debris, Terblanche and colleagues

(1973) devised a U tube which came to the outside and, therefore, could be washed out and replaced if necessary by 'railroading' a new tube through.

The common bile duct is opened in the usual way and a Bake's dilator is carefully passed up to locate the stricture. A choledochoscope can then be used to confirm the diagnosis and obtain a biopsy if possible. The stricture is dilated up to 5 mm into either the right or left hepatic duct and the dilator is passed up the duct and out through the surface of the liver. A thread is attached to the dilator, pulled back out through the choledochotomy and used to pull the firm-walled plastic tube (with side holes where it is to lie within the ducts) out through the liver. The choledochotomy is closed around the lower limb of the U tube and both limbs brought out through separate stab incisions onto the skin where they are connected via a Y connection to a sterile drainage bag (Fig 6.23). A corrugated drain is inserted. After a few days, the tubes allow bile to flow into the duodenum through the carefully placed side holes. Washing out the tube with antibiotic solution prevents infection.

Non-operative intubation of malignant bile duct strictures

In some patients in whom the bile duct carcinoma is clearly inoperable or in a secondary carcinoma, an operation can be avoided by introducing a tube by a

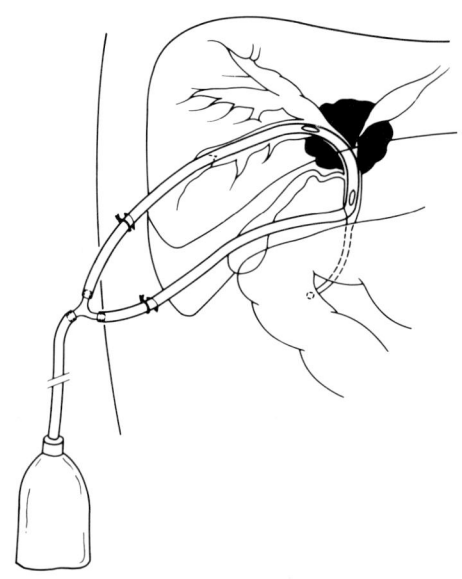

Fig 6.23 Diagram of U tube in position through an inoperable carcinoma of the hepatic ducts.

percutaneous transhepatic approach over a guide wire under radiographic control. A fine needle PTC will have identified the stricture.

If the stricture is very tight, the tube can be left in the proximal, dilated ducts to drain the bile externally. A further attempt at intubation can then be made through less dilated ducts. It has been suggested that this should be done before operation for retained stone or benign stricture to allow the liver to recover. However, patients should not be left so long before operation and collapse of the proximal ducts preoperatively makes identification at operation and anastomosis more difficult. Even if there is sepsis in the ducts, it is usually better to remove the stone and drain the duct thoroughly under antibiotic cover. Endoscopic intubation from below after a sphincterotomy is being evaluated in a few centres.

Choice of procedure for bile duct stricture

The surgeon must be familiar with all the above procedures so that he can choose the right one for the individual patient. The following scheme is a guide to the order of priorities (Table 2).

Table 2

Investigation	
Ultrasound	— to confirm dilated ducts
PTC	— to identify site of obstruction
ERCP (occasionally)	— to show the state of bile ducts below obstruction

Procedures

Benign strictures
  Hepaticojejunostomy at hilum
  Hepaticojejunostomy with liver split
  Hepaticojejunostomy with mucosal graft (Smith)
  Intrahepatic hepaticojejunostomy with resection
    (Longmire procedure)

Malignant strictures

Operative	*Non-operative*
Resection with hepatico-jejunostomy to opposite duct	Percutaneous transhepatic intubation if obstructive intrahepatic or due to secondary tumour
Palliative end-to-side hepaticojejunostomy	
U-tube intubation	
Internal tube through stricture	

Choledochal cysts

These are probably congenital and although they may not present until adult life, there is usually a history of symptoms in childhood. They are caused by increasing obstruction due to hypoplasia of the distal common bile duct. The bile in the cyst commonly becomes infected and stones may form. The classical presentation is pain, jaundice and a right hypochondrial mass. Diagnosis is by radiology and treatment is surgical as untreated cysts carry a poor prognosis – from biliary cirrhosis, recurrent cholangitis or occasional rupture. The easiest operation is a cystoduodenostomy or cystojejunostomy, but better results are claimed if the cyst is excised and a hepaticojejunostomy performed to the proximal duct.

Parasitic infestations of the bile ducts

Nematodes

Ascaris lumbricoides, the common round worm, may occasionally invade the bile duct and cause obstruction.

Trematodes

Clonorchis species are common in the East and parasitise the bile ducts. The life cycle is from the faeces of man via water snails and to the carp. The carp is eaten (raw) by man to complete the cycle. It is important for two reasons:

1 The worm may die in the duct and act as a medium for stone formation. In fact, 55% of the calcium bilirubinate stones seen in the East have a parasite at the centre.
2 There is a high incidence of carcinoma of the bile duct associated with the infestation.

Fasciola hepatica, the liver fluke, is transmitted to man by his eating contaminated watercress. The parasite invades the bile ducts and liver and causes obstructive jaundice. In any of these parasitic infestations there may be secondary bacterial infection.

Recurrent pyogenic cholangitis

Often known as Asian cholangio-hepatitis or Oriental cholangiohepatitis, it occurs in Korea, Vietnam, Malaysia, Singapore and Japan, but its cause is still not entirely clear. Many cases can be explained by infestation with one of the parasites listed above with secondary bacterial infection. There may not necessarily be stone formation although, as mentioned above (*see* p. 120), calcium bilirubinate stones are a common later finding.

The extrahepatic bile ducts may dilate due to obliteration, but the intrahepatic ducts may stenose giving rise to gross dilatation with stones deep in the liver.

The diagnosis is made by outlining the ducts by one of the methods already described, but special care must be made to differentiate it from viral hepatitis.

With the bacterial infection controlled by antibiotics, the aim of treatment is to decompress the duct and wash out the stones, parasites and debris. Although this can be done and a T-tube inserted, it is usually recommended to do a sphincteroplasty or choledochoduodenostomy to ensure free drainage of the bile duct.

References

Allison D.J. (1978). Therapeutic embolisation. *Brit. J. Hosp. Med*; **20:**707–15.

Anthony P.P. (1978). Tumours of the liver. In *Recent Advances in Histopathology*, No. 10 (Anthony P.P., Wolff N., ed) p. 217. Edinburgh: Churchill Livingstone.

Balasegaram M. (1970). Hepatic surgery: present and future. *Ann. R. Coll. Surg. Engl*; **47:**139–58.

Bismuth H., Malt R.A. (1979). Current concepts of cancer: carcinoma of the biliary tract. *New Engl. J. Med*; **301:**704–6.

Blumgart L.H. (1978). Biliary tract obstruction: new approaches to old problems. *Amer. J. Surg*; **135:**19-31.

Blumgart L.H., Drury J.K., Wood C.B. (1979). Hepatic resection for trauma, tumour and biliary obstruction. *Brit. J. Surg*; **66:**762–9.

Bouchier I.A.D., ed. (1973). Disease of the biliary tract. In *Clinics in Gastroenterology*, 2:1. London: W.B. Saunders.

British Medical Journal (1980). Editorial Brit. Med. J: **280:** 1155–6.

George, Phyllis A., Brown C., Foley R.T.E. (1981). Carcinoma of the hepatic duct junction. *Brit. J. Surg*; **68:**14–8.

Johnson A.G. (1975). Cholecystectomy and gallstone dyspepsia. *Ann. Roy. Cool. Surg. Engl*; **56:**69–80.

Lancet (1979). Non-invasive method for diagnosis of jaundice (leading article) *Lancet*; **ii:**18–9.

Longmire W.P., Trout H.H., Greenfield J. *et al.* (1974). Elective hepatic surgery. *Ann. Surg*; **179:**712–21.

Lund J. (1960) Surgical indications in cholelithiasis: prophylactic cholystectomy elucidated on the basis of long-term follow-up on 526 non-operated cases. *Ann. Surg*; **151:**153.

Mays E.T. (1976). Hepatic trauma. *Curr. Probl. Surg*; **13(11):**1–73.

Ong G.B., Chan P.K.W. (1976). Primary carcinoma of the liver. *Surg. Gynaecol. Obstet*; **143:**31–8.

Orloff M.J., ed. (1973). Surgery of the biliary tree. *The Surgical Clinics of N. America*; **53:**5. Philadelphia: W.B. Saunders.

Orloff M.J., (ed.) (1978). Retained and recurrent bile duct stones. *World J. Surg*; **2:**401-96.

Rob C., Smith R., (eds.) (1977). *Operative Surgery: Abdomen* 3rd edn. pp. 305–402. London, Boston: Butterworths.

Rubin R.H., Swartz M.N., Malt R. (1974). Hepatic abscesses: changes in clinical, bacteriologic and therapeutic aspects. *Amer. J. Med*; **57:**601–7.

Smith R., ed. (1974). *Surgical Forum – The Liver*. London: Butterworth.

Smith, R. (1979a). Obstructions of the bile duct. *Brit. J. Surg*; **66:**69–79.

Smith R. (1979b). Tumours of the liver. *Ann. R. Coll. Surg. Engl*; **61:**87–99.

Terblanche J. (1977). Liver tumours. *Brit. J. Hosp. Med*; **17:**103–14.

Terblanche J., Louw J.H. (1973). 'U' tube drainage in the palliative therapy of carcinoma of the main hepatic duct system. *Surg. Clin. North. Amer*; **53:**1254,5.

Triger D.R. (1981). *Practical Management of Liver Disease*. Oxford: Blackwell Scientific Publications.

Walt A.J. (1978). The mythology of hepatic trauma – or Babel revisited. *Amer. J. Surg*; **135:**12–8.

Whelton M.J., Petrelli, Mary, George, Phyllis, Young W.B., Sherlock, Sheila (1969). Carcinoma at the junction of the main hepatic ducts. *Qart. J. Med*; **38:**211–30.

Wood C.B., Capperauld I., Blumgart L.H. (1976). Bioplast fibrin buttons for the control of haemorrhage of the liver following biopsy and partial resection. *Ann. Roy. Coll. Surg. Ed*; **58:**401–4.

Further reading

Bengmark, S. (1982). Progress in the treatment of liver cancer. *World Surg*; **6:**1–85.

Blumgart L.H. (1982). *The Biliary Tract. Clin. Surg. Int*. Edinburgh: Churchill Livingstone.

7

Pancreas

C.W. IMRIE

Acute pancreatitis

Many aspects of the management of the initial phases of acute pancreatitis relate to intensive care and non-surgical methods of therapy, but the majority of patients present an initial differential diagnosis which comes within the sphere of surgical emergency practice (*see* chap 1). It is of the utmost importance that all should be aware of this condition which is, at least in one area of the UK, marginally more frequent in occurrence than perforated duodenal ulcer. The absolute incidence ranges from 40–200 cases per million per annum in different areas of Britain. Any disease with this incidence is of importance to all clinicians confronted with abdominal emergencies.

Classification

Patients are classified as having either:

1 Acute pancreatitis
2 Recurrent acute pancreatitis.

Recurrent acute pancreatitis occurs in those in whom the aetiological factor has not been removed, e.g. persistent biliary calculi or recurrent exposure to alcohol abuse. It is usual for such people to have completely recovered from a previous attack in terms of clinical status and pancreatic function. Occasional patients experience a 'spluttering recurrent pancreatitis', with episode upon episode when frequently multiple small biliary calculi are responsible.

In Great Britain biliary disease is the cause in 50–55% of patients, while alcohol abuse varies in incidence from 8–35%.

Clinical presentation and laboratory diagnosis

The clinical presentation invariably features acute upper abdominal pain which can be maximal in the epigastrium, left or right upper quadrants. On occasion the pain encircles the upper abdomen. Less than 5% of patients have pain in other locations, and a few are without pain. Vomiting is troublesome in 85–90% of patients and is absent in only 5%.

A definite diagnosis can be established at laparotomy where pancreatic swelling and flecks of fat necrosis are usually found together with free fluid within the peritoneal cavity. This fluid is rich in both amylase and albumin. In some severe forms both haemorrhage and areas of pancreatic or peripancreatic necrosis may be found. At the present time, it is much more common for the diagnosis to be based on the clinical picture and associated significant elevations of both serum and urinary amylase. Other biochemical markers have been used, but have been unsatisfactory because of the time-consuming nature of lipase tests and the lack of specificity of methaemalbumin (MHA) (McMahon *et al.*, 1980). Newer faster methods for measuring lipase have recently become available and serum trypsin measurements may prove valuable. Elevations of serum amylase above 1200 international units/litre (u/l) and urine amylase above 3000 u/l are diagnostic of acute pancreatitis in a patient with an appropriate clinical presentation. (Normal levels of serum amylase are 70–300 u/l and urine amylase up to 1500 u/l.) Amylase clearance values can be particularly valuable when the serum amylase level is in the grey zone between 300 and 1200 u/l and the presentation is suggestive, but not certain. Elevations of amylase clearance in excess of 4 ml/min support the diagnosis (Imrie and Whyte, 1975), while an amylase to creatinine clearance ratio (ACCR) in excess of 5% is also an indicator of the presence of acute pancreatitis. However, between 40 and 50% of patients with both strong biochemical and clinical evidence of acute pancreatitis may have normal or only marginally raised ACCR levels (Table 1).

Some additional emergencies occasionally present with confusingly high levels of serum amylase, but the natural history of those conditions is usually quite different from acute pancreatitis. Differences occur in preceding clinical history, radiological findings and clinical course. To explain hyperamylasaemia, there must be either an abnormally large source of amylase being released into the blood stream or some blockage to the renal excretion of amylase; therefore, it is difficult to include conditions such as acute cholecystitis or biliary colic. The major sources of amylase within the abdominal cavity are the pancreas, small intestine and Fallopian tubes.

Conditions which may mimic acute pancreatitis to the extent of associated hyperamylasaemia (Table 2)

1 *Perforated duodenal ulcer.* This is particularly true of perforation seen more than 24 h after onset; it is rare to find serum amylase levels over 1200 u/1 within 24 h of perforation.

2 *Dissecting aortic aneurysm or mesenteric vascular occlusion.* The history of the former is easily distinguished from acute pancreatitis, but in the latter one of the trickiest problems of differential diagnosis occurs. Needle aspiration of the peritoneal cavity may be helpful as an immediate Gram film will usually reveal organisms in the presence of mesenteric vascular occlusion. Where the likelihood of arterial embolisation is high, e.g. in atrial fibrillation, it is justifiable to proceed to laparotomy. Only by appropriate early surgical intervention, employing embolectomy, can any lives be saved from this condition. In one recent American

Table 1
DIAGNOSIS OF ACUTE PANCREATITIS

An appropriate clinical presentation accompanied by one or more

  a Serum amylase > 1200 u/l
  b Urine amylase > 3000 u/l
  c Amylase clearance > 4 ml/min
  d ACCR > 5%

Table 2
OTHER CAUSES THAN ACUTE PANCREATITIS WITH ACUTE ABDOMINAL PAIN AND HYPERAMYLASAEMIA

1 Perforated duodenal ulcer
2 Mesenteric vascular occlusion
3 Dissecting aortic aneurysm
4 Small bowel obstruction
5 Ectopic pregnancy
6 Renal failure
7 Macroamylasaemia

study 34 patients had their serum amylase measured and, although elevations were frequent, only 2 exceeded 600 u/l.

3 *Small bowel obstruction.* Abdominal x-rays are used to differentiate this condition from acute pancreatitis.

4 *Ectopic pregnancy.* This is an important diagnosis to remember, but usually the clinical history and findings will differ significantly from acute pancreatitis.

5 *Renal failure.* It is unusual for levels to rise above 800 u/l.

6 *Macroamylasaemia.* An unusual condition in which the circulating serum amylase is usually in the form of a molecule of approximately 4–5 times the molecular weight of normal serum amylase. This larger molecule does not filter through into the urine and urinary levels are minimal and amylase clearance very low.

Grading severity of acute pancreatitis

Until the 1970s the main objective signs of severe acute pancreatitis were hypotension and the development of major complications such as acute renal failure, pseudocyst or abscess formation, flank or periumbilical staining, or the death of the patient. Most of these signs took time to develop and sometimes merely reflected the inadequacy of fluid replacement, rather than the initial severity of the pancreatitis. More recently Ranson of New York introduced a valuable objective multifactorial analysis made after 48 h of admission (Ranson *et al.*, 1976). He used an 11-factor system with good statistical analysis and this has recently been simplified to a 9-factor system based on studies in Glasgow (Imrie *et al.*, 1978b). By both methods the presence of a minimum of three prognostic factors indicates severe acute pancreatitis and the greater the number of prognostic factors, the greater the risk of major morbidity and death. Using either method, it is possible to grade severe disease within a few hours of admission and always at 48 h. None of the factors measured are obscure and many contribute to the specific management of the severely ill patient. The 9-factor grading system is shown in Table 3. The criteria are more applicable to patients with a non-biliary cause and to improve the grading for all patients we would now recommend the exclusion of age as a criterion and doubling of the transaminase 'cut-off' to 200 u/l. Most recently analysis of peritoneal fluid obtained by a lavage catheter has been claimed to give a faster and equally accurate method of grading the severity of disease. Grading is partly based on the colour of the peritoneal or lavage fluid and claims that this approach is an improvement on the multi-factorial objective analysis are difficult to uphold because one of the most discriminating factors, LDH, was excluded from the comparison (McMahon *et al.*, 1980). There is also the possibility of trocar damage to viscera with this method, but in the very ill the perioneal catheter may be used for subsequent peritoneal lavage.

In a consecutive series of 205 patients with acute pancreatitis, the accuracy of objective assessment of disease with respect to death is illustrated in Table 4. It is possible to discriminate between one-third of patients, with severe disease who require intensive therapy, from the two-thirds with mild disease, who can largely be managed by less experienced medical and nursing personnel; such discrimination has obvious practical importance. Those with severe disease require careful and regular monitoring, especially during the first 36 h of admission, in a fashion analogous to the manage-

ment of the patient with a severe burn. It is important to appreciate that large volumes of intravenous plasma and electrolytes may be required as losses can exceed 5 l in the initial 24 h of hospitalisation. Patients with mild disease have very low mortality and the majority are quite well at the end of the first week of treatment. Trials of new approaches in therapy must be related to those with severe acute pancreatitis as any experimental therapies in patients with a mild form of disease and a mortality rate of under 1% are unjustified.

The main cause of death is multi-system failure in which respiratory failure is the major single problem. In 65% of the patients who died with severe acute pancreatitis quoted in Table 4, there was a failure to maintain a P_{AO_2} above 50 mmHg, despite supplementary oxygen therapy at the highest flow rate using a Hudson mask and humidifier. Hypercapnia is a rare problem in patients with acute pancreatitis and it is hypoxaemia which is the main respiratory abnormality.

Management of acute pancreatitis

The conservative management of severe acute pancreatitis is fundamentally an intensive care problem which must concentrate on the steps which will minimise the risks of failure in certain systems (Table 5).

Respiratory failure is the most frequent and troublesome problem. It is both unwise and dangerous to rely on a clinical assessment of respiratory insufficiency as it is particularly difficult to gauge the degree of hypoxaemia without measuring arterial blood gas levels.

Table 4
OUTCOME OF CONSERVATIVE TREATMENT (1975–78 GLASGOW ROYAL INFIRMARY)

	n	Deaths	
Severe acute pancreatitis	88	19	(21.6%)
Mild acute pancreatitis	167	1	(0.6%)
Totals	255	20	(7.8%)

Table 3
PROGNOSTIC FACTORS IN ACUTE PANCREATITIS

1 P_{AO_2} less than 60 mmHg (8.0 kPa)
2 Serum albumin less than 32 g/l (normal 41–53)
3 Serum calcium less than 2.0 mmol/l (normal 2.20–2.60)
4 White cell count in excess of 15 000/mm^3
5 Transaminase enzymes in excess of 100 u/l
6 LDH in excess of 600 u/l
7 Plasma glucose in excess of 10 mmol/l (in absence of diabetes)
8 Blood urea in excess of 16 mmol/l and not responding to intravenous fluid therapy
9 Age greater than 55 years

If, within the first 48 h of admission, three or more of the above nine factors are present, the patient has severe disease (Imrie *et al.*, 1978b).

Table 5
CONSERVATIVE MANAGEMENT OF ACUTE PANCREATITIS IS GEARED TO PREVENT OR MINIMISE

1 Respiratory insufficiency/failure
2 Renal insufficiency/failure
3 Myocardial insufficiency/failure
4 Haematological abnormalities
5 Biochemical abnormalities

Pleural effusions, atelectasis and pulmonary oedema, which occur more frequently in patients with acute pancreatitis, can be detected radiologically. Tachypnoea and the larger pleural effusions can be detected clinically, but the presence of hypoxaemia, and the degree of response to supplementary oxygen therapy requires measurement of the concentrations (Imrie *et al.*, 1977a). Although right to left shunting accounts for a large proportion of the hypoxaemia, other features must be present to account for the usual response to humidified oxygen therapy. Many explanations – interstitial pulmonary oedema, airways closure with gas trapping, and hyaline membrane formation – have been advanced. The well-documented, early loss of albumin from the intravascular space may facilitate the onset of pulmonary oedema especially if fluid replacement is over-enthusiastic. Recently it has been shown that airways closure plays little part in the development of respiratory insufficiency in acute pancreatitis (Murphy *et al.*, 1980). The same workers conclude that severe forms of respiratory insufficiency in this disease represent a variant of adult respiratory distress syndrome with certain unique features (e.g. pleural effusion).

In approximately one-third of patients the coagulation mechanism may be significantly activated to produce clotting time at least 6 s faster than controls. This may be a non-specific response, but it may also be an index of local intravascular coagulation in the pulmonary circulation. Significant degrees of activation of the complement system have been demonstrated in a proportion of those with severe disease. These two factors account for the shunts which develop. It has been claimed that peritoneal lavage minimises respiratory complications but, where respiratory insufficiency is present, it is wise with this technique to use one litre cycles rather than the customary two litre cycle. A poor response to the combination of oxygen and diuretics, especially when the P_{AO_2} remains below 50 mmHg, indicates the need for assisted ventilator therapy with PEEP up to 20 cm H_2O. This is a temporising measure in the hope that the process which has caused the respiratory failure will reverse during ventilatory therapy. Right-to-left shunts in excess of 25% of cardiac output have been measured in patients with acute pancreatitis, but follow-up measurements of respiratory function have indicated that a complete reversal of the abnormalities occurs by 3 months (Murphy *et al.*, 1980).

Acute renal failure was formerly a major hazard in acute pancreatitis, but attention to fluid replacement, to produce urine outputs of at least 30 ml/h, and to monitoring of central venous pressure, where required, significantly decreases the incidence of this complication (Imrie and Whyte, 1975). The most common cause of oliguria is inadequate fluid replacement; in the severely ill patient between 5 and 7 l of fluid may be

required within the first 24 h. If hypovolaemia has been reversed, but urine output remains inadequate a 20 g bolus of mannitol should be administered; the dose should be repeated 30 min later. Continued failure to produce urine in the next 15 min indicates that an intravenous bolus of frusemide should be given. Thereafter, a persistent absence of urine warrants immediate peritoneal dialysis. Problems may be encountered in overcoming renal physicians' reluctance to help in this regard until certain 'built-in thresholds' of blood urea and serum creatinine levels have been exceeded, but the intention is not only to provide early renal support, but also to 'wash-out' toxic material from the peritoneal cavity in these patients. By striving to maintain a minimal urine output of 30 ml/h the incidence of acute renal failure has been reduced from over 14% to just over 3% (Imrie *et al.*, 1978b).

Cardiac failure is a complication which has only recently been documented and may reflect the release of the much-debated peptide myocardial depressant factor (MDF) from the damaged pancreas. Whatever the exact mechanism, the finding of six myocardial infarcts amongst 14 patients who died is disturbing (Imrie *et al.*, 1978b). Specific therapy, after the restoration of blood volume and the correction of hypoxaemia, was to give digoxin or ouabain, but now low dose dopamine is also found to be a useful alternative.

Haematological abnormalities (including coagulation upsets) have been documented in patients with acute pancreatitis for many years (Murphy *et al.*, 1977). Falls in serial concentrations of haemoglobin, white blood count and haematocrit are partly accounted for by haemodilution, but other factors may be important (Trapnell, 1966). Retroperitoneal haemorrhage in and around the pancreas and bleeding from gastric erosions or stress duodenal ulcer may necessitate blood transfusion. Sporadic reports have also appeared of disseminated intravascular coagulation (DIC) occurring in acute pancreatitis. More recently, prospective studies have shown in more than one-third of patients an activation of the coagulation system, indicated by significant shortening of the kaolin cephalin clotting time (KCCT). In the 159 patients reported in one study (Imrie *et al.*, 1979), elevated fibrinogen degradation products were found in most patients, but levels over 40 μ/ml were uncommon. Levels of the large 'scavenger molecule' antithrombin 111 and alpha-2 macroglobulin fell slightly in the first 24 h, but thereafter returned to normal levels. Marked acute phase reactant changes were seen in fibrinogen, factor V, factor V111, alpha-1 anti-trypsin and C_1 inactivator levels. No patients developed the classic syndrome of disseminated intravascular coagulation (DIC) so that heparin therapy was not required. Nevertheless, acute pancreatitis was associated with non-specific acute phase reactant changes, possibly reflecting a moderate degree of intravascular coagulation. Thus specific measures to counteract these haemostatic changes are very rarely indicated. A minority of patients require blood transfusion and very few, heparin therapy, for DIC.

Biochemical abnormalities include acute hyponatraemia, hyperkalaemia and hypocalcaemia. These may co-exist in the same severely ill patient (Allam and Imrie, 1977) and the most effective management of this sick-cell syndrome, is to administer 50 ml pulses of 50% dextrose via a central venous catheter along with soluble insulin in 10 or 20 unit fractions each hour. Edmondson originally drew attention to hypocalcaemia in acute pancreatitis in 1942, and it was two years later he and his co-worker showed an incidence of apparent hypocalcaemia in 70% of patients. Almost 90% of those with apparent hypocalcaemia can be explained by associated hypoalbuminaemia causing a fall in protein bound calcium due to a primary loss of albumin from the intravascular space. Specific measurement of ionised calcium in patients with acute pancreatitis confirmed this explanation for the majority of patients (Allam and Imrie, 1977), although a more recent paper showed the correlation to be poor within the first 48 h of illness (Croton *et al.*, 1981). From a therapeutic standpoint, supplementary albumin, either in the form of plasma, purified plasma derivatives or commercial albumin, is necessary not only to restore blood volume, but also to replace albumin which has been lost into the pleural space, retroperitoneal and general peritoneal spaces.

In the most severely ill patients (less than 10% of the total) a true decrease in ionised calcium may occur. For a time, however, this finding was explained as a failure of parathyroid hormone (PTH) response, but very high levels of PTH were found in hypocalcaemic patients (Imrie *et al.*, 1978a). The typical type of response in severe acute pancreatitis with hypocalcaemia is illustrated in Fig 7.1. The precipitation of calcium in fat

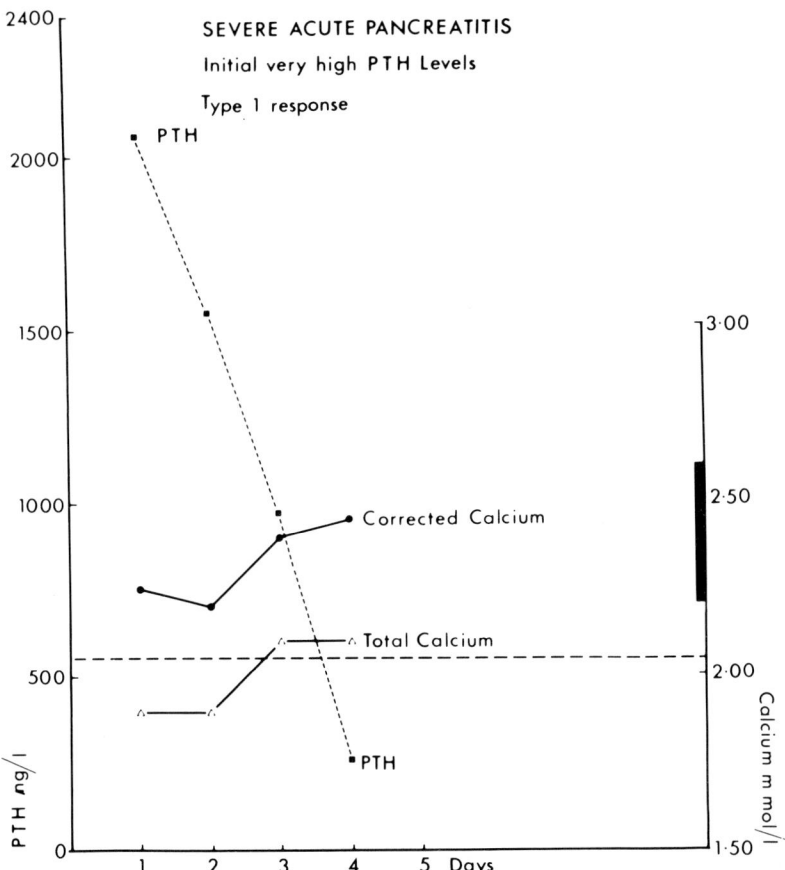

Fig 7.1 Plasma PTH levels in typical case of severe acute pancreatitis with hypocalcaemia. Horizontal dotted line = upper limit normal PTH. Solid vertical bar = normal range of serum calcium.

necrosis may be the initial stimulus to the PTH response which has occurred by the time the patient is admitted to hospital. The reason for previous confusion in the role of PTH related to a failure sequentially to analyse calcium and PTH levels in individual patients. In a recent study of 88 of 90 patients in whom both PTH and calcium were sequentially analysed, calcium homeostatic mechanisms were found to function remarkably well (Imrie *et al.*, 1978a). Therefore, supplementary PTH in the treatment of hypocalcaemia was shown to have little basis. An excellent response to 50% dextrose and insulin is documented (Allam and Imrie, 1977), suggesting a movement of extracellular ionised calcium into cells in some patients and, therefore, intravenous calcium gluconate is perhaps not necessary.

Additional drug therapy in acute pancreatitis

Antibiotics

There is little evidence that patients with acute pancreatitis routinely require antibiotic therapy. Only 3–4% of patients develop pancreatic abscesses. The use of prophylactic antibiotics may, in fact, increase the risk of abscess formation. Ampicillin has been used in two double blind American studies without benefit (Finch *et al.*, 1976; Howes *et al.*, 1975). It must be conceded that most of the patients in these studies had acute pancreatitis associated with alcohol abuse and a very small proportion with biliary disease. The evidence from the natural history of the disease is that the initial leucocytosis does not persist and in my experience of over 700 patients, only two succumbed from septicaemia, in each case *Cl. welchii* was the organism. On the present evidence, the author sees nothing to recommend routine antibiotic therapy in this disease.

Aprotinin (Trasylol)

After initial encouraging experimental work, this antiprotease drug was given in very low dosage with varying success in the 1960s. A fresh impetus to re-examine the evidence was given by a double blind study of high dosage in 105 patients in which a much lower mortality of 7.5% was found in the treated group compared to a control group with 25% mortality (Trapnell *et al.*, 1974). Two subsequent studies using the same dosage of Trasylol have failed to confirm these claims (MRC Multicentre Trial Study Group, 1977; Imrie *et al.*, 1978b). At the present time there is no case for the continual use of Trasylol in the recommended dosage

of approximately 4.5 million KI* units over 5 days. An even higher dose of 4 million KI units given within 4 h of admission has been used in a smaller double blind study (Imrie *et al.*, 1980) without clear benefit.

Glucagon

After an initial uncontrolled study, glucagon was suggested to benefit patients with acute pancreatitis. Again double blind trials have failed to bear out the initial promise of this treatment which can no longer be recommended (MRC Multicentre Trial Study Group, 1977).

A number of other therapeutic agents including calcitonin, somatostatin and epsilon-amino-caproic acid have been given to patients with acute pancreatitis, but proof of their efficacy is lacking.

Peritoneal lavage

Over the last 15 years peritoneal lavage has been used as an adjunct in the therapy of patients with severe acute pancreatitis in a sporadic fashion so that its value is difficult to assess (Ranson *et al.*, 1976). Ranson made an objective attempt to assess the clinicul value of lavage and came down in its favour in the conservative management of severely ill patients (Ranson and Spencer, 1978). The lavage was given for 48–96 h and a daily volume of 36–48 l of isotonic dialysis was used. All patients who entered this study had at least three of eleven prognostic factors positive (Ranson *et al.*, 1976). Twenty-four patients were subject to peritoneal dialysis and in 6 of these the catheters were placed at early laparotomy, while in 18 there was no early surgical intervention (Ranson and Spencer, 1978). Comparison in terms of mortality revealed no difference to a group of similar patients treated without peritoneal lavage. Nevertheless, there was an immediate clinical improvement found following lavage and no patient died within the first 10 days of onset of disease. This is to be compared with a mean period to death in our own experience of 8 days (Imrie *et al.*, 1978b). Late peripancreatic abscess formation, which was the major problem, not only contributed to morbidity, but also to death and resulted in no improvement in overall survival. It would, therefore, seem that peritoneal lavage offers hope for an improvement in outcome within this group of patients.

Two recent studies show conflicting results regarding the value of peritoneal lavage. The procedure was recommended by a team from Atlanta on the basis of a study of over 60 patients (Stone and Fabian, 1980). All had severe pancreatitis. These workers considered lavage of great benefit and added cephalosporin to the

*KI = Kallikrein inhibitor

lavage fluid. They had little trouble with abscess formation. On the other hand Ihse and his colleagues (Evander and Ihse, 1981) in Lund found lavage therapy to be without benefit in over 40 patients with severe pancreatitis.

What is the best conservative management for a patient with severe acute pancreatitis, irrespective of aetiology? Our practice would be to follow down the centre line shown in Fig 7.2 including peritoneal lavage and assisted ventilation. Should this therapy show no signs of stabilising the patient, surgical excision of necrotic tissue should be seriously considered in the younger patient. However, only one or two patients per year would fall into this class in our hospital out of the 70–75 new cases admitted over this time. Furthermore, although anecdotes abound, there is no unequivocal evidence that early surgical resection of peripancreatic necrotic tissue and any pancreatic necrosis reverses the course of the disease. Some surgeons believe that an even earlier laparotomy and surgical debridement of the pancreatic area is required, without a period of peritoneal dialysis or ventilation therapy. In the present stage of knowledge, especially when criteria for surgical intervention are so vague, it is difficult to support such an approach, despite the presence of enthusiastic reports in the literature.

Aetiology and its importance to the surgeon

To minimise the risk of recurrent acute pancreatitis, it is vitally important to identify the aetiologic factor in every case as early as possible. To this end, routine viral screening, especially for Coxsackie and mumps virus infection, is essential. A sample of serum is required soon after admission and at 10–14 days later. In this way around 3–4% of patients will be shown to have a probable viral cause (Imrie et al., 1977b). Hyperparathyroidism is a rare contributory factor to the onset of acute pancreatitis with an incidence of less than 0.2%, as has been shown by Trapnell (1966); we also have documented only two cases in over 700 patients monitored. Similarly, primary hyperlipoproteinaemia is a rare occurrence in our own experience, but in certain areas of the world, e.g. Kuwait, it may account for as many as 15% of patients. Exposure to particular drugs including steroids and azathioprine is important. Similarly on rare occasions, oral contraceptives or their analogues can be implicated. Finally, around 2–3% of patients may have acute pancreatitis associated with a primary adenocarcinoma in the head of the pancreas, a primary ampullary carcinoma or metastatic carcinoma in the pancreas.

The two major aetiological factors which account for 80–85% of patients in most prospective series, *alcohol abuse and biliary disease*, are found in differing frequencies not only in different areas of the world, but in different decades. Thus in the urban centres of the United States there is an incidence of alcohol abuse acute pancreatitis approaching 90–95% (Ranson et al., 1976), while in most of Europe and Scandinavia, it accounts for between 8 and 40% of patients. However, a more recent study from Scandinavia, has shown that the present Swedish incidence of alcohol-associated acute pancreatitis has risen to over 65% (Svensson et al., 1979). Alcohol abuse as the aetiology can be inferred when the attack occurs about 12–36 h after heavy alcohol intake. The association with alcohol tends to be made by excluding other causes. Up to 10% of patients may have more than one aetiological factor.

Timing of biliary surgery

The detection of gallstones early in the disease is highly desirable. Early cholecystography tends to be unrewarding, but ultrasonic scanning is of considerable benefit. Our practice is to scan all patients in the first week of illness to assess the degree of pancreatic swelling, to define any local collections around the pancreas, and to identify gallstones. Where stones are present and the disease is mild, the patient is put on the next appropriate elective operating list for biliary surgery. When the disease is severe, we prefer to keep the patient in hospital until respiratory function has stabilised and then to carry out the necessary operation during the same admission. This may mean a prolonged stay in hospital, but it is to be preferred to the alternative of allowing the patient home and a possible further attack of pancreatitis. Our approach is, therefore, similar to that described from New York (Ranson, 1979).

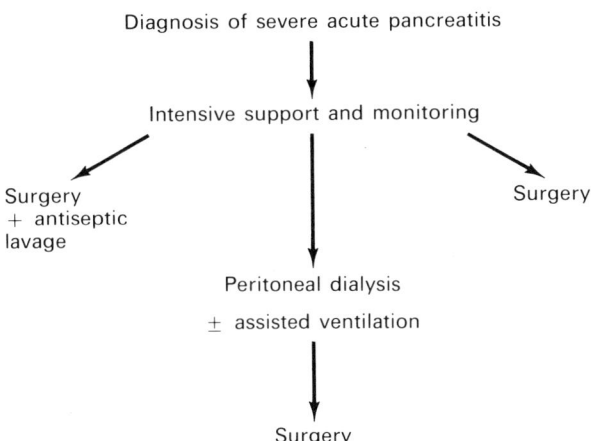

Fig 7.2 Treatment options in the management of severe acute pancreatitis.

There are some who have advocated immediate surgery in biliary-associated acute pancreatitis (Acosta *et al.*, 1978). In earlier work from Argentina the link of acute pancreatitis with the transient passage of small stones through the ampulla of Vater in patients with acute pancreatitis was well demonstrated (Acosta and Ledesma, 1974). If the stones are only transiently held up, is there a need for immediate surgery? Indeed, there is no good case for immediate surgery, both from our own experience and that of others (Ranson, 1979; Osborne *et al.*, 1981). Ranson has clearly shown that immediate, and unnecessary, surgical intervention in these patients is associated with a higher morbidity and mortality. It is preferred to carry out planned early operative intervention in patients with mild acute pancreatitis towards the end of the first week of illness, while in patients with severe disease, an individual approach is required, dependent on the respiratory status and general well-being of the patient. The sensible policy is to keep these patients in hospital until they recover from the most pronounced respiratory problems and then to remove their gallstones, but other major complications such as pseudocyst or abscess may necessitate earlier operation.

Similar arguments apply to immediate endoscopic sphincterotomy of the ampulla of Vater. Surgical and endoscopic treatment make much sense in the early phase of the relatively rare combination of acute pancreatitis and cholangitis, but the case remains to be proved in milder attacks.

Secondary acute pancreatitis

This term embraces postoperative acute pancreatitis, pancreatitis following blunt upper abdominal trauma and such investigations as ERCP and translumbar aortography. This group of patients can be separated from the remaining 90% who have primary acute pancreatitis by the history. Not only is the mechanism of induction different, but frequently the clinical course also differs, largely because of delay before the diagnosis is made. This fact alone probably accounts for much of the increased mortality and morbidity which is found in this form of the disease.

The operations which are known to be associated with immediate postoperative pancreatitis are procedures involving the ampulla of Vater, particularly the use of metal bougies to 'dilate' the sphincter and sphincterotomy or sphincteroplasty. The risk after partial gastrectomy and, to a lesser degree, after splenectomy has also been highlighted. Early diagnosis and conservative treatment by the same methods as outlined previously can result in a satisfactory outcome for the majority of patients (Imrie *et al.*, 1978c).

Where blunt upper abdominal trauma is followed by a clinical picture consistent with acute pancreatitis and hyperamylasaemia, laparotomy is indicated. The damage to the pancreas must be assessed and, if necessary, the distal part of the gland, which may have been completely transected against the vertebral column, may have to be resected. Blunt injury to the right side of the upper abdomen is a less common cause, but more dangerous than traumatic injury to the body of the pancreas, because injuries to other organs are frequent and the pancreatic damage may be more severe so that some drainage utilising a Roux loop may be necessary.

The danger of acute pancreatitis following ERCP has been well documented and, although most cases are infrequent and benign, this is not always so. Fatal cases are reported. Acute pancreatitis after translumbar aortography is sometimes due to the needle traversing the pancreas, but this is less common nowadays because the aorta is punctured at the level of the third and fourth lumbar vertebrae. The reason for the pancreatic inflammation in these patients, or those on cardiac bypass, is still uncertain but ischaemia is probably important.

Later complications of acute pancreatitis

The later complications of acute pancreatitis fall very much within the province of the surgeon. They tend to occur from 7 days onward in the illness and are listed in Table 6.

Pseudocyst of pancreas

This occurs in about 2–15% of all patients with acute pancreatitis. The highest incidence is found in those with alcohol abuse and, therefore, the condition tends to be less common in Britain. We have found an incidence of around 15% in alcoholics, but only around 4% in those with biliary disease.

A pseudocyst very rarely presents without a history of acute pancreatitis. Although the swelling may be gross, more frequently there is an epigastric fullness associated with anorexia, vomiting and weight loss. In addition, pain may be very troublesome and on rare occasions extrahepatic obstructive jaundice is caused

Table 6
MAJOR LATER COMPLICATIONS OF ACUTE PANCREATITIS

1 Pseudocyst
2 Abscess
3 Pancreatic duct stricture
4 Fistula formation
5 GI bleeding
6 Diabetes

by extrinsic pressure of the pseudocyst on the common bile duct. Upward retrogastric extension of the pseudocyst may so angle the oesophago-gastric junction that dysphagia occurs (Sankaran and Walt, 1975). A high level of clinical suspicion is necessary. The traditional investigation of a barium meal with lateral erect views has been replaced by ultrasonic scanning (Pietri and Sahel, 1979). The major advantage of ultrasonic scanning is that the progression and regression of a pseudocyst can be followed and the presence of multiple cysts and multilocular cysts can be well defined. A proportion of patients demonstrate biochemical findings which suggest persisting pancreatitis around the pseudocyst. In some, total serum amylase and urinary amylase are elevated, while in others the total serum amylase may be normal, but the thermolabile fraction is greatly increased.

Management of pseudocyst is conservative in the first instance and the traditional viewpoint has been to allow the pseudocyst to mature so that the wall reaches a thickness which will 'take' sutures. However, the recommended 42 days delay from onset of the attack may be overlooked where symptoms such as pain and jaundice become commanding. Obviously, when major gastrointestinal bleeding occurs within the pseudocyst, immediate surgical intervention is required. This is the most feared complication of pseudocyst and is most frequently caused by the erosion of the splenic artery or vein in its posterior wall. Rarely a vessel running across the central area of the pseudocyst may become so attenuated that it ruptures. The surgical problem is to secure the feeding vessel while considerable bleeding is taking place. Even in patients with no evident history of blood loss, it is wise at laparotomy to aspirate a pseudocyst before directly opening it with a knife.

The most popular and successful surgical procedure is direct drainage of the pseudocyst into the adjacent posterior wall of the stomach (cystogastrostomy). The length of opening in the posterior wall of the stomach should not be less than 5 cm and preferably near 8–10 cm. My own preference is to suture the edge of the stomach to the edge of the pseudocyst with interrupted PGA or chromic catgut. Peripancreatic or pancreatic slough in the depth of the pseudocyst should be removed. Cystojejunostomy, cystoduodenostomy and external drainage are alternative treatments. Internal drainage produces better results (Sankaran and Walt, 1975). In our experience, cystogastrotomy in over 30 patients has been associated with a mortality rate of less than 10%, while external drainage has been associated with 4 deaths in 8 patients due to a combination of sepsis and fistula formation.

An additional reason for delay in surgical drainage is that a considerable proportion will undergo spontaneous regression. Prior to the advent of ultrasonic scanning it was difficult to be certain whether one was dealing with an inflammatory mass or a pseudocyst. Spontaneous regression occurred in just under 50% of 38 patients primarily admitted to our own institution, a much higher figure than those quoted in earlier studies (Sankaran and Walt, 1975).

Pancreatic abscess

This, the worst surgical complication of acute pancreatitis, tends to occur more frequently in patients with biliary pathology and has a higher mortality rate than pancreatic pseudocyst. Without surgical drainage the mortality is claimed to be 100% (Trapnell, 1966) and the establishment of satisfactory drainage with a single operation can only be anticipated in a proportion of patients (White and Heimbach, 1976). No matter how many and how large the drains are at the first operation, further drainage procedures may be necessary. Retroperitoneal abscesses are notoriously difficult to evacuate. Diagnosis rarely presents a major problem as the signs of abscess are usually present. Ultrasonic scanning has been found of great value.

Main pancreatic duct stricture

This may occur after a single severe episode of acute pancreatitis of any aetiology. It tends to occur more commonly after trauma and alcohol abuse than in patients with gallstones. It is a relatively unusual complication, but an important one as the gland distal to the stricture will tend to become the site of chronic pancreatitis. An example of this abnormality on an ERCP is shown in Fig 7.3. Persistent local stricture with distal disease is best treated by distal resection.

Fistula formation

This may occur primarily and is most common around the splenic flexure of the transverse colon.

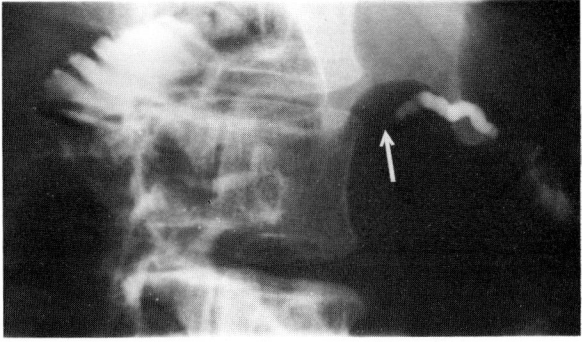

Fig 7.3 ERCP showing pancreatic duct stricture with dilation distal to arrow following a single severe attack of acute pancreatitis.

Secondary fistula formation following laparotomy is more common and this usually involves the transverse colon at or around the same site. Direct fistula formation from the main pancreatic duct may also occur and most of these fistulae respond well to intravenous nutrition. On rare occasions a colostomy or direct operation on the fistula may be required.

Gastrointestinal bleeding

All the common forms of GI bleeding such as gastric erosions and duodenal ulcer may complicate acute pancreatitis. These may represent a stress response, or on occasion, exacerbation of a previously known duodenal ulcer. Massive haemorrhage may occur into a pseudocyst and thereafter discharge along the main pancreatic duct into the duodenum.

Diabetes

This is a surprisingly rare complication of acute pancreatitis and, excluding preterminal diabetes, we have found it only in 2–4% of patients.

This is a deliberately curtailed list of complications of acute pancreatitis excluding rarities such as fat necrosis in unusual sites, e.g. bone marrow. Specific toxic confusional states have been attributed to acute pancreatitis (Trapnell, 1966), but it is difficult to distinguish this from alcohol withdrawal in some patients and severe hypoxaemia in others.

Chronic pancreatitis

According to the Marseilles classification there are two types of chronic pancreatitis which differ only in the frequency of major symptoms, especially pain.

1 Recurrent chronic pancreatitis (chronic relapsing pancreatitis)
2 Chronic pancreatitis

Both types come under the general heading of chronic pancreatitis and are typified by permanent functional and histological damage to the pancreas. The term recurrent chronic pancreatitis is a somewhat clumsy form of English and chronic 'relapsing' pancreatitis is a better description. This particular subdivision of chronic pancreatitis is represented by patients who have pronounced exacerbations of their symptoms, often against a background of discomfort or low-grade pain.

Patients with chronic relapsing pancreatitis differ from those who suffer recurrent acute pancreatitis in several ways. Firstly, in a clinical context those with chronic relapsing pancreatitis tend to have a progressive disease while the patient with recurrent acute pancreatitis returns to apparent normality and good health between attacks. Secondly, pancreatic calcification and pancreatic exocrine insufficiency, with or without diabetes, may be present in chronic pancreatitis, but not in recurrent acute pancreatitis. Finally the exacerbations of chronic relapsing pancreatitis may necessitate hospital admission, but are associated with moderate amylase elevations, while in recurrent acute pancreatitis the acute illness is usually much more severe and associated with marked hyperamylasaemia.

The foregoing implies that there is invariably a clear definition between recurrent acute pancreatitis and chronic relapsing pancreatitis, but this is not always so as a combination of clinical and radiological, biochemical and histological evidence combined with pancreatic function tests are used to categorise patients. A function grading might be satisfactory if the available function tests were more sensitive, but a gross degree of pancreatic insufficiency must be present for significant abnormalities to be detected using standard techniques such as the Lundh or secretin pancreozymin tests. A radiological grading based on the presence of calcification is most useful in Southern European countries where a calcified form of chronic pancreatitis is more common than in Northern Europe (including the United Kingdom) or the United States. This difference is partly explained by the traditions of wine drinking as opposed to beer and spirit intake in the latter areas.

The blurring of the margins between different categories of pancreatitis has been contributed to by the reluctance to carry out pancreatic biopsy because of the supposed dangers of haemorrhage and fistula formation. However, transduodenal biopsy is reasonably safe (Tweedle, 1979) and aspiration cytology either performed percutaneously or operatively has been successful. Thus, while a modification of the Marseilles classification will be employed in this description of chronic pancreatitis, it is important to be aware that different standards for the definition and description of chronic pancreatitis have been used by different authors. Pancreatic function tests currently being assessed may resolve these nomenclature problems. In this category are included tests which are time-consuming, often expensive, and have so far only been employed by a few groups of workers, e.g.:

1 Radioimmunoassay of lactoferrin in pancreatic juice
2 Dual isotope fat absorption tests
3 Para-aminobenzoic acid PABA (absorption and excretion test)
4 Pancreatic polypeptide response to food
5 Trypsin assays in blood, urine and faeces.

Clinical presentation

In the majority of patients epigastric pain is the major problem. However, a few patients present with pancreatic insufficiency of quite rapid onset and either minimal or no discomfort. The pain, characteristically epigastric, may radiate into either hypochondrium or through to the back and can, indeed, present primarily in any of these areas, depending on the part of the pancreas which is most affected by chronic inflammatory change. There is a tendency for disease, localised to the distal body and tail of the gland, to present with left upper quadrant pain and, in a similar fashion, disease confined to the head may only present with right upper quadrant pain. Pain is characteristically severe and may be helped by the patient leaning forward in the sitting position. In some patients the pain may be provoked by the intake of a large meal and tends to occur approximately 20–30 min after ingestion of food. Minor amounts of alcohol may precipitate an attack but, in some, even relieve pain. In others, the pain is of a constant nature, while some patients experience pain of unpredictable onset. Occasional patients have little or no pain.

Histological changes

These are characteristically sporadic throughout the pancreas, especially in the type of chronic calcifying pancreatitis described by Sarles and co-workers (Nakamura *et al.*, 1972). Diffuse changes may eventually supervene, but can also be present from an early stage of the condition. Furthermore, focal changes may occur distal to a single narrowing of a major pancreatic duct or the main duct itself, following a single attack of severe acute pancreatitis (Fig 7.3) especially of traumatic origin. In the typical lesions of chronic pancreatitis some lobules of pancreas can be severely abnormal while neighbouring ones are unaffected. There is intraduct deposition of protein precipitates or calculi with distal dilatation and periductal fibrosis and sclerosis. The exocrine elements are severely affected, while the endocrine tissue frequently escapes the fibrotic reaction until a late stage of the illness.

The role of surgery

Surgeons are usually called in when pain has become a major clinical entity, often requiring large amounts of analgesics for its control. It is essential that patients are assessed carefully in the hospital where alcohol intake can be controlled and the effect of abstinence assessed. A significant proportion will resolve without operation.

The efficacy of various analgesics can also be measured while the degree of impairment of pancreatic function and the extent of structural abnormality are assessed. Ultrasound scanning and computerised axial tomography have a place in the investigation of these patients, but the single most useful test is pancreatography (ERCP). Isotope scanning at present is virtually of no value.

The role of surgery in the control of pain in patients with chronic pancreatitis must be tailored to individual needs. The major guideline for most surgeons has been the appearance of the main pancreatic duct as outlined either endoscopically or preoperatively. It is undoubtedly helpful to have the pancreatogram obtained by preoperative endoscopic means as considerable time is saved during the operation. In addition a balanced clinical and radiological view of the situation for each patient can be reached before operation. Techniques of intraoperative pancreatography include direct needle puncture of the duct with the injection of 2–3 ml of radio-opaque dye; amputation of the tail of the pancreas with cannulation of the transected duct; duodenotomy with direct cannulation of the ampulla.

The long-term results of both *sphincteroplasty* and *coeliac ganglion excision or injection* give little cause for enthusiasm. Sphincter cutting procedures lack a rational basis; theoretically coeliac ganglion blockage seems attractive. A more recent approach has been the blockage of the pancreatic duct by intraductal injection of a latex-type material (Ethibloc), but this has only been employed in a small number of patients and the results are difficult to assess at present.

Two main therapeutic approaches are open to the surgeon. The first is some form of *internal drainage* of a dilated main pancreatic duct and the second is *resection of the most diseased part of the pancreas*. Where the disease is diffuse the surgeon may consider total pancreatectomy, but this radical treatment is followed by considerable long-term problems (Braasch *et al.*, 1978).

Pain in chronic pancreatitis: drainage and resection operations

The source of the pain in chronic pancreatitis is not fully understood, although there is good circumstantial evidence that stimulation of exocrine secretion against an obstruction is important. It was this concept which led Cattell in 1947 to drain an obstructed pancreatic duct of a patient with carcinoma achieving subsequently significant pain relief. As a result Duval (1954), Leger *et al.* (1974) devised various operative procedures which have become popular from the mid-1950s onwards (Figs 7.4, 7.5, 7.6). All these operative

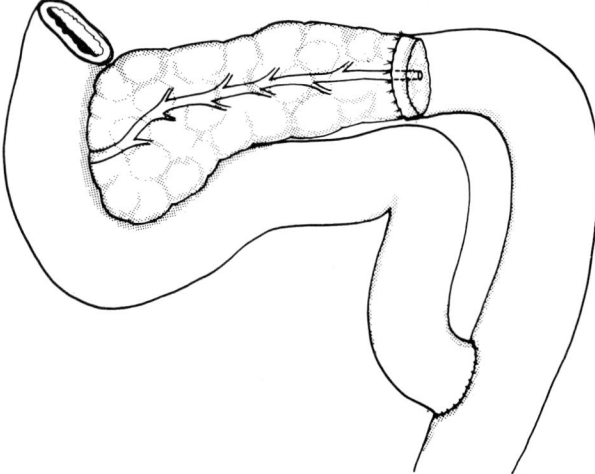

Fig 7.4   Caudal pancreaticojejunostomy (Duval).

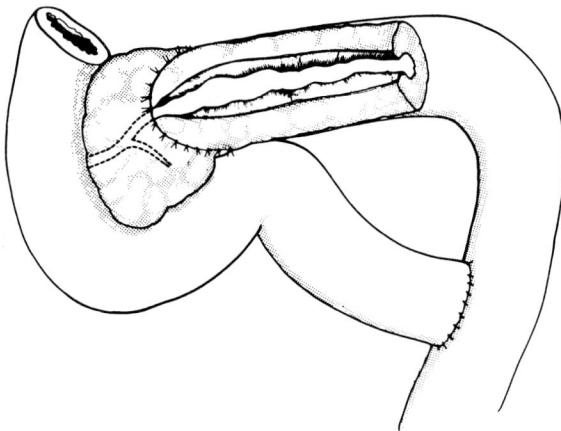

Fig 7.5   Longitudinal pancreaticojejunostomy with insertion of the distal pancreas into the Roux loop.

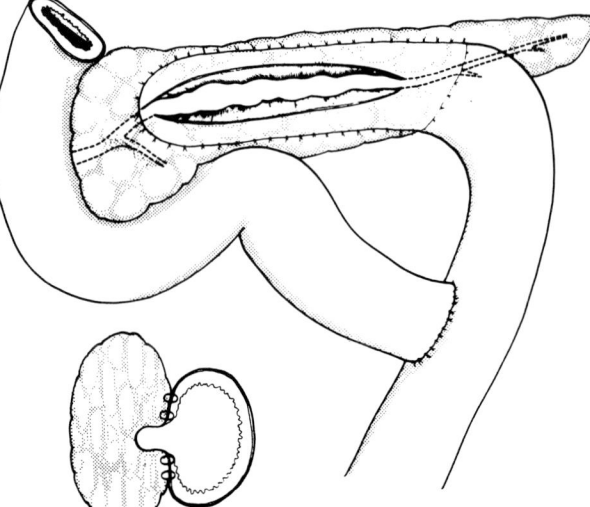

Fig 7.6 Side-to-side pancreaticojejunostomy which avoids splenectomy. Side view anastomosis shown in the insert.

procedures involve some form of drainage of the main pancreatic duct and the results suggest that pressure of pancreatic secretion in an obstructed duct or ducts plays a vital role in production of pain. In unsuccessful cases, the pain may be partly attributed to the envelopment of neural elements within the pancreas by fibrous reaction. No controlled study of pancreatic drainage procedures versus excision has ever been performed and, indeed, it is difficult to conceive of such a study as few centres see sufficient patients to enable statistically significant data to be accumulated. A multi-centre study in either France or the United States might provide the answer, but the frequency of chronic pancreatitis in the UK does not yet permit such an approach.

At least one study (Phillip *et al.*, 1978) has suggested that the natural history of chronic pancreatitis shows that approximately 30% of patients have progressively more severe pain, while the same number become stabilised with pain of constant intensity and approximately 40% experience a spontaneous disappearance of pain after a number of years. However, most authors contend that very few patients become spontaneously free of symptoms.

A review of recent papers indicates that the disease has been most intensively studied and surgically treated in two countries, i.e. France and the United States. Of the 15 papers cited in Table 7, only three do not derive from French or American hospitals. Some large series by very experienced surgeons have been excluded from Table 8. In particular, the work of Warren and associates at the Lahey Clinic in Boston (Warren *et al.*, 1967) recently quoted in the published discussion of the paper of Traverso *et al.* (1979) describes a total experience of over 200 resections, and Mercadier of Paris has a similar experience of over 200 major procedures not presented in detail. While all surgical experts agree that the operative procedure should be tailored to the needs of the particular patient, there are undoubtedly those who have a strong preference for drainage procedures in the form of some type of onlay side-to-side pancreatico-jejunostomy. This approach is particularly recommended by Jordan *et al.* (1977) from Texas, by Proctor *et al.* (1979) from North Carolina and J.C. Sarles of Marseilles (Sarles *et al.*, 1977). The strongest advocates of resection have been from the University of

Table 7
MAJOR PANCREATIC SURGERY FOR CHRONIC PANCREATITIS

		Drainage operations	Resections
F	Mercadier et al. (1968)	115	—
F	Guillemin et al. (1975)	—	103
F	Leger et al. (1974)	45	87
F	Ribet et al. (1975)	22	—
J	Sato et al. (1975)	24	17
A	Frey et al. (1976)	—	149
A	Jordan et al. (1977)	30	—
F	Sarles et al. (1977)	50	45
A	Prinz et al. (1978)	80	—
A	Braasch et al. (1978)	—	26
G	Phillip et al. (1978)	91	148
A	Proctor et al. (1974)	24	25
B	Trapnell (1979)	7	15
A	Traverso et al. (1979)	12	28
A	White and Slavotinek (1979)	55	30
	TOTAL	555	563

A = American: B = British; F = French; G = German; J = Japanese

Table 8
PANCREATIC RESECTIONAL SURGERY FOR CHRONIC PANCREATITIS

		Total pancreatectomy	Subtotal (85–95%)	Distal (L) (40–80%)	Whipple
F	Leger et al. (1974)	—	—	71	16
F	Guillemin et al. (1975)	—	—	—	103
F	Ribet et al. (1975)	—	4	—	23
J	Sato et al. (1975)	1	—	10	6
F	Mercadier et al. (1976)	—	31	—	—
A	Frey et al. (1976)	—	77	53	19
F	Sarles et al. (1977)	—	—	24	21
A	Braasch et al. (1978)	26	—	—	—
A	Proctor et al. (1979)	—	1	17	7
B	Trapnell (1979)	—	15	—	—
A	Traverso et al. (1979)	8	8	7	5
A	White and Slavotinek (1979)	—	9	16	5
	TOTALS	35	145	198	205

A = American; B = British; F = French; J = Japanese

Michigan (Frey et al., 1976) whose long-term follow-up and low in-hospital mortality and morbidity are admirable.

Alcohol is the main aetiological factor in most series, especially from France and the United States, but it was present in less than 30% of Japanese patients (Sato et al., 1975) and just over 50% in a smaller British series (Trapnell, 1979).

The mean age of patients in almost all series is just over 40 years which contrasts with that in studies of acute pancreatitis about a decade older. However, when one excludes the group of patients with biliary aetiology in acute pancreatitis, the difference between the mean age of patients for the two types is scarcely significant. This is an important observation as many contend that patients with recurrent acute pancreatitis rarely proceed to chronic pancreatitis while Trapnell found the opposite to be true, especially in those with a definite alcohol aetiology, as 32 of his 33 patients came into this category (Trapnell, 1979). Sarles considers that there is little evidence of progression from acute to chronic pancreatitis, and while this may be true of the South of France, it is not necessarily applicable in other areas. A further marked difference is the frequency of calcification which is present in approximately two-thirds of French patients, 56% of Japanese (Sato et al., 1975) and just over one third of American (White and Slavotinek, 1979). The incidence in Trapnell's series was even lower at less than 15% of 64 patients. This emphasises the difference in the disease from country to country.

From the analysis of the different types of pancreatic resection for chronic pancreatitis (Table 7) it is clear that few surgeons outside France have considered Whipples' procedure (pancreatico-duodenectomy) applicable to their patients. While this may be a reflection of surgical practice in France compared with the rest of the world, it is also likely that the disease behaves differently. The literature on pancreatic resection is dominated by the contribution from Frey et al. (1976) whose 77 subtotal resections comprise a very large part of the total. While their results are impressive, the majority of exponents of pancreatic surgery favour some form of drainage of the duct of Wirsung into a Roux loop as the initial operation, whenever pancreatography suggests this to be reasonable. Should such an initial procedure prove unsatisfactory, or at the first operation only a very narrow main pancreatic duct be found, then various alternatives are possible.

In a minority of patients, total pancreatectomy will be required and over 60 such operations have been recorded in the literature with 35 included in Table 7. We have obtained definite success in only 3 of the 8 patients who have undergone total pancreatectomy for chronic pancreatitis. Longer follow-up has emphasised the major problems of malnutrition, unemployability and drug addiction (Brasch et al., 1978). Thus while this operation is technically feasible and obviates the need for the difficult pancreatico-jejunal anastomosis, the long-term problems must not be underestimated. Patient selection is vital because acute hypoglycaemia can be rapidly fatal, as it was in one of our patients and in the experience of every group undertaking this type of surgery for chronic inflammation or carcinoma. It is now clear that the nutritional problem is not as simple as was previously thought, a point emphasised by Braasch. The problem of diabetes has been tackled by some groups by the use of autotransplantation at the time of total pancreatectomy. In this procedure the islets which are dissected earlier in the operation are reinjected along the portal vein and the development of this work is awaited with interest.

Cancer of the pancreas

Adenocarcinoma of the pancreas arising from the duct cells accounts for around 80% of tumours. Approximately 10% arise from acinar tissue, and occasional squamous cell carcinomas, cyst-adeno-carcinomas and a group of rarer tumours make up the rest. The incidence of the tumour is increasing worldwide and has overtaken gastric carcinoma in the United States, but not in Great Britain. This makes pancreatic cancer the second most common cancer of the alimentary tract in the United States after colorectal carcinoma, but in the UK the ratio is around 2.5:1 in favour of gastric carcinoma. Nevertheless, there has been a distinct trend for gastric carcinoma to become less frequent with each decade since 1910. The prognosis is appalling with a mean survival of around 6 months, very few patients surviving 5 years. Pancreatic cancer is more common in males with an international ratio of approximately 1.5:1, but ranging 0.39 among American Indians in New Mexico to over 3 in Malta. The tumour is more frequent in black Americans than white and in Jewish than non-Jewish patients in the United States. The mean age at which the carcinoma declares itself clinically is around 63 years, but many reports have highlighted the disease occurring in younger patients. The risk to cigarette smokers is approximately twice that of non-smokers and there is a similar ratio found in established diabetics compared to non-diabetics. No clear evidence regarding dietary habits (Cohn and Hastings, 1981) has been linked to the aetiology of this disease.

The clinical presentation is usually one of painless jaundice as most frequently the disease starts in the head of the pancreas. This location accounts for 65–75% of all pancreatic cancers, while tumours of the body and tail tend to present with central abdominal or back pain. The latter is found in approximately 10% of patients. Anorexia, nausea and weight-loss commonly occur and the rate of weight loss may be very great.

An apparent hypercoagulable state may result in venous thrombosis, arterial thromboembolism and migrating thrombo-phlebitis. Although such events can also occur in patients with carcinoma of the stomach, bronchus or ovary, they are more common in cancer of the pancreas.

There is great difficulty in diagnosing the disease before it is well advanced. Various tumour markers have been utilised in an attempt to identify the cancer at an early stage. Unfortunately neither carcino-embryonic antigen (CEA), alpha fetoprotein (AFP), nor pancreatic oncofetal antigen (POA) have fulfilled their early promise. CEA levels tend to be highest in patients with the most poorly differentiated tumours, but the test does not have sufficient reliability and AFP has been even more disappointing.

Pancreatic oncofetal antigen (POA) has been shown to be of little value in screening a population considered to be at risk of pancreatic cancer, but in individual patients, serial POA levels have been shown to fall abruptly following tumour resection. Recurrence of the tumour has been associated with rising postoperative levels in a similar fashion to CEA in patients with colorectal cancer. Patients with lung cancer tend also to have elevated levels of POA, but usually less pronounced than in pancreatic lesions. Ribonuclease has been found to be of no real value as a marker for pancreatic cancer.

Ultrasonography and endoscopic retrograde cholangio-pancreatography (ERCP) with cytology are the most reliable tests. Ultrasonography was found to be the best screening test for the presence of the disease, while computed tomography (CAT) scanning was most sensitive in detecting nonresectable cancer (Moosa and Levin, 1981). Selective angiography may be of value in determining non-resectability by the demonstration of 'encasement' of major vessels in and around the tumour, occasionally splenoportography may also be similarly valuable.

Percutaneous aspiration cytology techniques have been used in conjunction with PTC, ultrasound scanning and also CT scanning of the pancreas. A high degree of diagnostic accuracy has been reported from Austria, Denmark and Finland using this approach. Smaller studies have also been conducted in the UK and the United States with promising results.

Most frequently the role of the surgeon is restricted to one of palliation. In patients with obstructive jaundice whose tumours are non-resectable, the standard procedure is to perform by-pass using cholecysto-jejunostomy with a gastroenterostomy to minimise the risk of subsequent pyloric hold-up due to encroachment of the cancer on the duodenum. A jejunojejunostomy is usually added to minimise problems of reflux of food material in the gallbladder.

Should the patient be unfit for operation, the insertion of a T-tube in the common bile duct may palliate the major problems of obstructive jaundice. In patients in whom the preoperative diagnosis has been determined by transhepatic cholangiography (PTC), a drainage tube may be inserted to decompress the distended intrahepatic bile ducts and reduce the intensity of jaundice with the intention of possible surgical resection at a subsequent stage. However, should metastases be known to be present, a prosthesis can be inserted over the guide wire used for the PTC, thus avoiding surgical intervention at all. This method is to be commended in less fit patients and those only likely to survive a short time.

Operations to excise pancreatic cancer have changed from time to time. Only a very small percentage of patients are amenable to resection. Pancreatico-duodenectomy (Whipple's operation) has been favoured by some, although of the 80% surviving the operation, only occasional patients are alive 5 years later. This has inclined many to favour simple by-pass procedures and very few surgeons to perform total pancreatectomy. The best results published for pancreatico-duodenectomy for pancreatic cancer have been from the Mayo (Mongé *et al.*, 1964) and Lahey Clinics (Warren *et al.*, 1967) respectively. In both these studies of highly selected patients the 5-year survival exceeded 10%.

The rationale for total pancreatectomy is the evidence that from 15–25% of patients with pancreatic cancer have microscopic evidence of multicentric tumour in the gland. Operative mortality has been reduced to less than 10% by some experienced campaigners. One reason for the lower mortality compared to the Whipple operation is the absence of the pancreatic-Roux loop anastomosis which is most prone to leakage. Despite these advantages, there are certain long-term disadvantages of this operation. All patients are diabetic and, while many can be readily stabilised on insulin, there are occasional patients who are very prone to hypoglycaemic attacks and these are much more liable to prove fatal than in patients who have functioning pancreatic tissue. In addition the exocrine replacement therapy usually fails to restore the patient's weight and as a result several of these patients never recover a satisfactory degree of vigour.

Alternative forms of treatment with or without by-pass surgery have been uniformly depressing. Chemotherapy with or without radiotherapy has not been demonstrated convincingly to be helpful and radiotherapy alone likewise. Indeed, with such a short expectation of life, radiotherapy to the upper abdomen is rarely justifiable at the present time, except where very high energy machines are available.

Carcinoma of the ampulla of Vater

In contrast to the depressing picture of pancreatic cancer, carcinoma at the ampulla of Vater has a remarkably good prognosis. Approximately 70% of patients who present with this tumour are suitable for resection by Whipple's operation. Most of the tumours can be diagnosed endoscopically and the clinical presentation is one of obstructive jaundice which may fluctuate in intensity. The well differentiated tumours are associated with an excellent 5-year survival rate in excess of 60% (Akwari *et al.*, 1977) while tumours with an intermediate degree of differentiation have a 24% 5-year survival, but no patient with a poorly differentiated tumour survives this time. Palliation was found to be good in this study from the Mayo Clinic as the 2-year survival of 30% in the poor cytological type of tumour makes pancreatico-duodenectomy a reasonable procedure.

References

Acosta J.M., Ledesma C.L. (1974). Gallstone migration as a cause for acute pancreatitis. *N. Engl. J. Med*; **290**:484–7.

Acosta J.M., Rossi R., Galli O.M.R., Pellegrini C.A., Skinner D.B. (1978). Early surgery for acute gallstone pancreatitis: evaluation of a systemic approach. *Surgery*; **83**:367–70.

Akwari O.E., Van Heerden J.A., Adson M.A., Baggenstoss T.H. (1977). Radical pancreatoduodenectomy for cancer of the papilla of Vater. *Ann. Surg*; **184**:403

Allam B.F., Imrie C.W. (1977). Serum ionized calcium in acute pancreatitis. *Brit. J. Surg*; **64**:655–68.

Braasch J.W., Vito L., Nugent F.W. (1978). Total pancreatectomy for end stage chronic pancreatitis. *Ann. Surg*; **188**:317–22.

Camer S.J., Tan E.G.C., Warren K.W. (1975). Pancreatic abscess. A critical analysis of 113 cases. *Amer. J. Surg*; **129**:426–31.

Cattell R.B. (1947). Anastomosis of the duct of Wirsung: 'It's use in palliative operations for cancer of the head of pancreas'. *Surg. Clin. N.Amer*; **27**:636–43.

Cohn I., Hastings P.P. (1981). Pancreatic cancer – UICC. Technical Report Series Vol. 59.

Croton R.S., Warren R.A., Stott A., Roberts N.B. (1981). Ionized calcium in acute pancreatitis and its relationships with total calcium and serum lipase. **68**:241–4.

Duval M.K. (1954). Caudal pancreatico-jejunostomy for chronic relapsing pancreatitis. *Ann. Surg*; **140**:775–85.

Edmondson H.A., Berne C.J. (1944). Calcium changes in acute pancreatic necrosis. *Surg. Gynaecol. Obstet*; **79**:240–4.

Evander A., Ihse I. (1981). A double blind trial of peritoneal lavage in severe acute pancreatitis. *European Pancreatic Club* 1981.

Finch W.T., Sawyers J.L., Schenker S. (1976). A prospective study to determine the efficacy of antibiotics in acute pancreatitis. *Ann. Surg*; **183**:6.

Frey C.F., Child C.G., Fry W. (1976). Pancreateotomy for chronic pancreatitis. *Ann. Surg*; **184**:403–14.

Guillemin G., Vachon A., Berard P. *et al.* (1957). Traitement chirurgical de lay pancreatite chronique. Choix d'une technique. *Lyon Med*; **234**:65–84.

Howes R., Zuidema G.D., Cameron J.L. (1975). Evaluation of prophylactic antibiotics in acute pancreatitis. *J. Surg Res*; **18**:197.

Imrie C.W., Whyte A.S. (1975). A prospective study of acute pancreatitis. *Brit. J. Surg*; **62**:490–4.

Imrie C.W., Ferguson J.C., Murphy D., Blumgart L.H. (1977a). Arterial hypoxia in acute pancreatitis. *Brit. J. Surg*; **64**:185–8.

Imrie C.W., Ferguson J.C., Sommerville R.G. (1977b). Coxsackie and mumps virus infection in a prospective study of acute pancreatitis. *Gut*; **18**:53–6.

Imrie C.W., Beastall G.H., Allam B.F., O'Neill, Jennifer, Benjamin I.S., McKay A.J. (1978a) Parathyroid hormone and calcium homeostasis in acute pancreatitis. *Brit. J. Surg*; **65**:717–20.

Imrie C.W., Benjamin I.S., Ferguson J.C., McKay A.J., MacKenzie I., O'Neill J., Blumgart L.H. (1978b). A single centre double blind trial of trasylol therapy in primary acute pancreatitis. *Brit. J. Surg*; **65**:337–41.

Imrie C.W., McKay A.J., Benjamin I.S., Blumgart L.H. :1978c). Secondary acute pancreatitis: aetiology, prevention, diagnosis and management. *Brit. J. Surg*; **65**:399–402.

Imrie C.W., Walker I.D., O'Neill J., Davidson J.F. (1979). Haemostatic changes in acute pancreatitis. *Gastroenterol. Clin. Biolog.* **3**:291A.

Imrie C.W., McKay A.J., Campbell F.C., Gordon D.A., Lang J.A., O'Neill J. (1980). Short duration megadosage trasylol therapy in acute pancreatitis. *Gut*; **21**:A457–8.

Jordan G.L., Strug B.S., Crowder W.E. (1977). Current status of pancreato-jejenostomy in the management of chronic pancreatitis. *Amer. J. Surg*; **133**:46–51.

Leger L., Lenriot J.P., Lemaigre G. (1974). Five to twenty year follow-up after surgery for chronic pancreatitis in 148 patients. *Ann. Surg*; **180**:185–91.

McMahon M.J., Playforth M.J., Pickford I.R. (1980). A comparative study of methods for the prediction of severity of attacks of acute pancreatitis. *Brit. J. Surg*; **67**:22–5.

Mercadier M., Clot J.P., Regensberg C.L. (1968). Les drainages et derivations de canal de Wirsung dans le traitement de pancreatitis chroniques a propos de 115 observations. *Ann. do Chirugie*; **21**:673–80.

Mercadier M., Clot J.P., Eudel F., Colquillaud J.P., Richard J.P. (1976). Resultats eloignes de la chirugie des pancreatitis et leurs complications, 9th Congres Internationalle Gastroenterologie. *Arch. Francaises des Maladies de L'Appareil Digestif*; **61**:299c.

Mongé J.J., Judd E.S., Gage R.P. (1964). Radical pancreato-duodenectomy. *Ann. Surg*; **160**:711–24.

Moossa A.R., Levin B. (1981). The diagnosis of 'early' pancreatic cancer. *Cancer*; **47**:1688–97.

MRC Multicentre Trial Study Group (1977). Death from acute pancreatitis. MRC multicentre trial of glucagon and aprotinin. *Lancet*; **ii**:632–5.

Murphy D., Imrie C.W., Davidson J.F. (1977). Haematological abnormalities in acute pancreatitis. A prospective study. *Postgrad. Med. J*; **53**:310–4.

Murphy D., Pack A.I., Imrie C.W. (1980). The mechanism of arterial hypoxia occurring in acute pancreatitis. *Quart. J. Med*; **194**:151–63.

Nakamura K., Sarles H., Payan M. (1972). Three dimensional reconstruction of the pancreatic ducts in chronic pancreatitis. *Gastroenterology*; **62**:942–9.

Osborne D.H., Imrie C.W., Carter D.C. (1981). Biliary surgery in the same admission for acute pancreatitis. *Brit. J. Surg*; **68**:758–61.

Phillip J., Koch H., Rosch W., Bottisher R. (1978). Follow-up after ERCP guided therapy of chronic pancreatitis. *Acta Hepatogastroenterol*; **25**:463–9.

Pietri H., Sahel J. (1979). Ultrasonography of the pancreas. In *The Exorcrine Pancreas* (Howat, Sarles, eds.). Philadelphia: WB Saunders Co. Ltd.

Prinz R.A., Kaufman B.H., Folk F.A., Greenlee H.B. (1978). Pancreaticojejunostomy for chronic pancreatitis. *Arch. Surg*; **113**:520–5.

Proctor H.J., Mendes O.C., Thomas C.G., Herbst C.A. (1979). Surgery for chronic pancreatitis. *Ann. Surg*; **189**:664–71.

Ranson J.H.C. (1979). The timing of biliary surgery in acute pancreatitis. *Ann. Surg*; **189**:654–63.

Ranson J.H.C., Rifkind K.M., Turner J.W. (1976). Prognostic signs and nonoperative peritoneal lavage in acute pancreatitis. *Surg. Gynaecol. Obstet*; **143**:209–19.

Ranson J.H.C., Spencer F.C. (1978). The role of peritoneal lavage in severe acute pancreatitis. *Ann. Surg*; **187**:565–74.

Ribet M., Prost M., Quandale P., Wurtz A. (1975). Traitement chirurgical des pancreatites chroniques autonomes. *J. de Chirurgie*; **110**:25–38.

Sankaran S., Walt A.J. (1975). The natural and unnatural history of pancreatic pseudocysts. *Brit. J. Surg*; **62**:37–44.

Sarles J.C., Delecourt P., Castelo H. (1977). Le traitement chirurgical des pancreatities chroniques calcifiantes. *Arquiv. Gastroenterolog*; **14**:83–8.

Sato T., Saitoh Y., Noto N., Matsuno K. (1975). Appraisal of operative treatment for chronic pancreatitis. *Amer. J. Surg*; **129**:621–8.

Stone M.H., Fabian T.C. (1980). Peritoneal dialysis in the treatment of acute alcoholic pancreatitis. *Surg. Gynaecol. Obstet*; **150**:878.

Svensson J.O., Norback B., Bokey E.L., Edlund Y. (1979). Changing pattern in aetiology of pancreatitis in an urban Swedish area. *Brit. J. Surg*; **66**:159–61.

Trapnell J.E. (1966). The natural history and prognosis of acute pancreatitis. *Ann. Roy. Coll. Surg. Engl*; **38**:265–87.

Trapnell J.E. (1979). Chronic relapsing pancreatitis: a review of 64 cases. *Brit. J. Surg*; **66**:471–5.

Trapnell J.E., Rigby C.C., Talbot C.H., Duncan E.H.L. (1974). A controlled trial of Trasylol in the treatment of acute pacreatitis. *Brit. J. Surg*; **61**:177–82.

Traverso L.W., Tompkins R.K., Urrea P.T., Longmire W.P. (1979). Surgical treatment of chronic pancreatitis. *Ann. Surg*; **190**:312–9.

Tweedle D.E.F. (1979). Preoperative pancreatic biopsy. *Gut*; **20**:992–6.

Warren K.W., Veidenheimer M.C., Pratt H.S. (1967). Pancreatoduodenostomy for periampullary cancer. *Surg. Clin. N.Amer*; **47**:639.

White T.T., Heimbach D.M. (1976). Sequestrectomy and hyperalimentation in the treatment of haemorrhagic pancreatitis. *Amer. J. Surg*; **132**:270–5.

White T.T., Slavotinek A.H. (1979). Results of surgical treatment of chronic pancreatitis. *Ann. Surg*; **189**:217–24.

Further reading

Hollender L. ed. (1981). Treatment of acute pancreatitis. An international group of papers on pancreatitis. *World J. Surg*; **5**:301–400.

Howat H.T., Sarles J.C. (1979). *The Exocrine Pancreas*. Philadelphia: W.B. Saunders.

Keynes W.M., Keith R.G. (1981). *The Pancreas*. London: Heinemann Medical.

8

Portal hypertension and oesophageal varices

ROBERT SHIELDS

The normal pressure in the portal vein ranges from 5–10 mm mercury. When the portal pressure is consistently raised above 20 mmHg, there can be serious clinical consequences, particularly bleeding from oesophageal varices. Associated with the varices, and usually related to the underlying disease, there may be ascites, encephalopathy and hypersplenism.

Causes

Portal hypertension is usually the result of a blockage in the outflow of blood from the portal circulation (Table 1). Its chief causes can be regarded as presinusoidal, intrahepatic and postsinusoidal. This classification is of practical value because, in presinusoidal obstruction, liver function is usually preserved and hepatic failure is uncommon when the varices bleed. On the other hand, where there is parenchymal damage, as in cirrhosis, liver failure often complicates variceal haemorrhage and its treatment.

In practice, in Western countries, the commonest *intrahepatic* cause of portal hypertension is cirrhosis, usually related to chronic alcoholism. Other hepatic disorders include non-alcoholic nutritional cirrhosis, postnecrotic cirrhosis and primary biliary cirrhosis. In cirrhosis, portal hypertension is caused by a combination of (a) a reduction in the volume, and increase in the resistance, of the intrahepatic vascular bed produced by diffuse fibrosis of the liver, (b) compression,

Table 1
CAUSES OF PORTAL HYPERTENSION

A *Presinusoidal*
   1 Extrahepatic obstruction of the portal vein
     (a) intrinsic thrombosis following
         (i)   neonatal umbilical sepsis
         (ii) pyelophlebitis
         (iii) increased coagulability of the blood.
     (b) extrinsic compression due to
         (i)   pancreatic tumour
         (ii) pancreatitis
         (iii) enlarged lymph nodes in porta hepatis.
   2 Intrahepatic obstruction of the portal vein
     (a) schistosomiasis
     (b) congenital hepatic fibrosis
     (c) sarcoidosis
     (d) reticulo-endothelial disease
     (e) early stages of primary biliary cirrhosis

B *Intrahepatic*
   Mainly cirrhosis

C *Postsinusoidal*
   Obstruction of the hepatic venous drainage or of the inferior vena cava (Budd-Chiari syndrome)

D *Increased flow into the portal system*
   (a) Arteriovenous fistula
   (b) Increased splenic flow

distortion and attenuation of the portal venules, hepatic venous radicles and sinusoids by regenerating nodules, and (c) development of anastomoses between the hepatic arterioles and portal venules, so that arterial pressure is communicated to the venous system.

Presinusoidal block

This is of two main types:

Extrahepatic obstruction. This involves the main portal vein or one of its major tributaries, e.g. splenic vein. In childhood, sepsis is an important factor. In the neonate, umbilical sepsis may lead to thrombosis in the umbilical vein which spreads to the portal vein; in later childhood, portal vein thrombosis may follow appendix abscess or pyelophlebitis. Thrombosis of the portal vein may also complicate certain haematological disorders, e.g. polycythaemia and thrombotic thrombocythaemia. The portal vein may also be compressed by adjacent tumour, by a pseudocyst of the pancreas, or by enlarged lymph nodes in the porta hepatis.

Intrahepatic obstruction. As part of its complex life-cycle, the ova of schistosomiasis may come to lie in the portal zones of the liver and as a result of the granulomatous reaction (of a delayed hypersensitivity type) to antigen released from the egg, portal venous radicles are compressed. Other causes of presinusoidal obstruction within the liver include sarcoidosis, congenital hepatic fibrosis and various diseases of the reticuloendothelial system.

Postsinusoidal obstruction

Obstruction to the venous outflow from the liver (Budd-Chiari syndrome) is rare, but can produce a dramatic, and often fatal, illness. The syndrome is usually produced by occlusion of the major hepatic veins. This is in contrast to venocclusive disease where there is progressive obstruction of the small intrahepatic veins. In an individual patient the exact cause of the Budd-Chiari syndrome may remain obscure, but known causative factors include polycythaemia, leukaemia, primary and secondary tumours of the liver, and, recently, oestrogen-containing oral contraceptives. A variant, seen in Japan, is obstruction of the vena cava by a fibrous membrane or web at the level of the hepatic venous ostia.

Portal hypertension may also be seen in the absence of obvious obstruction and then may be the result of an *increased flow into the splanchnic system*. Arteriovenous fistula, between the hepatic artery and portal vein, or between the splenic artery and splenic vein, are rare. Increased blood flow through an enlarged, overactive spleen may be the cause, e.g. in chronic malaria, Felty's syndrome or metabolic disorders, e.g. Gaucher's disease, sarcoidosis, etc. These causes of portal hypertension are uncommon.

Pathophysiology
Oesophagogastric varices

In health, most of the blood which drains from the portal circulation passes through the liver and enters the systemic circulation by the hepatic veins. In cirrhosis, however, less than one-fifth of the portal blood flows in that direction; the great bulk of the blood leaving the splanchnic bed has to find its way back to the heart through collateral channels. Several groups of collaterals have been described (Fig 8.1), but the ones

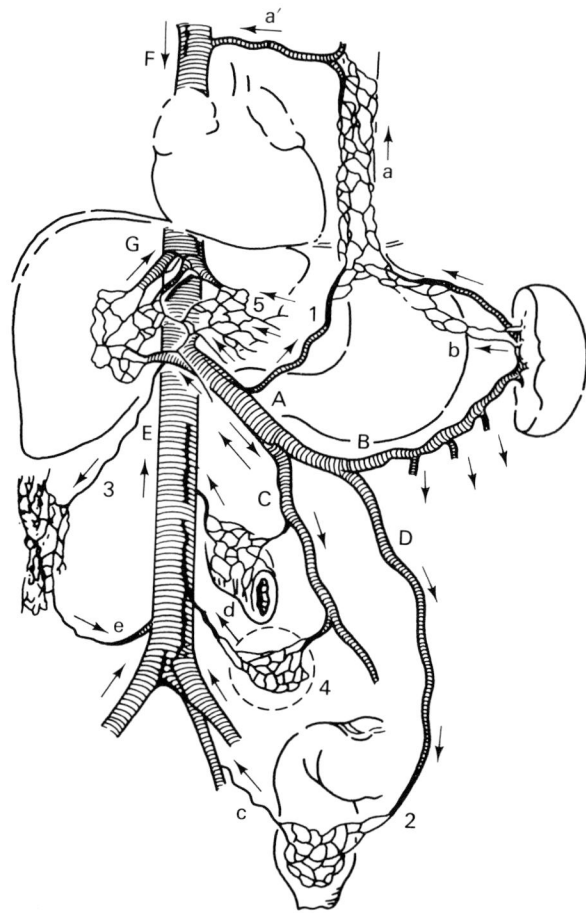

Fig 8.1 Collateral circulation. 1 = coronary (left gastric vein); 2 = superior rectal vein; 3 = paraumbilical vein; 4 = vein of Retzius; 5 = veins of Sappey. A = portal vein; B = splenic vein; C = superior mesenteric vein; D = inferior mesenteric vein; E = inferior vena cava; F = superior vena cava; G = hepatic veins. a = oesophageal veins; a' = azygos veins; b = vasa brevia; c = middle and inferior rectal veins; d = intestinal veins; e = epigastric veins. (From Seymour I. Schwartz, 1974, *Principles of Surgery*, New York and London: McGraw-Hill.)

of major importance are the large submucous varices which protrude into the lumen of the upper part of the stomach and of the lower end of the oesophagus, and which drain blood mainly from the coronary vein of the stomach into the azygos and hemiazygos systems of the systemic circulation. When these varices rupture, bleeding can be alarming, and frequently fatal. The immediate precipitating cause of haemorrhage is often unknown, but the actual height of the portal pressure, peptic oesophagitis, and laxity of the lower oesophageal sphincter are probably the main determining factors.

Dilatation of the umbilical and paraumbilical veins, which communicate with the superficial veins of the abdominal wall, leads to varicosity of the superficial and inferior epigastric veins to produce the caput medusae, which is found in less than one-fifth of patients.

In general the collateral circulation is haemodynamically ineffective. Diversion of the portal flow through these spontaneous shunts rarely alleviates the portal hypertension.

Ascites

Ascites in liver disease is still not fully understood, but is probably the result of several factors – portal hypertension, hypoalbuminaemia secondary to hepatic parenchymal damage, and secondary hyperaldosteronism. Portal hypertension *per se* is rarely the sole cause of ascites, but may be responsible for the localisation of the retained fluid within the peritoneal cavity.

Effective decrease of the portal pressure by a successful portasystemic shunt may reduce an intractable ascites. However, because of the efficacy of modern diuretics, shunt operations are rarely prescribed for ascites.

Spleen

Prolonged obstruction of the portal outflow may lead to congestion and enlargement of the spleen. The engorgement is most evident in the venous sinuses of the spleen and rarely involves the pulp spaces.

The enlarged spleen may sequestrate and destroy platelets and granulocytes and, as a result, thrombocytopaenia and granulocytopaenia may be found in about half of the patients with portal hypertension. The term 'hypersplenism' is often applied, incorrectly, to this combination of a reduction in one or more of the formed elements of the blood, and normal, or hyperactive, bone marrow. The reduced white cell count usually responds to inflammation; the granulocytopaenia rarely requires treatment.

On the other hand, thrombocytopaenia, particularly when associated with coagulation defects in cirrhosis, can increase the risk of haemorrhage. Severe thrombocytopaenia (platelets less than 45 000/dl) may very well frustrate necessary investigations such as splenoportography and liver biopsy unless corrected by platelet infusion.

Usually platelet and white cell counts improve after a successful portasystemic shunt, especially if splenectomy is included, e.g. spleno-renal shunt. Splenectomy alone is rarely required for these deficiencies and, indeed, should be avoided, because of the risk of thrombosis in the splenic vein spreading throughout the portal system and so preventing major shunt surgery in the future.

Hepatoportal encephalopathy

In severe liver disease, especially cirrhosis, there can be disorders of consciousness. The two basic requirements are a degree of hepatic insufficiency and the presence of large, natural, or surgically-created portasystemic shunts. The resulting syndrome is called hepatoportal encephalopathy. Many noxious agents have been incriminated in its causation including ammonia, short-chain fatty acids, methionine, but the pathogenesis of hepatoportal encephalopathy is complex.

Precipitating factors include gastrointestinal bleeding, high protein diet, infection, overprescription of analgesics and sedatives and hypokalaemia, which may be secondary to injudicious diuretic and steroid therapy. Encephalopathy is very liable to occur during and after haemorrhage. Moreover, shunt operations, which can reduce portal hypertension and prevent recurrence of the bleeding, may themselves induce, or aggravate, encephalopathy.

Clinical presentation

The clinical importance of portal hypertension is that oesophageal varices may develop and may bleed. About 30–40% of cirrhotic patients with varices will bleed from them at some time, usually within 2 years of initial diagnosis. When a patient has bled from his varices, he, or she, stands a 60% chance of having a recurrent haemorrhage – indeed in half of the patients bleeding recurs within 72 h. Mortality, when the cause of portal hypertension is extrahepatic, is much lower than in those with alcoholic cirrhosis, of whom 60–70% die within 1 year of haemorrhage.

When a child under 10 years vomits blood copiously, the source is usually oesophageal or gastric varices.

In adults, about 8–10% of patients admitted to British

hospitals with upper gastrointestinal haemorrhage have portal hypertension and oesophageal varices, but the incidence is rapidly increasing because alcoholism is becoming more common, especially in women whose liver seems more sensitive to alcohol.

Varices may be suspected as a source of gastrointestinal bleeding, because of the associated clinical features – jaundice, hepatosplenomegaly, ascites, caput medusa, or the presence of other stigmata of liver disease, e.g. spider naevi. There may be a suggestive history of chronic alcoholism. However, in a well-compensated cirrhotic, or in a patient with schistosomiasis, these features may be absent. Occasionally, slight clouding of consciousness after a brisk haemorrhage may be the only clue to the underlying cirrhosis and portal hypertension.

Diagnosis

The need to make a rapid and accurate diagnosis becomes crucial when the varices are bleeding or have bled.

Endoscopy

The most useful investigation is oesophagoscopy, at which the varices can be seen as bluish, tortuous protrusions of mucosa into the oesophageal lumen. Oesophageal varices are most clearly seen at, or just above, the cardio-oesophageal junction. Small varices, however, can be confused with mucosal folds and gastric varices may easily be missed unless a flexible oesophagoscope is carefully manipulated to view the fundus.

Apart from confirming their presence, the endoscopist must also determine that the varices are the source of bleeding. This is easy if active bleeding is evident, although skill and patience are required to obtain a good view in an alarmed and struggling patient. More usually bleeding has stopped. Other sources of upper gastrointestinal haemorrhage should be searched for and excluded e.g. oesophagitis, duodenal ulcer, Mallory-Weiss tear, gastric erosions. If other bleeding sites have not been found despite careful and expert examination, the varices are probably the source of the bleeding and subsequent treatment should be planned on this assumption. It is, however, quite wrong to assume that a cirrhotic who bleeds has oesophageal varices only, because in 50–70% of cases bleeding can occur from erosions and gastric ulceration. Endoscopic diagnosis is, therefore, essential.

Radiology

Barium studies

An alternative means of detecting varices is a barium swallow. Varices are seen as long worm-like indentations in a slightly dilated oesophagus (Fig 8.2). However, in about 25% of cases, oesophageal varices may be missed. Oblique views in different stages of oesophageal filling may show varices not otherwise apparent. Usually, if the radiologist considers that he has seen varices, they will be present. False negatives are the main source of error.

Angiography

Splenoportography and mesenteric arteriography are occasionally required to demonstrate the varices but are more usually employed to determine the patency of the portal vein and, therefore, the feasibility of major shunt surgery.

Splenoportography. Contrast medium is injected through a needle which has been passed percutaneously into the splenic pulp. The portal vein and collateral

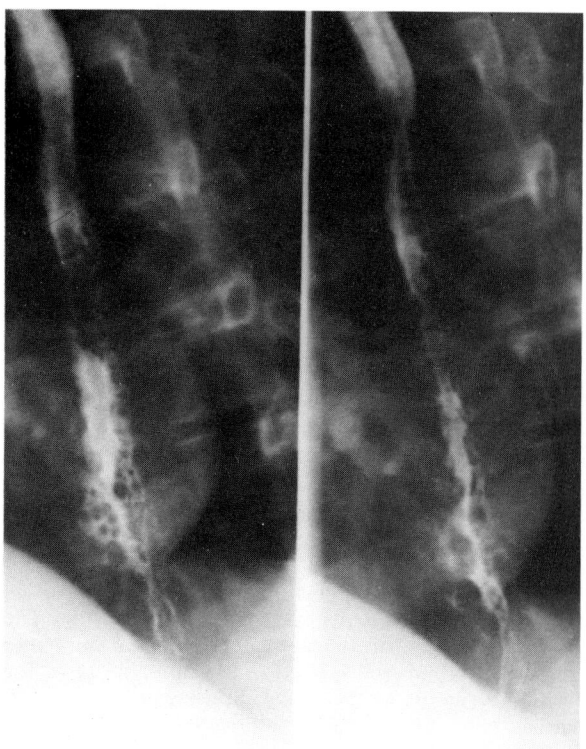

Fig 8.2 Barium swallow showing oesophageal varices.

circulation are usually well opacified (Fig 8.3). Varices can be demonstrated in about 90% of cases.

Contrast medium may leak from the spleen and cause abdominal pain. Rarely blood transfusion may be required. Contraindications include a low platelet count (less than 40 000/dl) and coagulation deficiency (with a prothrombin time of more than 5 s above control values). Failure to demonstrate the portal vein may mean thrombosis of the vein, but more usually the contrast medium has been diverted away from the vein through extensive collaterals.

During the examination, the needle can be attached to a manometer and the splenic pulp pressure recorded as a reasonable indicator of portal venous pressure.

Mesenteric angiography. Mesenteric angiography is used extensively in certain centres. Patients who have had a previous splenectomy, or who have thrombocytopaenia or hypoprothrombinaemia, can be studied by this technique. The coeliac axis is catheterised via the femoral artery and a bolus of contrast medium is injected rapidly. Splenic and portal veins can, therefore, be opacified. Contrast medium can also be injected into the superior mesenteric artery to visualise the mesenteric and portal veins.

A disadvantage of the technique is that occasionally the concentration of contrast medium in the portal vein is so low that the vein is not sufficiently opacified. However, the hepatic arterial system can be demonstrated and abnormalities, such as tumours, abnormal vessels, etc., are easily detected.

Umbilical vein catheterisation can provide a clear picture of the portal vein, but the technique is not easy and requires a minor operation.

Percutaneous transhepatic catheterisation involves the passage of a needle through the liver substance into the portal vein and subsequently a catheter is advanced along the portal vein into its tributaries. Portal pressure can be accurately recorded and clear venograms obtained following the injection of contrast medium. The technique, however, carries greater risks and requires considerable skill. It is usually used in conjunction with therapeutic sclerosis of gastro-oesophageal varices (*see below*).

Other radiological investigations

If major portasystemic shunts are being planned, other x-rays are required:

1 before a mesocaval shunt, patency of the inferior vena cava should be confirmed;
2 before distal splenorenal shunt (Warren operation), the left renal vein should be opacified to determine its patency, normality, and position relative to the splenic vein;
3 before any operation involving the renal veins, intravenous pyelography should be carried out.

Pressure recordings

If a patient is presumed to have portal hypertension, the actual height of portal venous pressure should be obtained. This may be done directly or indirectly.

Direct measurement of portal pressure

1 **Preoperative**
   (a) Percutaneous transhepatic technique (*see above*).
   (b) Umbilical vein catheterisation (*see above*).

2 **Peroperative.** By passing a catheter into a jejunal vein and threading it into the main mesenteric and portal trunks. During operation it is essential to demonstrate there has been an appreciable fall in pressure after shunting.

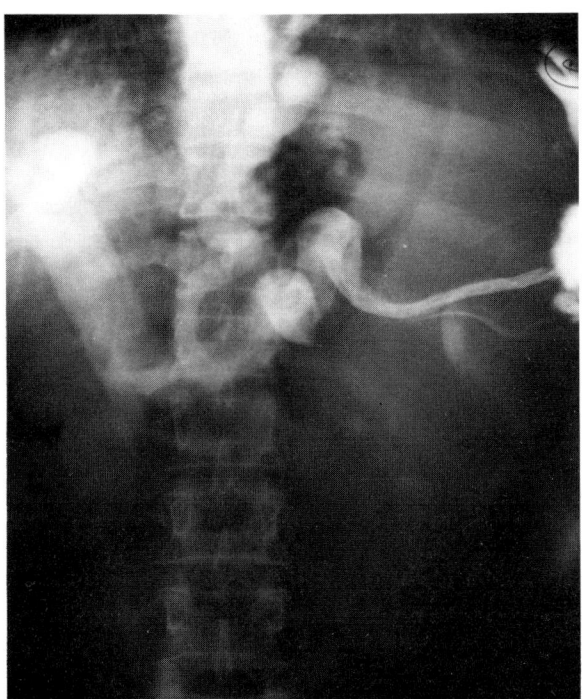

Fig 8.3 Splenoportogram showing patent portal and splenic veins with oesophagogastric varices.

Indirect measurement of portal pressure

1 Splenic pulp pressure (*see above*).
2 Wedged hepatic vein pressure. A catheter is passed from an arm vein down the superior vena cava into the hepatic vein and into a hepatic venous radicle until it can be inserted no further. The pressure reflects pressure in hepatic sinusoids, which is normally 10 cm saline. In conjunction with measurement of splenic pulp pressure, the wedged hepatic vein pressure can help determine the cause of portal hypertension. Thus, in obstruction of the main portal vein or in schistosomiasis, the splenic pulp pressure is increased, but hepatic sinusoidal pressure, that is wedged hepatic vein pressure, remains normal. However, in cirrhosis both splenic pulp pressure and wedged hepatic vein pressure are elevated.

Haemodynamic investigations

There have been many attempts to measure flow characteristics of the splanchnic circulation in portal hypertension. It is generally held, but by no means proved, that the ill-effects of a shunt operation are related to the abrupt reduction of the portal venous flow to the liver. It has been hoped that careful haemodynamic studies, e.g. measurement of portal flow, of total hepatic blood flow, etc., would enable the surgeon to predict those who would do well, or badly, after a shunt operation. Although several new haemodynamic investigations have recently been described, they have not yet earned a place for themselves in the routine investigations of a patient with portal hypertension.

Other investigations

Other investigations are required, not so much to make a diagnosis as to determine the degree of the hepatic insufficiency and the feasibility of further diagnostic and therapeutic measures.

Coagulation studies

In liver disease haemostatic mechanisms may be seriously disturbed. These defects often require correction, not only for operation, but for such important investigations as liver biopsy and splenoportography. Expert haematological help is necessary.

Biochemical investigations

Biochemical investigations are carried out to determine hepatic function and to assess the risks of opera-

tion. In this context no single biochemical test is useful, but the multiple clinical and biochemical system devised by Child (1958) (Table 2) is a reasonable indicator of operative mortality and short-term prognosis. Serum alpha-fetoprotein should be estimated if primary liver cell carcinoma is suspected.

Table 2
CLASSIFICATION OF CIRRHOTIC PATIENTS IN TERMS OF HEPATIC RESERVE

	Group A	Group B	Group C
Serum bilirubin (μmol/litre)	<34.0	34.0–51.0	>51.0
Plasma albumin (g/litre)	>35	30–35	<30
Ascites	None	Easily controlled	Poorly controlled
Encephalopathy	None	Minimal	Advanced coma
Nutrition	Excellent	Moderate	Poor
Risk of operation	Good	Moderate	Poor

(Modified from Child C.G. (1958). *Major Problems in Clinical Surgery*, vol 1. Philadelphia: Saunders.)

Histology

It may be helpful to obtain a sample of liver tissue, by percutaneous biopsy, to determine the activity of liver disease. Operation should be postponed in chronic hepatitis, for example, if the disease is particularly active.

Treatment

Treatment for oesophageal varices is required under two sets of circumstances (a) to control acute bleeding, (b) to prevent recurrence of haemorrhage after a previous bleed.

Acute variceal haemorrhage

General principles

On admission, the patient should be rapidly resuscitated by the transfusion of blood, preferably fresh. Adequacy of transfusion should be confirmed by monitoring the central venous pressure. A nasogastric tube should be passed into the stomach to remove blood and prevent its aspiration into the lungs and to detect any continuation or recurrence of haemorrhage. Measures should be immediately instituted to minimise or prevent encephalopathy (Table 3). Vitamin K_1 should be injected intramuscularly and the H_2 antagonist, cimetidine, given to reduce gastric acid secretion.

Since the management of bleeding varices differs quite radically from that of other causes of upper gastrointestinal haemorrhage, the diagnosis must be made on an emergency basis at this stage.

Table 3
MEASURES TO PREVENT ENCEPHALOPATHY

Rapid control of bleeding
Correction of water and electrolyte disorders, e.g. hypokalaemia
Treatment of infection
Enemas, e.g. magnesium sulphate
Antibiotics, e.g. neomycin
Careful use of sedatives

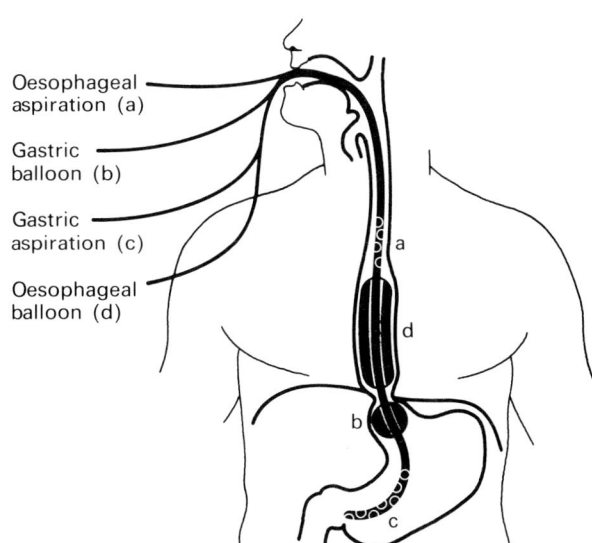

Fig 8.4 Sengstaken tube in position. (From Shields R., 1979, *Medicine*; **17**:876–83.)

Labels: Oesophageal aspiration (a); Gastric balloon (b); Gastric aspiration (c); Oesophageal balloon (d)

Vasopressin

If bleeding does not stop, or recurs, vasopressin is used as a powerful vasoconstrictor to reduce portal flow and pressure. Conventionally vasopressin is injected intravenously in a single bolus dose of 20 u in 100 ml dextrose over 10 min. Side effects, which are common, include abdominal colic and facial pallor. In addition, there is a risk of undesirable vasoconstriction of the coronary arteries leading to myocardial infarction. The bolus doses can be repeated at intervals of 2–3 h but repeated doses seem to become less effective.

More effective and with fewer side effects, is *continuous* infusion of vasopressin into a peripheral vein at a rate of 0.4 u/min until the bleeding stops or to a maximum of 24 h.

Direct infusion of vasopressin into the superior mesenteric artery has had a vogue, but controlled trials have not demonstrated any long-term benefit. A recently-described analogue of vasopressin is triglyceryl-hormogen (glypressin) whose action is more prolonged, but further evaluation is required. The use of somatostatin as an alternative to vasopressin is also being evaluated.

Vasopressin is moderately effective in stopping a brisk haemorrhage, but recurrence of bleeding is common and long-term survival is not appreciably affected.

Balloon tamponade

If bleeding is not controlled, or recurs despite vasopressin, the next step is to apply balloon tamponade. Several types of balloon are available, but probably the best is the Sengstaken-Blakemore tube (Fig 8.4). The high morbidity and mortality, reported initially, can be

avoided by meticulous attention to detail (Table 4). Particularly important is the use of a fourth channel (or separate tube) to aspirate pharyngeal and oesophageal contents accumulated above the oesophageal balloon.

In some patients, bleeding from the varices ceases in the early stages of the disease. If bleeding does not recur and no further emergency treatment is required, chances of survival are good. In contrast are the high morbidity and mortality in those who continue to bleed despite the above measures. Early cessation of bleeding is a valuable prognostic sign.

Continued bleeding, or its early recurrence, presents the clinician with a major therapeutic problem. Major operations, either a portasystemic shunt or a devascularising procedure, carry a high mortality in the emergency situation. Portacaval or mesocaval shunt

Table 4
HOW TO USE BALLOON TAMPONADE

1. Aspirate upper gastrointestinal tract with conventional tube before passing Sengstaken tube
2. Use new tube
3. Pass tube by mouth
4. Ensure that oesophagus and pharynx above balloon are continuously aspirated
5. Elevate bedhead
6. Inflate gastric balloon with air and pull up balloon until it impinges on cardio-oesophageal junction
7. Aspirate stomach continuously
8. Inflate oesophageal balloon to 40 mmHg
9. Deflate oesophageal and gastric balloons after 24 h of tamponade
10. Continue tamponade for only a further 24 h if bleeding continues or recurs

may have to be performed, because the patient is bleeding to death, but even in the best of hands, more than half of the patients die. Major devascularisation procedures, e.g. gastric or oesophageal transections (*see below*) also carry a high mortality when performed in an emergency, particularly in poor-risk alcoholics.

In this difficult situation of uncontrolled bleeding, injection sclerotherapy has been tried. Early results are promising.

Injection sclerotherapy

The varices are obliterated by the direct or indirect injection of sclerosants.

Direct injection. A rigid or flexible oesophagoscope, both modified slightly, is passed into the oesophagus with the patient under general anaesthesia or heavily sedated. A distended varix is allowed to protrude into the slot of the modified rigid oesophagoscope or into the slot of the flexible sheath which surrounds the flexible oesophagoscope. Ethanolamine oleate (3–5 ml) is injected into the varix. The oesophagoscope is immediately rotated to present another varix for injection and to compress the injected varix to promote sclerosis and prevent bleeding. In this way, several varices can be injected in one session. An alternative technique involves injecting the sclerosant in the submucosa in the vicinity of the varices.

Complications of the procedure are unusual, but they include ulceration at the injection site (more commonly after submucous, rather than intravariceal injection), stricture formation and, rarely, perforation of the oesophagus.

There seems to be little difference in results between the various techniques. The emergency control of acute haemorrhage is achieved in over 90% of patients. The value of injection sclerotherapy by the endoscopic approach is that it represents a relatively minor form of treatment which can be repeated and it does not carry the high mortality and morbidity of alternative therapies.

Later recurrence of bleeding from injected varices is common, but can be minimised by repeated sclerotherapy until all the varices are obliterated. Early results of controlled trials suggest that, with repeated sclerotherapy, survival of the patients is longer than in those not so treated.

Indirect injection. An alternative technique is percutaneous transhepatic obliteration of the varices. A catheter and needle are passed through the liver into the portal vein and the catheter further advanced into the veins supplying the oesophageal varices. The varices are obliterated with injection of human thrombin followed by a gelatin foam to stabilise the clot. Control of bleeding can be successful in the short-term, but

recurrence of bleeding is common 4–6 weeks after injection, because of reformation of varices. The technique requires considerable skill and expertise.

Prevention of recurrent haemorrhage

The predominant role of surgery in the treatment of portal hypertension is to prevent a recurrence of bleeding (*therapeutic* operation). The term *prophylactic* operation is applied to operations performed for varices which have not yet bled.

There are two basic types of operation for portal hypertension and oesophageal varices (a) *devascularisation procedures* in which the varices in the oesophagus and stomach are ligated or ablated, but there is no attempt to reduce the portal pressure, (b) *portasystemic shunting* in which the splanchnic circulation is decompressed by a major bypass between the veins of the systemic and portal circulation; of course, the underlying liver disease persists.

Devascularisation procedures

Several operations have been described directly to obliterate the oesophagogastric varices.

Transthoracic operation

The varices in the oesophagus may be individually ligated (Boerema-Crile operation), or the oesophagus is transected and immediately reanastomosed with closely-applied sutures to occlude the varices (Milnes-Walker operation). These operations can be carried out rapidly because thick vascular adhesions common in the abdomen are not encountered in the thorax. However, the contents of the peritoneal cavity cannot be inspected for other sources of haemorrhage which may require simultaneous treatment, e.g. duodenal ulcer.

Abdominal operations

Alone abdominal operations do not usually provide sufficient exposure. However, with an abdominal approach the oesophagus can be transected using a stapling gun which simultaneously divides and reanastomoses the oesophagus using multiple staples. The advantage of this operation is its simplicity because the gun can be passed, through a small gastrotomy incision, into the oesophagus. Early results indicate that this is a useful operation; recurrence of bleeding is prevented in many instances and even quite ill patients tolerate this less severe operation. Gastric varices, a source of recurrent bleeding after apparently successful endoscopic sclerotherapy can be ablated by plication with continuous sutures during this operation.

Occasionally splenectomy is successful, especially if only the splenic vein is thrombosed, for example after pancreatitis. However, a splenectomy alone should be avoided because of the risk of spreading venous thrombosis.

Thoracoabdominal operations

This approach is usually necessary for devascularisation procedures. These operations impose a considerable strain on an ill patient who has recently bled and who may be suffering from the general effects of hepatic insufficiency.

A high gastric transection (Tanner operation) requires the division of the upper part of the stomach close to its junction with the oesophagus and reanastomosis to occlude the varices in the gastric wall. Usually, an enlarged spleen has to be removed to permit access. Rebleeding after this formidable operation is, unfortunately, common.

More extensive devascularisations are popular in Japan and the Middle East, especially for schistosomiasis. The general principles are splenectomy, division of all extrinsic venous collaterals and resection of all, or part, of the stomach along with the lower end of the oesophagus (that is, the varix-bearing area) with, perhaps jejunal or colonic interposition.

With these operations the splanchnic circulation is left undisturbed and the liver is not deprived of its venous blood supply. However, complications are common and often serious, e.g. anastomotic leakage. A specific indication for a devascularisation operation is continued haemorrhage in a patient with portal vein thrombosis in whom some form of portasystemic shunt is not possible. Fortunately, this is an uncommon requirement because the patients, most of whom are young, can tolerate frequent haemorrhages and large transfusions; a collateral circulation may develop over several years and bleeding becomes less frequent. These operations may also be required in the very young with varices because the portal and splenic veins are too small for a portasystemic shunt. Once the child has grown, the calibre of the blood vessels may have increased, so that a portasystemic shunt can be performed if episodic bleeding continues. First choice is usually splenectomy and splenorenal shunt, provided the splenic vein is more than 1 cm diameter. Alternatively, an end-to-side mesocaval shunt (Marion-Clatworthy) can be performed because, better than adults, children can tolerate transection of the inferior vena cava which is anastomosed to the side of the

superior mesenteric vein. An alternative operation is a coronary-caval shunt (*see below*).

Devascularisation operations have been more popular in the United Kingdom than in the United States, France or South Africa, where portal hypertension is more prevalent. Our own practice is to avoid these operations, if at all possible, because of the high incidence of recurrent bleeding. Injection sclerotherapy may very well lead to their demise.

Portasystemic shunts

The aim of a shunt operation is a reduction of portal pressure to prevent recurrent bleeding. This objective can be achieved by a major anastomosis between a splanchnic and systemic vein. Unfortunately, the risk of hepatoportal encephalopathy and postoperative liver failure may be increased. Lesser procedures aimed at reducing the portal flow, e.g. splenectomy and hepatic arterial ligation, or attempts to create diffuse shunts, e.g. omentopexy, are doomed to failure.

End-to-side portacaval shunts

End-to-side portacaval shunt (Fig 8.5) has been performed for more than 30 years, and is still the yardstick by which all other operations must be compared. Rebleeding is rare—2–3%—but one-fifth of the patients suffer from encephalopathy after the operation. The overall mortality is about 15–19%—quite acceptable bearing in mind the parlous state of some of the patients. Long-term survival varies, but has been reported as high as 50% at 5 years.

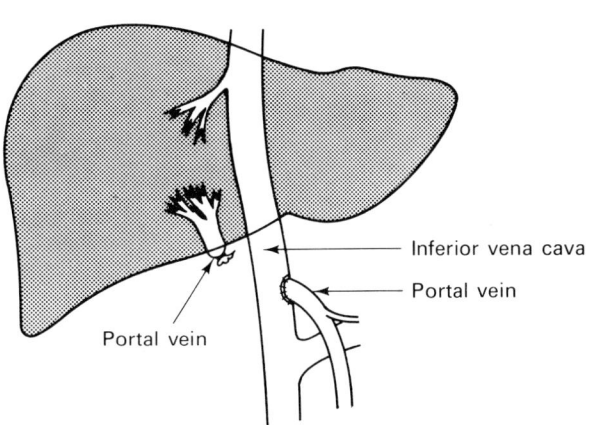

Inferior vena cava

Portal vein

Portal vein

Fig 8.5 End-to-side portacaval shunt. (From Shields R., 1979, *Medicine*; **17**:876–83.)

Technique

Details of the procedure should be sought from texts of operative surgery, or, preferably, by watching an experienced surgeon performing the operation. My own preference is to use a long subcostal incision, with the patient rotated somewhat to the left to expose his right flank. Thoracoabdominal incisions should be avoided because of the risk of leakage of ascitic fluid into the pleural cavity postoperatively.

The first step is to inspect the contents of the abdominal cavity, to ensure that there is no tumour of the liver nor other source of bleeding. Mesenteric pressure should be measured. The inferior vena cava is then exposed. After retraction of the liver cranially and mobilisation of the duodenum, the anterior and lateral aspects of the inferior vena cava are displayed, from the renal vein caudally up to the liver.

The portal vein is then exposed in the free edge of the lesser omentum. The bile duct is identified, mobilised, and retracted to the patient's left, by means of tape. A lymph node, which obscures the portal vein, should be carefully removed. The vein itself is then identified and carefully mobilised along its entire course. Caudally the junction of the splenic vein and superior mesenteric vein should be identified. Vascular clamps are applied to the portal vein close to its bifurcation in the porta hepatis, and the portal vein divided obliquely at the porta hepatis. The hepatic stump is ligated. The inferior vena cava is partially occluded by a side clamp placed on its anterior aspect. A small incision is made on the occluded segment of the inferior vena cava and a small portion of the vein removed to produce a window. The portal vein is then anastomosed to the inferior vena cava end-to-side, employing a continuous suture.

The clamp on the inferior vena cava should be removed first, so that, if there is free bleeding from the anastomosis, it can be quickly reapplied and the leak closed with a suture. The clamps in the portal vein are then removed.

The pressure in the mesenteric or portal vein should be measured again. There should be an appreciable fall in portal pressure, by at least 10–20 cm saline. If there is no fall, the anastomosis should be carefully inspected for some fault in its construction. If the fault cannot be easily corrected, the anastomosis is taken down and refashioned, or another type of portasystemic shunt established. To end the operation without producing a satisfactory fall in portal pressure means almost inevitably catastrophic haemorrhage within 4 days. Postoperative recovery is usually rapid and uneventful. Slight icterus after operation normally disappears at end of first week. Measures to prevent encephalopathy should be continued until patient leaves hospital. Recurrence of bleeding suggests thrombosis of shunt and is an indication for reoperation.

Factors affecting results of portacaval shunt

The results of portacaval shunt may be improved by attention to certain important factors:

Timing of shunt

Emergency shunts. Because of the high mortality of emergency shunting, most surgeons prefer to control bleeding in other ways, e.g. injection sclerotherapy or stapling. If, however, bleeding continues, an emergency operation may have to be performed to prevent the continuing and fatal exsanguination of the patient. Patients in Child Group C (*see below*) rarely survive this – or indeed any – form of major operative intervention and most surgeons experienced in the field avoid operation in this group.

In an emergency, the favoured operations are either end-to-side portacaval shunt or interposition mesocaval shunt.

Prophylactic operations. To operate upon a patient who has varices, which have not yet bled, is an attractive concept and was at one time widely practised. However, several well-conducted prospective trials have established beyond any doubt that there is no place for prophylactic operations. Variceal bleeding is prevented, but the survival is much less than a comparable group treated medically.

Therapeutic or elective shunts. The fact that almost two-thirds of patients who have had a major gastrointestinal haemorrhage will bleed again cannot be ignored. We have no sure means of predicting the fortunate 30–35% who will not bleed in the near future. The main indication for shunt operations is, therefore, a patient who has had a major haemorrhage from oesophageal varices. In the last few years, as a result of several 'controlled' trials, there has been a swing away from elective shunts. The pendulum may have swung too far and indeed on several counts the trials can be criticised. First, great emphasis has been placed on statistical significance which may be impossible to achieve in comparing groups made up of such complex heterogenous patients. Several of the trials contained a high proportion of older male alcoholics with marked impairment of liver function – probably no form of treatment would be effective in this group and their inclusion in a trial would lead to a lack of statistical significance between the results of treatment. Recently, several papers have shown that significantly better results can be achieved by operation, in young non-alcoholic patients, whose liver function is good, and who have had two or more episodes of variceal bleeding in the preceeding year.

Liver function

The Child classification (Table 2) forecasts with reasonable accuracy operative mortality and survival in the first year after operation. Of particular importance is the presence, or absence, of jaundice. Long-term survival is particularly related to the degree of wasting of the patient, and alcoholism.

Encephalopathy

After a shunt, encephalopathy is encountered in 20–30% of patients. However, encephalopathy also develops in many patients treated medically. Possibly the severity rather than the frequency of encephalopathy is affected by operation. Where a selective shunt has been performed (*see below*) the incidence of encephalopathy is possibly less.

Hepatic histology

The functional integrity of the hepatocytes rather than the type of liver disease seems to influence the outcome. Where liver disease is active, e.g. in aggressive hepatitis, the prognosis is particularly poor.

Side-to-side portacaval shunt

This operation has had its advocates, especially for treatment of intractable ascites, or in the Budd-Chiari syndrome. There is no firm evidence that the operation offers any particular advantage.

Splenorenal shunt

In this operation the spleen is removed and the cut end of the splenic vein is anastomosed end-to-side with the renal vein (Fig 8.6). The operation is indicated where removal of the spleen is required, e.g. severe hypersplenism. Otherwise, the operation does not offer any particular advantage and may present difficulties to the inexperienced surgeon. The incidence of encephalopathy may be lower than with end-to-side portacaval shunt, but recurrent bleeding is more common, probably due to thrombosis at the anastomosis between the vessels of smaller calibre.

Interposition mesocaval shunt

The portal system is decompressed through a wide-bore graft of synthetic material, or autogenous vein, inserted between the inferior vena cava and the superior mesenteric vein (Fig 8.7). The operation is easier to

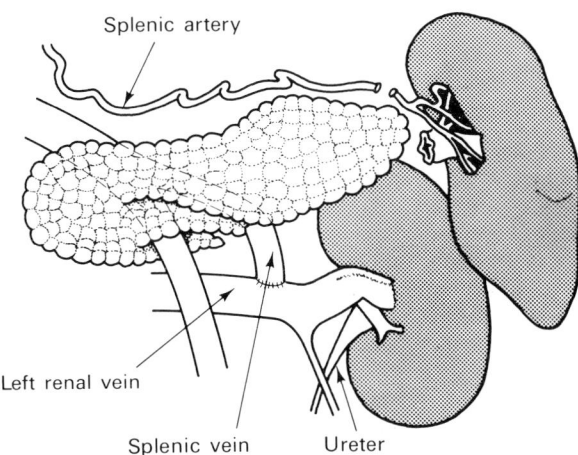

Fig 8.6 Conventional splenorenal shunt with splenectomy. (From Shields R., 1979, *Medicine*; **17**:876–83.)

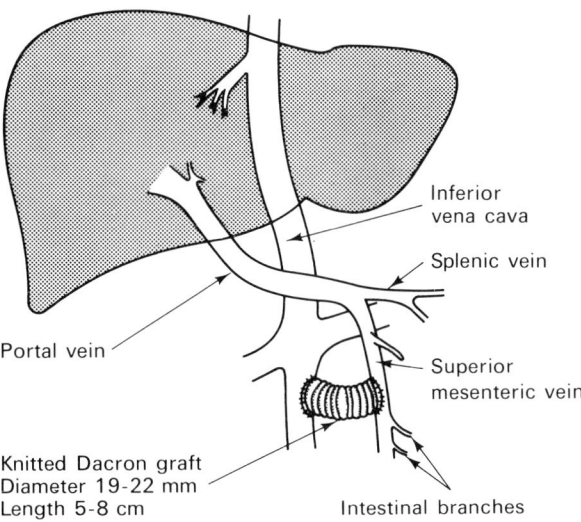

Fig 8.7 Interposition mesocaval shunt (From Shields R., 1979, *Medicine*; **17**:876–83.)

perform because the major dissection does not take place at the porta hepatis where large venous collaterals may impair access. Earlier claims that encephalopathy was less common have not been confirmed.

The abdominal cavity is opened through either a long mid-line vertical incision or, preferably in the obese patient, a transverse incision. The transverse colon is lifted cranially and the superior mesenteric vessels palpated at the root of the mesentery of the small intestine. The superior mesenteric vein is then exposed by incising the fat of the mesentery and mobilised from its jejunal tributaries until cranially it runs under the neck of the pancreas. The second and third parts of the duodenum are mobilised and retracted cranially. The anterior surface of the inferior vena cava is exposed in the depth of the wound and partially occluded by a clamp applied to its surface. A window of the inferior vena cava is excised. A wide-bore (18–22 cm) graft of synthetic material (Dacron or Gore-Tex) or an autogenous vein is anastomosed to the inferior vena cava using a continuous single suture. The other end of the graft or vein is anastomosed in an end-to-side fashion with the superior mesenteric vein, a segment of which has been isolated between vascular clamps. When the clamps are removed the mesenteric pressure should fall by more than 8–10 cm saline.

Distal splenorenal shunt (Warren selective shunt)

The theoretical advantage of this operation is that localised splanchnic decompression is achieved, but there is still a flow of blood to the liver. From the evidence of several controlled trials, the incidence of encephalopathy is much less after this selective shunt than after total shunts, e.g. portacaval and mesocaval. Moreover, this shunt seems to provide the same degree of protection from recurrent variceal haemorrhage.

The operation, (Fig 8.8) however, presents consider-

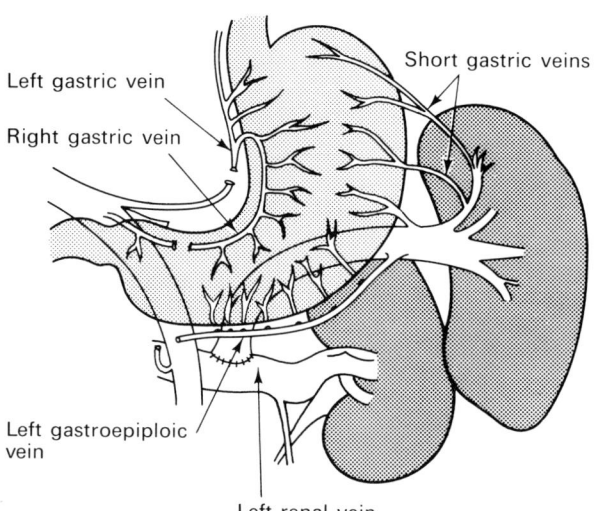

Left gastric vein

Right gastric vein

Short gastric veins

Left gastroepiploic vein

Left renal vein

Fig 8.8 Distal splenorenal shunt with partial devascularisation of the stomach. The extrinsic blood-supply of the stomach is divided, apart from the short gastric veins leading from the upper part of the greater curvature of the stomach to the spleen. The splenic vein is divided close to its junction with the superior mesenteric vein and anastomosed end-to-side with the left renal vein. (From Shields R., 1979, *Medicine*; **17**:876–83.)

able technical difficulties and the mortality rate among earlier series was rather high. It has two components: first, all the extrinsic venous collaterals of the stomach are ligated, except the short gastric veins which drain the lower part of the oesophagus and upper part of the stomach, and pass in the gastrosplenic ligament to the spleen; secondly, the splenic vein is detached from its junction with the superior mesenteric vein and anastomosed, end-to-side, with the renal vein.

Further long-term evaluation is required. It is by no means certain that the flow of blood to the liver will continue as further collaterals are opened up. This operation may not be suitable for patients whose varices have been injected.

Other shunts

Great ingenuity has been displayed in developing various shunts between the splanchnic and systemic veins to decompress the portal circulation (Malt, 1976). In general these shunts are of limited application, but a knowledge of them is of value because occasionally such unconventional shunts may be the only alternative in a patient with extrahepatic obstruction of the portal vein who requires operation for recurrent haemorrhage. In this context, of particular interest is the coronary-caval shunt where a segment of autogenous vein is anastomosed to the left gastric vein and the inferior vena cava. The Japanese surgeons who devised this operation claim a 90% patency rate without any encephalopathy.

Conclusions

Variceal bleeding is undoubtedly one of the most serious forms of haemorrhage into the upper gastro-intestinal tract. Patients usually present in poor condition, because of the deleterious effects of recurrent profuse bleeding and the ravages of the underlying disease.

There is little controversy about the early management of these patients. Rapid resuscitation is required with early attempts at diagnosis, particularly endoscopy, to determine if varices are present and if these are the source of haemorrhage. Attempts to control bleeding should be undertaken vigorously, initially by the intravenous infusion of vasopressin and, if this fails, balloon tamponade. If bleeding continues unchecked, emergency operation may have to be undertaken, but the results of such surgery are for the most part poor. Injection sclerotherapy through an endoscope may control massive bleeding in most patients, but long-term evaluation is desired. If bleeding continues despite apparently adequate sclerotherapy, the varices at the lower end of the oesphagus may be obliterated by stapling using an abdominal approach.

There are no clear guidelines, however, in the further management of the patient who has bled from varices and in whom the risks of further bleeding is high. Establishing the cause of the portal hypertension may provide guidance on further treatment. In children or adolescents, in whom an extrahepatic block is likely, operation should be avoided if possible and transfusions repeated if necessary. In time these children usually develop a collateral circulation and the bleeding episodes become less. If haemorrhage becomes life-threatening, operation may have to be undertaken. A devascularisation procedure, if necessary an oesophagogastrectomy, may have to be performed. Alternatively some form of portasystemic shunt may be possible.

If bleeding is due to a presinusoidal block, e.g. schistosomiasis, congenital hepatic fibrosis, and the haemorrhage is recurrent, operation may be required. End-to-side portacaval shunt is of value, although in schistosomiasis, devascularisation operations are popular in the Middle East. A selective shunt, e.g. a distal splenorenal shunt, is however preferable.

In the cirrhotic, careful evaluation of liver function is important. After a single haemorrhage, we should wait to see how the patient fares. Bleeding may not recur in one-third of the patients and, therefore, a major operation can be avoided. Moreover, this period of close observation will demonstrate whether the patient has continued to abstain from alcohol. If, after serious warnings and a major haemorrhage, a patient continues to drink, major operation should not be undertaken. One option is to continue conventional medical management, treating the haemorrhages as they occur. Devascularisation or disconnection procedures are unlikely to be of any long-term benefit. Of the portasystemic shunts, the two main ones to be considered are the distal splenorenal shunt, which has a lower encephalopathy rate but is technically difficult, or a conventional end-to-side portacaval shunt.

Alternatively, injection sclerotherapy can be repeated at regular intervals until all the submucous oesophageal varices are obliterated. The long-term benefits of this treatment are not known, but it offers the immediate advantage that a major operation has not been performed and, therefore, serious postoperative complications, such as postoperative liver failure or thrombosis of the shunt, with subsequent catastrophic haemorrhage, have been avoided. Moreover, at any time, a shunt operation can be carried out if it is thought necessary and if the patient is fit.

Further reading

Dykes P.W., Keighley M.R.B. (1981). *Gastrointestinal Haemorrhage*. Bristol, London: PSG Wright.

Galambos J.T. (1979). Major problems in internal medicine. In *Cirrhosis*, Vol. XVII. Philadelphia: Saunders.

Johnson G. (1980). Surgery for bleeding esophageal varices. In *Advances in Surgery*, vol. 14, pp. 85–105. Chicago: Year Book Medical.

Johnson G.W. (1982). Six years' experience of oesophageal transection for oesophageal varices, using a circular stapling gun. *Gut*; **23:**770–3.

Malt R. (1976). Portasystemic venous shunts. *New Engl. J. Med*; **295:**24–9.

Orloff M.J., Stipa S., Ziparo V. (1980). *Medical and Surgical Problems of Portal Hypertension*. London, New York: Academic Press.

Shields R. (1983). Bleeding oesophageal varices – a plan of management. In 'The Abdomen', *Operative Surgery*, 4th edn. (Rob C., Smith R., Dudley H. eds.) London: Butterworth.

9

Spleen

ROBERT SHIELDS

Anatomy

The spleen which, in the adult, weighs between 70–150 g, lies in the left upper quadrant of the abdomen, nestling under the protection of the ribcage and in close contact with the left dome of the diaphragm, the stomach, colon and left kidney. It is attached to these last organs by suspensory ligaments, e.g. gastrosplenic, splenocolic and splenorenal, so that its long axis corresponds to the tenth rib posteriorly. The gastrosplenic ligament contains the short gastric veins. The spleen receives its blood supply from the splenic artery which arises from the coeliac axis and is drained by the splenic vein which joins the superior mesenteric vein to form the portal vein.

The spleen is entirely organised around its blood supply. Blood flow is 150 ml/min, about 0.7 ml/g organ weight (cf renal blood flow 3.7 ml/g organ weight). The detailed intrasplenic circulation and its close relationship to the lymphatic sheaths, macrophages and other elements of the reticulo-endothelial system are not appropriate to this chapter, but the result of the complex arrangement is that blood passes through a macrophage-rich filration system. The splenic artery branches into five or six trabecular vessels, which supply segments of splenic tissue with little in the way of interconnecting vessels; consequently, there is an increased liability to infarction following arterial occlusion. These fine vascular pathways constitute some of the smallest vessels in the body which blood cells have to permeate. As a result abnormal, or fragile, cells are liable to be damaged. Removal of the spleen is, therefore, likely to be followed by an increased survival of these abnormal cells.

The spleen is also a secondary lymphatic organ with peri-arterial lymphatic sheaths, populated mainly by small-T-lymphocytes, concerned with the monitoring of antigens. The lymphoid follicles of the spleen are B-lymphocyte areas. In intermediate areas are mixed populations of B and T lymphocytes, probably responsible for cooperative cell interaction.

In up to one-fifth of patients, accessory spleens can be found, usually near the hilum of the spleen with which they can be in close contact, or related to the splenic vessels in the gastrosplenic or splenocolic ligaments, or behind the tail and body of the pancreas. The hypertrophy which they may undergo after splenectomy may be responsible for the return of the disorder, e.g. idiopathic thrombocytopaenic purpura, after an apparently successful splenectomy.

Physiology

The principal known functions of the spleen are:

1 *Production of blood cells.* Haemopoeisis in the spleen occurs normally in the fetus, but not after birth, except in disease, as a compensatory reaction or inappropriate metaplasia.

2 *Destruction of blood cells.* Destruction of senescent erythrocytes takes place in the spleen and in other parts of the reticulo-endothelial system. Because it is sensitive to slight abnormalities in cell shape, the bulk of cell destruction in certain diseases of the erythrocytes takes place in the spleen. The spleen is also a major site of platelet destruction, but neutrophils end their lives in other parts of the reticulo-endothelial system.

3 *Reservoir function.* The normal spleen holds only 20–40 ml red blood cells and, therefore, does not act as a reservoir for them. However, a high proportion of the red cell mass may be retained in an enlarged spleen. The organ can store platelets – up to one-third of the circulating volume – and some proteins including Factor VIII.

4 *Filtration and phagocytosis.* The narrow diameter of the splenic vessels and the slow rate of intrasplenic flow allow the spleen to filter off abnormal particulate matter, e.g. malarial parasites, bacteria, nuclear remnants of blood cells, which are then phagocytosed by the many free and fixed macrophages.

5 *Immune response.* The unique structure of the spleen and the presence of large numbers of T and B lymphocytes within it, allow it to respond vigorously to circulating antigens. The spleen contributes to antibody formation and probably to cell-mediated immune responses. Probably the increased risk of serious infections after splenectomy in children in the first three years of life is related to this function.

6 *Hormone production.* There is no evidence to substantiate the hypothesis that, by humoral mechanisms, the spleen can influence bone marrow activity.

Physiological consequences of splenectomy

In the adult no clearly identifiable disorders follow splenectomy for trauma. However, some haematological and immunological abnormalities may develop.

Haematological

1 *Transient.* Leucocytosis, thrombocytosis and increased longevity of erythrocytes are most marked between the second week and second month following splenectomy. These changes, which are not invariable, are followed by a return to normal levels in three months.

2 *More persistent.* Because of the loss of the spleen's property to remove intracellular nuclear material, red cells showing Howell-Jolly bodies, thought to be fragmented nuclei, can be detected in the peripheral blood.

Immunological

In man, splenectomy removes one-quarter of the total lymphoid tissue and a major mass of macrophages. Immunological abnormalities may develop, e.g. low concentrations of circulating antibodies, low concentration of IgM. These immunological changes along with impaired clearance of bacteria such as pneumococci and other particulate material, explain why some patients, especially children, are more prone to infection after splenectomy.

Defective spleen function

The major cause is splenectomy. However, defective splenic function may be found in the following conditions:

Congenital absence. A very rare condition and usually associated with other congenital anomalies, especially of the heart, often so severe as to preclude survival.

Splenic atrophy. A common accompaniment of coeliac disease. In Britain, if a hyposplenic blood film is unexpectedly discovered on routine screening, the diagnosis is likely to be asymptomatic coeliac disease.

The presence of these conditions may be recognised or suspected from the peripheral blood changes described above.

Splenic injury

The usual cause of splenic rupture is direct external violence, such as a blow to the abdomen or the left lower chest, or a fall on to a projecting object. Road traffic accidents are a common cause, e.g. a direct blow to the abdomen or a crushing violence (say, between a vehicle and a wall), or injury to a passenger in a severe side-swipe accident. In these accidents multiple injuries are common.

The force of violence to rupture a normal healthy spleen is substantial. A diseased spleen probably ruptures more easily, because it may be weakened by infarction, its capsule stretched by enlargement and the organ more vulnerable by enlargement below the costal margin. In certain conditions, e.g. infectious mononucleosis, the trauma can be so trivial that the rupture of the spleen is thought to be spontaneous.

Clinical features

The presenting features of splenic rupture depend upon the presence of associated injuries, the extent and rapidity of the intraperitoneal haemorrhage, and the interval between the injury and the time of presentation. Rupture may be acute or delayed.

In **acute rupture** there are signs of an intra-abdominal catastrophe and of internal haemorrhage. There is increasing pallor, tachycardia, and restlessness. The patient complains of abdominal pain, often generalised, but more pronounced in the left upper quadrant where there is tenderness and rigidity. Pain at the tip of the shoulder is an infrequent symptom, but may be induced by elevation of the foot of the bed. Occasionally shifting dullness may be present.

Delayed rupture is said to occur when, after a period of days or indeed weeks, but more usually under 7 days, the signs of splenic rupture, especially those of internal haemorrhage, suddenly appear. The apparent delay is usually related to a slowly-enlarging haematoma, ultimately rupturing the capsule, or renewed bleeding after transient haemostasis.

Investigations

Splenic rupture can be correctly diagnosed if the clinician is ever-mindful of the possibility in a patient with the signs and symptoms of left-upper quadrant abdominal injury.

1 A straight x-ray of the abdomen may reveal injuries associated with splenic rupture, e.g. fracture of the left lower ribs.

2 A radio-opaque mass of increasing size, gradually obliterating the psoas shadow or displacing the gas bubble in the stomach, is a sign of a large perisplenic haematoma. Other signs include reduced mobility of the left lobe of the diaphragm.

3 Splenic arteriography may show extravasation of the radio-opaque dye into the substance of the spleen, or into the peritoneal cavity. This technique, however, should be reserved for those patients where the diagnosis is obscure.

4 If there is some doubt about active internal haemorrhage, peritoneal lavage should be carried out. Catheters are introduced into the abdominal cavity which is irrigated with isotonic saline solution. The lavage fluid is drained by gravity through another tube. The effluent is examined for red cells. This technique is highly accurate for the diagnosis of intra-abdominal injury, in contrast to abdominal paracentesis by a single tap.

Treatment

The only reliable treatment is splenectomy. A left paramedian incision is the one of choice. Usually a copious volume of blood has to be evacuated from the abdominal cavity. Blood may continue to well up into the wound, so that the spleen has to be mobilised rapidly by dividing the posterior leaf of the splenorenal ligament. Powerful retraction should be applied to the left costal margin and the vessels in the splenic pedicle can be compressed between the fingers and thumb. The spleen is then removed, (*see below*). The abdominal cavity must be explored to determine damage to other intra-abdominal organs, especially kidney and liver.

Complications

The complications of splenic injury for rupture are related to the operation itself (*see below*) and the associated injuries. A most serious complication is that of infection, which particularly affects children under three years. Septicaemia may develop even up to three years after splenectomy. Splenectomy may be inevitable if the rupture is complete, and, therefore, penicillin should be given prophylactically to this age-group.

However, there is an increasing tendency to conserve the spleen, either by resuturing a divided spleen or performing partial splenectomy, removing devitalised tissue. Bleeding is controlled by suture and cautery and the raw surfaces are oversewn with omentum. Because of these infective problems after splenectomy in children, consideration should be given to conservative non-operative treatment, especially if the patient's condition has become stabilised with no evidence of continued bleeding.

Splenomegaly

Splenomegaly usually implies that the spleen is palpably enlarged and, to be so, the organ has to increase its volume two or three times. However, in a child, a spleen which is only slightly enlarged may easily be palpated.

Causes

Almost all diseases of the spleen cause it to enlarge. Conversely, splenomegaly usually indicates splenic disease and warrants exhaustive investigations to determine the diagnosis. Indeed splenectomy may, on occasion, be required to make a positive diagnosis because of the suspicion of an underlying lymphoma, reticulosis or infiltrative condition.

The causes of splenomegaly are listed in Table 1.

Table 1
CAUSES OF SPLENOMEGALY

	Condition	Degree of splenomegaly[1]	Indications for splenectomy[2]
1 Infective and inflammatory			
(a) bacterial	(i) acute	+	+/0
	typhoid and paratyphoid		
	septicaemia		
	acute bacterial endocarditis		
	(ii) subacute and chronic		
	brucellosis	+	+/0
	subacute bacterial endocarditis	+	+/0
	tuberculosis	+	++
	syphilis	+	+/0
(b) viral	infectious mononucleosis		0
	viral hepatitis		0
(c) protozoal	malaria	+++	+
	bilharzial disease	+	0
	Kala-azar	+++	+
(d) parasites	hydatid	++	+++
(e) inflammatory	systemic lupus erythematosis	+	+
	Felty's syndrome	++	+
(f) granulomatous disease	sarcoidosis	+	+
	berylliosis	+	0
2 Blood and reticuloendothelial disease			
(a) haemolytic	congenital haemolytic anaemia	+	+++
	acquired haemolytic anaemia	++	++
	thalassaemia	+	+
	paraxysmal nocturnal haemoglobinuria	++	+
(b) haematological malignancy	acute leukaemia	+	0
	chronic myeloid leukaemia	+++	+
	chronic lymphatic leukaemia	++	+
	lymphoma (Hodgkin's disease)	+	+++
(c) myeloproliferative disorders	polycythaemia vera	++	0
	myeloid metaplasia	+++	+
(d) thrombocytopaenic disorders	acute	+	+
	chronic	++	+++
3 Congestive			
(a) heart	congestive cardiac failure	+	0
	constrictive pericarditis	+	0
(b) portal circulation	portal hypertension		
	intrahepatic	+	+
	extrahepatic	++	+
4 Metabolic storage disease	Gaucher's disease	+++	+
	histiocytosis X	++	+
	amyloidosis	++	0
5 Neoplastic	angioma	++	+++
	cysts	++	+++
	metastases	+	0
6 Cryptogenic	tropical splenomegaly	+++	+
	non-tropical splenomegaly	+++	+++
7 Miscellaneous	megaloblastic anaemia	+	0

[1] Degree of splenomegaly: +++ = marked (below umbilicus); ++ = moderate (4–8 cm below costal margin); + = slight (4 cm – just palpable
[2] Indications for splenectomy: +++ = benefitted by splenectomy; ++ = often benefitted by splenectomy; + = splenectomy sometimes indicated

Pathophysiology

The diseased spleen frequently, but not invariably, enlarges. The consequences of splenomegaly include:

Hypersplenism. This tetralogy consists of:

1 anaemia, leucopaenia, and thrombocytopaenia
2 normal, or hyperactive, bone-marrow
3 splenomegaly
4 cure by splenectomy.

The term 'hypersplenism' is unsatisfactory because the syndrome is not the result of a single process and the demonstration of the first three elements of the tetralogy in a patient does not guarantee that the fourth will hold true; that is, cure by splenectomy will be inevitable.

Red cell destruction. A grossly-enlarged spleen may hold more than 40% of the total red cell mass. The concentration of these cells in the spleen without accompanying plasma results in dilution of red cells elsewhere in the circulation, i.e. anaemia. The splenic pulp with its low oxygen tension and low glucose concentration, and narrow blood vessels within the spleen, constitute an unfavourable environment for the red cells and thus damaged red cells are destroyed and removed from circulation.

Thrombocytopaenia. More than 90% of the platelets in the body may be sequestered in an enlarged spleen, especially in congestive forms of splenomegaly (e.g. in portal hypertension). In addition, platelets which are slightly abnormal, for example sensitised to auto-antibodies, may be destroyed excessively in the spleen so that the balance between production and loss is upset, leading to thrombocytopaenia.

Leucopaenia. In contrast to red cells and platelets, the relationship between white cells and the spleen is less well understood. Nevertheless, splenomegaly is often accompanied by leucopaenia.

Hypervolaemia. Increased blood volume is often a feature of splenomegaly and may be related to the high blood flow through an enlarged spleen.

Clinical features

As it enlarges, the spleen moves downwards along the line of the ninth, tenth and eleventh ribs, until it becomes palpable at the left costal margin. Further enlargement takes place downwards towards the right iliac fossa, but only rarely does the spleen traverse the mid-line.

The enlarged spleen presents as a left-sided abdominal mass, with the following characteristics:

1 The mass moves downwards on inspiration
2 The medial border is well defined
3 A notch may be palpable
4 It is not possible to get above the mass
5 There is dullness to percussion over the mass when percussion is performed along the line from the umbilicus to the left mid-axillary line.

Other masses which may be confused with an enlarged spleen are an enlarged left kidney, left lobe of the liver, colonic or gastric masses.

Special investigations

1 Plain x-ray films of the abdomen may demonstrate the outline of the spleen. In addition the left hemidiaphragm may be elevated and the gastric air bubble may be medially or caudally displaced.
2 Intravenous urogram, barium meal or barium enema may be helpful in excluding renal, gastric or colonic lesions and in showing distortion or displacement of these organs by the large spleen.
3 Radio-isotope scanning. Technetium (^{99m}Tc) sulphur colloid defines the size and shape of the spleen as well as of the liver. In addition, focal lesions, infarcts, absence or hyperplasia of the spleen can be demonstrated. Sequential estimates of splenic radioactivity after the injection of autologous red cells labelled with chromium-51 provide a rough estimate of red-cell pooling and destruction in haemolytic anaemias. Destruction in the spleen at a rate greater than red-cell loss in the liver, suggests that splenectomy may be beneficial.
4 Ultrasound. Although non-invasive, ultrasound does not greatly help in splenic investigations.
5 Computerised axial tomography. If available, this technique can produce excellent pictures of an enlarged spleen.

Splenectomy

Indications

Indications for splenectomy can be divided into absolute and relative (Table 1). The *absolute* indication is rupture of the spleen (*see above*) and primary tumours and cysts (rare).

Relative indications are difficult to classify because in these conditions there can be more than one reason why the patient would benefit. Thus a patient with a huge spleen may obtain relief not only from the dragging discomfort of the organ, but also from the haematological consequences, e.g. anaemia and thrombocytopaenia.

In the cytopaenias – hypersplenism – two facts must be established before splenectomy. First, the spleen must be shown to be the site of excessive destruction of red cells, by examination of the bone marrow and of the peripheral blood, as well as isotope studies using labelled cells to determine a shortened life of the cells in the bloodstream and excessive uptake in the spleen. Secondly, in the absence of the spleen, the marrow must be shown capable of producing sufficient new cells to correct the cytopaenia. If these conditions are not met, the cytopaenia may not be reversed after splenectomy and the patient's condition will continue to deteriorate.

Splenectomy for haematological disorders

Haemolytic anaemia

These anaemias are usually classified as congenital (due to intrinsic abnormality of red cells) or acquired (related to an extracorpuscular factor acting on a normal red cell).

Congenital haemolytic anaemia. (Hereditary spherocytosis). This disorder, transmitted as an autosomal dominant trait, has, as its basic abnormality, a defect in the erythrocyte membrane, which causes the cell to be smaller, thicker, and almost spherical, with an increased osmotic fragility. The spherocytic cells are unable to pass easily through the splenic pulp in which they are susceptible to injury. The cardinal features of the disease are anaemia, reticulocytosis, jaundice and splenomegaly. Usually, neither the anaemia nor jaundice is particularly severe, but periodic crises may occur with marked increase in the severity of the disease, occasionally with fatal outcome. More than half of the patients develop pigmented gallstones.

Diagnosis is confirmed by examination of the peripheral blood which shows spherocytosis and reticulocytosis, and by determination of the osmotic fragility of the red cells. The spleen should be removed. Provided the operation is delayed to the third or fourth year of life, the results are generally good, although the basic erythroycytic abnormality remains. Before and during the operation, a search should be made for gallstones, and if present, the gallbladder should be removed.

Hereditary elliptocytosis, whose clinical manifestations closely resemble spherocytosis, should also be managed by splenectomy. Patients suffering from hereditary non-spherocytic anaemia, e.g. pyruvic kinase deficiency, may benefit from splenectomy if the anaemia is severe.

Thalassaemia, primarily a defect of synthesis of haemoglobin, was, as its eponym (Mediterranean anaemia) implies, originally described in those from South Europe and the Mediterranean littoral. The disease is of great theoretical and practical importance and reference should be made to the appropriate haematological text. Rarely splenectomy is required to reduce the haemolytic tendency, to diminish transfusion requirements, and to relieve the patient of an abdominal mass. Operation does not alter the basic disorder in haemoglobin.

Acquired haemolytic anaemia *(Idiopathic auto-immune)*. In this condition the life-span of normal red cells is considerably shortened, presumably by an auto-immune mechanism. The cells, immunologically altered, may be sequestrated and destroyed in the spleen. Moreover, there is some evidence that the spleen may be the source of the offending auto-antibodies. The disease, which usually runs a mild course, typically, but not invariably, in the middle-aged female, is characterised by slight icterus, splenomegaly and, in about 30% of cases, gallstones. In severe cases haemoglobinuria may result in renal damage. The distinguishing feature of this form of haemolytic anaemia is the demonstration, by a direct form of Coomb's test, of auto-antibodies to the patient's own red cells. Occasionally no treatment is required. A good response is often obtained with steroids and blood transfusion. Splenectomy is indicated (a) if steroids are not effective or are required in high dosage, or if toxic reaction to steroids appears, and (b) if there is evidence from isotope studies of excessive splenic sequestration of the red cells, when a favourable response may be expected in 80% of cases.

Idiopathic thrombocytopaenic purpura

The cause of this condition is not known, but it is characterised by a low platelet count and a bone marrow containing normal or increased numbers of megakaryocytes. By definition the disease is not secondary to systemic disease, nor is it an idiosyncratic response to drugs, e.g. arsenicals, gold, etc.

The acute form of the disease is seen in children, affecting both sexes; the chronic form usually affects females. The excessive bleeding tendency shows itself as bleeding from trivial wounds, e.g. tooth extraction, easy bruising, purpura and ecchymosis. Although a platelet count of $150 \times 10^9/l$ is the lower limit of the normal range, spontaneous bleeding is rare until the count is below $50 \times 10^9/l$ and usually does not take place until the count is less than $20 \times 10^9/l$. Marked splenomegaly is unusual and suggests another cause for the platelet deficiency.

Diagnosis is confirmed by the low platelet count and the typical bone-marrow features.

Treatment consists of steroid therapy and

splenectomy. Considerable discussion remains on the timing of these two aspects of treatment: in general the results of splenectomy are good and it is particularly indicated when the disease is severe and relapsing. Since most patients have had steroids, a preoperative booster dose of cortisone and hydrocortisone is usually required before splenectomy. The operation may have to be covered by the infusion of platelets. The results are good and relapses, several months or years after splenectomy, suggest hypertrophy of an overlooked accessory spleen.

Thrombotic thrombocytopaenic purpura is a disease primarily of arteries, arterioles and capillaries, accompanied by haematological changes such as purpura, haemolytic anaemia, reticulocytosis, thrombocytopaenia and leukocytosis. The disease usually runs a rapid course terminating in intracranial haemorrhage and renal failure. The most successful treatment has been a combination of steroids and splenectomy.

Chronic leukaemia

Splenectomy is only rarely indicated, chemotherapy and/or radiation being the main forms of treatment. Removal of the spleen may be considered if there are severe symptoms due to perisplenitis, infarction, or, indeed, to the sheer weight and size of the organ. The results have been more favourable when cytopaenia is present.

Hodgkin's disease

Hodgkin's disease is usually diagnosed on histological examination of enlarged lymph nodes. The outlook for affected patients has been greatly improved with the staging of the disease and a planned programme of radiotherapy and chemotherapy. For the staging, the last decade has seen the increased use of laparotomy and splenectomy (Table 2). In addition to splenectomy, a liver biopsy is performed and nodes should be removed from the para-aortic chain, the intestinal mesentery, and from around the common iliac vessels.

Super-voltage radiotherapy, administered in adequate dosage to all involved areas, is the treatment of choice for early disease; combination chemotherapy is highly effective in controlling, and sometimes curtailing, advanced disease. The value of laparotomy is shown by the statistic that, in about one-third of patients thought on clinical grounds to have disease localised above the diaphragm, unsuspected disease is revealed in the abdomen. Moreover, for patients with known stage III disease, laparotomy will reveal unsuspected liver involvement in 20% of cases, making them stage IV.

Table 2
STAGING CLASSIFICATION OF HODGKIN'S DISEASE

Stage	Definition
I	Involvement of a single lymph-node region.
II	Involvement of two or more lymph-node regions on the same side of the diaphragm (II), which may be accompanied by localised involvement of an extra-lymphatic organ or site (II_E).
III	Involvement of lymph-node regions on both sides of the diaphragm (III), which may also be accompanied by involvement of the spleen (III_S) or by localised involvement of an extra-lymphatic organ or site (III_E).
IV	Diffuse or disseminated involvement of one or more extra-lymphatic organs or tissues, with or without associated lymph-node involvement.

The absence or presence of fever, night sweats or unexplained loss of 10% or more of body weight in the 6 months before admission are denoted by the suffix letters A & B respectively.

Diagnostic laparotomy and splenectomy are claimed to be justified because the surgical findings may lead to an alteration in the stage of the disease, and so to a change in therapeutic strategy. Splenectomy plays an important role, but it must be emphasised that the continuing value of staging laparotomy and splenectomy must await the proof that patients so staged survive longer than patients staged without laparotomy.

Children under the age of 15 years with suspected Hodgkin's disease require special care and their programmes should be suitably modified.

Myeloproliferative disorders

Splenectomy is rarely indicated for polycythaemia vera or essential thrombocythaemia. However, in myeloid metaplasia, a proliferative process affecting bone marrow, liver and spleen and lymph nodes, the spleen may be grossly enlarged and portal hypertension may develop. The splenomegaly may produce symptoms.

Pallor and an enlarged spleen are common physical signs. Diagnosis is made from a peripheral blood smear, which contains immature myeloid cells and shows a raised white count. Marrow biopsy shows replacement of the marrow by fibrous tissue and is confirmatory evidence.

In addition to correcting the anaemia by blood transfusion and using alkylating agents to which these patients are particularly sensitive, splenectomy may be required to control the anaemia and thrombocytopaenia, and remove the symptoms of splenomegaly. Operation for this condition, however, carries a high mortality.

Other indications for splenectomy

Iatrogenic

The spleen is liable to injury especially in the course of upper abdominal operations, e.g. vagotomy, partial gastrectomy, and mobilisation of the splenic flexure of the colon. Even simple exploration of the abdomen can tear splenic adhesions, leading to embarrassing haemorrhage. If the capsule only is torn and the underlying pulp is undamaged, the bleeding can be controlled by pressure and topical haemostatic agents. Only if the splenic pulp is severely damaged and bleeding uncontrolled, need the spleen be removed.

Felty's syndrome

Rheumatoid arthritis, splenomegaly and neutropaenia comprise Felty's syndrome. The last component of the triad, neutropaenia, may well be responsible for the increased susceptibility to infections which these patients demonstrate, and may be controlled by corticosteroids whose beneficial effect, however, may be only temporary. The haematological response to splenectomy is usually excellent and, although the benefit may occasionally be only partial or temporary, the susceptibility to infection diminishes. The arthritis is unaffected by splenectomy.

Gaucher's disease

In this familial condition, there is a storage of the abnormal cerebroside, kerasin, in the spleen and other parts of the reticulo-endothelial system. Massive enlargement of the spleen is accompanied by neutropaenia, anaemia and thrombocytopaenia. Splenectomy can relieve the haematological complications and the local symptosm due to splenomegaly, but the course of the basic disorder is unaffected by operation.

Massive splenomegaly

The spleen may be enlarged in a variety of disorders. Occasionally its removal is indicated by the need to establish the diagnosis, or to alleviate the symptoms due to its size and weight. The convincing indication, however, for its removal is the development of haematological problems.

Facilitative

Splenectomy is often performed as a facilitative measure in the course of some other operations, such as subtotal gastrectomy or pancreatectomy in which removal of the spleen has no direct connection with the patient's disease. However, because of the postoperative infective complications, removal of the spleen should not be undertaken lightly.

Technique for splenectomy

For the details of splenectomy, texts of operative surgery should be consulted, but certain principles could perhaps be set down with advantage. The management of the ruptured spleen has already been described.

Incision

In elective operations where the spleen is of normal size or barely palpable (e.g. idiopathic thrombocytopaenic purpura), a left subcostal incision should be used. In a staging laparotomy for Hodgkin's disease, a long left paramedian, or vertical mid-line from xiphisternum to below the umbilicus are probably most convenient.

For an enlarged spleen, a long oblique incision in the upper abdomen is advised, extending from the costal margin, at the level of the ninth rib, across the epigastrium to beyond the right rectus. For a very large spleen, greater access may be obtained by dividing the costal margin at the left extremity of the incision, although the pleural cavity need not be entered. Through this incision, a spleen of almost any size can easily be delivered. Rarely, in the United Kingdom, is it necessary to use a thoracoabdominal incision, which, however, may be required if there are many adhesions between spleen and diaphragm.

Procedure

After laparotomy, with inspection of the liver and gallbladder (exploration at this stage may be frustrated by the large size of the spleen) the spleen is drawn downwards and to the patient's right. Good retraction is applied to the left costal margin, and the splenorenal ligament is put on stretch and divided by long scissors not too close to the spleen. Attention should be directed then to its superior pole which is often tethered to the stomach. The short gastric vessels around the pole are separately ligated and carefully divided, care being taken not to damage the spleen or the greater curvature of the stomach. The spleen is now more mobile. The tail of the pancreas is identified and the splenic artery is trebly ligated and divided close to the hilum of the spleen. Only then should the splenic vein be ligated and divided. The remaining attachments are divided and the spleen removed. Any bleeding from the splenic bed or from the under surface of the diaphragm should be controlled. Only rarely is external drainage required after the operation.

Tough vascular adhesions between the diaphragm and the spleen may prevent easy mobilisation and delivery of the spleen. Under these circumstances, the first step in the operation should be to divide the gastro-splenic ligament and expose the splenic artery along the upper border of the pancreas, where it is ligated in continuity, using an aneurysm needle. A few light adhesions can be divided easily, but if there are many tough vascular attachments, the chest may have to be opened and the diaphragm divided, so that these adhesions can then be dealt with under direct vision.

Occasionally, when the spleen is grossly adherent to the diaphragm, an extraperitoneal approach may have to be adopted, but, in general this is not recommended. In this situation an alternative as a first stage, is simple ligation of the splenic artery to produce shrinkage of the spleen, but such is the inflow of blood into the spleen through the vasa brevia etc., that the spleen often remains well-nourished, of undiminished size and fully-functioning.

Where splenectomy is being carried out for causes other than rupture, and particularly for haemotological disorders, a careful search should be made for accessory spleens (*see* p. 172).

Postoperative management and complications

1 During and immediately after operation *haemorrhage* is a hazard. During operation bleeding can occur from divided adhesions, a tear in the splenic capsule, or from the splenic vessels or vasa brevia. Bleeding can also occur from around the tail of the pancreas.

After operation, bleeding may take place from the small vessels in the posterior abdominal wall and diaphragm. Haemostasis must be meticulous to prevent the development of a large haematoma, which may become infected.

2 *Abdominal distension* is usually due to acute dilatation of the stomach and invariably can be prevented by continuous suction through a naso-gastric tube.

3 *Subphrenic abscess* is not common. It may be caused by infection developing in a haematoma, or following a penetrating injury. A likely cause, however, is

perforation of the adjacent stomach or colon, perhaps due to an inexpertly placed ligature.

4 *Thrombocytosis and leukocytosis* begin after operation and reach a peak between the 7th and 14th day. No particular measures need to be taken unless these responses become intense, the exception being severe thrombocytosis after splenectomy for myeloproliferative disorders.

5 Occasionally overwhelming sepsis with disseminated intra-vascular coagulation may develop. A frequently infecting organism is *Diplococcus pneumoniae*. Most of these infection occur in the first three years after splenectomy and are more common in children. To prevent this complication, prolonged prophylactic treatment with antibiotics for at least three years has been suggested, but the measure is not uniformly successful. The spleen should not be readily removed, especially in the young.

Although splenectomy predisposes to bacteraemia in children and immunosuppressed patients, e.g. those receiving chemotherapy, evidence of its harmful effects in normal adults is minimal.

6 *Mortality* varies between 3 and 15%, depending upon the physical state of the patient and the condition for which the operation was performed – mortality is particularly high following splenectomy for myelosclerosis. In general, morbidity and mortality correlate with the size of the spleen so that, once symptoms or complications develop, operation should not be postponed.

Further reading

Cochrane J.P.S. (1980). The spleen – ruptured spleen. *Brit. J. Hosp. Med*; **25**:398–404.

Irving M. (1978). Contemporary surgery – splenectomy. *Brit. J. Hosp. Med*; **23**:623–9.

Leonard A.S., Giebank G.S., Baesl T.J., Krivit W. (1980). The overwhelming post-splenectomy sepsis problem. *World J. Surg*; **4**:423–32.

Macpherson A.I.S. (1980). The spleen – cyst and tumour. *Brit. J. Hosp. Med*; **25**:413–6.

Oakes D.D. (1981). Splenic trauma. In *Current Problems in Surgery*, Vol. XVIII. Chicago, London: Yearbook Medical.

Schwartz P.E., Sterioff S., Mucha P., Melton L.J., Offord K.P. (1982). Postsplenectomy sepsis and mortality in adults. *JAMA*; **248**:2279–83.

10

Small intestine

ROBERT SHIELDS

Anatomy and physiology

Gross anatomy

In the gastrointestinal tract, the small bowel is the one component which is essential for life – in its absence, survival is not possible, whereas a patient may survive the loss of the oesophagus, stomach, or the entire large intestine.

Surprisingly the length of the small intestine is not accurately known. At postmortem, the small intestine, separated from its mesentery, elongates; and its length has been quoted as between 6 to 8 m. Measurement at operation is difficult due to the elasticity of the tissues. However, when a fine tube is passed orally until its tip appears at the anus, only 3.5–4 m is taken up, suggesting that in life the small intestine is probably only 3 m long. The duodenum, *in situ*, measures 25 cm.

For a full description of the gross anatomy of the small intestine, appropriate texts should be consulted. Certain points, important to the surgery of the small bowel, however, should be emphasised:

1   The right-half of the transverse colon runs across the front of the second part of the duodenum and head of the pancreas. Usually, in a healthy subject, this relationship presents little difficulty, but in the obese patient, especially if the colon is diseased, care must be taken to avoid damage to the duodenum or pancreas during colonic operations. Moreover, during operations upon the duodenum, pancreas and lower biliary tract, the surgeon must begin by reflecting the hepatic flexure and adjacent colon out of the operative field.

2   The superior mesenteric vessels cross the third part of the duodenum. From this relationship certain important points arise: (a) slow emptying and dilatation of the third part of the duodenum have been ascribed to its compression between these vessels and the aorta (*see* duodenal ileus, p. 198); (b) more important, however, is the relationship between these vessels and the first part of the jejunum during operations upon the pancreas and the duodenum: the first few branches of the superior mesenteric artery supplying the jejunum are short and do not branch freely, and, therefore, care must be taken not to compromise the blood-supply of the proximal jejunum during operations at the duodenal-jejunal flexure; (c) the flexure is kept in position by the ligament of Treitz which attaches it to the left crus of the diaphragm; the first part of the proximal jejunum may be lengthened by dividing the ligament as far right as the superior mesenteric vessels.

3   Although the jejunum, which constitutes almost two-fifths of the small intestine, merges imperceptibly with the ileum, differentiation between them and identification of a specific segment of intestine can be of great importance. The differences between proximal jejunum and distal ileum are shown in Fig 10.1 and Table 1.

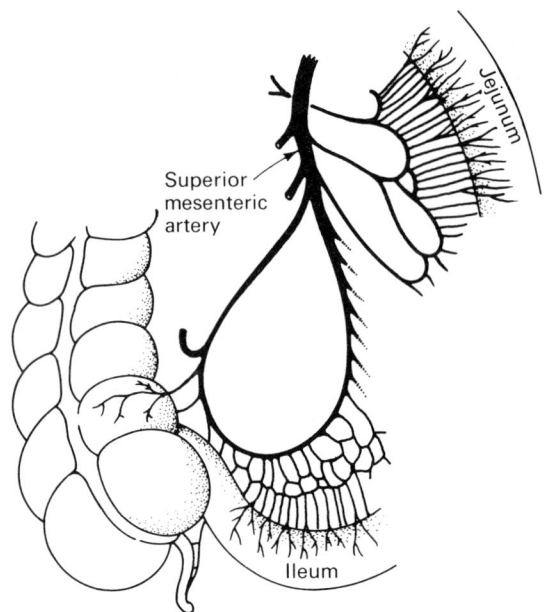

Fig 10.1 Blood-supply to jejunum and ileum (Adapted from Colcock B.P. and Braasch J.W., 1968, *Surgery of the Small Intestine in the Adult. Major problems in Clinical Surgery*, Vol. VII. Philadelphia: Saunders.)

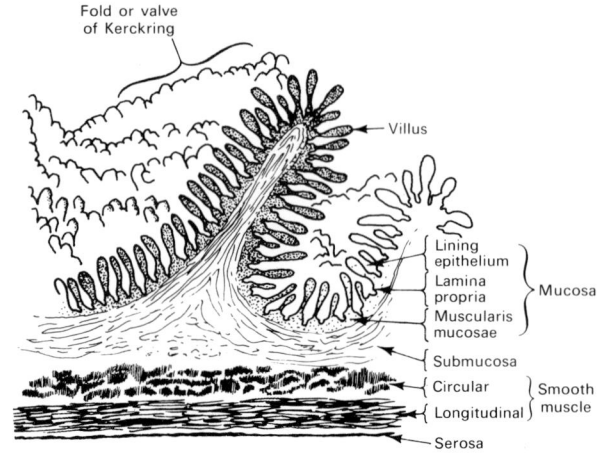

Fig 10.2 Layers forming wall of small intestine. Each squared area in Figs 10.2 and 10.3 is shown in greater magnification in succeeding figure (From Laster L. and Ingelfinger F.J., 1961, *New Engl. J. Med*; **264**:1138.)

Table 1
MACROSCOPIC DIFFERENCES BETWEEN JEJUNUM AND ILEUM

Feature	Jejunum	Ileum
Wall	Thick	Thin
Lumen	Wide	Narrow
Mesenteric fat	On mesentery	On bowel and mesentery
Valvulae conniventes	Prominent	Less prominent
Blood supply	Single arcades	Multiple arcades

Microscopic anatomy

To perform its primary function of absorption, the intestine must provide a large surface area to the luminal content. This is achieved (a) by throwing the lining mucosa of the jejunum into folds (valvulae conniventes or valves of Kerckring) (Fig 10.2); (b) by projecting villi into the lumen (Fig 10.3); and (c) by lining the luminal surfaces of the columnar absorbing cells with a brush border of microvilli (Fig 10.4).

The crypts of Lieberkühn, considered to be the source of new columnar cells, contain Paneth cells, argentaffin cells, etc. Diseases which destroy the entire

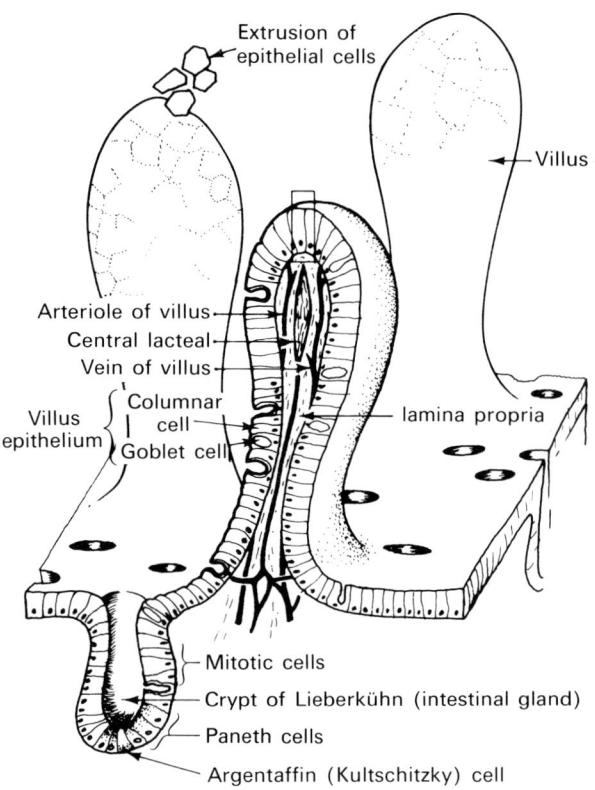

Fig 10.3 Villi and crypts of Lieberkühn. (From Laster L. and Ingelfinger F.J., 1961, *New Engl. J. Med*; **264**:1138.)

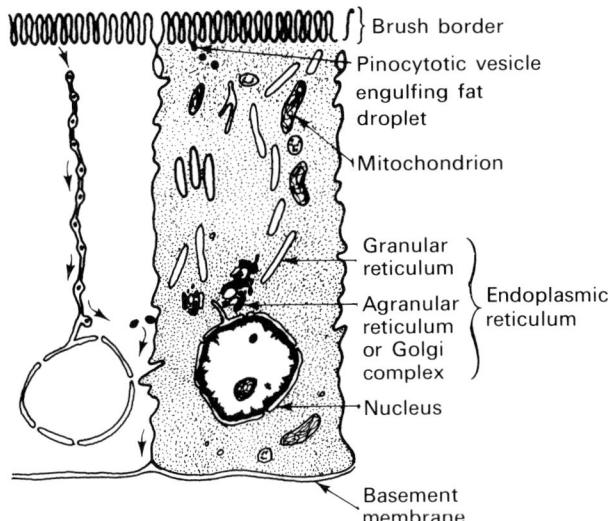

Brush border

Pinocytotic vesicle
engulfing fat
droplet

Mitochondrion

Granular
reticulum
Agranular   Endoplasmic
reticulum   reticulum
or Golgi
complex
Nucleus

Basement
membrane

Fig 10.4 Diagram of electron microscope appearance of
columnar cell. (From Laster L. and Ingelfinger F.J., 1961,
New Engl. J. Med; **264**:1138.)

structure of, or impair the function of, the villi and microvilli, e.g. coeliac disease, can be more devastating to
intestinal function than simple removal of even quite
sizeable lengths of intestine, because the large capacity
of the intestine to absorb nutrients depends almost
entirely upon the integrity of the villi and microvilli.

Physiology

For effective absorption, the partially-digested contents of the stomach are delivered, at a measured rate,
into the small intestine, where further digestive processes, in the lumen or within the intestinal membrane,
break down complex molecules into simpler forms for
transport across the intestinal cells into the lymph or
portal blood. To mix the intestinal contents with the
digestive enzymes, the small intestine shows complex
segmentation movements. The pumping action of the
villi facilitates absorption. Forward propulsive movements of peristalsis ensure that there is no undue hold-
up of the luminal contents which are yet allowed sufficient time to be brought into close contact with the
wide surface area of the intestine for absorption.

For the absorption of essential nutrients, complex
transfer systems have been developed in the intestinal
mucosa. Some are highly specific and active processes,
requiring work to be done by the intestinal cells; others
are less specific; for detailed description the appropriate physiological text should be consulted.

The bulk of absorption, especially of substances
which require to be absorbed in large amounts, e.g.

water, electrolytes, carbohydrates, proteins, etc., takes
place in the upper part of the jejunum. The reason is
that this is the first part of the small bowel encountered.
The lower jejunum and ileum, however, can take over
these functions if the upper jejunum has been removed
or involved in a disease process. There is an extremely
large reserve capacity in the intestine for the absorption
of these important substances. In contrast, other substances are absorbed at specific sites in the intestine, e.g.
bile salts and vitamin B_{12}, which are absorbed specifically and mainly in the terminal ileum; their malabsorption is likely to occur if the ileum has been removed or
involved in disease.

Perhaps, surgically, the most important substances
absorbed by the small intestine are water and electrolytes. In addition to a daily dietary intake of between
1–2 l of water and 150 mmol sodium, about 3–5 l of
isotonic electrolyte solution are poured into the upper
reaches of the gastrointestinal tract from the secreting
glands of the stomach, liver, pancreas and upper small
bowel. Almost all of this fluid is absorbed, so that only
100–200 ml are lost each day. Most of the absorption
takes place in the small intestine, for the volume of the
ileal effluent is, at most, one litre per day. This orderly
sequence of secretion and reabsorption can be easily
upset by diseases of the small intestine, especially
obstruction, fistula or diffuse mucosal disease e.g.
Crohn's disease. Not surprisingly, the commonest
causes of water and electrolyte depletion are gastrointestinal in origin.

Despite its impressive length and essential functions,
the small intestine is much less vulnerable to disease
than the stomach or colon. This is fortunate, because
until recently the small intestine has been relatively
inaccessible to non-operative diagnostic procedures.
Diffuse diseases of the mucosa, e.g. coeliac disease, can
be diagnosed by per oral capsule biopsy. Only the
duodenum and perhaps the upper jejunum and, occasionally, the terminal ileum, can be visualised directly
by fibreoptic endoscopy. Barium studies and mesenteric angiography do not have the same accurate and
reliable yield that they can have in the stomach or large
intestine.

Congenital anomalies

The complex intrauterine development of the intestine renders it susceptible to various congenital anomalies. The most severe of these – atresia and stenosis –
declare themselves usually as emergencies in the early
neonatal period (*see* Chapter 13). The developmental
anomalies, which present in adolescence and adult life,
are usually abnormalities of mid-gut rotation, the majority
of which are asymptomatic and remain undetected.
However, without a knowledge of the development

of the intestine, a surgeon may be baffled by the unexpected discovery of such anomalies at operation
and his ignorance can lead, for example, to such serious
errors as gastroileostomy following gastric transection.
Another important anomaly that may be the cause of
symptoms in adult life is Meckel's diverticulum.

Embryology of intestine

The primitive alimentary canal develops from the
endodermic vesicle of the zygote. The vesicle is, by a
constriction, divided into two parts – an intraembryonic
portion which becomes the future alimentary canal,
and an extraembryonic part, which becomes the yolk
sac. The constriction itself represents the future vitellointestinal duct. The duodenum down to the biliary
papilla, along with the stomach, forms the abdominal
portion of the *foregut*, which becomes fixed slightly to
the right of the mid-line. The blood-supply of the foregut comes from the coeliac axis. The *hindgut*, lying in
the mid-line of the abdomen, is fixed by a retention
band to the origin of the superior mesenteric artery,
ensuring that the upper end of the hindgut remains in
close proximity to the origin of the vessels. The hindgut, representing the distal one-third of the transverse
colon and the rest of the large intestine, is supplied by
the inferior mesenteric artery. From the two fixed
points (the duodenum at the biliary papilla and the
retention band at the upper point of the hindgut) there
is a narrow duodenal colic isthmus from which the two
limbs of the *midgut* are attached. The midgut is supplied by the superior mesenteric artery. The proximal
limb, cranial to the superior mesenteric vessels, is
called the prearterial segment. The segment caudal to
the superior mesenteric vessel is called the postarterial
segment.

Rapid growth of the midgut loop during the fifth
week causes it to form a large loop herniating into the
root of the umbilical cord with the vitellointestinal duct
at its apex. During subsequent weeks, as the peritoneal
cavity enlarges, the midgut returns to the abdomen,
rotating in a counter-clockwise direction around the
axis of the superior mesenteric artery, so that the
prearterial segment of midgut is placed inferior to, and
then to the left of, the superior mesenteric artery; and
the caudal limb, or postarterial segment, is placed
superior to, and then to the right of, the superior
mesenteric vessels. The duodenum is then placed
behind the transverse colon with the superior mesenteric artery in front.

With further rotation in a counter-clockwise direction, the caecum descends to its normal adult position.
The caecum, ascending and descending colon become
fixed. The base of the entire mesentery of the small
intestine is also fixed from the ligament of Treitz to the
ileo-caecal junction, so that the danger of volvulus is
eliminated. The leaves of the mesentery fuse at this
stage.

Four types of malrotation are recognised:

Non-rotation. Because the midgut does not rotate
after its reduction into the coelomic cavity, the small
bowel is on the right, and the large bowel is on the left,
of the abdominal cavity. The duodenum descends to
the right of the superior mesenteric vessels and the terminal ileum crosses the mid-line to enter the caecum
from the right. This is an uncommon anomaly.

Malrotation (or incomplete rotation). Rotation of
the midgut may be held up anywhere in its normal
course, so that the caecum may come to lie in the left
upper quadrant, in the subpyloric region (anterior to
the superior mesenteric artery), or in a subhepatic position. The malrotated caecum is usually fixed by peritoneal reflections, so-called 'Ladd bands', which may
overlie and compress the distal duodenum. Symptoms,
which usually begin in the neonatal period may not
declare themselves until early adult life, and consist of
copious vomiting of bile. Barium meal shows a dilated
stomach and proximal duodenum and on barium
enema, the caecum is in an incompletely rotated position. Treatment is by operation at which Ladd bands
are divided and the freed caecum is relocated in the left
lower quadrant of the abdomen.

A second problem associated with this anomaly is a
midgut volvulus, caused by a failure of fixation of the
posterior mesentery and consequent volvulus of the
intestine from the duodenal-jejunal junction to the mid
transverse colon. Early intervention is required to prevent strangulation of the small intestine. Diagnosis is
suggested on plain x-ray when jejunal loops with their
circular folds may be seen on the right side, and
smooth-walled ileal loops on the left side of the abdominal cavity. The anomaly may be suspected at operation by the right half of the colon being obscured by a
mess of small intestine. The small bowel is delivered
into the wound and the volvulus is untwisted. Caecal
bands should be divided and the caecum placed in the
left lower quadrant. The small bowel need not be fixed
– postoperative adhesions will attend to this. Resection
of gangrenous small intestine may occasionally be
required and can pose a major problem of the short
bowel syndrome (p. 196) in the early and late postoperative period.

Reversed rotation. The midgut rotates through 90° in
a clockwise direction around the axis of the superior
mesenteric artery. The descending colon comes to lie
on the left side and the ascending colon on the right
side of the abdomen. The transverse colon lies between
the superior mesenteric artery in front and the aorta
and inferior vena cava posteriorly. The duodenum lies

anterior to the superior mesenteric artery. This is a rare anomaly, but its importance lies in the fact that the opening at the base of the small bowel mesentery, through which the caecum and the transverse colon pass behind the superior mesenteric artery, is often so small that there is a risk of intestinal obstruction.

Paraduodenal hernia. In this form of internal hernia, the small intestine becomes encased in a mesenteric sac to the right, or left, side of the duodenum. The pre- or postarterial segment has rotated into the mesentery of, respectively, a post- or prearterial segment. The sac is transparent, the small bowel is much shorter than usual, and the terminal ileum extends out of the sac to empty into the caecum.

Trauma

Damage to the small intestine comprises about one-quarter to one-third of abdominal trauma, and may be caused by blunt (or non-penetrating) injury, or by penetrating wounds. Blunt injury is the more difficult to diagnose and carries the higher mortality. Injury to the duodenum presents the major problems and will be discussed first.

Duodenal injury

Damage to the duodenum following either blunt or penetrating injury presents one of the most challenging problems to the surgeon. Mortality in the region of 25–50% has been reported, but can be greatly reduced by early recognition combined with vigorous and skilled surgery.

Diagnosis

1   *Penetrating injuries* of the duodenum are frequently the result of gunshot wounds and, therefore, laparotomy is usually carried out. However, at operation, injuries to the duodenum, especially involving the third and fourth parts, may be missed, frequently because of inadequate exposure, hurried examination, or surgical inexperience. Exploration of the entire duodenum is essential, particularly (a) if the duodenum has been bruised, or (b) if there is a large haematoma near the duodenum, close to the head of the pancreas and extending on to the base of the transverse colon, or (c) if crepitations, blood, or bile-stained fluid are present in the retroperitoneal tissue beside the duodenum. The second part of the duodenum must be mobilised, and the third and fourth parts carefully explored. The surgeon encountering a periduodenal retroperitoneal haematoma must not leave the area unexplored and should call for expert assistance if necessary.

2   Following *blunt injury* of the duodenum, the clinical features are often unhelpful, at least in the early stages. Duodenal content more often leaks into the retroperitoneal tissue than into the peritoneal cavity. Initially sterile, duodenal content quickly becomes contaminated by bacteria and the tissues are extensively damaged by sepsis and by leakage of pancreatic secretion and bile. Diagnosis should always be suspected in those who have received an injury to the lower chest or upper abdomen in a car accident.

Several aids may help in the diagnosis. A considerable volume of blood (removed by paracentesis from the right upper quadrant), the presence of air under the right diaphragm or above the right kidney, and increasing elevation of the serum amylase, all suggest duodenal damage; but quite severe duodenal injury may be present in the absence of these signs. If there is any doubt, laparotomy should be undertaken, because delays in diagnosis and treatment are the two major factors which lead to unsatisfactory results.

Treatment

Blood transfusion, prophylactic antibiotics, careful fluid and electrolyte balance and first class anaesthesia are all important elements for success, but the essential ingredient is early operation.

Simple repair by suture without decompression of the duodenum is probably feasible only for small stab wounds in the first or second part of the duodenum. Closure of larger defects in this manner may lead to a narrowing of the duodenal lumen with a risk of fistula formation. In these circumstances, the duodenum can be cut across at the site of the injury and continuity re-established by end-to-end anastomosis. Alternatively, the duodenum can be divided, both ends closed, and gastroenterostomy carried out.

Alternatively, a large duodenal defect can be closed by applying a 'patch' of proximal jejunum, brought up behind the colon to the defect. The jejunum is sutured to the edges of the defect with a double layer of non-absorbed suture material. Larger duodenal wounds may be managed by anastomosing the open end of a Roux-en-Y loop of proximal jejunum to the duodenal defect. On rare occasions, a pancreaticoduodenectomy may be required, especially if the duodenum and pancreas are extensively damaged. However, the majority of injuries can be handled by adequate debridement and closure either by suture or by a patch technique.

With operations for duodenal rupture, certain important additional features must be mentioned:

1   If the ampullary region is damaged, the common bile-duct should be identified and a T-tube should be inserted. Occasionally reimplantation of the bile-duct may be required.

2 Adequate drainage during the postoperative period is required. Two or three Penrose drains should be led from the site of injury directly on to the anterior abdominal wall. External drainage is even more important if the pancreas has been damaged.

3 Because suture lines must be free from tension and duodenal obstruction should be avoided, the duodenum has to be decompressed. A jejunostomy tube should be threaded in an afferent direction towards the site of injury, to aspirate the large volumes of bile, duodenal and pancreatic juice, which will collect in the duodenal lumen. Further decompression may be achieved by inserting a gastrostomy tube, to aspirate gastric contents and decompress the lumen of the duodenum above the injury. A second jejunostomy tube can be inserted down the jejunum to assist in enteral feeding.

After operation the need for skilled care continues – to deal with sepsis and fistula formation, and to provide nutritional support. Oral feeding should not be begun until the second or third week after the injury, when contrast studies should be undertaken to show that the repair is intact and that there is a normal duodenal transit. At any time in the postoperative period further re-operation, debridement and drainage may be indicated.

Small bowel injury

Injuries to the small intestine are more common than those to the duodenum in a ratio of 8:1.

Non-penetrating trauma usually lacerates the small intestine at a fixed point, e.g. at the upper jejunum near the ligament of Treitz or in the lower ileum near the ileocaecal valve. A common cause is the compression of the small intestine between a car steering-wheel and the vertebral column.

Penetrating wounds of the small bowel in civilian practice are usually associated with stabbing or a knife wound. They carry a lower mortality, because of the reduced risk of concomitant injury and the shorter delay between the receipt of the injury and treatment. In contrast, in the battlefield, penetrating injuries of the small intestine, usually caused by gunshot wounds, carry a higher mortality.

Less commonly, penetrating injuries of the small intestine can be caused by laceration of the bowel inadvertently at operation, or during abdominal paracentesis. Occasionally, the bowel may also be damaged from within, due to an animal bone.

With injury to the small intestine, abdominal pain, guarding and tenderness are the cardinal features. The most reliable is tenderness, at first localised but becoming quickly diffuse and often referred to the patient's back and shoulder. An important investigation is a straight x-ray of the abdomen, with the patient in the upright position, which may show air under the diaphragm. Diagnosis may be difficult when there are other injuries to the chest or head, but abdominal rigidity and the absence of bowel sounds are clear signs of bowel injury and laparotomy should be undertaken. Various diagnostic aids – paracentesis, peritoneal lavage – may be helpful, but, if negative, should not delay a laparotomy if the signs of injury are present.

Treatment

The patient is prepared with nasogastric suction, antibiotics and adequate replacement of blood and fluid. At operation the contents of the abdominal cavity must be examined carefully. Small lacerations can be closed by a single-layer suture. Two small adjacent lacerations may easily be converted into a single larger one, which can be closed more easily. Larger lacerations may require resection of a segment of small intestine with end-to-end anastomosis. With multiple lacerations, it may be prudent to resect an entire segment rather than attempt multiple resections with several anastomoses.

Injuries caused by high velocity missiles may bruise the bowel widely, so that extensive debridement may be required to reach bowel which is viable, indicated by fresh bleeding. Injuries to the mesenteric side of the bowel, or avulsion of the mesentery, can often impair the blood-supply of a segment of intestine which may have to be resected. A denuded surface of bowel should be reperitonealised to minimise the risk of post-operative obstruction due to adhesions.

After operation, intravenous infusion of fluids and nasogastric suction should be continued until there is a return of bowel function. Fortunately, with such proper management, leakage from suture-lines is uncommon. Delay in operative intervention is the main reason for death following injury to the small intestine.

Radiation injury

Injury of the small intestine represents one of the most tragic complications of radiation of the pelvis or abdomen. Patients may die of this complication and its treatment, but more commonly, they become intestinal cripples with chronic partial intestinal obstruction and malnutrition.

With a usual therapeutic dose of 4000–6000 rad, severe gastro-intestinal symptoms may develop in 2–5% of patients. Mild symptoms may respond to antispasmodics, low residue diet, antiemetics, anti-diarrhoeals, as well as corticosteroids and cholestyramine. At most, however, medical treatment provides only temporary symptomatic relief. Unfortunately, surgical treatment, although potentially curative, is associated with a high mortality and morbidity rate.

Pathology

The effect of ionising radiation on the gastrointestinal tract is two-fold. Initially, direct damage affects mainly the mucosa, but can cause perforation. Later, there may be a progressive obliterative vasculitis with the slow development of chronic intestinal ischaemia developing many years after the initial radiation treatment.

The intestine becomes friable and easily damaged at operation. Fibrosis may be extensive, especially after irradiation of the pelvis; dissection in this region becomes hazardous, and often recurrence of carcinoma is mistakenly diagnosed. The bowel becomes gradually fibrosed and narrowed by strictures.

The dose, fractionation, degree of shielding and type of radiation therapy can all influence the degree and intensity of the intestinal injury. Although the small bowel is more sensitive to radiation than the colon (minimum and maximum radiation doses are from 4500 to 6500 rad in the small intestine and from 5500 to 8000 rad in the colon), the colon and especially the rectum are more vulnerable, probably because of their greater immobility. After abdominal surgery there is a higher risk of radiation injury to the small intestine, perhaps because of its fixation by adhesions. Patients with a history of previous abdominal operations should have a barium meal and barium enema studies before irradiation, to determine if the bowel is adherent in the pelvis.

Clinical features

The immediate response to excessive irradiation of the small bowel is diarrhoea with or without abdominal pain. These symptoms are self-limiting. Later, as strictures develop, the patient complains of cramping abdominal pain, bloating, alternating diarrhoea and constipation. Weight-loss is common and fistulas may occur. Bleeding and perforation are less common.

Diagnosis

The diagnosis of radiation injury should always be considered when a patient presents with abdominal symptoms after radiotherapy, even many years previously. Laboratory investigations are not especially helpful. Radiology of the gastrointestinal tract may show oedema of the small intestinal mucosa with areas of narrowing and stricture.

Treatment

Medical treatment is at best symptomatic. Before operation is undertaken, radiological studies should be carried out, including barium meal and follow-through, barium enema, fistulography, cystography, and intravenous urogram.

Preoperative nutritional support is required because many of these patients are severely anaemic and show marked hypoprotinaemia. Antibiotics should always be given prophylactically at the time of operation.

The choice of operation lies between resection with end-to-end anastomosis and bypass. In general, bypass operations seem to be safer, with a lower incidence of intestinal anastomotic dehiscence. There is, however, the risk of development of a blind-loop syndrome and malabsorption. When the radiation damage is extensive, bypass is clearly the treatment of choice.

On the other hand, resection should be performed when the disease is restricted. Wide resection may be required to ensure that only healthy bowel is anastomosed. The anastomosis should be protected by a temporary loop ileostomy or tube jejunostomy. Frequently, to decide whether the bowel is sufficiently healthy for anastomosis, microscopic examination of bowel after frozen section is undertaken.

Fistulas are especially difficult to treat. Partial or total exclusion of the fistula with bypass operation is generally successful. Failure-rate following resection and anastomosis is high in the presence of fistulas. Multiple operations may be required, because of the poor healing of irradiated bowel and the progressive nature of the intestinal damage.

Avoidance of the problem is ideal. In only a few cases has the dose of radiotherapy been excessive. Patients at risk of developing intestinal damage with an ordinary therapeutic dose of radiation are those who have had previous abdominal, and particularly pelvic, operations complicated by sepsis, those with cardiovascular problems including diabetes, and the group of thin, elderly female patients with a deep pelvis which may contain more small bowel than usual.

Tumours

Although the small intestine accounts for about three-quarters of the length of the gastrointestinal tract, only 3–6% of gastrointestinal tumours occur within it. Tumours of the colon, in contrast, are 40–60 times more common than those of the small intestine. Because of their rarity and, often, clinical innocence, tumours of the small intestine are frequently omitted from a differential diagnosis. Almost all the structures which compose the small intestine may give rise to benign or malignant tumours, and so the histological variety is great.

Benign tumours

Benign and malignant tumours are reported with almost equal incidence at operation, but autopsies show a very much higher incidence of benign lesions, indicating that many do not cause symptoms and are probably of little clinical significance. The frequency of these tumours increases progressively towards the ileum. Almost all ages are affected, with a peak incidence in the fourth decade.

TYPES

Epithelial tissue

Adenoma. These are benign neoplastic epithelial proliferations, most of which are polypoidal. The commonest presenting symptoms are intestinal obstruction, usually due to intussusception, or bleeding. Small lesions can be removed by excision through a simple enterostomy; larger lesions may require segmental resection.

Villous adenoma. These are rare tumours, occurring most frequently in the duodenum. Presenting symptoms are obstruction and bleeding. The copious leakage of mucus leading to serious electrolyte depletion, common with colonic villous tumours, is not reported in the small intestine. Because of their tendency to undergo malignant change, all villous tumours should be excised.

Hamartomas (Peutz-Jeghers syndrome). This is an uncommon familial disease, characterised by intestinal polyposis and melanin spots on the lips, buccal mucosa, fingers and toes. The condition is a genetically determined Mendelian dominant. Grossly, the lesions look like other intestinal polyps, but are thought to be hamartomas, probably arising from the abnormal overgrowth of muscularis mucosae. Malignant transformation is rare.

The polyps, found mainly in the jejunum and ileum, less commonly in the colon and stomach, may bleed or obstruct the lumen. Intussusception is the main cause of obstruction, which is rarely complete, frequently recurrent and usually resolves spontaneously.

The diagnosis may be suggested by the above clinical features. Contrast barium studies may be helpful, but more precise diagnosis can be made on endoscopy if the lesions occur in the stomach or in the duodenum. Alternatively, the diagnosis may be made at laparotomy. Management should always be conservative. Where surgery is required, operation should be confined, for example, to polypectomy or minimal resection. The wide distribution of numerous polyps precludes their complete removal.

Connective tissue

Leiomyoma. Benign neoplasms of smooth muscle may occur either within the wall of the small intestine, where they may reach a large size, or project into the lumen producing intussusception and bleeding secondary to mucosal ulceration. Occasionally great difficulty may be experienced by the pathologist in distinguishing between benign and malignant lesions. For this reason, treatment should always be by segmental resection.

Lipoma occurs most commonly in the ileum and, by projecting into the lumen, may produce the symptoms of obstruction and bleeding.

Neurogenic tumours. These may arise from the nerve sheath and be neurilemmomas or neurofibromas. Others may arise from the sympathetic nervous system as ganglion neuromas.

Vascular tumours (angioma). These may be true neoplasms or may represent developmental abnormalities and, therefore, be more correctly regarded as hamartomatous vascular malformations.

Haemangiomas are often small, but numerous, in the gastrointestinal tract and, in hereditary form, are known as Osler-Rendu disease.

Capillary and cavernous angiomas usually form polypoidal masses, sometimes small, often multiple and, in about two-thirds of cases, cause symptoms due to bleeding. Larger lesions may be detected by barium contrast studies. Occasionally a plain x-ray may disclose multiple calcium deposits due to calcification of a thrombosed haemangioma, but the most useful investigation is selective visceral angiography, which is often successful when bleeding is brisk. At operation, engorgement of mesenteric vessels can be a useful sign. Occasionally the lesion may also be seen by transillumination of the bowel wall, provided that the intestinal lumen is not filled with blood. They should be excised either through an enterostomy or by resection of an intestinal segment.

Malignant tumours

Adenocarcinoma

This is the commonest primary malignancy of the small intestine, occurring most frequently in the duodenum, where it has to be distinguished from malignant tumours arising from the ampulla of Vater. Symptoms will largely depend upon the site. Jaundice and chronic anaemia due to bleeding suggest a periampullary lesion. Lesions more highly placed can give rise to symptoms indistinguishable from pyloric stenosis; while those in the jejunum and ileum usually produce rather non-specific symptoms. The diagnosis is usually made on barium studies showing a lesion, accompanied by mucosal ulceration. High lesions may be biopsied using a flexible endoscope.

Treatment is by resection of the small intestine, with adequate removal of the adjacent regional mesenteric lymph nodes, because these tumours metastasise early. Tumours arising near the ampulla of Vater should be treated by pancreaticoduodenectomy, which offers the best chance of cure.

Carcinoid

These tumours have excited great interest because of the variation in growth-potential and the unusual syndrome associated with them. The term 'carcinoid' was coined because at the time, the tumours were thought to be benign, but resembling carcinoma morphologically. After much discussion they are now considered to arise from the granular chromaffin cells, and by 1954 were associated with an endocrinological disorder known as the *carcinoid syndrome.*

These tumours may arise from any part of the gastrointestinal tract, especially the appendix, ileum and rectum. Of slow growth, all have malignant potential especially in the small bowel. Spread takes place to the serosa, then to the regional lymph nodes and thence to the liver. According to an ability to reduce silver salts after fixation in formalin, they have been classified as argentaffin tumours which reduce silver salts, and argyrophil tumours which do not. Carcinoid tumours of midgut origin are both argentaffin and argyrophil and may be associated with the carcinoid syndrome. Tumours of fore- or hindgut origin are rarely associated with the syndrome.

The occurrence throughout the body of neoplasms which are associated with diffuse endocrinological abnormalities, and which are structurally and physiologically similar to carcinoid tumours, has given rise to the concept of an endocrine cell system of probable neural crest origin, known as the APUD system (amine precursor uptake and decarboxylation). Neoplasms arising from this group of cells have been called apudomas and include carcinoid tumours, all varieties of pancreatic islet-cell tumour, medullary carcinoma of the thyroid, oat cell carcinoma of the lung and pituitary adenomas (*see* Chapter 37).

Carcinoid tumours are, for the most part, asymptomatic and are encountered accidentally at operation. Symptoms are usually non-specific with obstruction due to the intussusception being the most common complication. Only rarely is a preoperative diagnosis made even when clinically suspect. Metastasis is common in 20–30% of cases. Up to one-third of patients with a carcinoid tumour may harbour a second primary malignancy of another type.

The *carcinoid syndrome* arises when a carcinoid tumour metastasises to the liver. Midgut carcinoids secrete serotonin (5-hydroxytryptamine (5HT)) which is the major biochemical cause of the syndrome. Foregut carcinoids secrete 5-hydroxytryptophane (5HTP) and histamine, resulting in an atypical carcinoid syndrome.

Serotonin, the major biochemical product of carcinoid tumours, is derived from exogenous tryptophane, whose usual metabolic pathway results in nicotinic acid. In the carcinoid syndrome up to 60% of the dietary tryptophane is diverted to serotonin, which is released into the plasma and rapidly bound to platelets. Free serotonin is rapidly catabolised in the liver and lungs to 5-hydroxyindoleacetic acid (5HIAA) which is excreted in the urine. The vasoactive secretions of small-intestinal carcinoid are inactivated mainly in the liver, so that the typical syndrome does not appear until there are significant hepatic metastases to overcome the detoxifying action of the liver.

The typical carcinoid syndrome is characterised by:

1 *Vasomotor* symptoms. Prominent flushing of the skin of the head and upper trunk, often precipitated by excitement and alcohol, is considered to be due to kinin peptides, e.g. bradykinin. The enzyme kallikrein, which forms bradykinin in the plasma, has been found in high concentration in hepatic metastases.

2 *Gastrointestinal* symptoms. Episodic watery diarrhoea due to serotonin causing small bowel contraction and hypermotility.

3 *Cardio-pulmonary* symptoms. (Asthmatic attacks and cardiac valvular lesions.) Bronchospasm is considered to be caused by histamine, serotonin and bradykinin; the cardiac lesions, involving mainly the tricuspid valve and characterised by the deposition of dense fibrous tissue, are attributed to the action of serotonin.

The syndrome should be suspected in any patient with diarrhoea, flushing of the skin and a palpable liver, and can be diagnosed by the detection of more than 20 mg 5HIAA in a 24-h specimen of urine, provided the patient has not recently eaten bananas or taken chlorpromazine. Typical attacks can be provoked by administration of a small dose of adrenalin (1–5 u) which produces the cutaneous flush in patients with the carcinoid syndrome.

Because all carcinoids are capable of metastasising and about a third actually do so, the tumours should be removed by wide segmental resection including adjacent node-bearing mesentery. The tumours show a tendency to involve contiguous loops of bowel, and under these circumstances all affected intestine should be removed *en bloc*. As much tumour as possible should be removed, preserving only vital structures such as the superior mesenteric artery. Because these tumours grow slowly, survival can be enhanced by such bulk removal.

In the treatment of the carcinoid syndrome, hepatic metastases should be removed as much as possible by enucleation of metastases, or even by partial hepatectomy. The distressing symptoms of the carcinoid syndrome may be greatly relieved by the judicious use of pharmacological agents aimed at the serotonin and kinin pathways. Flushing can be best controlled with phenoxybenzamine, and other alpha-adrenergic blocking agents that block the endogenous catecholamine stimulation of kallikrein. Diarrhoea and malabsorption may be controlled with methysergide, a serotonin antagonist. Asthmatic episodes must not be treated by adrenalin which will aggravate the bronchospasm. Inhalation bronchodilators are the safest means of control. Recently cyproheptadine which blocks serotonin and histamin H_1 receptors has been shown to cause regression of carcinoid tumours.

Cancer chemotherapy for inoperable metastases is currently under investigation and some relief is obtained by the combined use of cyclophosphamide, 5-fluorouracil and streptozotocin, a drug active against beta islet cells. Symptoms have also been relieved by complete dearterialisation of the liver. Good results have been reported by the use of selective catheterisation and embolisation of the liver via the hepatic artery.

Leiomyosarcoma

These are the commonest malignant connective-tissue tumours of the small intestine. They usually bleed following ulceration of the overlying mucosa. Treatment is by wide intestinal resection, but little attention needs to be paid to the mesenteric lymph nodes, because they rarely spread by the lymphatic route. Recurrence is common, but growth is so slow that complete removal should be attempted. The tumour is, unfortunately, radio-resistant, but residual tumour may respond to combined chemotherapy using such agents as cyclophosphamide, vincristine and adriamycin.

Malignant lymphoma

Lymphomas of the gastrointestinal tract are rare – commoner in the stomach than in the small intestine where they are more usually associated with systemic lymphomas. These tumours may develop in adult patients with long-standing coeliac disease. The lesion is usually a reticulum-cell sarcoma and may be related to, and perhaps caused by, prolonged antigenic stimulation.

Intestinal lymphomas can occur in children (where they are the commonest tumours of the gastrointestinal tract between the ages of 3 and 8) or after the sixth decade.

In patients of Mediterranean origin, the lymphoma appears commonly in patients in their twenties, in whom malabsorption is a common feature. The disease, commonly seen in the Middle East, is not limited to these regions and appears with a relatively high incidence among the Cape black population in South Africa. The term 'immunoproliferative small intestinal disease' is now applied to this condition.

The clinical features of intestinal lymphomas are weight-loss, anorexia, abdominal mass and constipation. Mucosal ulceration is common, often producing bleeding and anaemia.

The treatment of primary lymphoma of the small intestine is surgical, that is, wide excision of the primary lesion and removal of adjacent regional lymph nodes. If the lesion is considered to be incompletely resected, adjuvant radiotherapy should be considered. Adjuvant chemotherapy, using such agents as vincristine, methotrexate, cyclophosphamide etc., should also be considered for palliation.

Inflammatory disease of the bowel

The term 'inflammatory bowel disease' embraces diseases of several causes. The cause is known of some, e.g. tuberculosis, bilharzia, and, as effective medical treatment becomes available, surgery is rarely required. The cause of the two principal types of inflammatory bowel disease, ulcerative colitis and Crohn's disease, remains elusive and specific medical treatment is not yet available. Nevertheless, for both diseases medical management predominates, but operation is indicated in two main circumstances – failure to respond to medication and development of such complications as abscess, stricture, bleeding, fistula and toxic dilatation.

Although Crohn's disease (regional enteritis) may involve all parts of the gastrointestinal tract, the small intestine is frequently implicated, and so the topic will be discussed in this chapter.

Crohn's disease (regional enteritis)

This is a chronic granulomatous disease of the gastrointestinal tract of unknown aetiology. Viral, microbiological, psychosomatic, vascular and dietary factors have all been incriminated but its cause still remains a mystery.

Originally described by Moynihan in 1907 and Dalziell in 1913, the key description by Crohn, Ginsberg and Oppenheimer referred to 'terminal ileitis', but it was quickly recognised that any part of the small bowel, and indeed of the gastrointestinal tract, may be involved.

Incidence and epidemiology

Although information on the prevalence of Crohn's disease remains patchy, populations prone to the disease seem in general to be highly developed, with a predominance in North-western Europe, North America and Australasia. The disease has probably an incidence of 1–7 per 100 000 of the population and seems to be increasing in frequency in absolute and real terms.

The disease attacks male and female equally, and is seen in all age groups, but most frequently in young adults with the average age of onset being about 25 years. The disease is more common in urban rather than among rural dwellers, among Jews living in Europe and North America than among non-Jews, and seems to occur more commonly in families of sufferers. Whether this familial association is caused by a genetic predisposition or by common exposure to an environmental factor has not been settled.

Pathology

Segments of intestine involved in Crohn's disease are thick-walled, dull red, and rubbery in consistence. Involved segments become adherent to one another or to other viscera, and in the thickened inflammatory masses, fistulas are often present. The adjacent mesentery is thick, oedematous, laden with fat and contains enlarged lymph nodes. The affected mucosa shows a marked nodularity with intervening ulcers. The lumen is greatly narrowed and the submucosa is thickened.

In most cases (over 80%) the small bowel is involved, with the most frequent site being the terminal ileum. In many cases, it may be the only segment involved. In about one-third of the patients both small and large intestine are involved. The disease may be a continuous one extending from the lower ileum through the ileocaecal valve to involve the caecum and ascending colon. Frequently, there are skip lesions, that is, the disease is discontinuous, affecting separate segments of bowel with intervening segments of apparently normal intestine. Less commonly, the disease may be extensive, involving most of the jejunum and ileum. The duodenum and stomach may be afflicted, but usually in association with ileal disease; it is rare for the disease to affect the stomach and duodenum exclusively.

Microscopically, in the early stages of the disease, there is marked inflammation of the submucous layer, with oedema and hyperaemia. Later the mucosa becomes ulcerated and in the submucous layers fibrosis predominates. There is a diffuse infiltration by mononuclear cells and lymphocytes. In addition granuloma cells appear – multinucleate epithelioid giant cells in lesions which do not caseate nor contain tubercle bacilli. In later stages of the disease, fibrosis becomes intense and the mucosa almost denuded by ulcers, which may penetrate deeply through the intestinal wall, producing fistulous tracts.

Clinical features

The clinical presentation of Crohn's disease is extremely variable, but the two commonest complaints are abdominal pain and diarrhoea. In the 'classical' form of the disease, a patient in his or her twenties gives a 6–12 months history of anorexia, lassitude, colicky lower abdominal pain especially in the right iliac fossa, associated with diarrhoea and weight-loss. On examination, the patient is often thin and pale with a low-grade fever. Clubbing of the fingers may be found. The abdomen is often slightly distended, with tenderness, and perhaps a mass, in the right iliac fossa. Bowel sounds may be increased. There may be, in the anal and perianal region, fissures, fistulas, or oedematous blue discolouration of the perianal skin, or indeed ulceration. In such patients the disease pursues an intermittent course.

In a few patients, the onset of the symptoms may be dramatic, with severe abdominal pain localised in the right iliac fossa, mimicking acute appendicitis. Emergency operation is undertaken, at which the appendix is found to be normal, but the terminal ileum is reddened, thickened, and congested (so-called acute Crohn's disease). Crohn's disease of the colon is discussed in Chapter 12.

Less common presentations (but, nevertheless, important because of their serious effect upon the patient and their non-specific nature which may prevent early diagnosis) are widespread oedema (due to hypoproteinaemia), and growth retardation which may be the sole manifestation in children or adolescents.

Complications

Intestinal obstruction. Complete obstruction is rare. Usually the obstruction, the result of inflammation, fibrosis and stricture, is partial and responds to non-operative measures.

Fistulas may form between diseased intestine and other segments of bowel, urinary bladder or vagina. Enterocutaneous fistulas are rarely spontaneous, but are common after operation, whether or not an intestinal anastomosis has been carried out.

Perforation of the intestine is caused by the penetration of an ulcer through the intestinal wall to reach the serosa. However, free perforation into the peritoneal cavity is rare, but paraileal or paracaecal abscesses are common.

Anorectal complications (viz. fissures, abscesses, sinuses and fistulas) are very common. Anal lesions are more usually associated with colonic, than small intestinal, disease, and with other extraintestinal manifestations of Crohn's disease. Operations for apparently simple anorectal conditions should not be embarked upon, until Crohn's disease has been excluded by careful history and examination, including sigmoidoscopy. Moreover, all tissue excised during anorectal operations should be examined microscopically for evidence of Crohn's disease.

Anal and perianal disease presents usually as swollen oedematous areas with dusky red cyanosis, intervening ulceration and fissuring. These appearances have to be distinguished from those due to bacterial and fungal infections, skin disease (e.g. lichen planus) and neoplasm.

Extra-alimentary manifestation

1 *Anaemia.* This is usually of the iron-deficiency type, due to chronic blood loss in the stools, or to diminished erythropoiesis due to chronic infection. Folate deficiency is less common. Megaloblastic anaemia due to vitamin B_{12} deficiency is surprisingly rare in a disease which so frequently affects the terminal ileum.

2 *Electrolyte disturbances.* With severe and prolonged diarrhoea, the patient may become depleted of sodium, potassium and magnesium. Serum albumin may fall, often quite markedly, due to the loss of protein from the inflamed bowel and to defective synthesis in the liver.

3 *Malnutrition* is common and is the result of many factors, e.g. anorexia, vomiting, diarrhoea, impaired intestinal absorption, etc.

4 *Liver disease* occurs in about 10% of patients. The commonest lesion is fatty infiltration of the liver. Pericholangitis and hepatic necrosis may be seen in advanced disease. Cirrhosis of the liver is uncommon. Also associated with inflammatory bowel disease is sclerosing cholangitis, involving both the intrahepatic and extrahepatic biliary systems.

5 *Skin diseases.* Although various skin diseases may be found, the commonest is erythema nodosum.

6 *Eyes.* Anterior uveitis, conjunctivitis, keratitis are associated with Crohn's disease, but their cause is unknown.

7 *Arthropathy and ankylosing spondylitis.* The incidence of joint complications varies, but may be as high as 20%. Acute inflammatory synovitis affects the larger joints, especially in the lower limbs. Arthritis is usually related to the severity of the symptoms of Crohn's disease, disappearing during remissions. The arthropathy usually responds to such measures as injection of corticosteroids into the joint and to the general treatment of Crohn's disease.

Ankylosing spondylitis may begin before the intestinal symptoms, and, thereafter, its course and that of the Crohn's disease may be quite independent. The spondylitis also may not respond to the medical treatment of Crohn's disease, even surgical extirpation. There is an hereditary component through the linkage with HLA-B27 antigen.

Malignant change. An association between Crohn's disease and intestinal carcinoma is being increasingly recognised. Indeed, a twenty-fold increase in incidence of carcinoma in patients with Crohn's disease has been quoted. About one-third of the carcinomas occur in the large bowel and the remainder in the small intestine but, since the distribution in the small intestine follows that of the Crohn's disease, the terminal ileum is especially affected. Carcinomas tend to develop in excluded segments of bowel. Like malignant disease associated with ulcerative colitis, carcinoma tends to occur in patients with long-standing disease and may go unrecognised until it is well-advanced.

Diagnosis

Although the disease may be suspected on clinical grounds, a firm diagnosis requires radiological investigations. Depending on the site of the disease, barium meal with follow-through, small bowel enema or barium enema may be required. Features suggesting Crohn's disease include an abnormal mucosal pattern – cobblestoning, filling defects, dilatation of bowel proximal to the abnormal area and the well-known 'string sign'. A diffuse abnormal pattern suggesting malabsorption may be present in extensive disease, but single or multiple strictures give a clue to diagnosis. Although there are typical angiographic appearances of Crohn's disease, such studies are rarely necessary to make the diagnosis.

When the small intestine is involved, x-ray studies may be unhelpful and exploratory operation may be required to establish the diagnosis. Lymphoma, reticulo-sarcoma and intestinal tuberculosis are three conditions which may mimic Crohn's disease and require laparotomy for diagnosis. It is always important to consider tuberculosis in any case of apparent Crohn's disease in patients of Indian ethnic origin.

The appearances of the bowel at operation are characteristic – dusky red, marked inflammation of the serosa with a rigid mesentery and enlarged lymph nodes. The appearances of the bowel has been likened to 'an eel in the state of rigor mortis' (Dalziell, 1913). To confirm the diagnosis, tissue should be obtained for microscopic examination e.g. a lymph node.

Medical treatment

Since the cause of the disease is unknown, there is no specific treatment. The fluctuating activity of Crohn's disease makes assessment of short-term therapy particularly difficult. However, the initial treatment of Crohn's disease is medical. The aim of medical management is to palliate by suppressing symptoms or by moderating inflammation. Drug treatment can have a profound effect upon the course of the disease in an individual patient, but it should be emphasised that rest and improved nutrition can contribute greatly to a patient's improvement.

Anti-diarrhoeal treatment. The patient's most frequent, distressing symptom is diarrhoea. Codeine phosphate (from 15 mg b.d. to 60 mg q.i.d.) is the cheapest and most effective remedy and, being an opiate, may help in relieving pain. Other anti-diarrhoeal agents of proved efficacy are diphenodxylate (5 mg t.i.d.) and loperamide. If the diarrhoea seems to be the result of extensive ileal disease or resection, cholestyramine, a potent bile salt binding agent, should be given.

Antibiotics have probably no general role in the treatment of Crohn's disease except when there is gross sepsis.

Corticosteroids are probably unequalled for the rapidity and intensity of their effect upon the acute inflammatory phase of the disease. They are particularly effective in alleviating symptoms in the short-term, that is, say, in the first 20 weeks of treatment. In severely ill patients, a parenteral route, using hydrocortisone hemisuccinate or prednisolone 21 – phosphate, should be chosen. In some centres, corticotrophin (ACTH) is given intramuscularly, because it is thought to be more effective and to stimulate, rather than suppress, adrenal cortical function. However, neither of these premises holds up greatly on investigation.

In less severely ill patients, prednisolone is given by mouth in the dose range 40–80 mg/per day initially. The dose should be rapidly decreased within the next few weeks to avoid the severe side-effects of adrenocortical overdose. With improvement, which most patients show, the dose should be reduced to a maintenance one of 5–15 mg a day.

Sulphasalazine, a sulphonamide, has some beneficial effect especially in segmental disease of the colon. The dose is 1 g per 15 kg body weight.

Metronidazole – an antibacterial agent – and the immuno-suppressive agent, azathioprine, have also been used. Good, indeed spectacular, results have been reported in some patients, but the efficacy of these drugs is still to be proven in controlled trials. The beneficial effects are quite unpredictable. One of the main problems in assessing these drugs is that their adminis-

tration may be required over a long period of time – over a year – to demonstrate any benefit. Azathioprine is a toxic drug, with the risk of causing pancreatitis and depression of the bone marrow. Other immunosuppressive agents are currently being studied, e.g. 6-mercaptopurine.

Total parenteral nutrition. Weight-loss, with varying degrees of malnutrition, is a common feature in Crohn's disease. With intravenous feeding, weight can be gained and nutrition improved. Moreover, with the consequent rest to the gastrointestinal tract, diarrhoea can be reduced, discharge from fistulas decreased, and, in some cases, fistulas may close. Parenteral nutrition may be total, or may be used as a supplement to oral feeding.

Total parenteral nutrition has its drawbacks. First, there are the dangers of septicaemia, due to bacterial contamination of the indwelling catheter and the risk of pneumothorax by needle puncture in attempted catheterisation of the subclavian vein. Secondly, this form of treatment can only be employed in the short-term, because, with its cessation, the complications of the Crohn's disease often recur. Parenteral feeding can help to restore a patient quickly to a normal weight and state of nutrition, either until more specific treatment has its effect or in preparation for a major operation.

Elemental diets, which contain predigested nutritional substrates and are rapidly and efficiently absorbed with little residue, can also be used in Crohn's disease. They are particularly useful in distal ileal disease, because the diet will be absorbed almost entirely in the upper jejunum, if it is free of disease. Unfortunately, these diets tend to be hyperosmotic and, therefore, can provoke diarrhoea, a consequence undesirable in a patient with Crohn's disease.

Surgical treatment

Three features of Crohn's disease necessarily limit the therapeutic role of surgery. First, the whole of the alimentary tract is at risk from mouth to anus. Secondly, the disease shows a tendency to involve multiple sites. Thirdly, it is a disease with a high recurrence rate – about one-third of patients submitted to operation require further surgery later. The natural history of the disease implies that it cannot be cured by extirpative surgery.

The indications for operation may be listed as follows:

EMERGENCY
These indications are rare.

Colonic dilatation. This occurs in 1–2% of patients and should be treated in a similar manner to toxic dilatation of the colon in ulcerative colitis.

Perforation of the ileum or colon is uncommon. Simple closure should not be attempted. The affected segment should be resected.

Haemorrhage. This is a very rare complication.

Obstruction. While obstruction is common, it is usually partial and recurrent, and frequently responds to conservative treatment, viz. nasogastric suction, intravenous fluid and electrolyte replacement (especially potassium repletion).

Abscesses. These should be simply drained, even although a fistula may develop subsequently. Intestinal resection with anastomosis should be avoided in the presence of sepsis. Occasionally, a bypass operation can be performed with exclusion of the affected segment. The bypass should take place at some distance from the abscess which should be drained extraperitoneally.

ELECTIVE

Intractable disease, unresponsive to medical treatment, and some of the more severe complications of the disease constitute the major indications for elective operation. However, surgery for Crohn's disease must be looked upon always as second choice and should rarely constitute primary treatment. There is no place for attempts at aggressive extirpation of all known disease. Nevertheless, operations should not be unreasonably delayed if there is no obvious response to expert medical management. The commonest indication for resection is abdominal pain and diarrhoea which have not responded to conservative treatment.

Complications. Operation may be indicated for certain complications of Crohn's disease, but it must be emphasised that the mere presence of complications does not mean that surgery is required.

Persistent fistulas. Occasionally operation may be required for persistent fistulas. Enteroenteric and enterocutaneous fistulas may close with improved nutrition of the patient, rest to affected bowel and a remission induced by medical treatment. An enterovesical fistula represents an absolute indication for operation.

Obstructive uropathy. A large mass of Crohn's disease can, by extrinsic pressure, obstruct the ureter and lead to hydronephrosis. The obstruction and its effects may be detected only on a routine urogram. However, in many cases these patients have severe hip and flank pain associated with Crohn's disease. Operation should be performed for the Crohn's disease in its own right, but at operation care is required to identify and preserve the ureter.

Carcinoma may complicate Crohn's disease – often occurring in an excluded segment of intestine.

Anal abscesses. In many cases anal and perianal disease heals spontaneously. Operation should be deferred if at all possible, because healing is slow and the results of surgery can often be disastrous – e.g. faecal incontinence due to operative damage to the sphincter. A conservative policy should be adopted and the anal lesions treated as part of the general management of the Crohn's disease. At most, operations should consist of decompression of an abscess, or dilatation of anal stenosis.

Right iliac fossa mass. The patient presents with a mass in the right iliac fossa with the symptoms of peritoneal irritation, fever and leucocytosis. The lesion may only be an acutely active, but uncomplicated Crohn's disease. On the other hand, there may be a frank abscess beside the colon or ileum. Frequently, the signs will abate with conservative non-operative treatment – corticosteroids, antibiotics, nasogastric suction and intravenous fluid replacement. If the clinical signs of an abscess persist with increasing leucocytosis and fever, operation should be undertaken to drain the abscess.

Definitive operations

Small intestinal disease. There are two possible surgical strategies. Formerly, bypass surgery was popular because of its apparent lower mortality and morbidity. Over the years, however, its advantages have been eroded by improved preoperative management, including blood transfusion and antibiotics, and by the increased evidence of later morbidity due to progression of the disease in the retained affected segment. The disease in a bypassed segment does not subside.

As a result, resection is now favoured although the evidence for its superiority is not proven. There have been few good controlled trials comparing both strategies. Once he has decided to resect, the surgeon must judge how much intestine he should remove. There is no evidence that, with extensive resection, the prognosis is improved. Most surgeons leave a 10–15 cm margin of apparently healthy intestine on either side of the gross disease, in order to minimise the chances of leaving skip lesions. Two adjacent segments of Crohn's disease are preferably resected as one rather than separately, to avoid multiple anastomoses. However, in view of the tendency of the disease to recur, intestinal conservation should be the rule and classical cancer operations such as right hemicolectomy should be avoided. Only minimal lengths of ileum and colon should be resected. Moreover, the surgeon should remove only segments of intestine which are clearly diseased and which have formed the indication for the operation. It is quite in order to leave, say, an involved segment of jejunum or colon if the operation was undertaken for gross troublesome ileal disease.

There is no need to extirpate the mesenteric lymph nodes. Where adjacent viscera have been implicated with fistulas, they need not be resected either in whole or in part. Thus a small fistulous opening into the bladder, sigmoid colon or duodenum can be closed. Such treatment, however, is not appropriate where there is marked intrinsic disease of the bowel.

Colonic disease. This is dealt with in chapter 12.

Recurrence after surgery

The major problem of surgery for Crohn's disease remains the tendency for recurrence. Recurrence is particularly likely when operations are carried out in children and its frequency falls off with age. The disease probably recurs in 40% of patients after resection of the small intestine. A similar incidence has been shown in patients with large bowel disease, but the recurrence rate seems particularly low (about 10%) after total colectomy with ileostomy.

In the small intestine the usual site for recurrence is at, or just proximal to, the anastomosis, occurring within 1–2 years of the operation, although occasionally the recurrence may not be seen for 5–10 years after operation.

It is important, therefore, for the surgeon to realise that by embarking upon the operative treatment of Crohn's disease, he must assume the responsibility for a careful follow-up of the patient and for further operations if and when these become necessary. In spite of these disadvantages, with careful treatment many patients are able to lead satisfactory lives, and have long intervals without symptoms.

Diverticular disease

Diverticula of the small intestine can be considered under two headings:

1 Diverticula of the duodenum, jejunum and ileum
2 Meckel's diverticulum

Diverticulum of the duodenum, jejunum and ileum

Duodenal diverticula, diagnosed in 1–5% of patients undergoing barium studies of the upper gastrointestinal tract, are usually found along the pancreatic border of the second, third, and fourth part of the duodenum. They are usually only of passing interest. Complications, which are rare, are severe bleeding, perforation, biliary and pancreatic obstruction.

Obstruction may be brought about in several ways. A common duct draining directly into the diverticulum can become obstructed by biliary calculi. Alternatively, the bile-duct may be compressed in its intraduodenal portion by a diverticulum distended with duodenal content. Obstruction may be relieved by excising the diverticulum, but operative mortality may be high, because of the development of a duodenal fistula or impairment of pancreatic drainage. The preferred treatment of bile-duct obstruction is choledochoduodenostomy.

Perforation of a duodenal diverticulum is uncommon and is best managed by excision of the diverticulum, leaving sufficient cuff at the base to allow turning in of the edge without tension. Alternatively, the walled-off perforation can be drained and gastrojejunostomy performed.

Massive bleeding is extremely rare, fortunately, because these diverticula can be extremely difficult to localise at operation. A preoperative diagnosis may be made by endoscopy or arteriography and under these circumstances the diverticula should be excised in whole or in part with secure control of the bleeding point.

Jejunal and ileal diverticula

Apart from Meckel's diverticulum, these usually arise on the mesenteric border of the bowel and are composed only of mucosa and submucosa. They are found where blood-vessels penetrate the bowel wall, and slight injury may cause bleeding. Perforation is relatively rare. The triad of obscure pain, anaemia and dilated jejunal loops should alert the clinician to the possibility of jejunal diverticulosis.

Ileal diverticula may also be complicated by bleeding, perforation or obstruction and, as with jejunal diverticula, treatment is by local excision or by resection of the involved segment with primary anastomosis.

Meckel's diverticulum

Meckel was the first to associate the diverticulum on the antimesenteric side of the distal ileum with the embryonic vitellointestinal gut (p. 178). Atrophy and obliteration of the vitellointestinal duct occurs between the fifth and seventh week of intrauterine development.

Complete or incomplete persistence of the duct results in the following anomalies (Fig 10.5):

1 Meckel's diverticulum – the commonest
2 Complete, or incomplete, vitellointestinal fistula
3 Enterocystoma
4 Fibrous band joining umbilicus to mesentery of the small intestine
5 Strawberry tumour of umbilicus
6 Intussusception

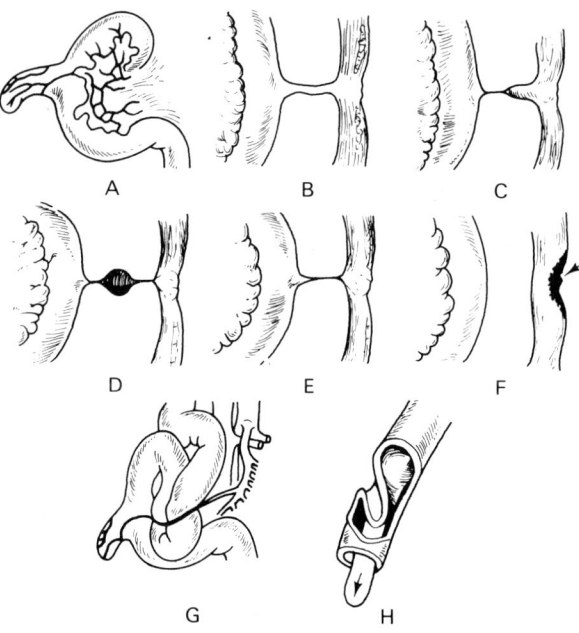

Fig 10.5 Anomalies of the vitellointestinal duct. A = Meckel's diverticulum; B = complete fistula; C = incomplete fistula; D = enterocystoma; E = band; F = strawberry tumour; G = internal tumour; H = intussusception. (From de Bartolo H.M., van Meerden J.A., 1976, *Ann. Surg*; 183:30.)

The incidence of Meckel's diverticulum at operation has been reported as between 0.14–4%. The size may vary from 1–56 cm in length. Most of these diverticula occur within 90 cm of the ileo-caecal valve.

Heterotopic tissue was first reported to be of pancreatic type. Later gastric, duodenal, colonic, rectal and endometrial tissue have all been described, but the importance of the Meckel's diverticulum lies in the development of peptic ulceration in association with aberrant gastric mucosa. Bleeding is a common complication, especially under the age of ten years. Haemorrhage may be copious with dark red clots being passed per rectum. A clinical diagnosis may be confirmed by abdominal scanning following the injection of radioactive technetium which is taken up, and secreted, by the ectopic gastric mucosa.

In adults, the common complication is intestinal obstruction due to volvulus, or kinking around a band leading from the diverticulum to abdominal wall.

The third complication, also in the adult, is inflammation of the diverticulum leading to its perforation in about 50% of patients.

Meckel's diverticulum should always be excised, provided that the operation can be done with safety. A narrow diverticulum can be excised directly, but a broad-based diverticulum should be removed by resection of the segment of ileum bearing it.

Enterocutaneous fistulas

Enterocutaneous fistulas are a major, but fortunately infrequent, complication of abdominal surgery. Mortality is high and they pose considerable problems in management. Over 90% of enterocutaneous fistulas follow a surgical operation, frequently an emergency procedure or reoperation. Less commonly, a fistula may be the result of intestinal disease (e.g. Crohn's disease, tuberculosis or cancer), or related to a congenital abnormality e.g. persistence of the vitellointestinal duct. Occasionally, there may be contributing factors such as radiotherapy, cancer chemotherapy, or mesenteric vascular disease.

Clinical features

The fistula may declare itself by the discharge of small intestinal contents through the wound or a drainage hole on to the surface of the skin. Frequently a fistula presents as a postoperative 'abscess', a tender red mass near the operation wound. The contents of the abscess are allowed to discharge and the fistula is established. Occasionally leakage from an anastomosis takes place into the abdominal cavity and generalised peritonitis develops and then a fistula is formed and the patient's condition improves temporarily.

Diagnosis

The diagnosis is rarely in doubt. On occasion, discharging pus may closely resemble small intestinal content, but the diagnosis of a fistula can readily be confirmed by giving the patient a drink of methylene blue or congo red and then checking for the appearance of the dye on the abdominal skin.

In making a diagnosis, several additional facts have to be established:

1 *The level of the fistula:* fistulas may be classified according to their anatomical position; (a) high, viz. duodenal or gastric fistulas from which fluid losses may be more than 1 l per day; (b) intermediate, viz. jejunal and ileal, whose losses approximate to 100–500 ml per day; (c) low, or colonic, fistulas whose output is commonly less than 100 ml per day. The problems are greatest with a high fistula – excessive fluid loss leading to water and electrolyte deficiency, erosion of the skin by digestive enzymes, and the loss of nutrients leading to malnutrition.

2 It is necessary to determine if there is distal obstruction because in its presence a fistula will not close spontaneously. Barium meal and enema studies will be required. An x-ray fistulogram should also be carried out to demonstrate the presence of a fistula and show its anatomical position; to identify distal obstruction; to determine if the fistula is multiple, involving several loops of bowel, or associated with the biliary and urinary tract; and, finally, to show if the fistula leads directly from the skin to the small intestine (and is, therefore, more easily dealt with), or if it is tortuous with an intervening abscess cavity.

Management

Factors favouring a good prognosis are:

1 A distal (ileal) fistula
2 An output of less than 500 ml per day
3 A young patient
4 Late occurrence of the fistula, that is, more than 15 days after the initial operation
5 A healthy small bowel
6 Absence of associated biliary or urinary fistulas
7 No associated dehiscence of the abdominal wall.

The treatment of a fistula is initially medical and any surgical intervention should be carefully timed. Early surgical closure is usually associated with a high mortality and should be avoided.

The important aspects of the management of a fistula are:

1 Care of the skin
2 Fluid and electrolyte replacement
3 Maintenance of nutrition
4 Control of sepsis
5 Surgical treatment

Care of the skin

An attempt should be made to collect all the fluid discharging from a fistula: not only will complete collection provide accurate information on the volume and nature of the discharge, and so aid in fluid and electrolyte management, but also the skin itself will be protected. In many cases simple drainage of the fistula may suffice, but where large volumes of irritating fluid are discharging from a high fistula, great skill is required to achieve a leak-proof seal around the fistula. Materials, such as Stomahesive and Karaya gum powder along with drainage-bags, are important aids for the collection of the discharge and protection of the surrounding skin. As soon as a fistula has been diagnosed, the skin should be immediately protected because its rapid digestion will prevent these appliances from being used. With such methods of fistula care, sump drainage, at one time the corner-stone of fistula management, is no longer required. Indeed, the presence of a tube within the fistulous drainage tract may impair healing and frustrate spontaneous closure of the fistula.

Fluid and electrolyte replacement

Depletion of water and electrolytes, particularly potassium, is very common with a fistula. The volume of fistulous discharge should be carefully measured, and samples should be sent frequently for biochemical analysis, so that the electrolyte losses can be accurately calculated.

Maintenance of nutrition

Before the mid-1960s the mortality from enterocutaneous fistulas ranged from 30–60%, with high fistulas having the worst outlook. The cause of the high mortality was mainly malnutrition.

The nutritional requirements of a patient with a fistula have to be calculated on an individual basis, depending chiefly upon energy requirements and the extent of muscle catabolism. The nitrogen requirements of a patient can be estimated by measuring the output of nitrogen in the urine and fistula. An approximation may be obtained by measuring the urea content in the urine and converting to an equivalent value of nitrogen loss, using the formula:

Urine urea (g/24 h) $\times$ 20/60 + 2g [urine urea (mmol/24 h) $\times$ 0.028 + 2g].

Normal individuals excrete about 5–7 g of nitrogen a day but the loss increases rapidly in the presence of sepsis. As a rule a patient should receive synthetic amino acids containing the equivalent of the nitrogen lost from the body, plus an additional 2–3 g. The calculation of a patient's energy requirements is difficult: one approach is to give 150–200 kcal (0.63–0.84 MJ) for every gram of nitrogen infused. There is a tendency to over-estimate a patient's requirements, and in general terms even the most septic patient will require little more than 2000 kcal, (8.4 MJ) per day.

Unless the patient's requirements are met, weight loss may be as high as 1.5 kg per day. Acute weight loss, amounting to 30% or more of body weight in 30 days, is usually fatal. In the past mortality was high in those who did not receive nutritional support (*see also* Chapter 51).

Although the need for increased energy and nitrogen intake has long been appreciated, the major difficulty has been in its provision. Increasing the oral intake merely augments the losses from a high fistula. The introduction of intravenous feeding led, however, to a marked reduction in mortality, because not only was the patient's state of nutrition maintained, but also volume of the discharge through the fistula diminished, often with its spontaneous closure. In addition, wound healing, immunological competence and resistance to infection are all enhanced.

Unfortunately, prolonged intravenous nutrition has its own problems – septicaemia arising from the infected tip of the feeding catheter and thrombophlebitis due to infection and to the irritating nature of the feeding solutions.

A recent advance has been the provision of protein and calories in an elemental liquid diet which contains balanced mixtures of essential and non-essential amino-acids, calories and minerals. Given by mouth or by feeding jejunostomy, they can meet most nutritional requirements with minimal need for digestion and hardly any residue. Compared to intravenous nutrition, elemental diets have the advantage of simplicity, low cost and minimal complications apart from diarrhoea, occasionally, because of their hyperosmotic nature.

Control of sepsis

The benefits of intravenous nutrition cannot overcome the devastating effects of uncontrolled sepsis, which is now the major factor in determining mortality. Two-thirds of patients with a fistula have serious sepsis, e.g. intra-abdominal abscess, septicaemia, wound-infection, cellulitis, etc. In one recent series, 70% of patients with a fistula and peritonitis died, while all those free of sepsis survived. The key to successful control of sepsis is careful selection of the most appropriate antibiotic, especially if there is cholangitis, or septi-caemia, and especially if an operation is imminent. However, if there is evidence that there is an intra-abdominal abscess, operation to drain pus should not be delayed.

Surgical treatment

With nutritional support, many enterocutaneous fistulas will close spontaneously. However, this does not mean that there is no place for direct aggressive surgery.

The indications for surgery are:

Drainage of abscess. Abscesses may prevent a fistula from closing by exerting pressure upon the intestine and have a marked deleterious effect upon the patient's nutrition. Some abscesses, e.g. subphrenic and pelvic, can be approached by an extraperitoneal route; however, an intra-abdominal abscess, associated with intestinal fistula, requires full abdominal exploration, for these abscesses are often multiple and are closely associated with viscera which could easily be damaged unless clearly exposed during access.

Defunctioning of diseased bowel. This type of surgery is particularly effective for a fistula complicating Crohn's disease, diverticulitis or radiation enteritis. An ileostomy or colostomy is established above the fistula. Alternatively the affected bowel is excised and, if possible, the bowel above is brought to the surface as an enterostomy, and the distal bowel may be closed or, alternatively, brought on to the abdominal wall as a mucous fistula. This approach is particularly appropriate where the fistula is the result of complete disruption of an anastomosis, and is applicable to low level fistulas.

Creation of an enterostomy. In the management of a prolonged chronic fistula, the nutrition of the patient can be greatly improved by establishing an entero-stomy, to avoid the problems of prolonged intravenous nutrition and the unpleasantness of a nasogastric tube. With at least 100 cm of jejunum or 150 cm of ileum, the patient can be nourished with an elemental diet, delivered by a fine tube jejunostomy. With a low level fistula, a simple gastrostomy can be established, initially for gastric drainage and, later, for the administration of an elemental diet and fluid and electrolytes. With a high fistula, a catheter can be inserted into the jejunum, below the fistula, not only for continuous infusion of the elemental diet, but also for the reinfusion of fistulous contents.

Definitive operation. There are three important reasons for a fistula not closing spontaneously:

1　Distal obstruction
2　A small fistula has leaked into a larger abscess cavity and then drained through a small cutaneous opening (under these circumstances, adequate drainage of the abscess may lead to spontaneous closure)
3　Fistulous opening of diseased bowel, e.g. Crohn's disease or carcinoma.

Surgical intervention is necessary, but should be delayed until the patient is well nourished, sepsis has been controlled, and the patient thoroughly investigated. The diseased segment of bowel is excised and continuity restored by an end-to-end anastomosis of healthy intestine.

Vascular disease

Anatomy

Arteries

1　The coeliac axis supplies only a short segment of the small intestine and, since it possesses a good collateral circulation, the results of its occlusion are trivial, rarely declaring themselves clinically.

2 The rest of the small intestine is supplied by the superior mesenteric artery, which has a poorer collateral circulation; its occlusion can readily produce serious, and indeed fatal, results.

Veins

The portal circulation begins in the mucosa of the small intestine. The emerging veins coalesce to form arcades, and subsequently form the superior mesenteric vein which drains the entire small intestine and the right half of the colon into the liver. This vessel lies anterior to the third part of the duodenum and joins with the splenic vein and inferior mesenteric vein to become the portal vein.

Pathology

Although *atheroma* may affect any small intestinal artery, the usual site is the superior mesenteric artery near its origin. Narrowing of a vessel may be gradual and partial but, with additional thrombosis, the occlusion can become acute and complete, especially when the clot propagates distally. A gradual occlusion of the superior mesenteric artery is relatively common in those over 55 years, but, if there is sufficient time for the development of a collateral circulation, the effects of the occlusion do not present clinically.

The superior mesenteric artery can also be obstructed by an *embolus*, originating from a cardiac mural thrombus, secondary to myocardial infarction, or associated with cardiac arrhythmias. The size of the embolus determines the site of the obstruction, which is often well beyond the origin of the artery, in one of its distal branches; under these circumstances the length of infarcted bowel is much less than with thrombosis, superimposed on an atheromatous obstruction at the origin of the superior mesenteric artery.

Occlusion of the *mesenteric veins* is not recognised frequently. It is difficult to say whether occlusion of the mesenteric veins is as frequent as that of the arteries, because at laparotomy both arteries and veins contain thrombus: primary occlusion of the one leads inevitably to a secondary formation of clot in the other. Mesenteric venous thrombosis may be associated with infection of the viscera, slowing of the portal venous flow, or blood dyscrasias with increased coagulability of the blood. In some cases at operation the mesenteric veins are seen to contain clots of various ages, suggesting that thrombosis occurs intermittently.

As a result of mesenteric vascular occlusion, arterial or venous, the affected portion of bowel goes into intense spasm. The mucosa becomes oedematous, then haemorrhagic, and the mucosal cells die. Later the more resilient muscular layers succumb to the effects of anoxia, and soon the entire thickness of the wall of the gut becomes gangrenous. In contrast, with partial occlusion, these changes may be limited to the mucosa only, which becomes ulcerated. With subsequent healing by fibrosis, the bowel is narrowed by the formation of strictures.

With an acute vascular occlusion the bowel becomes paralysed. The lumen is filled with blood-stained fluid, and at the same time there is a blood-stained exudate into the peritoneal cavity. The anoxic intestinal wall becomes permeable to the intestinal bacteria proliferating in the strangulated loops of bowel. Perforations and spreading bacterial peritonitis are terminal events. The anoxia of the bowel is aggravated by hypovolaemia and circulatory collapse caused by the loss of fluid and blood into the intestinal lumen. Haemoconcentration due to fluid loss further impairs mesenteric flow. Finally, the successful and rapid restoration of mesenteric circulation, following successful surgery to the superior mesenteric artery, may create further serious problems. The damaged blood vessels are dilated and permeable and, therefore, blood flowing into these vessels may leak into the intestinal lumen. Moreover, the ischaemic bowel produces vasoactive kinins which, with the restoration of blood-flow, become dispersed throughout the body to produce a widespread vasodilatation which will further aggravate the hypovolaemic shock.

Acute occlusion of the superior mesenteric artery

Aetiology. Sudden occlusion of the superior mesenteric artery is more often due to embolus.

Acute thrombosis alone rarely occurs in healthy vessels, but more usually develops on an atheromatous patch. The extent of the resulting intestinal infarction will be largely dependent upon the presence of a collateral circulation.

Clinical features. Typically a middle-aged or elderly patient, with a history of either previous coronary artery disease or cardiac arrhythmia, is suddenly afflicted by severe, diffuse abdominal pain. There may have been previous cramping abdominal pain. Uncommonly the patient may vomit blood or pass a blood-stained stool.

On examination the striking finding is that of extensive abdominal guarding, more than one would expect from the extent of the pain of which the patient complains. Guarding is never usually so marked as to be termed 'boardlike'. Bowel sounds may be hyperactive, but more usually the abdomen is silent.

Abdominal x-rays may show several dilated loops of bowel; in many cases, however, the x-rays are quite unhelpful, but the clinician should not be deterred from making the diagnosis. An important feature of the disease is a white-count which rapidly rises to between 15000–20000 cells/dl, highly suggestive of intestinal strangulation.

Deterioration in the patient's condition is usually quite rapid: abdominal tenderness becomes widespread, the pulse becomes rapid and thready and blood-pressure falls. Arteriography is not helpful because in more than half of the patients above the age of 55, occlusion of the superior mesenteric artery is present without symptoms.

Treatment. Laparotomy is urgent and only a short time should be set aside for resuscitation, which is required for the urgent correction of blood and fluid deficits. Quite large volumes of fluid may have to be infused. At operation, the extent of the intestinal infarction is identified and viable bowel is defined. The mesentery should be carefully palpated for vessel pulsation.

All non-viable bowel should be resected. There is clearly little problem where only one of the peripheral mesenteric vessels has been occluded and a relatively short length of segment is ischaemic. However, if the main vessel has been occluded at its origin, the entire small intestine, distal to the ligament of Treitz, and the right half of the colon will have to be resected. The immediate and late postoperative problems can be immense.

If the ischaemia of the intestine is thought to be reversible, and particularly if an embolus is considered to be the cause, relief of the vascular occlusion should be attempted. It is difficult to display the origin of the superior mesenteric artery, because it lies within a large plexus of veins around the neck of the pancreas and it is usually safer to expose the ileocolic artery at a distal site where it can accommodate a size 4F Fogarty embolectomy catheter. The common iliac arteries should be occluded by soft clamps to prevent any thrombus being dislodged into the lower limbs. The Fogarty catheter is then passed up the ileocolic artery which has been opened between tapes, to the origin of the superior mesenteric artery. It is important to establish that the catheter goes right into the aorta. The clot is then withdrawn. An attempt should be made to milk the clot out of the other branches into the major artery, which is then flushed from the aorta. Success is indicated by an obvious improvement in the colour of the bowel and a return of pulsation of the mesenteric vessels. If the clot has been dislodged into the aorta and is arrested in the common iliac arteries, it should be removed through a small arteriotomy.

Occasionally, if this technique fails, the origin of the superior mesenteric artery will have to be approached and an endarterectomy performed, with or without a patch graft. However, this is a difficult procedure and an alternative would be to perform a side-to-side anastomosis between the ileocolic artery and the right common iliac artery using a 1.5 cm arteriotomy. Unfortunately, the rate of success for these attempts at direct restoration of circulation of the ischaemic bowel is very low.

Mesenteric venous occlusion

Aetiology. The superior mesenteric vein is more frequently involved than the inferior mesenteric one. The venous thrombosis may be idiopathic, but more often is related to such predisposing factors as (a) infection secondary to intra-abdominal sepsis, e.g. appendicitis, diverticulitis, (b) increased coagulability of the blood, e.g. polycythaemia, and (c) slowing of the mesenteric flow, e.g. hepatic cirrhosis or occlusion of the mesenteric vein by extrinsic tumour. The venous thrombosis may either be acute or chronic in onset and is often extremely difficult to recognise.

Clinical features. The symptoms are usually very similar to those of occlusion of the superior mesenteric artery – sudden onset of severe abdominal pain, vomiting and circulatory collapse associated with bloody diarrhoea. Abdominal tenderness, guarding, and a marked leucocytosis are very often present. Radiology is unhelpful.

At operation it may be difficult to distinguish between mesenteric venous and arterial occlusion. With venous occlusion mesenteric arteries may be pulsating up to the intestinal wall and usually only short segments of the intestine are involved, compared to the much longer infarction with arterial occlusion.

Treatment. With obvious gangrene of the bowel, the affected segment must be resected and continuity of the intestinal tract re-established by end-to-end anastomosis. Unfortunately, breakdown of the anastomosis is common. If the thrombosis seems to extend beyond the limits of the infarction, the resection should include adjacent normal bowel and mesentery, until all thrombosed vessels are encompassed.

Anticoagulants must be given. Heparin should be delivered by intravenous infusion, and a transfer to oral anticoagulation should not be made until the intestinal tract returns to normal. Unfortunately, anticoagulants can cause problems, such as haemorrhage into the damaged bowel. Anticoagulants should be continued for some time, e.g. 6 months, because mesenteric venous thrombosis has a great tendency to recur.

Chronic intestinal ischaemia (intestinal angina)

With the analogy that pain may be experienced when the heart and calf muscles try to work in the presence of an impaired blood supply, the concept of ischaemic symptoms, arising from intestine functioning despite occlusion of a blocked mesenteric artery, has great appeal. Unfortunately, the symptoms, consisting of post-prandial abdominal pain, are imprecise. The patient may cease to eat because of the severity of the pain, and ultimately becomes markedly emaciated. There may also be diarrhoea and steatorrhea.

Formerly, it was thought that diagnosis could be confirmed by selective visceral angiography, but, unfortunately, stenosis or complete blockage of one, two, or even all three main visceral vessels can be observed in between one-third to one-half of apparently normal patients above the age of 45. The weight-loss of these patients is almost certainly the result of diminished food intake due to pain, rather than any impairment of absorption of nutrients by the hypoxic bowel. It is, therefore, very difficult to estimate the true incidence of chronic intestinal ischaemia. There may, indeed, be only a few patients whose abdominal symptoms can be directly attributed to chronic ischaemia, and in them a few may have to be operated upon because of the severity of the symptoms.

Treatment. The selection of patients for operation is difficult. First, it is necessary to eliminate the commoner causes of chronic abdominal pain. Secondly, the origins of the visceral arteries must be clearly displayed by biplane free and selective aortography.

Two types of operative procedures have been described. First, a direct approach may be made to relieve the obstruction at the origin of the superior mesenteric artery or, secondly, a bypass can be established. Because of the difficulties of a direct approach, the bypass procedure is being carried out more often. The splenic artery can be used, provided that there is no occlusion of the coeliac axis. Alternatively, a dacron graft or a graft of autogenous vein can be inserted between the aorta and the superior mesenteric artery distal to the obstruction. Another procedure is a side-to-side anastomosis between the superior mesenteric artery and the aorta.

Unfortunately, however, the number of patients who show a marked improvement following these operations is small. Careful selection for operation is vital.

Small intestine and severe obesity

Severe obesity is a disabling condition which shortens life. In this context the term 'morbid obesity' is used to describe the condition of an individual who is more than twice, or in excess of 100 lbs above, his or her ideal weight for age, height and sex, and who has maintained this level for 5 years, despite efforts to bring about effective and sustained reduction of weight to acceptable levels.

Medical treatment for obesity – dieting, psychiatric treatment, and anorectic drugs – has a poor record for success. Probably less than 1% of patients have a sustained weight-loss for a year or more. Because of this failure in long-term management, many patients turn to surgery.

The earliest operation, *jejunocolostomy*, was soon abandoned because of intolerable side-effects. Extensive *jejunal ileal bypass* was the operation widely used for morbid obesity; other methods are described below. The small intestine is shortened by anastomosing the proximal 36 cm of jejunum to terminal ileum and by joining the remaining blind jejunal loop to colon (Fig 10.6). The length of the small intestine remaining in continuity is critical – if too much remains, weight-loss is insufficient, and, if too little, diarrhoea and weight-loss are excessive. The ideal length in continuity lies between 45–50 cm.

To achieve a high rate of success, patients for operation should be carefully selected from the large group of obese patients who invariably present themselves to centres undertaking this form of surgery. The following criteria should be satisfied:

1 Obesity of twice, or 100 lbs over ideal weight
2 Failure of dietary efforts
3 Absence of correctable endocrine abnormality
4 Absence of unrelated disease which would increase the operative risk
5 The presence of certain complications, e.g. hyperlipidaemia, maturity-onset diabetes, hypertension
6 Assurance of the patient's cooperation in the postoperative evaluation and management.

Usually less than 10% of patients referred are submitted for preoperative evaluation, and, of these, almost a half will ultimately refuse operation.

The beneficial effects are said to include reduction in blood-pressure, improvement in respiratory function, reduction in serum lipids, improvement in glucose tolerance, along with psychiatric recovery. The results of a controlled trial in Denmark suggest that those patients who had the operation had significantly greater weight-loss and a much improved quality of life, compared to the control group without operation.

On the debit side, however, are several complications:

1 Early postoperative problems, e.g. wound and respiratory infections, deep-vein thrombosis and pulmonary embolism are found in 5%.
2 Diarrhoea, which always follows the operation and diminishes in severity with time, can, in a substantial proportion of patients, be severe, consisting of 5–15 loose bowel motions per day a year after operation.
3 Severe electrolyte disturbances are common in

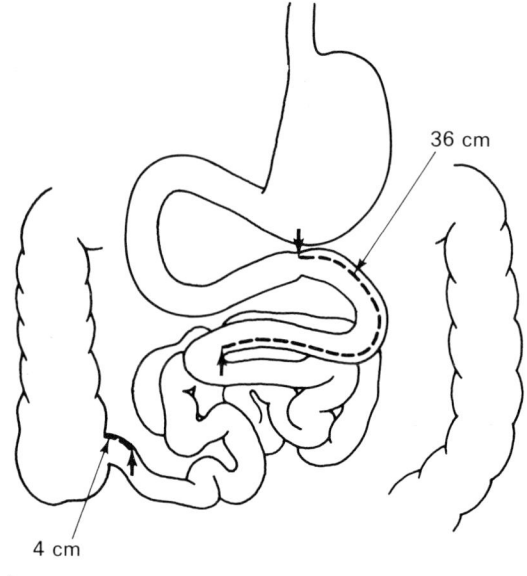

36 cm

4 cm

(a)

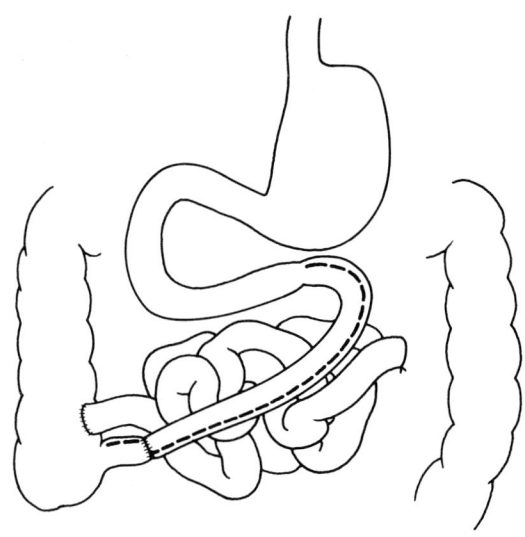

(b)

Fig 10.6 (a) The proximal jejunum is divided 36 cm from ligament of Treitz and ileum divided 4 cm from ileocaecal valve. (b) Restoration of intestinal continuity. (From Joffe S.N., Oct. 1979, *Hosp. Update*; p.869.)

the immediate postoperative period, including hypokalaemia, hypocalcaemia, and hypomagnesaemia.

4   Increased tendency to formation of gallstones and renal oxalate stones.

5   Abdominal bloating and pseudo-obstruction.

6   Arthritic symptoms due to circulating immune factors.

7   Liver complications are the most serious. Although most obese patients have fatty infiltration of the liver and show transient hepatic damage immediately after operation, in a few patients gross deterioration in liver function may lead to liver-failure and death. Alternatively, there may be a more indolent picture of portal fibrosis developing into micronodular cirrhosis.

The present opinion of most surgeons in this field is that jejuno-ileal bypass is no longer justified.

Other procedures

1   **Dental splintage** may produce a significant weight reduction, but the long-term results are unsatisfactory, since abnormal eating habits are resumed after dewiring.

2   **Operations on the stomach** aimed at reducing the size of the gastric pouch were introduced because of dissatisfaction with jejuno-ileal bypass, especially metabolic problems. Weight loss is achieved by reducing the patient's capacity to eat. The mortality of these operations is probably similar to that of jejuno-ileal bypass and is usually related to anastomotic leakage with peritonitis. Later complications include vomiting, rapid emptying of the gastric pouch, and stomal ulcer.

Careful selection of patients is important. After some initial success, many patients cease to lose weight. A variety of gastric operations have been described – bypass or partitioning – but time is required to assess which will produce the best results.

The surgical treatment of obesity should at present be confined to centres where there is a definite interest in the problem, and where there is the skill, time and resources to be fully committed to the effort and cost of this treatment.

Small intestinal insufficiency
('Short gut syndrome')

Total loss of the entire small intestine, by disease or surgical resection or both, is incompatible with survival. However, many patients not only have survived extensive resection, but have also enjoyed apparent good health without any measurable loss in intestinal function. There is considerable variation in the severity of the symptoms from patient to patient, related probably to individual capacity for functional adaptation and compensatory hypertrophy. The exact length of small intestine that is required for survival is unknown, but loss of more than 75% of small bowel causes rapid intestinal transit, leading to intractable diarrhoea and malabsorption. However, 30–60 cm seem to be necessary to maintain life, and 90–120 cm probably minimal for reasonable health.

Causes

The major reasons for massive intestinal resection include extensive internal strangulation, mesenteric vascular occlusion and inflammatory bowel disease. With those last two diseases, part, or all, of the colon may have to be resected aggravating the malabsorption, particularly of water and electrolytes. Loss of the ileocaecal valve seems to be important, because where it has been preserved, it may contribute considerably to adaptation by slowing transit of the small intestinal content into the caecum.

Pathophysiology

The immediate reasons responsible for the 'short bowel' syndrome are complex and includes such features as reduction in absorptive surface area, increased transit of luminal contents over remaining mucosa, and possibly deficiencies in digestion. There is some evidence that loss of the proximal small intestine is better tolerated than that of the ileum, partly because the transit time in the ileum is slower, (allowing more time for absorption) and partly because, from animal studies, the *distal* intestine is more capable of compensatory hypertrophy and functional adaptation after *proximal* resection than the converse.

Another cause for the diarrhoea is gastric hypersecretion induced by massive intestinal resection. Where this is a factor the diarrhoea can be controlled by vagotomy and drainage, or by oral cimetidine.

Copious watery diarrhoea may be caused also by the cathartic action on the colon of excessive quantities of bile acids, normally absorbed in the terminal ileum. Diarrhoea may also be due to excessive amounts of fatty acids entering the colon – fatty diarrhoea.

After massive resection, the remaining gut shows changes of adaptation – lengthening of the villi, thickening of the intestinal wall, dilatation and slowing of transit. Therefore, there is always a good chance of spontaneous recovery and it is necessary in the early days and weeks after the operation for careful and expert attention to be paid, particularly to nutrition, to maintain normal body functions, to replenish the depleted stores especially the negative nitrogen balance, and to supply the nutrients necessary for functional adaptation.

Clinical features

The deficiencies which may develop rapidly after massive intestinal resection are varied. Due to excessive losses of water and electrolytes in the stool, hypokalaemia, hypocalcaemia and hypomagnesaemia are particularly common. Fat absorption may also be greatly impaired with 80–90% of the ingested fat appearing in the stool, compared to less than 10% in healthy subjects. In contrast carbohydrate and amino-acid absorption are not usually impaired to a serious extent.

Deficiencies of vitamins A, B and C, iron and folic acid have all been recorded. The net result of the excessive diarrhoea and malabsorption is weight-loss, muscle wasting, osteoporosis, weakness and lassitude.

Treatment

The treatment of massive small bowel resection falls into two stages: (a) *early* – during the adaptative stage and (b) *later* long-term management.

Early phase

During the period of adaptation, the bowel may be unable to tolerate a conventional diet, even fluids. The patient's condition must be maintained by correcting fluid and electrolyte deficiencies. In this context it is most important that the diarrhoeal losses are carefully measured and samples sent for biochemical analysis, in order to determine and correct the exact electrolyte losses.

The main difficulty is maintenance of adequate nutrition. The survival rate has been greatly improved by intravenous feeding, the initial treatment of choice. Indeed, intravenous nutrition may be required in a few patients on a permanent basis. Elemental diets have also been introduced in the treatment of the short bowel syndrome and, compared to intravenous nutrition, have the advantage of fewer complications, easier management of vitamin and mineral deficiencies and the early introduction of food to the gastrointestinal lumen which may very well stimulate some of the adaptive changes. Cimetidine should be given to reduce gastric hypersecretion.

Later treatment

Most patients can be managed medically with a low-fat, non-residue diet with, if necessary, added medium-chain triglycerides. Cholestyramine may be used to bind bile salts. Diarrhoea can be treated successfully in most patients with such drugs as codeine phosphate or diphenoxylate (Lomotil).

Anaemia, usually due to iron-deficiency, but occasionally to lack of folate or vitamin B_{12}, will require appropriate treatment.

In the long-term there is a risk of osteomalacia and to make an accurate diagnosis bone biopsy may be required. Treatment is by parenteral vitamin D or 1-α-hydroxy vitamin D.

A few patients show little or no improvement with such treatment. Some good results have been achieved surgically by reversing a segment of small bowel in order to slow transit time. The length of small bowel seems to be critical – too little and there is no benefit; too much and the intestine may be obstructed. Usually a segment of between 7.5 and 14 cm is reversed. The most distal part of the remaining small bowel should be used in order to minimise the risk of developing a blind loop syndrome. Care must be taken during reversal to avoid twisting and occlusion of the vascular supply to the reversed segment.

Fortunately, the prognosis after small intestinal resection is much better than expected and only rarely are surgical procedures required, or is it necessary to put the patient on prolonged intravenous nutrition.

Duodenal ileus

('Wilkie syndrome')

Obstruction and dilatation of the duodenum by extrinsic compression by the superior mesenteric artery was originally described by Rotikansky in 1849 and studied in greater detail by Wilkie, who, in 1920, gave a detailed and accurate account of its pathophysiology. The latter described the characteristic symptoms of postprandial epigastric pain, eructations and fullness, frequently associated with vomiting. Symptoms were often of intermittent nature and Wilkie noted that the patient frequently obtained partial or complete relief in the knee-chest position or in a recumbent position on the left side.

Diagnosis is usually made on x-ray showing dilatation of the proximal duodenum as far as the mid-line, with an abrupt obstruction of the third part as it crosses the vertebra.

At operation there may be no significant findings. On the other hand, there may be an obvious compression of the third part of the duodenum by the superior mesenteric artery. Careful dissection often shows, underlying the vascular trunk, a fibrous band which itself may be producing the compression.

Nevertheless, considerable doubt exists if this syndrome forms a clinical entity. Medical treatment is rarely successful and surgical treatment by duodenojejunostomy, which would be thought to be effective in relieving all of the mechanical symptoms, produces relief only in a few patients and many others do not show any improvement. Severe vomiting is a sign of a poor prognosis. Gastrojejunostomy should not be performed because of the risk of developing a stomal ulcer.

In the majority of patients diagnosed as having duodenal ileus, relief by operation is usually only partial and transient.

Pneumatosis cystoides intestinalis

This rare condition is characterised by multiple gas-filled cysts in the wall and mesentery of the gastro-intestinal tract. The condition is seen at all ages, but occurs most commonly in middle-age. The cysts may be subserous or submucous, occurring most frequently in the jejunum, followed by the ileo-caecal region and colon.

In 85% of cases the gas cysts are associated with other lesions of the gastrointestinal tract, the most common being pyloric stenosis due to peptic ulcer, and intestinal obstruction. The gas is composed mainly of nitrogen. Careful inspection of the mucous lining of the affected bowel usually fails to show any break in the mucous membrane that would have permitted gas to permeate from the lumen into the tissues.

Symptoms are non-specific and are more usually related to the underlying disease.

Diagnosis may be made unexpectedly at operation or, occasionally, on a plain or contrast x-ray examination of the abdomen or intestine. Radiolucent areas in clusters and following the contour of the bowel are diagnostic.

No treatment is required unless one of the complications supervenes, e.g. rectal bleeding, cyst-induced volvulus or tension pneumoperitoneum.

Further reading

Alexander-Williams J., Irving M. (1982). *Intestinal Fistulas*. Boston, London, Bristol: PSG Wright.

Alpers D.H. (1983). Surgical therapy for obesity. *New Engl. J. Med*; **308:**1026–7.

Berardi R.S. (1980). Anomalies of intestinal fixation and position in the adult. *Surg. Gynecol. Obstet*; **151:**561–70.

Ellis H. (1981). Mechanical intestinal obstruction. *Brit. J. Surg*; **283:** 1203–4.

Golladay E.S., Byrne W.J. (1981). Intestinal pseudo obstruction. *Surg. Gynecol. Obstet*; **153:** 257–73.

Herbsman H., Westein L., Rosen Y. *et al.* (1980). Tumours of the small intestine. *Curr. Probl. Surg*; 121–82.

Hocking M. (1981). Duplications of the alimentary tract. *Brit. J. Surg*; **68:**92–6.

Jamieson W.G., Marchuck S., Rowsom J., Duranol D. (1982). The early diagonosis of massive acute intestinal ischaemia. *Brit. J. Surg*; **69** (Suppl): S52–S53.

Kerremans R.P., Lerut J., Penninckx F.M. (1979). Primary malignant duodenal tumors. *Ann. Surg*; **190:**179–82.

Khojasteh A., Haghshenass M., Haghighi P. (1983). Immunoproliferative small intestinal disease. *New Engl. J. Med*; **308**:1401–7.

Kinsella T.J., Bloomer W.D. (1980). Tolerance of the intestine to radiation therapy. *Surg. Gynecol. Obstet*; **151**:273–84.

Kirsner J.B., Shorter R.G. (1982). Recent developments in 'non-specific' inflammatory bowel disease. *New Engl. J. Med*.; **306**:775–85; 837–48.

Kyle J. (1982). Inflammatory bowel disease – surgery for Crohn's disease. *Brit. J. Hosp. Med*; **27**:482–7.

Marston A. (1977). *Intestinal Ischaemia*. London: Edward Arnold.

Martin J.K., Moertel C.G., Adson M.A., Schutt A.J. (1983). Surgical treatment of functioning metastatic carcinoid tumors. *Arch. Surg*; **118**:537–42.

Progress Symposium – Alimentary Tract Fistulas (1983). *World J. Surg*; **7**:445–501.

Surgical Treatment of Morbid Obesity. (1981). *World J. Surg*.; **Vol. 5.**

Williams R.S. (1981). Management of Meckel's diverticulum. *Brit. J. Surg*; **68**:477–80.

Williamson R.C.N., Welch C.E., Malt R.A. (1983). Adenocarcinoma and lymphoma of the small intestine. *Ann. Surg*; **197**:172–8.

11

Appendix

HAROLD ELLIS

Acute appendicitis

Acute appendicitis is the commonest cause of the 'acute surgical abdomen' in this country and accounts for some 40% of all operations carried out as emergencies in this situation. Since the disease is not notifiable, its exact incidence is not known, but it is estimated that some 125,000 patients are submitted to surgery for acute appendicitis each year. Approximately 500 deaths are notified annually as being due to appendicitis in England and Wales. It is interesting, in passing, to note that the death rate for acute appendicitis in the first half of the 20th century fluctuated between 2500 and 3000 cases, but there has been a progressive decline in the death rate since 1945. Appendicitis can occur at any age, but is rare before 5 and uncommon in the elderly. The disease has a world-wide distribution but its incidence does appear to be associated with a Western diet, although the reason for this remains a subject for debate. Although extremely common in Northern Europe, North America, Australia and among white South Africans, it is rare in most of Asia, Central Africa and among the Eskimos. When people from these areas migrate to the Western world or change to its diet, appendicitis becomes prevelant, suggesting that the distribution of this disease is environmentally rather than genetically determined. However, there is a familial predisposition in children with appendicitis (Andersson *et al.*, 1979).

Surgical anatomy

The appendix arises from the posteromedial aspect of the caecum approximately 2.5 cm distal to the ileocaecal valve. Both its size and position are extremely variable. Its length ranges from 1 to 25 cm and it may truly be said to be the only organ in the body without any constant anatomy. Usually the appendix lies in the retrocaecal position (75% of cases). If very long, it may extend behind the ascending colon with its distal portion lying extraperitoneally against the right kidney. In about 20% of cases the appendix lies in the subcaecal position or hangs down into the pelvis. Occasionally it passes in front or behind the terminal caecum and may even extend right across into the left iliac fossa, while rarely it lies in front of the caecum or in the right paracolic gutter. Dextrorotation of the heart may be associated with reversal of all the intra-abdominal organs and in such cases the caecum and appendix are situated on the left side of the abdomen. Most experienced surgeons will have seen a true left-sided appendicitis in such circumstances.

The mesentery of the appendix carries the appendicular branch of the ileocolic artery. This represents the entire arterial supply of the organ and runs first in the edge of the appendix mesentery and then along the wall of the appendix. Thrombosis of the terminal branches of this artery in acute appendicitis inevitably results in gangrene and subsequent perforation. This is in contrast to acute cholecystitis, where the rich collateral blood supply of the gallbladder, arising from the liver bed, accounts for the comparative rarity of gangrene in acute cholecystitis.

Structure

The layers of the appendix are the same as those of the rest of the intestine – serous, muscular, submucous and mucous. The serosal coat is complete except for the line of mesenteric attachment. The longitudinal muscle fibres form a thick, fairly uniform layer except at the base of the appendix where the longitudinal muscle becomes thickened at three points around its circumference which become continuous with the taenia coli of the colon. Indeed, in searching for a 'difficult' appendix, tracing a couple of taenia coli along the caecum until they meet is one well-known technique of identifying the appendix base. The circular inner muscle layer is thicker than the longitudinal coat and this, together with a thick submucous layer which contains numerous masses of lymphoid tissue that bulge into the appendix lumen account for the small size and irregular shape of its lumen. The mucous membrane is lined with a columnar epithelium with scattered goblet cells.

Pathology

Acute appendicitis is not associated with any specific bacterial, viral or protozoal invader, although claims in support of each of these have been made. The bacteriology of the inflamed organ is that of the normal bowel flora, suggesting secondary invasion of damaged tissues from the gut lumen.

The examination of a series of fresh specimens of acute appendicitis removed at operation will soon show that these fall into two groups. The first demonstrate a 'catarrhal' inflammation of the whole organ while the second, commoner, group demonstrate an obstruction of the appendix beyond which there is acute inflammation, distension with pus and, in later cases, progression to gangrene and later perforation.

Catarrhal appendicitis is initially a mucosal and submucosal inflammation. In early cases the external appearance of the appendix may be quite normal or may merely show hyperaemia. However, on slitting open the appendix, the mucosa is inflamed and may even demonstrate patchy necrosis. In more advanced cases, the whole organ may be inflamed and its serosa covered with fibrinous exudate. The probable aetiology of this condition is a bacterial invasion of the lymphoid tissue in the appendix wall and some cases are probably localised manifestations of a generalised enteritis. Because the lumen of the appendix is not obstructed, these cases rarely progress to gangrene and, indeed, in many instances the acute inflammatory attack will resolve spontaneously. In other cases, swelling of the lymphoid tissue in the appendix wall may lead to obstruction of the lumen and the condition may then proceed to obstructive appendicitis and gangrene. Repeated episodes of catarrhal appendicitis may result in adhesion formation and kinking of the appendix leading to a final episode of acute obstructive appendicitis. It is interesting that an episode of gangrenous appendicitis may well have been preceded by several milder resolving attacks.

Obstructive appendicitis may be due to a large number of possible causes. We have already noted that there may be inflammatory swelling of the lymphoid tissue in the appendix wall which may occlude the lumen. Kinks and adhesions may angulate the organ upon itself and these may result either from congenital bands or from previous episodes of inflammation. One or more faecoliths are commonly found within the appendix lumen in the normal organ, but it is a common finding (in about two-thirds of all gangrenous appendices) to discover a faecolith firmly impacted at the junction between the uninflamed proximal and gangrenous distal part of the appendix. Other foreign bodies such as food debris, worms and even a gallstone have been found to obstruct the appendix lumen. Rarely a carcinoma of the base of caecum has occluded the appendix which has then become acutely inflamed and perhaps the rarest cause of obstructive appendicitis is the appendix becoming strangulated within a hernial sac. Indeed, Sir Zachary Cope (1965) relates that the very first occasion on which an inflamed appendix was removed from a living patient was in 1736 when Claudius Amyand, of St George's Hospital, removed an appendix perforated by a pin encrusted with stone from a sinus in a right scrotal hernia in a boy of 11 years. The base of the appendix was ligated, the inflamed organ removed and recovery followed.

The relationship between obstruction of the appendix and gangrenous appendicitis was demonstrated by Wilkie (1914) who showed that death from acute appendicitis followed 24 h after ligation of the appendix in the rabbit. Wangensteen and his colleagues (Wangensteen and Bowers, 1937; Burge *et al.*, 1940) documented that combined obstruction and bacterial infection produces acute appendicitis, whereas if the appendix is washed free of faecal material and then ligated, a mucocele results as the goblet cells in the appendix mucosa continue to secrete mucus in to the bacteria-free lumen.

When the appendix becomes obstructed, the process of events is accumulation of normal mucus secretion, proliferation of contained bacteria, pressure atrophy of the mucosa which allows access into the deeper tissue planes of bacteria, inflammation of the walls of the organ with vessel thrombosis, leading to gangrene and then perforation of the necrotic appendix wall. On other occasions, bacterial invasion occurs through pressure erosion of the contained faecolith, which may actually discharge into the peritoneal cavity through the perforation.

The microscopic appearances in experimental studies of acute appendicitis in laboratory animals (Burge *et al.*, 1940) document the early minimal changes which progress to purulent inflammation, perforation and gangrene. Examination of the early case of acute appendicitis, histologically, demonstrates small collections of pus cells in the lumen with patchy mucosal desquamation and scattered polymorph leucocytes in the lamina propria, sometimes collected together in the form of crypt abscesses. Later, small submucosal abscesses, oedema and congestion are more obvious with polymorph infiltration of the muscle coats and overlying serosa. Later manifestations are necrosis, gangrene and the presence of thrombi in the intramural vessels (Morson and Dawson, 1972).

The appendix faecolith

Faecal material is commonly present in both the normal and the inflamed appendix. This should be differentiated from the true faecolith which is ovoid, usually 1 to 2 cm in length, and faecal coloured. Unlike ordinary faeces, the true faecolith shows a well ordered lamination in section. It is usually compressible between the fingers, but may occasionally form a hard 'appendix stone'. Shaw (1965), in an exhaustive study, showed that the great majority of appendix faecoliths are radio-opaque and prefers the term *appendix calculus*. In 10% of cases of acute appendicitis the stones contain sufficient calcium to show on a plain x-ray of the abdomen. They may be multiple and faceted. Appendix stones are not unlike gallstones on plain x-ray and to exclude the possibility of gallstones in a low-lying gallbladder, a cholecystogram may be needed. Ureteric stones do not show the lamination or ring structure typical of appendix stones and they are unlikely to be confused with calcified mesenteric nodes, phleboliths, or other common intra-abdominal calcifications. In Shaw's study of 240 cases of acute appendicitis, radiography of the removed specimen showed calculus in 33% of cases. When a faecolith was present, 77% of the specimens were gangrenous compared with 42% of gangrene when there was no evidence of calculus.

Clinical diagnosis

The patient with acute abdominal pain remains one of the last bastions of clinical medicine (Ellis, 1968). In no other common situation are clinical features, immediate decision and accurate diagnosis of such paramount importance. In most other fields an initially tentative, or even incorrect, clinical diagnosis is not necessarily harmful; we can wait until it is confirmed or refuted by laboratory and radiological investigation. But in an acute abdominal emergency, delays of even a few hours in initiating the correct line of treatment may make the difference between a smooth or a stormy course or, indeed, even place the patient in lethal danger. To leave, for example, an early case of acute appendicitis overnight undiagnosed and well sedated with morphia means missing the opportunity of achieving almost certain smooth recovery for this patient. Twenty-four hours later one may be faced with a seriously ill patient with advanced peritonitis from a perforated gangrenous appendix. Sir Heneage Olgilvie summed this up perfectly when he wrote that 'in the acute abdominal emergencies the difference between the best and the worst surgery is infinitely less than that between early and late surgery, and the greatest sacrifice of all is the sacrifice of time'.

In dealing with the patient with acute abdominal pain, the surgeon must steel himself to realise that he has to rely almost entirely on clinical features rather than on laboratory and radiological investigations. In recent years, he has become so used to being able to skimp on history and examination in other situations that it comes as something of a shock that, with the acute abdominal emergency, he has to depend on his own five senses. It is a very good aphorism that, in the diagnosis of the acute abdomen, the special investigations can only be used to reinforce a clinical diagnosis; seldom, if ever, can they establish or refute it. And this is particularly so in the diagnosis of acute appendicitis.

Acute abdominal pain is not only an important diagnostic problem, but it is also often a difficult one and it is important to remember that the pain may result from disease of almost any organ in the body. Apart from the abdominal and retroperitoneal viscera themselves, including, of course, the pelvic organs, one must also consider the chest, the central nervous system, and even the ears and throat. Metabolic disorders, particularly diabetes, may give acute abdominal symptoms and finally the psychological disturbance of the Munchausen syndrome provides us with a teasing diagnostic difficulty. It has been well said that nothing can be so simple nor yet so difficult as the diagnosis of acute appendicitis!

Symptoms and signs

The classical story of acute appendicitis is an onset of central, colicky abdominal pain situated in the region of the umbilicus. The patient may be nauseated or may vomit one or more times and after several hours the pain shifts to the lower right abdomen. It is now continuous and more severe so that the patient finds moving about uncomfortable and wishes to lie still, often with the legs flexed. With progression of the disease process, the pain becomes more diffusely spread over the abdomen. The explanation of the pain distribution in appendicitis is that the central colicky pain is the result of stretching of the appendix wall. When the inflammatory process extends to its serosa, the parietal peritoneum is involved and the pain shifts to the site of the appendix. Later diffuse spread of the pain corresponds with the development of diffuse peritonitis.

Occasionally there is no history of this classical shift of pain. The onset of central pain might have occurred during sleep or, because of its relatively mild nature, may be forgotten by the patient preoccupied by the much more intense lower right abdominal pain. The severity and time relationships of the pain are also very variable. Indeed, the patient may give a history of several previous mild attacks of what must undoubtedly have been appendicitis which were overlooked as mild 'stomach ache'. Rapid progression to gangrene and peritonitis may take place within 12 or so hours. In other instances, an acutely inflamed but non-perforated appendix may be removed after 3 or 4 days.

Usually there is constipation during the period of pain, but the patient may have a perfectly normal bowel action. In other instances there may be diarrhoea and this is said particularly to occur when the appendix lies in the retroileal position. It is the appendix tucked into this position which is likely to be deceptive. It will produce less overlying peritoneal irritation and less marked shift of pain than an appendix in one of the other more usual sites.

The clinical examination of the patient must commence with a careful general inspection and this is usefully combined with taking the pulse and the temperature. Both are usually raised in acute appendicitis and the rise progresses during the course of the disease. However, both the temperature and the pulse may be perfectly normal and this certainly does not exclude acute appendicitis. In adults, the usual finding is a temperature elevated about 1°C above normal; higher temperatures can be expected in children, but a very high pyrexia, although occasionally seen in acute appendicitis, suggests some other diagnosis such as a pyelitis or respiratory infection.

The tongue is usually coated and the breath foetid, but it is a good rule that there is no absolute finding in acute appendicitis, so one should not be surprised to find a patient with a perfectly clean moist tongue in this condition. An interesting study of 100 consecutive patients with acute appendicitis by Smith (1965) showed that only 60 had a temperature of 37.2°C or more and 75 had a coated tongue.

The patient is usually flushed and is in obvious pain, which is aggravated by movement. Palpation of the abdomen in early cases reveals localised tenderness, guarding and release tenderness over the region of the appendix. Usually, of course, this is the right iliac fossa but, if the appendix is lying in one of its less common positions, this localised tenderness may be in the right flank, low down in the abdomen, towards the umbilicus or even over in the left iliac fossa. In late cases with generalised peritonitis, the abdomen is diffusely tender and rigid, the bowel sounds are absent and the patient is obviously very ill. Later still, the abdomen is distended and the patient shows features of advanced peritonitis.

Rectal examination in the early case reveals tenderness only when the appendix lies in the pelvic position. However, if there is pus in the pelvic cul-de-sac tenderness is again a feature.

If the perforated appendix has become walled-off by surrounding structures into an appendix mass, the examinder can palpate the tender swelling in the right iliac fossa and may also detect a boggy swelling on rectal examination. However, the rest of the abdomen is soft with no evidence of generalised peritonitis and bowel sounds are present.

It should be stressed, of course, that the physical signs in acute appendicitis are those produced by local peritoneal irritation and by far and away the commonest cause of this in the right iliac fossa is the acutely inflamed appendix. But there are no specific physical findings confined to acute appendicitis; exactly the same clinical features are seen in other causes of lower right-sided inflammatory disease, for example, an acute Meckel's diverticulitis. The most constant and reliable signs of local peritoneal inflammation are tenderness and guarding; a completely soft abdomen is most unlikely to harbour any serious intra-abdominal catastrophe.

Special investigations

Acute appendicitis is essentially a clinical diagnosis and there is no laboratory or radiological test which is diagnostic of the condition.

White blood count

A polymorph leucocytosis is stressed by American authors as an important feature of acute appendicitis. Certainly the white cell count is raised above 12 000 in about three-quarters of patients with acute appendicitis. However, it is only slightly raised or entirely normal in the remainder and one must not discount the diagnosis under these circumstances.

Urine examination

This should, of course, be routine in every case of acute abdominal pain. The presence of glycosuria will raise the question of a 'diabetic acute abdomen' (*see under* differential diagnosis). Graham (1965) quantitatively analysed midstream urine specimens in 71 patients operated upon with a diagnosis of acute appendicitis. Of these, 62 had acute appendicitis and the remaining 9 had a normal appendix removed. Three of these had mesenteric adenitis and the other 6 had no abnormality detected. In the whole group of patients, microscopic pyuria was found in 9, all of whom were female, and one of whom also had haematuria. One male with acute appendicitis had microscopic haematuria. Graham points out that the distribution of microscopic pyuria was about that to be expected in the normal population. Significant haematuria should point to a urinary tract lesion, but, as indicated in this study, the presence of unequivocal clinical features should not deter the surgeon from proceeding to appendicectomy, when the inflamed appendix may be found to be adherent to the right ureter or to the bladder. If pus cells or red cells are found in the urine, certainly the clinical features should be carefully reviewed. If the surgeon is satisfied that appendicitis cannot be ruled out, operation under such circumstances is entirely justified.

Radiography of the abdomen

Plain films of the abdomen in the erect and supine positions are of particular value in the exclusion of lesions which may simulate appendicitis. Thus free gas may be demonstrated, suggesting a perforated peptic ulcer, or a right ureteric calculus may be obvious. There are a number of radiological signs which have been described in plain x-rays of the abdomen in patients with acute appendicitis (Brooks and Killen, 1965). These include:

1   Fluid levels localised to the caecum and to the terminal ileum, which indicate localised inflammation in the right lower quadrant of the abdomen.
2   Localised ileus, with gas in the caecum, ascending colon or terminal ileum.
3   Increased soft tissue density in the right lower quadrant.
4   Blurring of the right flank stripe, the radiolucent line produced by fat between peritoneum and transversus abdominis.
5   A faecolith in the right iliac fossa (which may be confused with a ureteric calculus, a gallstone or a calcified mesenteric lymph node).
6   Blurring of the psoas shadow on the right side.
7   A gas-filled appendix.
8   Free intraperitoneal gas (extremely rare).

9   Deformity of caecal gas due to an adjacent inflammatory mass. This is difficult to interpret because there may be disturbance of caecal gas from intraluminal fluid or faeces.

Saebo (1978) reports three cases of pneumoperitoneum associated with perforated appendicitis and notes that there are about 40 published reports of this situation. However, he points out that often appendicectomy is performed without x-raying the abdomen, so that more cases may actually occur than appear in published reports. I have personally not seen an example of this.

It is extremely rare for gas to be seen in a normal appendix or in the appendix distended as part of a large bowel obstruction. Killen and Brooks (1965) add five examples of a gas-filled appendix in gangrenous appendicitis to the four cases previously reported.

In a review of 200 patients undergoing laparotomy for acute appendicitis, these authors found that 54% of patients with acute non-perforated appendicitis had one or more of the signs listed above and the instance rose to 80% in patients with advanced appendicitis. Fifteen out of 41 patients who did not have acute appendicitis showed one or more of these x-ray appearances. Eight of these had another acute lesion in the right iliac fossa and three had no abnormality discovered at the time of operation.

The difficult case

Whilst the diagnosis of the straightforward case is usually obvious, difficulties are especially likely to be encountered in those patients who are unable to give a good account of their symptoms, the obese (where the subcutaneous fat disguises localised tenderness and guarding), those with an appendix in an unusual site, and in young children, the elderly and the pregnant.

Appendicitis in children

This is especially worrying. Because in the infant the appendix has a relatively wide lumen, appendicitis is rare under the age of 2 years (*see also* Chapter 13). However, it has been recorded in a baby aged 9 days (Coetzee, 1958), in another aged 15 days (Fields *et al.*, 1957) and even in a 12-day-old, 31-week premature infant (Ayalon *et al.*, 1979). From the age of 2, the incidence rises to a peak at about 11 years, declines gradually at 15 and then drops fairly rapidly thereafter (Lefall *et al.*, 1967).

Both the mortality and morbidity of appendicitis are

higher in preschool children than those over the age of 5. It used to be said that this poor outlook in infants was due to the fact that the omentum of the child is a filmy structure which is less well able to form a protective sheath around the inflamed appendix. However, a much more likely explanation is that delays in diagnosis are more prone to occur in infants, so that a higher percentage are admitted to hospital with the appendix already perforated.

In an important study from Newcastle, Jackson (1963) studied 313 children under the age of 12 years admitted to hospital with acute appendicitis. No less than 49.2% were perforated at the time of admission. Perforation was closely correlated with delay in the parents sending for the doctor. Details were available in 275 of these cases; in 63, delay was up to 12 h and 24% of these had perforated. In 80 the delay was up to 24 h and of these 42% had perforated. No less than 80 children did not reach hospital until the second day and 60% were perforated and a further 52 had delays of more than 48 h and of these, 83% had perforated appendices. It is interesting to note that one-third of the children were given purgatives by the parents and 62% of these arrived at the hospital with the appendix perforated compared with 43% of the unpurged group. There was fortunately only one death in the whole of this series (0.3%). Fields and Cole (1967) studied almost 7000 cases of acute appendicitis at all ages over a 10-year period from the Los Angeles County Hospital. Of these 22% had perforated by the time of admission and there was a 2.4% overall mortality. In the whole series, there were 30 examples of acute appendicitis in infants aged 3 years or less. No less than 18 of these had perforated and 4 more were gangrenous, but not yet ruptured. There were 2 deaths among these 30 children.

The picture of appendicitis in children is often not the classical one seen in older age groups. There may not be the early central abdominal colic and the shift of the pain to the right iliac fossa, so that the child frequently only complains of a generalised abdominal pain. Extreme patience is required when it comes to examining the abdomen of the ill, fretful and often crying child. It is a good rule that if there is localised tenderness and muscle guarding in the right iliac fossa in a previously healthy child, then the chances are very strong indeed that the appendix is acutely inflamed. In a group of 153 children in Aberdeen subjected to operation for acute abdominal pain, no less than 114 had proven acute appendicitis. A further 21 operated upon with a diagnosis of acute appendicitis were found to have a normal appendix and most of these had mesenteric adenitis. Of the remaining 18, 11 had intestinal obstruction (mostly cases of intussusception) and 7 had visceral injuries (Winsey and Jones, 1967; Jones, 1974).

Appendicitis in the elderly

In the elderly, appendicitis is undoubtedly a more serious situation than in younger patients. Peltokallio and Jauhiainen (1970), in an interesting study from Finland, showed that the clinical features in patients with acute appendicitis over the age of 60 years were quite similar as regards pattern and duration of the symptoms, the temperature changes and the leucocyte responses. However, there was a striking difference in the operative findings, since both gangrenous changes of perforation occurred five times as often in the older age group. These findings suggest that poorer localisation of the infection and diminished blood supply of the appendix are important factors in allowing rapid progression of the disease. Similar findings have been reported in other surveys. Andersson and Bergdahl (1978) found that half of their 68 patients with acute appendicitis over the age of 60 had perforations of the organ and there were postoperative complications in one-third of their patients. Owens and Hamit (1978) reviewed 68 appendicectomies in patients between 65 and 99 years of age. Four of these were normal, but the remainder had acute appendicitis and three-quarters of these had ruptured. Six of the patients with perforated appendices died, a mortality of 8.8%. In their study, 21 of the patients delayed 48 h or more before surgical consultation.

Other problems facing the surgeon in dealing with the elderly patient is the inevitable increased incidence of associated chronic disorders such as degenerative, cardiac, neurological and respiratory diseases. The number of alternative causes of intra-abdominal emergencies is greater in the elderly so that the differential diagnosis poses greater problems. Finally, there is little doubt that most elderly patients are less likely to complain of pain and other troublesome symptoms than younger people and their stoical attitude is probably a powerful factor in delay in seeking surgical help.

Appendicitis in pregnancy

This occurs not infrequently since the pregnant woman is no more nor less prone to appendicitis than a non-pregnant young adult. Diagnosis, however, is undoubtedly more difficult in the pregnant woman. In the first trimester, the history of amenorrhoea, together with the local physical signs, may lead to diagnosis of ruptured ectopic pregnancy. The nausea and vomiting may be put down to 'morning sickness' and delay diagnosis. As the pregnancy progresses and the uterus enlarges, the appendix is pushed upwards and more laterally than in the normal abdomen so that the pain, tenderness and guarding are situated in the mid or upper abdomen and may lead to confusion with pyelitis or cholecystitis. The stretched abdominal muscles in the late stages of pregnancy make the detection of guarding or rigidity very difficult.

In the advanced stages of pregnancy, differential diagnosis must be made from pyelitis, cholecystitis, degeneration of a fibroid and concealed accidental haemorrhage.

The prognosis with regard to survival of the fetus depends on the stage of the pregnancy and the degree of severity of the appendicitis. In the first three months of pregnancy there is an increased risk of abortion, but during the second trimester there is a good chance that the pregnancy will go through to successful conclusion providing appendicectomy is performed carefully and at an early stage in the disease. In the presence of severe peritonitis, there is a high risk of fetal death. In the advanced stages of pregnancy, appendicectomy may precipitate premature labour.

Differential diagnosis

We have already stressed that nothing can be so easy, nor anything so difficult, as the diagnosis of acute appendicitis. The tyro may smile indulgently at the long list of differential diagnoses given in the textbooks but, as year follows year, he will experience the chagrin of making most, if not all, these errors (see Ch. 1).

Of course, one is not too ashamed to make a diagnosis of appendicitis and to find, at laparotomy, that there is some other acute abdominal condition that itself requires urgent surgery, for example, a twisted ovarian cyst or an acute Meckel's diverticulitis. A small proportion of cases will be found to have a normal appendix and the exact diagnosis of the cause of the pain will probably never be found. Here too, provided the proportion is kept low, the surgeon will accept a small number of such negative laparotomies against the risk of leaving a possibly early acutely inflamed appendix within the abdomen. The tragedy comes when appendicectomy is performed in a patient with some medical condition, such as diabetes or pleurisy, where operation can only aggravate the condition.

It is convenient to consider the differential diagnosis systematically under the following headings:

1 Other intra-abdominal causes of acute pain
2 The urinary tract
3 In the case of female patients, acute pain of gynaecological origin
4 The chest
5 The central nervous system
6 Other medical conditions.

Other intra-abdominal diseases

Diseases which commonly simulate appendicitis are perforated peptic ulcer, acute cholecystitis, acute intestinal obstruction, gastroenteritis, acute diverticulitis, acute regional ileitis and, in children, intussusception, acute Meckel's diverticultis and mesenteric adenitis.

Urinary tract

Renal colic and acute pyelonephritis are included here. The urine must be tested for blood and pus cells in every case of acute abdominal pain but, as we have already mentioned, the presence of either of these abnormalities does not exclude acute appendicitis.

Gynaecological causes

These include acute salpingitis, ectopic pregnancy, a ruptured cyst of the corpus luteum and a twisted ovarian dermoid.

The chest

Basal pneumonia and pleurisy may give referred abdominal pain which may be surprisingly difficult to differentiate, especially in children. Jona and Belin (1976) found that 12 of 250 children who presented with acute abdominal pain had a basal pneumonia as the only cause. It is interesting that of these 12 children, 8 had only minor respiratory symptoms, 4 had none at all and only 2 had abnormal physical findings when the chest was examined. However, the abdominal pain was severe, sustained and was associated with abdominal tenderness and even, on occasion, with absent bowel sounds. These authors point out that a chest x-ray is valuable and should include a good lateral film, because consolidation may be hidden by the diaphragm in the usual posteroanterior film.

A coronary thrombosis may be accompanied by chronic marked epigastric pain, but generalised abdominal pain and rigidity are rare and the condition is only occasionally confused with an abdominal emergency.

Diseases of the central nervous system

These should just be kept in mind in the differential diagnosis. The lightning pains of tabes have all but disappeared from clinical practice in this country. Abdominal pain and local tenderness in the two or three days before the rash of herpes zoster appears may make some intraperitoneal disease suspected, but cases of unnecessary operation in this condition are unusual. In this category it is also proper to include simulated abdominal pain (the Munchausen syndrome) where the presence of multiple abdominal scars, a bizarre history and no fixed address should put the clinician on his guard.

Other medical conditions

Medical conditions which have been confused with acute appendicitis include infectious hepatitis, gastro-enteritis, sickle cell crisis (which should always be thought of in black children) and, very rarely, acute porphyria. The condition which must always be kept in mind is undiagnosed diabetes which undoubtedly may mimic an acute abdominal emergency, especially in children. Valerio (1976), for example, describes three children with acute abdominal pain which was the presenting feature of their undiagnosed diabetes. He stresses three important clinical clues which are, first a history of polyuria, polydipsia and anorexia which precede the abdominal pain, second deep, sighing, rapid respirations and third, severe dehydration. The abdominal pain is usually generalised in contrast to the localised pain and tenderness of acute appendicitis. It may be difficult to get a urine specimen to test for sugar, because of the dehydration and an important step in confirming the suspected diagnosis is to arrange an immediate blood sugar estimation. The abdomen will become pain-free and soft within a few hours of appropriate treatment for the diabetes, but obviously very close observation is required during this critical period.

Treatment

The treatment of acute appendicitis is appendicectomy – the sooner the better. There are four exceptions to this excellent rule:

1 The patient is desperately ill with advanced peritonitis. Under these circumstances, nasogastric suction, intravenous fluid replacement (including blood) and broad-spectrum antibiotic therapy are employed to get the patient fit for operation.
2 In those rare circumstances where no surgical facilities are available, for example, a small boat at sea, where one has to rely on a conservative regime in the hope that resolution or a local appendix mass will form. If available, morphia, antibiotic therapy and i.v. fluids are given.
3 The attack has already resolved. Here there is no need for urgency, but an elective appendicectomy is advised.
4 The inflammatory process has localised into an appendix mass (*see below*).

Operative technique

If the diagnosis is one of a straightforward acute appendicitis, no special steps need be taken apart from those of any routine abdominal operation. However, if a diagnosis of generalised peritonitis is made, then preoperatively a nasogastric tube is passed, i.v. fluid replacement commenced and broadspectrum antibiotic therapy initiated. Our own regime is to use gentamicin and metronidazole.

A right iliac fossa skin crease muscle-split incision is used, commencing just above and medial to the anterior superior iliac spine. It is a mistake to place the incision too medially, which brings the surgeon down onto the anterior rectus sheath and not over the oblique muscles. After splitting the oblique muscles in the lines of their fibres, moist packs are placed around the wound, the muscles are retracted and the peritoneum opened. There is usually little difficulty in delivering the acutely inflamed appendix by drawing the caecum through the abdominal incision. If difficulty is encountered in localising the appendix, it can be found by tracing the taeniae coli along the caecum to their junction at the appendix base.

The appendix mesentery may be long, in which case appendicectomy is a simple procedure, or the appendix may be found closely bound to the caecum by congenital adhesions which require preliminary mobilisation before one is able to deal with the vessels in the mesoappendix. The mobilised organ is held up by tissue forceps and the appendicular vessels ligated with thread. The base of the appendix is crushed with artery forceps, ligated with catgut and the stump surrounded by a catgut purse-string suture. The appendix is removed by incising between the ligated stump and the more distally placed artery forceps and the stump invaginated by means of the purse-string. A second purse-string suture invaginates the first and careful inspection is carried out of the mesoappendix to ensure haemostasis.

If the appendix is gangrenous or perforated, the purulent fluid is sucked away after first taking a swab for bacteriological examination. Great care should be employed in mobilising and removing the gangrenous appendix, because it is a simple matter to rupture the organ. Once delivered, the appendix should be wrapped in a moist swab to prevent further contamination. If found to be wrapped in omentum, the appendix is best removed together with adherent omentum which acts as a protective sheath. Occasionally, the caecal wall is so oedematous and thickened that invagination is impossible. Under such circumstances, simple ligation of the appendix stump without invagination should be performed. Occasionally the inflamed appendix in the retrocolic position is firmly bound down along the length of the ascending colon and cannot be delivered into the wound. It is then best to perform retrograde appendicectomy. The base of the appendix is freed and divided and then the rest of the appendix mesentery serially picked up and divided with artery forceps until the tip has been reached.

Closure of the muscle-split incision is simplicity itself. The peritoneum is closed with chromic catgut, the transversus and internal oblique muscles are left unsutured and one or two catgut sutures are used to appose the external oblique aponeurosis. The skin is sutured with interrupted nylon stitches. I use povidone iodine spray in the muscle layers of the wound, but other surgeons prefer topical antibiotic therapy.

Where there is a local abscess or there is gross peritoneal contamination, or where difficulty has been encountered in ligaturing or invaginating the appendix stump, a corrugated drain is passed down to the appendix base and brought out through the lateral extremity of the wound where it is left *in situ* for two or three days.

There are some who advise a lower right paramedian incision for appendicectomy, particularly if the diagnosis is in some doubt or, in female patients, where there is some question of a gynaecological cause for the acute abdominal pain. However, there is no doubt that the right iliac fossa incision gives the most direct access to the appendix even in the most difficult cases. Even if the diagnosis is incorrect, most other local pathologies can be dealt with through the right iliac fossa incision, especially if the skin incision is somewhat extended and then the oblique muscles divided or the rectus sheath opened medially. A ruptured ectopic pregnancy, an acutely inflamed Meckel's diverticulum or an acute caecal diverticulitis, for example, can be managed without any particular problem. If, however, it is found that the cause of the acute abdominal pain is out of reach of the right iliac fossa incision – a perforated duodenal ulcer for example – then the right iliac fossa incision is left open, the appropriate vertical incision performed, the emergency dealt with and both incisions then closed at the end of the laparotomy.

The appendix mass

Occasionally a patient will present who has walled-off his perforated appendix into an inflammatory mass, usually after at least a 4- or 5-day history of abdominal pain. This is probably being seen less commonly these days as a result of improved health education. Thus, Bradley and Isaacs (1978), in a review of 2621 patients with aute appendicitis treated between 1962 and 1976 in Atlanta, found that only 2% had an appendix abscess on admission, and here the average duration of symptoms was 9 days. The clinical features are a swinging temperature, with an elevated pulse rate. There is a tender mass in the right iliac fossa which can often also be palpated on rectal examination. However, there is no evidence of a generalised peritonitis in that the rest of the abdomen is soft and bowel sounds are present. In such cases, the initial treatment should be conservative. The patient is put to bed, maintained on fluids only, and a careful watch is maintained on his general condition, the temperature and pulse, and the size of the mass, which is marked out on the abdominal wall with a skin pencil. Antibiotics should be firmly avoided at this stage becuase they merely result in a honeycomb of chronic abscess cavities, the so-called 'antibioticoma' (Stammers, 1957). On this treatment, the majority of appendix masses resolve. However, in some 10% of cases, the swelling obviously enlarges over the next day or two, the pyrexia becomes more elevated, and in such circumstances it should be drained through a small incision over the apex of the mass. No formal attempt should be made at removing the appendix at this stage unless it 'delivers' easily into the wound.

Whether resolution occurs or whether drainage is required, elective appendicectomy should be recommended after an interval of about 3 months which allows the inflammatory condition to settle down. This is because of the significant risk of further episodes of acute appendicitis if the damaged appendix is left *in situ*. Useful reports of large series of cases have been published by Foran and his colleagues (1978) in adults, and by Gastrin and Josephson (1969) in children.

Occasionally the inflamed tip of the appendix may result in an appendicovesical fistula (Parton, 1958) or in an appendicocutaneous fistula (Hedner *et al*, 1978).

Postoperative complications

The enormous difference between the usually smooth postoperative course of appendicectomy in a case of an early acute appendicitis and the stormy postoperative recovery that so often accompanies the removal of a gangrenous perforated appendix with generalised peritonitis underlines the importance of early diagnosis and treatment.

Paralytic ileus

This is the invariable accompaniment of general peritonitis and is treated with the relief of pain by means of regular doses of morphia, gastric aspiration, careful fluid and electrolyte replacement by i.v. drip and antibiotic therapy guided by the bacteriological study of the peritoneal exudate. Careful watch must be maintained to differentiate from mechanical obstruction from adhesions, since continued ileus requires conservative therapy while a mechanical obstruction calls for urgent laparotomy to relieve the small bowel occlusions.

The differential diagnosis is based on the following:

An ileus rarely lasts for more than three or four days and persistence of symptoms after this time is always suspcious of mechanical obstruction. The presence of noisy bowel sounds indicates mechanical occlusion and may be accompanied by colicky pain. Recurrence of symptoms after the patient has already passed flatus or has had a bowel action makes the diagnosis of mechanical obstruction likely. An important investigation is a plain x-ray of the abdomen. Diffuse distribution of gas throughout the small and large bowel is indicative of paralytic ileus, whereas a localised loop or loops of distended small intestine with fluid levels and without gas shadows in the large bowel strongly favour mechanical obstruction.

Septic complications

A local wound abscess is a common complication of appendicectomy and is dealt with by removal of a suture and gentle probing of the wound to release the pus.

A pelvic abscess is particularly common after removal of a perforated gangrenous appendix. There is pyrexia and often diarrhoea with mucus discharge per rectum. Rectal examination reveals a tender pelvic mass which, in the majority of cases, drains spontaneously either into the vagina or the rectum. Occasionally, drainage needs to be performed through the rectum or the posterior fornix of the vagina under a general anaesthetic.

Subphrenic abscess is much less common after a perforated acute appendicitis than after peritonitis of upper abdominal origin. It usually occurs some two or three weeks after the general peritonitis, although if antibiotics have been used, abscess formation may be delayed for weeks or even months after the origianl episode of peritonitis. There may be no localising clinical features whatsoever, the patient merely presenting with malaise, loss of weight, anorexia, anaemia and a fever. However, there may be localising features of upper abdominal pain or pain in the lower chest or referred to the shoulder with localised tenderness and signs at the right lung base. The white count is usually raised. A chest x-ray demonstrates elevation of the diaphragm on the affected side, a pleural effusion, which is often accompanied by collapse of the lung base, and there may be gas and a fluid level below the diaphragm in about 75% of cases. Accurate localisation may be achieved by ultrasound or a CAT scan. Early cases may respond to a short course of broad-spectrum antibiotic therapy, but if resolution fails to occur rapidly or if there is radiological evidence of a localised abscess, then formal surgical drainage is required.

Neoplasms of the appendix

Tumours of the appendix are infrequent, a fact which probably reflects simply the small surface area of mucosa which is available for malignant change to take place. However, the distribution of tumour types is in rather sharp contrast to the rest of the large intestine. By far the commonest neoplasm of the appendix is the carcinoid tumour, which is found in about 1 in 1000 of all appendices examined and accounts for about 85% of all tumours of the appendix.

Benign tumours

These are rare, but include adenomatous polyps, mucous cystadenoma, leiomyoma and neuroma. The mucous cystadenoma may obstruct the lumen of the organ and distend the appendix to form a mucocele. The other benign lesions do not obstruct the appendix lumen, are rarely of clinical importance and are usually only detected as an incidental finding in the histological study of an appendicectomy specimen.

The malignant tumours comprise the carcinoid tumour, villous adenocarcinoma and what might be termed the colonic type of adenocarcinoma.

The carcinoid tumour

As already noted, this is the commonest tumour of the appendix and the only one likely to be encountered in routine surgical practice. It arises from chromaffin cells, has a characteristic yellow colour, and microscopically is composed of solid nests of tumour cells which stain with silver salts. In a detailed study by Moertel and his colleagues (1968), 71% occurred at the tip, 22% in the body and 7% at the base of the appendix. The tumour may occur at any age although it tends to affect middle-aged adults. Metastatic spread is rare and in the study by Moertel and his colleagues, metastases were present in only 1.4% of the cases and was practically confined to lesions which were larger than 2 cm in diameter.

The majority of carcinoids are incidental findings on histological study of appendices removed during the course of laparotomies for other procedures. Acute appendicitis is not commonly caused because the usual location is at the tip of the organ. However, occasionally the lumen may be occluded by a tumour at the base or the body of the appendix and such cases may present as acute appendicitis.

Villous adenocarcinoma

Villous adenocarcinoma of the appendix has a propensity to fill the appendix with mucus and differentiation from a benign mucocele may be difficult. If unruptured, the tumour rarely metastasises, but perforation of the malignant mucocele may result in pseudomyxoma peritonei.

Adenocarcinoma

Adenocarcinoma of the appendix resembles histologically similar tumours elsewhere in the large bowel, although mucus secretion is rather more prominent. Typically the tumour arises at the base of the appendix in patients over the age of 50. It may be an incidental finding or present as acute appendicitis or as an appendix abscess. If the tumour invades the caecum it may be very difficult to differentiate it from a primary carcinoma of caecal origin. in a useful study by Hesketh (1963) of a collected series of 95 cases, the majority presented as acute appendicitis, an appendix abscess or with chronic right iliac fossa pain. Fourteen percent were detected at incidental laparotomy and extensive carcinomatosa was found in 11% of patients. In not a single case had the diagnosis been made preoperatively.

Treatment

It is most unusual for the diagnosis of an appendix tumour to be made preoperatively. The usual situation is that the tumour is found either in dealing with an acutely inflamed appendix or as an incidental finding at abdominal exploration. If a confident diagnosis of carcinoid tumour is made and the lesion affects the tip or shaft of the appendix, careful search should be made for a carcinoid tumour elsewhere in the small intestine since occasionally these may be multiple. The regional nodes are examined and the liver carefully palpated for secondary deposits. In the great majority of cases these findings will be negative, and under these conditions, particularly if the tumour is less than 2 cm in diameter, nothing more is required than appendicectomy. In those rare cases where involved lymph nodes are found or where the tumour is more than 2 cm in diameter, the carcinoid should be treated by a right hemicolectomy. Where the tumour of the appendix is obviously malignant, then a right hemicolectomy should be performed.

In some circumstances the diagnosis of an appendix tumour is not established until the pathological examination of the operative specimen. If this proves to be a carcinoid tumour and the resection has been adequate, no further procedure need be performed. In the rare circumstances where the carcinoid involves the base of the appendix and resection has been incomplete, it would be reasonable to advise re-operation with excision of an adequate cuff of adjacent caecum. If the appendicectomy specimen shows the presence of an undoubted adenocarcinoma then, even if the resection has been adequate, it is wise to advise formal right hemicolectomy.

Prognosis

The majority of cases of carcinoid tumour of the appendix are cured by appendicectomy. The rare exceptions are those in which the carcinoid is more than 2 cm in diameter or where there is lymphatic or hepatic spread at the time of operation.

In a detailed paper concerning prognosis of carcinoma of the appendix, Andersson and his colleagues (1976) note that the prognosis of a malignant mucocele of the appendix is excellent following appendicectomy provided that perforation has not taken place, that the tumour is confined to the tip of the organ and the submucosa has not been invaded. In 6 cases treated by appendicectomy, all achieved five-year survival. In a review of 51 cases of primary adenocarcinoma of the appendix of the colonic type, 26 patients were treated by appendicectomy alone and 12 of these (46%) were alive five years later compared with 15 (60%) of the 25 patients subjected to right hemicolectomy.

References

Andersson A., Bergdahl L. (1978). Acute appendicitis in patients over sixty. *Amer. Surg*; **44**:445–50.

Andersson A., Bergdahl L., Boquist L. (1976). Primary carcinoma of the appendix. *Ann. Surg*; **183**:53–7.

Andersson A., Griffiths H., Murphy J., Roll J., Serenyi A., Swann I., Cockroft A., Myers J., St. Leger A. (1979). Is appendicitis familial? *Brit. Med. J*; **2**:697–8.

Ayalon A., Mogilner M., Cohen O., Luttwak Z., Schiller M. (1979). Acute appendicitis in a premature baby. *Acta Chir. Scand*; **145**:285–6.

Bradley E.L., Isaacs J. (1978). Appendiceal abscess revisited. *Arch. Surg*; **113**:130–2.

Brooks D.W., Killen D.A. (1965). Roentgenographic findings in acute appendicitis. *Surgery*; **57**:377–9.

Burge R.E., Dennis C., Varco R.L., Wangensteen O.H. (1940). Histology of experimental appendiceal obstruction. *Arch. Pathol*; **30**:481–90.

Coetzee T. (1958). Acute appendicitis in an infant. *S. Afr. Med. J*; **32**:890.

Cope Z. (1965). *A History of the Acute Abdomen*. London: Oxford Medical Publications.

Ellis H. (1968). Diagnosis of the acute abdomen. *Brit. Med. J*; **1**:491–3.

Fields I.A., Cole N.M. (1967). Acute appendicitis in infants 36 months of age or younger. 10-year survey at the Los Angeles County Hospital. *Amer. J. Surg*; **113**:269–72.

Fields I.A., Naiditch M.J., Rothman P.E. (1957). Acute appendicitis in infants. *Amer. J. Dis. Child*; **93**:287–9.

Foran B., Berne T.V., Rosoff L. (1978). Management of the appendiceal mass. *Arch. Surg*; **113**:1144–5.

Gastrin U., Josephson S. (1969). Appendiceal abscess – acute appendectomy or conservative treatment. *Acta Chir. Scand*; **135**:539–42.

Graham J.A. (1965). Urinary cell counts in appendicitis. *Scot. Med. J*; **10**:126–8.

Hedner J., Jansson R., Lindberg B. (1978). Appendico-cutaneous fistula. *Acta Chir. Scand*; **144**:123–4.

Hesketh K.T. (1963). The management of primary adeno-carcinoma of the vermiform appendix. *Gut*; **4**:158–68.

Jackson R.H. (1963). Parents, family doctors and acute appendicitis in childhood. *Brit. Med. J*; **2**:277–8.

Jona J.Z., Belin R.P. (1976). Basal pneumonia simulating acute appendicitis in children. *Arch. Surg*; **111**:552–4.

Jones P.F. (1974). Abdominal emergencies in infancy and childhood. In *Emergency Abdominal Surgery*. Oxford: Blackwell Scientific Publications.

Killen D.A., Brooks D.W. (1965). Gas-filled appendix: a roentgenographic sign of acute appendicitis. *Ann. Surg*; **161**:474–5.

Leffall L.D., Cooperman A., Syphax B. (1967). Appendicitis. A continuing surgical challenge. *Amer. J. Surg*; **113**:654–6.

Moertel G.C., Dockerty M.B., Judd E.S. (1968). Carcinoid tumours of the veriform appendix. *Cancer*; **21**:270–4.

Morson B.C., Dawson I.M.P. (1972). *Gastrointestinal Pathology*, pp.399. Oxford: Blackwell Scientific Publications.

Owens B.J., Hamit H.F. (1978). Appendicitis in the elderly. *Ann. Surg*; **187**:392–6.

Parton L.I. (1958). Appendico-vesical fistula. *Brit. J. Surg*; **45**:583–4.

Peltokallio P., Jauhiainen K. (1970). Acute appendicitis in the aged patient. Study of 300 cases after the age of 60. *Arch. Surg*; **100**:140-3.

Saebo A. (1978). Pneumoperitoneum associated with per-forated appendicitis. *Acta Chir. Scand*; **144**:115–17.

Shaw R.E. (1965). Appendix calculi and acute appendicitis. *Brit. J. Surg*; **52**:451–9.

Smith P.H. (1965). The diagnosis of appendicitis. *Postgrad. Med. J*; **41**:2–5.

Stammers F.A.R. (1957). Treatment of acute appendicitis. *Brit. Med. J*; **1**:225.

Valerio D. (1976). Acute diabetic abdomen in childhood. *Lancet*; **i**:66–8.

Wangensteen O.H., Bowers W.F. (1937). Significance of the obstructive factor in the genesis of acute appendicitis. An experimental study. *Arch. Surg*; **34**:496–9.

Wilkie D.P.D. (1914). Acute appendicitis and acute appendicular obstruction. *Brit. Med J*; **2**:959–60.

Winsey H.S., Jones P.F. (1967). Acute abdominal pain in childhood: analysis of a year's admissions (Royal Aberdeen Hospital for Sick Children). *Brit. Med J*; **1**:653–5.

12

Colorectal surgery

R.J. HEALD

Clues to the aetiology of colorectal disease

The large intestine of the African village dweller is rarely affected by the diseases which are discussed here. Within months of changing to urban life, appendicitis becomes common, and within 20 years the incidence of adenoma, carcinoma, diverticula, haemorrhoids and colitis approaches that of those who live in the West. We owe these basic observations to Denis Burkitt (1971), but 15 years of intensive research has failed to fill in essential detail. A decrease of dietary fibre probably leads to increased transit times, smaller harder motions and a tendency to strain at stool: it may thus be the cause of muscle hypertrophy and spasm, diverticula and haemorrhoids (Walker and Painter, 1972). However, a threefold increase in bowel cancer risk in Japanese migrants to Hawaii is accompanied by no change in transit time (Glober et al., 1977). A similar failure to correlate transit times with cancer risk in Danes (high cancer risk) and Finns (low risk) (Jensen and Michenham, 1979) leaves little doubt that one must look further than the bulk and transit time hypothesis to explain mucosal diseases such as cancer. It is possible that diet may influence the colonic microflora to induce carcinogenic degradation of bile acids, or that high fat, protein or meat consumption may themselves be contributory. It is even possible that nitrosamines, already implicated in upper gastrointestinal cancer, might be produced by bacterial action on dietary amines and be relevant in the lower bowel. The most diverse research has so far provided no convincing answers to the aetiology of colorectal cancer. Inflammatory bowel disease is similarly unexplained although abnormalities of the immune complexes and bacterial sensitivity are possibly implicated. There is some evidence that different factors may influence the aetiology of rectal as opposed to colonic cancer. Furthermore, it is probable that most of the current increase is in colonic tumours rather than in those of the rectum. Much of this may be related to the improvement in methods of detection by double contrast radiology and the colonoscope, but it is possible that there is a real change in the balance towards colonic cancer. It is interesting that Doll and Peto, (1976), in their classical prospective review of the consequences of smoking amongst doctors, observed that smokers had an increased risk of developing rectal though not colonic cancer. The reasons are unknown, but the patchy decline in smoking in Western countries might provide some explanation for changes in incidence.

All this points to an environmental and dietary aetiology with the refinement and processing of foods as the chief culprits. Furthermore, the approximately equal sex incidence in all major colorectal diseases argues against obvious occupational factors, and the genetic aspect reaches significance only in conditions such as adenomatosis. Nevertheless, the lesions in this last disease are identical to those which we regard as the usual precursors of colorectal cancer in the population as a whole, so that an interaction of environmental and genetic factors remains inherently probable. Although the consumption of bran and vegetable fibre remains the most sensible advice that we can offer our patients, it would be optimistic to suppose that this alone will have a widespread impact on the prevalence of these diseases.

Operative principles

Incisions for colorectal surgery

It is a common mistake in rectal surgery for the incision to be inadequate for proper mobilisation of the splenic flexure. A long midline incision from the pubic symphysis to within a few centimetres of the xiphisternum will permit any part of the large bowel to be mobilised and dealt with safely. A lower midline will suffice only for limited procedures such as those for diverticular disease or prolapse.

Preoperative preparation of bowel

The special dangers and complications of bowel surgery are a direct consequence of the contamination of previously sterile tissues by bacteria and the vegetable matter of the faeces.

The most immediate and serious possible sequel is bacteraemic shock, the most common is wound infection, and the most chronic is deep pelvic sepsis. Half of the weight of faeces is composed of anaerobic bacteria which outnumber the aerobes by over 100:1. Most of the septic complications are due either to a mixture of aerobes and anaerobes or to anaerobes alone. Probably all deep sepsis is fundamentally anaerobic and all foul smelling pus is certainly anaerobic. It is, therefore, mandatory to consider the anaerobe, but prudent also to budget for the Gram negative aerobes.

The dangers of sepsis are guarded against in three ways:

Surgical technique

Crushed and ischaemic tissue and collections of blood are fertile fields for anerobes. Gentle precise technique, the avoidance of tearing and crushing, and prevention of faecal spillage are the hallmarks of the successful colorectal surgeon. The so-called non-crushing clamp is either avoided or applied well away from bowel during anastomosis so as not to compromise the blood supply. Drainage of a pelvic space is a matter of great importance to avoid collections of blood which will inevitably become infected.

Physical bowel preparation

The safest colon is an empty one. However, the semi-liquid stool of the imperfectly prepared bowel is even more dangerous than that in the unprepared patient. Obstructed, or partially obstructed, bowel may be difficult or impossible to prepare by any method, especially the frail and elderly patient. Nevertheless, the quality of the surgical result depends in no small measure upon the determined application by special nurses of one or more of the following methods:

Non-residue diet. Large volumes of clear fluids for 5 days may be supplemented by elemental diets. The latter, however, reduce stool bulk only by about three-quarters.

Purgatives. These should generally be avoided on the night before operation, or their action may coincide with the operation.

Castor oil, 2 × 50 ml may be given if tolerated 24–48 h prior to operation. *Senokot*, 4 tablets given 2 nights before operation. *Magnesium suphate*, 5 g repeated hourly until it produces colic and diarrhoea, or three times a day on 5th, 4th and 3rd days before operation. *Mannitol* 10% (0.5–1 litre) is made more palatable if it is kept in a refrigerator and made acceptable with lemon juice (Hunt and Waye 1981). There is a theoretical danger in its preoperative use in that it provides a good medium for bacterial growth. If used, it should be followed by a wash-out from below.

Enemas and wash-outs. These can be given on the night before or morning of operation. The Henderson colonic lavage machine can give excellent results in skilled hands provided an hour, or even two, are set aside for the purpose. Various proprietary enemas such as Veripaque are effective.

Whole gut irrigation ('Hercules' Washout – he diverted the river to cleanse the stables of Aegeus). This technique involves the administration of 10–15 l of an electrolyte solution over 2–5 h via a nasogastric tube. The process may be made more tolerable by giving metoclopramide and by providing a comfortable padded commode and a good book. Some excellent results have been reported, but the technique is not possible in the obstructed patient and may induce cardiac failure or electrolyte problems in the frail. Grace (1983, personal communication) has recently demonstrated significantly superior results by including neomycin in the irrigant.

The colonic douche. If the above methods have failed, faecal loading should not be tolerated by the surgeon. After the end of the colon has been mobilised and divided, it can be hung over the patient's side into a suitable receptacle. A Foley balloon catheter is introduced via a tiny incision in the terminal ileum into the caecum, the balloon inflated and snugged back against the ileocaecal valve and several litres of fluid run through until the colon is quite clean.

The use and abuse of preoperative antibiotics

Attitudes to the crucial question of antibacterial usage in large bowel surgery are changing radically as emphasis shifts away from 'bowel preparation' towards a concept of 'patient protection'. For many years sulphonamides and non-absorbable antibacterials such as neomycin were administered for 5–7 days before operation to reduce colonic bacterial counts. Such medication can, however, be shown to favour pathogenic and more resistant organisms and may thus be harmful. Despite many trials, there has never been conclusive evidence that the observed reduction in bacterial counts had any beneficial effect upon the patient, except when absorbable antibacterials were present at the time of operation.

Current emphasis is shifting towards the concept of perfusing and protecting the patient from the effects of contamination which is inevitable. Thus the antibacterials are given systemically an hour or two before operation (e.g. with the premedication), continued during the operation and frequently for 24–48 h thereafter.

Because of anaerobes, the majority of surgeons in Great Britain use a combination of metronidazole with a broad-spectrum antibiotic such as ampicillin, gentamicin, or a cephalosporin.

The author's routine is as follows:

ANTIBACTERIALS

Cefamandole 1 g	Preoperatively
or	
Cephazolin 1 g	Intravenously on the operating table; and intravenously every 8 h for 24 h, or longer if necessary (500 mg 8-hourly)
Metronidazole	2 suppositories during the 8 h before operation; 1 g intravenously during operation and continued if necessary, (500 mg 8-hourly).

The newer β lactamase inhibiting cephalosporins such as moxalactam may provide a single agent alternative.

MECHANICAL

Fluids only 5 days.

Plus 4 'Trisorbon' sachets + 2 cans 'Ensure' per day to give 2000 cals.

Senokot tabs IV on 4th and 3rd nights preoperatively.

Henderson wash-outs (1–2 h each) 36 and 13 h preoperatively.

Stomas

Accurate skin to mucosal suture is the basic principle of all good stomas; attachment of the bowel to the parietal peritoneum is not essential, but guards against parastomal hernia. Eversion is essential for stomas which may leak liquid and stomatherapists argue that this implies that all colostomies should be everted to make attacks of diarrhoea more manageable.

Site

The surgeon should be guided by the stomatherapist and the skin marked with the patient standing and wearing an appliance before operation. A high site is chosen for the pelvic end colostomy in the fat person, low for a transverse colostomy so as to miss the costal margin. A wide flat area clear of bony points and scars is best and the waist must be avoided because an appliance interferes with clothing, adheres badly, and spoils the waistline of a young woman.

For an ileostomy a 2.5 cm spout should protrude through a 2.5 cm hole in flat skin at a site convenient for the wearing of an appliance which is usually half way between the umbilicus and the anterior superior spine.

To achieve the eversion, an initial 6 cm protrusion of ileum needs to be secured by sutures within the abdomen between the abdominal wall and the ileum and its mesentery. Goligher (1980) advises against picking up the inner tube with the skin to mucosa stitches as a method of securing eversion. If such sutures are used, special care is required to avoid deep bites through to the mucosa which carry a risk of skin-level fistulas.

The lateral space

There is much controversy about the dangers of intestinal strangulation in the lateral space. One school maintains that a somewhat medially sited stoma leaves such a large space that no such risk exists. Goligher, on the other hand, regards closure as mandatory, and has devised the extraperitoneal tunnel method of obliterating the space (Goligher, 1958). Most surgeons who perceive it as a danger prefer to close it by stitching the lower bowel to the parietal peritoneum lateral to the stoma, so as to retain the remainder of the ileum medial to it.

Loop ileostomy

The loop is brought out over a bar or rod. The incision in the bowel is made transversely and distally and folded back to create an everted proximal spout with a nearly flush distal one. Some surgeons prefer this form of temporary defunctioning to transverse colostomy on the grounds that there is little smell.

Loop transverse colostomy

With increasing sphincter conservation, this is becoming the most common of all stomas. It has been usefully and simply modified by Schofield to defunction more effectively by rotating the colostomy anticlockwise by about 100° (Schofield *et al.*, 1980). This brings the opening of the proximal bowel into a dependent position so that less 'spill-over' occurs.

The right transverse colon is usually the preferred segment. A soft plastic catheter is threaded round the bowel after cutting a small hole in the mesentery close to the bowel wall and well to the right of the middle colic artery. The catheter is used to draw the loop of bowel through a transverse incision made separate from the main wound: this must be adequately roomy to avoid oedema and obstruction later (2 loose fingers). The catheter can be left in place of the more traditional glass rod and made into a short circular retaining device which remains within this bag. Alternatively, one of the proprietary self-retaining bars can be used to stabilise the 'spur'. Skin to mucosa suturing is effected so as to leave the minimum gap for the bar or catheter. If the bar is flat, the bag may be fixed over it, or the base of the bag placed between bar and skin.

Split colostomy for complete defunctioning

A satisfactory and totally defunctioning colostomy can be created by dividing the bowel completely and bringing the distal limb to the skin several centimetres away from the main stoma.

Immediate fixation of appliance

An adhesive bag which can be cut to the exact size is desirable, Surgicare System 2 or Coloplast Comfeel beneath the MC2000 appliance are both excellent.

Loop colostomy closure

This operation is often much underrated. It should not generally be attempted sooner than 4–6 weeks after the loop colostomy was created, or the tissue planes will be difficult to identify. It requires great skill and care to dissect the stoma out of the abdominal wall without tearing or penetrating its muscle coat. This is best done with a small (e.g. No. 15) blade and fine dissecting scissors. Much is written about the differences between extra- and intraperitoneal closure. With a routine loop colostomy which has not been 'double-barrelled' this differentiation is somewhat artificial. Generally, the bowel is freed from the abdominal wall to the point where it can be closed and dropped back inside the abdomen without difficulty. If sufficient adhesions remain around the closure, it can be termed extraperitoneal, but usually the peritoneum has been entered via at least one point and the closure is technically intraperitoneal. The advantages of the extraperitoneal closure in no way justify a less meticulous operation. Perfect healing without leakage can be virtually guaranteed provided the edges are excised and accurate suturing effected with an inverting muscular layer ('natural' suturing).

Occasionally, it is necessary to resect the whole stoma and to perform an intraperitonal end-to-end anastomosis.

Complications of stomas

Prolapse

This tends to occur after a colostomy has been performed for obstruction. It requires excision of the prolapsing bowel and the creation of a new stoma.

Colostomy hernia

Mild degrees are common and require only a belt. If operation is required, it invariably involves re-siting of the stoma; the defect is then treated as an incisional hernia and closed separately.

Stenosis

This should not occur if the bowel has been sutured to the skin. If it does, it requires the creation of a new skin to mucosa union of adequate diameter.

Retraction of an ileostomy

If this occurs, it may lead to skin excoriation. It should usually be dealt with by the creation of a new everted stoma.

Skin problems with ileostomy

These embrace much of the specialty of stomatherapy. The essence of the surgeon's task is to provide a flat surface for the appliance and an everted spout to project into it so that ileal contents do not dissect their way between the skin surface and the appliance when the skin has become sore and moist. The solution to this problem is Stomahesive which was created for use in dentistry where adherence to a moist surface is also crucial. A square of this between the appliance and the skin permits adhesion to the moist skin within and to the appliance without. A new and more flexible material for the same purpose is Comfeel (Coloplast). A bag with this material incorporated is the MC2000 (Coloplast).

Management of the permanent colostomy

It was for many years considered unnecessary to use irrigation techniques for the patient with a long-term colostomy. In the United States at least one in two colostomists prefers the method, and it should certainly be offered to all active intelligent colostomists with suitable bathrooms as one of the available options. Good irrigation kits are offered by Hollister, Coloplast and Davol. These guard against perforation by providing a safe cone for insertion into the stoma, and a bag is worn for an hour or so after the fluid has been run in. Investment of an hour or more each morning enables many patients to abandon the use of an appliance during the day except in emergency situations.

Magnetic colostomy

This device was evolved in Erlangen (Hager *et al.*, 1976). In selected patients a magnetic ring can be buried on the rectus sheath around the terminal colostomy at the time of surgery. A corresponding magnetic plug or cap can subsequently be used to seal the stoma and may provide an acceptable degree of continence. The author's experience with the device suggests that the majority of patients can be satisfactorily managed by irrigation techniques alone. The buried magnetic rings have given little trouble and less than 10% have required removal. However, only a few of the patients have continued to make use of their caps, so that the method has not made a major contribution.

Magnetic ileostomy was also proposed by the German group, but is probably contra-indicated since it necessitates making a flush ileostomy. As a result, if continence is less than perfect, troublesome skin excoriation is inevitable.

Caecostomy

This still has many supporters. It has the advantages that it may be performed under local anaesthetic and that there is a good chance of spontaneous closure. It has the disadvantage that it will block unless it is washed through every 2 h, and it does not completely defunction the bowel. Goligher has condemned it because of a high incidence of septic fatalities, but these probably occur when the caecum is not adequately attached to the abdominal wall.

Anastomosis

Colonic and high rectal anastomosis

In skilled hands the risks of breakdown of an anastomosis of the colon or upper rectum are very small. Pulsatile blood supply is a prerequisite, bowel preparation is desirable and antibacterial protection of the patient to be preferred. Faecal spillage should be avoided and mobilisation should be adequate to avoid tension. An inverted anastomosis has been shown to be superior to one in which the mucosa is everted to the peritoneal aspect and the latter technique has now been largely abandoned (Goligher *et al.*, 1970). Provided these factors are respected and combined with precise and atraumatic suturing, it is of little importance what materials are used for the anastomosis, or indeed, in most cases, whether stapling or one or two layer stitching techniques are employed.

The conventional Lembert suture has stood the test of time. The author prefers to follow the submucosal groove for placement of a single layer of interrupted muscle stitches (00 Mersilene or linen thread). The latter groove provides a useful guiding line when the anatomy is otherwise obscured by a fatty mesentery. This method also has the theoretical benefit of avoiding any devascularisation of the submucosal layer by sutures. The importance of the submucosa in the healing process was originally emphasised by Halsted, and most conventional inversion techniques separate the submucosal layers.

Low rectal anastomosis

A different situation exists for anastomosis in the low extraperitoneal part of the rectum. As the anal canal is approached the risk of breakdown rises steeply, irrespective of the anastomotic technique used.

It is possibly true to say that almost all true coloanal anastomoses performed by any method would have at least transient radiological 'leaks' if serial x-rays were taken during the month after surgery. Thus there is a gradient of risk from almost zero at 12 cm from the anal verge to over 50% at 3 cm. Both Lockhart-Mummery (1960) and Goligher (1980) put the leakage rate below the peritoneal reflection at five times greater than when the anastomosis lies above it. Unfortunately the literature is unclear in defining what constitutes a low anastomosis; the term has been applied by some to anastomoses as high as 12 cm where the risk is negligible. At the other extreme, we limit it to cases where the lateral ligaments have been divided, the whole mesorectum excised and an anastomosis made in the lower one-third of the rectum – usually about 4–7 cm from the anal verge. In these patients late anastomotic leakage (7–28 days) is, in our hands, a significant clinical risk and consequently they should all be protected by a temporary loop colostomy. This is not closed until anastomotic integrity has been confirmed radiologically at about 3 weeks.

What is the reason for the unpredictable healing of the very low anastomosis? Clearly the bacteriological hazard is a major factor, but this is in no way confined to the low anastomosis. The colon has to be brought down a very long way, and pulsatile blood supply is not always easy to achieve. In particular, this applies when the surgeon has preserved the inferior mesenteric origin and not fully mobilised the splenic flexure. In our opinion the sigmoid vessels do not provide enough mobility for a tension-free anastomosis in the lower part of the rectum, although they are adequate for anastomosis in the upper rectum. In our series when the sigmoid has been used for an anastomosis almost 50% of the patients have developed leaks (Heald and Leicester 1981). Parks (1977) makes the same point about the unsuitability of the sigmoid colon for his endoanal technique of anastomosis.

The fullest mobilisation is achieved by dividing the inferior mesenteric artery close to the aorta above its first branch and the inferior mesenteric vein close to the splenic vein. In most cases, division of all the avascular structures which tether the left colon will then provide a viable and mobile upper descending colon which can lie without tension in the levator gutter. This is a prerequisite for anastomotic healing at a low level.

A further possible vascular factor is the blood supply of the lower or anorectal end. This is probably only rarely defective and leakage rates seem to be lower when the reservoir is larger and higher in the true colo-anal anastomosis. The reverse would be true if anorectal blood supply were a major factor.

The second potential danger is the size of the splinted cavity which is left by the wide pelvic clearance necessary for removing cancer. Every effort is made to fill this cavity with live colon and with omentum where possible. However, some 'late leaks' are due to the pointing of posterior abscesses or infected haematomas through or just above the anastomosis. The puddling of plasma around the anastomosis may impair adherence of viable surrounding tissue which are an important part of the healing. Thus drainage by suction, sump, or with the aid of irrigation, is probably extremely important.

The problem of healing in a low colorectal and colo-anal anastomosis remains one of the greatest challenges in this kind of surgery. It is likely to be solved only by specialisation with concentration on the technical details of ensuring blood supply, mobilising to eliminate tension, filling the pelvic space, good drainage and bowel preparation, and perhaps a continued need for temporary defunctioning colostomy. No doubt, further factors will be recognised as a low anastomosis is more widely used in patients who would formerly have undergone abdominoperineal excision.

Faecal fistula

Certain important principles govern the management of all fistulas. The track is initially lined by granulation tissue which has the proliferative momentum to occlude it. This process competes with the tendency of the epithelial surface at each end to line it and make it permanent.

If there is distal obstruction or a disease of the epithelial surface (e.g. cancer or Crohn's disease) this will perpetuate the fistula, thus dictating excision of the lesion and reapposition of healthy epithelium on each side. If an abscess cavity separates the two surfaces, this will need to be drained so that granulation tissue and consequent fibrosis will occlude it.

Thus four major factors prevent spontaneous closure of faecal fistulas:

1 Proximity of epithelial surfaces leading to early establishment of epithelial continuity (e.g. recto-vaginal fistula, rectovesical fistula).
2 Intervening abscess cavity.
3 Disease of the epithelium lined fistula (e.g. cancer or Crohn's disease).
4 Distal obstruction (e.g. diverticulitis or cancer).

Investigation thus involves using gastrografin or barium and x-ray of the bowel side of the fistula to establish the nature of distal obstruction or epithelial disease. A fistulogram may also be of value in excluding an abscess which may require drainage. Fistulas where epithelial continuity has been established are usually apparent because the track is short.

Surgical management is conservative provided none of the four primary factors is present. Nutrition in all its aspects is of paramount importance and may involve hyperalimentation, i.e. total parenteral nutrition and vitamin supplements by parenteral means. Surgery involves excision of a diseased segment, drainage of an abscess, or excision of an epithelial lined fistula with separation and reapposition of epithelial surfaces. The use of omentum or other mobile intact organs, such as the caecum, may be of value in separating the two surfaces.

Rectovaginal fistula

This used to be a complication of prolonged labour, but more commonly nowadays follows radiotherapy for uterine cancer or low anastomosis for rectal cancer or as a direct complication of Crohn's disease. Small obstetric fistulas may heal spontaneously and surgery should only be advised after failure to do so after 6 months. The other iatrogenic fistulas will not heal spontaneously, but should only be operated upon when the patient is in good health and all abscesses have drained and inflammatory oedema subsided – if necessary after a period of defunctioning.

If there is primary pathology it is usually rectal, and rectal excision of (for example) the bowel damaged by radiotherapy may be appropriate.

Most fistulas above 5 cm from the anal verge are probably best dealt with by an abdominal operation based upon the principles already ennumerated. In particular, omental or caecal interposition between the rectal anastomosis or closure and the vaginal wall may be used to separate the epithelial surfaces. Similar methods are appropriate for rectovesical fistula.

Fistulas through the lower 5–6 cm of the rectovaginal septum will be tackled from below. The aim is apposition of healthy viable vaginal mucosa without tension, similar apposition of rectal mucosa, plus separation of the two 'layered' closures. This may be achieved by sufficient mobilisation to allow inversion of the mucosal edges into vagina and rectum, by muscle interposition, by advancement flaps of vaginal or rectal wall, or by slight rotation of the mobilised organs in opposite directions. The approach may be vaginal, perineal, anal, rectal, by an anterior anoproctotomy created by opening and excising the fistula track, or by a formal York-Mason postero lateral anoproctotomy.

It should be remembered that the chances of breakdown are increased by the faecal pressure within the rectum so that proximal defunctioning colostomy is often a wise precaution. Failure makes surgery more difficult and is profoundly demoralising for patient and surgeon while temporary colostomy takes much of the anxiety out of the whole process.

Injuries to the colon and rectum

When war or violence strikes unexpectedly, unwary surgeons learn old lessons the hard way. Perhaps the relative safety of planned colonic operations on patients performed with antibacterial cover has diminished the respect of the modern surgeon for the lethal potential of faecal contamination. All too often primary suturing or anastomosis on torn or penetrated colon leads to serious septic complications. Just as the doctrine of excision and non-closure of the bullet wound needs re-emphasising, so does the colonic surgeon need warning of the dangers of unprotected intraperitoneal colonic suture-lines, and the value of the delayed primary colosure of the badly contaminated wound.

Penetrating injury

The high velocity weapon produces a small entry wound, a larger exit wound, and a pear-shaped 'cavity' of destruction due to the dissipation in the tissues of its kinetic energy (*see* Chapter 46). Into this cavity are sucked debris, clothing and other contaminants by the negative pressures in the wake of the bullet. Low velocity bullets and knives cause only direct trauma due to their prenetration.

Closed trauma

Seat-belt perforations, bursting and transection of the colon, and tears of the main colic vessels occur occasionally, in addition to the much commoner small bowel and other visceral injuries.

Principles of management

It is always safer to explore injuries of the abdomen in which there is any likelihood of bowel injury. In all cases it is sensible to anticipate septic contamination and to administer effective antibacterials systemically prior to and during surgery. In closed trauma the small bowel and mesentery are much more likely to be injured than the large, and in every patient each part of the gut must be painstakingly examined. A long midline or paramedian incision is a prerequisite to performing this adequately, and all mesenteries and other organs such as liver and spleen must be carefully inspected. The scheme of management for colonic injury must take account of the danger of contamination by faeces. The more distal the injury is in the colon, the more shattered and shocked the patient and the longer the contamination has been present; the greater the danger. Thus only very occasionally will a simple intraperitoneal suture-line be safe, when an injury is single, recent and uncontaminated. No absolute rules can be laid down, but the choice will follow basic principles:

Principles of management in large bowel injury

A Excision of necrotic gut.
B Re-establishment of integrity of the bowel wall by:
1 primary repair (early, clean, single);
2 resection and anastomosis (early, clean, single);
3 protection by:
   (a) simple end colostomy and delay of the anastomosis;
   (b) exteriorisation;
   (c) proximal loop colostomy;
   (d) thorough irrigation and emptying distal to the point of defunctioning.
4 mobilisation of the rectum for proper inspection, repair and adequate lavage and drainage of the retrorectal space.

Injury to the rectum

The management of rectal injuries frequently calls for ingenuity to match the extraordinary imagination of the people who inflict them. Sexual perversion, vibrators and accidents with sigmoidoscope or enema nozzle provide pitfalls for the clinician. One variant of the 'battered baby syndrome' is the insertion into the rectum of sharp foreign bodies such as needles, with no mark on the skin to provide a clue. Thus, if cause for the injury is absent, the doctor must pick his way through a fog of embarrassment or guilt to establish the truth.

Rectal examination on the conscious patient is of prime importance. Tenderness may be elicited, there may be blood on the finger, or a foreign body may be palpated. Air insufflation for endoscopy must be undertaken with caution. X-ray, including both an erect and lateral view, should never be omitted; it may demonstrate a foreign body high in the bowel or in the peritoneal cavity, and there may be subphrenic gas or extravasated barium. Haemorrhage is a potential danger, both as a consequence of the original trauma and of the manipulation to remove the foreign objects.

Operation

Unusual skill may be called for in the removal of a rectal foreign body. The lithotomy, Trendelenburg or the prone jack-knife positions are suitable for attempted removal from below. Relaxation and lubrication are major allies. Various tricks have proved valuable in

selected situations such as a catheter slipped beyond a rounded object to release the mucosal suction effect and obstetric forceps or a powerful magnet.

Anoproctotomy (York Mason procedure)

This will occasionally provide extra access for removal from below. The jack-knife position is required. The whole anal musculature is divided while each layer is marked with colour-coded sutures so that at the end of the procedure the whole mechanism can be reconstructed.

Laparotomy

This will be required if there is any question of perforation by the original injury or by the attempted removal of a foreign body. When rectal perforation has occurred by injury from below, the tear will usually be irregular with an extensive haematoma. Such lacerations can occasionally be sutured, but the most important surgical steps are:

1 defunctioning by colostomy as close as possible to the injury;
2 complete wash-through of all faeces distal to the colostomy;
3 adequate mobilisation and inspection of the rectum with repair when practical, plus drainage of the retro and pararectal areas.

Sometimes lavage and suction may be needed to clear away extravasated faeces or barium.

Diverticular disease of the colon

Incidence

Diverticula of the colon are common in all people who have eaten Western diets for many years. They are rare before 40 years, but occur with increasing frequency in both sexes thereafter. Only a small proportion of people so affected have any clinical manifestations. Nevertheless the disease is second only to cancer as an indication for colonic surgery.

Principles and pathology

It is an interesting observation, substantiated by surgical experience rather than scientific investigation, that the definitive procedure for complicated diverticular disease is the excision of approximately 15 cm of the most distal sigmoid colon. Diverticula are practically never found in the rectum, but often affect the colon proximal to this segment; nevertheless, they seldom cause trouble other than in the sigmoid colon and complications seldom recur after this conservative colectomy. The explanation is probably to be found in the other pathological process which is now recognised as a crucial part of the disease – muscle shortening and thickening confined to the lower left colon. This is essentially a concertina-like process, in which muscle wall thickening is matched by irregular narrowing of the lumen, producing the characteristic 'prediverticular' saw-tooth appearance on x-ray. Possibly the localisation of inflammatory complications within the sigmoid is a result of a change in diverticular shape due to this process, i.e. the open-mouthed diverticula found higher up are relatively innocuous, but lower down the narrow-necked diverticula may drain poorly or become liable to obstruction at their necks. The chronic symptoms of subacute obstructive pain are easily explained by this 'muscle-binding' of the sigmoid. The complications may occur in one of two ways – firstly, free sudden perforation due to areas of high pressure between segments of spasm, and secondly, inflammation in a poorly draining or blocked diverticulum. The former is rare and usually gives a picture of sudden generalised peritonitis with gas under the diaphragm, and the latter presents a whole range of syndromes analogous to those of appendicitis, indeed the condition once earned the title of left-sided appendicitis.

To these two complications can be added the prodigious capacity of diverticular disease for forming local abscesses and fistulas into adjacent organs. Faecal organisms play a crucial part in the dangerous sequelae of diverticular disease and effective antibacterial blood levels before surgery are a major part of their management. Metronidazole has, in the opinion of many surgeons, been a major step forward in this respect, although the author prefers to combine this anti-anaerobe with an antibiotic such as cefamandole or cephazolin sodium.

Chronic obstructive diverticular disease

This form of the disease is common in out-patients or 'office' practice – it is symptomatic diverticular disease without inflammatory complications. Cramping lower abdominal pains, distension, rabbit-like motions and bowel upsets of all kinds are typical. Rectal examination may reveal some tenderness at the fingertip and multiple faecoliths within diverticula like 'grape-pips'. Sigmoidoscopy may produce spasm and pain which is recognised as similar to the complaint. The surgeon's first duty is to exclude cancer by full investigation, and to remind himself constantly that bleeding of a recurring or persistent nature is rarely from diverticular dis-

ease (*see* Chapter 2). Colonoscopy is indicated in such patients in addition to proctosigmoidoscopy and barium enema.

Total obstruction is unusual although attacks of pain and distension due to subacute obstruction may force the surgeon towards a 'semi-emergency' situation. In such cases an actual inflammatory mass may be palpable and there is a risk of confusion with cancer. X-rays are often helpful in that the shouldered 'apple-core' or 'napkin-ring' malignant stricture differs markedly from the tapering stricture of inflammatory disease throughout which the mucosal pattern can be seen intact. Such observations are not, however, infallible and a persisting mass should be regarded as an indication for operation.

Medical treatment

A high fibre diet is the cornerstone of management. One to two tablespoons of unprocessed bran a day can be disguised on cereals, as gravy or soup thickening, or in cooking, and the importance of true wholemeal bread should be emphasised; most 'brown' breads are useless in this respect. In addition, the fibre containing vegetables are valuable – all the 'C's – cabbage, celery, carrots, cauliflower, cucumber, courgettes, chicory, chinese leaves, celeriac and corn. Various tablets such as bran with calcium phosphate (Fybranta) or methyl cellulose (Celevac) should be chewed or they may form soggy 'bulk-balls' and cause colic. Unfortunately, bran causes flatulence in many people although for most the problem settles after a few weeks' perseverance. Cellulose granules such as Isogel are less likely to cause this problem. The effect of drugs is unpredictable, mebeverine (Colofac) is worth a trial, but most of the traditional tablets and proprietary preparations are of little value.

Indications for surgery

A mass, persisting subacute obstruction, or fear of malignancy are the chief reasons for proceeding to operation in the absence of frank complications. It should be emphasised to the patient that the irritable bowel that predisposed to the condition will probably not return to a completely normal habit. For this reason, it is a mistake to advise surgical treatment in the hope of alleviating minor bowel disturbance. Most surgeons would regard two or more attacks of inflammatory 'diverticulitis' as proper reason for operating, but would treat the first attack conservatively provided it had not been life-threatening. The serious complications such as abscess and fistula, demand surgical correction except in the very frail.

Definitive surgery

In most cases the distal 15–20 cm of the sigmoid is resected. The vessels are taken midway between the inferior mesenteric bundle and the bowel wall. If necessary the bowel can be mobilised by developing the avascular retrorectal plane, but the superior rectal vessels should not be divided unless there is doubt about the diagnosis. Thus the correct diameter of upper rectum as it narrows down to the rectosigmoid can be used for the anastomosis, i.e. the colonic side and the rectal side should be approximately of equal size. The muscle wall on the upper side is thick and sometimes oedematous with a rather narrow lumen. This situation is not always ideal for a stapling gun, since the upper end may not slip readily over the anvil and may thus become split or crushed. The gun is also difficult to introduce around the sacral curve for a high anastomosis in some patients. The author's preference in this situation, therefore, is for a manual suturing technique which also produces no luminal narrowing.

Complications

These frequently occur in the absence of a prior history of chronic disease.

Peritonitis

This may be local, in the left or even right iliac fossa, or may be generalised and spreading. It may represent a purulent inflammation on the surface of the sigmoid colon or be a frank faecal perforation complicated by profound shock. Details of management are given in Chapter 1 on peritonitis, but certain principles will be reiterated here. If the patient is relatively fit and appendicitis or other potentially perforating condition can be ruled out, the treatment can be conservative in the first instance. A fluid intake combined with an effective antibacterial regime such as cephazolin sodium and metronidazole may suffice in the mildest cases. Failure to settle, however, or suspicion of faecal peritonitis, shock or general deterioration should lead to early exploration.

Laparotomy. Traditional management with a loop transverse colostomy and drainage has a high mortality. It is, therefore, essential in cases of frank faecal peritonitis that the septic focus be removed from the peritoneal cavity. Since the patient is unwell the operation should be achieved as simply and quickly as possible. A clamp is placed beyond the septic focus, if this is possible, and sufficient vessels are divided to bring out healthy bowel proximal to the lesion as an end colostomy – either separate from or through the wound.

The lower end is closed and the diseased bowel is removed and sent for histological examination. This procedure is usually referred to as a 'modified Hartmann's operation'. Alternatively, both ends may be brought to the surface so that the later reconnection is easier. If the faecal focus cannot be removed because the pelvis is a mass of matted purulent tissue – the so-called 'frozen pelvis' – a defunctioning colostomy proximal to the lesion is a reasonable alternative. The nearer this is made to the perforated segment, the more effective it will be. Thus a clamp is placed across the lowest accessible piece of bowel and this is brought to the surface as an end colostomy. There is probably some value in then opening the distal bowel and removing any faeces which may be impacted above the perforated segment, as this may perpetuate the faecal leak within the pelvis. When this has been done the end should be closed and the area drained.

Alternative methods. Resection and immediate anastomosis are occasionally appropriate for carefully selected patients in experienced hands. A Paul Mickulicz double-barrelled colostomy can be used when the sigmoid is long and mobile, thereby reducing the second operation to a relatively minor procedure. It is not, however, without problems in inexperienced hands, whereas the scheme that has been outlined is largely safe and can be followed in almost all circumstances.

A second planned colorectal anastomosis can usually be undertaken within 6 weeks if the colon with diverticulitis has been resected, but often not for several months if it is still within the peritoneal cavity. There is always a healthy rectum beyond the diseased area.

Abscess

A mass may be either phlegmon or abscess. If the patient is sick and shows a swinging fever, the latter is likely and drainage is desirable. Usually this must be performed suprapubically and preferably the septic focus removed by the so-called Hartmann's procedure at the same time. In some cases simple drainage of the abscess may suffice and later resection be undertaken only if there is recurrence despite a scrupulously observed high fibre diet regime.

Fistula

It is usually assumed that a diverticular abscess has pointed into the organ concerned, but a history of the acute attack is not always obtainable. Furthermore, evidence of the abscess is often absent so that operation may be simpler than expected.

Colovesical fistula occurs mostly in men because of the direct relation of the sigmoid to the bladder. Symptoms

Table 1

ULCERATIVE COLITIS	CROHN'S DISEASE
Distribution	
Never affects the small bowel	Common in ileum
Worst in the rectum	May affect any part of the gut
Affects whole colon in severe cases	Colon affected in 50%
Continuous extension proximally from rectum to top end of affected bowel	Segmental with skip areas
Anus	
Secondary excoriation is only typical manifestation	Specific anal lesions common
Appearance and gross pathology	
External appearance often normal (e.g. at operation)	Thick 'hose-piped' strictured segments
Fibrotic strictures only occasionally seen	Mucosa oedematous (cobblestoning)
Mucosa a granular red carpet of diffuse inflammation (e.g. at sigmoidoscopy or colonoscopy)	Deep penetrating serpigenous ulcers
Actual ulcers often absent	Mass often present and typically adherent to adjacent tissues (hence fistulas)
Palpable mass rare	
Radiological appearances	
Loss of haustration	Tapered strictures
Mucosal irregularity or oedema	'String-sign', cracks and fissures
Microscopic appearances	
No sarcoid lesions	*Sarcoid lesions diagnostic* but only present in 50%
Diffuse *mucosal* inflammation	Uneven submucosal and *transmural* inflammation with deep irregular ulcer
Crypt abscesses	
Goblet cell depletion	
Serious complications	
Acute fulminating attacks are the chief threat to life	Unusual, though increasingly observed in some areas
Toxic dilation, perforation haemorrhage are particular dangers	*Obstruction* – of a chronic or subacute type is common
	Fistula – may occur into any organ or to the skin or at the anus
Carcinoma	
A significant risk in this mucosal disease if it lasts over 10 years	Is described as a slight risk – but not clinically important
Widespread precancerous changes can be detected in some cases (colonoscopy)	Not seen
Symptoms	
Typically blood and mucus diarrhoea + colic and urgency	Unpredictable bowel upset with colic due to subacute obstruction
Anaemia, weight loss, inanition	Similar
Medical treatment	
1 Symptomatic	
Codeine, Loperamide, etc	Similar. Cholestyramine after resection
2 Specific	
*(A) Salazopyrine	
For long-term control in chronic disease 1 g 6-hourly reducing to half this dose as maintenance	Unpredictable, but probably same in distal small bowel and colonic Crohn's disease
(B) Steroids	
Mainstay of the treatment of the acute attack	Always worth a clinical trial particularly in fulminating disease
	(C) Dapsone
	Occasionally of value
	(D) Azathiaprine
	This is worth trying in chronic fistulating disease which is unsuitable for operation

Table 1—contd.

ULCERATIVE COLITIS	CROHN'S DISEASE

Surgery
Extent

Total proctocolectomy or colectomy especially to save life in fulminating disease	Resection of single segment disease causing obstruction or fistula End-to-side by-pass for obstruction in multisegment disease
Recurrence never occurs if all large bowel mucosa has been removed	Recurrence common though often long delayed Typically located just proximal to an anastomosis

Metastatic

Polyarthritis, sacro-iliitis, anklyosing spondylitis, episcleritis, iritis	Also occur simultaneously

Liver – pericholangitis, sclerosing cholangitis, II° biliary cirrhosis, bile duct cancer
Skin – erythema nodosum, pyoderma gangrenosum

*N.B. Minor side effects such as indigestion and headache are common. Enteric coated or suppositories may be useful. Regular blood pictures to detect occasional progressive aplastic anaemia. Sterility in males – reversible when discontinued. Agranulocytosis may occur suddenly.

may be obvious and disturbing i.e. the passage of wind with the urinary stream, or, (exceptionally) in the presence of prostatic hypertrophy, of urine per anum. Sometimes, however, the condition may be missed because there is simply a slight urinary frequency and the passage of 'tea leaves' from time to time. A granular area on the bladder vault, perhaps wrongly labelled 'cystitis cystica', should always alert the cystoscopist to the possibility of this important condition. An erect x-ray revealing an air-urine fluid level is often diagnostic. Surgery is usually indicated except in the very frail and elderly with minimal symptoms where careful observation may sometimes suffice.

Operation. There is usually adequate time for full bowel preparation in the hope that a one-stage resection will be practicable. As with all the complications of diverticular disease, the surgeon must be prepared to protect his anastomosis with a transverse colostomy if this seems wise, or to perform a Hartmann type of segmental excision if a friable-walled abscess is present and primary anastomosis appears hazardous. The abscess will need adequate drainage in addition to the defunctioning achieved by the end colostomy. Often, however, the adherent sigmoid can simply be 'pinched' off the back of the bladder, a one-stage resection undertaken, and the bladder drained for a week. The use of omentum, retaining its vascular pedicle, can prove invaluable in assisting healing and separating the two organs.

Other internal fistulas. These are managed on similar lines: drainage for an abscess, excision of the distal 15 cm of sigmoid if possible, immediate anastomosis if it appears safe, or defunctioning when necessary.

Bleeding in diverticular disease (see Ch 2)

This is quite separate from the inflammatory complications of diverticulitis which are seldom associated with bleeding. Diverticular bleeding is sudden, major, typically painless, and not usually associated with the passage of a stool. It occurs in the elderly and hypertensive and comes from tiny granulations or ulcers at the necks of diverticula anywhere in the colon, particularly from open diverticula in the right or transverse colon. In some patients the diverticula may be coincidental and the bleeding comes from angiodysplasia which also occurs in the elderly and is the commonest site of major haemorrhage. Fortunately, the majority stop bleeding spontaneously and in less than a third does the haemorrhage recur subsequently. Therefore, the treatment is primarily that of major haemorrhage; blood transfusion monitored by central venous pressure observation and the introduction of a urinary catheter. Emergency operation is rarely required but, if contemplated, must be preceded by gastroduodenoscopy to exclude gastric or duodenal haemorrhage, plus careful proctosigmoidoscopy and selective angiography. Barium enema should be avoided in the acute situation as it will frustrate angiography for several days. If angiography does identify the bleeding point, local resection may suffice, if not a subtotal colectomy and ileorectal anastomosis is the only procedure that can be relied upon to control the bleeding.

Non-specific inflammatory bowel disease (Table 1)

This term is customarily reserved for the two major conditions of unknown aetiology, ulcerative colitis and

Crohn's disease. Diagnosis usually rests on the exclusion of specific infective conditions by stool microscopy and culture and then the establishment of a composite clinical picture pointing to one or other disease. Errors and overlap are common and, in contrast with tumour management, it is the clinician rather than the histopathologist who generally has the last word. Table 1 is dedicated to this clinical tug of war and attempts to list the most important characteristics of each condition. It must be borne in mind, however, that the only incontrovertible diagnostic features are the presence of involved ileal segments and the recognition of sarcoid-like granulomas – either of which exclude a diagnosis of ulcerative colitis.

Indications for operation in ulcerative colitis (Table 1)

In colitis confined to the rectum and distal left colon, the patient is seldom very ill and seldom requires surgery. Thus severe disease is usually widespread, and it is this total colitis which most concerns the surgeon. Surgery may be performed to save life during an acute attack, or it may be considered as an interval procedure for recurrent severe attacks or for 'metastatic' distant complications. Monitors of progress include (1) the clinical state, (2) the pulse rate, (3) the girth and the diameter of the transverse colon on x-ray, (4) abdominal tenderness.

This disease can be cured by total excision of the colon and rectum. The 300–400 deaths which occur each year in the UK are, therefore largely preventable and are almost entirely deaths due to acute fulminating disease. An insidious onset is, perhaps, the most common pitfall, so that high dosage steroids, nutritional support and blood transfusion – the cornerstones of medical management – become delayed for perhaps days or weeks. Timely admission to hospital is essential, and failure to improve after a week (occasionally less) of intensive medical treatment indicates that operation may not be safely deferred.

Crile compared the acute attack of ulcerative colitis to 'an enormous third degree burn with a faecal poultice'. When progressive distension occurs it is the harbinger of doom, because this toxic dilatation reflects a failure of the intrinsic nerve plexuses to maintain normal propulsive tone in the gut. Faecal perforation with the great danger of death is not far away and immediate operation is indicated. The clinician must not be misled by a reduction in stool frequency which may simply reflect the breakdown of peristaltic activity. Straight x-ray is valuable and may be repeated to follow progress when the dilated colon (more than 6 cm in diameter at mid transverse colon) is outlined with gas, and the mucosal islands of oedematous colonic mucosa are characteristic. Haemorrhage is another serious complication. While blood and mucus are the hallmarks of the disease, the passage of fresh blood in volumes of over a unit during an acute attack constitute an indication for emergency operation.

Complications and the cancer risk

Pyoderma gangrenosum is usually cured by excision of the colon and rectum, as is arthritis of the large joints, erythema nodosum and the eye complications. Cirrhosis may not respond at all and careful consideration is required in each individual patient.

The cancer risk has probably occupied more space and led to the sacrifice of more colon than it justifies. It is never a significant factor unless there is total colitis which has been clinically apparent for at least ten years. Thus the colon should seldom be removed purely for its cancer risk without seeking at least one second opinion. The chronic ulcerative colitic is usually easy to colonoscope and precancerous changes may be widespread and detectable by random biopsy before invasive cancer appears. Thus regular colonoscopy every 2–3 years and prompt investigation of new symptoms may often be adequate. The true risk is probably almost nil in the first ten years, about 5% in the second ten years, and may approach 25% by the end of thirty years. Thus particular care is required in the small latter group, but there is adequate time in most people to await further results of the efforts currently directed towards cancer avoidance by predictive endoscopic biopsy (Lennard-Jones et al., 1977). Pseudopolyposis is not an indication of possible malignancy, but is often related to regeneration and recovery.

Childhood

The usual problem with children who have ulcerative colitis is a failure to thrive, grow and develop. A difficult balance exists between the tendency towards creating a Cushing syndrome by steroid treatment and the desirability of avoiding ileostomy at school age. Usually a firm decision to operate pays the highest dividends.

Pregnancy

Where possible drug therapy is avoided in the first trimester. Otherwise the disease is treated as it would be in the absence of pregnancy. Sometimes spontaneous regression of disease occurs in pregnancy with reversal after delivery.

The operation in ulcerative colitis

The extent of resection

The definitive operation for ulcerative colitis is the complete removal of the colon and rectum. It is usually a mistake to resect only part of the colon, and early activity in the remainder is the common sequel. The excellent results of Aylett (1966) in his cases of ileorectal anastomosis have not been generally repeated by other workers, although the Cleveland Clinic group is currently advocating it as the initial operation of choice in most cases. Although worthy of a trial in certain patients who are anxious to avoid ileostomy, it is often followed by recrudescence of disease in the residual mucosa, i.e. the rectal stump. This must always be carefully monitored remembering the long-term cancer risk.

Modern alternatives to ileostomy

The question of anal preservation is likely to become important in the future following some promising early results from Parks et al., (1980) with the creation of an ileal reservoir anastomosed to the anus at the level of the dentate line. This is a logical development of the Kock (1969) internal reservoir. In both procedures the lower 30–40 cm of ileum are converted into an nonexpulsive reservoir. The metabolic consequences have been fully investigated in Kock's unit and are not severe. In the Kock technique, the pouch is protected by a complex nipple valve situated deep to the anterior abdominal wall. The patient catheterises the pouch through a flush ileostomy and is thus spared the wearing of an appliance – an advantage which many ileostomists would question.

The Parks' pouch is much simpler to create with no trouble-prone valve required. It is anastomosed to the dentate line and, therefore, requires the retention of the anal sphincters which render the pouch continent. In some cases spontaneous defaecation of relatively normal motions has been achieved, although somewhat high stool frequencies of 6–10 motions per day sometimes ensue. So far the operation has been performed only as a primary procedure and the pouch usually protected by a loop ileostomy for 6–8 weeks. The possibility exists, however, that the primary operation might be to excise the colon and rectum from above, followed in selected and well motivated patients by a secondary procedure in a special centre to create the pouch and join it to the anal 'stump'.

With this ultimate hope in mind the author preserves the lower anal canal and sphincters when operating for ulcerative colitis, although the value of doing so remains unproven.

Total proctocolectomy and ileostomy

The ileostomy site should be marked by the stomatherapist prior to surgery. Total removal of the colon should be carried out without devitalising large bunches of mesenteric tissue which may lead to band obstruction later; full mobilisation prior to ligation of the vessels minimises this problem. The transverse colon should be dissected out of the greater omentum which is preserved as a pelvic filler. Its blood supply is derived almost entirely from the anterior layer and is not compromised. Excision of the rectum can be most expeditiously achieved in the female by following the plane posterior to and outside the mesorectum right down into the levator gutter keeping close to the rectal and mesorectal surface. Here it will lead to a clean anorectal ring where the rectum may be cross clamped and pulled up into the wound before cutting it off through the upper part of the anal canal – within the anorectal ring of muscle (author's method). Alternatively, a perineal operator may, with the aid of dilute adrenaline solution, dissect out the whole 'inner tube' of anus in the plane between the external and internal sphincters. In either of these procedures the levators, the external sphincters, the anorectal ring, and the nerves in the pelvic fascia are preserved. To this end also the dissection in the male, where potency should be a high priority, is kept close to the muscle wall within the mesorectum. This adds to the difficulty, because numerous vessels passing forwards into the rectum from the superior rectal bundle must be divided. It is, however, generally believed to safeguard the autonomic plexuses to the maximal extent and the residual mesorectal tissue may also be of some value in filling the pelvis. For this reason many surgeons prefer the same technique in the female. Continuous closed suction drainage is instituted for 5–7 days as necessary.

Subtotal colectomy with ileostomy and mucous fistula

It is a prevalent and reasonable compromise to preserve the lowest part of the sigmoid and the rectum to minimise operative trauma. If this is done, however, the end must be brought out as a mucous fistula, because closure and replacement of the diseased bowel may lead to a local abscess. In most cases the lower end will have to be excised later and, in a few, haemorrhage or persistent disease will cause serious trouble. It is probably better, therefore, if the patient's condition permits, to remove the whole large intestine at the first operation.

Ileostomy and blow-hole colostomies

Some lives have undoubtedly been saved by multiple colostomies when a patient has been in extremis (Turnbull and Schofield, 1970). Ileostomy plus one or more blow-hole colostomies may occasionally be appropriate, especially if there is a walled-off perforation. This is, however, extemporising and should be followed by elective resection in due course.

Indications for surgery in Crohn's disease (Table 1)

In most patients Crohn's disease is probably a generalised gut disease and is almost always more extensive than it first appears. The radical excision of cancer surgery should not, therefore, be followed in Crohn's, because operations are directed against symptoms and will seldom eradicate the disease.

Their danger lies in the fact that an ill-conceived suture line through actively diseased tissue may leak or lead to fistula and the situation thus be made worse. Unnecessary sacrifice of small intestine may also worsen the patient's lot since malabsorption and inanition are his long-term plight.

Operation is of greatest value in the relief of obstruction or fistula, particularly when this is of long standing and due to single segment disease. Indeed, the results from the common terminal ileal resection (usually with conservative hemicolectomy) have been so good at the five- and ten-year point as to lead some surgeons to believe that they have indeed 'cured' a half to two-thirds of their patients. Longer follow-up, however, eventually uncovers many patients with a recurrence just proximal to the suture-line. The reason for this is by no means apparent and no drug therapy is known that reduces it.

When surgery for single segment obstructive disease is undertaken and there is no visible disease elsewhere the question is how much to remove? Some have recommended as much as 25 cm and some as little as 1 cm, while a compromise of around 2–3 cm would probably seem reasonable to most in the absence of hard evidence one way or the other. Where multiple segments make removal of all visible disease impractic-

able, opinions differ between palliative by-pass of an obstruction and local segmental excision. Where by-pass is undertaken it should probably be of the end-to-side variety with a mucous fistula on the distal side above the obstructing segment.

Single segments of large bowel disease, especially solitary granuloma of the caecum, frequently do well after excision. Large bowel disease has a common association with anal lesions, and both excision of the proximal disease and defunctioning by colostomy may have some beneficial effect on the anal lesions.

Acute Crohn's disease

The patient with a short history suggestive of appendicitis, but appearances at laparotomy of Crohn's disease, usually does not have true Crohn's disease. A varieity of infective agents such as *Yersinia* can produce a thick inflamed segment of bowel and resolution will occur without resection which should, therefore, be avoided.

Anorectal manifestations of Crohn's disease

In 1949 Crohn reported anal lesions in 17.5% of his own patients, but little attention was paid to the anal disease until the papers of Lockhart-Mummery and Morson (1960, 1964). For many surgeons the anal lesions not only are a common and integral part of the clinical syndrome of Crohn's disease, but have become the diagnostic tag and their progress often reflects the state of the disease within. Histological confirmation by discovery of sarcoid-like granulomas from the anal lesions is claimed in two-thirds of the St Mark's series although this requires careful searching for granulation tissue from a suitable crevice. Anal lesions occur in around one-third of those with ileal Crohn's, two-thirds of those with colonic, and almost all of those with frank rectal Crohn's disease – all of these figures applying to follow-up over many years (Lockhart-Mummery, 1972).

The lesions most characteristically seen are as follows:

Fissures which are really anal ulcers are not necessarily specific to the anterior or posterior position. These produce soreness rather than the pain so characteristic of simple fissure, or they may be painless. They are deep, undermining and penetrating ulcers which are indolent. They may be deep and cavitating, sometimes internal to the sphincters.

Oedematous cyanotic skin tags, often ulcerated and inaccurately called by some, the ulcerated pile complex. Mechanical complications of these ulcers include the following:

1 Abscess
2 Fistula   (a) *High fistula* due to cavitating ulceration through the wall above the sphincters. The external opening may be far away through the scrotum.
                  (b) *Low fistula* due to faecal penetration of the undermined edges of an ulcer often producing multiple openings.
3 Stricture   This may be very difficult to differentiate from carcinoma.
4 Rectovaginal fistula.

Differential diagnosis

This includes simple fissure and tuberculosis, malignancy and lymphogranuloma.

Treatment

Control of proximal disease is of paramount importance. Active surgical intervention in Crohn's ulceration is best avoided by the surgeon as the wounds may not heal and the disease may progress. Surgical management of the mechanical problems of certain fistulas, however, may be rewarding provided the actual disease process is quiescent or controlled.

The most difficult decision is when to advise abdominoperineal excision. Up to half of the perineal wounds in most series fail to heal for a year or more so that a reasonable alternative is to avoid proctectomy at the time of colectomy. Goligher (1980) has pursued this policy in his own series for some years and estimates that only half of such patients require subsequent rectal excision because of persisting trouble from the stump. This suggests a new conservative approach to management in which the rectal stump is only excised if it gives trouble, despite control of proximal disease and faecal diversion.

Specific infections and disorders

Amoebiasis

It is a disaster to treat amoebiasis as ulcerative colitis with steroids and colectomy and the patient is likely to die of anastomotic breakdown. Entamoeba histolytica is sensitive to metronidazole 2–3 g per day for one week and most of the unpleasantness of former treatments is now avoided. The problem is largely one of awareness.

The typical disease after 1–2 weeks incubation is acute dysentery with a tendency to relapse or become chronic when it can be confused with colitis or Crohn's disease. A short course of metronidazole is, therefore, a wise precaution. Liver abscesses and amoeboma are occasional clinical problems. Men are affected more often than women. Diagnosis depends upon the examination of warm stools or mucus or pus from endoscopy for trophozoites or cysts. The fluorescent antibody titre may help in the diagnosis.

Bacillary dysentery (Shigella group)

This is a contagious bloody diarrhoea with an incubation period of a few days. It may be mild (*Sh. Sonnei*) or severe (*Sh. Shigae*). Sigmoidoscopic appearances vary from diffuse hyperaemia to membrane formation, ulceration and even necrosis. Shigella is isolated from the stools. Treatment is by fluid replacement plus either tetracycline, ampicillin or chloramphenicol.

Schistosomiasis

Particularly prevalent on the African continent, this disease is most important for its hepatic and urological manifestations. However, schistosomal polyps and ulcers may produce symptoms and signs similar to rectal cancer. Stools must be examined for ova and biopsy must also be reviewed with the schistosome in mind. Treatment is with niridazole (Ambilhar).

Tuberculosis

This is common throughout India and Pakistan. The ileocaecal region is the most frequent location where a mass may occur and closely mimic carcinoma. Multiple ileal strictures are also seen in some patients. Tuberculous peritonitis with ascites is a further possibility. Treatment is by antituberculous drugs.

Giardiasis

This is by no means rare as a cause of bowel upset in Britain. Careful stool study should make the diagnosis, and the condition is treated by metronidazole.

Actinomycosis

This may occur in the rectum, the sigmoid colon or in the caecal region. A woody pericolitis and a frozen pelvis or iliac fossa are typical. Multiple fistulas make the diagnosis obvious, but are not invariably present. Diagnosis is by biopsy and treatment is by penicillin in very large doses until resolution occurs.

Campylobacter

This is a widespread cause of an acute painful attack of diarrhoea with bleeding. Erythromycin is effective, but probably unnecessary.

Pseudomembranous colitis

This condition caused great confusion in the past and sometimes caused death in sick patients on treatment in hospital with clindamycin or lincomycin. It is now realised that the cause is an overgrowth of the anaerobe *Cl. difficile* and usually occurs during treatment with antibiotics, most particularly those that have some effect against some anaerobes. Severe diarrhoea and a white membrane on sigmoidoscopy are characteristic. The condition may develop suddenly and dangerously and may require intensive general supportive therapy – specific treatment is with metronidazole.

Other infective conditions

Readers are referred to *Colorectal Disease* edited by Thomson, J.P.S. *et al.* (1981).

Radiation enterocolitis and proctitis

Pelvic irradiation by an uterine implant is the usual culprit and the nearby rectum or a loop of ileum tethered by adhesions is the usual victim. More recently the use of dosage above 5000 rads has led to similar problems from external radiation – indeed, transient diarrhoea and colic are almost invariable during the early weeks after heavy pelvic irradiation. The true problem, however, is a long-term ischaemic fibrosis of the bowel wall and enfeeblement of the mucosa which is progressive for many years after the irradiation has ceased.

The mucosa appears pale, thin, telangiectatic and sometimes ulcerated. Fistula into the vagina or elsewhere is common.

There is no treatment apart from excision, and this has a high risk of anastomotic failure and stricture. The Parks' sleeve technique has been successfully modified by Cook with excellent results in Johannesburg where rectovaginal fistula from this cause is common (Cook and de Moor, 1981).

Ischaemic colitis

Though only recognised in the last two decades, this condition is not rare. Ischaemic sloughing of the mucosa of the colon occurs quite suddenly. Usually this leads to transient infection and resolution, but sometimes to sacculation and stricturing of the affected segment most commonly at the splenic flexure. Occasionally the ischaemia is so severe as to produce full thickness damage with faecal peritonitis. The condition may follow inferior mesenteric artery ligation performed as a part of aneurysm surgery, particularly if an internal iliac artery has also been ligated, when a rectal stricture can occur. However, it more commonly occurs spontaneously and large vessel blockage by thrombosis or embolus is usually not apparent. It is thus necessary to postulate a fall in flow below what is required for mucosal viability.

The condition should be suspected when an elderly person, particularly one with hypertension or atherosclerosis, develops sudden abdominal pain followed by bloody diarrhoea. Though there may be appreciable blood loss, the attack is usually self-limiting and settles in a few days. Pyrexia and leucocytosis are usual, but abdominal signs are generally slight except with the severe full-thickness variety. It can be differentiated from diverticular and angiodysplastic bleeding because these are generally painless without leucocytosis or pyrexia.

The stricturing variety is recognised on a subsequent barium enema by the tapered hunting horn stricture and by antimesenteric sacculation which is due to bulging of weakened areas of bowel wall. Mucosal oedema and protrusion produces a characteristic thumbprinting along the affected bowel. The colon may be severely damaged and produce obstructive pain that dictates operation. It is surprising how much functional improvement occurs despite marked x-ray changes and the general policy should be conservative.

Operation may be required in the acute phase because the patient's condition deteriorates and signs of peritonitis develop. In such patients patchy yellow areas of necrosis are observed at laparotomy and it is usually obvious how much bowel must be removed. The anastomosis is generally best delayed and the two ends are initially brought to the surface as colostomies.

If surgery becomes necessary for the stricturing variety, this may be preceded by bowel preparation and a primary intraperitoneal anastomosis undertaken.

Pneumatosis cystoides intestinalis

This is a curious condition in which multiple gas cysts occur along the wall of the large or small intestine. It produces symptoms of mucous diarrhoea and colic and the gas cysts provide a dramatic x-ray appearance. The coexistence in many cases of obstructive airway disease has led to the suggestion that gas tracks retroperitoneally from the mediastinum into the wall of the bowel. A more credible idea is that the cysts form in dilated obstructed lymphatics, although the cause is not known.

Since the gas is predominantly nitrogen, the breathing over several days of high concentrations of oxygen may result in its resorption. Surprisingly, recurrence is not invariable and the condition is relatively benign.

Cathartic colon–melanosis coli

The long-standing habit of ingesting senna leads to pigmentation of the colonic mucosa with lipofuschin. This is of little clinical significance although the true cathartic colon may become virtually functionless and ahaustral on x-ray with characteristic slowly moving 'pseudo-strictures'. Rarely the functional effect may be severe with diarrhoea and electrolyte loss.

Idiopathic megacolon and megarectum

This term implies chronic large bowel distension without an obvious obstructive cause. It thus overlaps with some causes of adult Hirschprung's disease where the agangliomic segment requires identification by full thickness biopsy of a strip of muscle just above the anorectal ring under anaesthetic (Todd, 1977).

Such cases are generally free from any anal leakage or soiling which helps to differentiate them from the truly idiopathic variety. Treatment in the adult is by ultra-low anterior resection with special care being required to avoid autonomic nerve damage.

The truly idiopathic variety of megacolon poses great problems for the surgeon. The 'paper-thin colon' affects females more than males and is managed by Epsom salts or liquid paraffin in most cases. If surgery has to be advised in the occasional intractable case, then colectomy and anastomosis of the mobilised right colon to the top of the rectum is probably the most satisfactory measure available.

Volvulus

This occurs with a long mobile sigmoid colon; it produces total obstruction for gas and the condition is often recurrent. Typically, it occurs with a geographical distribution in certain racial groups and also on diets largely composed of fibre. A recurrent variety of subacute obstruction and distension is occasionally seen in young women and may be accompanied by changes in heart rhythm.

Ischaemic necrosis of the bowel wall is fortunately rare and carries a poor prognosis. The condition is suspected because of the enormity of the distension and recognised by the gross dilatation of a huge sigmoid loop on x-ray. Where possible the loop is deflated sigmoidoscopically and in most cases managed definitively by planned sigmoid resection since no form of fixation has ever been shown to be reliable.

The deflation may be achieved by the sigmoidoscope itself or may require a 7 mm rubber tube which, well lubricated, is passed through it. The point of obstruction is usually around 25 cm from the anus. In the occasional patient in whom strangulation has occurred, this will generally not succeed. Other pointers to laparotomy are severe pain, signs of peritonitis and a leucocytosis. Immediate resection and proximal-end colostomy will usually be appropriate with anastomosis at a second operation some weeks later.

Caecal volvulus also occurs as an occasional complication of malrotation of the gut with an unduly mobile caecum. X-ray is characteristic and management is by resection or by fixation which can be achieved with a caecostomy.

Large bowel polyps

Adenoma

The common benign neoplasm of large bowel epithelium is the adenomatous polyp which presents as a pedunculated tubular adenoma like a raspberry on a stalk. At the other end of the range is the sessile carpet of villous tumour, and between these extremes intermediate forms of tubulo-villous adenoma are recognised. Malignant potential is first observed as cytological changes and typically variation in nuclear size and shape with deeper staining and an increase in mitotic figures. The term carcinoma *in situ* is sometimes wrongly used and it is important to reserve the term carcinoma in this situation for those cases where invasion of the muscularis mucosae occurs.

The malignant potential of any lesion is proportional to its size and its position on the tubular to villous spectrum. Thus a purely tubular adenoma of less than 1 cm diameter has a 1% chance of having developed malignant invasion and one of over 2 cm a 10–35% chance: the same figures for villious lesions are 10% for a 1 cm lesion and 40–50% for one in excess of 2 cm. This explains the common disappointment of finding that an apparently villous lesion has already developed into invasive cancer (Fig 12.1).

Treatment. The treatment of adenomatous polyps is not to biopsy them but to remove them completely. If, as it commonly is, the malignant change seen on microscopy is of well differentiated type and the stalk at the point of division is not invaded, the risk of more distant spread is less than 1% and careful follow-up is all that is required. This risk rises to 10% for the poorly differentiated and much rarer lesions, so that more radical surgery is then indicated. The removal of villous lesions sometimes provides a considerable technical challenge to the surgeon. They are commonest in the rectum where large or circumferential lesions can be managed most readily and most safely by low anterior resection, which seems justified because of the risk of

malignancy. Biopsy is unreliable unless it is specifically sampling an area detected as hard by digital examination. If the upper limit of a large lesion cannot be felt digitally, it is safer to manage it as if it were malignant. Small and intermediate villous lesions can be removed transanally or by anoprototomy using the technique advocated by Parks of raising the mucosa off the rectal wall by dilute adrenaline solution. These lesions often have an assocaition with other benign or malignant tumour elsewhere in the bowel, so that colonoscopy or a good double contrast enema is mandatory. Careful and thorough follow-up is required for the same reason and also because recurrence after local excision is common. If perfect visualisation of the whole colorectal mucosa has been achieved, it is probably reasonable to defer the next investigations for three years. It is impossible to state with certainty when follow-up can safely be discontinued.

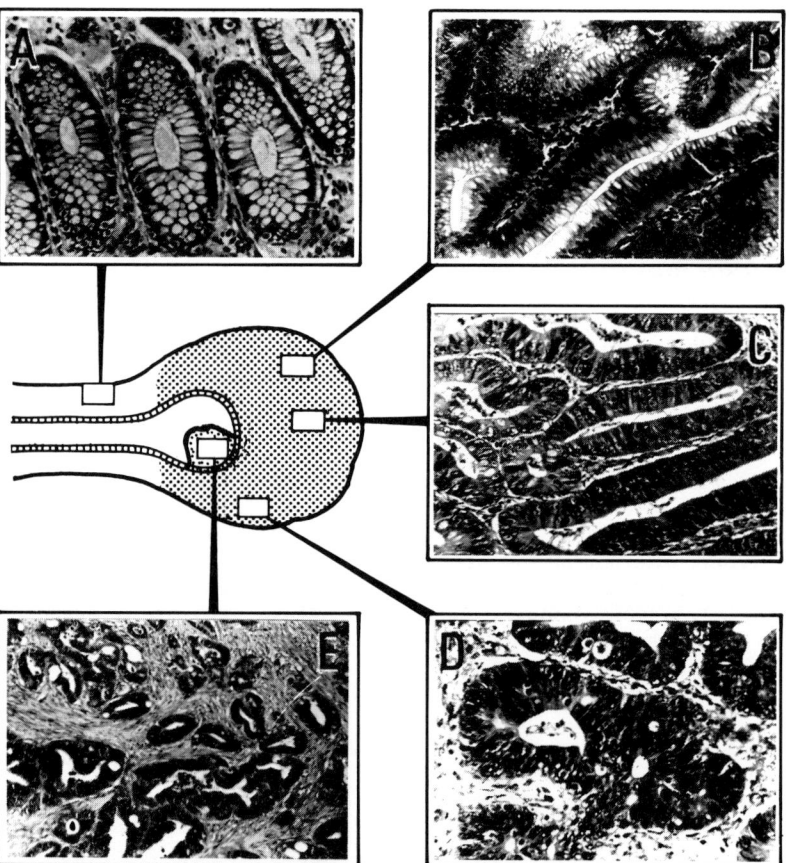

Fig 12.1   Morphology of adenoma – adenocarcinoma sequence. A. Normal epithelium. B. Mild dysplasia. C. Moderate dysplasia. D. Severe dysplasia. E. Invasive carcinoma. (From *Colorectal Disease*, Thomson James P.S., Nicholls R.J., Williams Christopher B., eds., Fig 8.3, p. 242 by courtesy of the Editors.)

Other polyps

Metaplastic polyps

These are common lesions with a watery appearance, usually under 1 cm in diameter and typically without a stalk. They are harmless. The rare metaplastic polyposis, therefore, does not justify colectomy.

Juvenile polyps

This is typically a bleeding prolapsing red cherry in a child. It may require excision or it may autoamputate. It has no tendency to become malignant and, therefore, in the rare occurrence of juvenile polyposis there is no justification for colectomy and the tumours should be managed one by one. It is microscopically quite different from an adenoma, being a hamartoma covered by normal mucosa and containing cystic spaces – the so-called mucus retention polyp.

Lymphoid polyps

The commonest type is found particularly in the rectum and is a benign lymphoma. There is a possibility of the polyp which is removed by a snare being misdiagnosed on histological grounds as a lymphosarcoma and major ablative surgery being undertaken unnecessarily. Lymphosarcoma does occur occasionally and there is also a rare lymphosarcomatous variety of polyposis. However, the much commoner simple lymphoma requires no special treatment, even if it has been incompletely excised.

Submucous lipoma

This may occur anywhere in the gut, but is rather rare in the rectum, though well recognised in the caecum.

Leiomyoma and leiomyosarcoma

These may be intramural or they may project into the lumen as a polyp and erosion of the overlying mucosa leads to haemorrhage and their recognition.

Familial adenomatosis

Familial polyposis is a Mendelian dominant with an 80% penetrance so that about 40% of each generation of either sex is affected. This risk applies as much to the offspring of new mutations without a familial history, as to members of established families. The polyps start to appear at the age of about 10–12 years and always affect the rectum. Thus sigmoidoscopy only is required for screening which should start during the teens. A total of between 200 and 2000 adenomas or villous lesions may be expected in the whole of the large intestine. The average age at which cancer develops is 40 years and almost 50% of patients with cancer will have two lesions by the time of operation, compared with only 3.5% in non-polyposis patients. The essential tragedy of the disease is that two-thirds of those who present with symptoms have already developed carcinoma. Thus a programme of family screening and ablative surgery at a socially acceptable time in the twenties can be expected to save many lives.

Since familial adenomatosis is a disease of the rectum and colon, its complete cure requires total excision of the whole of the large bowel. Until recently this has meant total proctocolectomy with rectal excision and permanent ileostomy. We can now add the alternative of the ingenious mucosal proctectomy, with ileal reservoir and anal sleeve anastomosis (Parks *et al.*, 1980). Parks now regards this operation as the procedure of choice in polyposis, but reasonable results have been obtained by the compromise procedure of ileoproctostomy which is likely to remain the favoured treatment in many centres. In sparing one patient a permanent stoma, it probably saves more lives of siblings to whom a colectomy thus becomes acceptable than it loses because of cancer in the rectal stump. It appears from the St Mark's experience that the total cumulative rectal cancer risk due to the retained rectum will prove to be around 6–10% provided careful monitoring is carried out. A much higher incidence is reported by the Mayo Clinic, which is probably a reflection on its vast catchment area, but also underlines the potential danger. Thus the surgeon who advises colectomy with ileorectal anastomosis has a clear responsibility to monitor and control the patient's rectal stump for the remainder of his life.

A well recognised variant of adenomatosis is Gardner's syndrome in which mesodermal tumours, osteomas of the jaws, epidermoid and sebaceous cysts and a variety of other tumours occur. This extraordinary syndrome demonstrates that large bowel adenomas can be part of a complex connective tissue and epithelial disorder, which includes many other abnormalities, in particular the other soft tissue tumours, but also carcinoma of the ampulla of Vater and a variety of small bowel lesions. One practical importance is that the visible skin lesions may precede the polyps and thus make family control easier. In addition, there is a surprising tendency towards the formation of desmoid tumours in the abdominal wall or retroperitoneum after excision of the colon. Although these tumours are not frankly malignant and progress very slowly, they may become impossible to control by surgery or by any other form of treatment because of local infiltration and the eventual involvement of such vital organs as the ureters. This is important because it may produce the occasional lapse in the otherwise constructive business of cancer prevention in multiple polyposis.

Cancer

General considerations

Probably the greatest challenge in colorectal cancer surgery is that three out of four patients who undergo average investigation and treatment still die of their disease (Slaney, 1971). Against this bleak fact must be weighed the achievements of specialised surgeons in centres whose overall 5-year survival figures often exceed 50% and approach 60–70% in 'radical' cases, although selection of cases may be partly responsible.

The majority of tumours are relatively well-differentiated adenocarcinomas whose biological nature is markedly favourable when compared with tumours arising higher in the gut. Most of them appear to spend years confined to the wall of the bowel, initially as adenomas and then as carcinomas of Dukes A type when cure is comparatively easy (*see* Fig 12.2). They are probably confined within pericolic tissues or lymphatics for many further months or years where skilled radical excision may yet salvage the patient. In most series less than 20% are obviously incurable due to liver metastases or peritoneal spread at the time of their first operation. Unfortunately, at the time of presentation even fewer are early 'A' lesions confined to the wall of the bowel, and this clearly calls for effort towards earlier diagnosis in the future.

Lymphatic spread is of prime importance. Although reported in one-third or less of the cases in many series, and 45% at St Mark's Hospital, Gilchrist (1959) showed that there are involved nodes near to the tumour in two-thirds of all cases resected for cure if sufficient time is spent looking for them. Thus at present more than 3 out of 5 patients operated upon pose a real opportunity for surgical virtuosity and merit the widest lymphatic clearance that can be achieved. Adherence to adjacent organs is due to microscopically malignant disease in only 50% of cases and even then does not warrant undue pessimism. Size and adherence are never a contraindication to surgery and seldom profoundly adverse to prognosis. Indeed, the very large tumour which has not metastasised is often prognostically favourable, because it has a lower malignant potential. In every respect, treatment of these tumours repays the determined surgeon or oncologist with a special interest in the subject. There is great danger for the future in the surgical nihilism which spreads from breast oncology where cancer is regarded as a systemic disease. Each patient with bowel cancer deserves the

surgical consideration due to a lethal disease which remains technically resectable for a remarkably long time.

By the same token, bowel cancer offers the greatest challenge also in the field of prophylaxis and screening which should be primarily directed to the discovery of lesions when early diagnosis is manifestly valuable.

Histopathology of bowel cancer

More is known about bowel cancer than most other malignant tumours. This is not only because of the relatively orderly behaviour of the tumour, but because better documentation and classification has been combined with extensive follow-up at specialised institutions. There is, therefore, reluctance in Great Britain to alter or modify the classification of adenocarcinoma so successfully introduced by Dukes at St Mark's Hospital which remains for the most part internationally recognised. Dukes was a pathologist and therefore the A, B and C represent the staging of the pathology specimen and not the patient (Fig 12.2). Thus to obtain the prognostic picture, it is also necessary to know whether liver secondaries, peritoneal secondaries, or more distant spread were detected. Perhaps this situation justifies a D category.

It is also necessary to know the malignant potential of the tumour as measured by the histopathological grade, usually expressed in Britain as High = poorly differentiated, Average = moderately differentiated, and Low = well differentiated. Other variations are observed such as mucoid or colloid (mucin secreting) carcinoma, signet-ring cell carcinoma, and small cell carcinoma. All of these can be of varying degrees of differentiation, but are difficult to grade satisfactorily. They all tend to carry a worse prognosis and are best regarded as poorly differentiated if there is doubt.

The incidence of the various stages varies somewhat in different series according to the centre and the time available in the laboratory for the tedious dissection of nodes. This explains the low incidence of 'C's from laboratories with no special interest in large bowel cancer. In most series only about 15% are 'A' tumours with about equal numbers of 'B's and 'C's, whilst 60% are of average grade with equal numbers of 'high' and 'low' grade lesions.

Recently much emphasis has been placed on extramural thick walled vein invasion by tumour as a prognostic indicator. It has a more adverse value, particularly on distant metastasis, than nodal involvement, and might perhaps, therefore, be used for selection of cases for systemic adjuvant therapy.

The number of nodes also has a profound influence on prognosis. A C_1 case with one node involved has over 60% chance of survival, a C_2 with over 10 nodes

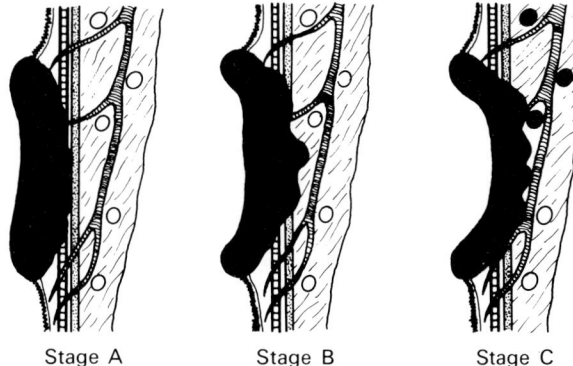

Stage A   Stage B   Stage C

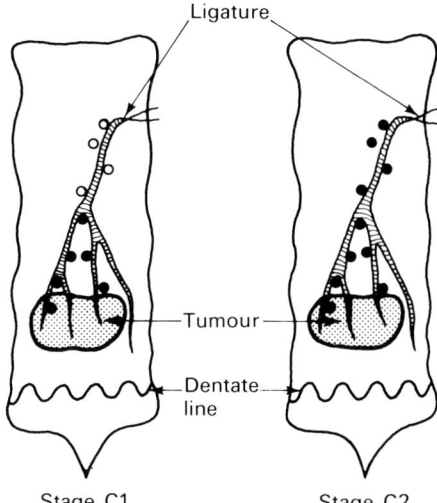

Ligature

Tumour

Dentate line

Stage C1   Stage C2

Fig 12.2 Dukes' classification. The stages of the Dukes' classification are: A. Spread by direct continuity into submucosa or muscle, but not beyond, and without lymph node involvement. B. Spread beyond the muscle coat into pericolic or perirectal tissues, but without lymph node involvement. C. As stage A or B but with metastasis to regional lymph nodes. Stage C is subdivided into: C1 where involved nodes do not extend up to the point of surgical ligature of the vascular pedicle; C2 where the node at or immediately below the ligature is involved. (From *Colorectal Disease*, Thomson James P.S., Nicholls R.J., Williams Christopher B., eds., Fig 8.5, p. 249 by courtesy of the Editors.)

less than 2%. These are St Mark's figures with specialised histopathology and a high 'C pick-up rate'.

Symptoms and signs

Surprisingly, there is no correlation between the duration of symptoms before surgery and prognosis which is relatively good with a very large localised slow growing tumour. In any individual case, however, there can be no doubt that earlier treatment will give a greater chance of cure.

Bleeding

This is the cardinal symptom of rectal cancer. Everyone with rectal bleeding must be investigated and cancer eliminated. The 'red-herring' of haemorrhoids is a constant confusion, but haemorrhoidal bleeding is seldom mixed with the motion and often squirts into the pan during the passage of a stool which is itself normal. Another pitfall is diverticular disease which is not an acceptable explanation for 'little and often' bleeding. In every case where bleeding is not satisfactorily explained a first class double contrast enema or a colonoscopy must be undertaken.

Spurious diarrhoea

Spurious diarrhoea of mucus and blood is highly significant, and tenesmus is a classical symptom.

Bowel upset

Any change of bowel habit which persists for more than a month demands sigmoidoscopy and barium enema examination. Occult or overt bleeding or anaemia require that the matter be pursued to colonoscopy or double contrast radiology.

The fallibility of the average barium enema

This only detects large tumours or malignant strictures such as the classical 'apple-core' or 'napkin-ring'. It is particularly likely to miss caecal carcinoma because of the size of the caecum, or to overlook sigmoid carcinoma because of overlapping loops of bowel. It must never lull the clinician into a false sense of security, and must be followed by colonoscopy or high grade double contrast radiology if necessary.

The haemoccult slide is of value in sorting out cases of diverticular disease or irritable colon from cancer in which some positive results are likely on repeated testing. It is not, however, infallible and is no substitute for comprehensive endoscopy and radiology.

Patterns of spread

The most valuable information about colorectal cancer comes from the interpretation of observed patterns of spread during, and recurrence after, various operations. Thus our basic philosophy of radical surgical excision is relevant because four out of five cancers are free of obvious distant spread at the time of initial surgery. Similarly transcoelomic implantation is relatively rare since less than 2% of rectal cancer and 5% of colon cancer have peritoneal nodules at the time of surgery, even though ulceration of the primary into the peritoneum is common in both.

That rectal cancer is very different from gastric cancer was apparent in the very low incidence of rectal stump recurrence after Hartmann's operation (Dixon, 1936). Though never widely popular this operation produced 'good' results. Conversely, limited procedures for rectal cancer performed from below have all eventually been discredited because of high local recurrence rates.

These facts suggest that upward and lateral lymphatic spread is most relevant to the surgeon. Miles' lateral and downward spread perhaps only occurs after blockage of the 'easier' upward pathways and is thus only found in the advanced case. This at least is the theoretical basis for orthodox anterior resection.

In the case of rectal cancer we are entering a decade where the possibilities of extending anterior resection will occupy colorectal surgeons more and more. Clinical experience, however, warns that this operation alone in colorectal cancer surgery is associated with suture-line recurrences which are rare after operations for colon cancer (Rosenberg, 1979). These recurrences are virtually untreatable in most cases, and the surgeon must never permit a patient to pay this penalty for the avoidance of a stoma, however great the initial pressure upon him may be.

Whereas pelvic wall recurrence probably relates to inadequate lateral and posterior clearance which might occur in any operation, suture-line recurrence may be the direct consequence of the choice of operation. Thus any surgeon who embarks on a policy of sphincter conservation must examine the staple or suture-line regularly during the follow-up period.

Similar signposts from past clinical experience may be relevant. The author believes that wide lateral clearance and completeness of excision of the mesorectum will become recognised as an essential of sphincter-saving procedures (Heald *et al.*, 1982). The importance of lymphatic satellites is implied by the fact that local and suture-line recurrences are found commonly only after the excision of 'C' tumours. A suture-line recurrence is usually the tip of an iceberg due to growth of an initially extrarectal fragment of tumour, usually posteriorly. Most interestingly the three well tried procedures where this mesorectal tissue is completely removed all enjoy similarly low local recurrence rates, abdominoperineal excision, Hartmann's operation, and the 'pull-through' operation.

The implication is that preventable suture-line and local recurrence is a consequence of residual mesentery left behind in the region of an anastomosis. It lends further weight to the view that lymphatic spread, particularly to perirectal and pericolic nodes and vessels a few centimetres distal to the tumour, has great practical importance in the surgical control of this disease. The internal iliac nodes are untouched by our standard dissection, but it is the belief of most British surgeons that their involvement is almost invariably a part of a situation which is essentially incurable.

Blood stream spread is the final route to disaster in most fatal cases and at least a half of all patients currently die with liver metastases. Attempts to study this aspect, however, have produced confusing results. Many observers have demonstrated circulating cancer cells and clumps of malignant cells in the peripheral blood at various times, particularly at the moment of ligation of a main vessel. No correlation is, however, seen with the subsequent course of the disease, and the administration of peroperative chemotherapeutic cover to destroy these cells has largely fallen into disrepute. Although interesting and important, it is not yet possible to draw any practical conclusions regarding the spread of the tumour via the blood stream. Despite this, valuable steps are being made towards perfusion of the liver with the aim of destroying hepatic micrometastases (Taylor, 1981).

The lesson of the second tumour – synchronous and metachronous lesions

The St Mark's experience (Lockhart-Mummery and Heald, 1972) indicates that 3.5% of patients undergoing surgery for one cancer have a second malignant tumour present at the time (synchronous cancer). A further 3.5% of those who survive, develop a second lesion an average of 10–15 years later (metachronous cancer). Synchronous adenomas occur in more than 20% of patients and the risk of a metachronous cancer developing is observed to be doubled in such patients. About 30–40% of patients after any adenoma or carcinoma has been excised will develop further adenomas. Thus long-term exhaustive follow-up would seem to be of value. A number of interesting clinical observations emerged from the St Mark's series – the prognosis as measured in mean survival months was the same whether one, two or three cancers were present synchronously. Even if two 'B' tumours or a 'B' and a 'C' tumour coexisted the prognosis remained that of a single lesion (Heald and Bussey, 1975). A similar somewhat favourable factor applied to the metachronous lesion. Possibly the most useful aspect of cancer follow-up is the detection metachronous lesions, both benign and malignant. Far from being gloomily accepted as an inevitable harbinger of doom, the second lesion should be sought and treated with enthusiasm. There is some controversy regarding the extent of resection appropriate to multiple lesions. Wangensteen (1949) and others have advocated total colonic or colorectal excisions on the grounds that these minimise the risk of further cancers developing. St Mark's policy has, however, been to treat each lesion on its merits and to conserve and subsequently observe the large bowel mucosa that remains. Results of this policy (Heald and Bussey, 1975) have been excellent and most British colorectal surgeons would regard the unnecessary sacrifice of significant lengths of large intestine as unjustifiable.

One other important message emerges from a clinical study of second tumours. It is essential never to operate on the colon without first performing a good sigmoidoscopy, or operate on the rectum without proper visualisation of the whole colon. There is no substitute for complete colorectal investigation prior to major surgery on any individual part of it.

Operation for colorectal cancer

Preoperative assessment

The patient should be fully investigated locally, i.e. the colon and the rectum with colonoscope and x-rays from end-to-end to exclude synchronous lesions. The general assessment relates to the patient's fitness for surgery and to the presence of metastases and follows orthodox lines. Liver scans may be unreliable and should never be taken as sole evidence of inoperability. Isotope scans and ultrasound are both valuable in skilled hands and may aid the planning of adjuvant therapy when appropriate, but the CAT scan of the liver is probably the best single determinant of metastatic involvement. The IVU should never be omitted since it demonstrates function in the two kidneys in case one must be removed, it helps to differentiate between malignant and inflammatory ureteric involvement and provides information about congenital anomalies and the state of the bladder. The latter may be invaded, as may the prostate which may prove relevant later. A base-line figure for CEA is of some value if this investigation is used in the follow-up clinic.

Preoperative physiotherapy is a useful prelude to the postoperative period when a long midline incision will significantly impair the vital capacity and the patient's ability to clear the bronchi of mucus plugs. Bowel preparation and antibacterials are essential.

Heparin prophylaxis of thromboembolic complications. All major bowel cancer surgery, especially deep pelvic dissections, are in the high risk group for deep vein thrombosis. Our routine is to give Heparin 5000 u subcutaneously with the premedication and 5000 u.b.d. until mobile (*see* Chapter 33).

Operative details

As previously stated, a long midline incision is usually suitable. The bowel is examined completely and the liver carefully palpated. Some confusion between solitary liver nodules and various other lesions sometimes occurs: a calcified or fibrosed tape worm is a special mimic, but the geographical history may help. If in doubt, a biopsy must be performed before proceeding to a partial hepatic resection, and this should be done with care to avoid spillage or the contamination of the main operative field. The decision as to when to proceed to such a major additional operation should only be taken after an assessment has been made of the success of the excision of the primary and the condition of the patient. It is probably wise to defer hepatic resection until a CAT scan has excluded other deposits and an angiogram has defined the hepatic vascular anatomy.

Colon resection

Right hemicolectomy

Excellent results were attributed by Turnbull and Schofield (1970) to their technique of ligating the vessels initially and carrying the dissection laterally – the so-called 'No touch' technique. Few other surgeons believe that the order of the operation is important and many interpret the excellence of their results as being due to wider lymphatic clearance. However, an initial approach to the superior mesenteric artery and vein with early ligation of the ileocolic and right colic vessels is an entirely sastisfactory method for right hemicolectomy.

All of the tissue to the right of the superior mesenteric vein is cleared laterally in a block and dissected off the duodenum and the structures of the posterior abdominal wall so that a good cancer operation is guaranteed.

Transverse colectomy

This follows general principles and involves ligation of the middle colic vessels at their origin from the superior mesenteric vessels. Both flexures must usually be mobilised.

Left hemicolectomy

Radical left hemicolectomy is the most satisfactory procedure for most tumours of the left colon. It involves near flush-ties of the inferior mesenteric artery and vein and necessitates removal of the whole left colon, so that anastomosis is between the transverse colon and the top of the rectum at the point where its diameter is suitable. In the frail, sick or elderly a conservative segmental left colon resection may be appropriate. This involves preservation of the main inferior mesenteric vessels and individual ligation of the vessels supplying the tumour, with removal of as many nodes as possible.

Emergency operations in colon cancer

Right hemicolectomy

This may generally be carried out in the emergency situation, although leakage may occur in inexperienced hands. An alternative, therefore, is immediate ileo-transversostomy (antiperistaltic) followed later by a staged resection with closure of ileum and colon just to the right of the anastomosis. This routine is much to be preferred to an inadequate clearance of the tumour when adequate facilities and skills are not available.

Operations for obstruction

Obstructing lesions occur most commonly in the sigmoid colon or more proximally. Rectal cancer only rarely obstructs. The patient's abdomen is often distended, but he is in little pain, appears deceptively well and it is important to recognise that he will require skilled and lengthy surgical care to survive. Not only are the complications of operation rather common, but prognosis in terms of cancer cure is less good than in the non-obstructed patient.

Various alternatives exist, but they must all include an incision large enough to confirm the diagnosis.

Emergency right transverse colostomy

Followed by staged resection emergency right transverse colostomy is the orthodox plan of management and is certainly the most satisfactory in average or inexperienced hands. If it appears necessary to decompress the bowel in order to close the abdomen, then this must be done with great care. It is all too easy to become engulfed in copious quantities of liquid faeces. Thus, if possible, the loop colostomy is only opened after the main wound has been closed.

Immediate colon resection

This sounds easier than it may prove to be if the bowel is greatly distended. If it can be conducted in a radical manner, it may possibly increase the chances of achieving permanent cure of the tumour (Fielding and Wells, 1974). Savage (1967) and others have reported good results from a one-stage operation, although there is widespread fear that the distended oedematous stool-laden proximal bowel is unsuitable for anastomosis. Immediate total colonic lavage to empty bowel is desirable if anastomosis is contemplated.

Delayed anastomosis

A safe compromise which has many supporters is for the resection to be carried out in a radical manner and the end of the proximal bowel to be brought out as a colostomy (Sames, 1960). The distal end is then either closed and tethered in a spot where it can be found later, or brought out as a mucous fistula. A formal second operation is required for intraperitoneal anastomosis.

Immediate total colectomy and ileorectal anastomosis

This has been supported by Hughes (1966) on the grounds that the whole distended and loaded segment is resected and that the ileum for anastomosis is not itself oedematous or distended. In experienced hands it is an excellent answer to a difficult problem, but the long-term functional results are not always as good as with the more conservative approach.

Juxta-lesion colostomy

This should not be performed for cancer if a right transverse colostomy well away from the lesion is practical. It is, however, acceptable for growths in the transverse colon if they are not considered suitable for immediate resection. Like the Paul Mickulicz double-barrelled colostomy method, it may carry a risk of local recurrence of tumour in the colostomy wound.

Caecostomy

This operation has its advocates, but it is essential that it is carried out in a unit with experience of the method as the occasional operation is dangerous because of sepsis and leakage of faeces laterally between caecum and abdominal wall.

Tumour 'markers' in colorectal cancer

The carcino-embryonic antigen test (CEA) is becoming widely used in follow-up clinics. It is of little value for screening, since it lacks specificity and it requires large volumes of tumour. The test is a radioimmune assay capable of detecting antigen in the serum. It is raised in a variety of other tumours and is, therefore, of value only as a sequential follow-up tool. One particular pitfall is the fact that heavy smoking can raise the figure as high as 20 units (upper limit of normal = 10 units). Its main application is for the early detection of metastases and trials are under way to see if the treatment of such presymptomatic metastases with cytotoxics is of any value.

A rise in the CEA is regarded by some as an indication for a 'second look' laparotomy or at least for CAT scanning of the liver in the hope of a curative lobectomy or tri-segmentectomy. In the author's opinion its lack of specificity makes it undesirable that treatment should be based solely on a rise in CEA, but should simply dictate strenuous attempts to localise the source of the rise. All of this does, however, cause much anxiety to a symptomless patient and hard evidence of its value is as yet lacking.

Occult hepatic metastases

Finlay has recently drawn attention to the predictive value of CAT scanning of the liver in the prognosis of colorectal cancer (Finlay *et al.*, 1982). It is already apparent that palpable hepatic metastases are the major determinant of prognosis. Finlay's small series suggests that 80% or more of the 'radical' cases who are not cured by surgery are incurable because they do, in fact, have occult hepatic metastases. When this group is excluded, the results with operation alone in the remainder without these occult metastases is excellent. This, therefore, raises doubts as to whether cytotoxics should ever be used as adjuvant therapy without selection by the CAT scanner.

Orthodox selection of operation

The primary treatment of rectal cancer is surgical. In most centres the choice lies between abdominoperineal excision and some form of sphincter-conserving anterior resection. Before either operation, good biopsies for grading of the tumour are essential. The distance from the anal verge and the size and degree of fixity on palpation are the two other major determinants.

A few small mobile tumours may be suitable for management by local excision followed by careful histological assessment of its completeness and by long-term follow-up. For the majority, however, the choice will be between the two major procedures. Traditionally, all poorly differentiated tumours, all fixed tumours, and most lesions below a sigmoidoscopic height of 12 cm in a man and 10 cm in a woman are selected for abdominoperineal excision. For a fat patient with a narrow pelvis 2–3 cm must be added to these measurements. The final decision is taken at operation as a variable number of extra centimetres of length are gained in the process of mobilisation of the

rectum out of the hollow of the sacrum. Traditionally, a clear margin of at least 5 cm of bowel wall was allowed beyond a differentiated tumour, and no poorly differentiated lesion was considered for a restorative procedure.

The current challenge to orthodoxy

Abdominoperineal excision remains the most commonly performed procedure in most centres, and all surgeons who deviate from it for tumours below the upper third (i.e. about 12 cm) of the rectum must monitor most carefully the results they are achieving. Anderson reviewed the literature in 1981 and gave the 5-year local recurrence rate after restorative excision as 12–20% in reports from special interest centres and about 40% in general surgical practice. If this is true, it suggests that at least the latter group should be returning to more abdominoperineal excisions. Others believe that the anal sphincters and the levators are only rarely involved by rectal cancer and can usually be preserved. To spare them safely, however, without compromising excision of the tumour is a difficult task. It demands changes in technique which are still the subject of argument, and the widespread use of staplers to attempt lower resections may yet prove to have been a disaster.

A policy for selection

The author has used the staplers for 5 years in all differentiated cancers where a clear margin of 2 cm or more exists between the anorectal ring and the lower edge of the tumour. About twice this length is required for a poorly differentiated tumour, and all doubtful cases are monitored by frozen section in the operating theatre.

All cancers of the middle third of the rectum (7–12 cm) and some of the lower third have thus been managed by 'low' or 'ultra-low' anterior resection. Some male patients with difficult build have required abdominoperineal excision, because the clamp could not safely be applied beyond the tumour. In every case great emphasis has been placed on wide clearance and total excision of the mesorectum. Preliminary results (Heald *et al.*, 1982) with regard to local recurrence are extremely promising and at least as good as previous abdominoperineal results. The wide clearance, however, creates a huge splinted cavity and this may explain why anastomotic leakage remains a significant problem. All anastomoses below 7 cm are, therefore, at the present time protected by temporary colostomy in our unit. Other writers on the subject of low stapled anastomosis have better results with anastomotic healing, but few series have included so many coloanal or near coloanal cases. The management of the pelvic cavity and many other aspects of stapling technique have yet to be standardised. Useful and sometimes near normal function is usually achieved by the patient with the very low anastomosis. A small number of patients, however, have such poor control or such frequent bowel action or urgency that it has become necessary to revert to a colostomy.

Surgeons who perform only occasional rectal cancer excision, but are attracted by these principles have the alternative policy of the Hartmann procedure. If a proper wide clearance of a tumour can be achieved from above, there is little purpose in sacrificing the levators or the anus. The latter may be closed and the patient later referred to a surgeon with an interest in low anastomosis for a second stage reconnection. This is greatly to be preferred to desperate and unsatisfactory low anastomosis by any method, and this routine may find an occasional place in surgical practice in the future.

Excision of the rectum for cancer

The patient is catheterised and placed in the lithotomy-Trendelenburg position with Lloyd-Davies split stirrups. A long midline incision right down to the pubic bone facilitates full assessment of the tumour. Only if there is no question of a restorative operation should the perineal operator start work before the rectum has been fully mobilised. The majority of the dissection should be performed in all cases from above. This is because stripping of the pelvic fascia off the sacrum is more apt to occur if the lower third of the rectum is mobilised from below – with consequent damage to the inferior hypogastric plexus.

Ligation of the inferior mesenteric vessels

Miles recommended ligating the vessels at the aortic bifurcation. This is still a reasonable option in the elderly, although it is not as radical as can easily be achieved by a 'high tie'. As described previously when discussing the low rectal anastomosis separate 'high ties' of the inferior mesenteric artery and vein allow the greatest possible length of left colon to be released, mobilised, and brought down for anastomosis near to the anus. In most patients, in the absence of visible glands around the origin, it seems sensible to preserve the autonomic nerve plexuses and thus divide the artery about 1 cm from the aorta and the vein 1 cm from the splenic vein. The lengthy mobilisation of the splenic flexure and left half of the colon that is necessary for restorative procedures is carried out at this stage – i.e.

before the plane around the mesorectum is carried down into the pelvis.

Mobilisation of the rectum

The rectal mobilisation is performed by sharp dissection under direct vision in the plane between the rectum and mesorectum (within) and the presacral and hypogastric nerve plexuses (without). Proper pursuit of this plane is a delight for the proctologist, since it is avascular except where it is crossed by the middle rectal vessels and the 'stalks' laterally. These are cut directly and only occasionally require to be tied or diathermied. More often they need only be packed and dealt with, if necessary, after removal of the tumour. This plane leads ultimately to the anorectal ring and because it encompasses the rectum and its mesorectum both will lift naturally out of the levator gutter. Throughout this procedure, care is taken to avoid digital extraction of the tumour or rectum since this may tear into tumour planes or start uncontrollable venous bleeding. At the same time the main parts of the autonomic nerve plexuses are preserved as far as possible, particularly low down where they are near the midline and passing forwards across the levators.

High anterior resection

This is an entirely orthodox procedure which differs only a little from a low sigmoid colon resection. The rectum should be partially mobilised without dividing the lateral 'stalks'.

A full 5 cm clearance of bowel wall and mesorectum should be taken with the tumour, so that the mesorectum must be divided well below the tumour and its vessels ligated. Ideally high ties and full splenic flexure mobilisation will be a prelude to either a manual or a stapled anastomosis.

Local invasion of pelvic walls

It is very rare for the tumour to invade the levators. This is fortunate since Goligher (1980) comments on the feebleness of the advertised 'disc' of levators on most abdominoperineal specimens. Serious problems, however, are met a few centimetres higher where invasion of the pelvic walls laterally and of the prostate and bladder anteriorly are common enough. It is in such tumours that preoperative radiotherapy may perhaps offer hope; this is why their detection because of size and fixation preoperatively may be of some value. At all events the surgeon has little room for manoeuvre: he can remove part of the iliac vessels and some muscle laterally, but such endeavours are apt to be haemorrhagic as is the stripping of the pelvic wall to remove internal iliac nodes. It is, in the author's opinion, unlikely that any cases where these nodes are involved are within the scope of surgical cure.

Genitourinary involvement

In either sex, a disc of bladder may require excision with a high tumour, and in a middle third lesion in a male a slice may have to come off the back of the prostate. A more common problem is the vaginal vault – part of which may be excised in the female, with or without the uterus. The formal removal of the whole posterior vaginal wall as part of abdominoperineal excision is occasionally appropriate, but need not be routine. When ultra-low anterior resection has been combined with excision of part of the vaginal wall, every effort must be made to keep the anastomosis separate from the vaginal epithelium to avoid epithelialisation of the track creating a permanent fistula in the event of leakage. Usually the anastomosis retracts well down behind the vaginal wall, but an omental overlay is a useful extra precaution in this situation. An adherent loop of ileum should be excised when necessary before commencing the deep pelvic dissection.

The final decision

This may be made preoperatively because the lesion is too close to the anus or at operation because a clamp cannot safely be placed across the rectum beyond the tumour. If this can be done and the surgeon feels happy that proper and adequate clearance has been achieved, then the addition of a perineal dissection probably has little to offer the patient.

The surgeon has a choice of:

a low stapled anastomosis;
a transanal or perineal technique;
a low manual anastomosis;
Hartmann's operation with the option of a second stage anastomosis.

Anastomosis with circular stapling devices

Three main machines are currently available, the Russian SPTU Gun which is the cheapest to use, but requires obsessional and individual maintenance, the EEA with disposable cartridges and now as a totally disposable unit, and the Ethicon disposable intraluminal stapler. The author's perference is for the last of these because of the clean cut-off of the 'doughnuts' within the gun.

The importance of these anastomotic devices is that the purse-string stitch can be inserted low down in the rectum by a simple manoeuvre, the cross-clamped rectum is drawn up out of the pelvis and the purse-string inserted in the anterior wall before the posterior wall is cut. In this way a satisfactory circumferential gathering stitch may be inserted as low as the anorectum itself in favourable (particularly female) patients. In any patient the practical lower limit for satisfactory anastomosis is extended by several centimetres in the hands of most surgeons.

Preparation of bowel ends for stapling. *The anorectum.* Provided that the plane outside the mesorectum is followed right down to the pelvic floor and the lateral ligaments are divided correctly, the plane around the muscle of the anorectum is entered naturally. It is important that there is about 1–2 cm of muscle clean and proud of the levator gutter. The blood supply of this end is never a problem.

A right-angled clamp is placed across the bowel beyond the tumour so giving adequate clearance. A second clamp positioned in the opposite direction prevents leakage from the extreme end if the rectum is wide at this point. The distal stump is then washed thoroughly via the anus.

The gathering stitches. The two clamps are next drawn up into the wound so as to gain access to the anterior wall, which is divided first with a knife and then with scissors. (O) Prolene is used as a gathering suture over-and-over. A thin line indicates the end of the muscle tube and only 2 mm or so of this should be picked up or there will be too much tissue gathered into the gun. After dividing the anterior wall, the clamps are angled and the lateral wall is cut and sutured similarly. The cut is next extended along the posterior wall and the gathering stitch continued round the full circle. If any mesorectum has been left at the back, this should be cut away at this point. The levator gutter and pelvis should be empty of perirectal lymphovascular tissue.

A 1.5 cm length of bowel proximally must be cleaned of mesentery and a similar gathering suture inserted. If the purse-string instrument is used, this step is done quickly by-passing the straight needle back and forth through the clamp.

Firing the gun. The device, liberally coated with K-Y lubricating jelly, is inserted with one hand carefully guiding progress from within. Particular care is required for a high anastomosis as it is possible to damage the lower part of the rectum while negotiating it. The gap is then opened, the gathering stitches are tightened and the gun pushed into the patient while its periphery is checked for freedom from excess tissue. A gap of about 2–2.5 mm is usually appropriate. After firing, the gap is opened and the gun wriggled out gently. The integrity of the anastomosis is checked by ensuring that the 'doughnuts' are complete and also by washout with suitably coloured water.

Filling the pelvis. Provided that the necessary redundancy has been achieved by separate high ligations and extensive mobilisation, the excess colon is then folded into the pelvis with the lowest coil lying without tension in the levator gutter. A soft silicone drain or a suction system is inserted behind it and brought out anteriorly to be connected to a bag.

Is a transverse colostomy necessary? It must not be forgotten that an anastomosis just proximal to the anus is probably the most prone to dangerous complications that a surgeon ever attempts. There should be over 90% certainty of healing by first intention if there is a pulsatile blood supply, redundancy of colon, no dead space, and good bowel preparation, together with a short-course of high dose antibacterial. However, if any of these aspects is less than perfect, it is good and safe practice to protect the join with a transverse colostomy. Alternatively, there must be special vigilance during the second week and readiness to perform one if it becomes necessary. The author now uses a colostomy to protect all anastomoses below 7 cm as a routine (Heald and Leicester, 1981).

Postoperative care. The absence of the perineal dissection usually means that there is not as much postoperative shock in the frail and the elderly, and less worry about the patient's general condition. Also, the impression is that the catheter can often be dispensed with earlier than after an abdominoperineal dissection. We usually remove it at about 7–10 days, but one patient pulled his out on the fourth day and did not need it replacing. If the pelvis has been well filled with redundant colon, the drainage dwindles rapidly and it is probably safe to remove the drain on the 4th or 5th day. There is a temptation to leave it in place until the end of the dangerous period i.e. 8–14 days after operation when leakage may occur. If every aspect of the anastomosis has been satisfactory at operation and the drainage has fallen off rapidly, then the drain is better removed.

In these circumstances it seems probable that the relatively tacky coils of bowel will adhere and surround the anastomosis with the safest of all sealers – viable tissue.

Gastrografin enema. We can see little purpose in performing this if the patient is clinically fit and well. However, it is indicated if there is a fever or any anxiety regarding possible dehiscence. If a colostomy has been made, it is useful to confirm integrity of the anastomosis before closing it. Only those with a large dead space, usually posteriorly, will require prolonged protection (6–12 months) with a colostomy. Occasionally such a space may need to be opened up under anaesthesia to facilitate epithelialisation.

Other methods of low anastomosis

Coloanal sleeve anastomosis (Parks). The St Marks series of this operation performed for cancer approaches 100 patients. The technique involves dividing the rectum a few cm above the anorectal ring and denuding it of mucosa. The prepared colon is then brought down within the sleeve of rectal muscle and anastomosed transanally to the dentate line. Clearly the tumour must be high enough for adequate clearance to the point of muscle section (Parks and Percy, 1982).

Abdominoanal pull-through. Most centres in the world where this was practised with enthusiasm have abandoned it in favour of the circular staplers.

Ultra-low manual anastomosis from above

The advantage of the stapler depends upon the anatomical distortion achieved by retraction and sequential cutting and stitching. This same trick can be used to lay stitches through the muscle and muscularis mucosae of the rectum. These can then be completed by passing the needle through the corresponding layers of the mobilised colon which is then 'rail-roaded' down on to the anorectum. Thus a single layer of 'natural' or 'sero-submucosal' interrupted sutures can be used in place of the stapling gun anastomosis, if preferred.

Abdominoperineal excision

The perineal dissection. If the tumour is too close to the anorectal ring for sphincter conservation to be considered, the perineal dissection may proceed synchronously. If there is doubt, then the abdominal operator will defer the mobilisation of the splenic flexure until the deep pelvic dissection has been completed. The final decision is then based upon whether a clamp may sensibly be placed beyond the tumour, and ultimately upon the confirmation that the cut end is free of tumour on frozen section.

Two perianal purse-strings are inserted to prevent faecal spillage. The incision is deepened posteriorly to the coccyx, and laterally through the ischiorectal fossae to the levators, and anteriorly close to the vaginal wall or periurethral muscles in the male.

It is a major disaster to tear the tumour or perforate the bowel, and the disc of levators is best cut through with both surgeons working together.

Postoperative management

Colostomy

If a colostomy has been performed, the appliance is attached in the operating theatre. A defunctioning rod or bar is generally removed after 10–14 days although it should be retained if there is anxiety regarding the anastomosis.

The posterior space

The American routine of packing has been completely abandoned in Britain and indeed in many parts of the United States. Considerable differences exist, however, on the question of whether to preserve enough pelvic peritoneum for closure. This will exclude a large space which then collects sero-sanguineous fluid and takes many weeks to obliterate. In the author's opinion a preferable routine is to cut a wide hole in the pelvic peritoneum initially and to make no attempt at closure. The skin is closed primarily and either the omentum or the caecum and right colon are mobilised and swung down to obliterate the space. It is important to realise that the small bowel cannot safely be allowed to prolapse into the pelvic depths to fill space left by the surgeon, because this may lead to intestinal obstruction and the retrieval of bowel at a subsequent operation may be both difficult and hazardous. It is, therefore, a matter of high priority that viable filler of some kind be devised in both abdominoperineal and anterior resection and also that proper drainage for the sero-sanguineous fluid be provided.

In the case of abdominoperinal resection a closed sterile bag or suction drainage or a corrugated drain through a primary perineal skin closure is appropriate.

Urinary function

A urinary catheter is required for 5–15 days according to the height of the tumour, the extent of deep pelvic dissection, and the general state and progress of the patient after operation. Pre-existing prostate obstruction and the amount of damage to the hypogastric plexuses are the most important determinants of long-term urinary function. In some patients catheterisation may be necessary for as long as a month, thereafter transurethral resection or retropubic prostatectomy may be required in the male and manual expression plus occasional bladder-neck resection in the female. It must be remembered that approximately one in four patients after low wide pelvic dissection, particularly abdominoperineal, have permanently and totally denervated bladders. With suitable encouragement plus surgery to their outflow tract, even males will generally achieve reasonable function in the long term.

Posterior anoproctotomy (The York Mason procedure)

This procedure was originally devised for exposure of a rectoprostatic fistula. It is perhaps the best method for improving access to the lower half of the rectum. Thus it facilitates removal of superficial tumours such as villous lesions or small mucosal carcinomas or carcinoids, where the transanal approach seems inadequate and yet radical excision is considered unnecessary. York Mason (1974) has emphasised the importance of careful preoperative digital assessment of mobility of the lesion and of palpation for mesorectal nodes close to the tumour. Clearly the fundamental drawback of any local excision for carcinoma is the complete failure to remove such nodes, although protaganists of the method claim a low incidence of extrarectal spread in small mobile mucosal differentiated lesions.

For anoproctotomy, the patient is placed in the prone jack-knife position and the buttocks are strapped apart. After local infiltration with dilute adrenaline the whole sphincter mechanism is divided and each layer is carefully marked by colour-coded sutures for reconstitution at the end of the procedure.

The incision is carried up on one or other side of the sacrum and the wedge shaped incision in the ischiorectal fossa retracted to provide excellent access to the lower reaches of the rectum. Either submucosal or full thickness excisions can be undertaken, although the author is doubtful whether the small cancer which requires full thickness excision should ever simply be resected locally.

The author prefers to cover this procedure with a loop colostomy, though this is not considered necessary by York Mason. Little impairment of sphincter function is encountered and the procedure can readily be tackled by a surgeon with limited experience in the field.

Adjuvant therapy for colorectal cancer

R.D.H. RYALL

Surgery remains the most effective and radical treatment for patients with colorectal cancer. A recent reawakening of interest in adjuvant therapy accompanies the realisation that it can broaden the scope of surgery and improve the results of treatment in high risk cases. Contrary to some early reports, radiotherapy can be a useful treatment for colorectal cancer. It was first used in the 1920s and reintroduced in recent years as radiotherapeutic technique improved and as the limitations of surgery have become more clear.

Radiotherapy

Radiotherapy can be used to treat colorectal cancer with radical or palliative intent and as a single modality or combined with surgery preoperatively or postoperatively. Until now radiotherapy has most commonly been used in an attempt to reduce the risk of local pelvic recurrence following operation. Postoperative radiotherapy is unsatisfactory since surgery will have damaged the vascular bed leading to areas of anoxia, which will protect surviving tumour cells from the effects of radiation. In addition, radiotherapy delays wound healing and cannot therefore be commenced until after healing is complete. In patients recovering from abdominoperineal resection of the rectum, this may take up to 3 months. Such a long delay is not generally acceptable.

Trials of modest doses of prophylactic preoperative radiotherapy have failed to show significant effects on survival. Some reduction in the percentage of patients with node involvement after treatment, however, has led to claims that secondary tumour in nodes near to the primary can be destroyed or neutralised. If the dose is increased to around 5000 rad further possibilities exist for the prevention of local recurrences – perhaps because of this effect on nodal deposits in the nearby mesentery.

Cytotoxic drug therapy in colorectal cancer

For the most part cytotoxic drug therapy has proved very disappointing in colorectal cancer. Partial response rates of 15% are usual for a wide range of chemotherapeutic regimes accompanied by median survival times of a few months in palliative cases and little evidence of improved performance. 5-fluorouracil has been extensively researched by Moertel et al. (1975) and Hahn et al. (1975) and is the most effective agent available for this disease. We are unimpressed by the systemic use of cytotoxic drugs and can provide no evidence that they influence the prognosis of our patients. However, a recent specialised development shows promise.

Irving Taylor et al. (1979) have pointed out that colorectal liver metastases develop due to malignant cells entering the portal venous circulation. They performed a randomised prospective clinical trial to assess the value of adjuvant umbilical vein perfusion with 5-fluorouracil following surgical removal of the primary tumour. Initial results are encouraging. At the time of publishing their paper, there had been 23 deaths in the control group and only 7 in the perfusion group. Liver metastases were present in 13 of the controls and only 2 of the patients receiving hepatic perfusion. There was a total of 154 patients in this study and the results justify further investigation.

A recent paper comparing the results of computerised axial tomographic (CAT) scanning of the liver for metastases compared with isotope liver scans (Finlay et al., 1982) shows that CAT scanning is a sensitive technique for selection of those patients with a poor prognosis in whom cytotoxic regimes may be justifiable.

At the Basingstoke Bowel Cancer Clinic we believe that improvement in survival for some patients with colorectal cancer may be achieved by adjuvant therapy. This can only occur if patients are carefully selected for the treatment available, according to the extent of their disease after clinical and pathological staging and following the accurate collection and processing of the data obtained.

Our preliminary experiences with apparently low local recurrence figures after surgery with wide lymphatic clearance have led us to a selective approach. Thus, only large fixed and apparently inoperable tumours are considered for preoperative radiotherapy, and doses of over 5000 rad in 20 fractions over 5 weeks are used. Similar regimes are used for truly inoperable lesions after marking of the full extent of the tumour at laparotomy; a defunctioning colostomy is also performed to cover the period of treatment. If marked reduction in size occurs, or if excision is considered possible after treatment, this is timed for about 6 weeks after completion of the radiotherapy.

The anorectum

Anatomy

The anorectum extends from the anorectal ring to the anal margin. The anal canal is regarded by some as synonymous with this, by others only as that part distal to the pectinate line.

The muscle rings (Fig 12.3)

The outer tube of voluntary external sphincters is readily defined by digital examination in the conscious patient. Its powerful upper limit is the anorectal ring which corresponds with the puborectal sling around the lower rectum. An effective and adequate ring of muscle at this level is essential for continence.

The inner-tube or internal sphincter is the thickened downward extension of the circular muscle layer of the rectum. This can be divided in whole or in part without significant consequences, provided there is an adequate anorectal ring. The intersphincteric groove is

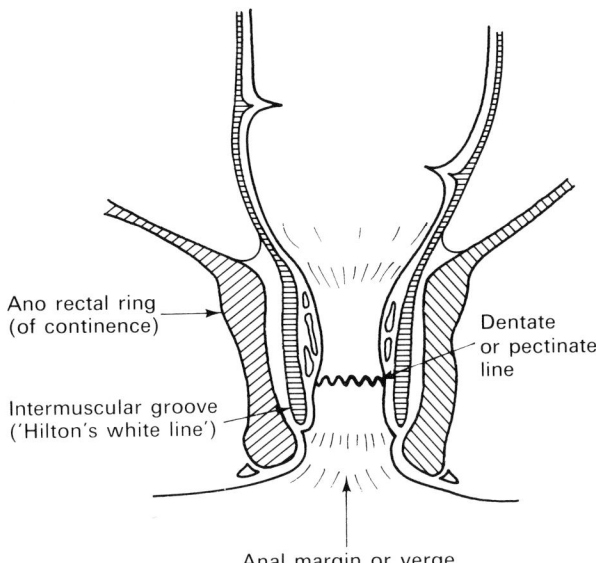

Ano rectal ring
(of continence)

Dentate
or pectinate
line

Intermuscular groove
('Hilton's white line')

Anal margin or verge

Fig 12.3 The anorectum. Two palpable and one visible 'ring' landmarks.

readily palpable in most patients and is important to the surgeon. It is somewhat drawn up within the anal canal in the conscious patient due to contraction of the lower end of the external sphincter.

Mucosal lining

The most important endoscopic landmark is the pectinate or dentate line. This separates essentially visceral epithelium above (columnar epithelium, inferior mesenteric blood supply and lymphatic drainage, autonomic nerves) from skin below (pain-sensitive nerves, lymphatic drainage to the groins). The pecten is the zone just distal to the dentate line, lacks the hairs of the anal margin and forms an intermediate watershed zone. A variable distribution of squamous, columnar and transitional epithelium exists in the region just above the pecten.

Anal glands drain via anal ducts into crypts at the distal end of the corrugations known as the columns of Morgagni, i.e. at the dentate line. They are somewhat concentrated posteriorly and they often extend through the internal sphincter into the intersphincteric region. Infection in these glands is probably the starting point for most fistulas and abscesses.

Spaces below the levators of relevance to the surgeon

Perianal	From intersphincteric groove distally: perianal abscess, haematoma, fistula.
Ischiorectal	Lateral to anorectum and levators: abscess, fistula.
Submucous	Deep to mucosa above dentate line: internal haemorrhoids.
Intersphincteric	Anal glands, intermuscular abscess, fistula.
Deep postanal	Between coccyx, levators and back of external sphincter, deep to its superficial part: horseshoe abscess and fistula, viz. the communicating plane between the ischio-rectal fossae.

Haemorrhoids

These have been defined in many ways from varicosities of the submucous venous plexus to vascular erectile cushions.

Perhaps everyone has them, certainly they are so common as to be almost normal and experience teaches that they vary in respect from week to week. They are the commonest cause of rectal bleeding, the greatest red-herring in the diagnosis of bowel cancer, and they provide the most persistent treatment controversies in proctology.

Degrees

These refer to the degree of prolapse:

First degree	Do not prolapse
Second degree	Prolapse, but return spontaneously
Third degree	Prolapse, require manual reposition but remain 'up' until the next motion.
Fourth degree	Prolapse on exertion or hang out continuously.

As the degree of prolapse becomes more marked, the stretching and laxity of the tissues involves more perianal skin forming interoexternal haemorrhoids.

Symptoms

Bleeding and prolapse are characteristic. Difficulty in cleaning the area is extremely common and minor degrees of soiling often occur due to failure of anal sealing. Similar irritation and dampness of the anal skin may occur due to mucous discharge. This is usually due to an associated fissure, a perianal haematoma which is common due to the laxity of the perianal skin, or to strangulation of one or more prolapsing haemorrhoids. A careful history is thus crucial in the proper planning of treatment.

Treatment

The first duty of the surgeon is proper investigation to exclude serious causes of bleeding. In every case where local treatment fails to eliminate bleeding, the whole colon and rectum must be fully visualised by sigmoidoscopy plus colonoscopy or good quality x-rays. As a general measure a high fibre diet is usually of benefit.

First and second degree. Sclerotherapy remains the most popular minor local therapy. 3–5 ml of phenol in arachis oil are injected submucosally in the main piles well above the dentate line. Rubber band ligation is a suitable alternative and may be more effective in prolapse of purely internal haemorrhoids. Care must be taken to avoid involving skin in the strangulating band.

Cryotherapy enjoys some supporters. It usually requires 2–4 min application to produce a useful volume of tissue destruction. Many surgeons prefer, therefore, to deal with one pile at a time with 6 weeks between sessions.

Stretching (Lord's manoeuvre). There is little doubt that the extensive anal stretch advocated by Lord (1975) and followed by regular dilatation is often of considerable value in the symptomatic management of haemorrhoids. There is equally little doubt that third and fourth degree haemorrhoids do often recur despite the most extensive stretching activities, though this may represent a failure to dilate regularly. There is also some danger of causing incontinence in the elderly patient.

Haemorrhoidectomy. This remains the choice of most surgeons for third and fourth degree haemorrhoids. In Britain most surgeons stretch the sphincter and excise each haemorrhoid leaving three oval open wounds and three bridges of skin to mucosa across the dentate line as recommended by Milligan and Morgan. In the United States closed or semi-closed techniques are favoured, which involve preservation of more mucosa and skin, with slight undermining and apposition to cover the defects.

Various technical points deserve comment. Firstly the position on the table. In the UK the lithotomy position is favoured and has the advantage of not requiring endotracheal intubation. In the US the prone jack-knife position gives superior access and visualisation and allows blood to drain away from the field, but the general anaesthetic is more complex. The method is, however, particularly suitable for a combination of Diazepam (Valium) and local infiltration with a long acting local anaesthetic and adrenalin, possibly with the addition of hyalase. The use of this method does reduce the amount of bleeding and is extremely safe. It is probably to be preferred for the closed technique.

A gentle four finger stretch or an internal sphincterotomy are good pain preventing measures. The avoidance of muscle fibres in the ligature for the base of the haemorrhoid is also important in this respect. Indeed, the precise dissection down to a small discrete vascular base is essential to avoid secondary haemorrhage which formerly dominated postoperative management and dictated long hospitalisation. This occurred when a large volume of tissue which had been strangulated in a mass ligature, separated a week or more after operation. No pack should be left in place as its removal was often the most painful part of the entire procedure. The preservation of adequate skin 'bridges' is the essence of prevention of stenosis. If the wounds are to be closed, it is essential that the inner (mucosal) end be carefully approximated over the ligature because it is all too easy to close the skin end so as to pleat the anus and provide a faecal cul-de-sac above it.

Usually haemorrhoidectomy requires excision of the three primary piles – i.e. left lateral and right anterior and posterior. Sometimes however only one, or perhaps two, pile complexes are prolapsing and in such patients an excellent result is obtained with minimal discomfort by a limited operation sparing the more normal segments.

If these guidelines are followed and particularly if the area is infiltrated preoperatively with a long acting local anaesthetic such as bupivacaine (Marcain) the patient will generally be comfortable in the first few postoperative days. The avoidance of extensive preoperative bowel preparation and the early administration of stool softeners also help with the one problem that does remain, the first bowel action. Local pain, anxiety, fear, packs and interference with the normal bowel pattern due to operation all militate towards deferring bowel function, sometimes to the extent of faecal impaction and even occasionally urinary retention. The prophylactic use of diazepam (Valium) or chlorpromazine (Largactil) for the first week is often helpful.

Strangulation. Since the advent of systemic antibacterial protection, the most satisfactory management of strangulation is probably early operation and this is particularly true if great pain is present from a large single strangulated pile complex. When all three piles are strangulated, the all important skin bridges are sometimes difficult to preserve, or they may necrose later with subsequent risk of stricture. In such cases an anal stretch may make the patient more comfortable. If no procedure is undertaken, bed rest, elevation and analgesia may be necessary for days or weeks.

Fissure

Fissure is the characteristic lesion which produces anal pain related to defaecation. It is a longitudinal tear of the anal skin overlying the distal rim of the internal sphincter. It may thus be recognised most readily if the patients everts his anal canal voluntarily, i.e. withdraws the outer tube of voluntary sphincter. It is most commonly seen in the midline posteriorly, or , occasionally in women and children, anteriorly. Lateral fissures should be suspected of being neoplastic or due to Crohn's disease. If the fissure becomes chronic, a hypertrophied anal papilla or so-called fibroma may develop above the fissure, while the heaped up oedematous skin found below it has been dignified by Brodie with the name of sentinel pile. An abscess or low fistula are occasional complications.

Many fissures heal spontaneously or with the aid of bulk stool softeners and local analgesia. It is doubtful whether the time honoured dilator has much effect. Those that merit it may be dealt with by a general anaesthetic and anal stretch, or by a later internal sphincterotomy. The latter produces the most certain results with rapid healing and with minimal risk of seepage or incontinence later. This did sometimes occur after the older fissurectomy operation or as phincterotomy performed through the floor of the fissure due to a leaking posterior groove or keyhole deformity. This is generally not amenable to any form of surgical correction.

Subcutaneous lateral internal sphincterotomy

The lateral part of the internal sphincter must be put on the stretch by a retractor or the assistant's fingers while the skin is drawn taut and the intersphincteric groove identified by palpation. Then, after infiltration between the sphincter with bupivacaine (Marcain) and adrenaline, an incision is made lateral to the groove. The lowest 2 cm of the internal sphincter is then divided with a knife by feel, or scissors under direct vision. Generally the wound does not require sutures. Presumably the operation works by changing permanently the shape of the anal canal, removing the 'step' of internal sphincter over which tearing of the skin has led to fissure formation.

A problem is sometimes posed by concomitant haemorrhoids. Where possible these should be excised or injected at the time of the sphincterotomy.

Perianal haematoma – external pile

Constipation, straining and the lax skin associated with haemorrhoids predispose to this condition. An acute painful cherry-like swelling appears at the anal margin. The pain is self-limiting after a few days and the swelling subsidies into an anal tag over a few weeks. A very painful early lesion occasionally justifies deroofing under a local anaesthetic. This results in the extrusion of a small subcutaneous clot of blood and produces rapid relief of pain.

Abscess and fistula

Most abscesses and fistulas probably start as infection in the anal glands, usually between internal and external sphincter at the level of the dentate line. The internal opening of a fistula is thus likely to be along the duct of a gland, i.e. at the dentate line and most commonly posteriorly. The external opening is on the perianal skin where an abscess has pointed.

In the great majority of both abscesses and fistulas the muscle ring of external sphincter above the dentate line need not be divided (Fig 12.4). Thus adequate opening and drainage may be achieved without threat to continence. Most high internal openings are made by the injudicious use of the probe by a surgeon, less commonly, delay in drainage of pus results in upwards burrowing and medial pointing with a similar consequence.

The surgeon who is in any doubt about the relationship of the opening to the anorectal ring should not hesitate to refer to a colleague with a special interest in this area. In making the assessment, the position of the anorectal ring is most reliably made *in the conscious patient*. It is a common error to anaesthetise and paralyse a patient without having first established this crucial aspect of the anatomy.

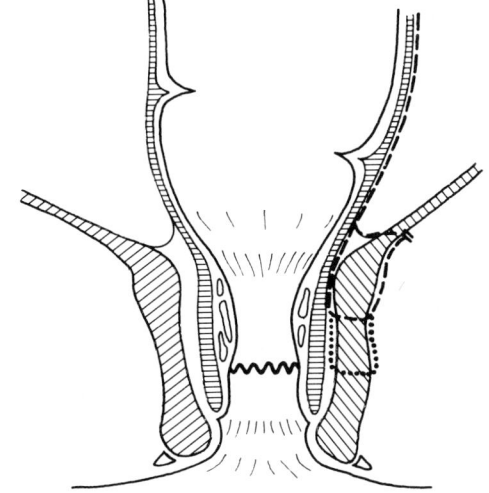

Fig 12.4 All complex fistula surgery is directed towards avoidance of a communication between the bowel and the ischiorectal fossa above the anorectal ring, i.e. the dotted line ---- must never be breached by pus or by the surgeon.

Permissible drainage

Figures 5, 6 and 7 indicate the directions of drainage which do not threaten continence. Note that the internal sphincter may be divided as required and also that part of the external sphincter below the dentate line.

Acute abscess

There is a real risk of missing deep intersphincteric (Fig 12.5) and occasionally even ischiorectal (Fig 12.6) suppuration which may not be obvious externally. Always heed a history of a sleepless night of deep throbbing pain which announces not cellulitis, but suppuration, and demands expeditious drainage, both to relieve the pain and to avoid irreversible damage to the sphincters. Antibiotics have little place in this situation and are no substitute for surgery. Examination under anaesthetic is always justified and the abscess should be drained adequately without any unnecessary division of the sphincteric apparatus. Fistulotomy should usually be deferred until the acute inflammation and oedema have settled or valuable anorectal muscle may be lost by necrosis. In addition, further separation of sphincter fibres occurs if a fistula is opened during the acute stage, since useful splintage is achieved by subsequent fibrosis. Intermuscular or the usually wrongly called submucous abscess should be drained into the lumen carrying the incision right down to the bottom of the

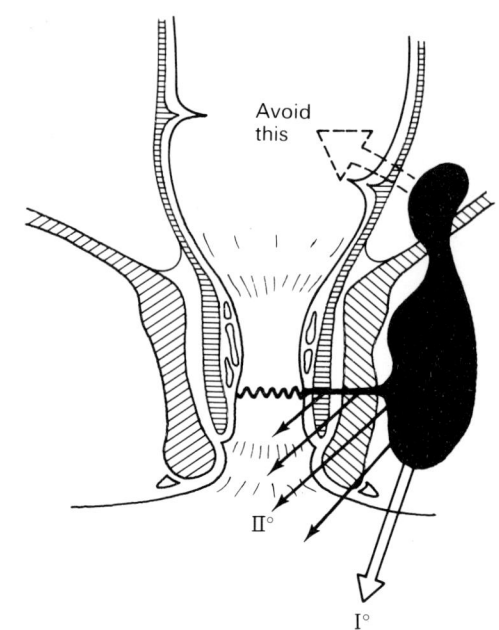

Fig 12.6 Ischiorectal abscess with a supralevator extension. Ischiorectal suppuration is another cause of severe anal pain which is commonly missed. Expeditious primary drainage through the skin will prevent the uncommon upward extension. This must *never* be opened into the rectum or an *extra* sphincteric fistula will result.

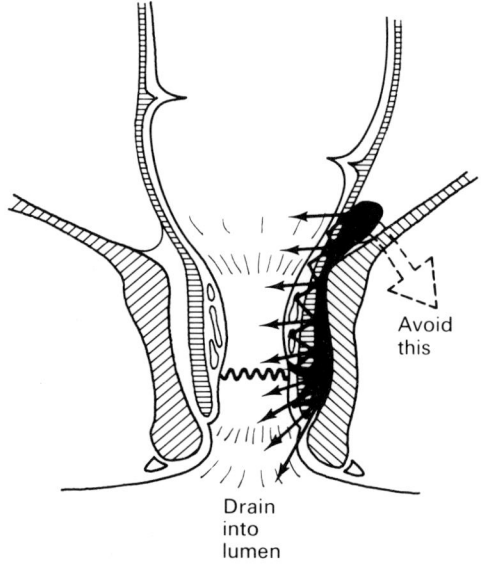

Fig 12.5 Deep intermuscular abscess. A cause of severe anal pain commonly missed for several days. Managed by long open internal sphincterotomy. *Never* open through the perineum or a *suprasphincteric* fistula will result.

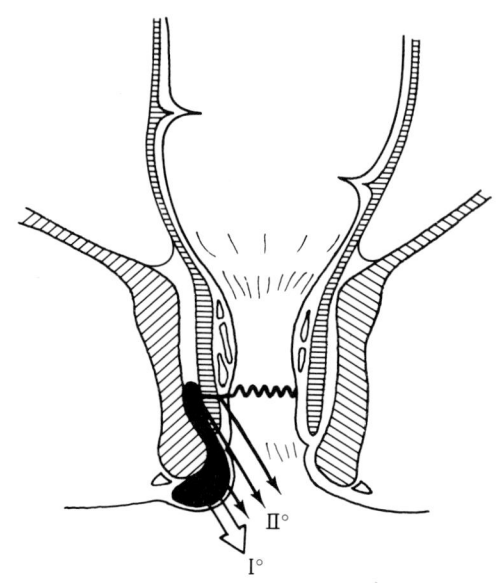

Fig 12.7 The commonest: intermuscular fistula and perianal abscess.

internal sphincter and up as far as the abscess cavity extends (Fig 12.5). A ring of residual internal sphincter below the cavity may result in great chronicity or even extension of the abscess due to lateral faecal burrowing above it. For those abscesses drained through the perineum, adequate opening at skin level is essential and should obviate the need for painful packing by a nurse, a practice which should be relegated to history (Figs 12.6, 7).

Two stage management. Some abscesses, usually due to staphylococci and without undue odour, are not connected with fistulae and do not require a second operation. Those which grow gut organisms and produce foul smelling pus are probably associated with a fistula. A definitive second operation for EUA and laying open of the fistula is, therefore, appropriate after about 2 months (Grace *et al.*, 1982).

Supralevator abscess. If this occurs due to upward extension of an intersphincteric abscess it should be drained by a long internal sphincterotomy into the lumen (Fig 12.5). If it follows extension of an ischiorectal abscess (Fig 12.6) it should be drained externally through the skin. In either case, the wrong route of drainage will result in a high supra or extrasphincteric fistula which will be a major problem in management. If it follows bowel or pelvic disease (Fig 12.8) it is often preferable to drain it suprapubically; each case, however, must be considered on its merits and definitive surgery for the underlying disease (e.g. diverticulitis or Crohn's disease) may be appropriate. It is never relevant to divide any part of the external sphincter unless the track is demonstrated to pass through it.

Practical points regarding fistula

Palpation of the indurated low track is valuable in defining its limits and detecting circumferential extensions. Goodsall's law is useful; it states that anterior fistulas are single and straight and run to the nearest crypt, whilst circumferential multiple tracks are usually posterior with the internal opening in the midline communicating with the deep postanal space.

Detailed diagrams and classification of complicated fistulas can be found in the paper by Parks, (Parks *et al.*, 1976). However, most patients can be managed on basic principles. The definitive procedure is the laying open of the track from the internal opening distally on to the skin (Fig 12.7). It is of little importance whether the track is excised, marsupialised or simply deroofed.

If the track passes through the muscle this may be cut, provided it does not disrupt the upper half of the external sphincter. This is best identified with the patient awake. The internal sphincter may be divided as high as necessary, always avoiding a distal intact

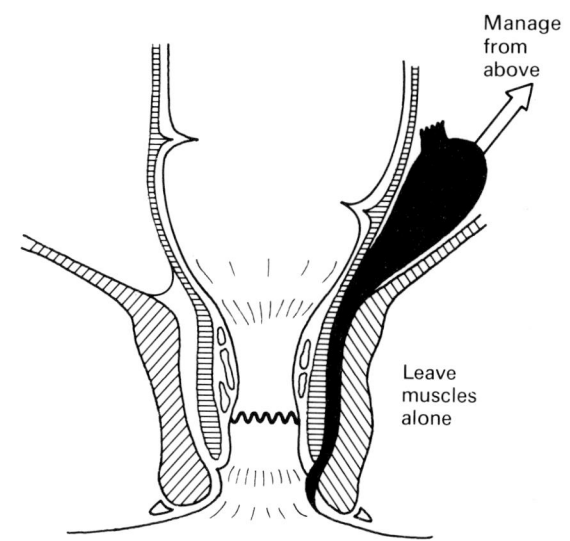

Fig 12.8 A supralevator abscess usually requires attention to its primary cause within the abdomen plus suprapubic drainage. It is then not relevant to divide the sphincter mechanism at all unless the track passes through the muscle.

ring, i.e. the sphincterotomy must extend at least from the internal opening to its lower end.

Upward extensions must be identified as being either within or outside the crucial 'outer tube' of external sphincter. Within the tube an intersphincteric upward extension is drained by a long open sphincterotomy (Fig 12.5). Outside it an upward extension of an ischiorectal abscess is drained via the perineum (Fig 12.6), i.e. the surgeon's efforts are directed to avoiding an iatrogenic or suppurative communication between an ischiorectal fossa or postanal space and the bowel above the anorectal ring.

Horseshoe fistula is managed by multiple lateral incisions or a circumferential incision plus opening of the primary causative internal end of the fistula, which may best be done by opening up the T track in the deep postanal space. It is usually not necessary to sever the anococcygeal ligament although this is not disastrous.

High fistula. If a high fistula is due to injudicious probing it may be cured by conservative measures. The true internal opening and the lower part of the track are laid open by internal sphincterotomy. The upper false passage is cored out and the sphincter stretched to faciliate drainage. If the top end seems likely to accumulate faeces, then an effective defunctioning colostomy and distal limb wash-out are prudent additional measures. In other high fistulas proper drainage within or without the anorectal ring plus defunctioning are appropriate. Occasionally a seton offers the best chance of cure.

Use of the seton. If a muscle is divided 'per primam', it retracts a significant distance. If there is time for fibrosis the ends become tethered and this distance is reduced. A seton works by transecting the sphincter slowly and gradually so that the ends do not retract to the extent that incontinence results. In addition the stitch can be moved back and forth while the patient soaks in the bath, so that drainage is facilitated. Furthermore, the patient may be examined without anaesthetic and progress of the salvage of sphincter function monitored while the seton is tightened distally.

Braided nylon is a suitable material. An alternative is a rubber band which is sequentially tightened over several weeks so as to maintain the pressure.

Pruritus ani

This symptom is one of the most difficult to manage in proctology. Investigation is directed towards exclusion of local treatable causes and also to the consideration of generalised skin disease. The causes are legion and only a few common pitfalls will be mentioned here.

Antibiotics may lead to anal candida infection, pediculosis and scabies must be looked for, threadworms may affect adults as well as children – they are seen only if the anus is examined in a good light, true fungal infection may occur in the natal cleft, dietary excess such as coffee may occasionally be relevant. Candida is recognised by the numerous satellite spots around the periphery of the central red area. Erythrasma is brown and fluoresces in ultra violet light while psoriasis and taenia both have characteristic margins.

In most cases no convincing primary cause is found and the cracked sore oedematous skin is a chronic source of irritation. The patient is advised against the use of toilet paper, and washing with baby soap or aqueous cream BP is preferred. Cool clothes, cotton underwear and dusting with baby powder may prevent the aggravation of sweating, and the loss of some weight may also help in this regard. Haemorrhoids, skin tags and other local conditions are dealt with as indicated and specific skin conditions treated by a dermatologist. Short courses only of steroid creams, preferably hydrocortisone cream, should be recommended and local anaesthetic or antihistaminic creams will lead eventually to local allergic rashes which make the situation worse.

Condyloma acuminata – anal warts

These are similar to warts seen on the vulva and the penis and are generally supposed to be venereal in origin. Occurring most commonly in males, they are usually associated with homosexual practice. They are, however, sometimes seen in normal young children of normal families so it would be wrong to attribute a venereal origin to every case.

The transmissible agent is a slow papilloma virus with an incubation period of many months or even a year or more. The greater frequency of warts in the recipient anus when compared with the transmitting penis probably reflects the favourable enironment of the warm moist anal canal and natal cleft for their growth. They vary from a few tiny projections to a mass of radially arranged columns which may totally obscure the anus and surrounding skin. The anal canal itself may also be the site of many of these warts.

Management

The diagnosis usually presents little difficulty, although the condyloma lata of secondary syphilis must not be forgotten. Coexistent gonorrhoea must be watched for and appropriate cultures set up. Ideally these should be plated out immediately onto a selective culture medium. Alternatively microscopy of a smear may be diagnostic or a suitable transport medium used for early transfer to the selective plate. The author's treatment is scissor excision of the warts which are raised by extensive subcutaneous injection with dilute adrenaline. Often the radial arrangement is a help in the preservation of normal skin between the raised lesions so that large defects can be avoided. Extensive use of diathermy is apt to cause painful wounds and sloughing, while cryosurgery is painless but rather difficult to control precisely.

Proctalgia fugax

This condition is typically a complaint of doctors and professional people, males more often than females. The history is diagnostic in that pain in the anorectum awakes the patient during the night. Sometimes it also affects him during the day and this calls for more careful investigation to exclude rectal disease. The deep searing anal pain is sometimes associated with tenesmus, but never with bleeding, mucus, or other important symptoms of organic disease. It settles after 15 min or less and only occasionally recurs on the same night. Indeed, it is unusual for it to occur more often than about half a dozen times a year. Simple reassurance usually suffices, after exclusion of serious disease by digital examination and sigmoidoscopy. Diazepam, hypnotics, quinine, opiates and suppositories all have their supporters, but the simple process of waking up is probably what cures the pain. Reassurance can be reinforced by encouragement and the information that it only happens to intellectual people. A high fibre diet is certainly worth trying in refractory cases.

Pilonidal sinus

Controversy continues to surround the aetiology of this common condition. A few are undoubtedly congenital pits. In most, hairs shed from higher on the trunk appear to work their way, perhaps by rolling off the buttocks, into the skin of the natal cleft. The latter explanation rests on the discovery of hairs pointing inwards: it also fits with the high incidence in hirsuite individuals and particularly men. The alleged associated with repetitive trauma – 'jeep driver's bottom' – would also fit with this explanation. Comparable sinuses between the fingers of barbers provide an interesting experimental model, and the rarity of the condition in the Chinese who have relatively little sacral hair lends further support to this theory.

The clinical condition is seen particularly in dark, hairy, obese males between 15 and 30 years, but seldom continues to cause trouble in middle or later life. It is therefore important to avoid operations which may inflict more suffering than the condition itself which will improve with time. Abscesses must be drained in continuity with the pit, and nests of hairs be removed by the most conservative approach available. If little trouble has occurred, it may suffice simply to pull out accessible hairs with forceps. In others simple opening of the track will be appropriate. The author avoids wide deroofing procedures and has seen abscesses undermining the flaps of the Z plasty operation. It is likely that recurrence rates are similar after major and minor procedures. Some authors have claimed excellent results with excision and primary suture, but it is important that no dead space is left over the surface of the sacrum. It must be admitted that even the conservative approach outlined does leave a few incompletely healed wounds and that the condition remains a significant cause of morbidity and lost work. The avoidance of undermined wounds and the control of chronic sepsis are probably the essence of management and chronic granulations may need to be curetted. Shaving the lower half of the back and regular bathing are probably of some value.

Hidradenitis suppuritiva

This is a rather uncommon inflammatory condition of the apocrine glands of the perianal skin. It starts as a nodule which progresses to abscesses, sinuses and areas of induration and oedema. If it becomes a problem the area must be excised down to the deep fascia and grafting may be necessary. It may cause confusion with fistula *in ano*, but has no communication with the anal canal.

Cancer of the anorectum

Rectal adenocarcinoma is more than twenty times commoner than anal cancer. The mucosa lining the anorectum is of three types, rectal mucosa in the upper third, squamous in the lower third, and transitional with varying admixtures of each in the central area around the dentate line.

Squamous carcinoma

The commonest neoplasm is a squamous carcinoma occurring in the lower or middle zones and producing an indurated anal ulcer. Characteristically this is painful and may cause confusion with a simple fissure. There should be no hesitation in advising examination under anaesthesia, and multiple deep biopsies should be taken. The procedure may need to be repeated and mistakes are by no means rare.

The management of squamous lesions poses problems. Abdominoperineal excision is frequently not essential, but the penalty for inadequate local excision or radiotherapy may be an incurable local recurrence and spread to the groins. In general, the smaller more superficial lesions under 2 cm at the anal margin can be managed by local excision or by radical radiotherapy, and the results are excellent. If recurrence develops, there should be no further delay in advising abdomino-perineal excision. Prophylactic groin excision is not called for, but inguinal dissections may be needed for involved lymph nodes.

Squamous lesions are radiosensitive and radical radiotherapy for the larger, deeper, or recurrent lesions has much to offer. Anaplastic lesions and large, deep or recurrent infiltrative, differentiated squamous lesions demand either radical radiotherapy with a temporary defunctioning colostomy, or an abdominoperineal excision. If the former is adopted, careful monitoring for recurrence is essential. 5-year survival figures are between 25% and 50% which has led some to combine radical radiotherapy with an aggressive cytotoxic regime. They currently claim considerable success and regard abdominoperineal excision unnecessary in a high proportion of patients.

Rare tumours of the anus

Basal cell carcinoma may occur at the anal margin and has a good prognosis. Perianal Bowen's disease causes confusion with idiopathic pruritus ani. Similar confusion may occur with perianal Paget's disease. Melanoma in this site has a hopeless prognosis; although abdominoperineal excision is usually advised, it is almost never successful.

Of great histopathological interest are the lesions of the transitional zone, cloacogenic, basiloid or epidermoid carcinomas. From the practical viewpoint they are managed exactly like squamous lesions, taking account of their size and degree of infiltration.

Temporary colostomy

In general a radical course of radiotherapy is best tolerated if the areas has been effectively defunctioned. Without this a very sore moist anus is likely to make the patient uncomfortable.

Colorectal tumours other than adenocarcinoma

Carcinoid tumour

These fall into two groups: small superficial lesions under 2 cm in diameter with a good prognosis, and larger lesions which behave like cancers. They are seldom secreting tumours, the blood level of 5HIAA is not raised and the carcinoid syndrome with flushing and borborygmi does not occur.

The commonest type is a solitary mobile umbilicated submucosal nodule about 1–2 cm in diameter, usually occurring in the lower rectum. Treatment is by local excision of the small nodules and abdominoperineal excision of the large ones. Histology does not greatly help differentiating between them, so careful follow-up is mandatory after local excision.

Lymphoma

Lymphosarcoma may be solitary or multiple and may mimic carcinoma or single or multiple polyps. A solitary lesion is resected like a carcinoma, possibly with adjuvant radiotherapy, while multiple lesions tend to be subjected to cytotoxic therapy. In general prognosis is poor, but long-term survival has been reported even after incomplete excision.

Leiomyosarcoma

This is rare and often radio-resistant.

Retrorectal tumours

A long list of extremely rare tumours can be compiled for this site (Goligher, 1980). Teratoma usually occurs in infancy, is commonly visible, has a high risk of malignancy and should be excised. A soft tumour in an adult woman is probably an enterogenous cyst, a firm bone-destroying one in a man a chordoma and a more laterally placed solid tumour may be a neurofibroma. It is seldom wise to use a transrectal approach to a cyst, since infection and incomplete excision may ensue. Low lesions are traditionally approached by a post-rectal incision with the patient in the prone jack-knife position. The coccyx is excised and the levator muscle divided to gain access to the retrorectal space from below. Higher lesions are approached through the abdomen by mobilising the rectum fully from above.

In the author's opinion all lesions which occur above the levators in a female can be best approached by this upper route. The blood supply of the cysts normally comes from above and full postrectal mobilisation in a wide female pelvis provides safe access and control.

A combined abdominosacral approach may be necessary for a chordoma, for which radiotherapy may also have some value.

Anal incontinence

'False' incontinence due to faecal impaction occurs postoperatively and in bedridden elderly patients. It requires faecal disimpaction and a period of re-education with enemas.

True anal incontinence may follow obstetric trauma or fistula surgery. It is important to state that these patients can be cured by surgical reconstruction in most cases. The belief that they are incurable is still widely held and many patients remain imprisoned as recluses by their condition and their lives ruined unnecessarily because they were formerly given a hopeless prognosis.

Major neurological incontinence is confined to cauda equina lesions since paraplegics do develop an automatic defaecation based on anal canal stimulation with suppositories. Idiopathic anal incontinence is probably due to a local neuropathy and this type is being increasingly recognised with lax sphincters and loss of the anorectal angle.

Anal reconstruction

Despite division, the anal muscle mass remains potentially functional for many years. Its severed ends must be identified in the conscious patient. At operation the incision curves round the anus from one end to the other, the muscles are dissected out of the fibrous tissue and overlapped. The intervening scar having been excised, the anal canal is reconstructed in layers. A protective colostomy provides reassurance when this procedure is performed for the first time.

Postanal repair

Parks has described an operation (Lytle and Parks, 1977) which is based upon access to the postanal levators by opening up the bloodless intersphincteric plane behind the anus. The internal sphincter is dissected off the outer tube of skeletal muscle posteriorly and laterally, and a lattice of non-absorbable sutures is places via this incision between the levators to restore the anorectal angle and lengthen and tighten the anal canal.

Disorders of the act of defaecation

Straining at stool is our heritage from the Victorian belief that 'regularity' was a virtue and milling to remove the fibre from the grain has compounded the issue. Denis Browne once described rectal prolapse in children as 'a complaint of the mother and an achievement of the child', thus putting some of these problems into perspective.

However, a whole range of important syndromes does arise from the breakdown of coordination of expulsive voluntary and involuntary muscle activity with pelvic floor and sphincter relaxation. The most obvious is full thickness rectal prolapse with a stretched and defective anal sphincter adding incontinence to the patient's problems. More obscure and incomprehensible is the syndrome of the descending perineum where the struggle to produce a non-existent stool often dominates the patient's daily life. While rectal prolapse can be satisfactorily controlled by surgical means, the associated incontinence, constipation and a whole range of 'straining syndromes' constitute some of the most refractory problems in proctology.

Rectal prolapse

Straining, constipation and incoordinated defaecation are the obvious causes of this condition and it has been reported in the earliest medical literature. The commonest sufferer is a thin, elderly middle-aged woman, who is often nulliparous. Thus the condition is quite different from vaginal prolapse with its clear association with childbearing.

Porter (1962) made the fundamental electromyographic observation of prolongation of the suppresssion of pelvic floor and sphincter tone that occurs in response to rectal distension. However, the observed prolapse starts in the anterior wall of the middle third of the rectum which turns itself inside out carrying the more distal rectal wall out with it. Thus a finger inserted at the anal margin around the fully prolapsed rectum, does not detect a groove – which differentiates it from an intussusception. As prolapse occurs the rectum straightens and comes forward out of the hollow of the sacrum. Most abdominal operations for prolapse are directed towards fixing it back there.

The symptoms of prolapse include varying degrees of anal incontinence which is partly primary and is partly secondary to stretching of the sphincters by the prolapse. Diagnosis is made by seeing several centimetres of prolapse with concentric mucosal folds, and feeling two thicknesses of bowel wall between finger and thumb. If only 1–2 cm of prolapse is seen by the surgeon, a problem exists in deciding if it is simply mucosal prolapse. The mucosal furrows or folds are helpful: in full-thickness prolapse they are circumferential whereas in mucosal prolapse they are radial (i.e. more like piles). Furthermore if 1–2 cm of mucosal prolapse is visible the anus itself will be everted in continuity with the mucosa and if it is the advancing head of a prolapse a groove will be palpable around it.

Indications for surgery

In infancy, it is generally necessary only to treat the child's constipation or predisposing cause and the mother's preoccupation with her offspring's bowel. Predisposing causes include urinary obstruction, wasting diseases, diarrhoea and laxative abuse. Ocassionally injection of phenol into the prolapse is required, and exceptionally a rectosigmoidectomy may be required for a strangulating full-thickness prolapse.

Abdominal operation for prolapse

Most adults who are fit enough are probably best treated by an abdominal operation.

In Britain the wrapping of polyvinyl sponge (Ivalon) around the mobilised rectum has become extremely popular (Wells, 1959). In the USA the Ripstein Sling operation (Ripstein, 1972) has become almost universal.

Both these operations involve various combinations of the following surgical steps:

1   *Posterior mobilisation* in the avascular plane between nerve plexuses and mesorectum – to beyond the coccyx.
2   *Anterior mobilisation* between rectum and vagina – to the anorectal ring.
3   *Division of the lateral ligaments.*
4   Various procedures for *fixation* of the rectum *in*

the hollow of the sacrum, e.g. Ivalon (Wells), Ripstein sling, suturing.

5 Various procedures to *buttress the levator muscles*, e.g. the original Ripstein 'trouser-graft', puborectal anterior approximation with stitches, or alternatively postrectal approximation.

6 Reconstitution of the divided peritoneal edges lower down so as to *draw* and fix *the rectum* and sigmoid *within* the *peritoneal cavity*.

The general trend has been towards procedure for sacral fixation and away from those designed to buttress the levators. This undoubtedly makes the operation easier, safer and quicker.

In the Ivalon sponge operation step 1, plus steps 2 and 3 if desired, are followed by retrorectal insertion of a 10 × 15 cm rectangle of Ivalon. This is stitched transversely to the presacral fascia with its lower margin as near to the level of the coccyx as is practicable. It is wrapped and stitched around the rectum and trimmed so as to leave the anterior surface uncovered. It is then excluded from the peritoneal cavity in any way which seems convenient. The Ripstein (Mark II) procedure (Ripstein, 1972) does not attempt such a low insertion of foreign material, but uses a 5 cm sling of Teflon or other suitable material around the rectum to tether its upper part to a point about 5 cm below the sacral promontory.

Each of these operations produces good results with recurrence rates below 10%. In the 'Wells' operation (Wells, 1959) the rectangle of Ivalon is wrapped around the mobilised rectum and mesorectum leaving the anterior surface free – it probably works both by fixing and by stiffening the rectal wall so that it cannot turn inside out. It is excluded from the peritoneal cavity by closing the peritoneum over it. Large volumes of buried Ivalon, however, do sometimes lead to postoperative faecal impaction. Furthermore, Ivalon sponge has few other established uses in surgery and is almost impossible to remove since it fragments and tends to disappear in time. If the Teflon sling of the Ripstein operation is fixed too tightly around the anterior surface, occasional cases of erosion through the rectal wall have occurred.

It seems probable that sacral fixation due to post-mobilisation fibrosis, perhaps enhanced by Ivalon or other foreign material, is usually all that is necessary. Some surgeons, therefore, prefer to mobilise the rectum thoroughly down to the anorectal ring anteriorly and posteriorly and then simply fix it with non-absorbable sutures within the hollow of the sacrum. They then reconstitute the peritoneal attachments lower down so as to retain the rectum within the abdomen. The lateral ligaments are much stretched and it is often possible to mobilise down to the anorectal ring without dividing them. They then can be hitched up and back to help retain the rectum by stitching to the sacral periosteum. The author also feels that there may be some importance in a full anterior mobilisation and in stitching the anterior wall to the vaginal wall since this does not usually prolapse with the rectum and may provide useful extra fixation.

Resection of the redundant sigmoid has also been practised in association with rectal mobilisation, but this is a much larger procedure for an elderly person. It is appropriate when there is, in addition, associated diverticular disease, and many American surgeons regard it as necessary to reduce recurrence. Low anterior resection was also successfully practised by Muir but this also is a major procedure with significant morbidity and mortality.

The dominant postoperative problem after any operation for prolapse is persisting incontinence. However, some improvement is likely for up to a year due to cessation of repeated stretching by the prolapse, and in some cases can be clearly identified as being due to residual mucosal prolapse. The latter may be injected or excised with improvement in both incontinence and mucous soiling. Sphincter exercises by 'perineal shrugging' may be of some value while bulk purgatives and a high fibre diet may also be helpful. Occasionally, however, bran may actually make the incontinence worse and aggravate the problem with flatulence.

Perineal operation for prolapse

Thiersch wire. Wire, braided nylon, monofilament nylon or prolene, half-inch folded mersilene slings, silicone rubber and various other non-absorbable materials have been used as a subcutaneous anal support introduced through two tiny incisions from below. A significant recurrence rate, the risk of postoperative faecal impaction, occasional extrusion of the foreign material and virtually no improvement in the incontinence are the main disadvantages. Despite these, the Thiersch procedure has a definite place in the management of prolapse in feeble and aged patients.

Perineal and transacral operations. A variety of procedures has been devised to buttress the levators behind the anorectum or to fix the rectum to their upper surface, or to the sacral hollow by dividing them behind the anus from below. Rectosigmoidectomy from below has largely been discredited due to high recurrence rates in many centres. None of these operations has become widely accepted, and none can be recommended for occasional use.

Excision of the rectum and permanent colostomy. Occasionally this is carried out when the patient's life has become permanently and hopelessly dominated by the impossible quest for defaecatory satisfaction. It is essential to take a second opinion before this irrevocable step and such patients are often in need of psychiatric help.

References

Anderson J.M. (1981). Chemotherapeutic prevention of recurrence after stapled anastomosis in rectal cancer. *Scot. Med. J.*; **26**:21–3.

Aylett S.O. (1966). Three hundred cases of diffuse ulcerative colitis treated by total colectomy and ileo-rectal anastomosis. *Brit. Med. J.*; **1**:1001.

Burkitt D.P. (1971). Possible relationships between bowel cancer and dietary habits. *Proc. Roy. Soc. Med*; **64**:964.

Cook S.A.R., de Moor N.G. (1981). The surgical treatment of the radiation damaged rectum. *Brit. J. Surg*; **68**:488–92.

Dixon C.F. (1936). Cancer of the recto-sigmoid: resection without permanent colostomy. *Proct. Staff Meet. Mayo Clinic*; **11**:384, 1936.

Doll R., Peto R. (1976). Mortality in relation to smoking: 20 years observation in male British doctors. *Brit. Med. J*; **2**:1525–36.

Fielding L.P., Wells B.W. (1974). Survival after primary and staged resection for large bowel obstruction caused by cancer *Brit. J. Surg*; **61**:16.

Finlay I.G., Meek D.R., Gray H.W., Durant G., McArdle C.S. (1982). Incidence and detection of occult hepatic metastasis in colorectal carcinoma. *Brit. Med. J*; **284**:803–5.

Gilchrist R.K. (1959). Lymphatic spread of carcinoma of the colon. *Dis. Co. Rect*; **2**:69–77.

Glober G., Nomuts A., Kamiyama S., Shunada A., Abba B. (1977). Bowel transit time and stool weight in populations with different colon cancer risks. *Lancet*; **ii**:110.

Goligher J.C. (1958). Extraperitoneal colostomy or ileostomy. *Brit. J. Surg*; **46**:97.

Goligher J.C. (1980). *Surgery of the Anus, Rectum and Colon*, 4th edn. pp. 570–4. London: Bailliere Tindall.

Goligher J.C., Morris C., McAdam W.A.F., de Dombal F.T., Johnston D.A. (1970). Controlled trial of inverting versus everting intestinal suture in large bowel surgery. *Brit. J. Surg*; **57**:817–22.

Grace R.H., Harper I.A., Thompson R.G. (1982). Anorectal sepsis: microbiology in relation to fistula in ano. *Brit. J. Surg*; **69**:7, 401–3.

Hager T., Schweiger M., Botticher D. (1976). *The Erlangen Magnetic Closure System for Colostomies and Ileostomies*. Paper presented to the International Society of University Colon-Rectal Surgeons, 6th International Congress, Salzburg.

Hahn R.G., Moertel C.G., Schutt A.J. *et al.* (1975). A double blind comparison of intensive course 5-Fluorouracil by oral vs. intravenous route in the treatment of colo-rectal carcinoma. *Cancer*; **35**:1031–5.

Heald R.J., Bussey H.J.R. (1975). Clinical experiences at St Mark's Hospital with multiple synchronous cancers of the colon and rectum. *Dis. Col. Rect*; **18**:1.

Heald R.J., Husband E.M., Ryall R.D.H.R. (1982). The mesorectum in rectal cancer surgery – the clue to pelvic recurrence? *Brit. J. Surg*; **69**:613–6.

Heald R.J., Leicester R.J. (1981). The low stapled anastomosis. *Brit. J. Surg*; **68**:333–7.

Heald R.J., Lockhart-Mummery H.E. (1972). The lesson of the second large bowel cancer. *Brit. J. Surg*; **59**:16.

Hughes E.S.R. (1966). Cancer of the right colon, upper left colon and sigmoid colon. *Aust. N.Z. J. Surg*; **35**:183.

Hunt R.H., Waye J.D. (1981). *Colonoscopy – Techniques, Clinical Practice and Colour Atlas*. London: Chapman and Hall.

Jensen P.M., Michenham R. (1979). Dietary factors and colorectal cancer in Scandinavia. *Israel J. Med. Science*; **15**:329.

Kock N.G. (1969). Intra-abdominal reservoir in patients with permanent ileostomy. *Arch. Surg. Chicago*; **99**:223.

Lennard-Jones J.E., Morson B.C., Ritchie J.K. (1977). Cancer in colitis: assessment of the individual risk by clinical and histological criteria. *Gastroenterol*; **73**:1280–9.

Lockhart-Mummery H.E. (1972). Anal lesions of Crohn's disease. *Clinics Gastroenterol*; **1**:377.

Lockhart-Mummery H.E. (1982). *Crohn's Disease*. Presidential address to the St Mark's Association.

Lockhart-Mummery H.E., Heald R.J. (1972). Clinical experience with metachronous cancer of the large intestine. *Dis. Col. Rect*; **15**:4–17.

Lockhart-Mummery H.E., Morson B.C. (1960). Crohn's disease of the large intestine and its distinction from ulcerative colitis. *Gut*; **1**:87.

Lockhart-Mummery H.E., Morson B.C. (1964). Crohn's disease of the large intestine. *Gut*; **5**:493.

Lord P.H. (1968). A new regime for the treatment of haemorrhoids. *Proc. Roy. Soc. Med*; **61**:935.

Lord P.H. (1975). Conservative management of haemorrhoids: 2 – Dilatation treatment. *Clin. Gastroenterol*; **4**:60;–8.

Lytle, Parks A.G. (1977). Intersphincteric excision of the rectum. *Brit. J. Surg*; **64**:413.

Mason A. York (1972). Transsphincteric exposure of the rectum. *Ann. Roy. Coll. Surg. Engl*; **51**:320.

Mason A. York (1974). Transsphincteric surgery of the rectum. *Prog. Surg*; **13**:66–97.

Moertel C.G., Schutt A.J., Hahn R.G. *et al.* (1975). Therapy of advanced colorectal cancer with a combination of 5-Fluorouracil, methyl-1,3-cis (2-chlorethyl)-1-nitrosourea, and vincristine. *J. Nat. Cancer Inst*; **54**:69-71.

Parks A.G. (1977). The endoanal technique of low colonic anastomosis. *Surg. Tech. Illus*; **2**:2.

Parks A.G., Nicholls R., Bellivean P. (1980). Proctocolectomy with ileal reservoir and anal anastomosis. *Brit. J. Surg*; **67**:533–8.

Parks A.G., Gordon P.H., Hardcastle J.D. (1976). A classification of fistula-*in-ano*. *Brit. J. Surg*; **63**:1.

Parks A.G., Percy J.P. (1982). Resection and sutured colo-anal anastomosis for rectal carcinoma. *Brit. J. Surg*; **69**:301–4.

Porter N.H. (1962). A physiological study of the pelvic floor in rectal prolapse. *Ann. Roy. Coll. Surg. Engl*; **31**:379.

Ripstein C.B. (1972). Procidentia – definitive corrective surgery. *Dis. Colon Rect*; **15**:334.

Rosenberg I.L. (1979). The aetiology of colonic suture-line recurrence. *Ann. Roy. Coll. Surg. Eng*; **61**:251–7.

Sames C.P. (1960). Resection of Ca. colon in the presence of obstruction. *Lancet*; **ii**:948.

Savage P.T. (1967). Immediate resection with end-to-end anastomosis for carcinoma of the colon presenting with acute intestinal obstruction. *Proc. R. Soc. Med*; **60**:207.

Schofield P.F., Cade D., Lambert M. (1980). Dependent proximal loop colostomy: does it defunction the distal colon? *Brit. J. Surg*; **67**:201–2.

Slaney G. (1971). Results of treatment of Ca. colon and rectum. In *Modern Trends in Surgery 3* (Irvine W.T. ed.) pp. 69–89. London: Butterworth.

Taylor I., Rowling J., West C. (1979). Adjuvant cytotoxic liver perfusion for colorectal cancer. *Brit. J. Surg*; **66**:833–7.

Taylor I. (1981). Studies on the treatment and prevention of colorectal liver metastases. *Ann. Roy. Coll. Surg. Eng*; **63**:270–6.

Todd I.P. (1977). Intractable constipation and adult megacolon. In *Operative Surgery*: Colon, Rectum and Anus, 3rd edn. pp.268–70. London and Boston: Butterworth.

Turnbull R., Schofield P.F. (1970). Choice of operation for the toxic megacolon phase of nonspecific ulcerative colitis. *Surg. Clin. N. Amer*; **50**:1151.

Walker A.R.P., Painter N.S. (1972). Effect of dietary fibre on stools and transit times and its role in the causation of disease. *Lancet*; **ii**:1408.

Wangensteen O.H. (1949). Cancer of the colon and rectum. *Wis. Med. J*; **48**:491.

Wells C. (1959). New operation for rectal prolapse. *Proc. Roy. Soc. Med*; **52**:602–3.

Further reading

Cotton P.B., Williams C.B. (1980). *Practical Gastrointestinal Endoscopy*. Oxford: Blackwell Scientific.

Heberer, G. ed. (1982). Current management of rectal cancer. *World J. Surg*; **6**:501–95.

Thomson J.P.S., Nicholls R.J., Williams C.B. (1981). *Colorectal Disease*. London: Heinemann Medical.

Todd I.P. (1978). *Intestinal Stomas*. London: Heinemann Medical.

13

Paediatric and neonatal surgery

A.W. WILKINSON

Inguinal hernia

In childhood, as in older patients an **oblique inguinal hernia**, is due to persistence of a patent processus vaginalis of the testis and may be bilateral.

There is often a tendency to delay operation on an inguinal hernia, especially in babies, because it is thought this involves less risk than immediate operation. Inguinal herniotomy in babies and young children is a simple operation in the absence of incarceration, obstruction or strangulation. These complications result in oedema of the delicate coverings of the sac and the structures of the cord and make a usually easy operation very difficult indeed.

When a baby with an inguinal hernia is seen as an outpatient, early, if not immediate, admission for operation should be advised, especially if the history suggests that it has ever been difficult to reduce. When a hernia in a baby cannot be reduced, the child must be admitted at once. The legs should then be slung in a gallows splint so that the buttocks are just off the bed and 0.1–0.2 mg morphine per kg body weight should be injected i.m. If the hernia reduces spontaneously, the baby should be kept in the splint for 3 days to allow oedema of the coverings to subside before operation. If the hernia does not reduce within 2 h, operative reduction must be done. The obstruction is usually due to the tight grip of the external ring on the contents of the sac and division of the external ring usually allows reduc-

tion of the contents of the sac. If during operation the sac is greatly torn, the incision must be enlarged and the inguinal canal must be opened widely and the neck of the sac, which is probably not oedematous, must be found and drawn together with an 00 silk suture.

In the baby and infant the inguinal canal is shorter and less oblique than later in life and the lateral border of the external ring is only just medial to the medial border of the deep ring. For this reason the whole of the sac can readily be exposed through a transverse incision over the external inguinal ring and there is no need to open up the inguinal canal by splitting the fibres of the external oblique aponeurosis. The transverse incision is made in the suprapubic skin crease immediately cranial to the point at which the vas deferens can be rolled with the finger on the pubic ramus. Forceps are placed on the subcutaneous fat on each side in the centre of the incision and the deep fascia is divided. By blunt dissection the cord and coverings are identified and cleared so that the testis can be drawn out into the wound. The cord is rotated so that an area of the coverings is exposed away from the vessels and this is taken up in forceps on either side and put on the stretch; the coverings are then carefully incised with a scalpel and the hernial sac is identified and cleared of the ductus, the vessels and the coverings to its neck which is identified by a conical blob of fat. Having made sure the sac is empty, it is transfixed with an 00 black silk suture on a round bodied needle and ligated. The excess is cut away and the testis is returned to the scrotum. The skin is closed with a subcuticular continuous stitch of 00 catgut. A dry gauze dressing is applied for 24 h and then removed and the wound is sprayed with collodion. If the patient is well, he is sent home. The procedure in a girl is the same except that there is not a testis to be mobilised and the round ligament is the landmark instead of the ductus.

A **direct inguinal hernia** is due to a protrusion of peritoneum and extraperitoneal fat through a small opening in the transversalis fascia in the posterior wall of the medial half of the inguinal canal. It is very rare in childhood. All that is needed is to close the fenestration in the transversalis fascia with a black silk stitch (00).

Hydrocoele of the tunica vaginalis of the testis

This also is due to the persistence of the processus vaginalis of the testis and is due to the collection of fluid in the processus. This may be caused in various ways, such as minor injury to the testis, inflammation of the testis as in epididymo-orchitis, or for no obvious reason at all. In childhood, a hydrocoele almost always subsides spontaneously and it should be left alone to do so. When emptied by aspiration, it usually rapidly refills and aspiration may cause a haematocoele; excision is commonly complicated by the formation of a scrotal haematoma. On the other hand in the *communicating type of hydrocoele* there is a narrow channel at the upper end which communicates with the peritoneal cavity, through which the fluid can be slowly expressed, in this way establishing the diagnosis. This type is usually treated as if it was an inguinal hernia by herniotomy. If discomfort is associated with a large hydrocoele in older boys, they should be advised to wear tight underpants as a support. An encysted hydrocoele of the cord is a small hydrocoele 1 to 2 cm in diameter and it should be excised because of the anxiety it causes, and this holds also for the same condition involving the round ligament in girls, (hydrocoele of the canal of Nuck).

Varicocoele

This is uncommon in childhood and when it causes symptoms, the effect of wearing tight underpants should be tried in the first place and if this is not effective the veins should be divided as in older patients.

Femoral hernia

This also is rare in childhood. It is best treated by excision of the sac by the retropubic extraperitoneal approach through a transverse suprapubic incision.

Testis

For those who are not accustomed to handling and examining small boys the distinction between the normally placed, the retractile, the ectopic and the undescended testis may sometimes be very difficult.

The retractile testis

This is a normally descended testis with a very active cremasteric reflex, so active that on exposure of the lower half of the body, the testis is at once drawn up out of the scrotum into the subcutaneous inguinal pouch. This may happen even at bath-time and the testis may not come down even after 10 to 15 min in a warm bath. It will certainly happen if the child's napkin or pants are taken down some minutes before he is examined, and if the examiner has cold hands the testis will stay retracted. If the trousers or napkin are taken off only immediately before the child is to be examined and the examiner's hands are warm, the testis can almost always be gently pushed down into the scrotum. If it does retract, it does so slowly and not suddenly as an ectopic testis does. When the testis has been pushed down to the scrotum, this must be demonstrated to the parents and moreover they must be shown that it is staying in position. They should be firmly reassured that it is normal and does not need any surgical treatment and the same sentiments should be conveyed to the general practitioner.

The ectopic testis

This is one which has gone off the normal line of descent of the testis from the lower pole of the kidney to the scrotum. The gubernaculum passes down the inguinal canal and at the external inguinal ring divides into five parts. One goes on down into the scrotum, the normal line of descent of the testis. The other four pass out, one to the suprapubic region, one to the femoral triangle, one to the perineum, and one to the surface of the external oblique in the lower quadrant of the abdomen. This last is believed to be the attraction for by far the commonest type of ectopic testis, the 'inguinal ectopic' lying in the subcutaneous inguinal pouch on the surface of the external oblique aponeurosis above and lateral to the external inguinal ring.

An inguinal ectopic testis cannot usually be pushed down further than the pubic tubercle and when released jumps immediately back to its original position on the elastic recoil of its attachments. An ectopic testis will never descend spontaneously into the scrotum. It must be dissected free from its fibrous attachments and usually the coverings also must be divided before it can be placed in the scrotum. Sometimes, it will not reach the scrotum and then it should be left where it will lie. It is usually worth-while trying again to bring it down at a second operation after an interval of a year. For this reason the parents should be warned at the out-patient consultation that, although an operation is essential, it may not be possible to get the testis all the way into the scrotum and that a second operation may be necessary.

Undescended testis

An undescended testis is one which is on the normal line of descent, but which has not reached the scrotum. About 10% of undescended testes are still within the peritoneal cavity hanging on the lateral wall of the pelvis by their mesentery. About 10% are at the deep inguinal ring, sometimes in the ring and sometimes just in the peritoneal cavity. The remainder are in the inguinal canal, or at the external ring or between it and the pubic tubercle. It is often difficult to feel a testis in the inguinal canal, yet in a well-relaxed child it is sometimes possible to feel a testis at the deep inguinal ring or even on the lateral wall of the pelvis near the ring (Figs 13.1, 2).

The treatment of undescended testis is by operation. Hormones are useless except as substitution therapy after bilateral orchiectomy. The parents should always be clearly warned at the outset that because of the shortness of the blood vessels it may not be possible to get the testis down to the scrotum either at the first or even at subsequent operations, but the only way to find out is to try to bring it down. If there is any doubt about whether the testis can be felt, they should be told this and they should be warned that the testis may be intra-abdominal and permission should be obtained to proceed to a laparotomy at once after exploration of the inguinal canal if the testis is in the peritoneal cavity and cannot be reached or found.

At operation, the testis, ductus and vessels should be cleared of all their coverings and gently stripped clean

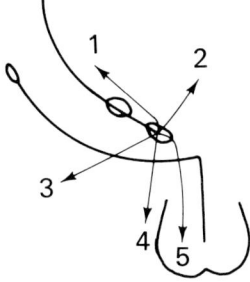

Fig 13.1 To show five divisions of the cremasteric fascia. 1 = iliac; 2 = abdominal; 3 = femoral; 4 = perineal; 5 = scrotal.

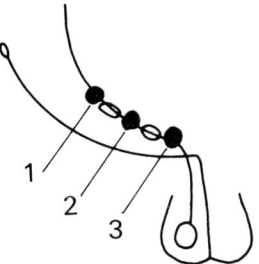

Fig 13.2 Failure of descent of the testis. 1 = nitroabdominal; 2 = in the canal; 3 = in the subcutaneous inguinal pouch.

of all fibrous bands. This should be carried right up to and into the deep inguinal ring, but not much further length is gained by stripping the vessels in the iliac fossa. If there is a hernial sac, this must be cleared and ligated at its neck and completely freed from the vessels and ductus. The testis is then laid in its bed. If it can be placed in the scrotum, the fat and fascia anterior to the ductus and vessels in the root of the scrotum should be approximated with catgut stitches to stop the testis retracting out of the scrotum. If the testis will not reach to the scrotum, it should be allowed to lie where it will reach and the external oblique aponeurosis is closed over the ductus and vessels. If the testis is intra-abdominal, it is unlikely to be of any functional value and even less likely to come down further than the uppermost part of the inguinal canal and is better removed. It must be examined histologically and the parents should be told why it was removed and about the histological findings.

Anorchia

This is very rare, but when it occurs the parents must be told frankly. They must also be told that normal growth and development can be assured by substitution hormone treatment. They should also be told that after puberty silastic testicles can be implanted in the scrotum, with usually great psychological benefit to the patient. This should be done also in those boys who have had orchiectomy for an intra-abdominal testis. Great care must be taken, however, to ensure that the scrotum is not overstretched by the prosthesis. It is better to put in one and wait a year before putting in the other so as to avoid pressure gangrene of the scrotum with sloughing of the skin and the discharge of both prostheses.

There is much controversy about when an undescended testis should be operated on. If there is an evident hernia, or a history suggestive of one, operation should not be delayed. The hernia should be dealt with and if the testis can be brought down this should be done. If a boy with an undescended or ectopic testis complains of pain on the same side, this also is an indication for early, if not immediate operation, because of the risk of torsion of the testis.

There is a good deal of evidence that for normal development of the testis, it should be brought down to the scrotum by the age of five years. Since many testes do not come down to the scrotum at the first operation and a second is necessary, it is advisable to operate on undescended testes at the age of four years.

There has been much argument about fixation of the mobilised testis in various ways. Most forms of fixation involve holding the testis in position against the pull of the blood vessels and in a proportion of patients this causes spasm of the vessels and infarction of the testis. If the testis will not stay in the scrotum without fixation, it is safer to let it lie at a higher level without tension. The most that should be done is to put one or two cat-gut sutures in the neck of the scrotum to narrow it.

The results of operations on undescended testicles are bad, but this is usually evident only when both are undescended and the cause of infertility is investigated. Very, very few men who had bilateral undescended testes are fertile and biopsies show poor development of the tubules, a low fertility index and impaired motility and structure of any spermatozoa they may produce.

Torsion of the testis

A testis may twist on its pedicle wherever it may be lying, but this is more common in the so-called 'bell-clapper' testis which is fully descended in the scrotum, but lies more transversely than the normal testis. The onset of torsion is indicated by severe pain in the groin, scrotum or abdomen and the testis becomes swollen and acutely tender to touch. It is sometimes possible to untwist the testis by gentle manipulation and success in this results in reduction of both pain and tenderness. It is usually wiser to explore the testis under general anaesthesia and this should be done as soon as possible. After 12 h the chances of saving the testis are poor. If the exposed testis is black and the colour does not improve when the pedicle is untwisted, a small incision should be made in the tunica vaginalis. If any arterial blood is seen, there is still hope of recovery but, in any case, it is probably worth putting the testis back in the scrotum. If it does not recover, it will shrink and can then be removed at another operation.

Torsion of a hydatid of Morgagni

Torsion of a hydatid of Morgagni causes the same severe pain usually in the scrotum or groin as torsion of the whole testis. There is less swelling of the scrotum, the cord is not usually oedematous and if the testis is very gently palpated, it is usually possible to localise the acute tenderness to a small area near the upper pole of the testis on one side and so to make the diagnosis. It is, however, always wiser to operate on the testis than to wait for the pain to subside, as it commonly does after about 12 h when the hydatid becomes gangrenous and sloughs.

Umbilical hernia

This type of hernia is due to the persistence of the primitive peritoneal protrusion into the umbilical cord at about 7½ weeks of gestation. The size of the hernia varies greatly from being barely perceptible in some babies to a protrusion 10 cm from the abdominal wall with a neck 5 cm in diameter. The neck of the true umbilical hernia is circular and has a sharp, well-defined margin. The contents are usually bowel and omentum and the latter may become adherent to the sac wall and the hernia is then irreducible. There may be wide separation of the rectus muscles with a soft linea alba which bulges forwards, so-called divarication, which extends from the umbilicus to the xiphoid process.

Umbilical hernia is very common in the negroid races but most, except the very large ones, subside spontaneously as they do in the children of most other races. In general up to the age of 2 years umbilical hernia should be treated conservatively. Strangulation and incarceration are very uncommon and only occasionally has perforation been recorded.

If the parents insist that some form of treatment is undertaken, the first option is reduction of the hernia and its retention by the firm application of three strips of waterproof strapping 8–10 cm wide which overlap each other and extend from the anterior axillary line on one side to the same line on the other side. This strapping should be renewed every 2 weeks. This method is inconvenient and the child can only be washed and not bathed, but it works if continued long enough.

Operative treatment consists in making an incision in the actual edge of the lower half of the umbilical scar and then dissecting the sac away from the skin. When the sac is clear, the fascia round the neck at the opening in the linea alba is divided circumferentially, the neck of the sac is cleared, transfixed with a silk stitch (00) and ligated, the excess is cut away and the opening in the linea alba is closed transversely with 3 interrupted silk stitches (00) and skin edges are also closed with silk stitches.

Supraumbilical hernia

This is a protrusion through an elliptical opening in the linea alba about 1 cm above the true umbilical scar and can be clearly distinguished on clinical examination from an umbilical hernia. A supraumbilical hernia never closes spontaneously and should always be treated by operation in the same way as a true umbilical hernia.

Epigastric hernia

Like a supraumbilical hernia, an epigastric hernia is due to the protrusion of a small pouch of peritoneum through a gap in the decussating fibres of the linea alba, most often in its middle third. It most often causes symptoms in older children when omentum becomes incarcerated in the sac. The child complains of upper abdominal midline pain towards the end or just after a meal and of local tenderness over the small knob about 1 cm in diameter in the midline of the epigastrium. It should always be treated by operation in the same way as a supraumbilical hernia.

Exomphalos (omphalocoele)

This is a very large umbilical hernia. The inner layer of the sac is peritoneum and the outer layer is fibrous tissue which was originally continuous with the amniotic membrane. It may be only a few centimetres in diameter or may involve a third of the anterior abdominal wall and contain most of the intestines and part of the liver; the reduction of the contents may then be very difficult because of the small size of the abdominal cavity relative to the bulk of the contents of the sac. Alternatively, it may appear as a herniation of bowel into the umbilical cord with a narrow pedicle, a type in which the contents may be reduced into the peritoneal cavity. If completely clear the base of the cord can be tied in the usual way.

About half the patients with exomphalos have other severe associated anomalies which are the chief cause of the high mortality rate (40%). The most lethal are anomalies of the heart and great vessels, but others may occur in the genitourinary tract, the worst of which is vesicointestinal fistula. Malrotation of the midgut and other intestinal anomalies are common and should always be looked for at operation before the sac is closed. Immediately after the birth of the baby, the sac should be covered with gauze soaked in 0.9% saline, 0.5% hibitane in water or a 2% aqueous solution of mercurochrome and the abdomen should then be wrapped in thin polythene film to prevent evaporation and

cooling and the baby should, if possible, be transferred to a specialist surgical unit.

Conservative treatment has been used, without much success, in the hope of reducing the high mortality rate. It consists in painting the sac several times a day with a 2% aqueous solution of mercurochrome or some similar antiseptic until a dry crust forms under which epithelium spreads in from the margins of the defect. This takes from 8 to 12 weeks. The resulting large ventral hernia is closed later. If another intestinal anomaly is present operation is unavoidable.

It is sometimes possible to free the skin round the margins of the sac and undermine the skin widely and then sew the edges together over the sac. In some babies, there is so much of the abdominal contents in the sac that when these contents are forced back into the abdominal cavity, they cause such pressure on the diaphragm that its movement, on which most of the respiratory exchanges depend in the neonate, is so reduced that respiratory acidosis develops. In this circumstance, warning of which should be given by the anaesthetist, a silastic bag should be made as is described for gastroschisis. Some surgeons have enlarged the abdominal cavity by forcibly stretching the abdominal wall with their fingers until it will accommodate all the contents of the hernia. Others have cut the rectus muscles transversely at the level of the umbilicus. After operation, apart from respiratory difficulties which may require ventilation, it is usually necessary to feed the baby intravenously for a week or more until gastrointestinal motility is good enough for oral feeds to be tolerated.

Gastroschisis

In this condition there is a small defect in all the layers of the anterior abdominal wall just to the right of a normal umbilical cord. This defect appears days or weeks before birth, its cause is not known, and through it all of the alimentary tract from the middle third of the stomach to the rectum may prolapse. The prolapsed bowel is matted together by firm fibrous adhesions. Immediately after birth, the prolapsed bowel should be wrapped in gauze soaked in warm 0.9% saline and put into a plastic bag and the baby should be transferred in a warm incubator; even so, most arrive at the surgical unit with the body temperature well below normal.

When the baby has been warmed, a transverse incision is made on either side of the opening dividing both rectus muscles with the skin. An artificial hernial sac, large enough to contain the bowel which cannot be comfortably accommodated in the abdominal cavity, is made out of reinforced silastic sheeting which is sewn to the edges of the peritoneum and cut muscles and aponeurosis with silk stitches. This sac is suspended from the top of the incubator and each day some of the contents are squeezed back into the abdominal cavity. When reduction is complete the skin edges are closed. Intravenous feeding is usually necessary for 10 to 14 days because transit through the matted mass of intestine is so poor. The adhesions should not be interfered with at operation as they subside completely if left alone and attempts at separation cause unnecessary damage.

Urachus

During the early stages of its development from the urogenital sinus, the bladder has a long conical extension to the umbilicus, the urachus. As the bladder migrates to the pelvis, the apex of this projection may retain its attachment to the umbilicus and its lumen may not be completely obliterated. The whole channel may remain patent and urine may be discharged from an opening in the lower border of the umbilicus. If the urinary tract is otherwise normal, the patent tract is excised and the opening in the apex of the bladder is closed. If, however, there is a distal obstruction in the urinary tract the urachus offers a convenient means of draining urine until the distal obstruction has been treated. The urachus may disappear partially leaving a cyst in the central part or a diverticulum of the apex of the bladder; both should be excised.

Neonatal intestinal obstruction and other anomalies of the alimentary tract

Diaphragmatic hernia

There is no doubt that some babies with large left-sided diaphragmatic hernias constitute the most urgent surgical emergencies of all in the first 24 h after birth and are still subject to a mortality rate of 60% or more.

The commonest and most important type of diaphragmatic hernia is that through the patent pleuroperitoneal canal (Bochdalek). This causes trouble on the left side more often than on the right, where the liver blocks off all but very large hernias. This hernia is predisposed to by the return of the midgut from the hernia in the cord and the unfixed and unrotated intestine passes up into the chest. The presence of the intestines and the spleen and, perhaps, the left lobe of the liver and the stomach in the pleural cavity interferes with the normal development of the lungs, especially the left one. The resulting hypoplasia of the lungs can be recognised by the small size of the left one when seen at operation on the hernia and is the cause of the respiratory insufficiency which persists after the reduction of the contents of the hernia and in spite of artificial ventilation. In addition, major cardiovascular anomalies may be associated and the right lung also may be smaller than usual.

In a newly-born baby, cyanosis, difficulty in starting respiration, and dextrocardia should suggest the diagnosis of a large left-sided diaphragmatic hernia. A plain radiograph of the chest will show loops of bowel in the chest with a shift of the heart to the right. The most important cause of confusion is a lung replaced by air-filled cysts.

Survival depends on immediate treatment. An endotracheal tube is passed and gently insufflated with oxygen; forcible ventilation will rupture the hypoplastic lungs. A gastric tube is passed, the stomach is emptied and continuous aspiration is established. Oxygen should never be administered by a face-mask nor should oxygen be given by an intragastric tube, because both will distend the stomach and, if the stomach is in the chest, this will increase the mediastinal shift and respiratory embarrassment. Cardiac arrest should be treated by external cardiac massage.

If the baby is to be transferred to another hospital for treatment, an anaesthetist should accompany the baby in the ambulance because deterioration is so common and controlled ventilation may be necessary. If the condition of the baby remains poor, it may be wiser to operate without transfer. Operative relief is urgent and it is unwise to delay while blood is being cross-matched. This and volvulus of the midgut are the only neonatal surgical emergencies of which this can be said.

The abdomen should be opened through a long transverse incision above the umbilicus from the left costal margin to the outer border of the right rectus muscle. The herniated bowel is drawn out of the chest on to the abdominal wall and wrapped in warm packs and the orifice of the hernia is inspected. It is almost always possible to find enough diaphragm to close the defect. The posterior lip of the hernia is usually thick, because the sheet of muscle has rolled up on itself. This can be undone by careful dissection after dividing the overlying peritoneum and will then almost always provide enough muscle to close the defect. It is sometimes necessary to use a piece of reinforced silastic sheet to close the gap. A drain with an underwater seal should be inserted into both pleural cavities for 24 h because the incidence of spontaneous pneumothorax on the opposite side is so high. Before the bowel is returned to the abdomen, it should be searched throughout for other anomalies, especially malrotation. If the capacity of the abdominal cavity is too small to contain the alimentary tract, a temporary hernial sac of silastic sheeting should be made as for a gastroschisis. Gastric aspiration should be continued for at least 48 h and parenteral feeding may be necessary. The main post-operative problem is likely to be respiratory insufficiency which is the commonest cause of death; some babies just do not have sufficient lung to provide enough ventilatory capacity on which to survive.

A baby with a diaphragmatic hernia which does not cause a clinical disturbance within 24 h of birth has a much better prognosis and the mortality rate in this type is less than 20%.

The anterior type of diaphragmatic hernia (Morgagni) seldom causes trouble in the neonate or infant. The hernia is small and usually has a sac. When the sac is absent, bowel may herniate into the pericardium and treatment is then required.

Hiatus hernia

An abnormally wide oesophageal hiatus in the diaphragm allows the cardiac end of the stomach and the cardio-oesophageal junction to lie above the diaphragm. Occasionally, and especially in older infants, a considerable part of the fundus of the stomach may be above the diaphragm and very rarely two-thirds of the stomach may herniate through the hiatus and bulge into the right pleural cavity. In the para-oesophageal type, the fundus of the stomach herniates in front of the oesophagus with a sac of pleura and peritoneum. Reflux is common only in the first of these types which is the commonest and most important in the infant. This reflux of acid gastric juice causes severe inflammation of the lower third of the oesophagus and bleeding may be so heavy as to require transfusion in the first week or two after birth.

The most important sign of hiatus hernia is the effortless vomiting of gastric juice and feeds which may start soon after birth and commonly occurs when the baby is laid down in the cot after a feed. Radiological examination after the baby has swallowed a radio-opaque feed usually shows the hernia, with or without reflux, and thick folds of gastric mucosa lying above the diaphragm. Pyloric obstruction can also be excluded.

Treatment is primarily conservative. The feeds are thickened, small and frequent, and if the baby brings back a feed, another should be given at once. The child is nursed sitting almost upright in a hiatus hernia chair or box. Aluminium hydroxide, or magnesium trisilicate if the baby is constipated, should be given after every feed to reduce gastric acidity. In 95% of patients such treatment results in subsidence of the disturbance.

Rarely, if the reflux persists, it is necessary to operate on the hernia. This should be done through the left eighth intercostal space; the pleura over the oesophagus is slit longitudinally, the oesophagus and herniated stomach are mobilised, the herniated peritoneum is divided all round the uppermost part of the fundus of the stomach and, through an incision in the left dome of the diaphragm, the cardio-oesophageal junction is drawn down into the abdomen. The two crura of the oesophageal hiatus of the diaphragm are then brought snugly together behind the oesophagus with a strong silk suture (Fig 13.3).

If a stricture forms in the lower oesophagus, it should be dilated through the oesophagoscope. Rarely it is necessary to resect a stricture and if end-to-end anastomosis is not possible, a segment of colon must be brought up to join the stumps of the oesophagus together.

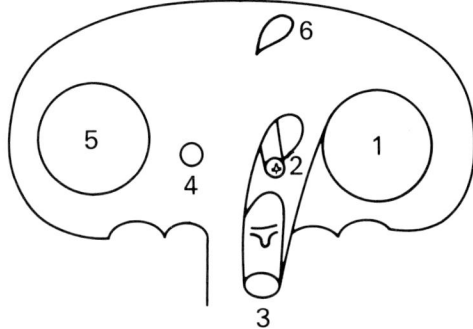

Fig 13.3 Diaphragmatic hernia. 1 = left posterolateral type (Bochdalek); 2 = oesophageal hiatus; 3 = aorta; 4 = vena cava; 5 = large hernia of right cupola; 6 = anterior or Morgagni type.

Oesophageal atresia

Oesophageal atresia most commonly occurs at the junction of the upper and middle thirds of the oesophagus, a junctional zone of the blood and nerve supply, the musculature and the mucous membrane. The five different types of anomaly and their frequency and associated mortality in a personal series are shown in Fig 13.4. In type A the lower oesophagus is very short and there is not a fistula with the trachea. In type B there is a fistula between the upper pouch of oesophagus and the trachea, but the lower piece of oesophagus is very short. Type C is the commonest form of the anomaly and occurs in over 80% of patients. The oesophagus ends blindly at the lower end of the upper third and the lower oesophagus communicates with the trachea by a tracheo-oesophageal fistula. There may be a gap of up to 4 or 5 cm between the two pieces of oesophagus or they may overlap and appear to have a continuous muscle coat. There may be fistulas to the trachea from both pieces of oesophagus (type D); the upper fistula is often not diagnosed in the early stages, even when a search is made for it at operation and there are recurrent attacks of bronchopneumonia. Finally, the oesophagus may be normal apart from a fistula to

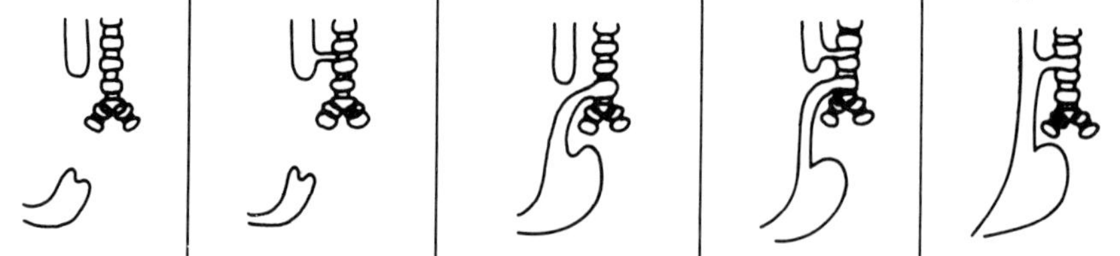

Type of anomaly

	Type A	Type B	Type C	Type D	Type E

	Type A	Type B	Type C	Type D	Type E
1959–67	6 (6.4%)	4 (4.3%)	76 (81.7%)	2 (2.1%)	5 (5.3%)
1967–76	4 (4.8%)	2 (2.4%)	78 (81.9%)	6 (7.2%)	3 (3.6%)
TOTALS	10 (5.6%)	6 (3.4%)	144 (81.8%)	8 (4.5%)	8 (4.5%)
Mortality	4 (40.0%)	5 (83.3%)	52 (34.3%)	3 (37.5%)	— —

Fig 13.4 Types of oesophageal anomaly (personal series). A = atresia without a fistula; B = atresia with fistula to upper pouch; C = atresia with fistula to lower oesophagus; D = atresia with fistula to both portions of oesophagus; E =tracheo-oesophageal fistula without atresia.

the trachea (type E); this type is usually diagnosed at an early stage and is readily treated by ligation of the fistula.

Other major anomalies of the heart and great vessels, the urinary tract and the intestine commonly complicate oesophageal atresia (40%) and 45% of babies with oesophageal atresia are premature and small in size. It is very important that the chances of survival of the individual baby should be assessed immediately after admission. This is done primarily on a basis of birth weight and the resulting grouping is modified according to whether other anomalies are present or the baby has pneumonia (Table 1). This risk group classification can be used for most other anomalies in the alimentary tract, but is of less value in Hirschsprung's disease. It is unfortunate that a number of major cardiac anomalies do not always produce any clinical signs

in the first days or even weeks of life and become evident only after operation on the atresia. The importance of the risk group classification is that there is no urgency to operate on a baby with oesophageal atresia and preoperative treatment of pneumonia by vigorous physiotherapy, chemotherapy and aspiration of the trachea and bronchi and the upper pouch usually produces great improvement in the general state of the child and is always worthwhile.

If in all newly born babies an attempt to pass a stiff catheter into the stomach was a routine part of the immediate postnatal examination, the diagnosis of oesophageal atresia would be made almost without exception. As it is, in more than 25% of babies with oesophageal atresia the diagnosis is not made for more than 24 h after birth. It is only when on trying to feed the baby chokes, coughs and becomes cyanosed that the diagnosis is suspected. It can be confirmed by x-raying the child in the upright position with the catheter in the upper pouch; the upper abdomen should also be included so that air below the diaphragm, which indicates the presence of a tracheo-oesophageal fistula, is also seen in the film. No other diagnostic procedure is necessary. Because there is no immediate urgency for operative treatment, babies with oesophageal atresia should always be transferred in a heated incubator to a specialist neonatal surgical unit, as they have been in the past by air from Singapore and Central Africa to the United Kingdom. The baby should be accompanied in the ambulance by an experienced nurse. The upper pouch should be kept clear by repeated suction during transfer.

Tracheo-oesophageal fistula without atresia causes coughing and spluttering in a baby who is taking normal feeds. There are repeated bouts of pulmonary infec-

Table 1

CLASSIFICATION INTO THREE RISK GROUPS ON THE BASIS OF WEIGHT AT BIRTH AND PRESENCE OF ANOTHER ANOMALY OR A COMPLICATION

Group A	Birth weight 2.5 kg (5½ lbs) or more. No other anomaly or complication
Group B	Birth weight 1.8 to 2.5 kg (4 to 5½ lbs). No other complications or anomalies
or	*Group A* with another anomaly or complication of moderate severity
Group C	Birth weight less than 1.8 kg (4 lbs)
or	*Group B* with another anomaly or complication of moderate severity
or	*Group A* by weight with another severe anomaly or complication

(After Waterston *et al.*, 1962).

tion. These signs persist even when the feeds are thickened and are accompanied by unusual distension of the stomach during feeds. The fistula is usually in the neck and is readily diagnosed when the baby is screened while being fed with opaque medium which escapes upwards into the trachea and bubbles of air are seen in the oesophagus. The fistula is approached through an incision 1.5 cm above the left clavicle. The dissection passes over the anterior border of the sternomastoid muscle and behind the left lobe of the thyroid gland to the interval between the oesophagus and the trachea. It is probably safer to transfix and ligate doubly the fistula with silk ligatures and not to divide it. Any child who has had oesophageal atresia and tracheo-oesophageal fistula treated successfully and later develops repeated severe pulmonary infections should be suspected of having either a second unrecognised primary tracheo-oesophageal fistula, or a recurrence of the original fistula.

Stomach

Spontaneous perforation of the stomach is rare. Its cause is not known. It most often involves the greater curvature or the posterior surface and leads to peritonitis, abdominal distention and quite a severe general disturbance. A plain radiograph of the abdomen in the upright position shows gas under the diaphragm. At laparotomy through a transverse upper abdominal incision, a long ragged perforation with grey sloughing edges is seen. It may be necessary to open the lesser sac below the greater curvature of the stomach to make the diagnosis. This perforation should be closed with interrupted seromuscular mattress stitches of 000 silk. The sloughing edges should be turned in and should not be excised. An antibiotic should always be given after operation.

Volvulus of the stomach very occasionally occurs in the neonate and usually can be untwisted. Fixation is not necessary, but gastric aspiration should be maintained for several days.

Duplication of the stomach is also rare and requires partial gastrectomy.

Pyloric atresia is very rare and causes complete obstruction of the gastric outlet with huge distension of the stomach. It should be treated by resection of the pylorus and part of the antrum and the first few centimetres of the duodenum with end-to-end anastomosis. Gastrojejunostomy, although simpler, is unsatisfactory and should not be done.

Duodenum

Duodenal obstruction may be intrinsic and complete due to an atresia or a membrane, or partially due to stenosis. It may be extrinsic, which is usually due to volvulus of the midgut in association with malrotation and Ladd's bands, or to external pressure by a large hydronephrosis or choledochal cyst. Intrinsic obstruction is three times more common than extrinsic and is most often due to atresia.

More than a third of atresias are above the level of the ampulla of Vater, but the commonest site is at or just below the ampulla. It is very unusual to find a gap between the two blind ends of the atretic duodenum. Obstruction due to a diaphragm is complete unless there is a hole in it, when small quantities of intestinal content may pass through. Very rarely a patient with a duodenal diaphragm with a hole in it has survived until middle age before the diagnosis was made.

Duodenal stenosis also is most common at the level of the ampulla and may then be associated with a ring of pancreatic tissue which encircles the stenotic duodenum, the 'annular pancreas'. This ring of pancreatic tissue is not the cause of the obstruction and if it is divided a stenosis or even an atresia will be found in the duodenum. The pancreatic ring should never be divided as not only will this not relieve the obstruction, but a pancreatic fistula may result.

Associated anomalies are common such as malrotation of the midgut (28%), Down's syndrome (20%), anomalies of the heart and great vessels (18%) and atresia of the oesophagus (12%) and more than one may occur at a time. At least half the babies with duodenal lesions are premature or weigh less than 2.5 kg. In the presence of severe associated anomalies the mortality rate is over 50%.

Repeated vomiting is the most important sign and begins within a few hours of birth. When the obstruction is above the ampulla of Vater the vomitus is not bile-stained unless there is an accessory pancreatic and bile duct opening above the obstruction. Any newly-born baby who repeatedly vomits bile-stained fluid must be suspected of having an intestinal obstruction until this has been specifically excluded. The epigastrium may be full, there may be visible gastric peristalsis, but the rest of the abdomen is not distended. One or two normal meconium stools may be passed, but if operation is delayed the usual change in the stools does not occur. Complications of pregnancy and especially hydramnios are common.

The diagnosis of duodenal atresia is made by the demonstration in an erect radiograph of the abdomen of a fluid level and gas shadow in the stomach and a smaller gas shadow and fluid level in the obstructed duodenum to the right of the midline, but gas is absent in the rest of the abdomen. If the stomach has been aspirated, the gas shadow may be small or absent and 10 to 15 ml of air should then be injected into the stomach and another film taken after a short interval. In duodenal stenosis, air passes on into the small intestine whether the cause is a true stenosis, a diaphragm with a hole in it, or compression by a cyst or hydronephrosis. Valuable further information and an exact diagnosis can then be obtained by radiological examination after an opaque meal.

Sometimes newly-born babies are allowed to go on vomiting bile-stained fluid for a week or more before the diagnosis is made and they may lose up to a third of their birth weight, mainly from starvation. Metabolic acidosis may be severe and if the negative base excess is more than 15 mmol it should be corrected. Improvement in the general condition of the baby depends on relief of the obstruction and the institution of feeding by an indwelling transanastomotic tube. If the peripheral circulation is poor, it should be restored by the infusion of large molecular weight (150 000) dextran in 0.9% saline after blood has been drawn for cross-matching. Delay should be permitted only while compatible blood for transfusion is obtained.

Under general anaesthesia the abdomen is opened through a long transverse incision just above the umbilicus. The stomach and duodenum are examined to establish the level of the obstruction and then the entire alimentary tract is examined for other anomalies, especially for malrotation and Ladd's bands which may be an additional cause of obstruction of the duodenum. Ladd's bands, if present, must be completely divided to free the right colon and duodenum which must be completely cleared. The simplest way to relieve the duodenal obstruction is to make an opening in the transverse mesocolon near the right flexure and draw the first loop of jejunum up through this opening and anastomose it to the front of the lower part of the obstructed duodenum with a single layer of interrupted mattress sutures of silk (00). If convenient a duodeno-duodenostomy may be preferable. Just before the anterior layer of the anastomosis is completed, a stab incision is made in the anterior wall of the stomach into which is put a 20 F catheter as a gastrostomy tube and beside this an 8 F soft Portex tube is passed through the pylorus and the upper jejunum and across the anastomosis for 15–20 cm into the distal limb of the jejunum. Both tubes are fixed to the stomach wall with a purse string stitch and the stomach is sewn subsequently to the peritoneum of the anterior abdominal wall (Fig 13.5). The duodenojejunal anastomosis is then completed.

After operation all the fluid which is sucked off the stomach and upper duodenum should be injected into the jejunal tube; this can be started 24 h after operation and small feeds of full strength milk (5 to 10 ml) 4 h

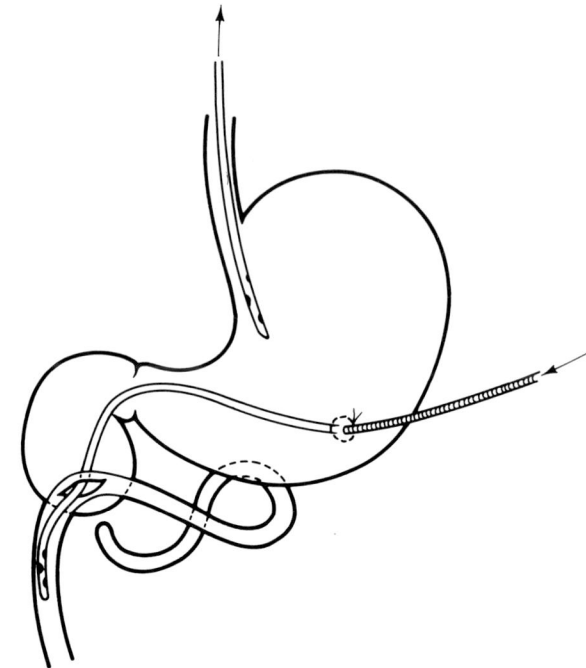

Fig 13.5 Duodenal atresia to show the arrangement of intragastric tube for aspiration of gastric secretions and transgastric and transanastomotic tube for injection of aspirated gastric secretions and milk feeds into the jejunum beyond the duodeno-jejunal anastomosis.

later. Gastric aspiration may have to be continued for 10 to 14 days after operation because of disordered peristalsis in the hypertrophied and dilated stomach and proximal duodenum which at first do not empty satisfactorily.

Malrotation of the midgut

Originally the intestinal loop lies in a vertical axis in the median sagittal plane, but when it is in the omphalomesenteric duct from the 4th to the 10th weeks' gestation, it rotates through 90° in a clockwise direction on the axis of the artery of the midgut which is to become the superior mesenteric artery; the duodeno-jejunal junction then lies to the right of the axis (Fig 13.6). After the 10th week as the intestine returns to the coelomic cavity, it continues to rotate and the duodeno-jejunal junction passes below and to the left of the axial artery. The caecum and ascending colon pass through 270° from below the axis to lie in the right side of the abdomen below the liver and eventually in the right iliac fossa (*see also* Ch. 10).

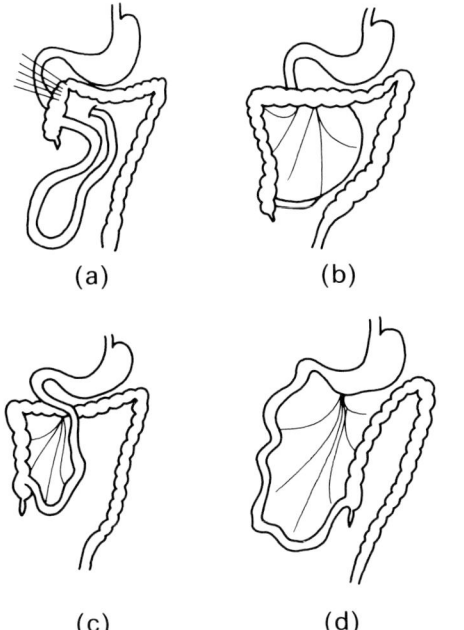

Fig 13.6 (a) Incomplete rotation of midgut with Ladd's bands; (b) Small intestine lying behind mesocolon; (c) Reversed rotation of midgut; (d) Failure of rotation of midgut and of fixation of colon.

Very rarely this rotation may not take place, usually in association with a large exomphalos, and then the small intestine lies on the right side and all the colon is on the left. Rotation may be arrested at the first stage, but the commonest type of malrotation is when it is arrested at 180° with the duodenum behind or to the right of the superior mesenteric artery and the caecum and ascending colon lie in front of the duodenum, bound together and to the undersurface of the liver, the gallbladder and even the abdominal wall by adhesions, 'Ladd's bands'.

Rotation may be normal, but the usual fixation of the colon to the posterior abdominal wall does not occur and the mesocolon may envelop the small intestine as in a sac, the so-called mesocolic hernia. Alternatively, the unfixed midgut may twist on its axis, the root of the mesentery being unusually narrow and the whole or part of the midgut may be strangulated and much of it may become gangrenous. Rotation may be reversed and then the duodenum lies across the front of the transverse colon instead of behind.

Whenever rotation and fixation of the midgut is abnormal or incomplete there is a risk of the whole midgut twisting on its pedicle, producing a volvulus around the root of the mesentery. This causes obstruction of the second part of the duodenum due to compression by Ladd's bands and of the duodeno-jejunal junction by kinking. The child vomits bile-stained fluid, there is some abdominal distension, but there is usually no characteristic appearance of intestinal obstruction in the plain upright radiograph of the abdomen. There are scattered gas shadows throughout the intestine but seldom any fluid levels. If the twist of the mesentery is sufficiently tight to occlude the venous return, but not the arterial inflow, the child bleeds into the obstructed venous circulation of the strangulated bowel and the general state rapidly and progressively deteriorates. This is another of the rare neonatal emergencies when immediate laparotomy may offer more chance of survival than transfer to a specialist unit. Blood must be obtained for cross-matching, but if deterioration continues, it is better to open the abdomen and untwist the volvulus than to wait for blood for transfusion. It is essential to use a long transverse incision above the umbilicus from costal margin to costal margin using the cutting diathermy. The twisted bowel should be completely delivered out of the abdomen and untwisted and wrapped in warm packs. It is also essential, after a pause to let the trapped blood drain out of the volvulus, to make quite certain that all the adhesions of Ladd's bands have been completely divided, that the liver and gallbladder are free and to clear the caecum, ascending colon, right flexure and the right half of the transverse colon so completely that they hang down on the mesocolon and the mesentery to the left of the midline.

If the bowel is gangrenous, it must be resected, but as much as possible must be saved. The length of the small intestine in a 3.5 kg baby is about 250 cm. Although babies have survived with less than 50 cm, the chances of doing so are poor, and better if it is terminal ileum than any other part. If all the ileum must be resected then vitamin B12 deficiency will certainly occur later as well as disturbances of bile-salt metabolism and fat absorption.

Atresia of the small intestine

Atresia of the small intestine is usually due to some kind of vascular occlusion during intrauterine life such as incarceration in an umbilical hernia, volvulus or intussusception. The bowel becomes gangrenous and sloughs and in the sterile conditions of the fetal coelom the ends seal off. The proximal stump of bowel is dilated by the accumulation of its contents and the muscular wall is hypertrophied by the peristaltic attempts to force the contents onwards. The distal bowel is of normal size, but empty, and contracted on its lumen. Prematurity and other anomalies are much less commonly associated with atresia of the jejunum or ileum than with duodenal atresia.

The repeated vomiting of bile-stained fluid is the

most important sign of obstruction of the small intestine due to atresia and the higher the obstruction the sooner vomiting begins. Abdominal distension varies in degree with the level of the obstruction and is inconspicuous in high jejunal atresia, but may be very marked when the obstruction is low in the ileum. The impression of peristaltic waves may be seen on the abdominal wall. Normal meconium may have been passed before admission from the bowel below the atresia. A plain radiograph in the upright position usually shows fluid levels with gas shadows in loops of bowel of different sizes and this is diagnostic of intestinal obstruction.

A nasogastric tube should be passed and the stomach is emptied and repeatedly aspirated. Blood should be obtained for cross-matching and operation should be delayed until compatible blood is available. An intravenous infusion of balanced electrolyte solution should be started, but no attempt should be made to replace all the fluid which it may be guessed has been lost by vomiting. If the peripheral circulation is poor, it may be improved by the injection of high molecular weight dextran (150 000) 6% in 0.9% saline.

The usual long transverse upper abdominal incision above the umbilicus is made with the cutting diathermy as for all laparotomies in the neonate, for no other incision gives such good access to as much of the abdominal contents. The whole intestine is examined from the stomach to the rectum. Whether it is a jejunal or an ileal atresia, the proximal dilated and hypertrophied segment of bowel is resected to where the calibre of the intestine approaches normal. The distal blind end of bowel is also resected. The large difference in calibre of the two ends of bowel makes anastomosis difficult. The easiest solution is to anastomose the end of the proximal bowel to the antimesenteric border of the distal limb, the end of which is brought out as a terminal jejunostomy or ileostomy (Bishop-Koop, Fig 13.7). An alternative method is to slit the antimesenteric border of the distal bowel until the opening fits the wide proximal stump. In either case the contents, air and fluid, of the proximal bowel should be sucked out before the abdomen is closed.

The stomach should be aspirated every half hour for the next 24 h and then when the aspirate is no longer bile-stained, hourly feeds of 5 ml of milk may be started. Fluid sucked off the stomach can be injected into the enterostomy. In this way fluid loss is minimal and the need for intravenous infusion is diminished or avoided.

When there are multiple atresias of the small intestine, these are best recognised by injecting 0.9% saline into the upper end of the distal bowel and milking this fluid distally along the gut. The main object in dealing with multiple atresias is to preserve as much intestine as possible while resecting all obstructions. If possible not more than three anastomoses should be made but it is

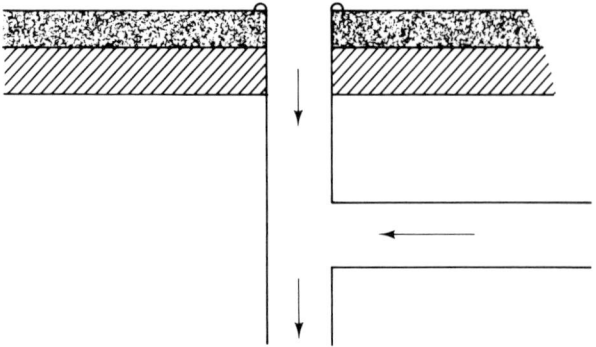

Fig 13.7 An end-to-side enterostomy.

also better to make several temporary enterostomies if in this way more bowel can be saved.

Sometimes, in association with a jejunal atresia, the gut beyond the atresia is carried on a very narrow mesentery which has a very short attachment to the posterior abdominal wall. The bowel lies in short curled loops, the so-called 'Christmas Tree' or 'apple-peel' deformity. This is very liable to twist and become gangrenous. This must be dealt with by the Bishop-Koop type of enterostomy which fixes the distal segment and prevents it from twisting.

Milk plug obstruction

Some mothers mistakenly make up reconstituted dried milk feeds much too strong in the belief that this will be better for the baby than the ordinary strength. The undigested curds become impacted, usually in the lower ileum and sometimes in the colon, and produce intestinal obstruction. The impacted masses are readily recognised in the plain radiograph. It may be possible to disimpact them with a gastrografin enema, but more often they have to be removed by enterotomy. They should not be squeezed on into the colon, because they may cause obstruction of the descending colon.

Meconium obstruction

In mucoviscidosis the mucus secreting glands of the pulmonary air passages, the pancreas and the lower small intestine may all be abnormal, although usually one system is more seriously affected than the others. When the intestine is involved the meconium in the distal ileum becomes thickened to the consistence of firm rubber and forms into tough pellets which are adherent to the mucosa. This causes obstruction of the terminal 20–25 cm of the ileum and less viscid, but still very thick, meconium accumulates higher up and causes dilatation and hypertrophy of the intestine as in an atresia. This dilated piece of intestine may undergo volvulus and may become gangrenous, perforate and discharge meconium into the peritoneal cavity, causing meconium peritonitis and later calcified plaques may form amongst the adherent loops of bowel.

The intestinal obstruction due to the impacted meconium plugs causes repeated vomiting of bile-stained fluid and abdominal distension. The impression of distended loops of bowel can be seen on the abdominal wall and the loops of intestine loaded with meconium can often be felt in the right iliac fossa. The rectum is usually empty, but sometimes pale khaki-coloured beads of meconium may be felt or be passed.

In the plain upright radiograph of the abdomen, there is marked distension but there may be few fluid levels. There is usually a grayish mottled or granular appearance especially in the right side and sometimes calcification. The use of a gastrografin enema usually demonstrates the pellets in the terminal ileum, and provided enough gastrografin can be run into the ileum, it will loosen the pellets and they will be evacuated with the enema and the viscous meconium from higher up the ileum. It is essential, however, to have an intravenous infusion of balanced electrolyte solution running before the enema is started, because the hygroscopic effect of the gastrografin may draw so much secretion into the bowel as to cause rapid depletion of the extracellular fluid volume and circulatory collapse. Because of the risk of perforation during the enema, preparations for laparotomy, if necessary, must also have been made.

If the gastrografin enema is not used or is unsuccessful, the abdomen is opened through the usual transverse incision. The dilated and hypertrophied segment of ileum is resected and enough of the pellets in the distal stump of the ileum are picked out to allow the construction of a Bishop-Koop type of end-to-side anastomosis and distal ileostomy.

Because of the risk of pulmonary complications, the intravenous infusion should be stopped when blood replacement, if necessary, has been completed. Pancreatic extract should be injected into the stomach through the nasogastric tube and into the enterostomy and milk feeds (5 ml at first) should be started 24 h after operation. There is usually no discharge from the enterostomy, but it should be left for 2 or 3 months. Prophylactic antibiotics should be started at once and the baby should soon be transferred to a pediatrician for the care of the mucoviscidosis or cystic fibrosis.

Atresia of the colon

This is extremely rare and is usually diagnosed only at laparotomy for a low intestinal obstruction. The atretic segment is resected and because of the very great difference in size of the colon above and below the atresia the ends should be brought out as a colostomy. When the proximal bowel has shrunk sufficiently, a formal end-to-end anastomosis should be made.

Functional intestinal obstruction in the neonate

The three classical signs of intestinal obstruction, the repeated vomiting of bile-stained fluid, abdominal distension and the failure to pass normal meconium may also occur in the absence of any organic lesion of the bowel, because of a temporary disturbance of peristalsis or when the meconium is abnormally viscid. This disturbance is known as 'functional intestinal obstruction' and occurs in one in five of all neonates admitted with the suspected diagnosis of intestinal obstruction. Half of these babies are admitted within three days of birth and the rest within a week, two-thirds weigh 3.5 kg or more at birth and four out of five are born after uncomplicated pregnancies and deliveries. Some of these babies suffer from respiratory distress and the mothers of some of them have been heavily sedated before delivery. The abdominal distension subsides spontaneously and some of these babies pass a plug of meconium after a rectal examination. Functional obstruction may also be associated with cannulation of the umbilical vein and the infusion of 10% glucose solution into it; in other babies it is associated with exchange transfusion.

A plain radiograph in the erect position shows gas throughout the bowel without fluid levels. About 6% of normal babies do not pass meconium for more than 24 h after birth. Functional obstruction should be treated conservatively and usually subsides within 24 h of admission. This condition is liable to be confused with meconium obstruction or Hirschsprung's disease. In the former, there are usually the characteristic shadows of inspissated meconium or calcification in the radiograph and the loaded terminal ileum may be palpable, whereas in Hirschsprung's disease there are usually the signs of low small intestinal obstruction, gas filled loops of bowel with fluid levels. In either case, patience is normally rewarded by resolution of the abdominal distension or a gastrografin enema excludes both meconium obstruction and Hirschsprung's disease. The other only important possibility is hyperthyroidism, the clinical features of which may sometimes resemble those of Hirschsprung's disease.

Neonatal necrotising enterocolitis

This is a disease of the neonatal period and in 90% of patients begins in the first 10 days of life and seldom occurs after the first month. It most often affects the terminal ileum and the ileocaecal region and is patchy with apparently normal bowel between segments of bowel which are obviously necrotic. Histological examination shows ischaemic necrosis which first affects the mucosa with haemorrhage, oedema and ulceration, which spreads through all layers of the bowel in the affected areas unlike the enterocolitis of Hirschsprung's disease, which is confined to the mucous membrane that sloughs extensively leaving large areas of the haemorrhagic submucous layer exposed. Bubbles of air may also be seen in the wall on microscopic examination in necrotising enterocolitis.

There is abdominal distension in 90% of patients, vomiting in 70%, bloody loose stools are passed by 60%, and 90% weigh less than 3.5 kg with 70% weighing less than 3.0 kg, which is also unlike Hirschsprung's disease. Most babies are flaccid and inactive and apnoea is common. As the disease progresses, the abdomen becomes tense and tender. In the upright radiograph of the abdomen, gas bubbles can be seen in the thickened wall of the intestine in more than half the patients with enterocolitis and gas can be seen in the biliary tract in more than a quarter. Free gas in the peritoneal cavity indicates perforation of the bowel. In a baby who has a tender, distended abdomen, vomits bile-stained fluid and passes blood in loose stools, the most likely diagnosis is necrotising enterocolitis. The severity of the disease varies widely and in the less severe forms conservative treatment is usually satisfactory and the disease subsides spontaneously. The stomach should be aspirated regularly and if necessary the aspirated fluid should be replaced with an equivalent volume of a balanced electrolyte solution. If the blood loss is large, it should be replaced by transfusion. If conservative treatment must be maintained for more than three or four days, the baby should be fed intravenously.

If the general condition of the child deteriorates or if there are signs of perforation of the bowel, the abdomen should be opened. Necrotic and perforated bowel should be resected. Even when only one segment is resected, it is better to bring both ends to the surface as enterostomies than to risk further necrosis at the anastomotic suture line. When there are multiple areas of gangrene multiple enterostomies should be made through stab incisions in the abdominal wall. When areas of damage of the intestinal wall which do not progress as far as gangrene heal, strictures are quite common.

The cause of this disease is not known and its incidence varies widely between countries and districts in the same country. It may occur in almost epidemic form in a single institution and there is some evidence that it may be due to infection by the *Clostridium butyricum*.

Anorectal anomalies

This group of anomalies can be classified anatomically on a similar basis to that originally used by Ladd and Gross (Table 2). Other more complicated classifications are confusing and less closely applicable to the clinical problems.

Table 2

Lesion	Boys	Girls	Total Number	%	Deaths Number	%
Anorectal stenosis	9	6	15	7.6	2	13
Covered anus	36	7	43	21	2	4
Anorectal atresia in lower third	69	74	143	70	34	23.7
Perineal fistula	4	12	16	7	1	6
'Low' vaginal fistula	—	52	52	25	13	25
'High' vaginal fistula	—	6	6	3	1	16
Rectourethral fistula	38	—	38	19	6	16
No fistula	27	4	31	15	13	41
Anorectal atresia in middle third	1	1	2	1		
Total	115	88	203		38	18.7

(Personal series, unpublished).

Figure 13.8 a and b show the normal anatomy of the pelvis in full term babies. These diagrams were traced from sagittal sections of the pelvis of a normal boy and girl. The only arbitrary additions are the curved broken line which indicates the levator ani muscle and the thick solid line which represents the puborectalis part of the levator in this and subsequent diagrams.

Anorectal stenosis

In anorectal stenosis (Fig 13.8c) the only abnormality is a fibrous ring in the anal canal somewhere between the anal orifice and the anorectal junction. Everything else is normal and treatment consists in dilating this fibrous area, at first under general anaesthesia; subsequently, daily dilatations are carried out by the child's mother at home. Provided the anal canal is kept dilated for 5 or 6 months bowel function will be normal. Unfortunately, because of the normal appearance of the anus, stenosis may not be diagnosed for some days or even weeks after birth. It is then noticed that the baby is straining to pass a stool and that the

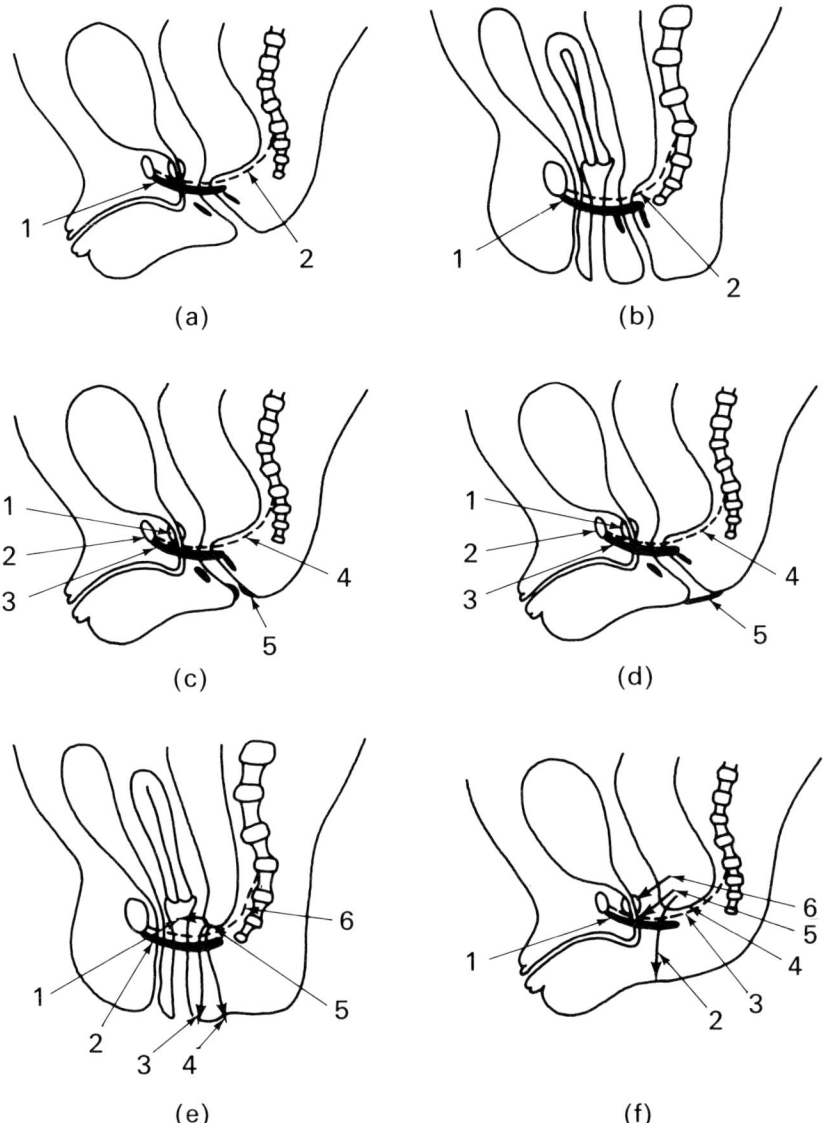

Fig 13.8   (a) Median sagittal section of the pelvis of a boy, still-born at term. 1 = puborectalis muscle; 2 = levator ani muscle. (b) Median sagittal section of the pelvis of a girl, still-born at term. 1 = puborectalis muscle; 2 = levator ani muscle. (c) Median sagittal section of the pelvis of a boy, still-born at term on which an anorectal stenosis has been superimposed. 1 = prostate; 2 = symphysis pubis; 3 = puborectalis muscle; 4 = levator ani muscle; 5 = anorectal stenosis. (d) Median sagittal section of the pelvis of a boy, still-born at term on which a covered anus (5) has been superimposed (1–4 as in 'c'); (e) Median sagittal section of the pelvis of a girl with anorectal atresia who died. The puborectalis (2) and levator ani muscles (6) have been superimposed and also lines to show a high-level rectovaginal fistula (1) a low-level rectovaginal fistula (3) a rectoperineal fistula (4) and the blind end of the rectum (5). (f) Median sagittal section of the pelvis of a boy with an anorectal atresia on which the puborectalis (1) and the levator ani muscles (3) have been superimposed and also lines to show the line of a rectoperineal fistula (2), the blind end of the rectum (4) and a fistula into the membranous part of the urethra (5) and the prostatic urethra (6).

bowel is loaded and only then on rectal examination for the first time is the stenosis found. Very rarely, the fibrosis is so extensive that excision and a pull-through operation to bring the rectum itself to the perineum is the only satisfactory form of treatment.

Covered anus

In the covered anus (Fig 13.8d) everything is normal except that the anus is closed by a lid of skin. There may be a roll of skin as the cover and this may already have perforated by the time of birth. In another type a tortuous channel in the skin, containing meconium or yellowish material, runs forward from the anus across the perineum and along the median line of the scrotum. The lid of skin over the anus should be cut off with scissors and the scrotal track, if there is one, should be laid open and the edge of the mucous membrane lining the anal canal should be sewn to the skin edges. The anus should be dilated daily at first for two weeks, and often enough thereafter to keep the opening wide. Function is normal but, as the subcutaneous and superficial anal sphincters do not work after this operation, there is usually a slight leak of faecal-stained mucus.

Anorectal atresia

Anorectal atresia involving the lower third of the rectum accounts for 70% of all anorectal anomalies. The rectum ends blindly above the pelvic floor and may or may not be associated with a perineal fistula in either sex, or a high or low rectovaginal fistula in a girl, or a rectourethral fistula in a boy. The frequency of each type in a personal series is shown in Table 2.

Rectoperineal fistula

A rectoperineal fistula (Fig 13.8e, f) opens in the perineum in front of the anal dimple and since it is not surrounded by sphincters is patulous and will always leak a little mucus. It should be treated by repeated dilatation. Because it passes through the puborectalis sling, continence and bowel function will be normal.

A **high-level rectovaginal fistula** (Fig 13.8e) opens into the posterior fornix of the vagina and is accessible only by a transabdominal approach. It is best treated with the atresia by an abdominoperineal pull through operation which should be delayed until the child weighs 10 kg at about 1 year old. A transverse colostomy should therefore be made in the neonatal period.

A **low-level rectovaginal fistula** (Fig 13.8e) opens at the posterior border of the vulva or the lowest part of the vagina. In the past, mainly because of unsatisfac-

tory anaesthesia, this kind of fistula was treated by local enlargement by the 'cut-back' operation, in which one blade of the scissors was placed in the fistula and one on the perineal skin. The resulting cut enlarged the orifice of the fistula but, if it was made too deeply, also divided part or the whole of the puborectalis sling and the child was incontinent. As with high rectovaginal fistulas, by far the best form of treatment is by transverse colostomy in the neonatal period and a pull-through operation at a year. The cut-back operation sometimes gives a good result, but in some girls the faeces are passed partly into the vagina and this is not tolerable, especially after puberty. Dissection of the fistula out of the vagina and transplantation of it to the site of the true anus is seldom, if ever successful, because the anal ring is farther from the puborectalis sling than the original site of the orifice, and the transplanted fistula tears away from its new site and retracts.

Rectourethral fistula

A rectourethral fistula runs forward from the blind end of the rectum to open into the prostatic or membranous parts of the urethra (Fig 13.8f). This type of fistula can be satisfactorily dealt with only by an abdominal approach which should logically be part of the abdominoperineal pull-through operation at about the age of a year. In the neonatal period a transverse colostomy should be made to relieve the intestinal obstruction due to the atresia and the distal bowel should be repeatedly washed out until it is clean. If this is done, there is little likelihood of urinary infection from the fistula.

In the absence of any fistula, the intestinal obstruction due to the rectal atresia should be relieved by a transverse colostomy.

Diagnosis of these various types of anorectal atresia depends first on careful inspection of the perineum, scrotum or vulva. Meconium may be passed from a vaginal fistula or per urethram in a boy and may be seen on the napkin and a careful examination of the perineum may not be made. A rectourethral fistula should be confirmed by a urethrogram or by injecting opaque medium into the distal limb of the colostomy. The bony pelvis should always be x-rayed because bony defects suggest there may also be neurological deficits and poor function of the pelvic floor, and in their presence a guarded prognosis should be given about future continence. All patients with anorectal anomalies, regardless of their severity, should be x-rayed after intravenous urography as a routine during their first admission because the incidence of associated anomalies in the genitourinary tract is probably about 40%.

Atresia of the middle third of the rectum

This is almost certainly caused by a vascular accident similar to those which cause some forms of atresia higher in the alimentary tract and is by far the rarest type of anorectal anomaly. The anus, anal canal and lower third of the rectum are normal and there is usually a gap where the middle third should be and the upper end of rectum ends blindly in the hollow of the sacrum. This type of atresia is not associated with fistulas and should be treated by a transverse colostomy in the neonatal period. At the age of a year the blind ends should be excised and continuity restored either by direct anastomosis or by some form of pull-through operation.

Colostomy

The chief purpose of the colostomy is to relieve the partial or complete intestinal obstruction associated with all forms of anorectal atresia. The best site for the colostomy is in the right half of the transverse colon. With the diathermy the abdomen is opened through a transverse incision above the umbilicus from close to the right costal margin to just across the midline. The transverse colon should be carefully identified and drawn out and cleared of omentum for about 10 cm. An opening is made in the transverse mesocolon and two crushing clamps are applied and the bowel is divided between them. The gas in both pieces of colon is sucked out through a needle inserted close to the clamps. The mesocolon is divided sufficiently to allow the pieces of bowel to lie comfortably at each end of the wound where they are sewn to the peritoneum and rectus sheath with interrupted silk stitches (000) and the wound is closed in layers with similar stitches (00). The clamps are left in position for 24 h.

A sigmoid colostomy should not be used because it reduces the scope for mobilisation of the rectum at the pull-through operation; when the rectum has been dissected out of the pelvis it may be found that the bowel will not reach to the perineum. To gain mobility the superior rectal pedicle must be divided and this may result in the blood supply of the distal third of the rectal stump deteriorating. Further mobilisation of the rectum will then be necessary and sometimes the whole rectum must be sacrificed. There is obviously much more possibility of obtaining viable bowel if the colostomy is in the transverse colon.

If the ends of the colon are not widely separated as described above, faeces will cross over into the distal limb of the colostomy and pass down to pack the blind end of the rectum, which becomes even more dilated and hypertrophied than it was at birth and a potential source of contamination at the pull-through operation

and of the urinary tract if there is a rectourethral fistula. It is an important part of the treatment after a colostomy is established to wash out the distal colon until it is completely clean. A loop colostomy is quite unsatisfactory whether there is a skin bridge or not. The two ends of colon should be so widely separated that a Karaya gum ring and bag can be fitted to the proximal stoma clear of the distal stoma, which should be covered simply with a paraffin gauze dressing.

It is important that the baby's mother is fully trained in the management of the colostomy and the use of the bags before she takes the baby home. The introduction of greatly improved colostomy apparatus has transformed the management of colostomies, but it is still important to ensure that anaemia does not insidiously develop because of bleeding from the exposed colonic mucosa.

There is no justification for carrying out the definitive pull-through operation soon after birth and certainly none for doing it without a colostomy. At this time the dissection in the pelvis is much more difficult. Continence depends on the accurate placing of the bowel within the limbs of the puborectalis sling without damaging that muscle and this is much easier at a year than soon after birth.

The pull-through operation should be done through a left lower paramedian incision displacing the rectus muscle laterally. The rectum is mobilised by dividing the peritoneum of the mesorectum on each side and mobilising the posterior two-thirds of the circumference of the rectum from its accommodation space in the hollow of the sacrum. The lateral ligaments on each side are divided, and in atresia there is seldom any bleeding from middle rectal vessels. The dissection of the blind end of the rectum is carried downwards on all sides with scissors, cutting on the wall of the rectum. If there is a rectourethral fistula, it is dissected to the urethra, in which there is a metal sound, and is divided flush with the posterior wall of the urethra which is not sutured. The rectal end is closed with a stitch.

A low level rectovaginal fistula is dissected out from below when the rectum has been mobilised so that it can be cleared from the posterior wall of the vagina and drawn up into the pelvis; the open end is ligated.

The perineum is stimulated in the midline with the diathermy needle and an incision 3 cm in length is made in the midline centred at the point of maximum response. A blunt dissection is then made with forceps at an angle of 45° in the bloodless median plane towards the index finger of the left hand in the pelvis, placed at the apex of the prostate in a boy or the upper end of the vagina in a girl. As the forceps approach the finger, the plane between the prostate or vagina and the puborectalis sling is developed and the forceps passes in front of the sling into the pelvis. This pathway is dilated with Hegar's dilators until it will comfortably accommodate the rectum when it is pulled down.

If necessary, the rectum is further mobilised by division of the superior rectal pedicle at a higher level. If the rectum is unusually enlarged and hypertrophied, it may be better to excise it completely and bring down the pelvic colon. When this has been done bowel function has always been good and often better than in children where the rectum was preserved. The rectum is pulled down to the perineum, the stump is removed and, if bleeding from the cut edge is satisfactory, it is controlled and the muscle wall of the rectum is sewn to the edges of the perinal incision.

The new opening of the bowel in the perineum nearly always needs trimming to remove redundant mucosa, and dilatation or a V excision of scar tissue to maintain an adequate passage for faeces. Only when such adjustments have been made should the colostomy be closed. The baby should be kept under close supervision for at least a year after discharge from hospital and be reviewed every three months for several years.

Nearly all the deaths associated with anorectal anomalies are related or due to the associated anomalies and low birth-weight. Some babies die before any treatment can be started and the mortality rate associated with colostomy in the neonatal period may be high for the same reasons. The mortality rate related to the abdominoperineal pull-through operation is low and should be well under 5%.

The functional results of treatment are good. In stenosis and covered anus continence, sensation of fullness, warning period and control of flatus are all normal and the same applies to rectoperineal fistula, although there is usually some leakage of faecal stained mucus in both rectoperineal fistula and covered anus. When allowance is made for the small number of patients with associated ectopic bladder, sacral defects and myelomeningocoele, the long-term results of the pull-through operation for anorectal atresia are remarkably good and often function is barely distinguishable from normal, apart from slight leakage of mucus. It must be realised by the surgeon, the patient and the parents that control of urine and stools may take longer to achieve than in a normal child. The sensation of fullness of the bowel is not normal and it takes the child longer than normal to realise the significance of what sensation there is, but when they do, progress is usually rapid. Unfortunately, the warning period may at first be too short to allow the child to reach the lavatory in time. Some children become so preoccupied with play or work that they pay no attention to the warning and are persistently dirty.

The long-term management of children with anorectal anomalies requires much patience and persistence and should properly remain the responsibility of the surgeon who did the operation. If he is not pre-

pared to undertake this task, the operation should be done by someone who is. Some children seem to have an aversion to cleanness; they can obtain much more attention while they remain dirty and for them unremitting care is essential, combined with great sympathy for their mothers in the severe social and economic burdens they must bear in caring for a persistently incontinent child whose clothing is repeatedly soiled seven days a week.

In these circumstances the surgeon must be sure of the accuracy of his dissection of the pelvis at the pull-through operation and that the pulled-down bowel is in a proper relationship to an undamaged puborectalis sling. Then he can confidently and repeatedly reassure the discouraged and frustrated mother and the child that eventually continence and control will be established. Some further help can be given by persuading the parents to help the child to acquire a regular bowel habit with a single or at most two bowel actions per day by the use of a hot drink first thing in the morning and dietary variation to suit the bowel.

When a child is incontinent because a misguided attempt was made in the neonatal period to find the atretic rectum from the perineum and the puborectalis sling and the levator ani muscles have been divided, only a pelvic floor repair offers any hope of continence. Before this operation is attempted, a proximal defunctioning colostomy should be established. The results of repairs of the pelvic floor are not encouraging, but a repair should always be attempted before a permanent colostomy is advised.

Hirschsprung's disease

Hirschsprung's disease is due to congenital absence of the ganglion cells of the plexuses of Meissner and Auerbach and abnormality of the associated nerve trunks, which may replace the ganglion cells, but are usually present in large numbers in the submucosal layer. It is now also recognised that there is an abnormal and variable distribution of both adrenergic and cholinergic fibres in the muscle layers. The lesion extends upwards from the lower border of the internal sphincter of the rectum. In two-thirds of the patients a varying extent of the rectum and pelvic colon is involved, the 'short segment' type of the disease. In the other third, the aganglionic segment extends beyond the pelvic colon through a varying distance in the colon and occasionally into the ileum; in about 1% of patients the whole of the large and small intestine may be involved. As a result of these neurological defects a coordinated peristaltic wave cannot be transmitted distally through the aganglionic segment which does not relax in the normal way in front of any peristaltic wave of contraction that may be generated, and the result is intestinal obstruction. Bowel contents accumulate in the normal bowel above the aganglionic segment. The normal bowel becomes dilated and, in futile attempts to force the accumulated contents onwards, the longitudinal and circular muscle layers hypertrophy.

Hirschsprung's disease is one of the commonest causes of intestinal obstruction in the newly born; the short segment type affects boys four times more often than girls, but there is no sex difference in the incidence of the long segment type, which is now recognised to be commoner than it was formerly thought to be. Sibs of a child with long segment disease are more than usually likely to develop Hirschsprung's disease and, if they do, are also likely to have the long segment type.

Babies born with Hirschsprung's disease have been obstructed for weeks *in utero* as shown by the hypertrophied dilated bowel proximal to the aganglionic segment which is found at laparotomy within a day or so of birth. The diagnosis ought to be made soon after birth, but it is only within the last 15 or 20 years that this has been at all common. No doubt before that time the clinical picture was obscured by the prevalence of gastroenteritis.

In over 90% of babies in whom the diagnosis is made within a month of birth there is abdominal distension, repeated vomiting of bile-stained fluid and some abnormality in the passage of meconium or stools. Three quarters of the patients feed poorly and do not thrive. They have a characteristic appearance, a thin wrinkled face with a frowning and worried expression and dull grey skin. On rectal examination the anal canal and lower rectum may be narrow or seem to be of normal calibre, but when the finger is withdrawn there may be an explosive discharge of liquid faeces of a greyish yellow colour and much gas. This may produce relief of some of the abdominal distension, but it may also be followed by peripheral circulatory collapse as the result of the discharge of a large volume of liquid faeces from the bowel. This is more likely if there are repeated bursts of rather foul-smelling liquid faeces, especially if there are streaks of blood in the stools, which should immediately suggest that the baby is suffering from that form of enterocolitis which is associated specifically with Hirschsprung's disease.

In this type of enterocolitis, there are severe vascular changes in the mucosa of both the aganglionic and normal colon. The mucosa becomes haemorrhagic, bleeds and extensive areas of it may slough. There is little change in the muscle layers. Large volumes of exudate are lost into the lumen of the bowel and when this is released by a digital examination of the rectum or the passage of a tube, there is a large increase in the volume of blood in circulation in the wall of the colon as soon as compression of it by distension is relieved. This leads to a sudden large redistribution of the blood in active circulation in the body and peripheral circula-

tory collapse. Enterocolitis may occur soon after birth and cause death within 48 h of birth. Half the deaths in the first month associated with Hirschsprung's disease are due to enterocolitis. It should also be recognised that enterocolitis is often recurrent and one attack should be taken as a warning of what may happen again at any time. The cause of enterocolitis is not known.

Enterocolitis must be treated by immediate and energetic resuscitation; 100 ml of 0.9% saline should be rapidly infused at once, followed by 6% large molecular weight dextran (150 000) in 0.9% saline while compatible blood is being obtained. The volumes to be given should be judged by the response of the baby as shown by the state of the peripheral capillary circulation in the finger-tips and the colour of the skin and the rate at which colour returns after compression, the normal being 3 s.

In the uncomplicated patient, a radiograph of the abdomen in the erect position usually shows a good deal of gaseous distension and there may be fluid levels. In long segment disease the appearances are those of low small intestinal obstruction. The absence of gas in the pelvis is very suggestive and so is an isolated grossly distended segment of intestine.

Most help will be obtained by examination after an opaque enema which should show the narrow segment and the conical transitional zone above it. Another film 24 h later may provide additional confirmation if barium has not been completely evacuated. Few paediatric radiologists would give a firm opinion if the bowel has been washed out within 5 days of the radiological examination. When there is enterocolitis the mucous membrane has a characteristic ragged appearance.

In the end, diagnosis depends on the demonstration of the characteristic histological features of the disease in a biopsy taken from the wall of the rectum. The introduction of the punch biopsy of the mucosal and submucosal layers has made this a much easier and far safer procedure than the former open biopsy of the rectal wall which required general anaesthesia. A punch biopsy must be taken from above the normally hypoganglionic zone which is 2 cm above the sphincter. The biopsy should be taken at a level at least 3 cm above the anocutaneous margin. When ganglia are found, this excludes Hirschsprung's disease. When ganglia are absent, staining the section with cholinesterase may show marked uptake in the mucosa as well as large nerve trunks in the submucosal plexus, and these appearances are diagnostic of Hirschsprung's disease.

When a baby is admitted with gross abdominal distension and the history and radiological findings suggest that the cause is Hirschsprung's disease, the sooner the obstruction is relieved the better. The usual transverse upper abdominal incision should be made and, if the disease is of the short segment type, grossly dilated and hypertrophied sigmoid colon is likely to present in the wound. The bowel should be decompressed by suction through a needle and a transverse colostomy should be made as described for anorectal atresia. If the colon is contracted above the sigmoid loop this indicates a long segment type of disease and the conical transitional zone should be sought more proximally in the colon. In the long segment type, an ileostomy should be made, the bowel being cut across and the ends being brought out separately, a separate incision being made for one end. When the disease extends into the ileum it is often very difficult to judge by the gross appearance where the aganglionic bowel ends and a piece of ileum should be taken from the site of division of the bowel for histological examination. An emergency operation for acute intestinal obstruction is not the time for deliberate diagnosis of the exact extent of the agangliosis by the histological examination of frozen sections of a number of biopsies of the intestinal wall which must wait until the definitive pull-through operation.

The purpose of a colostomy or ileostomy is primarily to relieve the acute intestinal obstruction in the neonatal period. It has also the very important secondary function of making it possible to wash out the distal bowel immediately and to keep it clean, so that the risk of infection at the definitive operation is reduced as far as possible. In addition, by diverting the faeces during the postoperative period until after the suture line is healed, it reduces the risks of leakage at the suture line. For these reasons a pelvic colostomy which is disconnected at the pull-through operation is contraindicated. The dangers and complications of ileostomy in the neonatal period and infancy have been greatly exaggerated.

Whatever type of definitive operation is chosen, it is essential that the extent of the aganglionic segment should be established by the examination by a pathologist, who is accustomed to this procedure, of frozen sections of biopsies taken at operation. If this service is not available, the child should be transferred to a pediatric surgical unit where it can be done.

The definitive operations for Hirschsprung's disease are nearly all variants of the original rectosigmoidectomy described by Swenson and Bill in 1948; (Fig 13.9a) this was the first operation for this disease in which the aganglionic segment was excised rather than the dilated normal more proximal bowel. In this operation, when the aganglionic segment as defined by rectal biopsy has been excised, the stump of aganglionic rectum 1 to 2 cm in length is anastomosed to normally innervated colon or ileum In the Duhamel modification (Fig 13.9c,d) of this operation, after the upper two-thirds of the rectum have been resected, a pouch is made of the lower third of the rectum and the normally innervated colon is brought down behind this pouch within the puborectalis sling to an opening in the mid-

dle hird of the anal canal. The adjacent walls of colon and rectum are then crushed, usually with a stapling clamp, thus creating an opening from the colon into the anal canal. The object of this operation is to provide some anterior rectal wall for 'sensation' and to prevent obstruction by dividing the circular muscle of the rectum and part of the internal sphincter; it also avoids dissection of the anterior wall of the rectum behind the bladder and seminal vesicles in boys. In other modifications (Fig 13.9b) the mucous membrane of the aganglionic stump of the rectum and the anal canal is excised and colon is then pulled down through the aganglionic muscular cuff to the anal canal, the so-called 'endorectal' pull-through operation.

Swenson's operation has given satisfactory results in some hundreds of patients. Duhamel's operation may be a little safer than Swenson's and also gives good results. The overall mortality of both these operations should be about 5% and the incidence of complications is about the same with both, but the kinds of complication vary with the operation. If too much aganglionic rectum is left behind in Swenson's operation, there will be constipation, which may be so severe as to need

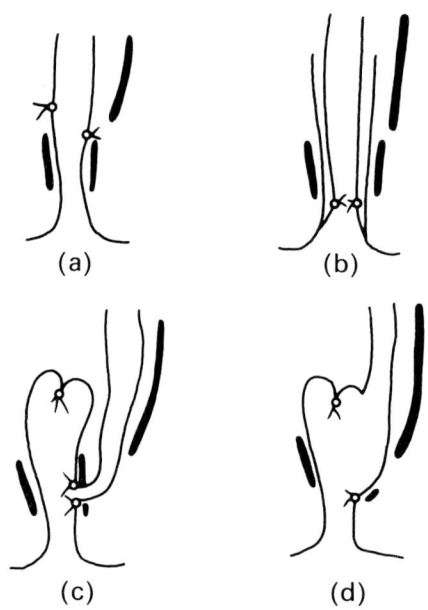

Fig 13.9 Operations for Hirschsprung's disease. (a) Swenson's rectosigmoidectomy. (b) Soave's operation in which the anorectal mucosa is excised down to the middle of the anal canal and the colon is pulled down and sutured to the mucosa of the anal canal. (c) Duhamel's operation showing the closed stump of the rectum and the normal colon brought down to the anal canal. (d) The effect of crushing the spur, formerly the posterior, wall of the lower third of the rectum and the anterior wall of the pulled-down colon.

sphincterotomy. If sphincterotomy is too extensive it may cause incontinence. After Duhamel's operation, if the rectal pouch is not divided sufficiently high, faeces collect in the fundus of the pouch, whereas if the colon is brought out too low in the anal canal there is a constant leakage of faecal-stained mucus. There is a risk of stricture after all these various operations which is worst after the endorectal type of pull-through operation.

The most serious complication of Hirschsprung's disease is enterocolitis which has already been described. It is very important indeed to realise that enterocolitis may be recurrent after colostomy and recto-sigmoidectomy and even in children who have been discharged from hospital for months or even years and whose bowels have been functioning normally. In any child who has had Hirschsprung's disease the onset of diarrhoea should always raise the possibility that it is due to enterocolitis and if possible the child should be referred immediately to hospital.

Leakage from the anastomosis is more common and has more serious consequences when the suture line is not protected by a proximal colostomy or ileostomy at the time of operation. There is no longer any justification for rectosigmoidectomy for Hirschsprung's disease of any kind being done without a proximal 'ostomy. A drain should always be left in the pelvis at the end of the operation, but even with this precaution a pelvic abscess and a faecal fistula are not uncommon complications and are very difficult to clear up; the colostomy must be maintained for a much longer time and the chance that a stricture will form at the suture line is much increased.

In the first place a stricture, which is more common after the endorectal type of pull-through operation, should be treated by repeated dilatation under general anaesthesia. When a stricture resists repeated dilatation, excision and reanastomosis may be tried, but is extremely difficult and usually reactivates the infection which followed the original leak. An alternative is to excise the mucosa from distal segment and pull the colon down to the anal canal, but this too may be followed by a stricture. In the last resort it may be necessary to make a permanent terminal colostomy in the left iliac fossa.

Duplication of the alimentary tract

In the alimentary tract a duplication may be found anywhere from the tongue to the lower rectum. It may be spherical or tubular and be intimately associated with the alimentary tube, or a cyst in more or less close association with it. The dorsal non-vitelline enteric malformations have a different embryological origin to those associated with the vitellointestinal duct and

about half present within a month of birth and two-thirds in the first year. Lesions in the mediastinum usually cause disturbances of respiration due simply to the large size of a cystic duplication; there may also be ulceration and perforation of the cyst into the pleural cavity, the oesophagus or the bronchus. Tubular lesions of the intestine may be associated with unexplained bleeding from the bowel and spherical duplications often cause intestinal obstruction. A congenital malformation of the vertebral column is often found in association with an intestinal duplication and in a few cases there is an associated lumbar myelomeningocoele with a plaque of intestinal tissue on its surface. It has been suggested that when a cause cannot be found for rectal bleeding in a child, it is worth while to x-ray the whole of the vertebral column to exclude a spinal malformation.

The most common site for intestinal duplication is the small intestine and the most common type is a cyst, either closely involved with the intestinal wall and projecting into the lumen or lying in the mesentery. Tubular duplication may be found in both small or large bowel and may involve long lengths of bowel. Both cystic and tubular types may contain gastric or pancreatic tissue and are liable to ulceration, bleeding or perforation. Oesophageal duplications are found in the mediastinum, but often extend through the diaphragm and involve the stomach and duodenum. They may be associated with both but be separate from them. Duplications of the colon are often associated with duplications in the upper urinary tracts. The diagnosis of a duplication is difficult. In the chest the most common sign is a large shadow in the mediastinum in the plain radiograph of the chest, and in the abdomen there are clinical signs and radiological evidence of subacute intestinal obstruction.

The only effective treatment is excision which may be difficult, dangerous and incomplete. In the oesophagus, the cyst may be closely adherent to the oesophagus or share a common muscular coat with it; excision may then involve the dissection of most of the cyst wall from the oesophagus and of the mucosal lining of the cyst from the oesophageal muscle wall. It may be necessary to trace a fistula from the cyst to a vertebral body, but the complete excision of the fistula is difficult and sometimes impossible and meningitis may subsequently develop. A mediastinal duplication which extends through the diaphragm should be removed in stages.

A duplication of the stomach must be treated by partial gastrectomy which is simple and well tolerated in infancy. A duplication in the first part of the duodenum can seldom be excised and partial gastrectomy is necessary; it is very rare in the rest of the duodenum.

In the small intestine, usually the normal bowel and the duplication share a common muscular coat and cannot be separated. If the length of the duplication is short, both it and its associated bowel should be resected. If the length is too great for resection to be well tolerated, an opening for drainage should be made at the lower end of the duplication with the associated normal bowel. A duplication cyst in the mesentery which is separate from the intestine should be resected. The same principles apply in the colon.

Congenital hypertrophic pyloric stenosis

This affects boys four times as often as girls and occurs about once in every 200 babies born. It may occur at any time during the first 4 months, but is most common in the first 4 weeks. The baby vomits towards or at the end of each feed. The vomitus is projected several feet from the child and consists of the feed, some of which may be curdled, but it is never bile-stained. As vomiting continues, the baby becomes constipated, thin and wizened in appearance and fretful and restless from hunger. On examination during or towards the end of a feed the pyloric tumour may be felt as an ovoid hard lump just to the right of the lateral border of the right rectus muscle midway between the umbilicus and the costal margin. Usually also contractions of the pyloric antrum may be felt, waves of peristalsis may be seen on the abdominal wall and then the baby vomits. If the history suggests pyloric stenosis and there is any doubt about the presence of a tumour, then the baby should be screened during an opaque swallow and meal. This will show whether there is a hiatus hernia and a pyloric tumour.

The medical treatment of congenital pyloric stenosis with Eumydrin and other drugs based on atropine is now out of fashion and most babies with pyloric stenosis are referred to the surgeon without much delay. These babies now seldom require any preoperative treatment, apart from washing out the stomach with 0.9% saline an hour or two before operation. In the rare patient in whom the diagnosis, or the decision to seek surgical advice, has been delayed there may have been severe starvation and loss of gastric secretion. The resulting extracellular fluid depletion requires treatment by the intravenous administration of 0.9% saline before operation, but it must be recognised that there have been large losses as well of potassium and magnesium because of tissue catabolism and intracellular dehydration. It is desirable therefore to use instead of, or as well as, 0.9% saline, balanced electrolyte solution (Plasmalyte) which more closely resembles extracellular fluid than does 0.9% saline. The metabolic alkalosis which also exists is best corrected by the addition of potassium chloride to the intravenous infusion and magnesium chloride should also be added.

Modern paediatric anaesthesia provides excellent conditions for both patient and surgeon, but when it is not available local analgesia in the line of the incision and as a subcostal block remains the best alternative; the anaesthetic solution should not contain adrenaline. The paramedian incision should start at the costal margin and extend to 2.5 cm above the umbilicus and the rectus muscle is split in the line of its fibres. This high incision has the advantage that when the abdomen is being closed the right lobe of the liver shuts off almost the whole incision and prevents prolapse of the intestines. The liver is pushed up and the pyloric end of the stomach is drawn out of the wound. The pylorus is rotated so that its upper surface is exposed and a longitudinal incision is made through the whole length of the hard tumour down to the submucosal layer, avoiding the vessels on the anterior surface of the pylorus. The incision is then enlarged with artery or special forceps. The contents of the duodenum are squeezed against the pylorus to make sure the duodenal mucosa has not been perforated. If it has, the hole is closed by a catgut stitch through all the layers. Bleeding from the cut surfaces of the pylorus usually stops with pressure from dry gauze. The pyloric antrum is dropped back and the wound is closed in layers.

The baby can be fed from 4 h after operation and should be discharged after 24 h.

Biliary obstruction

The commonest cause of jaundice in the young child is the so-called 'physiological jaundice of the newly born'. This is due to the rapid destruction of red blood cells during the first week of life and is most severe 3–5 days after birth and disappears within a month; the stools are a normal colour, but the urine is usually dark. Jaundice may also be caused by neonatal hepatitis or by maternal blood group incompatibility. The commonest cause which directly concerns the surgeon is atresia of the bile ducts which is more common in the Japanese and Chinese races than in any others and probably occurs about once in every 10 000 births in the British Isles. Jaundice may also occur in association with pyloric stenosis, but is then usually due to starvation and loss of gastric secretions. Jaundice due to pressure by a large hydronephrosis or duodenal duplication is extremely rare. Blockage of the extrahepatic bile ducts by inspissated mucus or bile has been described, but is very unusual.

There are broadly two types of biliary atresia. In extrahepatic atresia some part of the extrahepatic biliary duct system is absent and this is the only kind of atresia which offers any real hope of long-term relief by operation. In intrahepatic atresia either the intrahepatic ducts are absent or they are so small as to be incapable of transmitting bile in sufficient quantity to cope with the volume produced by the liver. There is increasing support for the idea that intrahepatic atresia is part of a progressive infective process, the varying severity of which accounts for the variable degrees of damage to and size of the intrahepatic ducts.

Jaundice appears soon after birth, persists and becomes more severe, but the rate of progression is very variable. Although obstructive jaundice due to atresia can usually be distinguished biochemically from that due to haemolytic disease or non-obstructive hyperbilirubinaemia, the only way to distinguish it from jaundice due to hepatitis or hepatocellular disease is by the histological examination of a liver biopsy. Needle biopsy of the liver is not always as satisfactory and seldom as certain as open biopsy, which has the great advantage that the extrahepatic ductal system and gallbladder can be examined and cholangiography can be done. Regardless of the cause of the jaundice, cirrhotic changes begin early and if jaundice has persisted and increased in severity for 4 weeks after birth the abdomen should be opened and the ducts explored. With modern paediatric anaesthesia the former objection that anaesthetic agents would adversely affect the liver no longer holds to anything like the same degree. After 4 weeks cirrhosis is almost always present and the prognosis which was poor anyway becomes worse as the delay in operating increases.

Anaemia should be corrected by the transfusion of whole blood several days before operation and vitamin K should be administered. The upper abdomen should be opened by a long transverse or slightly oblique incision centred to the right of the midline. If the gallbladder is present, a polythene tube should be tied into its fundus, the gallbladder aspirated and cholangiography should be done with a water-soluble radio-opaque medium. A large wedge of liver should be taken for histological examination. In extrahepatic obstruction the cholangiogram should give a good indication of what can be done. It is better to implant the dilated proximal duct into a Roux-en-Y loop of jejunum than to anastomose it or the gallbladder directly to the duodenum, so as to minimise the risk of ascending cholangitis.

In intrahepatic obstruction or atresia some surgeons proceed at once to dissect the porta hepatis and to search for dilated intrahepatic bile ducts whether any bile is seen or not. After dissection of the porta the end of a Roux-en-Y loop of jejunum is anastomosed to the porta hepatis. There are several versions of this operation and the tendency now is to isolate the segment of jejunum which is anastomosed to the porta and to bring its distal end to the surface of the abdominal wall, so that any bile drainage there may be, can be seen, and also to reduce the risk of cholangitis. This loop of jejunum is subsequently joined to the rest of the jejunum.

Unfortunately, the results of these operations for intrahepatic biliary atresia are not good. The immediate mortality is high, cirrhosis almost invariably develops within 18 months to 2 years in the survivors and cholangitis is very common, no matter what kind of anastomosis is made. Some children may survive for 10 or 15 years with intrahepatic atresia without any anastomotic operations, but with cirrhosis, ascites and portal hypertension and usually die of haematemesis from oesophageal varices. The average length of survival is a matter of months.

Choledochal cyst

This anomaly is rare but important, because it may appear as a large, round swelling in the right upper quadrant of the abdomen and be mistaken for a hydronephrosis or a duodenal duplication. The most common form is a large cystic dilatation of the common bile duct with normal ducts above and a normal segment of common duct below and a normal gallbladder. Sometimes there is a large fusiform dilatation of the whole of the common bile duct and very rarely there may be a large cystic diverticulum of the common bile duct. It is much more common in girls than in boys and is usually diagnosed late in childhood, but a few are found during infancy.

The clinical features are very variable and most choledochal cysts are diagnosed at laparotomy. The cyst may cause jaundice or obstruction of the portal vein, intermittent pain and, if infected, cholangitis, chills, fever and jaundice. The severity of the symptoms and signs depend on the age of the child. Intravenous cholangiography is not of much value unless the opaque medium is given slowly overnight in 5% glucose solution administered by intravenous infusion. The cyst may be shown by displacement of the duodenum after an opaque meal, but pyelography is usually necessary to exclude a large hydronelphrosis.

At laparotomy, the cyst should be dissected free and then either excised completely with anastomosis of the ends of the common bile duct, which is by far the best form of treatment, or the cyst wall should be resected until a common bile duct of near normal size can be made by suture of the remaining part. Excision of the cyst and anastomosis of the stump of the bile duct to the duodenum or to a Roux-en-Y loop both carry a high risk of cholangitis. The former practice of anastomosing the cyst directly to the duodenum, while the simplest and easiest procedure, almost always is followed by severe cholangitis, even when a very wide opening is made, and should not therefore be done.

Acute intussusception

Acute intussusception is second only to acute appendicitis amongst the acute abdominal emergencies of infancy and childhood. An obvious cause such as a tumour or polyp or the inversion of a Meckel's diverticulum is seldom found. Moreover, small loose intussusceptions are not uncommonly found at laparotomy for other causes in infants and children. The invagination is usually isoperistaltic and most often begins in the terminal ileum and the intussusception may pass through the ileocaecal valve or push it in front into the caecum and colon. How far the intussusception progresses in the large bowel depends on how well the colon is fixed to the posterior abdominal wall. As the invagination progresses, tension on the mesenteric vessels causes the intussusception to become curved and also interferes with the blood flow to and from the invaginated bowel.

About two-thirds of the patients are boys. About three-quarters of all patients are aged less than 1 year and it is commonest between 3 and 8 months and the peak incidence is at 5 months. The onset is sudden in a patient who has been doing well and the baby screams in a characteristic way which once heard is never forgotten and draws up his legs. After repeated bouts of pain, at regular intervals, there is an interval when the exhausted baby drops off to sleep only to be awakened by another bout of colic and pain. The baby may vomit a recently-taken feed and pass several normal stools and there may be some blood in the stools, or in about two-thirds of patients lightly blood-stained mucus may be passed or found on the finger after a rectal examination. The diagnosis should be, and usually is, made long before there are any signs of intestinal obstruction. Between the spasms the baby lies limply, looks grey, there is often a bluish tinge to the eyelids and the pulse is rapid. On examination of the abdomen between the spasms, the typical sausage-shaped curved tumour may be felt, concave towards the umbilicus. It may be difficult to feel the tumour because it is under the right lobe of the liver. Palpation of the tumour may cause contraction of the intestine and another spasm of pain. Tenderness of the tumour suggests that the sheath may be becoming gangrenous.

It is important to examine the sleeping baby in whatever position he may be, in his mother's arms or on her lap and if possible without waking him. If a tumour is felt there is no real need to examine the rectum. The intussusception rarely progresses so far that it can be felt with the finger and in any case this would be obvious from palpation of the abdomen.

Reduction of an acute intussusception by hydrostatic pressure with an opaque enema under visual control with the image-intensifier is being increasingly used, and is successful in about two-thirds of the patients in which it is used. It is most likely to succeed when the history is short, i.e. less than 24 h. It is very important to be quite certain that reduction is complete. If there is any doubt the abdomen should be opened. It is essential that the surgeon who will operate on the child if reduction is not achieved should be present with the radiologist when hydrostatic reduction is attempted.

Before operation, compatible blood should be available in case the intussusception is irreducible and must be resected. A low mortality largely depends on the surgeon's willingness to use blood transfusion freely and without hesitation. An intravenous infusion should always be set up before operation, indeed most anaesthetists would now rightly insist on this for their own purposes.

At operation the kind of incision which is made depends on where the tumour lies. If it is in the caecum, or ascending or right transverse colon, a right gridiron incision is usually satisfactory if the history is of less than 24 h duration and the baby is aged more than 6 months. Otherwise it is better to use a suitably situated paramedian or transverse incision. The apex is found by palpation and is pushed back with two fingers. The first part of the reduction is usually easy and when the caecum is reached, the bowel, which is mobile, is delivered from the abdomen and the final stage of the reduction is completed under vision. It may be necessary to apply pressure to reduce the oedema of the bowel wall before the reduction of the last part of the bowel can be achieved. The dimple at the apex must be gently eased out. If there is any obvious cause for the intussusception, it should be dealt with. The appendix should not be removed.

When, even with external pressure, the intussusception cannot be reduced or if, when it is reduced, the bowel is not viable, the surgeon must decide whether to resect the affected bowel and make a primary anastomosis, short-circuit the bowel above and below the intussusception which is then exteriorised, or resect the intussusception and bring the open ends of the bowel to the surface as enterostomies. There is no doubt that resection and anastomosis is the method of choice provided the condition of the baby is good enough and the surgeon has adequate experience of intestinal anastomosis in babies.

The anastomosis should be made in bowel which is not oedematous. The difference in size of the ends of the ileum and colon can be overcome by cutting the colon across transversely and the ileum obliquely. The anastomosis should be made with a single layer of 00 black silk mattress sutures. A side-to-side anastomosis should never be used, because of the risk of a subsequent blind-loop disturbance.

The best alternative to resection and primary anastomosis is excision of the intussusception and exteriorisation of the ends of the bowel. The loss of intestinal secretions from the proximal ileum can be minimised by stopping all oral intake and feeding the baby intravenously for a week and then reopening the abdomen and anastomosing the ends of the bowel. This is the method of choice in the baby in poor condition with a long history of delayed diagnosis and intestinal obstruction.

After uneventful simple reduction of an intussusception, the intravenous infusion can be stopped when blood replacement, if necessary, has been completed, gastric aspiration is usually not needed and the baby can be fed after 12 h. The same programme can be adopted even when resection and anastomosis has been done, because the suture line is in the lower ileum.

Meckel's diverticulum

The vitellointestinal duct normally disappears by the end of the seventh week of intrauterine life. When it persists, it is most commonly as a blind diverticulum 5 to 10 cm in length arising from the antimesenteric border of the ileum between 20 and 54 cm above the ileocaecal valve. A remnant of the axial artery of the midgut usually runs across the surface of the ileum from which the diverticulum arises on to the sac wall. The diverticulum may be attached to the deep surface of the umbilicus by a fibrous cord or may be almost completely obliterated in continuity with the cord. There may be no attachment at all to the bowel, the remains of the diverticulum being a cyst attached to the umbilicus by a fibrous cord. Rarely there is instead of a diverticulum a patent vitellointestinal duct which runs between the ileum and the umbilicus where it opens on the surface as a fistula and discharges intestinal contents.

In a Meckel's diverticulum there may be, singly or in combination, gastric, duodenal or intestinal mucosa or pancreatic tissue. Gastric tissue may give rise to a peptic ulcer, usually near the base of the diverticulum, which may bleed or perforate. The diverticulum may be inverted by abnormal peristalsis and become the leading point of an intussusception. Torsion round a Meckel's diverticulum which is attached to the umbilicus by a fibrous cord, or by adhesions to another intraabdominal structure, is a rare complication.

The commonest symptom associated with a Meckel's diverticulum is pain in the umbilicus or near it. The diverticulum is rarely seen on radiological examination after an opaque meal. It is most often found incidentally at laparotomy for another lesion. If it is associated with a perforation of an ulcer in its wall, it should be removed. When a diverticulum is found during the course of another operation, it should be removed only if this will not affect the outcome of the primary operation. For example, if it is not involved in an intus-

susception, it should be left alone and the same is true if it is found during the removal of a gangrenous appendix, or at operation on an intestinal atresia. When a diverticulum is removed, the bowel should be closed with a single layer of interrupted mattress sutures of silk.

Infection in the neonatal period and infancy

The commonest site for infection in the neonatal period is the umbilicus and while much infection in this site is not usually serious and subsides without specific treatment, some umbilical infections have grave short- and long-term implications.

Thrombophlebitis of the umbilical vein is rare, but may spread upwards to the liver and cause a septic hepatitis with liver abscesses and ultimately fibrosis and later cirrhosis of the liver and portal hypertension. The umbilical vein is commonly used for exchange transfusion and a catheter is very frequently passed through the umbilical vein so that blood may be withdrawn from the vena cava for measurements of the blood gases; such a catheter may be left *in situ* for several days and is a potential cause of severe infection and septicaemia. The umbilical vein cannula is also used for the intravenous feeding of very small premature babies. Especially when laparotomy is required, the umbilical vein should not be used for prolonged infusions. There is, however, one occasion when the umbilical vein is of very great value and this is when a neonate needs rapid resuscitation before a laparotomy. Under local anaesthesia the umbilical vein should be exposed through a short transverse incision in the site of the proposed later laparotomy incision, the linea alba is opened and the umbilical vein is cleared and lifted into the wound and the cannula is inserted into the vein and tied in position. When later at operation the abdominal wall is painted with antiseptic the cannula also is painted and is then passed to the anaesthetist before the towels are applied; in this way resuscitation can be continued without interruption.

Superficial abscesses in the skin and regional lymph glands may be due to *Staphylococcus aureus* and may progress to septicaemia and septic arthritis, most commonly in the shoulder, hip or knee joints or to osteomyelitis of the end of one of the long bones. The diagnosis of such arthritis or osteitis is usually the result of the observation, most often by one of the nurses, that the affected joint is not being moved as the others are or that whenever the affected limb is moved or handled the baby cries with pain. The tenderness over the end of a long bone is similarly first noticed in this way before there is swelling of the limb or redness of the overlying skin. A blood culture should always be made, but the baby should also be given a large dose of ampicillin-cloxacillin (500 mg) by intramuscular injection without delay and this dose should be repeated in 4 h and thereafter 250 mg should be given every 4 h while waiting for the result of the blood culture. The affected limb should be immobilised in a suitable splint with light traction. Aspiration of the joint may be helpful. If signs of localisation of the infection in the end of a long bone appear, such as swelling and redness of the skin or localised tenderness, the subperiosteal abscess should be opened and the bone should be drilled, pus should be sent for culture and the incision completely closed without drainage.

Abdominal tumours

Benign

Amongst the benign tumours is the mesenteric cyst which is not an intestinal duplication, but more often arising from the lymphatic system; this cyst, which may be very large, can usually be readily removed. Benign teratomas arising from the posterior abdominal wall may reach a large size before being found, usually by the mother when she is drying the child after a bath. These also can usually be completely removed. Teratomas also arise in the ovary and the commonest, sacrococcygeal teratoma, arises from the deep surface of the sacrum or coccyx and usually grows downwards into the perineum, but sometimes there may also be a large retroperitoneal extension upwards into the pelvic cavity and the abdomen. Large angiomas, bile cysts and hamartomas occur very rarely in the liver and should be excised if necessary by anatomical lobectomy.

Malignant

More children aged less than 5 years die of malignant disease than of any other single cause, even accidents. Acute leukaemia is still the commonest kind of malignant disease under the age of 5 years, followed by malignant disease of the central nervous system, neuroblastoma and nephroblastoma. In children malignant disease arises almost entirely from embryonic tissues rather than from epithelial cells. More than half the abdominal masses in children are due to enlargement of the liver in association with leukaemia, storage disease or Hodgkin's disease, or to enlargement of the spleen. Less than half the masses are due to causes which can be relieved by surgical treatment and two-thirds of these are in the upper urinary tract and half of these are

benign and are cysts or due to obstruction of the upper urinary tract.

Nephroblastoma

This tumour accounts for about 5% of all malignant tumours which occur under the age of 15 years, or about 80 each year in Great Britain. About a third are diagnosed before the age of 2 years, a third between 2 and 3 years, and a third in older children. In the first year of life, many tumours of the kidney are not nephroblastomas, but benign mesenchymal hamartomas.

The first sign of the disease is an abdominal mass which is found by the mother of the child or on a general routine examination of the abdomen by a doctor. An abdominal mass is nearly always palpable on admission to hospital. Only about a third of the patients complain of abdominal pain and in less than a quarter are there general symptoms such as pyrexia, loss of appetite, lassitude or blood-stained urine. The mass is usually smooth, firm and lies deep in the flank and may displace the liver or spleen and extend across the midline.

It is often not easy to distinguish between nephroblastoma and neuroblastoma. The most important investigation is intravenous urography. In nephroblastoma there is usually gross distortion of the caliceal pattern, but the kidney may not be displaced. There is usually some excretion and concentration of the medium even when the kidney is extensively involved. In neuroblastoma the caliceal pattern is not much disturbed, but the whole kidney may be displaced by the tumour. In infants, it may be necessary to use concentrated opaque medium and the upper urinary tract may be shown satisfactorily only in delayed films.

When it is suspected that a large abdominal mass is a nephroblastoma only one person should examine the abdomen, the surgeon who is to operate on the tumour, because of the risk of disseminating the disease. Needle biopsy of the tumour should never be done. The resection of a nephroblastoma should always be regarded as a surgical emergency and delay should be allowed only for intravenous urography and the provision of compatible blood for transfusion. When there is real doubt whether the tumour is a neuroblastoma or a nephroblastoma the operation should be delayed for a 24 h collection of urine for a VMA estimation, but only when the balance of evidence suggests that the tumour is a neuroblastoma. Some surgeons have preferred to reduce the size of a very large tumour by irradiation before operation. This involves very undesirable delay and if the diagnosis is wrong reduces the chances of ultimate success.

The best results are obtained when the tumour is confined to the kidney without metastases and the whole kidney and tumour can be completely excised. To reduce the risk of dissemination during the operation whenever possible the first procedure should be to ligate the renal vein and artery, and until this has been done the tumour and kidney should be handled as little as possible. The best approach to the kidney is through a transverse incision below the costal margin on the affected side running forwards to the midline or beyond. This allows good transperitoneal access to the renal pedicle when this is not so overlain by the tumour that it cannot be reached as a first step in the operation or without some mobilisation of the kidney.

The prognosis is based on the staging of the tumour after laparotomy and depends on the observations of the surgeon and the findings of the pathologist. In stage I the tumour is confined to the kidney and both are completely resected. In stage II the tumour has extended beyond the kidney, either by local infiltration, along the renal vein, or the para-aortic glands are involved but macroscopic removal of these extensions is complete. In stage III the tumour extended beyond the renal capsule and was not completely removed at operation, or the operation field was contaminated by tumour spilled at operation. In stage IV there are distant metastases in liver, lung, bone, brain or elsewhere. In stage V both kidneys are involved. A recent MRC trial has shown that the best results of treatment were obtained in hospitals which treated the largest numbers of children with this tumour and according to well-defined protocols which take into account the age of the child and the stage of the tumour, and which include a full course of maintenance chemotherapy. The overall mortality for patients who were included in the trial was 23% and for those who were eligible, but were not included it was 45%. There is a very good case for referring children with nephroblastoma to specialist children's hospitals for treatment.

In the case of benign mesenchymal hamartoma and patients with stage I tumours, especially those less than a year old, there is no indication for either radiotherapy or chemotherapy.

Neuroblastoma

This tumour arises from the primitive cells of the sympathetic nervous system and adrenal medulla in the retroperitoneal area in the abdomen and in the mediastinum and neck. It consists of small round or polygonal undifferentiated cells which may be arranged in rosettes. The incidence of this tumour is uncertain, but more than half the total arise in the abdomen, but it is less common there than nephroblastoma. If those in the neck and mediastinum are included, neuroblastoma is a little more common than nephroblastoma. The commonest age of onset is 18 months and like nephroblastoma the first sign of the disease is usually the discovery of an abdominal mass; subsequent inquiry, however, often reveals that for a week or two the child has not been as well as usual. The mass is nodular and fixed and is situated more often in the midline than the flanks and in the region of the umbilicus rather than under the ribs. Sudden enlargement of the tumour may be due to bleeding into it, but sometimes the first symptom is pain in a bone, or proptosis due to a metastasis in the orbit may be the first sign.

A plain radiograph of the abdomen should show the size and site of the tumour by the displacement of gas shadows in the bowel. There may be calcification in the capsule or in the centre of the tumour. Intravenous urography shows normal caliceal and pelvic outlines in both kidneys, but any deformity is extrinsic rather than intrinsic; the kidneys may be displaced from the normal position or rotated. The whole skeleton must be x-rayed for metastases and the bone marrow should be examined. The 24 h output of VMA in the urine must be measured.

The tumour has often so extensively invaded the structures on the posterior abdominal wall that it cannot be removed and then a generous biopsy should be taken and the capsule of the tumour carefully closed. Subsequently x-ray therapy and chemotherapy may reduce the size of the tumour sufficiently to justify another laparotomy to see if the residual tumour can be resected. In the first year of life, if the tumour can be removed, the prognosis is so good (about 85% survival) that radiotherapy and chemotherapy are not indicated. Neuroblastoma which arises in the mediastinum or neck has a very much better prognosis than when it arises in the abdomen, especially with modern long-term chemotherapy; the prognosis is also better when it arises in the pelvis than in the abdomen. When staged in the same way as nephroblastoma the prognosis is similar, but poorer in all stages.

Ganglioneuroma is a solid tumour which also arises from the sympathetic nervous ganglia in the abdomen or the mediastinum. It is benign and radio-resistant and must be excised. The prognosis is good. It is important to realise that the urinary output of VMA may be raised also in the presence of a ganglioneuroma.

Rhabdomyosarcoma

This is a highly malignant embryonic tumour of striped muscle. It is most common in the urinary bladder, but also occurs in the prostate, spermatic cord, vagina or broad ligament. More rarely it may occur in the pharynx, palate or middle ear. Treatment is by surgical excision combined with radiotherapy and chemotherapy and the prognosis has been much improved with repeated courses of multiple chemotherapy.

Hepatoblastoma

All tumours of the liver are very uncommon, but the hepatoblastoma is the commonest especially in the first two years of life. There is a large, usually smooth swelling more often in the right lobe than the left; later multiple knobs may be felt. There is usually no general illness or disturbance until the mass is felt. The only treatment is excision of the anatomical lobe which is affected. The best approach is by a high transverse incision which may be extended round the costal margin to the neck of the twelfth rib; a thoracoabdominal incision does not have the advantages which have been claimed for it. After dissection of the porta hepatis and ligation of the branches of the portal vein, hepatic artery and bile ducts of the affected lobe, the liver is incised and the hepatic vein of the lobe is ligated and divided. Even small infants survive this operation well, provided the blood loss is accurately and immediately replaced. Formerly the results of treatment were very poor, but there are signs that with more intensive multiple chemotherapy some improvement is being made.

Angiomas

The **port-wine stain** cutaneous angioma does not respond well to any kind of treatment and is best managed in older children, especially girls, by the use of suitable 'make-up'.

The **capillary angioma** usually starts as a small lesion not more than a centimetre in diameter at birth and then, especially on the face, may grow rapidly and extend over much of the face, the so-called 'spreading angioma of infancy'. Whenever a small capillary angioma of the face is seen, it should be treated at once by the application of carbon dioxide snow under light general analgesia. The stick of snow is applied to the angioma for 40 s and this should be repeated as often as is needed to freeze the whole lesion. A blister will appear and be followed by a scab which drops off in 2 to 3 weeks. It is well-known that capillary angiomas grow for a time and then spontaneously regress; what it is important for the surgeon to realise, however, is that in the early stages they can be controlled by the simple measure of applying carbon dioxide snow and the development of a huge unsightly lesion can be prevented. Multiple angiomas of the face should be treated by repeated applications of carbon dioxide snow, if necessary under general anaesthesia. Capillary angiomas in other parts of the body can be treated conservatively and allowed to subside spontaneously and the parents should be firmly reassured that this will eventually happen.

The **cavernous angioma** does not always need to be treated, but when it involves the face, the large swelling causes great distress to the parents and should be treated actively by the injection of 30% saline into the central part of the angioma under general anaesthesia. The needle should be inserted and as much blood as possible should be pressed out of the angioma before the saline is injected into the compressed angioma. If the injection is too superficial the overlying skin may slough. The injection should be repeated about once a month until the angioma is controlled. Mixed capillary and cavernous angiomas should be treated by a combination of carbon dioxide snow and injections of hypertonic saline.

A 'giant limb' may be due to a variety of combinations of arterial, venous and lymphatic anomalies. A single arteriovenous communication is very rare indeed in childhood. Occasionally multiple small arteriovenous communications are found so widely distributed in the subcutaneous tissues and muscles as to be untreatable. Injection with hypertonic saline is of very limited value and some form of compression is more effective than anything else, especially when parts of the lymphatic system are absent. The vascular anomalies are commonly distributed in a segmental fashion following the spinal nerve territories. One form of giant limb which does respond well to surgical excision is the large segmental lipoma, but this is rare.

Lymphangiomas

The most important lymphangioma in infancy and childhood is the cystic hygroma of the face and neck. This may exceed in size the baby's head. A hygroma consists of many cysts filled with clear fluid which extend widely in the neck and usually across the midline behind and between the oesophagus and trachea and amongst the great vessels and the nerves. Operation on a cystic hygroma is not to be undertaken without good reason at any age. The swelling may suddenly enlarge because of bleeding into one or more of the cysts. Aspiration and the injection of sclerosing solutions are of no value. A prime indication for operation is respiratory distress and a tracheostomy should if possible be the first step in the operation because endotracheal intubation may be impossible. Complete excision is seldom possible and in emergency operations in the newly born, as much of the hygroma as is reasonably possible, consistent with relief of the respiratory difficulties, is all that it may be wise to deal with.

An angioma, lymphangioma or a mixture of both may cause considerable enlargement of the tongue and this is best treated by the injection of 30% saline under general anaesthesia. Careful observation and nursing on one side or almost face down is necessary after operation.

The central nervous system

Encephalocoele, myelomeningocoele and hydrocephalus are the conditions which most often need treatment in the neonatal period and infancy.

An encephalocoele is due to the protrusion of the meninges through a defect in the skull, and sometimes, but not always, of the overlying skin as well. It seldom contains any brain tissue. The most common sites are occipital or suboccipital and much less often in the nasofrontal or vertical regions. An encephalocoele should always be closed. If it is covered by skin this should be dissected off and reduced so that when it is sutured the meninges are flush with the bone edges. The meninges should never be opened. When there is a defect of the skin, the edges should be dissected away from the protruded meninges and the scalp should be mobilised enough to allow the skin edges to be closed over the meninges. Hydrocephalus is very seldom a complication.

The treatment of myelomeningocoele is now very much more conservative than it was a few years ago. Active treatment should be avoided if there is paraplegia below the first lumbar segment, gross hydrocephalus, or severe spinal deformity. On these criteria Stark and Drummond found that 80% of the babies who were not treated died within 3 months and 70% of those who were treated were alive after 6 years with much less severe mental and physical handicaps than those reported in earlier series of more actively treated patients. The decision whether to treat a child with myelomeningocoele or not should be made in the hospital where the treatment will be carried out, preferably after the activities of the muscles below the lesion have been tested and charted. This is a decision which must be made by doctors and they should then explain the position fully to the parents and give them firm advice. The parents should not be asked to decide, although they may override the medical advice.

If a baby survives in spite of the original decision to treat the child conservatively, not a great deal will have been lost because of the criteria on which that decision was made. When long-term survival seems likely hydrocephalus must be controlled by the insertion of a Spitz-Holter valve and thereafter the child should be treated as if it had been decided to treat the child actively from the first.

Dermoid cysts

The scalp

The most important dermoid cyst of the scalp is the one which lies in the midline of the vertex or near to it because this cyst commonly has an intracranial extension which is larger than that part which is in the scalp. What is more important still is that the intracranial extension is very often closely related to the superior sagittal sinus. It may be possible to demonstrate in a radiograph of the skull that there is a bony defect which should be taken as an indication that there is an intracranial extension. The wiser and safer course then is to refer the child to a neurosurgeon.

The nose

A dermoid cyst in the midline of the nose, especially if it is situated over the junction of the nasal bone and the cartilage usually has a deep extension in the midline along the nasal septum which may extend as far as the ethmoid bone. If the whole of this extension is not removed the cyst will recur. It is as well to warn the parents that there may be a deeper extension to the innocent minor-looking lesion on the nose and that it may recur after operation.

Further reading

Apley J. (1975). *The Child with Abdominal Pain*, 2nd edn. Philadelphia: JB Lippincott.

Gross R.E. (1953). *The Surgery of Infancy and Childhood.* Philadelphia: WB Saunders.

Jones P. ed. (1976). *Clinical Paediatric Surgery*, 2nd edn. London: Blackwell Scientific Productions.

Judson G.R. (1979). *The Injured Child.* Chicago: Year Book Medical Publishers.

Potter Edith L., Craig J.M. (1976). *Pathology of the Fetus and Infant*, 3rd edn. Chicago: Year Book Medical Publishers.

Stark G.D. (1977). *Spina Bifida.* London: Blackwell Scientific Publications.

Waterston D.J., Bonham Carter R.E., Aberdeen E. (1962). *Lancet*; **i**:819.

Wilkinson A.W. (1963, 1969, 1975). *Recent Advances in Paediatric Surgery.* Edinburgh: Churchill Livingstone.

Wilkinson A.W. (1973). *Body Fluids in Surgery*, 4th edn. Edinburgh: Churchill Livingstone.

14

Surgery in tropical countries

DOUGLAS ROY

Surgery in tropical countries is not so much concerned with treating exotic conditions as with treating common conditions in exotic surroundings. In each country and within each country the epidemiology of surgical disease varies; in each area there will be a relatively small number of surgical conditions which cause the most disability, threat to life or economic handicap.

Essential facilities can be very simple (Fig 14.1). In western countries devoted to the 'disposable' economy in medicine, it is not appreciated that most disposables can be resterilised and reused. 'Disposable' surgical gloves can, for instance, be reused on average about eight times. Open windows are better and safer ventilators than expensive air conditioning systems, which often cannot be maintained and space is as valuable as expensive equipment.

In tropical countries many surgical procedures are performed by physicians who have not received a full postgraduate training in surgery. Their surgical supervision is derived from the specialist surgeon in the provincial or area hospital who must regard his responsibilities as extending beyond his own hospital to embrace all the district hospitals in his area.

There is variation in the prevalence of disease from area to area. Most is due to environmental factors and only in a few situations is it due to genetic or racial differences. The people of central and eastern Africa are not protected from atheroma because they are Bantu,

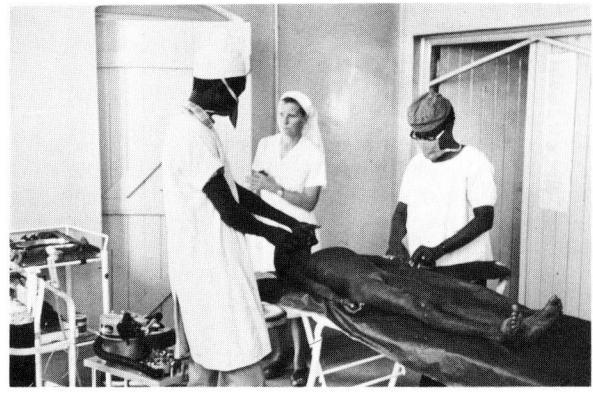

Fig 14.1 Surgery in a district hospital. Anaesthesia being given by a medical assistant using the EMO apparatus. The patient has a hydatid cyst of liver.

Nilotic or Hamitic, but because their diet and pattern of life inhibits its development.

Surgical care in tropical countries can be considered in three categories – background diseases, not specifically surgical, occurring in surgical patients; cosmopolitan diseases occurring in tropical countries and specifically tropical diseases of surgical interest. This chapter is concerned primarily with the first and third groups.

Background disease in surgical patients

Malnutrition

Malnutrition is widespread in the tropics, particularly in urban areas but only a minority of the millions who live there are affected. Worst affected are the children and, while frank starvation is easily detected, the surgeon must be careful to detect the minor degrees of protein deficiency characterised by oedema, so that the child appears to be of normal weight. It often exists synergistically with gastroenteritis which itself requires treatment.

In adults, gross malnutrition is rare except in famine conditions and vitamin deficiency is uncommon. Ascorbic acid deficiency only occurs when the individual lives in very artificial surroundings with unusual dietary habits. Deficiency of vitamin B complex is more common, but usually in association with obvious starvation, presenting as one of the forms of beri-beri.

Anaemia

Anaemia is common in tropical countries. Mostly it is an iron deficiency anaemia, the end result of low intake of dietary iron and folic acid aggravated by repeated pregnancy, abnormal blood loss as a result of parasites such as hookworm or increased blood destruction by diseases like malaria. It is wise to give both iron and folic acid to correct these anaemias before operation, as well as treating the underlying cause. There is no advantage in raising the haemoglobin above 10 g per 100 ml.

In the Mediterranean area, the Indian subcontinent and South East Asia thalassaemia, an inherited abnormality of the haemoglobin molecule, is a frequent cause of anaemia but, more important to the surgeon, in countries with large negro populations (Africa, West Indies, North and South America) sickle cell anaemia is relatively common and causes both anaemia and symptoms suggestive of surgical disease. The disease is due to the inheritance of an abnormal haemoglobin (haemoglobin S) from one or both parents. If from both, the child has homozygous disease (SS) and is unlikely to survive to puberty. However, the heterozygote (AS) has milder symptoms and is protected to some extent against infection with malaria and thus having a better chance of survival, maintains the abnormality in the population. The heterozygote is said to have the sickle cell trait.

The abnormal haemoglobin is insoluble in the reduced form and this distends the cell into the shape of sickle. These cells are more readily haemolysed and resist the deformation necessary for flow through capillary beds. Consequently, microinfarctions may occur in various organs and tissues. These changes are precipitated by hypoxia.

The surgeon may be concerned with this disease in several ways:

1 Microinfarctions in the wall of the intestine may cause acute abdominal pain simulating an acute abdomen.
2 Anaesthesia, if associated with hypoxia, may provoke a 'sickling' crisis with severe haemolysis and pulmonary microvascular obstruction.
3 Microinfarction in bone may cause bone pain and, in children, lead to osteomyelitis, characteristically, with salmonella typhi as the infecting organism.
4 Superficial ulcers on the medial aspect of the leg above the malleolus appearing in older children and adults are said to be commoner in people affected by this trait.

The diagnosis can be confirmed by electrophoresis which demonstrates the abnormal haemoglobin. There is also a simple side room test in which the addition of 2% sodium meta bisulphite, a reducing agent, to red cells on a slide will cause them to sickle.

Hypoxia must be avoided at all times. During a sickling crisis isotonic saline, by i.v. infusion, reduces the viscosity of blood and improves capillary flow; oxygen should also be given. Infection must be treated promptly and if osteomyelitis is suspected, the assumption can be made that the organism is salmonella typhi and treated accordingly. It is obvious that the mistaken diagnosis of an acute abdomen in a 'sickler' might lead to unnecessary laparotomy, hypoxia during anaesthesia and death from a sickling crisis.

Blood transfusion

Blood transfusion is as necessary in tropical countries as it is elsewhere, but blood is less easy to obtain so that electrolyte solutions and blood substitutes need to be used when possible. Gelatin solutions are popular in many countries, they are cheap, keep well and are no more liable to anaphylactic reactions than other more costly preparations. In many urban areas blood transfusion services have been established, despite local prejudices against the giving of blood, while in rural areas transfusion from relatives is commonly used. When no blood is available, it is surprising how seldom the need for it is felt.

In elective surgery, autogenous transfusion (Brzica *et al.*, 1976) is valuable providing the patient is not anaemic or the anaemia has been corrected. The patient is bled of up to one litre of blood which is stored, is given iron and folate and a good diet and the operation performed between 2 and 3 weeks later. In the emergency situation autotransfusion is applicable in cases with severe intra-abdominal or intrathoracic bleeding providing no viscus has been damaged and the exterior wound, if present, is not large. Quite simple apparatus without elaborate filters is sufficient, consisting of a trap on a suction line containing an appropriate anticoagulant. The value of this method outweighs the possible disadvantages arising from defibrination of the blood, although the dangers of this must be recognised.

Resuscitation

Every surgical unit can have an area set aside for intensive care even if no sophisticated equipment is available. ECG tracings are almost always available. Simple biochemical estimations of serum electrolytes and urea can be obtained. Urine flow, concentration and specific gravity are easily measured while central venous pressure measurements can be had by combining two intravenous giving sets with an appropriate cannula and a measuring stick. Control of respiratory failure is more difficult as oxygen is not often available. Respiration can be supported mechanically, if necessary, for considerable periods by a series of assistants compressing the bellows or bag of a simple anaesthetic apparatus.

Endemic infections and infestations

Tuberculosis

Tuberculosis is still common in the tropics and must always be a major consideration in differential diagnosis (Stoll, 1978). It is most important to the surgeon in the following circumstances:

1   Hypertrophic ileocaecal tuberculosis is particularly common in the Indian subcontinent as a cause of intestinal obstruction or of a mass in the right lower abdomen. It must be distinguished from Crohn's disease which is rare in most tropical countries.
2   Tuberculous enteritis (Pujari, 1979) may, if the patient recovers, lead to stenotic lesions causing small bowel obstruction. These stenotic lesions are usually multiple and are best treated by an enteroplasty rather than resection.
3   All the manifestations of genitourinary tuberculosis are seen in developing countries and every effort must be made to make an early diagnosis and confirm it, if possible, by positive culture of the organisms.
4   Tuberculous pericarditis with cardiac tamponade is not uncommon and constrictive pericarditis can be confused with cardiomyopathy if the lesion has not acquired its characteristic calcification.

5   Tuberculous infection of cervical lymph glands in children and adults is common and must be considered in the differential diagnosis of lymphadenopathies.

Treatment

Surgical procedures may still be necessary in some of these cases, but the main cause of failure in the treatment of tuberculosis is the defection of the patient from treatment. Recent work by the British Thoracic and Tuberculosis Association and the East African and British Research Councils has defined shorter, more effective regimes, based on rifampicin which should increase patient compliance and can be completed in 6 months.

Typhoid fever

Typhoid fever is not specifically a tropical disease, but it is very common in the tropics and its major surgical complication, perforation of the small intestine (Welch and Martin, 1975), is a frequent emergency. The patient has usually been ill for some days with a fever, but may not have had any diarrhoea. The perforation, occurring as it does in a patient already damanged by toxaemia, presents a serious problem. A toxic myocarditis is always present and replacement of fluid requires careful judgement in order to avoid congestive cardiac failure. Central venous pressure should, therefore, be measured during resuscitation. The infection is treated with chloramphenicol, amoxycillin or cotrimoxazole, but response is usually slow. Formerly it was advised that typhoid perforation should be treated conservatively because of the high mortality of surgical intervention. More recently, however, careful resuscitation and prompt surgical intervention has reduced the mortality rate from 50% to 20%. The perforated ulcer should be excised by wedge excision, a single area of diseased bowel may be resected or, in a very ill patient, exteriorisation of the small bowel may be the best procedure.

Leprosy

Advanced cases are usually the concern of the orthopaedic surgeon and those concerned with the rehabilitation of the crippled patient (Browne, 1968). However, early diagnosis may save the person from becoming a cripple. In some areas up to 15% of people may suffer from some form of this disease. The surgeon should be alert for:

1   Any unusual rash if it shows areas of hypopigmentation or hypoaesthesia.

2   Superficial ulcers which may be trophic in origin.

3   Thickening of subcutaneous peripheral nerves, e.g., the ulnar at the elbow or the cervical nerves (Fig 14.2).

Malaria

The importance of malaria needs no emphasis. Patients in most tropical countries, except for a few fortunate islands like Mauritius and Jamaica, are likely to be infected with one or other of the two main species (*Plasmodium falciparum* or *P. vivax*). The surgeon must take account of this disease in the following circumstances:

1   As a cause of postoperative pyrexia. A thick and thin blood smear stained with Field's stain will confirm the diagnosis, but treatment should be commenced on suspicion.

2   Malaria can be transmitted by blood transfusion (British Medical Journal, 1976) and therefore it is wise to give antimalarials prophylactically to patients receiving more than a litre of blood.

3   Splenectomy in children and adolescents will diminish their resistance to future infection with malaria and, therefore, splenectomy should be avoided. Where it is unavoidable it follows that the patient should be advised to take long-term prophylaxis.

4   Tropical splenomegaly is a condition in which an abnormal immune response to endemic malaria leads to great enlargement of the spleen. This usually shrinks with long-term antimalarial chemotherapy but, in a few cases, the spleen remains large and splenectomy is indicated to relieve the hypersplenism, portal hypertension or discomfort of the very large spleen.

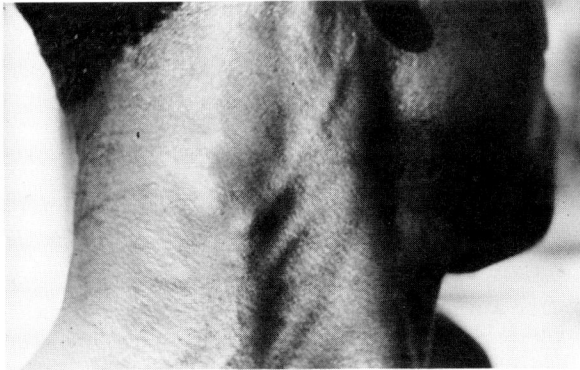

Fig 14.2   Thickened superficial nerves of the cervical plexus in a patient with leprosy. (Photograph by Prof Harold Rodgers.)

Falciparum malaria is the most dangerous of the two species as it presents atypically and may lead to cerebral malaria especially in non-immune patients. Treatment of both is effective and simple once the diagnosis has been made, although chloroquine resistance is becoming a problem in some areas (Hall, 1976).

Amoebiasis

Entamoeba histolytica is another protozoal parasite which is wide-spread in tropical countries and both amoebic colitis and amoebic hepatitis may concern the surgeon.

The symptoms of amoebic dysentery may be indistinguishable from those of ulcerative colitis (British Medical Journal, 1978). In areas where *E. histolytica* is endemic, ulcerative colitis is underdiagnosed while the reverse happens in areas where it is uncommon. The only way in which amoebic colitis can be differentiated from ulcerative colitis is by demonstrating, in the faeces or on rectal biopsy, the presence of the vegetative forms (trophozooites) of *E. histolytica*. Where doubt remains, a course of metronidazole is justified before treating a patient with steroids for ulcerative colitis. Studies in the past two decades make it clear that ulcerative colitis is not a rare disease in the tropics nor is amoebic colitis rare in Western Europe or North America.

Amoebomas are a rare complication of amoebic colitis and have to be differentiated from tumour, granulomatous colitis and ileocaecal tuberculosis. If the patient is excreting active amoebae, the diagnosis is likely although not certain.

Perforation of the colon is an uncommon, but serious, complication of amoebic dysentery in infants and children. Surgical procedures carry a high mortality, as in typhoid perforation, but in patients who are not already moribund the perforated bowel should be exteriorised or resected with a proximal colostomy. Metronidazole is active against both the amoebae and the inevitable Gram negative anaerobic infection.

Amoebic hepatitis is a common complication of amoebic infection. After the initial invasion of the liver, softening soon occurs producing an area of softened necrotic liver with amoebae invading the surrounding tissue. The parasites are in the wall of the abscess, not in the brownish pus. If untreated or unresponsive to treatment, the abscess will usually expand towards the bare area of the liver, penetrate the diaphragm and produce an empyema. Less commonly it may point on the abdominal wall or burst into the peritoneal cavity. The expansion of the abscess towards the diaphragm causes a very typical appearance on a chest radiograph with elevation of the dome of the diaphragm and inflammatory changes in the lower lobe (Fig 14.3).

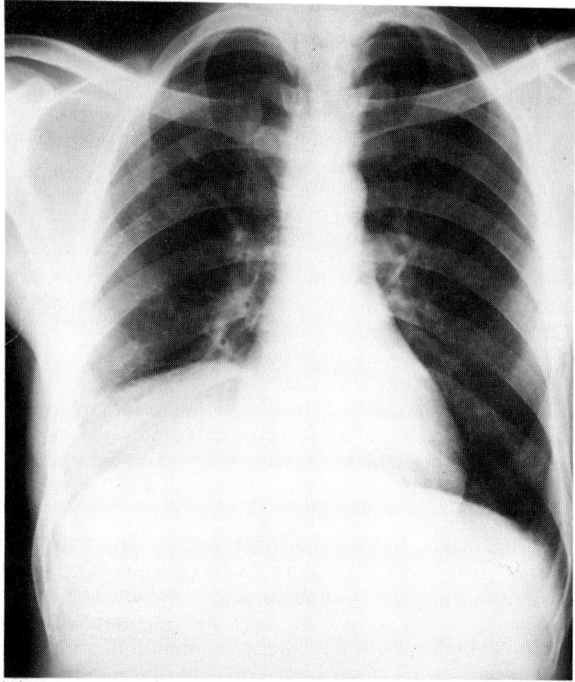

(a)

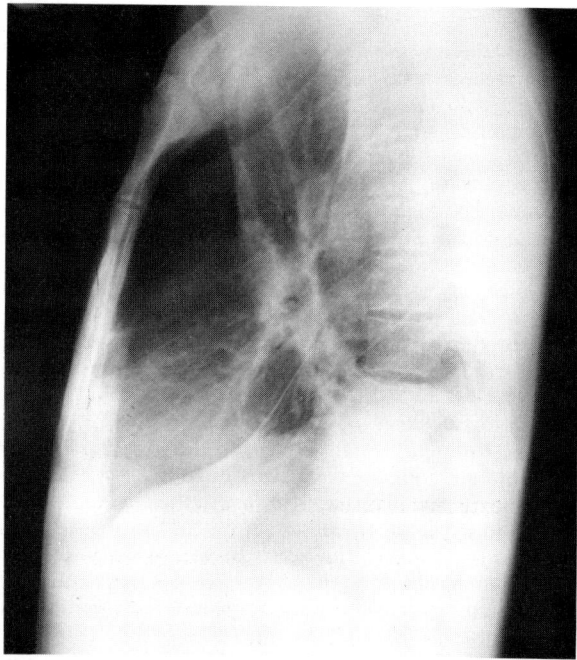

(b)

Fig 14.3a, b Amoebic liver abscess. The chest radiograph shows the peaking of the diaphragm and inflammatory changes in the lower lobe. (Radiograph by Prof Leslie Whittaker, Nairobi.)

Diagnosis is not difficult in endemic areas. The characteristic abdominal tenderness, fever and enlargement of liver is accompanied by leucocytosis and the radiological appearances described above. Aspiration of the abscess will not confirm the diagnosis as no amoebae will be seen although the pus is characteristic. Stool examination is often negative so the diagnosis is clinical. Serological tests may be of assistance if they are available, but take time and are expensive. The cellulose acetate precipitin (CAP) test is probably the best indicator of active disease.

Treatment begins with adequate doses of metronidazole (in adults, 400–600 mg t.d.s. for 5 days) although emetine may occasionally be required. The physical signs may then settle without further treatment. If they persist or if the liver enlargement increases, the abscess should be aspirated on one or several occasions as required. Open drainage has no place in the management of this condition except when a large amoebic empyema has to be drained.

Chagas's disease

This disease is due to chronic infection with *Trypanosoma cruzi*, a protozoal parasite transmitted to man by triatomine bugs. It is widespread in South America extending into Central and even Southern North America. Its surgical importance is that it results in an intestinal neuropathy as a consequence of destruction of ganglia and nerve fibres in the wall of the intestine. It presents as megaoesophagus, megacolon or a pseudo-obstruction due to distension of the small intestine. Local surgical intervention may be required to relieve symptoms.

Schistosomiasis

Schistosomiasis (Symposium, 1978) is the result of infestation with the worms *Schistosoma haematobium*, *S. mansoni* or *S. japonicum*. *S. haematobium* is widespread in Africa, the Middle East and the Islands in the Indian Ocean. *S. mansoni* is more focal in its distribution, but extends from Africa into the Middle East and Central and South America. *S. japonicum* is confined to the Far East. There is evidence of changing prevalence in many areas. In Egypt, for instance, *S. haematobium* is becoming less common and *S. mansoni* much more common.

The worms of *S. haematobium* are found in the pelvic venous plexuses around the bladder. The eggs penetrate the bladder wall to be discharged in the urine to begin its life cycle. The patients present with terminal haematuria or the consequences of the granulomatous reaction in the bladder wall and ureters resulting in dilatation of the upper urinary tract. Only in Egypt has it been convincingly shown to lead to an increase in bladder cancer and this might well be the result of another synergistic factor.

Examination of the deposit after centifugation of the terminal urine will reveal the characteristic ova. Plain radiography of the pelvis may show calcification in the bladder wall while i.v. urography may demonstrate dilatation of the upper urinary tract.

Praziquantel (40 mg/kg single dose) is the drug of choice for treatment of the infection. In children and young adults the changes in bladder and ureters can often be reversed by treatment of the infection, but in older patients it may be necessary to deal with ureteric fibrosis by reimplantation of the ureters or other plastic procedures utilising, if necessary, short loops of small intestine. Reinfestation almost inevitably occurs when the patients return home.

In the mansoni form of the disease the worms, after maturing in the large abdominal veins, migrate to the mesenteric veins especially those draining the colon. The ova penetrate the bowel wall to be shed in the faeces, but some may also be swept by the portal blood flow into the sinusoids of the liver where release of foreign protein results in an immunological reaction leading to the characteristic fibrosis of the portal tracts described as 'pipe stem' fibrosis. The consequence is portal hypertension.

The initial infection with *S. mansoni* may be symptomless, bowel symptoms occurring in only a small proportion of those who are infected. Pseudopolyps may form in the colonic mucosa and episodes of diarrhoea may occur, but it is often difficult to separate these symptoms from those caused by other endemic bowel infections. Intestinal schistosomiasis may, however, cause colonic strictures especially in the rectum and, if these are symptomatic, they may require to be resected. They must be differentiated from carcinoma of bowel, tuberculosis and granulomatous colitis. The diagnosis of mansoni infestation is best made by taking a snip of rectal mucosa, crushing it on a slide, and examining it under a microscope when the ova will be seen in the tissues. Serological tests, the best being of complement fixation or indirect fluorescent antibody, will only confirm exposure to infection.

Japonicum infestation closely resembles that of *S. mansoni*, but is usually more severe and the central nervous system may also be affected by the reaction to ova reaching the systemic circulation.

Cosmopolitan surgical disease

A detailed discussion of cosmopolitan diseases occurring in tropical countries would be irrelevant to this chapter which will only discuss special features of presentation or management of such conditions in tropical countries.

The prevalence of disease is not a static phenomenon. It is likely that the rapid changes in social and economic circumstances that have occurred in the last three decades have produced equally significant changes in the prevalence and diagnosis of certain diseases. So it is that in 1947 hardly any patient with duodenal ulceration was diagnosed amongst Kenyan Africans while in 1970 a prevalence of duodenal dyspepsia equal to that in the United Kingdom could be reported from Nairobi.

Gastrointestinal disease

Peptic ulceration

Duodenal ulceration is common in many tropical countries (Tovey, 1979) and requires a definite policy for treatment in relationship to the conditions under which the people live. The majority of patients do not require surgical treatment. When it is indicated, the choice is between proximal gastric vagotomy and truncal vagotomy with either gastroenterostomy or pyloroplasty. In circumstances where follow-up is unreliable, where recurrent ulcer must be avoided at all costs and where surgical expertise is limited, truncal vagotomy and gastroenterostomy is the best technique to teach.

Ulcerative colitis and Crohn's disease

It is probable that ulcerative colitis occurs in most tropical countries. Where colectomy is indicated, the question arises as to whether ileostomy is tolerable in these special circumstances. A vegetable diet with a high residue results in an ileostomy output of up to one litre a day. Light clothing, hot climate and poor availability of appliances all make the management of an ileostomy more difficult and the cost of appliances may be an intolerable burden. For all these reasons ileorectal anastomosis should be considered as the preferred operation and ileostomy only performed when the rectum is extensively diseased with stricture formation.

Crohn's disease is rare in Africa and probably so in most other tropical countries where tuberculosis is the common granulomatous lesion. Between 1965 and 1972 in Kenyatta National Hospital in Nairobi no cases of Crohn's disease in Africans were seen and the only case seen by the author in this period was an African physician who developed the disease whilst living and working in Europe. Nevertheless, it is very likely that this will be an emerging disease in many countries and its diagnosis must never be discounted.

Intestinal obstruction

In almost all tropical countries intestinal obstruction is the commonest surgical emergency. The three commonest causes of obstruction are volvulus, external hernia and adhesions (Table 1).

Table 1
CAUSES OF INTESTINAL OBSTRUCTION IN GOVERNMENT HOSPITALS IN KENYA (1971–72)

			%
Volvulus		117	35
Sigmoid colon	63		
Large intestine (excluding sigmoid)	6		
Double volvulus of colon	7		
Small intestine	41		
Adhesions		81	25
Strangulated external hernia		61	19
Intussusception		39	12
Roundworms		13	4
Tumours		6	2
Mesenteric thrombosis		5	1.5
Congenital atresia		2	0.5
		324	

Population about 8 000 000.
(From *East Afr. J. Med. Res*; **1**: 265–72. Wambwa, 1974.)

In strangulated volvulus (Rennie, 1979) of the pelvic colon, operation is urgent. Many texts have, in the past, recommended a Paul-Mikulicz resection when the bowel is not viable. This can be dangerous when the blood supply to the distal limb of the double-barrelled colostomy resulting from this resection has been jeopardised by thrombosis of mesenteric vessels (Fig 14.4). It is, therefore, better to perform a formal resection of the infarcted bowel with anastomosis and proximal colostomy or to close the distal limb and fashion the proximal limb as a single colostomy. Later the bowel can be reconstructed.

Small intestinal obstruction by round worms (ascaris) is a relatively common cause of obstruction in children. The diagnosis rests on the demonstration on a plain abdominal radiograph of evidence of small bowel obstruction and of soft tissue shadows of the packed bodies of the worms in the terminal ileum (Fig 14.5); sometimes the masses can even be felt. Operation is seldom necessary, usually i.v. fluids and nasogastric suction will lead to relief of the obstruction and the worms treated later with piperazine citrate. Occasionally, laparotomy is required to milk the worms into the large bowel and sometimes a worm is found to have penetrated the intestinal wall and to be lying in the peritoneal cavity. This is not usually associated with peritonitis and the perforation is often difficult to find.

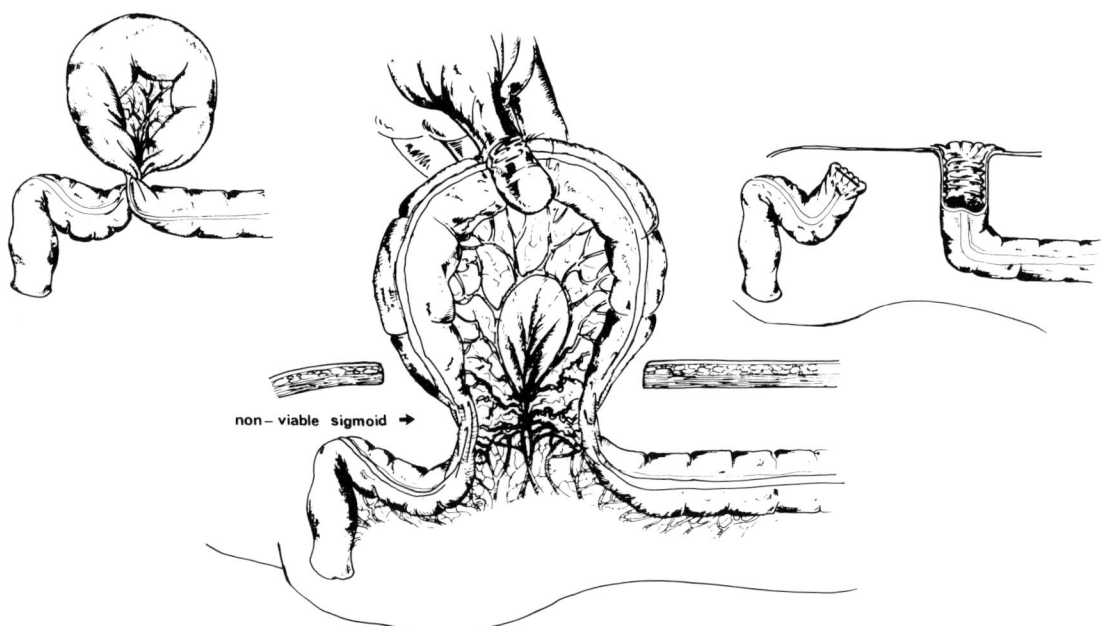

non– viable sigmoid →

Fig 14.4 Strangulated volvulus of the sigmoid colon. The infarction can extend to the recto-sigmoid junction and a Paul-Mikulicz resection may be hazardous. (Prepared by Mr B Ellis, Department of Medical Illustration, Royal Victoria Hospital, Belfast.)

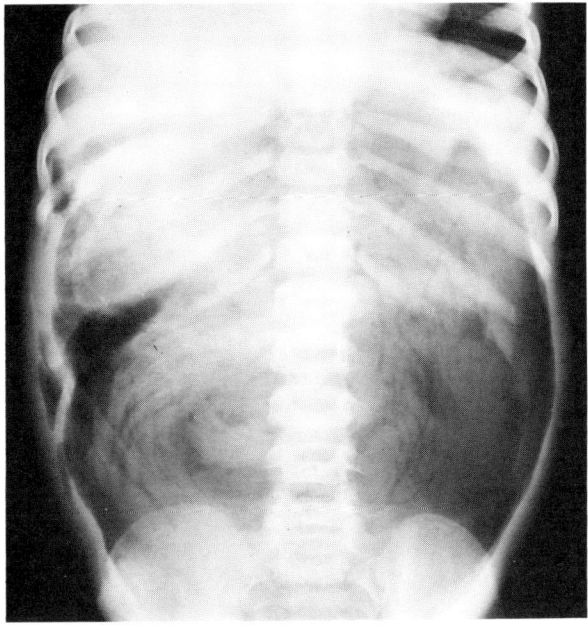

(a)

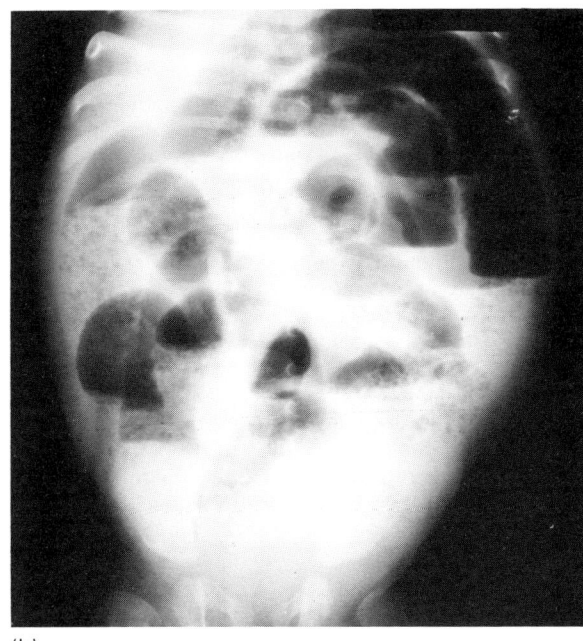

(b)

Fig 14.5 Round worm obstruction. (a) The bodies of the worms can be seen, some as linear areas of translucency and others in cross-section. (b) Complete obstruction with masses of worms seen in cross-section. (Radiographs by Prof Leslie Whittaker, Nairobi.)

Liver, gallbladder and pancreas

Portal hypertension is a common problem in most tropical countries. There are three important causes:

Alcoholic cirrhosis
Schistosomal fibrosis
Primary portal vein thrombosis, usually due to umbilical sepsis in the neonate, but also to spontaneous thrombosis in the course of severe febrile illness like malaria or typhoid fever.

The results of portosystemic shunting in the first two groups are disappointing while the third group are best treated conservatively with the expectation of gradual improvement as the patient grows older.

The acute episodes of bleeding should be controlled by Sengstaken tube or pitressin followed by injection of the varices through a rigid oesophagoscope. The simple technique of oesophageal transection using the SPTU automatic circular stapling 'gun' is likely to have a wide application in developing countries.

Hepatoma and cholangio-carcinoma are both more common in tropical countries. Associated with alcoholic cirrhosis and hepatitis certainly, and possibly related to the ingestion of toxins (aflatoxin) and infestation of the biliary tree with clonorchis sinensis, it is seldom that an opportunity for resection arises.

Infestation with the trematode *Clonorchis sinensis* is most common in South China, but occurs in many areas of the Far East. It leads to a secondary pyogenic cholangitis requiring surgical drainage of the biliary tracts.

Vascular system

Occlusive vascular disease with disease of the vessel wall is seldom seen in the indigenous people of tropical countries. Spontaneous arterial and venous thrombosis has, however, been reported from several centres in Africa. It affects two groups of people. Infants may be born with part or whole of the foot or lower leg already gangrenous. Pulses are normal down to the gangrenous area while histological examination reveals no intrinsic disease of vessel wall. Young women, often pregnant, present with acute ischaemia resulting from occlusion of both arteries and veins of one, or, sometimes more, limbs. Abnormalities of fibrinolysis can be demonstrated in both infants and adults and there may also be an increase in plasma fibrinogen, factor V and factor VIII. No cause has been determined, but the ingestion of herbal remedies has been considered a possibility. When thrombectomy has been attempted recurrence is usual.

Breast

The prevalence of breast cancer varies widely in tropical countries. Some people, for example the Parsis in India, have a high prevalence of the disease probably because of late marriage within a closed community while others, like most African negro people, have a low prevalence. There is an understandable reluctance among many women to have a mastectomy and particularly in communities where evidence of fertility and femininity are important in the family. Therefore, only a proportion of women with breast tumours are, in fact, seen by the conventional health services. In areas where this applies, a policy should be pursued of excising early tumours of breast by segmental resection preserving the nipple and the outline of the breast. Radiotherapy is seldom available but adjuvant therapy with tamoxifen or perioperative cyclophosphamide can be given in both early and late cases. The benefits of such a policy would be to increase the willingness of affected women to come for treatment at an early stage.

Genitourinary system

The surgeon in the tropics must be an expert with urethral sounds. Urethral stricture, which has largely disappeared from temperate countries, remains a major surgical disease in most tropical countries. The cause is, of course, gonococcal infection, but the severity of the stricture is greatly increased by inadequate treatment of the primary urethritis and by unskilled dilatation of early strictures. False passages are common, periurethral abscess leading to multiple perineal sinuses frequent and carcinoma may arise in these sinuses.

Burns

Burnt children are one of the tragedies of the tropics. In hot climates most food is cooked on open fires in simple open bowls and pans. Some tropical countries are cold for part of the year and open fires are set in the middle of the hut. Children fall into these fires or pull bowls of hot water or food over themselves. They sustain burns which may not be treated immediately, become infected and lead to terrible contractures and deformities. There is an urgent need to provide early treatment for all burnt children by doctors or auxiliaries skilled in managing the initial fluid problems and in performing simple split skin grafting at an early stage.

As a result of both burns and lacerations severe keloid formation is seen in Negroid races. True keloid must be differentiated from hypertrophic scars which are usually hyperaemic and tender and will regress over a period of 6 months to 1 year. It is only if the raised thickened tissue persists beyond this time that it can be classified as a true keloid. The problem of treating keloids has still not been solved. Excision of the keloid may be followed either by injection of hydrocortisone into the scar or a single dose of soft x-rays if available.

Hydatid disease

This is a cosmopolitan disease which is now largely confined to tropical countries where sheep are associated with dogs. Jackals may also act as hosts to this parasite. Examples of countries with a high incidence of hydatid disease are the northern areas of Kenya amongst nomadic tribes and many areas in the Middle East. This disease is preventable either by separating the dog (the primary host) from the infected offal of sheep or by separating infested dogs from close human contact, the sheep and man being the intermediate hosts.

The eggs are ingested, hatch into larvae and penetrate the bowel wall to enter the portal system. About 50% of the cysts which develop from the larvae will form in the liver (Fig 14.6), 30% in the lungs and the rest in other parts of the body including the central nervous system. If they die they usually calcify and can be left alone, but they usually grow to cause symptoms by pressure or, in the abdomen, may rupture with widespread dissemination of cysts often leading to the death of the patient. In the lung the cyst may rupture into a bronchus and the contents be coughed up.

The cysts stimulate an immunological reaction which may be used for serological diagnostic tests none of which is very accurate, but the complement fixation test becomes negative with cure of the disease and so can be used to assess treatment. Rupture of a cyst may provoke a severe immunological reaction causing death and this may also happen during operation on a cyst. It is therefore wise to give hydrocortisone by injection 12 h before, during and for a day after any surgical procedure.

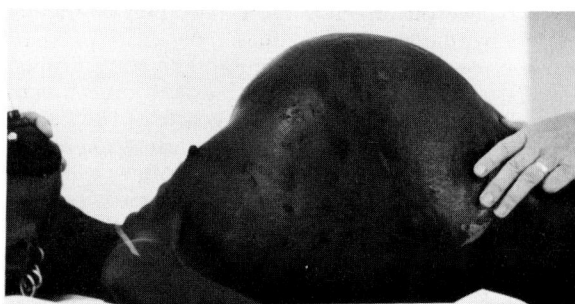

Fig 14.6 A large hepatic hydatid in an adolescent girl from Northern Kenya.

The cysts must be removed without disseminating daughter cysts or scolices from the inner lining of germinal epithelium. In order to kill these elements, it is usual to inject a scolicidal fluid into the cyst before mobilising it. There is no general agreement on which fluid is best and a choice between diluted formalin, hypertonic saline and cetrimide solution should be made. Sufficient should be injected, after aspiration of cyst fluid, to achieve a reasonable concentration and should be left for 5 min. Mobilisation of chitinous layer from the capsule formed by the host is usually easy unless the cyst is infected.

In the liver, the large cavity remaining should be drained if it is infected and any fistulae into bile ducts should be closed. If the cavity is not infected, it should be filled with normal saline and closed, a drain being inserted down to the line of closure; with this technique primary healing is usual. In the lung, the cyst can usually be enucleated if intact. If it is infected or communicates with a bronchus, a segmental resection may be necessary.

Recently studies have been undertaken to assess whether these cysts can be treated with mebendazole alone. Preliminary studies are encouraging in selected cases.

Tetanus

Tetanus assumes a particular importance in tropical countries as few people are immunised in childhood, many soils are heavily infected and injury to exposed limbs frequent. When it occurs adequate facilities for treatment are often not available. Quite trivial injury can lead to severe tetanus; indeed, in areas of heavy soil contamination cases can occur as a result of infestation of the feet with Chigoe flea (jiggers). Even the most trivial injuries must, therefore, be followed by adequate prophylaxis against tetanus. A special form is neonatal tetanus, the result of the application of cow dung to the umbilicus of the new-born child. The mortality rate is very high and yet could be totally prevented by the active immunisation of all pregnant women.

Specifically tropical diseases

There are probably no diseases that are entirely confined to tropical countries, all can be exported to any part of the world by air travel. They are the diseases that rarely appear spontaneously except in a tropical climate or cannot be transmitted except in tropical countries.

Tropical ulcer

The organisms that have been isolated from these ulcers are ubiquitous. They are *Fusiform fusiformis* and *Borrelia vincenti*, common commensals in the mouth and yet in the tissues capable of producing a fulminating cellulitis. Tropical ulcers are almost always on the lateral aspect of the ankle and leg and probably the consequence of trauma, from grasses and thorns, on the legs of those who walk barefoot along tracks between villages. They are prevented by wearing long trousers and simple shoes. The organisms may be passed from person to person on infected thorns or derive from saliva applied to superficial abrasions. The consequent cellulitis is severe and leads to ulceration. What is not clear is why the ulcer often does not heal and becomes chronic. They may persist for months or years and undergo malignant transformation. This is often preceded by healing of the ulcer with a depigmented scar and when it breaks down again the whole ulcer is malignant. It is essential, therefore always to biopsy a chronic ulcer before treatment.

In the acute phase of the ulcer (the first 4 weeks or so) healing can be achieved with a 10-day course of penicillin. Chronic ulcers should be excised and the resulting defect covered with split skin grafts. If malignant, it may be possible to perform a wide local excision if the bone is not involved. If it is, then amputation will be required.

Buruli ulcer

Although named after a district in Uganda where it is common and where it was first described by Sir Albert Cook, it was in Australia that it was first shown to be due to an infection of the superficial tissues, usually of the limbs, with *Mycobacterium ulcerans* (British Medical Journal, 1970). It has been reported from many other tropical countries in Africa, South and Central America, Malaysia and the South Pacific. The organism is closely related to tuberculosis and is characterised by having 35°C as its optimum temperature for growth. This probably explains why deep invasion is not seen, the lesion always lying superficial to the deep fascia. The infection spreads in the superficial fascia undermining the skin to produce an indolent ulcer, lined with pale granulation tissue and extending far beyond the apparent limits of the ulcer (Fig 14.7). There is a tendency to spontaneous healing, but they often extend to become very large. They are usually painless.

Early lesions detected when small and before they ulcerate can be excised and sutured, but larger, ulcerated lesions require wide excision of the diseased subcutaneous tissue down to the deep fascia followed by grafting. Some of the undermined skin can be used as a

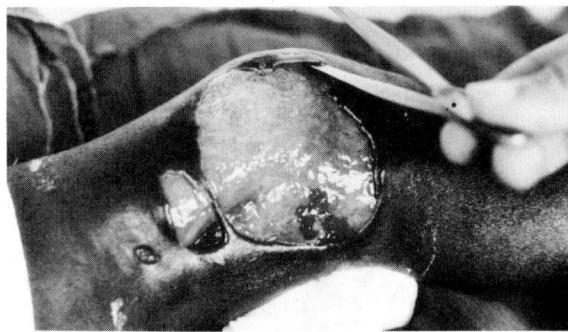

Fig 14.7 Buruli ulcer showing the undermined skin and pale granular base.

free graft providing the edges adjacent to the ulcer are discarded and the deep surface is denuded of all subcutaneous tissue. Rifampicin is of value to supplement surgical excision.

Ainhum

This is a curious condition which can be regarded as a deep narrow ulcer which encircles the fifth toe and ultimately amputates it. It is usually very painful, often bilateral and no one has suggested any good reason for its occurrence. It is not very common, affects only people who walk barefooted for part of the day at least and has been reported from all parts of the tropical world in both black and white people. The indication for treatment is pain and the best procedure is amputation of the affected toe.

Tropical myositis

This is predominantly a disease of children and young males with wide distribution throughout the tropics (Taylor and Henderson, 1972). It is probable that the initial muscle lesion is viral in origin leading to necrosis which is invaded by *Staphyloccocus aureus* to produce typical pyogenic abscesses. These may be multiple and affect any muscle in the body. The diagnosis is easy if it affects a large muscle mass such as quadriceps femoris. If, however, it affects a muscle near the joint in a child, it must be differentiated from osteomyelitis or septic arthritis. If it affects a visceral muscle like the diaphragm, it must be distinguished from an empyema or a subphrenic abscess. The iliopsoas is not uncommonly affected and so are the intercostal muscles. The toxaemia may be severe and lead to renal damage, myocarditis, endocarditis or pericarditis.

Abscesses should be drained adequately. Most of the organisms are sensitive to penicillin which may be combined with cotrimoxazole if antibiotic sensitivities cannot be quickly obtained. Cloxacillin or tetracycline are suitable alternatives. This is a serious infection requiring prompt treatment; the patients are often anaemic and may require blood transfusion.

Deep mycosis

Although surgical procedures play only a small part in the treatment of these conditions some of them are usually referred for surgical care and the most important of these will be considered (Mahgoub, 1977). The terminology in this field is bewildering. It is littered with neologisms and complex arguments about the naming of individual fungi. For simplicity two groups will be considered, phycomycosis and mycetoma.

Subcutaneous phycomycosis

This is caused by the organism *Basidiobolus haptosporus* which is widespread in soil and the faeces of reptiles. It is a disease of hot arid countries where the people are usually nomadic. Subcutaneous tissues of body or limbs are affected producing a woody induration which spreads slowly, raising the skin which rarely becomes ulcerated. Although usually confined to a well-defined area, in some cases venous invasion occurs with a dissemination of the infection leading to death of the patient.

The diagnosis can be made from the typical appearance and can be confirmed by biopsy and culture of the organism. Treatment is not yet clearly defined. Potassium iodide has traditionally been regarded as of therapeutic value and, more recently, cotrimoxazole. A related fungus, entomophthora coronata, causes a similar lesion affecting nasal sinuses and the tissues around the nose which must be differentiated from tumours of the paranasal sinuses.

Mycetoma

These lesions, which occur predominantly in the feet of peasant cultivators and pastoral people in tropical and subtropical countries, may affect any of the superficial tissues (Lancet, 1977). They are due to the penetration of the skin by either of two groups of organisms, aerobic actinomycetes (*actinomycetoma*) or fungi (*eumycetoma*). Penetration is a result of trauma and the agents are widespread in the soil. There is a distinct geographical distribution for each organism, so that in any given area there will be a predominant organism and the diagnosis can often be made without laboratory facilities. The distribution of organisms probably depends on rainfall and vegetation. The lesions consist of a chronic granulomatous invasion of subcutaneous tissues with small abscesses and sinus formation (Fig 14.8). They are progressive and bone is sooner or later involved. Tendons, muscles and nerves resist invasion and continue to function. Pain is not usually severe. The condition is slowly progressive with no tendency to spontaneous resolution and disability slowly progresses. Nevertheless, it is often possible for a patient to continue to use the limb for many years after the onset of the disease and amputation, if necessary, can be delayed until disability warrants it. Dissemination of the infection does not occur.

Each infection produces characteristic granules in the thin pus discharged from the sinuses. The fungi produce grains that are black, brown, white or yellow while the actinomycetes those that are red, white or yellow. The granules are aggregates of the organisms and can be stained, examined and cultured to identify the precise organism involved.

The best therapy is probably a combination of streptomycin, 1 g daily for one month and then on alternate days plus either diamino-diphenyl sulphone 100 mg twice daily or cotrimoxazole, two tablets twice daily; sulphadoxine/pyrimethamine and rifampicin are more expensive, but effective, if the lesions do not respond to the streptomycin combinations. These drugs cured 60% of patients, controlled the disease in others and only failed in about 5% of cases. Treatment extended over 4–24 months.

In the eumycetoma, it is possible to cure the condition if the disease is still confined to superficial tissues, by excision and grafting. Once the bone has become involved cure is not possible. Amputation should be delayed until disability warrants it, a peasant cultivator is gravely disadvantaged by amputation and should retain his diseased limb as long as he can.

Filariasis and lymphoedema

Chronic lymphoedema of the legs and scrotum is quite a common condition throughout the tropics. It is usually regarded as being due to filariasis (due either to *Wucheria bancrofti* or *Brugia malayi*) but it also occurs in areas not affected by these parasitic worms which are transmitted by mosquitos. In people who go barefoot, repeated trauma to the feet and ankles followed by sepsis can lead to fibrosis of the lymphatics, gradually progressive over the years, until a permanent state of chronic lymphoedema is produced. In addition to the thickening of subcutaneous tissues, hypertrophic changes in the skin produce an appearance well described as 'mossy' feet. Whether the cause is filariasis or chronic sepsis, the appearances are similar.

The diagnosis of filariasis is made by examining peripheral blood taken at night when the micro filaria appear in superficial vessels (presumably so that they can colonise biting mosquitoes to continue their life cycle). The filaria can often also be demonstrated in the fluid from hydroceles. It can be treated effectively with diethylcarbamazine, but reinfestation is common.

The surgical problem is the same whatever the cause. In the early cases control of oedema by elastic bandaging is possible; in the late cases only an excision of the subcutaneous tissues with the replacement of skin as a full thickness graft is of any value. When the scrotum is predominantly affected, the simple procedure of excising the excess scrotal skin and subcutaneous tissue is effective. In most rural tropical areas both forms of treatment for the legs are difficult to apply to the large number of cases that occur and prevention must be the hope for the future.

Guinea worm

The tropical world is prodigal with its parasites and one of the strangest is the Guinea worm (*Dracunculus medinensis*). It is widespread except in the Far East. The adult female may be up to a metre long living in the superficial tissues of man. In response to cooling, the worm penetrates the skin discharging eggs into water; there the larva invade a water flea (cyclops). When man swallows the flea in water the mature larvae penetrate the wall of the intestine to complete the cycle.

The penetration of the skin may lead to a local cellulitis due to secondary infection especially if the worm dies before being extruded or is broken whilst being extracted. Tetanus may also be a complication (similar to the Chigoe flea).

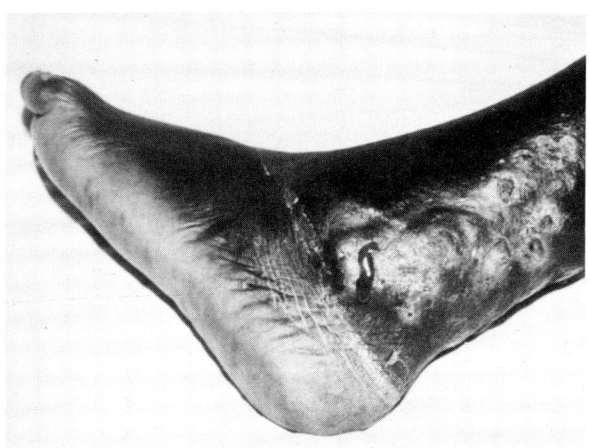

Fig 14.8 Mycetoma of foot showing an early lesion with sinus formation. *Note* its resemblance to early Kaposi's sarcoma (Fig 14.14).

The worms can be killed by diethylcarbamazine while those that have penetrated the skin can be removed by winding them carefully on to an orange stick. Prophylaxis for tetanus is essential.

Conditions of local importance

There are many very localised specific conditions, often quite disabling, of which a surgeon working in the tropics must be aware. He learns of them from his colleagues, who will usually have devised a simple treatment. Two examples will suffice to illustrate this.

Kikuyu bursa

The Kikuyu people of central Kenya live in a mountainous land. Women, who carry all the heavy loads, do so by means of a strap round the forehead supporting a load on the lower lumbar and sacral areas. Older women often develop a large chronic bursa in this area which the newcomer may mistake for a lipoma or soft tissue tumour. Excision is not acceptable as they then have a painful scar which precludes the carrying of loads. Instead the bursa should be padded to protect it from further trauma.

Tumoral calcinosis

This condition produces calcified swellings round the shoulder and hip girdles in the subcutaneous tissues usually in young people (Fig 14.9). The swellings contain radio-opaque, chalky material and are not the result of any known parasite nor are they new growths. They grow to a large size and may ulcerate. Excision is not followed by recurrence.

Bites (animal and snake)

In some rural hospitals the commonest cause of trauma is animal bites. For example, at Mandera in Northern Kenya a few years ago crocodile bites were far more common than road traffic accidents. All animal bites produce typical lacerated wounds, sometimes with fractures as well. Their treatment is no different from that of any other wound and delayed primary suture should always be employed as they are all heavily infected.

Snake bite is only marginally a surgical problem, although all surgeons should know the poisonous snakes present in their area that are likely to bite human beings and the correct treatment for each (Reid,

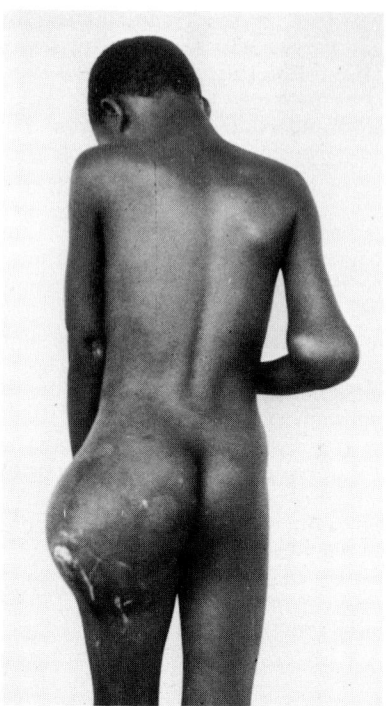

Fig 14.9 A 12-year-old girl with tumoral calcinosis over her left hip and right elbow.

1970). It is essential to remember that venom is injected in less than half the cases of snake bite and treatment with antivenom is indicated only when there is clear evidence that venom *has* been injected. It is sound management to wait until signs of envenomation appear before giving antivenom. 'The bite of a poisonous snake is *not* synonymous with snake bite poisoning' (Reid, 1970).

The surgeon is particularly concerned with viperine and some cobra bites in which the venom has a local cytotoxic effect producing a severe local reaction which may proceed to tissue necrosis (Fig 14.10). If, as is usual, it is a limb that is bitten it should be immobilised, the bite cleansed with soap and water or other mild antiseptic and either a venous tourniquet applied or, more safely, a firm crepe or elastic bandage applied to the limb to restrict venous and lymphatic flow in the superficial tissues. Local injection of antivenom is not of value, but systemic antivenom must be given if there is clear evidence of envenomation.

If necrosis occurs, a wide excision should be undertaken followed by split skin grafting. Tendons, muscles and nerves are not affected unless by secondary infection and can usually be preserved. Prophylaxis for tetanus should always be instituted.

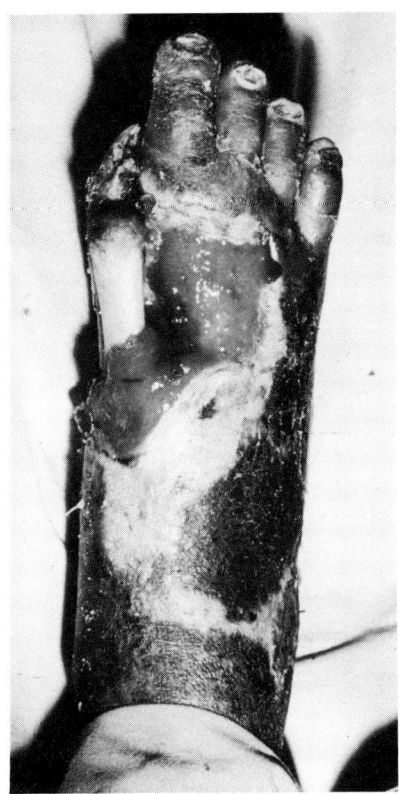

Fig 14.10 Bite by a puff adder with wide necrosis of superficial tissues exposing metacarpals.

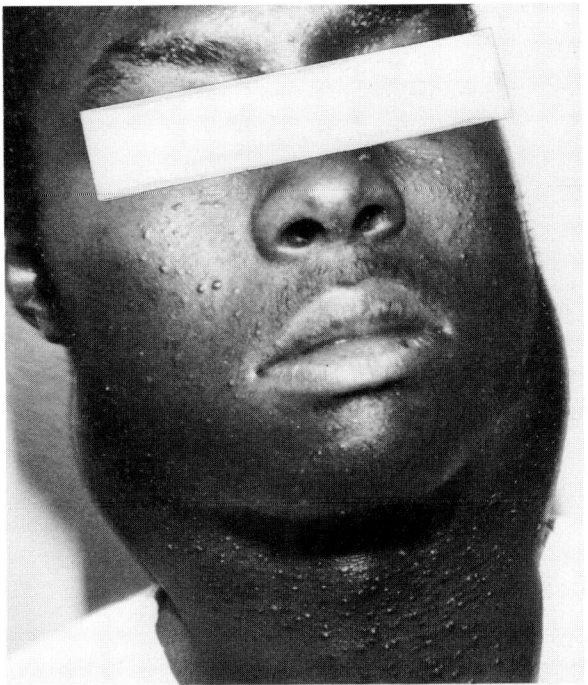

Fig 14.11 Bilateral enlargement of cervical lymph glands secondary to nasopharangeal carcinoma.

Some particular tumours

Nasopharyngeal tumours (Postnasal space tumours)

These are common in many tropical and subtropical countries. Areas of high prevalence include East and Central Africa, Southern China and in the Chinese population of south-east Asia. It is a terrible tumour rapidly involving the base of the skull to produce cranial nerve palsies and metastasising to the cervical glands at an early stage (Fig 14.11), often before the primary is apparent. Surgery plays no part in the management of the primary lesion except for biopsy. Secondary deposits in the cervical lymph glands enter into the differential diagnosis of lymphadenopathy in countries where tuberculosis is also common. These tumours are commonest from the end of the second decade onwards, an age at which tuberculous lymphadenopathy is becoming less common.

Treatment is most unsatisfactory. Radiotherapy can produce dramatic remission of symptoms, but recurrence is the rule. Cytotoxic drugs, in various combinations, have produced only short-term remission in a proportion of cases.

Burkitt's lymphoma

This tumour is particularly associated with Africa, but occurs in all tropical countries where malaria is endemic and sporadically in temperate countries. There is an extensive literature concerning its aetiology with the present consensus seeming to be that it arises in response to infection by the Epstein-Barr virus in susceptible children who have been immunosuppressed by endemic malaria. The commonest site for the tumour is the mandible or maxilla, but extra facial tumours are common either as apparent primaries or as secondary deposits (Figs 14.12 and 14.13). These may occur in bones, central nervous system or abdominal viscera where they become the concern of the surgeon. Burkitt originally suggested that cyclophosphamide alone is the drug of choice and, although many combination regimes have been tried, it still produces results comparable with them. Ziegler recommends six doses of cyclophosphamide, 40 mg/kg i.v.,

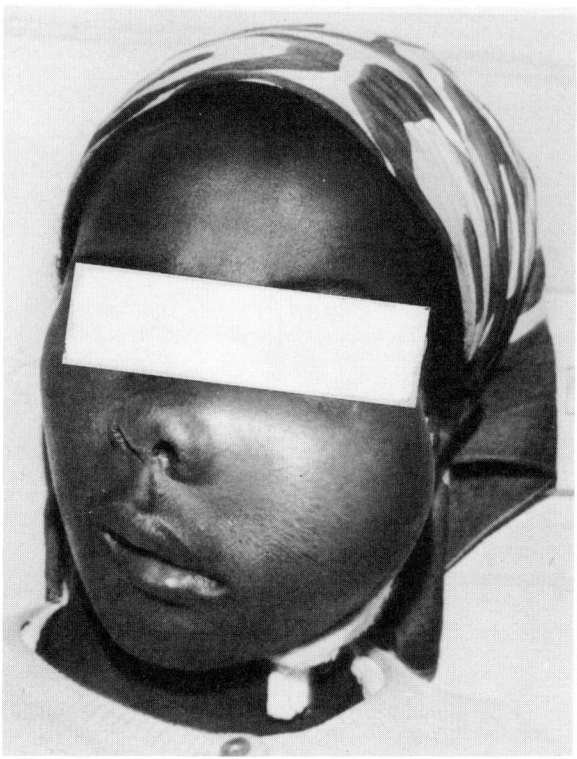

Fig 14.12 Burkitt's lymphoma in a 14-year-old girl.

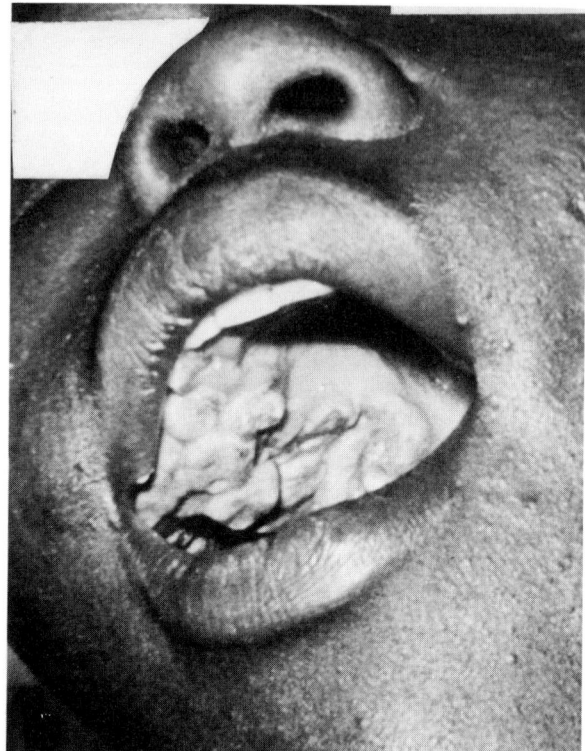

Fig 14.13 Burkitt's lymphoma in a 12-year-old boy show-ing the characteristic displacement of teeth by the expanding maxillary tumour.

every 2–3 weeks with intrathecal methotrexate for overt central nervous system disease.

With facial tumours alone (stage A) a high remission rate (60% at a year) can be achieved, but when abdominal tumour is present this may fall to 10%. The abdominal organs most often affected are the ovaries in girls and kidneys in both sexes. The initial presentation may be with an abdominal tumour the diagnosis only being made at operation. Magrath and his colleagues (1974), in a small series, show that removal of as much abdominal tumour as possible can improve the remission rate close to that for the stage A cases (Ziegler *et al.*, 1979).

When taking a biopsy of a suspected tumour an 'imprint' preparation should always be made; that is, the tissue should be firmly pressed on to a clean glass slide and the imprinted material allowed to dry on the slide before staining. The imprint preparation facilitates the identification of the typical lymphoid cells.

Kaposi's sarcoma

This tumour probably arises from vaso-formative cells, has a predilection for males rather than females and is a particularly African tumour although it has been reported from all parts of the world. It produces a very characteristic subcutaneous tumour on legs and arms which coalesce and later ulcerate. It may also cause lymphoedema. The nodular form must be differentiated from pyogenic granuloma, leprosy, multiple angiomata and the early lesions of mycetoma (Fig 14.14).

In adults, it is usually slow progressive over many years, ultimately invading the regional lymph glands and finally the intestinal wall causing severe intestinal haemorrhage. In children, the phase of peripheral nodules often does not occur, the child presenting first with lymphadenopathy and soon after with the intestinal lesions, death following within a year.

Surgery has little to offer apart from biopsy to confirm the diagnosis, and occasionally the amputation of a useless limb may be indicated. Extended field radiotherapy will usually cause remission of disease, but whether it extends survival is not known. Several cytotoxic drugs, singly or in combination, have been shown to control local disease in a similar way.

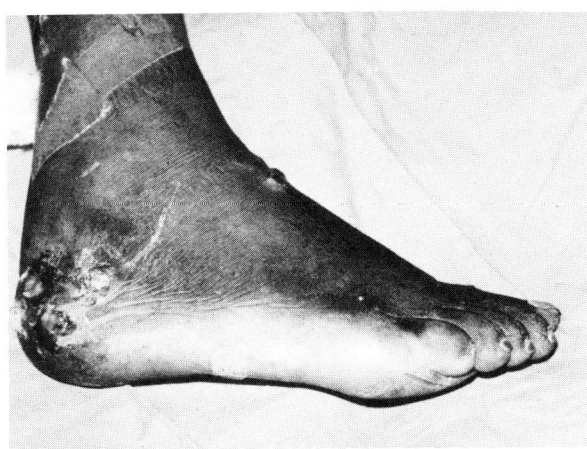

Fig 14.14 Kaposi's sarcoma. Early nodules closely resembling the early lesions of mycetoma. There are no sinuses.

Melanoma and other skin tumours

Melanoma is not uncommon in dark skinned races occurring, when it does, on the soles of the feet which are the least pigmented part of the body. Skin pigmentation protects strongly against skin tumours due to sunlight. Albinos, therefore, in tropical countries are at a grave disadvantage and unless they protect themselves with wide brimmed hats, long trousers and sleeves, are certain to develop multiple skin tumours at an early age.

Conclusion

Surgery in tropical countries requires flexibility both in clinical management and in operative techniques.

The principles of care, however, remain the same and the challenge for the future is to provide simple, efficient surgical care available to all who need it.

References

Browne S.G. (1968). Leprosy. *Brit. Med. J*; **3**:725–37.
British Medical Journal (1970). Buruli ulcer (editorial). *Brit. Med J*; **2**:378–9.
British Medical Journal (1976). Transfusion malaria in developing countries (editorial). *Brit. Med. J*; **1**:542.
British Medical Journal (1978). Misdiagnosis of amoebiasis (editorial). *Brit. Med. J*; **2**:379–80.
Brzica J., Pineda A.A., Haswell H.F. (1976). Autologous blood transfusion. *Mayo Clin. Proc*; **51**:723–37.
Hall A.P. (1976). The treatment of malaria. *Brit. Med. J*; **1**:323–8.
Lancet (1977). Treatment of mycetoma (editorial). *Lancet*; **ii**:23–4.
Magrath I.T., Lwanga S., Carswell W., Harrison N. (1974). Surgical reduction of tumour bulk in management of abdominal Burkitt's lymphoma. *Brit. Med. J*; **2**:308–12.
Mahgoub E.S. (1977). Mycosis of the Sudan. *Trans. Roy. Soc. Trop. Med. Hyg*; **71**:184–8.
Pujari B.D. (1979). Modified surgical procedures in intestinal tuberculosis. *Brit. J. Surg*; **66**:180-1.
Reid H.A. (1970). The principles of snake bite treatment. *Clin. Toxicol*; **3(3)**:473–82.
Rennie J.A. (1979). Sigmoid volvulus. *Roy. Soc. Med*; **72**:654–6.
Stoll H. (1978). The treatment of tuberculosis in developing countries. *Trans. Roy. Soc. Trop. Med. Hyg*; **72**:564–9.
Symposium on Schistosomiasis (1978). *Trop. Doct*; **8**:3–24.
Taylor J.F., Henderson B.F. (1972). Tropical myositis. In *Medicine in a Tropical Environment* (Shaper A.G., Kibukamusoki J.W., Hutt M.S.R., eds.) pp. 33–44. London: British Medical Association.
Tovey F.I. (1979). Peptic ulcer in India and Bangladesh. *Gut*; **20**:329–47.
Welch T.P., Martin N.C. (1975). Surgical treatment of typhoid perforation. *Lancet*; **i**:1078–80.
Ziegler J.L., Magrath I.T., Olweny C.L.M. (1979). Cure of Burkitt's lymphoma: ten-year follow-up of 157 Ugandan patients. *Lancet*; **ii**:936–8.

Urogenital tract and transplantation

Introduction

The inclusion of a section on urological surgery in surgical practice is entirely in keeping with the current trend for the development of urology as a specialty. Nowadays, almost all surgeons develop their particular interests as reflected by the authors of the various chapters in this book. However, not only must surgeons learn their surgery in general, but they must retain a basic knowledge of related surgical topics for, according to circumstance, they will surely need this knowledge from time to time.

The non-endoscopic part of urological surgery has a surgical practice and expertise that employs many standard surgical techniques, instruments and often involves the same anatomical areas. For example, both the general surgeon and the urologist have good reasons for exploring the retroperitoneal space, dissecting in the pelvis or operating through a loin incision. Thus surgical knowledge can never be, nor should be, wholly compartmentalised even although surgical practice often appears today to be evolving towards this.

In this section on urology, the introductory chapters are substantial contributions on the methods and range of the investigation of the urinary tract. Subsequent chapters cover the current approach to surgical problems and the generally accepted procedures recommended by most British-trained urologists. Sometimes the management recommended may not mention known alternatives, but there are very few decisions in surgery, or indeed medicine, which cannot be debated. Many of these debates, however, are not helpful to the practising surgeon and urologist, so they have been omitted.

More relevant to the general surgeon is to know the correct sequence for the initial diagnosis and investigation of a urological problem, so that the patient is not left without a 'plan of action'. Equally relevant is to know how to set about the initial management of a urological complication in a general surgical patient just as the urologist must know how to approach the surgical complications in urological cases. Once these initial steps have been resolved, there is time to assess the next step, either with or without the assistance of a colleague.

Some chapters in this section are undeniably in the realms of surgical super-specialisation. The problems of the infertile couple are now an important part of urological practice and reflect a major change in social attitudes in the past ten years. Organ transplantation has likewise expanded as a major commitment in most surgical centres. The emphasis on renal transplantation in Chapter 27 reflects the fact that this now plays a regular part in the management of patients with end stage renal failure. Transplantation of the heart, liver and pancreas have also made substantial progress within the past decade, but detailed reference to these has been omitted and the interested reader should follow their progress in current medical journals. Finally, the chapters on obstruction, malignancy and trauma closely reflect the problems of the aged and of trauma which are the sources of so much modern surgery.

G.D.C.

Urogenital tract and transplantation

15

Assessment of renal function

C.S. OGG

The kidneys play a crucial role in the excretion of non-volatile products of metabolism, the regulation of the volume and composition of the 'milieu intérieur', and in the production and metabolism of several hormones. In health, these functions provide the patient with a wide margin of protection from a variety of insults but, in disease, gross metabolic disturbances can arise very quickly and it is vitally important that the surgeon be aware of any defects that may exist.

Fortunately for the clinician, most facets of renal function usually decline in parallel and it is possible to gain a great deal of information by studying only one aspect – that of excretion. This means that, for most clinical purposes, tests of renal function are surprisingly simple.

Tests of excretory function

Blood concentrations

Urea is quantitatively the most important end product of protein metabolism and it is hardly surprising that it may accumulate in the body of patients with renal disease. Furthermore, its concentration can be measured quickly and accurately and this measurement is widely used, its level depending on a balance between production and excretion; in turn, production depends on protein intake and on the balance between protein anabolism and catabolism, while excretion

depends on the combination of glomerular filtration and tubular function. At normal levels of renal function and hydration, urea levels do not begin to rise until renal function has been reduced to about half of the normal level, so that a normal blood level does not exclude the presence of substantial renal damage (Fig 15.1).

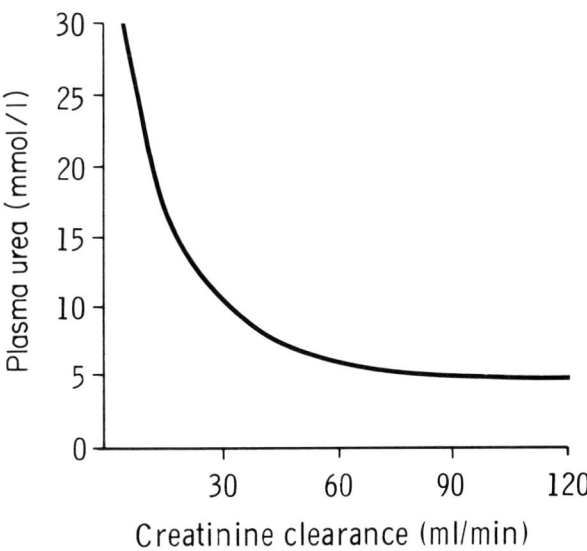

Fig 15.1 The relationship between plasma urea concentration and creatinine clearance.

Creatinine production is fairly constant in an individual, being related to his muscle mass, although a large meal of cooked meat (goulash!) may increase blood levels significantly. Excretion is largely by glomerular filtration although a small proportion is also secreted in the renal tubules. Again, accurate measurement is readily automated and there is much to be said for abandoning the routine measurement of blood levels of urea in favour of those of creatinine. Largely because of its dependence on muscle mass, the plasma creatinine level is higher in men than in women and in adults than in children, who may have plasma levels that are low enough to cause problems of measurement in many laboratories. Nevertheless, the problems of urine collection and clearance measurement (*see below*) in young children are such that considerable effort has been paid to the derivation of tables correlating creatinine levels and glomerular filtration rates in patients of differing sizes (Kampmann *et al.*, 1974).

Clearance measurements

The valuable concept of clearance was introduced to renal physiology 60 years ago. It represents the notional volume of blood that would have had to have been cleared of a substance to account for the amount that appears in the urine during a certain time. It is described by the simple formula:

$$\frac{U \times V}{P}$$

where U and P are the concentrations of the substance in urine and plasma respectively whilst V is the rate of urine flow. Clearance measurements are useful in that they are not influenced by variations in production of the test substance (unless there are gross variations in plasma concentration during the study) and are altered only by changes in excretion.

Measurement of urea clearance is no longer in clinical use since the quantity of urea reabsorbed by the tubules depends critically on urine flow rate – something which is more often affected by hydration than by renal function. However, creatinine clearance is a much more stable measurement and is one of the most useful renal function tests (normal range 80–120 ml/min).

An important practical problem concerns the difficulty of obtaining accurate timed urine collections. The use of 24-h collection periods has the advantage of minimising errors due to incompleteness of bladder emptying and minor mistakes with timing, but greatly increases the chances of incomplete urine saves. Many units rely instead on a series of short (2–4 h) consecutive collection periods and express the final result as an average of 2 or 3 clearances. Problems are, of course, magnified in small children in whom clearance calculations can be based on consecutive urine samples provided that the time at which micturition occurs is observed and complete collection is achieved.

Glomerular filtration rate (GFR) may be determined as the clearance of a substance which passes freely through the glomerular filter (i.e. has a relatively small molecule and is not protein bound) and which is neither reabsorbed nor secreted by the tubules. Since only a small proportion of the creatinine in plasma is protein bound and little is secreted in the tubules, creatinine clearance usually approximates fairly closely to GFR. However, under certain circumstances the approximation breaks down and GFR can then only be measured as the clearance of an exogenous substance which satisfies the above criteria. Conventionally, inulin is used as the standard against which potential agents are judged. It is infused intravenously to produce a constant plasma level, but problems arise because the infusion technique is cumbersome, collection periods are necessarily short (implying a need for bladder catheterisation) and chemical measurement is tedious. The method is, therefore, unsuitable for routine clinical use.

More recently it has been appreciated that GFR can be calculated from the concentration/time plot obtained 2 to 6 h after an i.v. injection of a bolus of a labelled substance that is handled by the kidney in the appropriate manner and is neither metabolised nor excreted by any other oute. Suitable agents include ethylene-diamine-tetra-acetic acid (EDTA) labelled with ^{51}Cr and sodium iodothalamate labelled with radio-iodine. The correlation with inulin clearance obtained using classical techniques is extremely good except in patients who are grossly oedematous. Three blood samples must be taken, but urine need not be collected and in many renal units this has now become the standard method of determining GFR.

Finally, GFR can also be measured by infusing any of the above agents at a constant rate until a contant blood level is achieved. At this point the rate of infusion must match the rate of excretion (i.e. $U \times V$) and all that is required is a determination of the plasma concentration (P). Whatever clearance technique is used, the result must be expressed in a form that takes account of the size of the patient. This is usually achieved by multiplying the result by a factor of 1.73 (the surface area in square metres of an 'average' man) divided by the patient's body surface area (expressed in square metres and obtained from a nomogram).

Tests of tubular function

Many of the tests that appear in physiological texts have either no relevance to the practising clinician or only a very limited role in the study of specific diseases. Thus glucose threshold will seldom need to be determined by any method more precise than that associated with the routine glucose tolerance test. Tubular phosphate reabsorption, urinary acidification and excretion of amino acids may need to be assessed in patients with renal stones and in the investigation of small children with some of the rarer defects in tubular function.

Measurements of renal plasma flow (normal 600 ml/min approximately) are hallowed in tradition, but are seldom used clinically. The classical technique involves measurement of the clearance of para amino hippuric acid (PAH), a substance which is filtered by the glomerulus and secreted by the tubules, so that, at low concentrations, plasma is almost completely cleared by a single passage through the kidney. Again the method is cumbersome and is not always reliable since clearance may be incomplete. On the rare occasions that absolute measurements of renal blood flow are clinically necessary, it is now more usual to use invasive techniques involving dye dilution, thermodilution or electromagnetic flow meters. It is much simpler, and usually more useful, to compare the perfusion of a kidney with either the opposite kidney or a neighbouring artery. This is usually achieved using isotopic methods, the most valuable of which involves the i.v. injection of a single bolus of diethylene triamine penta acetic acid labelled with technetium (^{99m}Tc DTPA). Perfusion is assessed using a gamma camera and a mini computer and the technique has a major place in the investigation of possible cases of renal artery stenosis and in the diagnosis of renal transplant rejection. It is also valuable in the investigation of patients with acute renal failure due to acute tubular necrosis (ATN), since perfusion is well preserved despite the absence of urine production.

The patient's ability to conserve salt and water is extremely important in surgical practice. With normal renal function, urinary sodium excretion may vary through an enormous range (less than 10 to more than 1000 mmol/day) according to the requirements for sodium balance dictated by variations in intake and extrarenal losses. It follows that the concept of a 'normal' urinary sodium excretion, oft quoted in laboratory tables, is fallacious and is merely a comment on the mean dietary salt intake of the community studied. More correctly, a particular level of sodium excretion should simply be regarded as either appropriate or inappropriate to a patient's current needs. In disease of other systems, urinary sodium excretion may be determined by factors other than external sodium balance – particular examples include heart failure and hypovolaemia due to hypoalbuminaemia, where sodium excretion may be low even in the presence of oedema, and uncontrolled diabetes mellitus where urinary sodium excretion may be high in the presence of saline depletion.

In renal disease, the capacity to vary sodium excretion is progressively limited, so that maintenance of sodium balance is increasingly dependent on extrarenal factors. Gross reductions in intake, whether the product of disease or doctors or increase in extrarenal (usually gastrointestinal) losses, are not followed by renal sodium conservation, so that saline depletion develops rapidly with the production of hypovolaemia, decreasing renal perfusion and further deterioration of renal function. Conversely, the administration of more sodium than can be excreted will lead to saline overload with venous congestion, dependent oedema and pulmonary oedema.

Defects in water conservation may be due to renal disease or to a variety of other causes including a deficiency of antidiuretic hormone (ADH), a rare inherited resistance to ADH, hypercalcaemia, and to an osmotic diuresis. The consequences, though severe, tend to be less critical than those of salt depletion, since the deficiency is spread through the total body water (rather than confined to the extracellular space). Concentration tests vary from the simple measurement of the specific gravity (SG) of either an early morning urine sample, or a sample produced after a prolonged period (24 h or sufficient to produce a 5% weight loss) of fluid deprivation (when an SG of 1.022–1.032 should be produced), to the formal assessment of the urine osmolality either 12 h after the i.m. injection of an oily solution of pitressin tannate or 4 h after the subcutaneous injection of an aqueous solution of pitressin (normal 800–1200 mosmol/l) (Monson and Richards, 1978). The ability to produce a dilute urine is relatively well preserved and its assessment is seldom necessary clinically.

Renal control of potassium balance is not nearly as complete as that of sodium balance, so that even in states of potassium depletion (the usual problem for the surgeon) excretion seldom falls much below 20 mmol/24 h). Renal disease diminishes even this ability so that potassium depletion may develop rapidly, particularly when there are abnormal gastrointestinal losses. Other factors such as an osmotic diuresis (diabetes mellitus), diuretics and corticosteroids are important causes of urinary potassium loss. To some extent, plasma levels may be maintained by the release of potassium from damaged tissues, but replacement is frequently necessary.

Proteinuria

Normal urine is virtually protein-free (less than 100 mg/24 h), so that the discovery of proteinuria should prompt formal renal investigation. The converse, that patients with significant renal disease have proteinuria, is not invariably true, so that reliance on

Albustix (R) and similar tests for screening patients for renal disease will inevitably lead to errors. The quantity of proteinuria is usually assessed either by measurement of the protein concentration in a single urine sample or by measurement of the total amount excreted per day. In certain circumstances (usually children with the nephrotic syndrome) it may be more useful to express glomerular 'leakiness' as the ratio between the clearances of albumin and creatinine; this measurement is independent of urine flow rate (this appears in both halves of the fraction and cancels out) and takes into account the reduction in albuminuria attributable to a fall in serum albumin or in creatinine clearance. Because of its relatively high plasma concentration and small molecular weight (compared with other plasma proteins) albumin virtually always predominates – particularly when proteinuria is due to glomerular disease. In only a minority of patients with proteinuria (i.e. those with the nephrotic syndrome) is the protein loss sufficient to be significant in its own right.

The urinary sediment

Microscopic examination of a clean fresh unspun specimen of normal urine reveals only a few red and white cells (less than $10/mm^3$) and occasional hyaline casts, often with epithelial cells from the lower urinary tract. These numbers may increase after severe exercise or with fever and may then be associated with finely granular casts. The appearance of large numbers of red or white blood cells nearly always indicates the presence of disease of the urinary tract. Cellular casts imply the presence of renal disease; active pyelonephritis is associated with the excretion of white cell casts and proliferative glomerulonephritis with coarsely granular and red cell casts. Epithelial casts may imply the presence of severe glomerulonephritis or interstitial nephritis, but may also be seen during recovery from acute tubular necrosis.

It has recently been recognised that, if fresh urine is examined by phase contrast microscopy, red cells coming from the glomeruli may be distinguished from red cells coming from the lower urinary tract. Application of this knowledge may frequently save the patient from a cystoscopy.

Divided renal function tests

It may be necessary to ascertain the contribution of each kidney to overall function in two different circumstances. The first concerns the patient with bilateral renal disease in whom renal surgery is being considered and in whom it is necessary to know what renal function will remain if one kidney has to be removed. The second concerns the patient with hypertension and renal arterial disease whose blood pressure cannot be readily controlled by medical means and in whom it is necessary to predict whether surgical correction of the arterial lesion will lead to cure of the hypertension.

Formerly this information could only be obtained from the analysis of separate timed urine samples from each kidney. Fortunately, these tests are no longer necessary. The separate contribution of each kidney can now be determined isotopically using the radio-pharmaceutical agent dimercapto-succinic acid (DMSA) labelled with radioactive technetium (^{99m}Tc). This is given intravenously and taken up by renal tubular epithelium with little urinary excretion, so that errors do not arise because of the accumulation of isotope in a dilated pelvicaliceal system (Fig 15.2). The accumulation of isotope in each renal area can be assessed using a gamma camera and a mini computer and, after expression of the uptake by each kidney as a fraction of the total, individual renal function may be calculated by multiplying each fraction by the total GFR or creatinine clearance.

The progressive introduction of potent and relatively non-toxic hypotensive drugs had led to a dramatic decrease in the number of patients with renovascular hypertension who require surgery (and therefore invasive investigation). Furthermore, the response to surgery can be predicted more surely, although not with certainty, by measurement of the renal vein renin concentrations. A satisfactory outcome is likely if the renin concentration in the blood draining from the suspect kidney is raised and is at least 1½ times that drain-

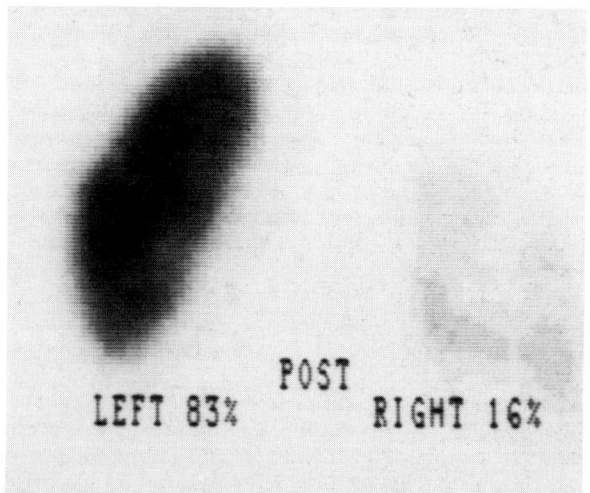

Fig 15.2 The distribution of renal function between the two kidneys assessed using ^{99m}Tc DMSA. *Note* the thin rim of functioning tissue remaining in the hydronephrotic right kidney and the small cortical scar in the left kidney.

ing from the contralateral (presumed normal) kidney which may even have a low venous renin concentration.

The renal response to stress

It has already been pointed out that the normal kidney responds to hypovolaemia or to diminished perfusion by conserving salt and water. Urine flow may fall to 20–30 ml/h and urine sodium concentration may fall to levels that are undetectable; urine specific gravity, osmolality and urea concentration all rise sharply (Table 1). The oliguria is associated with increased tubular reabsorption of filtered urea so that, even in the presence of normal renal function, blood urea levels may rise substantially. When a patient in this condition is seen for the first time, the unwary may interpret the oliguria and raised blood urea level as signs of the presence of acute renal failure. Analysis of a urine sample should quickly clarify the real situation since the urine passed by a patient with acute tubular necrosis has quite different characteristics. The urine flow rate may be equally low (although this is not invariable) but the sodium concentration is much higher (30–60 mmol/l), and the osmolality and urea concentration much lower (Table 1). Hypovolaemia and diminished renal perfusion may, of course, lead to acute tubular necrosis and confusion may arise when the patient is studied during the transition from the normal physiological response to renal failure. However, this progression can still be halted while the urine osmolality is significantly higher than that of plasma (more than 1.1 to 1), provided the underlying cause can be corrected. Once this has been done (or at least started), it is reasonable to administer a test dose of i.v. diuretic using either mannitol (25 g) or frusemide (40 mg). Obviously, the former should not be given if the patient is overloaded (implying the presence of either established ATN or heart disease), nor should the latter be given to the patient who is grossly dehydrated.

Inappropriate release of antidiuretic hormone (ADH)

Antidiuretic hormone is normally released only in response to a rise in the osmolality of blood entering the hypothalamus. However, a number of situations

Table 1
THE DISTINCTION BETWEEN PRERENAL URAEMIA AND ACUTE TUBULAR NECROSIS (ATN)

| | *Urine* | | *Urine/plasma ratio* | |
	Volume	*Sodium concentration*	*Osmolality*	*Urea*
Prerenal uraemia	< 600 ml/day	< 10 mmol/l	> 1.1	> 10
ATN	Usually < 600 ml/day	> 30 mmol/l	< 1.1	< 5

that are encountered by the surgical patient may lead to its release in a manner which may seem inappropriate. These include pain and the administration of morphia and anaesthetic agents. The normal renal response is a reduction in water excretion and if, at the same time, the patient is given a water load either orally or intravenously, this will accumulate, leading to a fall in serum sodium concentration and, in extreme cases, to neurological symptoms and signs of fluid overload with oedema. In itself this response is seldom sufficiently gross to cause the patient much harm, but danger does arise if the clinician interprets the hyponatraemia as a sign of salt depletion and, instead of simply restricting water intake, treats the patient with large volumes of normal saline.

In conclusion, despite the complexity of renal function, a simple measurement of the plasma creatinine concentration will provide an assessment that is sufficient for most clinical purposes. Although a normal result does not exclude the presence of significant renal disease, it does indicate that the patient has renal function that is good enough to sustain him through anything except the most severe crises. Conversely, an abnormal result should always be taken seriously, is an indication for further investigation, and should be taken as a warning that the patient's fluid and electrolyte balance will require close supervision.

References

Kampmann J., Siersbaek-Nielsen K., Kristensen M., Mølholm Hansen, J. (1974). Rapid evaluation of creatinine clearance. *Acta med. Scand*; **196:**517–20.
Monson J.P., Richards P. (1978). Desmopressin urine concentration test. *Brit. Med. J*; **1:**24.

16

Radiology

THOMAS SHERWOOD

Several new ways of making images of the urinary tract have arrived in clinical practice over the last decade and these new imaging techniques represent considerable advances, but have inevitably made sensible diagnostic tactics that much more difficult. They also exert subtle, but important, changes on the way surgeons and radiologists work together. In the past the surgeon rightly wanted to judge the evidence for himself, and the duty of an investigative department was sometimes seen as simply providing the best possible x-rays for the surgeon's eyes. It is probably still sound advice that 'nephrectomy should never be carried out without the relevant x-rays in the operating theatres . . . it is better to postpone the operation' (Blandy, 1979).

However, with a complex, highly operator-dependent technique like ultrasound, the surgeon can no longer be expected to master detailed interpretation – he would have to perform the scans himself. He may now have to manage a patient on a radiologist's ultrasound report, not the primary evidence, e.g. 'characteristic renal cyst on ultrasound and IVU – there is no need to puncture this lesion'. This approach can only work if there is close cooperation between surgeon and radiologist, so that each understands the other's problems.

Radiological tools

The intravenous urogram (IVU)

This is now the preferred term to IVP, emphasising that much more is seen than just a pyelogram (outline of the urine collecting spaces).

Contrast media

The standard preparations are all benzoic acid derivatives containing three iodine atoms. The radio-opaque iodine is tightly bound into the benzene ring, and the amount of free iodide present is minimal. The reactions occasionally encountered with these compounds have nothing to do with 'iodine sensitivity'. A non-opaque cation, either sodium or meglumine, is also present:

Cation	*Anion*
Sodium *or* meglumine	Diatrizoate *or* iothalamate, metrizoate, iodamide

Manufacturers put up combinations of these possible constituents under various trade names. The number at the end of the trade name now commonly designates the iodine concentration, e.g. Urografin 325 contains 325 mg I/ml; 300–600 mg I/kg body weight is the usual dosage.

Newer contrast media have been developed in an effort to make these substances less intensely hyperosmolar. This may be achieved by variations on linking two benzene rings together as a dimer (e.g. ioxaglate), or on non-ionic compounds (e.g. iopamidol). The new media are considerably more expensive. Despite this their use is now well established in certain fields, e.g. angiography.

Fast i.v. injection of a bolus of contrast medium is the standard procedure. If a drip is already in place, then drip infusion is, of course, a convenient alternative. The point of fast injection is that a high plasma contrast medium level will produce the best possible nephrogram (opacification of the renal parenchyma). There is a circumstance where fast injection should be *avoided*: patients with known heart disease, who may be at risk from cardiac dysrhythmias.

Renal failure

Ultrasound is the imaging test of choice and has displaced the IVU for initial assessment of the kidneys. If doubt remains and an IVU is called for in renal failure, care is needed with technique. The renal failure IVU is a *special examination*, demanding large doses of contrast medium and tomography (an x-ray technique of seeing only one plane in focus). There are important *contraindications* where the examination may do harm:

Absolute:	correctable prerenal uraemic factors, e.g. hypotension, dehydration, salt and water depletion.
Relative:	diabetes
	myeloma
	infants in renal failure.

Reactions

Reactions to contrast medium are much feared because they are sudden and potentially lethal. There is as yet no satisfactory scientific hypothesis embracing all reactions, and treatment is therefore on an insecure basis.

Most reactions are minor and need little active intervention, e.g. urticaria or 'stuffy eyes and sinuses'. Most patients feel uncomfortably hot during the first few minutes of the investigation because of vasodilatation induced by the contrast medium. Major reactions involve circulatory collapse or intense bronchospasm. Intravenous hydrocortisone is the hallowed, but unproven, stand-by: standard general resuscitative measures for cardiac arrest are of obvious importance.

In the problem of contrast medium reactions there is much speculation and little established fact. Guidelines are:

1 With any previous reactor there should be careful discussion on the need for a new IVU. If the examination is essential, the patient should probably be pretreated with steroids (Siegle and Lieberman, 1978).

2 Retrograde examinations are no certain protection against the reaction risk, since contrast medium is absorbed across the urothelium. However, reactions under the general anaesthesia are distinctly uncommon.

3 This highlights the fact that there is an undoubted psychological component to the problem: anxious patients and rough doctors will experience more reactions.

Ultrasound scan

This safe, painless technique produces sectional echo maps of the body. Because solid/fluid interfaces are easily mapped, renal cysts can be differentiated from solid masses (Figs 16.1) and dilated calices picked up in obstruction (Fig 16.2). Residual bladder urine can also be monitored.

Retrograde uretero-pyelogram

The best indication for this examination is inadequate information from the IVU. A bulb catheter gently wedged in the lower ureter, with contrast medium injection observed by fluoroscopy, makes for the best retrogrades.

Ascending urethrogram

This is a good examination for studying structural details of the urethral interior e.g. in suspected strictures. A normal urethrogram excludes a stricture. If in doubt go on to:

Micturition cystourethrogram (MCU)

A functional study of bladder and urethra, good for looking at vesicoureteric reflux.

Computed tomography (CT)

This major advance in radiological technique of the 1970s has brought about many insights into previously

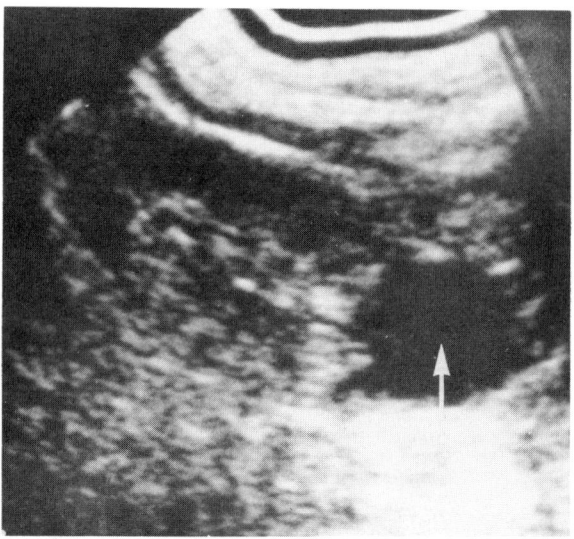

Fig 16.1a   Longitudinal ultrasound scan. There is a sharply demarcated echo-free lesion in the lower renal pole – a cyst (arrow).

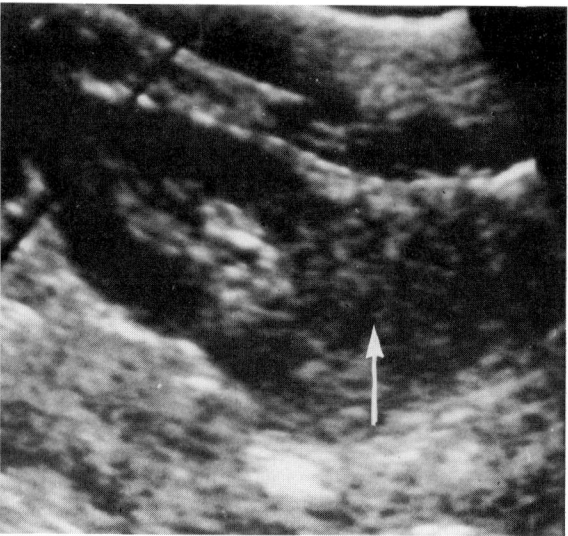

Fig 16.1b   Longitudinal ultrasound scan. *Note* the mass at the lower renal pole distorting the renal outline and filled with echoes – a carcinoma (arrow).

dark territories. The early diagnosis of retroperitoneal fibrosis and adrenal tumours, or the accurate staging of testicular tumours are some examples in urology. Renal masses are of particular interest. The differentiation of a likely cyst from carcinoma is still properly the preserve of ultrasound: cheaper and quicker. When a solid or indeterminate lesion is found, however, CT is now

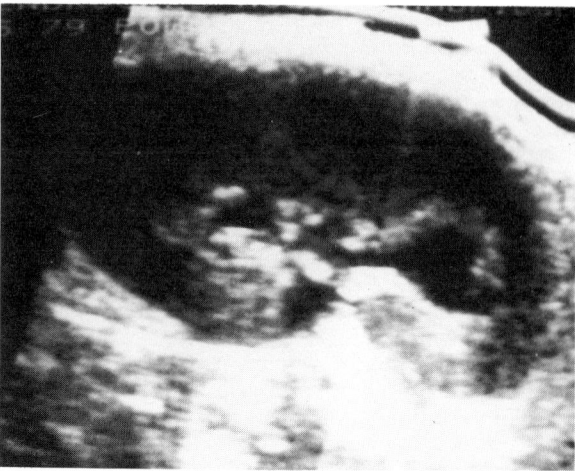

Fig 16.2   Longitudinal ultrasound scan. The renal sinus echoes are not tightly packed – echo-free spaces here outline dilated calices. *See* Fig 16.4.

the best next investigation. It can show the probable carcinoma, exclude involvement of the renal vein or inferior vena cava, and demonstrate a normal contralateral kidney (Fig 16.3).

Arteriogram and venogram

Far fewer angiograms are now done as ultrasound and CT units have spread. Every renal carcinoma no longer needs an arteriogram. The development of arterial embolisation as a therapeutic adjunct has ensured that the technique will not go under in the renal tumour field. Dilatation of renal artery stenoses (percutaneous angioplasty) has provided a further boost to angiography.

Antegrade (percutaneous) pyelogram and surgery

Needling the pelvicaliceal system of a kidney that cannot be shown adequately on the IVU is a good alternative to retrograde pyelography. Suspected obstruction is the common indication (Fig 16.4). Percutaneous urinary drainage ('a radiologist's nephrostomy') can be established during the same manoeuvre (Fig 16.5). The mere technical fact that a nephrostomy can readily be done in this way is never a sufficient justification: for example, whether a patient with an inoperable pelvic tumour stands to gain anything from the procedure is a moot point. Very careful discussion between surgeon and radiologist is essential for proper

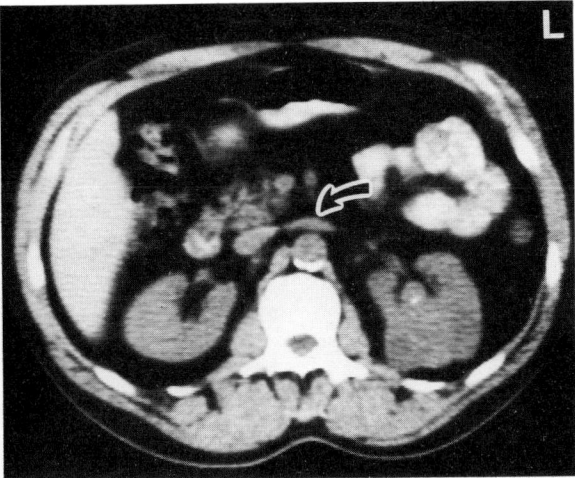

(a)

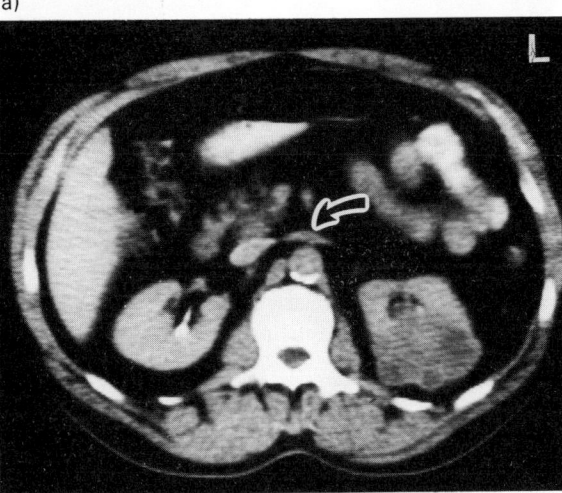

(b)

Fig 16.3 Two CT scans of a patient with a left renal carcinoma, before and after the injection of intravenous contrast medium. Note the large posterior mass in the left kidney, the normal left renal vein (arrow) and inferior vena cava. Computer manipulation of the images allows the different density levels in these vessels before and after contrast medium to be shown, confirming patency. The right kidney is normal.

selection and management of patients under this heading. Antegrade puncture approaches to the kidney have been further developed to allow the extraction of renal stones by this route. Similarly ureteric strictures can be dilated or bypassed with a stent.

Lymphogram, vasogram, cavernosogram

These special examinations are beyond the scope of this chapter.

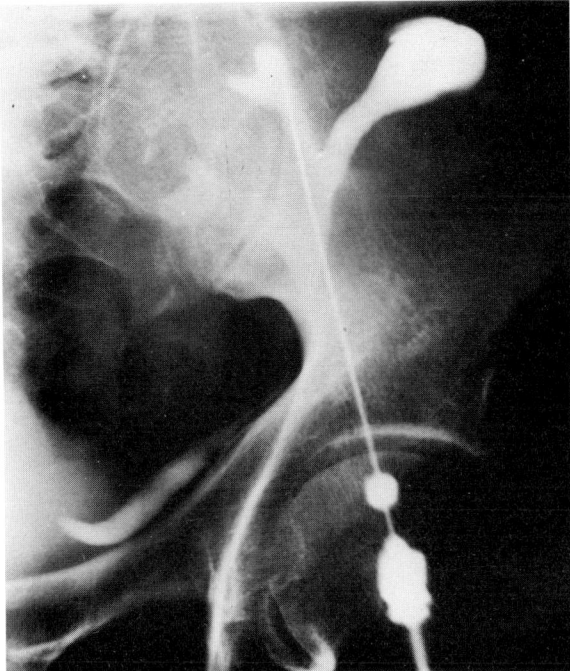

Fig 16.4 Antegrade pyelogram of transplant kidney also shown in Fig 16.2. The puncturing needle is entering a dilated calix, but *note* free flow of contrast medium down to the bladder. Although calices are a little distended, there is no obstruction here.

Nuclear medicine studies

The excretion of technetium labelled glomerular (e.g. DTPA) or tubular (e.g. DMSA) substances provides *functional* images which can be quantified for reliable assessment of individual renal performance or impairment. Questionable nephrectomy or doubtful ureteric obstruction are examples of functional questions which such studies should be called in to answer. Because of better resolution, x-ray studies are generally appropriate where *structural* information is sought, but the far smaller radiation cost of radioisotope examinations may make them investigations of first choice even for structural purposes, e.g. for repeated cystography in following up children with ureteric reflux.

Upper urinary tract investigation

Haematuria – is there a tumour in the upper urinary tract?

This presenting symptom/sign covers a wide range, from the doctor's chance microscopy finding of a few

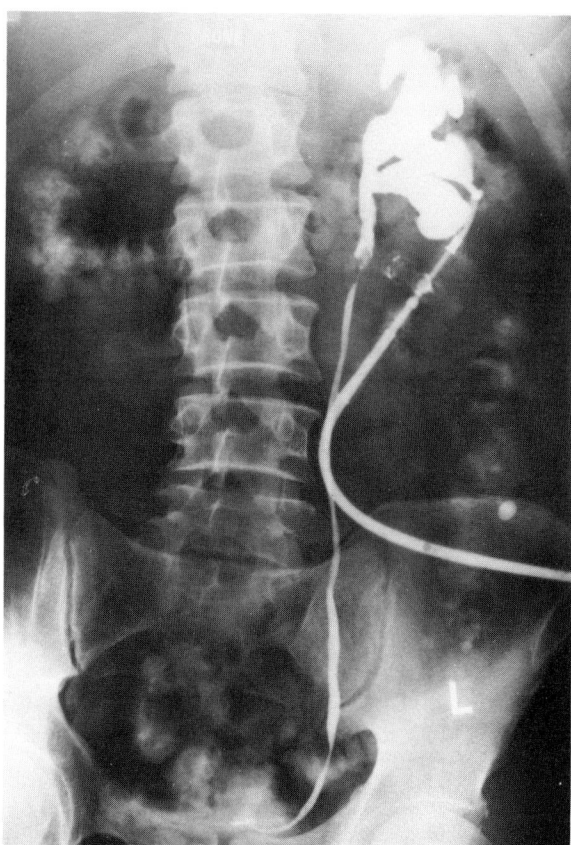

Fig 16.5 Radiologist's nephrostomy. There is an obstructive radiolucent (uric acid) stone lying in the upper ureter. This patient presented in acute renal failure, because this is his only kidney. *Note* contrast medium in the gut from the IVU carried out earlier (hepatic excretion, important in renal failure). The nephrostomy allowed a breathing space for the patient to recover from his renal failure, followed by an elective operation when he was fit.

red cells to the alarmed patient passing bloody urine. In any event an IVU will be needed to exclude a renal or urothelial tumour. Often ignored truisms are:

1   The IVU is a good *upper urinary tract survey*; it is not a reliable look at the bladder. A normal IVU never excludes a bladder tumour, the most important cause of haematuria in adults. Cystoscopy is the necessary sequel to the normal IVU in this group.
2   The IVU cannot diagnose glomerulonephritis. In the right clinical setting, attention to such medical causes of haematuria is obviously more appropriate than waiting for a surgical cause to declare itself on repeated IVUs.
3   The old triad of haematuria, flank pain and palpable mass has little to do with diagnosing renal tumours

in the 1980s. We expect to find these lesions at a much earlier stage on the IVU, so suspicion must be high. Many tumours will be chance findings on IVUs done for quite different indications (Fig 16.6).

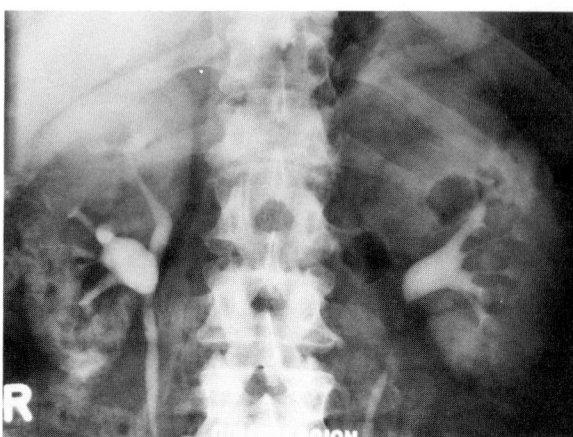

Fig 16.6 IVU carried out because of hypertension with renal impairment. There is a large mass in the left upper renal pole. *See* Fig 16.9.

Renal mass

This IVU finding may occasionally have unmistakable signs that a tumour is present, e.g. central amorphous calcification in the mass (Fig 16.7). More commonly the question 'cyst or carcinoma' will arise.

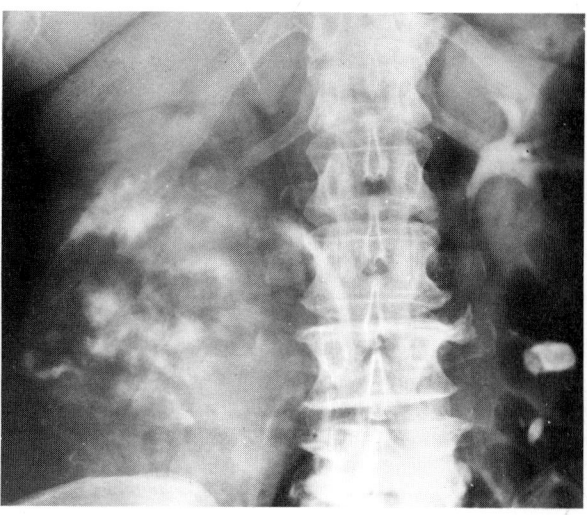

Fig 16.7 IVU done because of haematuria. There is a large mass destroying the right kidney, with extensive amorphous calcification – a renal carcinoma.

There is now a well tried investigative pathway involving immediate ultrasound examination of the patient (Sherwood, 1980). This will sort out whether the lesion is cystic or solid.

Renal cyst

These are common lesions in autopsy series, and now a frequent chance finding on an IVU, ultrasound or CT scan. Thus discovered in elderly patients, with wholly characteristic signs on imaging, the diagnosis need not be driven any further. However, this is not so if:

1   IVU or ultrasound findings do not satisfy strict 'simple cyst' criteria;
2   the patient is young, when renal cysts are uncommon;
3   haematuria continues unexplained;
4   there is any shadow of doubt clinically or radiologically.

CT is then the next step. Cyst puncture can be carried out to confirm the diagnosis. This is a straightforward outpatient procedure under local anaesthesia (Fig 16.8).

Renal carcinoma

Once an ultrasound scan has shown a renal mass to be solid, the usual advice was to confirm the cancer suspicion by arteriography. This advice need no longer be followed. Whilst the majority of renal carcinomas have floridly abnormal arterial patterns (Fig 16.9), this picture is neither entirely specific nor sensitive. A lesion with abnormal vessels can occasionally be benign (e.g. a renal abscess), and some few renal carcinomas are avascular. Angiography still has a useful place at times, because it excludes the 5–10% likelihood of a second tumour in the contralateral kidney, the chance of renal vein occlusion, and can also be used for therapeutic embolisation.

Where available, CT is now the investigation of choice in all solid or indeterminate renal masses. It can answer all the diagnostic questions asked of the arteriogram and stage the tumour preoperatively.

Renal cyst and carcinoma in the same kidney

This double lesion is a well-known diagnostic nightmare. The only common occurrence is the chance one of a cyst found at a distance from the same kidney's carcinoma. It emphasises that each renal lump of several should always be diagnosed on its own merits. Carcinoma may, of course, be necrotic with cystic debris contents – a fact readily appreciated on ultrasound and 'cyst' puncture. The apparently simple cyst arising because of a tiny carcinoma at its base is a finding of

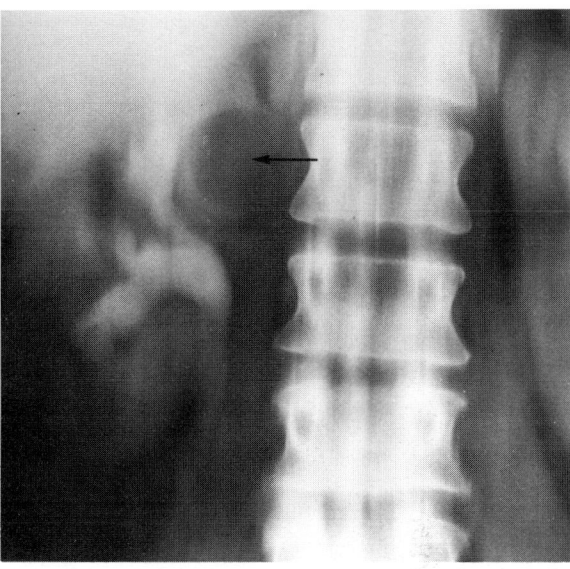

Fig 16.8a IVU showing a well defined cyst on the medial border of the right kidney (arrow).

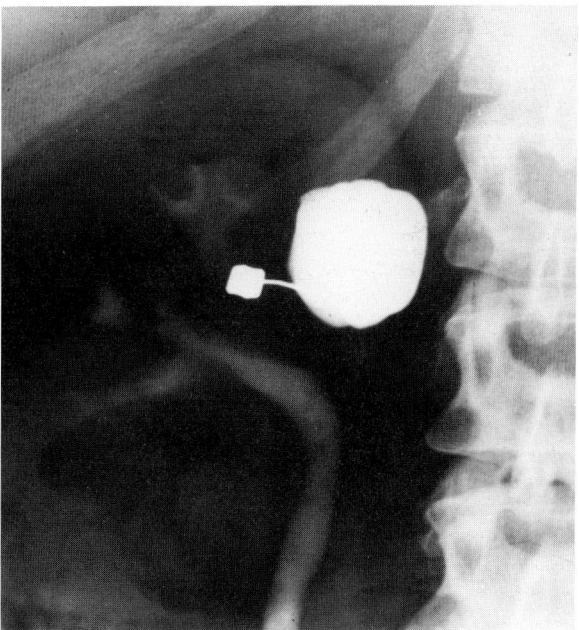

Fig 16.8b Cyst puncture, yielding clear fluid, and accounting for the whole lesion.

great rarity. If it were to dominate clinical management by recommending surgical exploration of all renal cysts, the resulting morbidity and mortality would far outweigh any benefit. However, it is proper that worry

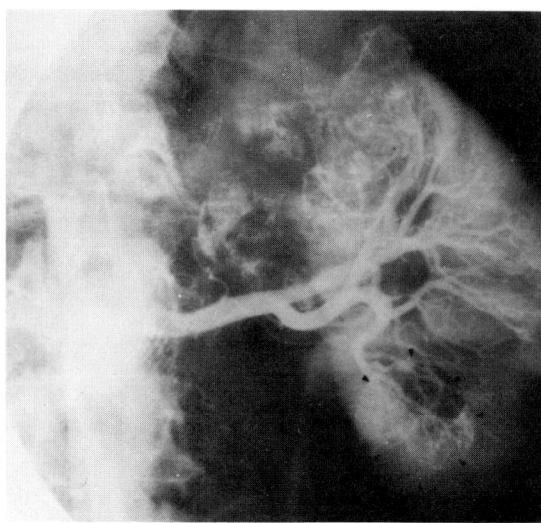

Fig 16.9 Selective renal arteriogram – there is an extensive abnormal vascular pattern in a mass at the left upper renal pole. This is the same patient as in Fig 16.6. *Note* that he has a second carcinoma in the lower renal pole (arrowheads).

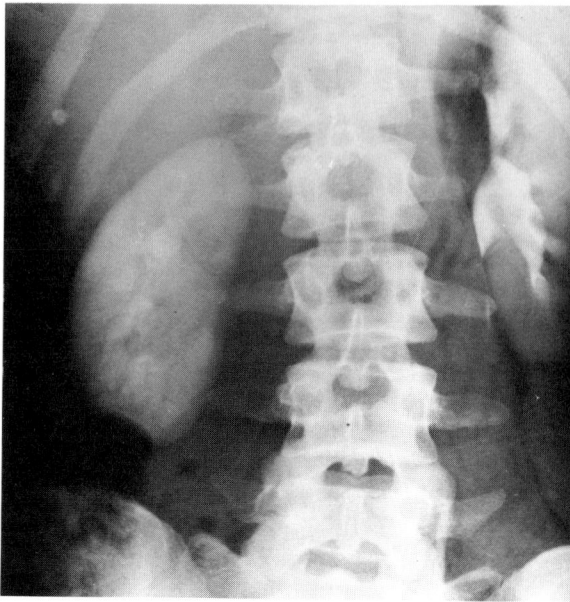

Fig 16.10 IVU in acute ureteric obstruction by a stone. *Note* dense right nephrogram with delayed opacification of dilated calices.

over the double lesion should keep surgeons and radiologists lively and anxious when dealing with the common renal cyst.

Loin pain – is there a stone or other cause of obstruction?

Acute obstruction

Most renal stones are radio-opaque, with the important exceptions of uric acid and matrix stones. Seeing an opacity along the ureteric course on the plain film of a patient with ureteric colic is, therefore, suggestive, but by no means conclusive. An immediate short IVU, with a single 15–20 min film taken immediately after micturition (to move opacified bladder urine out of the way) is needed to nail the diagnosis. The characteristic IVU signs of *acute* obstruction are:

1 increasingly dense nephrogram (Fig 16.10);
2 delayed pyelogram, with late opacification of the ureter down to the obstruction site (films delayed for several hours may be needed for this).

Particularly in right-sided ureteric colic, with perhaps clinical doubt concerning acute appendicitis, the diagnostic certainty provided by a short IVU can be very helpful. A normal IVU rules out acute ureteric obstruction as the explanation of the patient's symptoms.

Intermittent acute obstruction

Pelvi-ureteric junction obstruction is the best example of this state (Fig 16.11). Because the IVU is a good test of acute, but not chronic, obstruction, it should, if at all possible, be carried out during an attack of pain. If this cannot be arranged, the aim is to stress the urinary transport system by an i.v., fast-acting diuretic (e.g. frusemide). The patient may develop characteristic pain, and the IVU show acute obstruction.

Chronic obstruction

Chronic dilatation of the upper urinary tract on the IVU is often equated with obstruction. This *may* be right, but there are two other important states which may be responsible: vesicoureteric reflux and ureteric muscle failure (e.g. prune belly syndrome). Clinical and radiological evidence may point to obstruction as the likely cause of a distended ureter (Fig 16.12). In doubtful cases pressure studies of the upper urinary tract via antegrade pyelography are most helpful (Whitaker, 1982). Radioisotope studies are also of value here (Britton *et al.*, 1979).

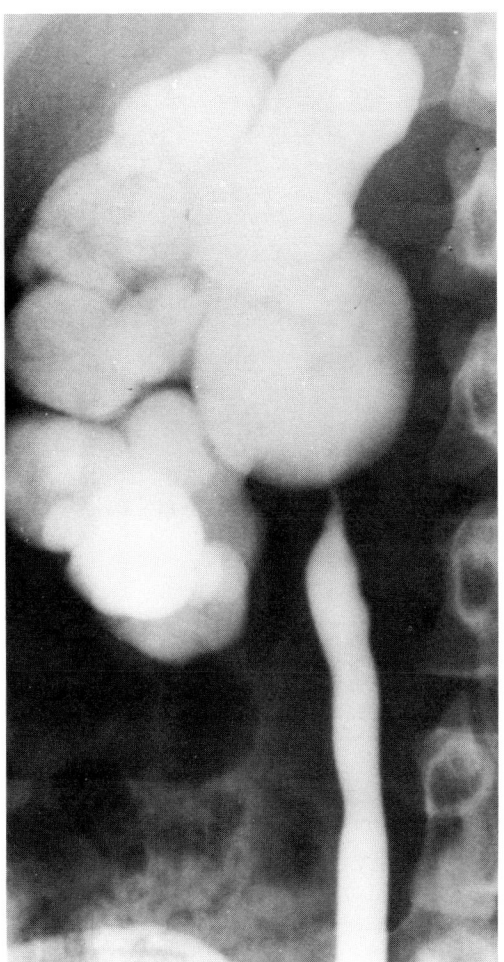

Fig 16.11 Characteristic picture of pelvi-ureteric junction obstruction, here obtained by a retrograde study.

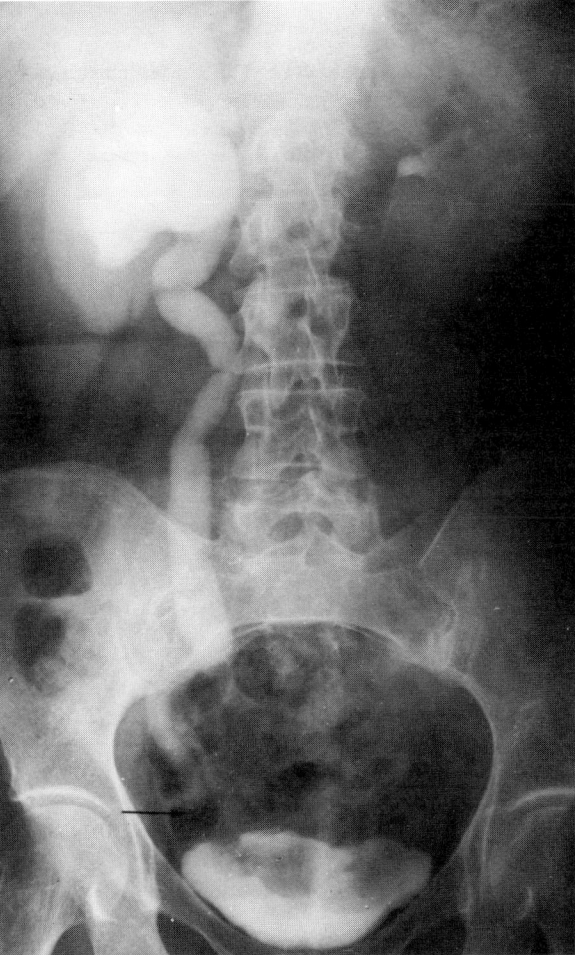

Fig 16.12 There is obvious dilatation of the right upper urinary tract to a point just above the bladder (arrow). This was a sequel to hysterectomy – the right ureter had been caught in a ligature.

Infection – children v. adults

Age is an important watershed for this topic: children deserve early investigation of a *proved* urinary infection. In adults, the rewards of investigating such infections are meagre and doubtful. This is particularly so for the problem of *recurrent cystitis* in women: there is no place for the routine IVU here, because it will not help. However, renal stones or papillary necrosis may be the background to adult urinary infection, and are clearly worth finding. There are three obvious IVU indications here: (1) loin symptoms; (2) sterile pyuria pointing to possible renal tuberculosis; (3) *Proteus* infections, with likely renal stones.

Renal tuberculosis

Most general hospitals will see one or two new cases each year. Erosion of papillae/calices is the early IVU sign, accompanied perhaps by ureteric strictures and a small bladder (Fig 16.13). Lesions at multiple sites in the urinary tract are a hallmark of the disease. Note that careful follow-up by short IVUs is needed in the early months of drug treatment, to detect the ureteric hold-up which may develop.

Renal stones and papillary necrosis

Calculi vary from large staghorn structures to tiny concretions and need little further comment. Most are

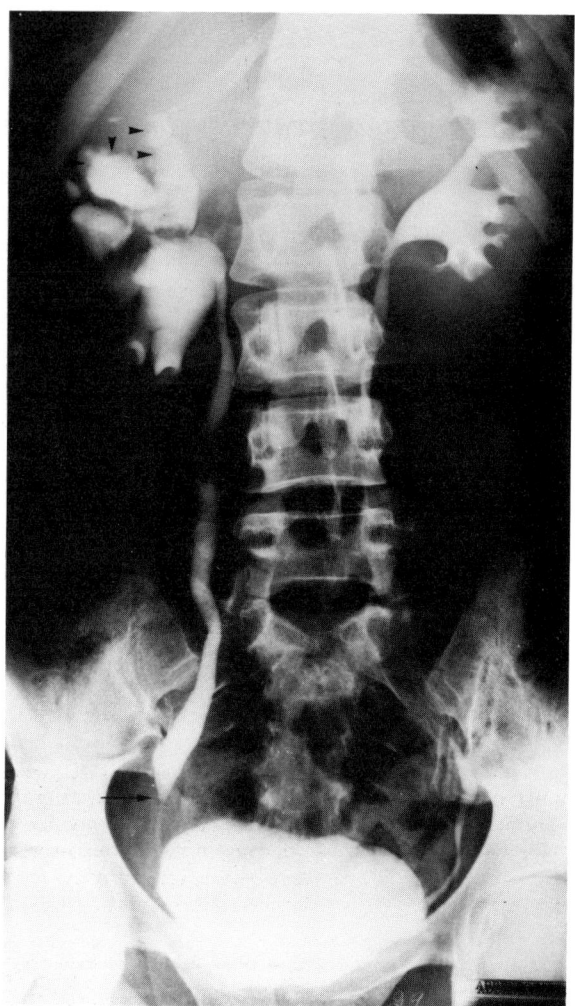

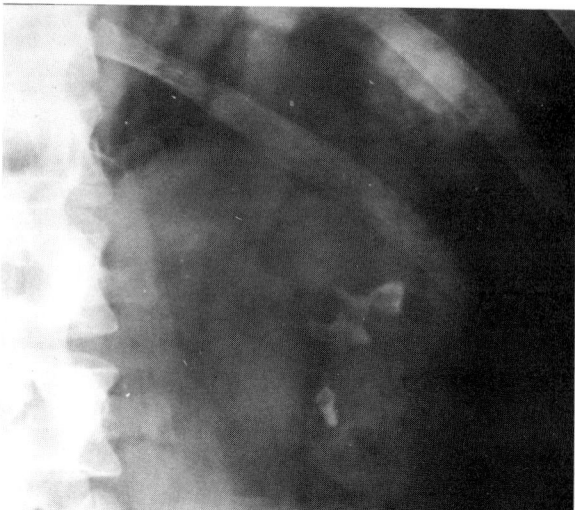

Fig 16.14 Plain film of left kidney. These 'stones' have radiolucent centres and irregular (triangular) shapes – they are necrotic papillae.

Fig 16.13 IVU in urinary tract tuberculosis. *Note* eroded, distorted calices (arrowheads) and ureteric stricture (arrow) on the right side. The left side is normal.

opaque; uric acid and matrix stones are the most important radiolucent examples. Radio-opaque objects in renal calices are not always stones: if they are odd shapes (triangular) with radiolucent centres, necrotic papillae must be suspected (Fig 16.14). Papillary necrosis is common and underdiagnosed. Papillary erosions or cavities are seen in this disease, and ureteric obstruction by the cast-off papillae is not rare.

Chronic pyelonephritis

This is a specific radiological diagnosis and must not be used as a dustbin for gathering in any kidney that looks misshapen. It is a disease determined in early childhood by the combination of vesicoureteric reflux, urinary infection and intrarenal reflux (Ransley and Risdon, 1978). Papillary shape decides whether intrarenal reflux occurs as part of vesicoureteric reflux: refluxing papillae are found predominantly at the upper renal poles, and so scar formation is seen here first and foremost. This is, therefore, a patchy renal disease of predictable distribution (Fig 16.15).

Renal failure

For the patient admitted in this state, the following radiological information is important:

1 What size are the kidneys, and where (in case of renal biopsy)?
2 Are they obstructed?
3 Is a cause evident?

Ultrasound (together with a plain abdominal radiograph) is the investigation of choice to answer these questions. Since it is a structural study independent of the severity of renal impairment, no special preparation or precaution is required. The only important hazards are misinterpreting the scan and forgetting the plain film of the abdomen. The radiograph is vital for detecting the renal stones which can be missed on ultrasound.

Renal size is of obvious value in deciding whether

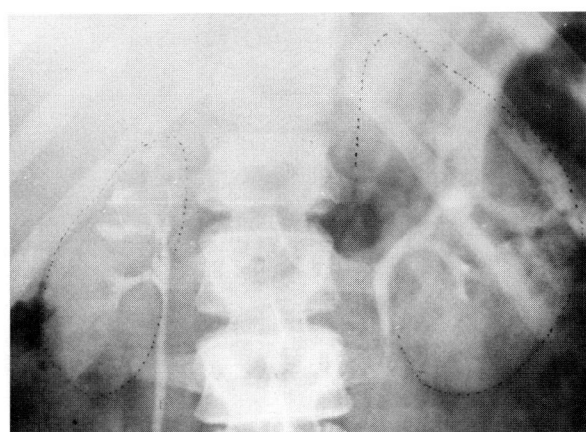

Fig 16.15 IVU in a symptom-free young girl, carried out because of her family history of chronic pyelonephritis. The left kidney is normal but the right is small, with severe scarring at the upper pole. She too has chronic pyelonephritis on the right (vesicoureteric reflux runs in families).

end-stage renal failure (shrunken kidneys) or a potentially reversible state (normal size or large kidneys) is present. Obstruction will be shown on ultrasound by finding the distended calices and renal pelvis. It is only when diagnostic doubt remains, particularly on the all important question of obstruction, that other imaging methods will have to be used.

Obstruction will also be detected by the IVU providing a nephrogram occurs: once this much contrast medium has entered the nephron, the obstruction will be revealed by careful follow-up films showing dilated calices or ureter. The distended non-opacified calices may be seen at once on early films as a 'soap-bubble' nephrogram. Obvious causes like obstructing stones or papillae need no comment. In acute tubular necrosis there is usually a dense, long-lasting nephrogram.

The IVU in renal failure is a special examination, only to be done after full clinical assessment. It is hazardous in:

1   dehydration – this should *never* be part of IVU preparation in *any* patient with renal impairment;
2   any other prerenal uraemic state;
3   infants;
4   diabetes, which is more important than the well-known myeloma contraindication.

Plain films of the abdomen (stones), chest (pulmonary oedema) and hands (osteodystrophy as a clue to chronic renal impairment) are the emergency films on admission; to be followed at once by ultrasound screening. If obstruction is found, immediate percutaneous drainage by antegrade nephrostomy (*see above*) may be considered.

Lower urinary tract investigation

Adult symptoms: frequency, incontinence, 'prostatism'

The micturating cystourethrogram (MCU) is an overrated investigation in this field, and will not usually answer any of the important questions to be asked about such patients. It is particularly useless in stress incontinence. The first need here is to determine whether the bladder is stable (behaving normally) or unstable (producing uninhibited contractions). This can be done by simple cystometry in the first instance. Complex patients may need full urodynamic assessment with combined structural (x-ray) and functional (pressure/flow) studies, outside the scope of this text (Turner-Warwick and Whiteside, 1982).

A young man presenting with difficulty in micturition will obviously need different management from the elderly with prostatic problems. He may have a urethral stricture and a *urethrogram* is an excellent way of checking on this suspicion (Fig 16.16).

Haematuria

A bladder tumour may be obvious on the IVU, but it must be stressed again that the IVU (or cystogram) cannot exclude this diagnosis. The IVU is needed in patients with this disease, because it will detect ureteric obstruction and upper tract urothelial tumours which may complicate management of the bladder lesions.

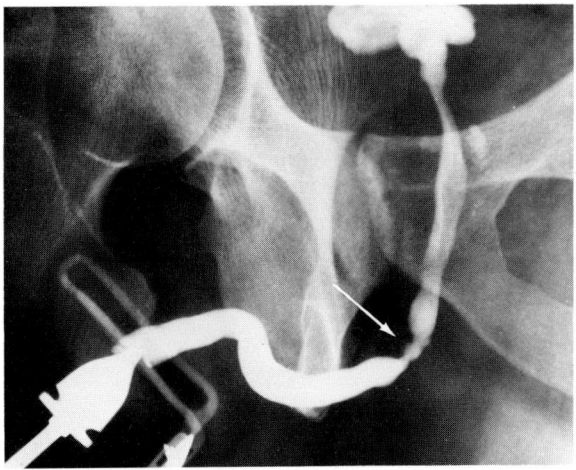

Fig 16.16 This young man with prostatic calcification complains of difficulty in voiding – the urethrogram shows a urethral stricture (arrow).

Infection in children

The MCU allows the diagnosis of *vesicoureteric reflux* and has, therefore, become a hallowed early investigation for children presenting with their first infection. The fact that all likely renal damage has usually occurred already at this stage throws doubt on this policy, and indeed on the whole field of antireflux surgery (Ransley, 1978). For the present, the young child below the age of 5 years should have an IVU (or perhaps plain film and ultrasound or radioisotope renal scan) after his first *proved* urinary infection, to look at the upper urinary tracts for a remediable cause (e.g. stone, ureterocele, megaureter, etc.). A single infection in a girl with a normal IVU probably does not call for an MCU, but it is an apt investigation in most others. If vesicoureteric reflux is found, any follow-up studies are better done as radioisotope cystograms: the radiation cost is less, and poor resolution of no moment.

A policy of cystography need not apply as strictly to girls as to boys, in whom *urethral obstruction* must also be excluded. Urethral valves produce a characteristic picture on the MCU (Fig 16.17), and are well worth finding.

The *ectopic ureterocele* is an IVU diagnosis in children presenting with infection (Fig 16.18).

Incontinence in children

The *ectopic ureter* draining outside the urinary tract usually has a characteristic clinical story: girls with this lesion are always slightly damp, not occasionally incontinent of urine. The key to the diagnosis is *not* a cystogram, but a careful IVU to find the upper moiety of the duplex kidney which is the background to the condition (Fig 16.19). Once this has been determined, the precise anatomy of where the abnormal ureter enters the

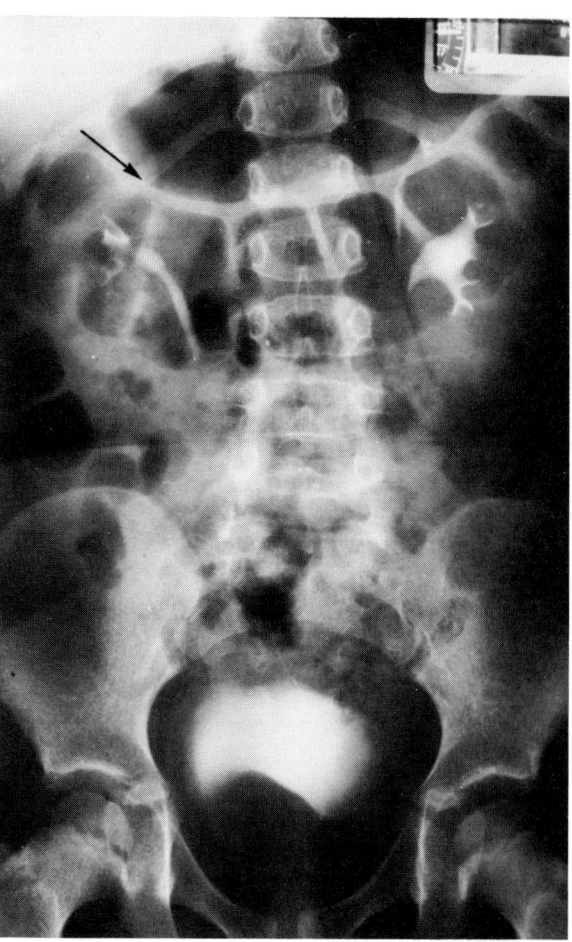

Fig 16.18 IVU of ectopic ureterocele in a young girl presenting with urinary infection. There is a duplex left kidney which is normal. She also has a duplex right kidney with a grossly dilated upper moiety, but this cannot be directly seen (arrow). The non-excreting upper segment of this kidney has to be inferred from the appearance of the lower moiety. Together with the obvious large filling defect in the bladder this makes a complete diagnosis.

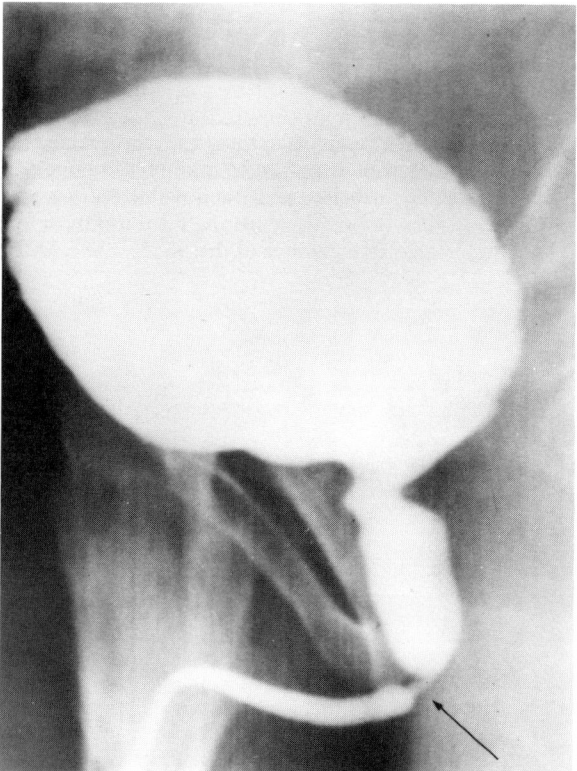

Fig 16.17 MCU in a boy with a urethral valve. *Note* distension of the posterior urethra down to the obstructive valve (arrow).

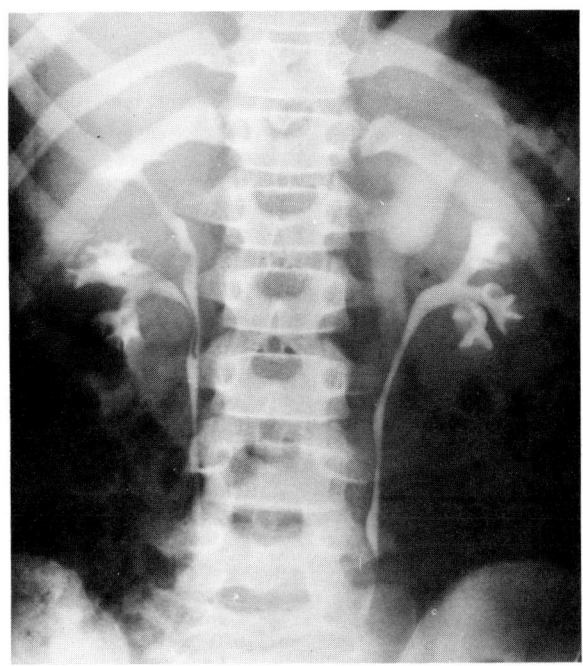

Fig 16.19 IVU in a girl who is always slightly damp. The right renal pelvis is bifid – this upper urinary tract is normal. Her left duplex kidney has a normal lower moiety, but the upper moiety is sick, with obvious caliceal and ureteric distension. This is an ectopic (vaginal) ureter – she can be cured by a left heminephrectomy.

vagina is of little practical interest, and in any event not detectable by cystography.

The *neuropathic bladder* problem is, of course, not confined to children, but the radiological discussion is similar to that in adults. There are no pathognomonic features of bladder shape toward this diagnosis, nor can the upper motor neurone lesion be distinguished reliably from the lower motor neurone one on cystography. IVUs to look for the effects of ureteric obstruction or reflux are the radiologist's more important contribution to the problem, short of full combined lower tract urodynamic assessment.

Critical diagnostic pathways

There are two approaches to investigating a patient:

1 Do every test which might be useful, and review the evidence (the diagnostic work-up);
2 Make an informed guess at the likely diagnosis, and choose investigations as critical tests of that hypothesis.

Scientific method might seem to support the blunder-

buss grapeshot method under (1). In fact, science is a persuasive argument for diagnostic sharpshooting under (2), in addition to those of humanity and economics (Sherwood, 1978). *Urinary tract trauma* will be used as an example.

Renal trauma

Traffic injuries are now the commonplace cause. There is continuing debate on how to investigate patients with haematuria following loin trauma. Documenting the renal injury in full will call for an IVU, radioisotope renogram and scintigram, ultrasound scan, arteriogram (and a CT scan?). These excellent demonstrations of any structural or functional renal impairment will have no impact on how most of these patients are managed: by masterly inactivity based on clinical signs. Aggressive investigators will answer at once that rewarding opportunities for conservative surgery are lost without a full diagnostic workup, e.g. evacuation of a silent perirenal haematoma.

Various clinical groups can be picked out from this jungle:

1 The badly hurt patient who has to be taken to theatre at once because of intra-abdominal bleeding. There may not even be time for a plain film of the abdomen in the casualty department, but the patient should have an i.v. injection of urographic contrast medium there. A radiograph can then be taken on the operating table, directed principally at demonstrating a normal contralateral kidney. This piece of information is of obvious vital moment to the surgery of the bruised organ: nephrectomy must be avoided if it is the patient's only 'good' kidney. Hypotension is no contra-indication to this plan. Providing it is not gross, nephrograms will be present for judging renal size.

2 The patient in whom there is time to carry out an immediate IVU, showing a non-excreting kidney on the side of injury. He should have an *arteriogram* at once to look at the cause – torn renal artery or parenchyma, haematoma, etc. This information will probably be very helpful in deciding further management.

There is one exception to this course: where there is obvious discordance between the alarming finding of a non-excreting kidney and the mildness of the injury. An *ultrasound* scan should then be done. This is because a long-standing renal disarray is sometimes fortuitously brought to light by trauma, e.g. a hydronephrosis or a congenitally absent kidney.

3 If the IVU is normal in the mildly injured patient, there is no argument. This starts up when minor unilateral renal damage is shown, e.g. contrast extravasation from a torn calix. All patients with a loin injury and haematuria probably deserve either a brief

IVU or a radioisofope scan – this may be carried out the next morning in the appropriate clinical setting. Either investigation makes a good baseline for the all important proof of a functioning contralateral kidney, and for monitoring progress on the injured side (British Medical Journal, 1979). This policy is directed at the uncommon event of progressive changes, demanding surgical action. The great majority of patients in this paragraph will need no further investigation, and be able to leave hospital shortly.

Bladder and urethral trauma

Bleeding from the urethra is the leading clinical sign; a fracture of the bony pelvis is the almost invariable radiological accompaniment. The IVU is a good initial investigation for checking on the integrity of the upper urinary tracts, and also for looking at the bladder. There may be an obvious vesical tear or a compression deformity of the bladder by a haematoma. With a suspected urethral injury, investigation will depend on the favoured school of management. In any event, attempts at passing catheters before x-ray studies are unwise. At the conservative end, suprapubic drainage will be done, with later leisurely investigation of the urethra by cystography. If immediate repair of a torn urethra is envisaged, a urethrogram with simple (watery) urographic contrast medium should be carried out first. This will show the site and severity of injury, e.g. dislocation/rupture of the prostate/urethra from the bladder base.

References

Blandy J.P. (1979). Nephrectomy. *Brit. J. Hosp. Med*; **21**:302–10.

British Medical Journal (1979). Haematuria after closed trauma. *Brit. Med. J*; **1**:841–2.

Britton K.E., Nimmon C.C., Whitfield H.N., Hendry W.F., Wickham J.E.A. (1979). Obstructive nephropathy: successful evaluation with radionuclides. *Lancet*; **i**:905–7.

Ransley P.G. (1978). Vesicoureteric reflux: continuing surgical dilemma. *Urology*; **12**:246–55.

Ransley P.G., Risdon R.A. (1978). Reflux and renal scarring. *Brit. J. Radiol. Suppl*; **14**.

Sherwood T. (1978). Science in radiology. *Lancet*; **i**:594–5.

Sherwood T. (1980). *Uroradiology*. Oxford: Blackwell Scientific Publications.

Siegle R.L., Lieberman P. (1978). A review of untoward reactions to iodinated contrast material. *J. Urol*; **119**:581–7.

Turner-Warwick R., Whiteside C. Graham (1982). Urodynamic studies and their effect upon management. In *Scientific Foundations of Urology*, 2nd edn. (Chisholm G.D., Innes Williams D., eds.) London: Heinemann Medical.

Whitaker, R.H. (1982). Pathophysiology of ureteric obstruction. In *Scientific Foundations of Urology*, 2nd edn. (Chisholm G.D., Innes Williams D., eds.) London: Heinemann Medical.

17

Investigation of urinary calculi

GEOFFREY D. CHISHOLM

Stones in the urinary tract are no respecters of persons: the symptoms can present at any time, often the most inconvenient. The patient may then be seen by and referred to almost any member of the profession. Thus, a patient with renal/ureteric colic is often admitted to hospital under the care of either a physician or surgeon and not necessarily a urological surgeon. Provided that symptomatic relief is achieved and basic investigations are instituted, then which doctor manages the case need not be a matter of debate since this is an area of medicine any doctor might be called upon to treat.

Familiarity with the problem does lead to more rapid decisions. In a study in Newcastle, 62% of patients with renal and ureteric calculi admitted to the urological department, but not requiring an operation, stayed 2 days or less; in contrast, only 26% of similar patients in general surgical units were discharged in 2 days or less. So the question – how much investigation is needed for the patient with a stone is of relevance to all physicians and surgeons.

All patients with renal/ureteric stones ask the same question 'What can I do to prevent another stone?' The question is justified since 20–50% of patients with stones have > 1–2 symptomatic episodes and half of these with recurrent stones will have either a structural or a metabolic cause. Thus the purpose of stone screening is to find a cause which can be treated, so preventing further stones from developing. This purpose is often frustrated by the number of investigations that prove negative, but with the increase in understanding of the metabolic factors concerned in stone formation, the opportunity to give effective treatment is gradually increasing.

Types of stone

Stones may be classified by their chemical composition, either by broad groups or by precise crystalline structure. The former gives the best guide to both the types and incidence of stones in the urinary tract (Table 1). However, if urinary stones are considered either 'infective' or 'metabolic', then it is easier to understand the basic approach to the screening for a cause of these stones.

Table 1
COMPOSITION, CAUSES AND FREQUENCY OF STONES IN THE URINARY TRACT

Composition	Cause	Frequency
Calcium oxalate/ phosphate	Metabolic Idiopathic	Up to 80%
Magnesium ammonium Phosphate with or without calcium	Infection High urine pH	Up to 14% in females 6% in males
Uric acid	Metabolic Low urine pH Low urine volume	5%
Cystine	Metabolic	1–4%
Xanthine	Metabolic	Rare
Matrix material	Infection	Rare

(Adapted from Anderson, 1980.)

Stones of an 'infective' origin are usually phosphatic stones (either apatite, basic calcium phosphate, or struvite, magnesium ammonium phosphate, with hydroxyapatite as the main type). These stones are found typically in an alkaline infected urine and are the type seen in large renal (often staghorn) stones; they are often mixed with a proportion of calcium oxalate. Stones of 'metabolic' origin are mainly composed of calcium oxalate though these, too, may have a variable proportion of calcium phosphate. (Calcium oxalate stones account for approximately 75% of all renal stones.) Cystine or uric acid stones are rare; more usually they are mixed with calcium oxalate or phosphate.

It follows that screening for infection and its cause (usually stasis), as well as calcium, phosphate, urate and cystine will provide the main clues in the aetiology of most stones. There are also important epidemiological aspects of stone disease. Phosphatic stones with or without urinary infection are predominant in those parts of the world where the level of nutrition and overall standard of living are low. Metabolic stones, and especially uric acid stones, are more common in areas of affluence and especially where red meat is a major part of dietary protein (Blacklock, 1982).

Stone screening

History

A careful history is essential since this will often guide the extent of subsequent investigations. The recurrent stone forming patient tends to be subjected to more detailed investigations, but this is largely because it is thought uneconomic to do little more than the simplest tests on the new patient. This would be true if the patient had to be hospitalised for a metabolic assessment, but this must be regarded as unnecessary except for those centres with special stone research programmes (Boyce and Resnick, 1979).

The age of the patient can be a guide to the likely cause. Thus, primary hyperoxaluria and cystinuria are more common in children than in adults. Idiopathic hypercalciuria and hyperparathyroidism are rare before puberty.

It is important to determine if the patient has unusual dietary habits such as drinking excessive quantities of milk. The patient may be taking excessive quantities of milk *and* alkalis for dyspeptic symptoms. A history of recumbency or dehydration is relevant. Although 30% of recurrent stone formers give a family history of stones, only a small proportion are associated with an inherited metabolic disorder.

Investigations

The extent of any investigations will be dependent on the facilities available. All patients should undergo the following *minimal screen:*

Intravenous urogram (IVU). In addition to defining the site, size and lucency of the stone, this may also reveal an anatomical cause for stones. Approximately 2% of patients with symptomatic stones will also have interstitial calcification – nephrocalcinosis. This is a strong indication for further investigation because 90% of patients with nephrocalcinosis are found to have a metabolic disorder (Table 2).

Table 2
CAUSES OF NEPHROCALCINOSIS: CLASSIFICATION ACCORDING TO RADIOLOGICAL APPEARANCE

	Nephrocalcinosis	
Orderly calcification		Patchy calcification
Cortex	Medulla	Tuberculosis
Acute cortical necrosis	*Medullary sponge kidney	Renal carcinoma
	*Primary hyperparathyroidism	Hydatid disease
	*Renal tubular acidosis	
	Papillary necrosis	
	Vitamin D poisoning	
	Milk alkali syndrome	
	Sarcoid	
	Hyperoxaluria	

* These three account for 70% of all cases of nephrocalcinosis.
(Adapted from Sherwood, 1980.)

Mid-stream specimen of urine (MSU). Culture and sensitivity will indicate the presence of significant infection.

Serum calcium (normal values: 8.5–10.5 mg/100 ml, 2.1–2.6 mmol/l). A random sample taken without venous stasis may be used, but if it is high or borderline-high, then it should be repeated when the patient is fasting. Since the ionised calcium is the important factor, the serum albumin must also be checked and the calcium corrected for any protein abnormality. The principal causes of hypercalcaemia (Table 3) show that hyperparathyroidism is an important cause of this abnormality. However, only about 5–10% of all cases of calcium stones are the result of primary hyperparathyroidism (Harrison, 1982).

Any abnormality of these minimal tests will lead to a more detailed assessment of renal function, microbiology and parathyroid metabolism.

Table 3
CAUSES OF HYPERCALCAEMIA

Malignant disease	55%
Hyperparathyroidism	40%
Vitamin D intoxication, sarcoidosis, thyrotoxicosis, immobilisation and milk alkali syndrome	5%

Further investigations

In *addition* to the above, the blood urea, electrolytes, including bicarbonate, and the following serum and urinary measurements should be done where possible:

Serum phosphate –   2.5–4.3 mg/100 ml
(0.8–1.4 mmol/l)

Alkaline phosphatase – 3–13 KA/100 ml (30–300 iu/l)

Serum uric acid:
  male   – 4.0–8.5 mg/100 ml (0.24–0.50 mmol/l)
  female – 2.5–7.5 mg/100 ml (0.15–0.44 mmol/l)

Urinary calcium:
  male   – not more than 350 mg/24 h (not more than 8.75 mmol/24 h)
  female – not more than 300 mg/24 h (not more than 7.5 mmol/24 h)

Urinary oxalate – 20–45 mg/24 h (0.2–0.5 mmol/24 h)

Urinary uric acid:
  male   – not more than 900 mg/24 h (not more than 5.33 mmol/24 h)
  female – not more than 800 mg/24 h (not more than 4.73 mmol/24 h)

Urinary cystine – qualitative (nitroprusside) test

These normal values vary from place to place and depend on local laboratory techniques and, more importantly, on local population dietary habits (Rose, 1982b).

Except for special investigative reasons, the patient should be instructed to make the urine collections as an out-patient on his or her normal diet; a disadvantage is that the patient may not make complete 24 h collections, but this error can be minimised by making two collections and by measuring the urinary creatinine.

It is relatively common (50–60%) to find a raised urinary calcium as an isolated abnormality – i.e. idiopathic hypercalciuria (Rose, 1982a). However, there is debate about the definition of this term and its significance. It is disappointing that even when measures are taken to reduce calcium excretion, further stones may develop, but this is only an indication that stone formation is a multifactorial problem (*see* Risk factors *below*). Urinary oxalate is probably of more importance in stone aetiology than urinary calcium, but this is a difficult substance to measure and is, therefore, often not included in the routine assessment. Similarly,

the role of urinary uric acid is now recognised as being important (Coe *et al.*, 1975).

Stone analysis

It is important to have a urinary stone analysed for its chemical composition. Crystallographic analysis has provided some interesting information on both the constituents and the incidence of stones in different countries. The constituents may be uric acids, urates, oxalates, phosphates and rarely, cystine and xanthine. Studies have shown that as standards of living improve, so the incidence of bladder stones decreases, renal stones increase and the composition changes towards more oxalates and phosphates (Sutor, 1980). Detailed stone analyses are not generally available and most clinical chemistry laboratories in the UK, will provide only a qualitative analysis and report the presence or absence of calcium, phosphate, ammonium, oxalate and urate.

Renal tubular acidosis (RTA)

A variable degree of interest has been expressed in this condition and in its relevance to stone formation. Patients with RTA have a specific distal tubule defect wherein the tubule is incapable of efficient transport of hydrogen ion, the urine is more alkaline than would be expected and there is a low plasma bicarbonate and often hypokalaemia. This is the complete form of renal tubular acidosis. In some patients where there is a normal plasma bicarbonate and no acidosis, a diagnosis of the incomplete form of RTA is made.

Patients with RTA have a tendency to develop nephrocalcinosis and renal calculi. It is important to make this diagnosis since renal calcification and osteomalacia may disappear with long-term alkali therapy.

It had been thought that RTA was uncommon, but this is more likely to have been because it is not often looked for; in studies where the abnormality has been sought, the incidence is approximately 20% (Williams and Chisholm, 1975). The measurement of the pH in a fasting specimen of urine provides a simple guide to this possible diagnosis; a pH of > 6.0 is an indication to check the pH response to an acid load. The normal response to oral ammonium bicarbonate (0.1 g/kg body weight) is to lower the urinary pH to 5.3 or below. Failure of this response indicates abnormal distal tubule function.

Risk factors

It has long been evident that there are many factors involved in the mechanisms that result in the formation of a stone. None of the measurements already discussed can be interpreted in isolation. The two main chemical events which seem to determine the risk of forming calcium-containing stones are the degree of saturation of urine with calcium oxalate and calcium phosphate and the level of protective inhibitory activity against the crystallisation of calcium oxalate. The concept of risk factors refers to a group of the components associated with these stone forming mechanisms. Thus there appears to be five such components in the urine which influence the risk of calcium oxalate stone formation; calcium, oxalate, pH, acid mucopolysaccharide and uric acid (Robertson *et al.*, 1978).

The measurement of these factors can identify those patients who are at risk of forming stones. It is now hoped that with this information, the clinician will be able to rationalise the treatment for the patient and so give a sensible reply to the question 'what can I do to prevent another stone developing?'

References

Anderson C.K. (1980). Stones: pathogenesis. In *Urology: Tutorials in Postgraduate Medicine* (Chisholm G.D., ed.) London: William Heinemann Medical Books.

Blacklock N.J. (1982). Epidemiology. In *Scientific Foundations of Urology*, 2nd edn. (Chisholm G.D., Williams D.I., eds.). London: William Heinemann Medical Books.

Boyce W.H., Resnick M.I. (1979). Biochemical profiles of stone-forming patients: a guide to treatment. *J. Urol*; **121**:706–10.

Coe F.L., Lawton R.L., Goldstein R.B., Tembe V. (1975). Sodium urate accelerates precipitation of calcium oxalate *in vitro* (38928). *Proc. Soc. Exp. Biol. Med*; **149**:926–9.

Harrison A.R. (1982). Hyperparathyroidism. In *Scientific Foundations of Urology*, 2nd edn. (Chisholm G.D., Williams D.I., eds.). London: William Heinemann Medical Books.

Robertson W.G., Peacock M., Heyburn P.J., Marshall D.H., Clark P.B. (1978). Risk factors in calcium stone disease of the urinary tract. *Brit. J. Urol*; **50**:499–54.

Rose G.A. (1982a). Calcium metabolism; normal and abnormal hormonal control. In *Scientific Foundations of Urology*, 2nd edn. (Chisholm G.D., Williams D.I., eds.). London: William Heinemann Medical Books.

Rose G.A. (1982b). *Urinary Stones: Clinical and Laboratory Aspects*. Lancaster: MTP.

Sherwood T. (1980). *Uroradiology*. Oxford: Blackwell Scientific Publications.

Sutor D.J. (1980). Stones: epidemiology and composition. In *Urology: Tutorials in Postgraduate Medicine*. (Chisholm G.D., ed.). London: William Heinemann Medical Books.

Williams G., Chisholm G.D. (1975). Stone screening and follow-up are necessary? *Brit. J. Urol*; **47**:745–50.

18

Instrumentation

J.G. GOW

The endoscope

The present-day endoscope is a precise instrument. No longer do we depend on a sheath whose source of illumination is an unreliable, insufficiently bright, small filament lamp situated at its tip, and a telescope which transmits inadequate light. The modern instrument which has been developed in the last three decades consists of a selection of sheaths and a telescope which contains glass fibres for transmitting the light and rod lenses for conveying the image to the observer.

Light source

The outstanding advantage of the external light source is that a lamp of high intensity can be used. For routine examinations a quartz iodine lamp of 150 watts is the standard fitting, since this gives a better colour spectrum than the normal tungsten filament bulb. This lamp would seem unnecessarily powerful, but it has to allow for loss by absorption in the glass fibres and at the various connections.

The glass fibre cable

The first great advance to revolutionise all forms of endoscopy was the discovery by Hopkins and Kopani of how to make glass fibres of a small diameter and to bind them into bundles. There are two types of glass fibre bundles – the coherent and incoherent. Coherent bundles are those in which the fibres are arranged so that the position of the fibres at the entrance and exit of the bundle are identical and consequently will transmit an image. They are used in instruments for gastrointestinal examinations and for the fibreoptic dual viewing attachment. They are extremely expensive and delicate.

Incoherent bundles are those in which the fibres are arranged in any order and are used only for conveying light, so that there is no need for the fibres to be arranged as precisely as those in the coherent bundles. The light cables for endoscopy are made of a bundle of incoherent fibres covered with a protective sheath of which there are two types: a flexible and a semi-rigid sheath. The flexible type is thinner with less protection, easier to use, but prone to fibre damage leading to poor light transmission; the semi-rigid type lasts longer, but is more difficult to use.

The telescope

The development of the Hopkins rod lens system for rigid endoscopes was the second great advance which transformed urological endoscopic procedures. The difference between the traditional and the Hopkins system is shown in Fig 18.1. The traditional system uses a group of lenses commencing with an objective, which is followed by a series of relay systems and field lenses which take the image to the eyepiece where it is

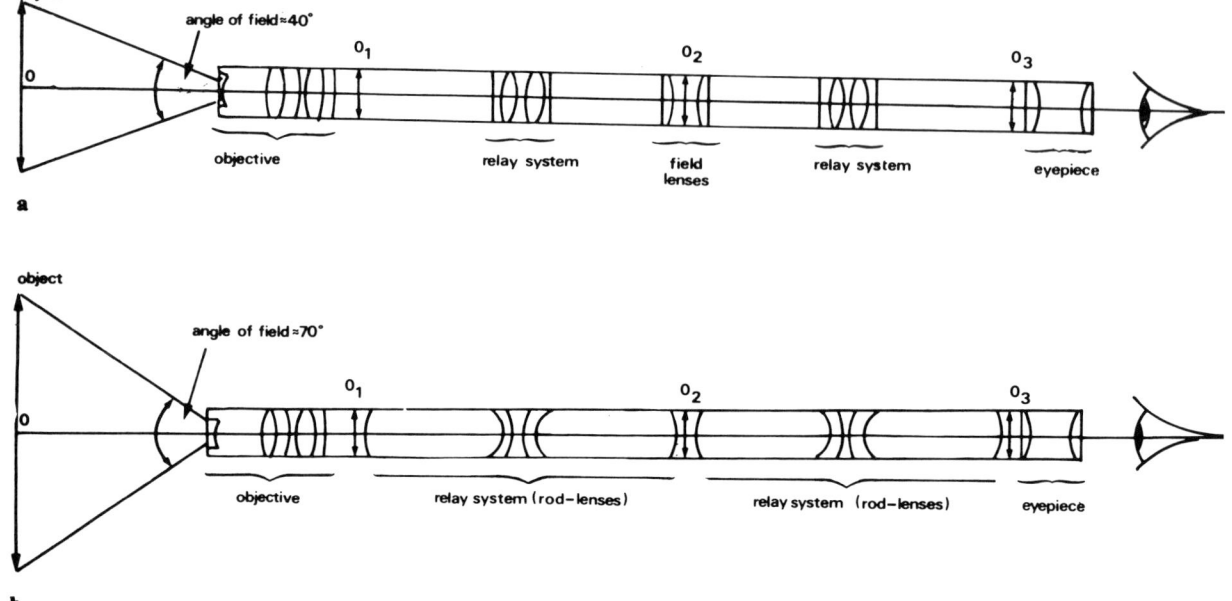

Fig 18.1 Comparison between the traditional and the new Hopkins rod lens system.

magnified before being seen by the observer. In the Hopkins system the image is relayed by a series of five rod lenses from the objective to the eyepiece, both of which are identical in the two systems.

Thus the difference between the two systems is that the traditional design consists of a tube of air with glass lenses, while the Hopkins system consists of a tube of glass with lenses of air. The effect of this change in design is two-fold. First, most of the space in the telescope is glass rather than air, and the amount of light transmitted is proportional to n^2 where n is the refractive index of the space. As n is 1.5 for the type of glass used as opposed to 1.0 for air, the increase in the light transmitted is $(1.5)^2 = 2.25$. Second, total light transmission is proportional to r^4 where r is the radius of the clear aperture; since it is technically easier to mount the rod lens in the telescope, it is possible to use a greater diameter for the lens for a given outer diameter of the telescope. This increase was a factor of 1.4 which gave an improved transmission of $(1.4)^4 = 3.8$. Taking these two factors together, there is an increase in the transmission of light of about nine times. Furthermore, by using this new system it is possible to increase the field of view to 70° in water compared with 40° for the traditional design.

The third important factor which contributed to the brightness and contrast of the image is the adoption of multilayer antireflection coatings of each lens. Without this, the amount of light lost would be unacceptable

and with the lens so treated, only 10% of light is lost during transmission through a system of 40 air/glass surfaces.

Modern telescopes are available in four different angles: 0° direct, 30° foreoblique, 70° lateral and 120° retrograde (Fig 18.2). All have a field of view of 70° under water and are fitted with adaptors on the light pillar so that each telescope can accept the different fibre cables that are available. It is rare for the 120° telescope to be required, or with the wide angle view all of the bladder can be seen with the 30° and 70° telescopes.

Cystourethroscopy

Position

The best position of the patient is supine with hips flexed and abducted to an angle of 45°. Lloyd-Davies supports are excellent as they can be adjusted to suit each patient. The lithotomy position is incorrect: it rotates the pelvis and urethra upwards and makes the endoscopic position awkward. Also, the lithotomy position can cause acute postoperative discomfort in the lumbar spine, especially for day-stay patients. The patient should never be examined flat, for in this position it is impossible to study the roof of the bladder, especially close to the bladder neck.

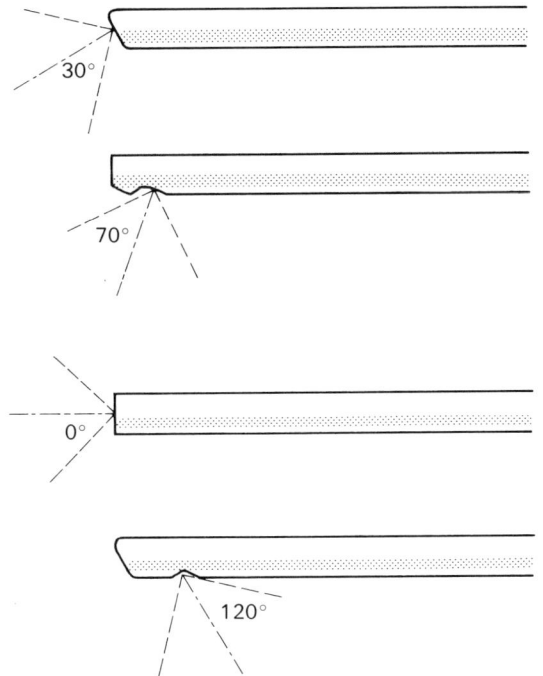

Fig 18.2   Diagram of four different types of telescopes.

Preparation of the urethra

It is important in all endoscopic procedures to reduce the risk of lower urinary tract infection to the minimum and an antiseptic lubricant is recommended. Hibitane 1 in 2000 in glycerine or KY jelly are common lubricants, but the former has to be prepared and the latter is not antiseptic, especially after it has been opened. A sterile disposable prepacked syringe filled with Hibitane and a lubricant is now available in a 'peel-pack' and is ideal for urethral preparations.

Anaesthesia

A local anaesthetic is adequate for many endoscopic procedures, especially in the female; 2% lignocaine with a lubricant gel is a common preparation but the 'peel-pack' syringe described for the preparation of the urethra is available with lignocaine added. For patients who are apprehensive 5 or 10 mg of i.v. Valium can be given. In the male 20 ml of solution will be required and a penile clamp should be placed over the penis for 10 to 15 min before the sheath is introduced. General

anaesthesia will always be required if a bladder biopsy or resection of tumours is required.

The examination

The procedure begins with the examination of the whole of the urethra by direct vision, a urethroscopy, and then the instrument is advanced into the bladder for the cystoscopy. With modern instruments it is never justified to pass the cystoscope 'blindly' as serious damage to the urethra can occur. A cystourethroscopy should not be considered an isolated investigation, but as part of a much wider study which could involve ureteric catheterisation, biopsy of suspicious areas, removal of small stones or foreign bodies, or resection of a bladder tumour. The surgeon must be prepared to deal with an unsuspected stricture of the urethra.

The initial examination is performed using a 16.5 or 17 F sheath cystoscope and a 30° telescope, and a detailed study of the urethra, prostate and bladder carried out. Routine examination of the bladder requires the use of both the 30° and 70° telescopes. The examination technique must be a personal preference for each individual surgeon, but it is essential that the routine should be repetitive and used for every examination, so that all areas of the bladder are always inspected. The roof, especially close to the bladder neck, is a danger zone and inspection of this area will be improved by suprapubic pressure on the dome of the bladder. It is also useful to watch the bladder while filling with irrigation fluid, for small lesions on the roof and the fundus may be more easily seen.

The initial urethroscopy may reveal a urethral stricture, in which case the examining sheath should be withdrawn and replaced by a panendoscope sheath. The panendoscope sheath is similar to the examining sheath, except that it has no beak and is used when endoscopy and urethral surgery are required. When a urethral stricture is discovered a linear incision (urethrotomy) is made at the 12 o'clock position using the optical urethrotome. Formerly, such a stricture would have been dilated by bougies, but these tear the tissues and can provoke further strictures. Bougies, however, still have a place in the treatment of patients with chronic urethral stricture who have been attending for regular bouginage for many years.

Strictures in the female are rare, but distal urethral stenosis is occasionally seen. Hegars dilators are used to dilate the urethra, or alternatively the Otis urethrotome (Fig 18.3) is used, making two incisions at the 3 and 9 o'clock position. Hegars dilators can also be used to dilate the urethra of patients with urethrotrigonitis.

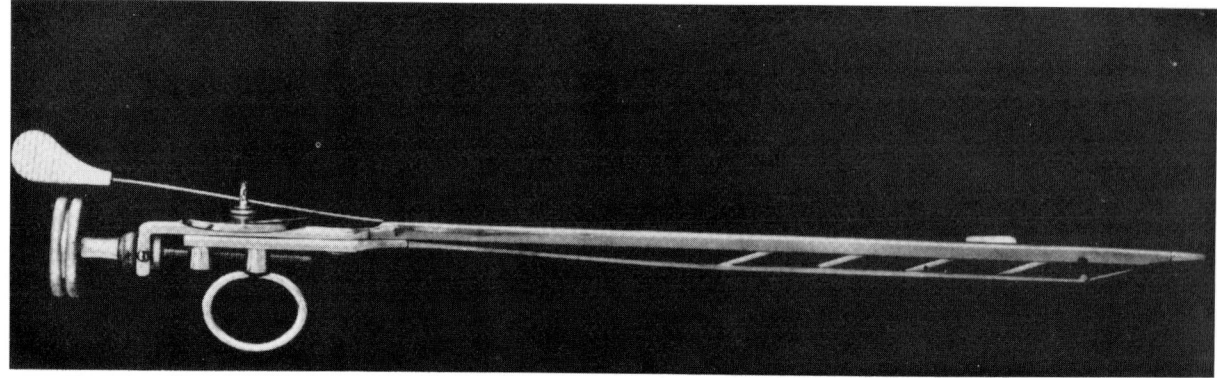

Fig 18.3 The Otis urethrotome.

Special techniques

Bladder biopsy

Any unusual appearance in the bladder mucosa is an indication for a biopsy using biopsy forceps which can be introduced through any sheath larger than 20 F, using a 30° telescope. Multiple biopsies are always taken from both the suspected area and other areas. Because some areas are difficult to reach with the bladder fully distended, the initial biopsies should be taken with only a small amount of irrigating fluid in the bladder.

Transurethral resection

If at cystourethroscopy, a further procedure requiring diathermy excision of the prostate or a bladder tumour is necessary, the cystoscope sheath is changed to a resectoscope sheath. These sheaths are either completely insulated tubes made from woven glass fibres bonded by epoxy resin or metal sheaths with an insulated tip which is bonded to the metal sheath. All of the sheaths can have either short or long beaks, depending on the preference of the operator and they are made in three different sizes (24, 26 and 28 F).

It should be standard practice to insert the resectoscope sheath under direct vision but occasionally, even under direct vision, it is not possible to direct the beak over a prominent middle lobe and an obturator is required.

Ureteric catheterisation

Ureteric catheterisation for a retrograde uretero pyelogram is now an uncommon procedure. However it may be required in the investigation of a suspicious area in the upper urinary tract, an obstruction or for the removal of a ureteric stone. Either a 20 or 22 F cystoscopic sheath is used and a ureteric catheter deflector inserted. Either a 30° or 70° telescope can be used, but 70° is preferred, especially if the ureteric orifice is of the stadium type, i.e. ureteric bar with prominent sides. A size 5 ureteric catheter should be tried first, but in some cases it will not pass and has to be substituted for a size 4. If a uretero pyelogram is to be carried out a Braasch bulb catheter is wedged into the urethral orifice and the x-ray contrast injected through the catheter.

If ureteric catheterisation is used to investigate and possibly remove a stone in the ureter, a Dormia stone basket (Fig 18.4) is passed up the ureter in the same way as a ureteric catheter until it has passed beyond the stone. The basket is then opened and the catheter slowly withdrawn, using a rotating movement to engage the stone. No force should be used since it is easy to damage the ureter. This manoeuvre should be carried out under general anaesthesia with radiographic control.

Stone or foreign body forceps

Cystoscopy may reveal small stones or foreign bodies. These are best removed by small forceps (Fig 18.5) using a 30° telescope. If the stone is too large to pass through the urethra without causing trauma, it can first be crushed and the pieces removed by the instrument or through an evacuator. Large stones up to 2.5 cm in diameter can be crushed by a cystoscopic lithotrite and evacuated in the same way.

Urethral catheters

For haematuria

Haematuria can be complicated by clot retention which can be evacuated through a large Foley or plastic

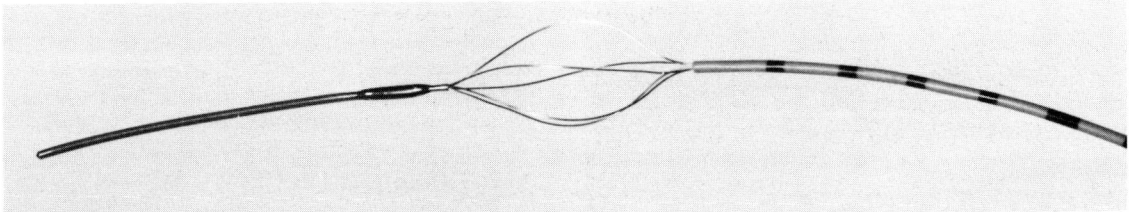

Fig 18.4 Dormia stone extractor.

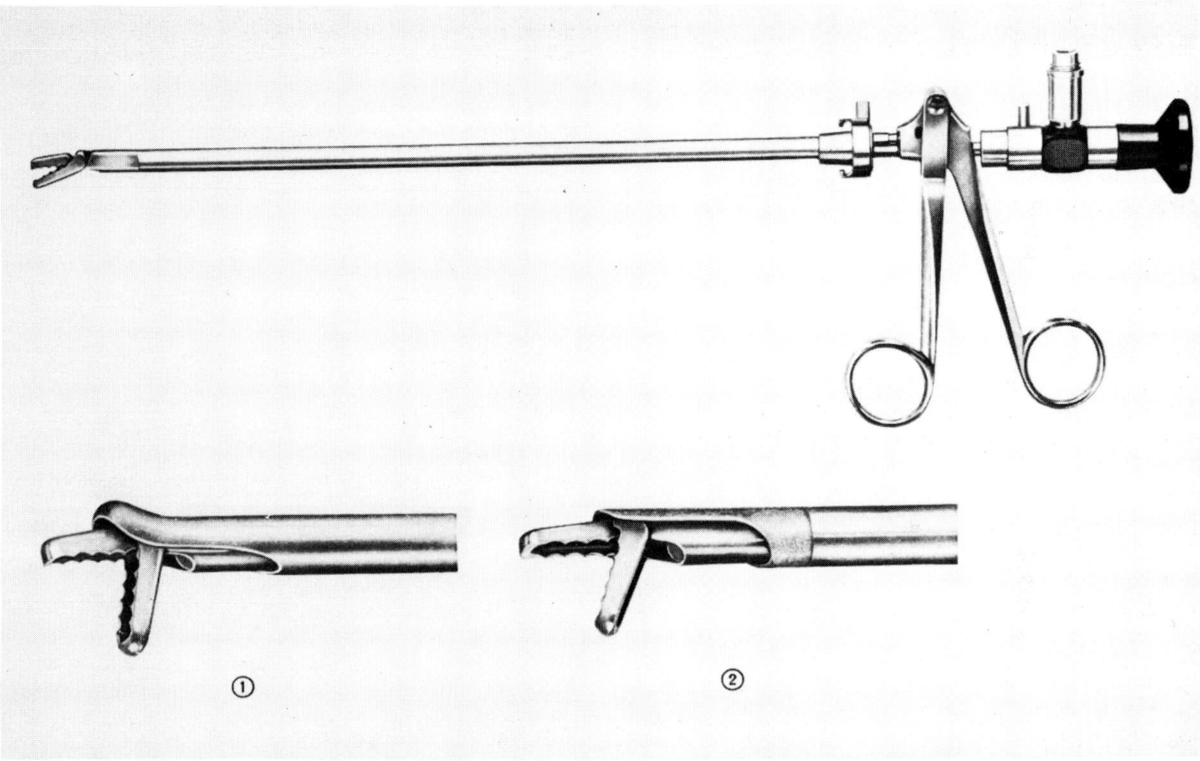

Fig 18.5 Stone and foreign body forceps.

indwelling urethral catheter. If this is unsuccessful, a haematuria catheter (Fig 18.6) can be tried. This is a latex catheter with a large terminal eye which is reinforced with nylon and does not easily collapse, with strong suction. Often this technique will be unsuccessful and the use of a Bigelow or other evacuator is needed and usually requires general anaesthesia.

For acute retention

Acute retention in the male requires urethral catheterisation using the same standard of preparation as described for endoscopic surgery. A 14 or 16 F latex Foley catheter is introduced and the bladder slowly drained over a period of 2 h. Alternatives are the Gibbon or Gow-Gibbon catheters. The Gow-Gibbon has the advantage that the wings can be adjusted to accommodate any length of urethra so that the catheter can be accurately placed at the tip of the penis. Sometimes it is difficult or impossible to pass a urethral catheter in patients with acute retention and rather than persist with catheterisation a suprapubic tube (Fig 18.7) should be inserted. Catheterisation with an introducer can cause considerable damage in an unanaesthetised patient and should not be attempted.

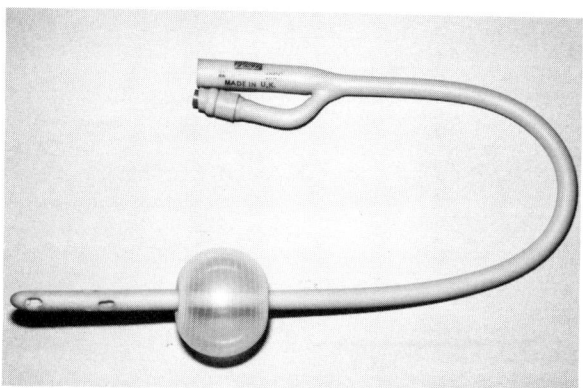

Fig 18.6   Haematuria catheter.

A suprapubic tube is available in presterilised disposable kits, is simple to use and involves no risk of trauma to the urethra; consequently this form of drainage has an important place in the management of acute retention in the male.

Acute retention in the female is rare and a Foley latex catheter gives satisfactory drainage.

Postoperative catheter care

After most open or endoscopic procedures involving the bladder, an indwelling urethral catheter is required. The details for the management of these catheters and the types of catheter may vary between surgeons and between hospitals but the principles are the same:

The prime objective is to avoid urinary tract infections and the introduction of the catheter must be made with full aseptic precautions. The catheter must be attached to a closed drainage system (Fig 18.8) which remains untouched and intact, apart from emptying the bag, until the catheter is removed. If, for example, the drainage system is open for a bladder wash out, full aseptic precautions must be taken.

A Foley latex catheter is satisfactory for routine postoperative drainage. If long-term urethral catheterisation is expected, a silastic catheter should be used as this does not require changing for at least 4 weeks.

Sterilisation of instruments

It is accepted that heat is the only safe way of guaranteeing absolute sterility. Unfortunately, this ideal is not applicable to all urological instruments, for many are too large; others are too delicate or will disintegrate under the intense heat of the high pressure steam autoclave. Sterility implies the destruction of all organisms, spores and viruses, but is this high ideal really necessary in urology? As it cannot be always achieved, the standard should be relaxed and disinfection – the destruction of harmful organisms but not bacterial spores – accepted, as there are many situations in urology when bacterial spores do not create a problem and in these situations sterilisation is not vital, but disinfection is mandatory. It cannot be stressed too often that if disinfection is being employed, a very high standard of instrument cleaning is essential.

The *high pressure steam autoclave* should be used to sterilise metal instruments such as sheaths, catheter deflectors, biopsy forceps and resectoscopes (the complete cycle takes 15 to 20 min), but some other system is necessary for the delicate and expensive telescopes and fibreoptic equipment. Two methods are available: chemical disinfection or low pressure steam with and without formalines. There are two chemical disinfectants in common use: glutaraldehyde and chlorhexidine.

Glutaraldehyde is a buffered dialdehyde solution and is active in up to 20% serum, has a low toxicity for living cells and once activated remains active for a week. It has no effect on optical cements or chemical substances and kills common organisms within 5 min. It is probably the best solution for immersing instruments, but it has the big disadvantage that it causes local contact reaction, including dermatitis, conjunctivitis and

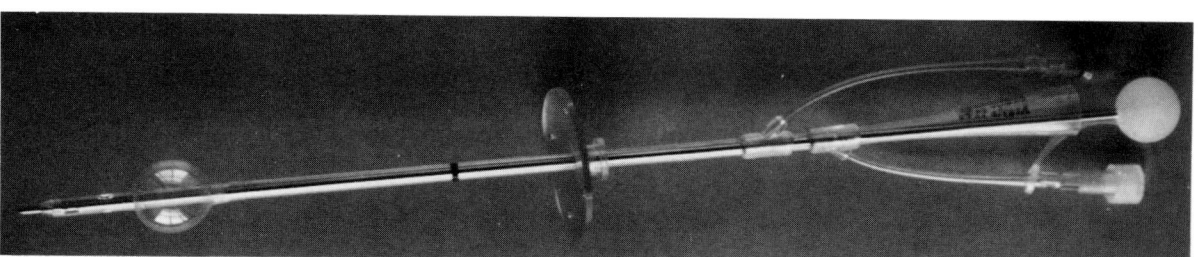

Fig 18.7   Suprapubic catheter set.

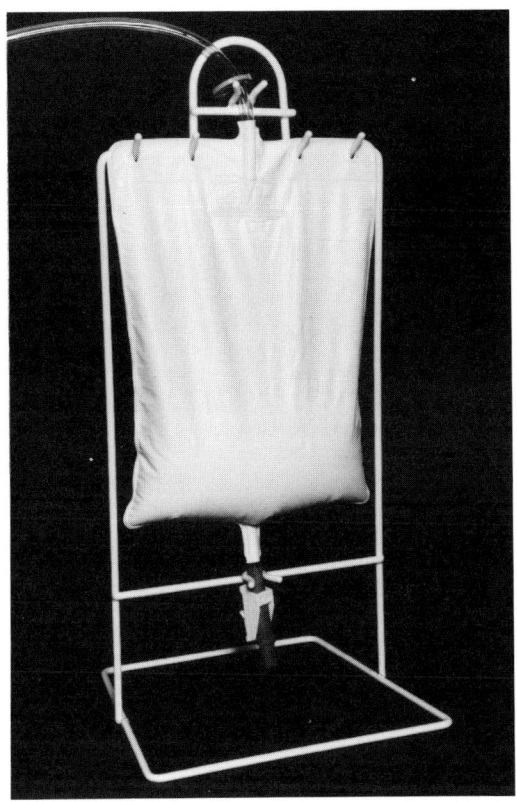

Fig 18.8   Closed bladder drainage system.

1% solutions it will kill most organisms found in urological practice within 10 min. It is, however, inactivated in the presence of blood or serum. If it is employed for sterilsing instruments, users must appreciate that if it is dissolved in alcohol, it can damage cements used in the construction of telescopes and that the use of steam sterilisation after immersion in hibitane in spirit is absolutely contraindicated, as it will almost certainly be followed by damage to the optical system due to softening of the optical cement. Hibitane should always be prepared fresh and discarded after use.

In *low pressure steam autoclaves*, the steam is injected into a chamber where the pressure has been reduced to half an atmosphere and the temperature is about 80°C; this can be tolerated by the delicate telescopes without risk of damage and if formaldehyde is added, it is undoubtedly the best way of sterilising these optical instruments. However, the cycle is long (1–1.25 h) which is unacceptable if a series of endoscopic examinations are required in quick succession, unless several sets of instruments are available. Nevertheless, low pressure steam without formaldehyde will disinfect telescopes and is an acceptable method for use between cases if the equipment is available. It is suggested, therefore, that sets of instruments should be sterilised by low pressure steam and formaldehyde at the end of a list, but that while a list is in progress the delicate telescopes should be disinfected between cases either by low pressure steam or immersed in glutaraldehyde or hibitane in 70% spirit and the other equipment by the high pressure steam autoclave.

peripheral inflammation, so that many operators are unable to use it.

Chlorhexidine is active against a wide spectrum of organisms, but it is only active against mycotuberculosis if dissolved in 70% alcohol. The speed of activity depends upon the concentration and in 0.5 or

Further reading

Gow J.G. (1978). *Handbook of Urological Endoscopy*. Edinburgh: Churchill Livingstone.
Mitchell J.P. (1981). *Endoscopic Operative Urology*. Bristol: John Wright.

19

Urodynamics

ERIC S. GLEN

Urodynamics involve the study of the transport of urine from the kidneys to the exterior, including the storage and voiding phases of bladder function. At present the upper and lower urinary tracts are usually considered separately, the dividing point being the uretero-vesical junction. Study of the upper urinary tract remains mainly a project for research and has not yet become applicable in routine clinical practice. Present techniques for studying innervation, motility and pressure changes in renal pelvis and ureter are invasive; new methods may be developed as a result of these. Controversy continues as to the role of renal scan and pressure measurements in the assessment of hydronephrosis and much depends on the expertise of the team and the facilities available. In the meantime, urodynamic studies of the lower urinary tract do provide information of clinical value and will be dealt with first.

Urodynamics of lower urinary tract

The commoner urodynamic investigations are outlined in Table 1. These investigations have the following uses:

1 Elucidation of disorders of micturition affecting storage, voiding or both.
2 Continuing research into the basic physiology of normal and disordered bladder and urethral function.

Table 1

Basic clinical urodynamic investigations
  1 Cystometry
  2 Urine flow studies
  3 Estimation of urine loss in incontinence

More complex investigations
  1 Combined pressure flow studies
  2 Combined pressure flow studies plus synchronous voiding cystourethrography
  3 Urethral closure pressure profile measurement
  4 Electromyographic studies of pelvic floor, urethral and periurethral muscle

There is still considerable dispute about the nature and significance of bladder and urethral innervation, and great scope for pharmacological studies leading to improved treatment.

Urodynamic procedures should be kept in perspective and should be used only after routine clinical assessment, ensuring that the full spectrum of interacting symptoms and conditions can be taken into account. For example, many women approaching the menopause and younger women on the pill succeed in persuading doctors to prescribe a diuretic for supposed fluid retention, described as a feeling of being increasingly bloated or distended as the day goes on. This coupled with the common high intake of tea or coffee will lead to frequency and urgency of micturition, possibly going on to urge incontinence. Change or cessation of diuretic therapy may restore normal function without recourse to urodynamic investigations. Many conditions including urinary tract infection, bladder tumours, neurological and psychiatric disorders may also affect bladder function.

A detailed history and examination are important parts of a urodynamic assessment (Table 2). Current

Table 2
MINIMUM REQUIREMENTS FOR INITIAL ASSESSMENT PRIOR TO URODYNAMIC INVESTIGATION

1   Full clinical history including:
      General health
      Current medication
      Previous history including neurological conditions
      Frequency and pattern of micturition
      Fluid intake including alcohol
      Mental state etc.
      Social and family history
2   General examination including neurological assessment
3   Urine culture and testing for glycosuria
4   Excretion urography including postvoiding film:
      Essential only when abnormalities of upper tract are suspected or must be excluded e.g. in presence of recurring urinary infections, neurological disorders, or when previous surgery may have jeopardised the urinary tract.
5   Cystourethroscopy

medication and its possible effects on the bladder and urethra should be considered. If possible, cholinergics and anticholinergics should be stopped and the patient reassessed before proceeding to urodynamic investigations. A high level of suspicion, attention to detail and wide clinical experience is necessary if these investigations are to be of value. It is not productive simply to refer a patient for urodynamic investigation expecting a report like an ECG. The overlap of interests and the need for liaison are shown in Table 3.

Table 3
RANGE OF SPECIALIST INTERESTS

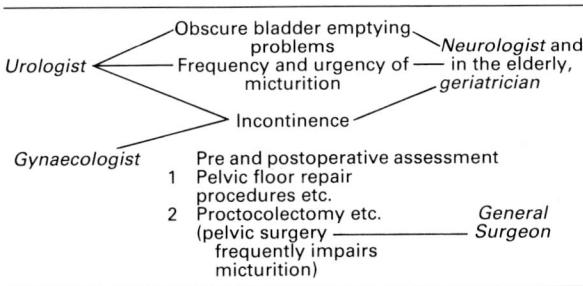

N.B. Close collaboration with a physicist or bio-engineer is essential.

Cystometry

This is a method of measuring pressure changes relative to volume of fluid in the bladder. Measurement may be made:

1   during filling;
2   at relatively constant volume;
3   during procedures designed to provoke bladder activity either as the bladder is filled or at static volume;
4   during attempted voiding. The measurement may then be combined with measurement of voiding flow rate, flow time and pattern of voiding (Fig 19.1)

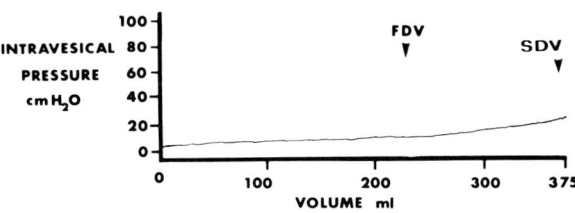

Fig 19.1a   FDV = First desire to void; SDV = Strong desire to void. At this point the patient is asked to inhibit detrusor activity. Subsequently cystometry can be continued during voiding or attempted voiding. Various provocative measures such as coughing, may be used to elicit abnormal detrusor activity that the patient may or may not be able to inhibit on demand. Sensation may be absent in neurological disorders, e.g. paraplegia. However, increase in depth and frequency of respiration is usually noticeable when the bladder is stretched to capacity. There may be profound alterations in blood pressure in these individuals.

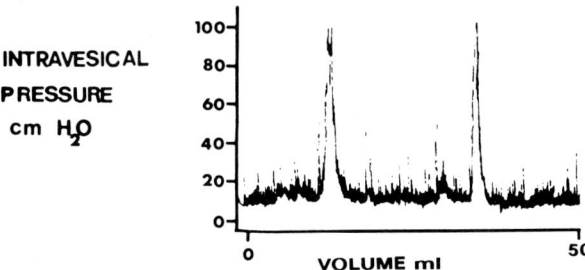

Fig 19.1b   Example of gross uninhibited bladder activity. Leakage of urine occurred with each of the high spikes of pressure.

If measurement is continued over a period of time, allowance should be made for the volume of urine entering the bladder, particularly in individuals with a tendency to diuresis.

Cystometry was first performed in the middle of the 19th century using water as the filling medium. However, the advent of transducers has revolutionised many measurements and cystometry is no exception. Pressure changes in the bladder are conducted to the transducer by a fluid-filled catheter and connecting line. Movement in the transducer is converted into electric signals by a strain gauge and these signals are amplified and displayed on a recording device. Usually a double lumen urethral catheter is employed although, alternatively, a suprapubic cannula from a cystotomy pack may be used. Measuring intravesical pressure in this way is preferable during voiding studies leaving the urethra free of tubes.

Care should be exercised in choosing the type of catheter or cannula. The sensitivity of the system decreases as the internal diameter of the tube decreases and as its length and compliance increase. A double lumen urethral catheter can be used for cystometry combined with urethral closure pressure profile measurement (Fig 19.2). Urethral catheters bearing microtransducers are becoming more popular as their reliability improves, but they remain relatively expensive.

Gas cystometry

Some workers prefer gas as a filling medium in cystometry. It has the advantage of avoiding spillage of water once the bladder is empty and is, therefore, easier for the clinician in a consulting room. Gas is unsuitable for accurate and repeated investigations and is less physiological than water or saline.

Technique

The International Continence Society Standardising Committee has produced recommendations, and some of these are summarised in Table 4.

It is essential to calibrate the system to avoid artefact. Although measurement of intravesical pressure during normal day-to-day activity is ideal, the systems available impose severe restrictions. For example, it is difficult to vary the zero level (upper margin of symphysis pubis) to take into account even simple movement such as sitting up or standing. Vibration affects the fluid manometer lines and catheter and produce characteristic interference changes. Changes of pressure occur when the patient moves, talks, coughs etc. due to alterations in intra-abdominal pressure. The patient should be observed throughout the procedure, and events such as movement or vibration should be entered on the trace.

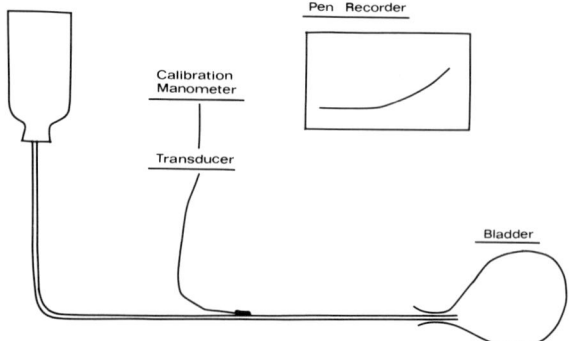

Fig 19.2a Schematic representation of technique for cystometry. Pen recorders have good response characteristics and give clear permanent records. They are preferable to those systems using ink jets or ultraviolet light sensitive paper.

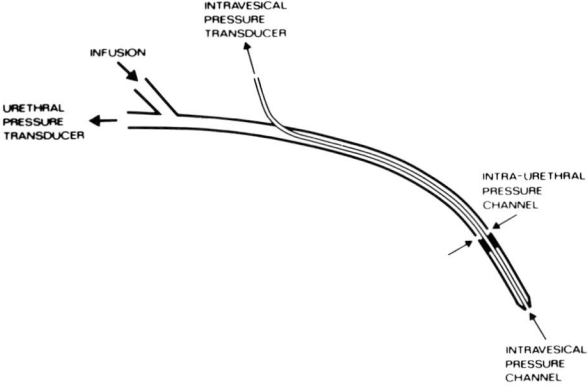

Fig 19.2b Double lumen catheter with Y connector enabling cystometry to be continued during UCPP measurement. Portex Ltd of Hythe, England, now make available a presterilised disposable catheter to our design (Ref. No. 499/042/001/010).

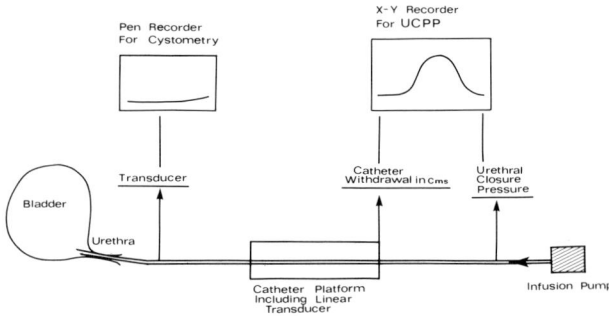

Fig 19.2c Cystometry and urethral closure pressure profile measurement.

Table 4
FROM RECOMMENDATION OF STANDARDISING COMMITTEE OF INTERNATIONAL CONTINENCE SOCIETY RELATING TO CYSTOMETRY

Table 4

FROM RECOMMENDATION OF STANDARDISING COMMITTEE OF INTERNATIONAL CONTINENCE SOCIETY RELATING TO CYSTOMETRY

1 Zero reference for pressure is the level of superior edge of symphysis pubis.
2 Residual urine should be measured before filling starts.
3 In reports, specify:
    (a) Access (transurethral or percutaneous).
    (b) Medium (liquid or gas).
    (c) Temperature of medium (in degrees Celsius). Ice cold water can be used for detrusor provocation.
    (d) Position of patient: supine, sitting or standing.
    (e) Filling (continuous or incremental). The precise filling rate should be stated. When incremental filling used, the volume of increment should be stated.
    (f) Type of catheter e.g. Single or double lumen catheter or multiple catheters, transducer tipped etc. Name of manufacturer, and size of catheter.
    (g) Type of measuring equipment.

Without this information, it is impossible to compare results from different clinics.

Table 5

ROUTINE QUESTIONS SPECIFIC TO BLADDER FUNCTION

Frequency of micturition by day and night
Fluid intake – 1   Volume
             2   Nature e.g. strong tea, coffee, alcohol
             3   Timing of intake
Concomitant therapy e.g. diuretic
                        anticholinergic
Degree of urgency of micturition
Hesitancy
Force of flow
Prolonged flow and relation to volume voided
Continuous or intermittent flow
Spraying, jet or dribble
Terminal dribbling after main stream
Feeling of incomplete voiding
Encores i.e. The need to void a second time within minutes
Sensation: Awareness of bladder when full
                   Pain related to degree of bladder distension
Incontinence: Frequency and degree
The duration of symptoms and variation in severity should be recorded

To avoid some of these errors, the intra-abdominal pressure should be subtracted from the cystometric pressure – called the subtracted pressure. The subtraction is made electronically and the result recorded on an additional channel. Intra-abdominal pressure is measured by means of an intrarectal fluid-filled cannula.

Measurement of bladder emptying

Many factors influence the way in which we void, such as environment, volume in bladder, medications, infections, caffeine and stress etc. Observation of our own micturition patterns over the course of a week or so will demonstrate the futility of drawing conclusions from a single measurement of flow rate even if it is combined with bladder and intra-abdominal pressure recording. The patient's own account of micturition and bladder awareness provide essential background when the right questions are asked (Table 5). More accurate information can be obtained by recording the maximum flow rate, flow time, volume voided and pattern of flow. Multiple measurements are required before drawing conclusions.

Some attempts must be made to determine whether there is residual urine, either by radiology or by catheterisation. Simple catheter drainage, even when assisted by aspiration, can be misleading since, for example, a flaccid large capacity bladder may not drain readily, while aspiration may suck the bladder wall onto the eyes of the catheter and occlude it. Over-enthusiastic use of lubricating jelly during catheterisa-

tion may also impede drainage initially since the commoner lubricants are water miscible not soluble.

Clinicians in the past have suggested that observation of micturition in a natural environment is as good, if not better, than interpretation of a flow meter recording. None has satisfactorily described how females can usefully be observed in action. The common inhibition experienced when asked for a specimen of urine emphasises that there will be problems when individuals are asked to void while under direct observation. Non-invasive techniques that allow for the measurement of the urinary flow rate in privacy are increasingly popular.

Flowmeters

A variety of techniques has been devised to measure the urinary flow rate (Table 6). The flowmeter made by Disa is widely used in urodynamic centres (Fig 19.3). It is simple to operate by an attendant in another room allowing privacy. Alternatively, the patient can operate it by pressing a button prior to voiding. Fewer mistakes are made if an attendant operates the mechanism, and the act of micturition can be performed without the patient worrying about the mechanisms of the device. Although this instrument has been shown to be reliable in urodynamic units, artefacts are likely when used in routine clinics or primary care surgeries for screening purposes. The apparatus requires calibration at the start of each session. The expertise of a physicist in monitoring its performance is essential, although this may not be possible on a day-to-day basis.

Table 6
SOME METHODS FOR RECORDING BLADDER EMPTYING FLOW

1 *Rotating disc.* A special disc tends to slow down when urine flow strikes it. The amount of electrical energy required to maintain the disc velocity is proportional to the urine flowrate. In practice this is not linear, but the difference is minimised by electronic compensation in the device. The Disa flowmeter uses this method.

2 *Air displacement.* Urine flow is funnelled into a closed vessel, displacing air. The volume displaced is measured by a constant temperature anemometer or by a pneumotachograph.

3 *Gravimetric.* The increase in weight of urine collected during micturition is plotted against time.

4 *Radioisotope.* The clearance of a radioisotope from the bladder during micturition can be measured and recorded.

5 *Drop spectrometer.* The urinary stream breaks up into drops within a short distance of the external urethral meatus. The drop sizes and velocities are measured and the instantaneous flow rate computed. This is costly, involving a computer.

6 *Peakometer.* This consists of a plastic disposable device that measures peak flow rate and volume voided. The maximum flow rate (peak flow) is recorded on an indicator strip without recourse to electronics. The strip changes colour as the level of urine rises in the chamber and by this dip stick effect registers volume voided. Flow time and pattern of voiding cannot be detected by this apparatus, but it does offer a simple test of voiding function. An added advantage is that a sample of the voided urine can be used for urine culture, the apparatus being sterile.

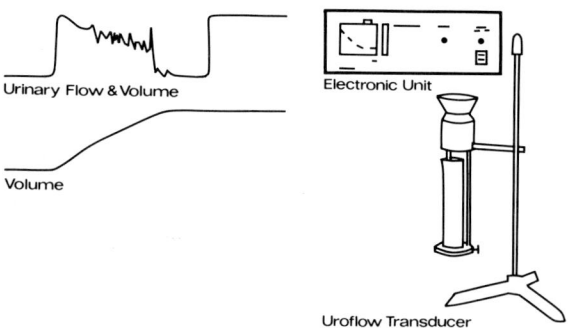

Urinary Flow & Volume

Volume

Electronic Unit

Uroflow Transducer

Fig 19.3   The Disa mictiometer.

Combined pressure flow measurements

In order to obtain more detailed information about bladder function during micturition, it is necessary to measure intravesical pressure, and derive detrusor pressure by subtraction of abdominal pressure. This measurement is more important during attempted micturition when abdominal straining may be used in individuals with outlet obstruction or defective bladder and urethral innervation. Despite some possible objections, most clinicians fill the bladder by means of a urethral catheter, enabling more accurate control of rate and volume of filling. Some prefer to use a second suprapubic cannula, or a double lumen suprapubic catheter. In any event, it is important that pressure recording is made by a separate channel when filling rates exceed 2 ml/min, otherwise distortion will result from the effect of the filling medium. Obviously, none of these procedures is physiological and every effort should be used to minimise the number of tubes and devices.

Combined pressure flow studies with filling and voiding cystometry and the measurement of detrusor pressure will differentiate between voiding resulting from detrusor contraction and voiding produced by abdominal straining. These measurements will determine whether high, normal or low pressures are produced, and correlate these pressures with resulting bladder emptying flow rate, volume voided, voiding time and pattern of voiding. Management of the patient can then be based on these measurements and may involve drugs to stimulate the detrusor, or surgery to relieve outlet obstruction.

A high pressure system associated with poor voiding may result from detrusor-sphincter dyssynergia or physical obstruction. Micturating (or voiding) cysto-urethrography (MCU) is required to differentiate between these conditions and it may be performed separately or simultaneously with combined pressure studies. In addition, the examination should determine the presence or absence of reflux into the ureters. The stress cystourethrogram favoured by gynaecologists in the past to demonstrate the vesicourethral angle is now known to be of little value. Response to straining can be more usefully assessed before asking the patient to void for an MCU.

Synchronous pressure flow-voiding cystourethrography

The development of this procedure began in 1953 and has extended to the present stage where the MCU is recorded on video tape with synchronous recording of pressure flow measurements and flow pattern side by side, or as a superimposed image, by means of an electronic mixer (Fig 19.4). Superimposed images sometimes lack clarity, and it is usually better to record MCU and pressure studies side-by-side.

The technique gives a complete and, if necessary, permanent record while involving the minimum of radiation. Unfortunately, the optimum equipment is not available in many x-ray departments; in the absence of this facility it is probably better to perform combined pressure flow measurements as a separate procedure in females, since this can easily be done while the patient is seated.

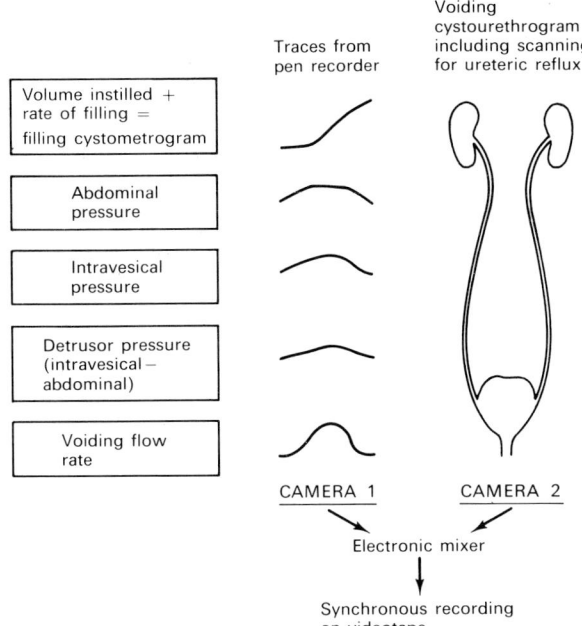

Traces from pen recorder

Voiding cystourethrogram including scanning for ureteric reflux

Volume instilled + rate of filling = filling cystometrogram

Abdominal pressure

Intravesical pressure

Detrusor pressure (intravesical – abdominal)

Voiding flow rate

CAMERA 1   CAMERA 2

Electronic mixer

Synchronous recording on videotape

Fig 19.4 Synchronous pressure flow – voiding cysto-urethrography. It is helpful to include sound recording so that instructions to patients such as the command to void etc. can be included in the synchronous record for future reference and possible comparison with subsequent studies. The videotape is also useful for teaching purposes and comments about artefacts, interpretation of findings and proposed management are helpful in this context.

The main use of synchronous pressure flow MCU is to determine whether or not detrusor-urethral dyssyngergia exists. Note that this condition can be sub-divided into detrusor-sphincter dyssynergia, when the striated sphincter is involved, and detrusor-bladder neck dyssynergia, when the smooth muscle of bladder neck is involved. If distal urethral smooth muscle is involved, it is suggested that this should be specified as detrusor urethral (distal smooth muscle) dyssynergia. These defintions are based on discussions leading to the Fourth Report from the ICS Committee on Standardisation of Terminology (1981). The definitions are given here because of the importance in identifying the structure concerned. The word 'sphincter' is used frequently in a loose way, and should be reserved for the urethral and periurethral striated muscle when discussing detrusor-sphincter dyssynergia. Dyssynergia between detrusor and the various components of the closure mechanism involves simultaneous contraction, preventing flow. Normal micturition involves relaxation of the urethral mechanisms, this relaxation usually occurring just before the onset of detrusor contraction

although some women void with little or no detrusor activity. Dyssynergia is most readily identified when synchronous studies reveal high detrusor pressure and sustained bladder neck and/or urethral closure preventing flow. Detrusor pressure will depend on the state of the detrusor itself, and may be low if decompensation has occurred. Dyssynergia is probably overdiagnosed at present, the diagnosis requiring careful and detailed investigation by experienced clinicians.

Electromyography

The recording of electrical activity of muscle can be invaluable provided the active muscle is identified and extraneous interference is kept to the minimum. The limitations when applied to clinical urodynamics are obvious, although efforts are being made to improve techniques. Target areas are levator ani and periurethral muscles, external urethral spincter and external anal sphincter. EMG can be recorded by means of either surface or needle electrodes.

Surface electrodes

Adhesive discs on the skin represent the least invasive approach, but they are not acceptable for critical measurement.

Anal plug. This device is used to measure EMG activity of the anal sphincter. It has been said that anal sphincter EMG activity reflects that of the urethral sphincter, but Nordling and his colleagues found that only 58% of 53 patients studied had identical reflex activity when the two sphincters were compared. EMG measurement is of particular interest in patients with known or suspected neurological disorders. Unfortunately, insertion of the anal plug may stimulate reflex such as leg spasm, voiding or defaecation, while any movement of the plug is liable to create electrical interference sufficient to obscure muscle activity.

Needle electrodes

There are two types: (a) monopolar using a single core needle in the muscle and an indifferent electrode to complete the circuit, and (b) bipolar (coaxial) and this is the most popular needle.

Insertion of needle electrodes into levator ani, periurethral muscle and external anal sphincter can be relatively accurate, but uncomfortable in patients with normal sensation. Insertion into the external urethral sphincter is not so easy although several methods have been tried.

Urethral closure pressure profile (UCPP)

There are several methods for the measurement of UCPP (Fig 19.5). The profile measures, urethral length and the pressure exerted along that length (Fig 19.6). Urethral closure pressure profile is an accurate name now recommended by the ICS Standardising Committee.

UCPP tends to alter as the bladder fills and for this reason it is essential to know the volume in the bladder. The normal urethra may show an increase in its functional length and/or the pressure exerted along that length as the bladder fills (Fig 19.7a). A urethra with defective closure mechanisms may show deterioration in either or both components of the UCPP (Fig 19.7b), and a fibrosed inelastic urethra may show a poor UCPP

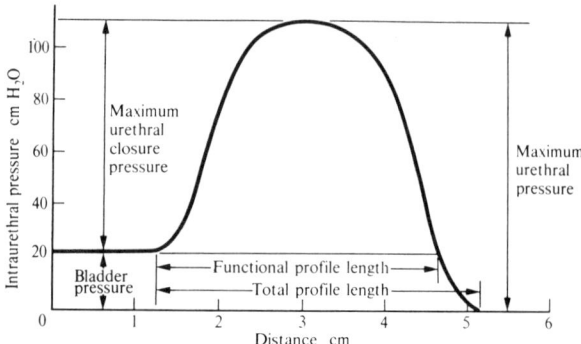

Fig 19.6   A schematic representation of the urethral closure pressure profile.

with little or no change as the bladder fills. It is, therefore, best to measure UCPP when the bladder is almost empty and again when the bladder is filled to near its functioning capacity. Uninhibited detrusor activity can produce deterioration of UCPP as voiding is initiated. Measurement of UCPP involves movement of a catheter or other instrument along the urethra, and such movement commonly provokes detrusor activity when there is an abnormality of innervation e.g. multiple sclerosis. For this reason, it is best to use a double lumen catheter to permit simultaneous recording of intravesical pressure and UCPP (Fig 19.2). Although these urethral changes resulting from alterations in bladder volume and from detrusor activity have been described by Enhorning and others, it is still common for UCPP measurements to be made without either measurement of the volume of water in the bladder or simultaneous cystometry; it is for this reason that the value of UCPP has not been fully appreciated. More accurate assessment is possible when stress tests are imposed and intravesical pressure is subtracted electronically to give the closure pressure.

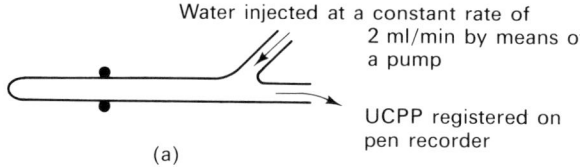

(a)

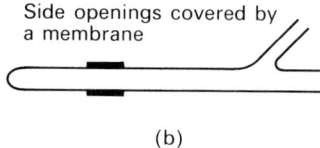

(b)

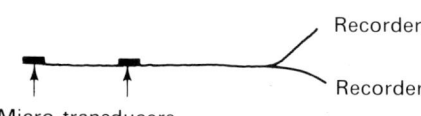

(c)

Fig 19.5   Various types of catheter systems for measuring urethral closure pressure profile. (a) Urethral catheter with two opposing side holes. The catheter is withdrawn either by hand or mechanically and a linear transducer registers accurately the withdrawal in centimetres. (b) This catheter has one or multiple urethral measuring points covered by a membrane. The system is filled with water which allows transmission of pressure change to the transducer (and recorder). (c) This device represents an ideal; present models are both expensive and fragile.

Recording nappy

Measurement of the degree of incontinence suffered by patients is difficult and usually highly subjective. Standards of hygiene are variable. Questions should include how often underwear is changed and if protective pads are worn, how many pads are used per day and how wet are they on removal.

A man who changes his underpants two or three times per week does not require urodynamic investigations for incontinence, although one such individual referred to our clinic still complains of this. Improved hygiene, the use of cotton rather than nylon pants with more frequent changes should remove this problem.

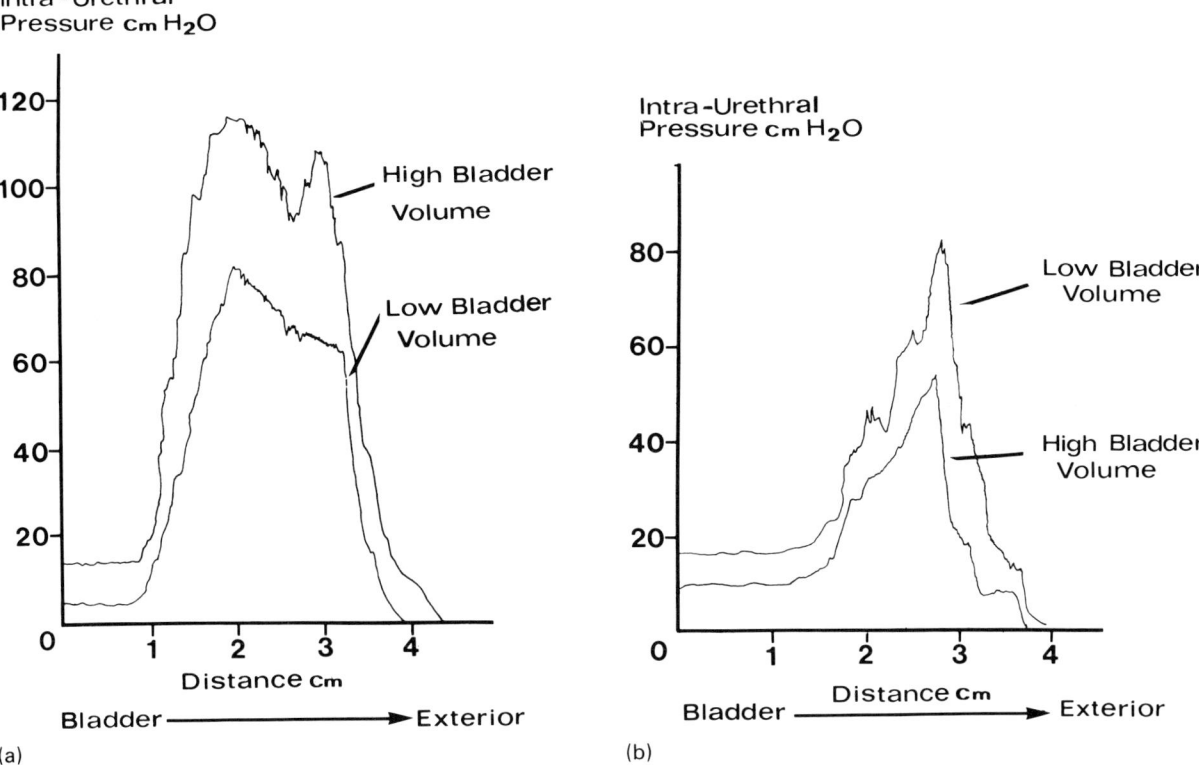

Fig 19.7(a) One variety of normal UCPP showing increase in pressure and length as the bladder fills. *(b)* UCPP showing deterioration as the bladder fills.

The Sphincter Research Unit in Exeter have introduced many innovations to the assessment and treatment of incontinence, not least of which is the concept of using a recording nappy. The nappy consists of a sensor pad impregnated with dry electrolyte that enables the recording of volume of urine leaked and number of episodes of leaking. Caldwell has combined this investigation with intravesical pressure recording results by means of a fine transducer. The patient can move within the limits of long leads connecting the nappy and transducer to the recorder. Telemetry has been tried without much success. The version available commercially is less accurate and is of variable reliability. Nevertheless, it is of value in clinical assessment when the history of incontinence is in doubt.

Urodynamics of the upper urinary tract

The upper urinary tract is less accessible to urodynamic studies involving pressure and EMG measurement,

and until recently most of the literature was concerned with animal experiments.

Investigations include:

1 intravenous urography including high dose contrast and diuresis;
2 micturition cystoureterography;
3 retrograde ureterography;
4 antegrade urography;
5 isotope clearance;
6 ultrasound;
7 frequency of contraction in ureter;
8 manometry of renal pelvis and ureter;
9 EMG.

In recent years improved techniques have provided much higher quality intravenous urography and include the use of high dosage of contrast, fluid loading and tomography. When renal function is so poor that even these techniques fail, ultrasound can be used to obtain more information about the kidneys and renal pelvis. Retrograde catheterisation is seldom required now, but when it is necessary to demonstrate ureter and renal pelvis in this way, the image intensifier provides maximum information with minimum radiation, including some indication of the activity in the ureter. Intravenous urography employing the image intensifier can be used to demonstrate speed of transit from renal pelvis and ureter into bladder, further reducing the need for retrograde studies. Micturition cystoureterography may be required to distinguish between vesicoureteric reflux and ureters obstructed at bladder level.

Manometry has been advocated, but is not widely accepted. It involves the percutaneous insertion of a fine cannula into the renal pelvis. The technique is most likely to be useful when it is suspected that renal function is deteriorating due to postrenal obstruction, or when pain may relate to a high pressure system, despite apparently normal radiology. However, the flow of fluid advocated is unphysiological and interpretation can be difficult.

Urodynamics of the upper urinary tract at present is of value in the experimental study of urine transport through calix into renal pelvis, ureter and thence into bladder. Our understanding of the physiology and pathophysiology is increasing, and from this may develop techniques that are more acceptable in clinical practice. In the meantime, it is useful to remember that size and frequency of the urine bolus in the ureter increase with diuresis, until the ureter can no longer coordinate peristalsis, and flow becomes disorganised. In other words, diuresis or injection of fluid may overcome the ability of the normal ureter to transport urine to the bladder. Diuresis intravenous urography may, therefore, give a misleading impression of ureteric obstruction.

Renography may be affected in the same way. Studies comparing the hydrated and dehydrated states claim to have shown over-diagnosis of obstruction in those with greatly dilated upper urinary tracts and under-diagnosis in those with early obstruction. However, the techniques against which renography was assessed are not universally accepted.

Measurement of transit time between renal parenchyma and the collecting system can be made using radioactive isotopes. Increased transit time is found in obstructive nephropathy, but whether this can be used as an index of obstruction is debatable since other factors influence transit time. More work is required before any of these tests can be accepted in clinical practice and it may be the answer will be found in some new technique.

In the meantime, intravenous urography and micturition cystoureterography are of proven value, supplemented by antegrade pyeloureterography, ultrasound and possibly renography. The increased emphasis on conserving kidneys, and bolder attempts at reducing obstruction even in kidneys with little apparent func-

tion has led to clinical evidence that the kidney has greater potential for recovery than might have been expected. What we still need is an accurate method for the prediction of recoverable renal function so that conservative surgery may be based on sound functional criteria.

Ureteric stents are now available, and can be inserted either endoscopically or by percutaneous nephrostomy, placing one end in the renal pelvis and the other in the bladder. It is possible to use these stents in the assessment of borderline hydronephrosis at one extreme, and in gross hydronephrosis at the other. When relief of renal angle pain follows insertion of a stent and the collecting system returns to more normal calibre, the diagnosis is certain. When gross hydronephrosis is present, drainage by this relatively atraumatic procedure permits accurate assessment and preservation of residual renal function. Now that reliable ureteric stents can be left in the ureter for many months, the treatment of hydronephrosis requires reassessment.

Further reading

British Journal of Urology (1981). Fourth report on the standardisation of terminology of lower urinary tract function. *Brit. J. Urol*; **53**:333–5.

Caldwell K.P.S. ed (1975). *Urinary Incontinence.* Tunbridge Wells: Pitman Medical (Sector Publishing).

Cantor E.B., Thomas C.C., eds. (1979). *Female Urinary Stress Incontinence.* Illinois: Springfield.

Johnston J.H. (1969). The pathogenesis of hydronephrosis in children. *Brit. J. Urol*; **41**:724–34.

Kaufman J.J., Raz S. (1978). Male incontinence. In *The Urologic Clinics of North America*, Vol. 5. No. 2. Philadelphia: W.B. Saunders.

Lupton E.W. *et al.* (1979). Diuresis renography and morphology in upper urinary tract obstruction. *Brit. J. Urol*; **51**:10–14.

O'Reilly, P.H. *et al.* (1981). The dilated non-obstructed renal pelvis. *Brit. J. Urol*; **53**:205–9.

Rowan D. (1976). The study and control of bladder – urethral function. In *References of Literature Published in the English Language* 1976 onwards.

Schulman C.C. (1981). *Advances in Diagnostic Urology.* Berlin: Springer-Verlag.

The Journal of Urology (1979). The Standardisation of terminology of lower urinary tract function: collation of first 3 reports from the International Continence Society Standardising Committee. *J. Urol*; **121**:551–4.

Turner-Warwick R., Whiteside C.G. (1979). Clinical urodynamics. In *The Urologic Clinics of North America*, Vol. 6. No. 1. Philadelphia: W.B. Saunders.

Whitaker R. (1979). Clinical application of upper urinary tract dynamics. In *Clinical Urodynamics. The Urologic Clinics of North America*, Vol. 6. No. 1. (Turner-Warwick R., C.G. Whiteside, eds), pp. 137–41. Philadelphia: W.B. Saunders.

Whitfield H.N. *et al.* (1981). The obstructed kidney: correlation between function and urodynamic assessment. *Brit. J. Urol*; **49**:615–19.

20

Infection

C.A.C. CHARLTON

Definitions

Bacteriologically, an infection of the urinary tract is defined as the isolation of an organism in a number which exceeds an arbitrarily stated concentration, i.e. greater than 100 000 organisms per ml. This is also termed a *significant* bacteriuria, because lesser concentrations of organisms are almost always due to urethral contamination. In recognition of this likelihood of contamination, the initial 5 ml of voided urine is identified as the urethral washout specimen (or voided bladder specimen 1, VB1); this may or may not be wanted for separate examination (this will be discussed later).

The mid-stream specimen of urine (MSU or voided bladder specimen 2, VB2) represents the uncontaminated bladder sample and is the usual specimen sent to the laboratory for microscopy and culture. In the female it may be difficult to obtain an uncontaminated MSU due to contact of the urine with the labia.

If there is difficulty in establishing the significance of an infection, i.e. due to possible contamination, then a suprapubic aspiration is undertaken. Cooperation of the patient is essential since no urine is voided until the bladder can be palpated above the symphysis pubis. The skin is cleansed (pubic shaving may be necessary) and urine aspirated with a sterile hypodermic syringe and dispatched to the laboratory.

The collection of urine specimens for bacteriological examination by means of a urethral catheter is to be discouraged, since the catheter undoubtedly displaces the urethral flora in to the bladder and may precipitate a significant urine infection. If a suitable urine specimen is not available (e.g. in the presence of an ileal conduit), then the strict criteria employed for defining a urinary tract infection have to be relaxed, and it is best simply to recognise that if a Gram-negative rod is isolated from the blood of an ill patient with an abnormality of the urinary tract, then it is almost certainly culpable. In this context it had been hoped that measuring the titre of serum antibodies of the urinary bacterial antigens would provide evidence of an infection. Unfortunately, difficulties arise with the specificity of the results in any one patient and with non-typable coliform bacilli. The microbiological aspect of identifying and culturing other urinary pathogens, e.g. virus, Tric agents, tuberculosis, or the growing of organisms in a carbon dioxide medium, will not be discussed in this chapter.

Urinary infections may be classified in clinical terms as symptomatic and asymptomatic, and the investigative aspects of these two groups are included in this analysis and discussion.

Symptomatic urinary tract infection

In the adult female

About 50% of all women will have at least one bout of what has been called cystitis in their life. Clinically they have an episode of frequency and dysuria which may resolve spontaneously or respond to a number of different treatments.

Mechanisms

Many studies have been made to determine the mechanism responsible for the symptoms. There is no doubt that enterobacteria can migrate from the anus across the perineum and, in the case of women, populate the introitus. There are a number of defence mechanism which may inhibit these organisms moving across the vestibule and into the region of the external urinary meatus, But under certain conditions the enterobacteria will ascend the urethra and enter the bladder (O'Grady *et al.*, 1970). There is little doubt that this movement of organisms is facilitated by the trauma of sexual intercourse (hence the term 'honeymoon cystitis'), in those who are socially unclean and unhygienic, in the presence of a vaginal infection or discharge (which may be secondary to the contraceptive cervical cap or intrauterine device) and in those who use irritant vaginal douches, deodorants and bubble baths. Some women identify the onset of the frequency and dysuria to the time of adopting modern tights or following swimming. Hence women seen with this symptom complex require careful history taking in the first place. Physical examination is almost invariably negative, although one must always seek causes for the establishment of urinary tract infection, such as a stagnant pool of urine, as seen in chronic retention secondary to obstructed or atonic bladders, cystocele, etc. Constipation may also be a precipitating factor in this disorder.

Initial investigation and management

The patient seen in a hospital out-patient department has often had a course of antibiotics, the symptoms have resolved and the urine specimen will be sterile. Patients with a history of bouts of frequency and dysuria should be given a dip slide or filter strip to keep with them, and this is used to inoculate the culture medium with urine at the time of the symptom. At the time of this interview patients are instructed in the value of a high fluid intake, effective bladder emptying, perineal hygiene and toilet, correcting any particular precipitating factor related to the onset of frequency and dysuria, e.g. changing the type of contraceptive used, adopting different coital positions or avoiding bubble baths, etc. In the majority of these women who have had an occasional (once a year) bout of frequency and dysuria, the symptoms do not recur after adopting the above advice and there is no advantage in investigating them further. Furthermore, a patient whose urine specimen is infected at the time of symptoms

should have the urine re-cultured a month after the completion of treatment, to ensure that the urine is sterile.

Further investigation

The persistence of an infection, whether it is relapsing, (i.e. the same organism) or recurring (a different organism) and with or without symptoms, demands further investigations by an intravenous urogram (IVU). The number of abnormal IVUs is 23% and 55% in symptomatic and asymptomatic bacteriuria respectively (Table 1).

Table 1
PERSISTENTLY BACTERIURIC PATIENTS
Radiological findings
(Expressed as %)

Radiology	Asymptomatic (19 Patients)	Symptomatic (61 Patients)
Normal	40	65
Congenital abnormality	5	12
Obstructive uropathy	15	8
Chronic pyelonephritis	10	5
Other intrarenal disease	30	5
Increased bladder residue only	0	5
	100	100

An IVU should also be requested in those adult female patients with a history of frequency and dysuria who have had an associated systemic illness and perhaps loin pain with malaise, etc. The quality of an IVU during a bout of acute pyelonephritis may be very poor, due to the dye not passing down the nephron as a result of intratubular blockage of debris, and so there is a failure to reabsorb salt and water and the dye is not concentrated. In such a situation, with a severely ill patient who fails to respond to conservative treatment, more active intervention may be necessary, since an obstructed pyonephrosis may be present. To define the problem further and establish whether the cause is stone disease, pelviureteric junction obstruction, retroperitoneal fibrosis or a necrotic papilla, it is necessary to proceed to a retrograde ureterogram. This will delineate the presence of an obstruction and the level of the obstruction, which must be known before proceeding to relieve the condition by early operation.

Women who have more than two bouts of isolated urinary tract infection in a year, despite having sterile urine after treatment, require an IVU, since about one-third will show abnormal radiological signs (Table 2).

Table 2
PERSISTENTLY SYMPTOMATIC PATIENTS
Radiological findings
(Expressed as %)

Radiology	Abacteriuria (91 Patients)	Abacteriuria and Bacteriuria (75 Patients)
Normal	85	53
Congenital abnormality	10*	14
Calculus disease	0	11
Other intrarenal disease	0	3
Increased bladder residue only	5	19
	100	100

*Anatomical variants	4
Caliceal cysts	2
Medullary sponge	2
Polycystic	1

Significance of haematuria

Haematuria associated with frequency and dysuria must be treated with suspicion. A month after the infection has been treated and the urine shown to be sterile, cytological examination of the urine should be undertaken. The significance of abnormal cells is difficult to interpret if the examination is undertaken within a month of an infection. A woman under 50 years of age with haematuria which is concurrent with an isolated bout of urinary tract infection, and who subsequently has no symptoms and normal urine cytology (and with no increased white or red cells), does not need an IVU or cystoscopy. However, in the presence of abnormal urinary cytology an IVU is mandatory irrespective of the age of the woman in question. Similarly, any woman over 40 years of age who has haematuria, with or without concomitant symptoms, must undergo an IVU and a cystoscopy.

Other infective causes

In women with a history of persistent frequency and dysuria, despite treatment, investigations other than urine culture should be carried out for infective causes. If sterile urine specimens show white and red cells to be present, then tuberculosis has to be considered and the appropriate examination requested. Agents such as *Chlamydia*, Tric agents and other rarer organisms require specialist laboratory help and this should be sought in these intractable cases.

Other pathological causes

Conditions which may give rise to symptoms suggestive of an infection, which do not, however, have organisms and rarely cells, are the contracted bladders of interstitial cystitis, postradiation cystitis, cases following ingestion of cyclophosphamide and even submucosal carcinoma. In all of these conditions an IVU is called for, not only to confirm or refute the suggestion of a small bladder, but also to establish the condition of the upper tracts (e.g. upper tract distension or tuberculosis).

Indications for cystourethroscopy

The need to examine the bladder endoscopically in urinary tract infection is not as frequent as was previously thought. As indicated above, all women with haematuria, except in the case of the younger woman under 40 years of age whose symptoms undoubtedly occur at the time of proven bacteriuria, need a cystoscopy. Similarly, all women who have persisting symptoms despite treatment must have the bladder examined (and often a biopsy of the mucosa) and have a bimanual examination under an anaesthetic to exclude any extravesical pathology (e.g. colonic, uterine or ovarian). In addition, those women who are unable to empty their bladder satisfactorily may benefit by having the outflow resistance reduced. It is wise to cystoscope them and do an examination under an anaesthetic before proceeding to urethral dilatation or urethrotomy.

Summary

The only regular investigation required for adult women with a bout of frequency, dysuria and bacteriuria is a urine culture about one month following treatment. Absence of further symptoms and sterile urine terminate the incident.

An IVU must be requested in those women with additional or recurrent symptoms or with persisting urinary abnormalities as seen in the laboratory (cells and organism). If the kidneys demonstrate tissue damage in that they are decreased in size and show clubbing of the calices with overlying scarring of the cortex, the term pyelonephritis is used. This disorder does not develop *de novo* in the adult and is almost certainly the result of vesicoureteric-intrarenal reflux in the growing kidney.

Progressive deterioration in function can be halted by the judicious use of chemotherapeutic agents, and there is no place for contemplating ureteric reimplantation, and hence no justification or need to submit the patient to micturating cystourethrography. Similarly, there is no need for women with a urinary tract infection and associated stress incontinence and prolapsing bladder base to have a cystogram.

It is clear that to eliminate the residual urine (which provides the stagnant pool as a suitable medium for infection) the hernial defects through the pelvic floor must be repaired and the bladder returned to its normal intra-abdominal position. It does not require a cystogram to make the diagnosis and plan the appropriate treatment. Doubts which might exist as to the effectiveness of detrusor activity and the ability to empty the bladder are best resolved by urodynamic measurements.

In the adult male

Infection of the urinary tract in the male is much less common than in the female. Possibly this can be attributed to the remoteness of the bladder and prostatic urethra from the bacterial flora which populate the external urethral meatus. In addition, there is some evidence that prostatic fluid has a bactericidal function (Stamey *et al.*, 1968) and so acts as a barrier to the ascent of any organisms which may migrate from the anterior urethra towards the bladder neck.

Mechanisms

The search for an underlying reason to account for the infection is often rewarded with finding an abnormality of the urinary tract. Following bacteriological examination of the urine, the next investigation which must be undertaken is an intravenous urogram.

The commonest abnormality detected is postmicturition residual urine, which implies relative stagnation of a pool of urine, which by virtue of a reduced 'turnover' of urine permits a rapid mutliplication of organisms and so the establishment of an infection. In the older age group in particular, this is attributable to an increase in the outflow resistance, and this is commonly due to prostatic pathology. This obstruction may be complicated by the formation of a vesical diverticulum, which itself perpetuates infection. The absence of covering bladder muscle over the diverticulum leads to this cul-de-sac being continually full of stagnant urine, which is a cause of urinary tract infection. In these circumstances the IVU will not only demonstrate these abnormalities, but also outline concomitant obstruction of the upper urinary tract.

Other causes of urinary tract infection also identified by an IVU are stone disease of the upper tract, pelvi-ureteric junction obstruction and ureteric obstruction. In the diabetic patient, or the patient who has ingested large amounts of phenacetin-like compounds, the possibility of papillary necrosis as a cause of infection must be borne in mind. Renal stone disease, with a distorted collecting system and a *Proteus* infection, should suggest a diagnosis of xanthogranulomatous pyelonephritis.

Clinical presentations

Systemic illness with a urinary tract infection in the male is relatively common. This may be associated with an epididymo-orchitis, which is presumably the result of the reflux passage of infected urine along the length of the vas deferens. The epididymis and testicle are exquisitely tender and the vas deferens is also involved – funiculitis – and is easily felt as a thick cord at the scrotal neck. An IVU may indicate the cause of what is primarily a vesical infection, e.g. some degree of chronic retention of urine, stone disease, or in the younger age group the rarer ectopic opening into the prostatic region. However, in the middle-aged and younger male the development of epididymo-orchitis in the presence of a normal IVU may suggest prostatitis as a primary source of infection.

Prostatitis. In the acute stage, the prostate gland is very tender and soft, whereas in the more chronic stage the gland, which is invariably small, soft and non-tender, will have the consistency of putty.

The diagnosis of prostatitis is difficult to make in an objective manner and requires a very thorough search for the pathogen. The following procedure (Meares and Stamey, 1968) is reserved for the time when the acute phase of the prostatitis has resolved, and the prostate is non-tender and the patient without any systemic disorder. A urethral washout urine specimen (VB1) and bladder specimen (VB2) are collected in the usual manner, and care is taken to make sure the patient does not empty his bladder completely. The prostate is then massaged by a finger in the rectum, and as a result of this activity some prostatic fluid may be milked into the prostatic urethra which can then be collected into a sterile container or, if available, on to a culture plate. This is known as the expressed prostatic secretion (EPS). Finally the bladder contents are voided, and it is reasonable to suppose that the organisms found in this specimen (VB3)represent organisms expelled from the infected prostate into the urethra which has been washed out by the urine. If the VB3 has a similar bacterial population to that of the EPS, which, in turn, differed from that of VB1 and VB2, it is logical to assume that a prostatic infection has been identified. On the other hand, a significantly greater count in VB1 as compared to EPS and VB3 indicates a urehritis, whereas similar high counts in VB1, 2 and 3 tend to implicate the bladder as the source of infection.

In recent years organisms other than enterobacteria have been implicated in causing prostatitis, particularly *Chlamydia*. Investigations centred on the microbiological aspects of urethritis are in the province of the venereologist (or physician in genitourinary medicine) but inevitably there is some overlap. The prostatic infection is accompanied by a systemic illness, with some milky or mucoid white discharge, frequency, dysuria and possibly some initial (at the beginning of the stream) haematuria. The patient often complains of low back pain and an ache in the perineum and back of thighs.

Urethritis. The patient with non-specific or venereal urethritis will often give a history of a recent sexual contact, a purulent discharge, scalding micturition and the lips of the external meatus look red and oedematous. The urologist will seek other causes of a urethritis, such as the unusual presence of a urethral diverticulum, which will lead to infection in this stagnant pool with the symptoms of urethritis. If this situation is suspected an ascending and descending urethrogram are indicated, so as to outline the lesion and also to demonstrate any associated urethral stricture and possible residual urine.

Indications for cystourethroscopy

Endoscopic examination as part of the investigations of urinary tract infection in the male should, if possible, be combined with any definitive treatment which may be contemplated. It seems judicious to limit the number of anaesthetics to a minimum and, furthermore, it is more economical in time for both the patient and surgeon to have one rather than two general anaesthetics. Endoscopic examination under local anaesthesia is an uncomfortable and often incomplete investigation, and if an adequate bimanual examination is required a general anaesthetic is necessary.

Cystourethroscopy is mandatory in those patients who have had haematuria associated with urinary tract infection, and also in those who have persisting symptoms following treatment. There is no advantage in examining the urethra and bladder endoscopically when prostatitis is the diagnosis.

Tuberculosis. It is unwise to use instruments in a patient in whom the diagnosis of tuberculosis is being considered, since a mucosal abrasion of the urethra with loss of continuity of the epithelium will, if bathed with urine infected with the *Mycobacterium*, be followed by a stricture. The diagnosis is suspected if symptoms persist after standard antibiotic treatment, particularly with frequency and dysuria, or less commonly epididymo-orchitis. Classically the urine specimens are sterile, but contain white and red cells and the IVU may show renal involvement with calcification and excavation of the calices, strictures of the urinary tract, etc. If the IVU is normal, a Mantoux or similar test is often helpful. The laboratory should be asked to stain organisms with the Ziehl-Neelsen method if there is a high index of suspicion, but commonly they prefer to inoculate and culture the organism before providing an answer.

In the child

Clinical features

Urinary tract infection in babies may present with vomiting, failure to thrive, malaise and fever or haematuria. It may also be uncovered as a result of noting a large bladder and/or kidneys. There is no doubt that those who have been proven to have bacteriuria should have an IVU. In over one-half, the IVUs will show an abnormality, e.g. abnormal kidneys and ureters, duplication of the tracts, and girls, in particular, may show obstructed upper tracts caused by ectopic ureteroceles. In this age group, if the kidneys and ureters look normal on the IVU, then any degree of reflux will be slight and the need for a micturating cystourethrogram (MCU) is doubtful.

Vesicoureteric reflux

It can be argued that it is important to establish the presence or otherwise of vesicoureteric reflux in these children, since long-term chemotherapy is indicated in the presence of reflux and urinary tract infection. It has been shown that, provided the urine is kept sterile, renal function increases with age to an equal extent in both the antireflux operation group and those managed conservatively (Smellie and Normand, 1968). However, if there is failure to control an infection, or persisting symptoms or difficulty in managing antibiotics (e.g. allergies), then reimplantation of refluxing ureters may be necessary. At such a time the presence of complicating pathology such as bladder outflow obstruction and diverticula must be sought for and corrected at the time of reimplantation, and so a MCU and cystoscopy are indicated.

Management

a In those children between the ages of 1 and 5 years who present with repeated infections (more than one bout per year), most paediatricians require a MCU with an IVU before deciding on management. All children are encouraged to drink large volumes of fluid, practise 'double' micturition, to ensure complete bladder emptying, and also avoid constipation. Long-term low-dose chemotherapy for 6 to 12 months is necessary. In the absence of urinary tract obstruction, kidney growth will proceed normally. This latter is monitored by repeated renal function tests and the presence of scarring is sought on the nephrogram phase of the radiological examination. Vesicoureteric reflux in mild and moderate cases ceases spontaneously in 70% of cases, although this resolution falls to under 30% in the gross examples; however, no further improvement occurs after the age of 12 years, and so continuous chemotherapy may be necessary up to that age.

b   In children who first develop urinary tract infection after the age of 5 years, an IVU must be undertaken. If this is normal, then they should be managed on the basis of careful bacteriological supervision and using the same protocol described above. If the infection recurs soon after stopping chemotherapy, cystourethroscopy is indicated to exclude congenital urethral and bladder abnormalities, e.g. minor degrees of valves, diverticula, fistulae and ureterocele, in addition to foreign bodies passed into the bladder, etc. If the IVU shows scarred kidneys or dilated ureters, then a MCU must be done to help plan treatment in the same way as outlined above.

Asymptomatic urinary tract infection

Population screening

Asymptomatic urinary tract infection can only be identified as a result of screening of population. This should be undertaken routinely in neonates, but the cost effectiveness of screening schoolchildren is less conclusive. In a study of 23 000 children (O'Donnell, 1974; personal communication) 1.8% were found to have asymptomatic bacteriuria, and in those (with bacteriuria) in whom an IVU was undertaken, about one-quarter had abnormal radiological findings. As stated above, those children with scarred kidneys or dilated ureters on IVU should have a MCU, since it will determine further management. In approximately one-half of these vesicoureteric reflux is present, although to a mild degree in about 60%, and the indications for operative intervention in the remaining severer cases are as outlined above.

Association with pregnancy

Evidence of urinary tract infection is also routinely sought for in pregnancy. About 4% of these women have asymptomatic bacteriuria and treatment should be prescribed to avoid the increased incidence of pyelonephritis which occurs at this time. Radiological examination is postponed until after delivery, unless there are difficulties in eradicating the infection. If this latter proves to be the case, a very limited (3 or 4 plates) IVU may be necessary, although the exposure to radiation may be further reduced by one plain abdominal x-ray and a renal isotope function test.

Routine medical screening

Asymptomatic bacteriuria may be detected in those having routine medical examination. The incidence of abnormal IVUs is considerable, and further management is planned in the usual manner as determined by the nature of the abnormality, e.g. stone disease, papillary necrosis, etc. As stated earlier, the incidence of abnormal IVUs in asymptomatic bacteriuria is high (Table 1). Occasionally, there is the problem of establishing which of two possible aetiological factors is responsible for an infection, e.g. a stone in the lower calix of a kidney, and/or the presence of a diverticulum in a previously obstructed bladder neck.

Localisation of infection

When there is a choice of two sites for the source of an infection, it is helpful to localise this site and so plan treatment appropriately. A modification of the method described by Stamey et al. (1965) has been employed. After suitable preparation, including full hydration, the patients are cystoscoped and a bladder urine sample obtained. The bladder is then rinsed with 4 consecutive litres of sterile saline and a sample from each litre sent to the laboratory. Ureteric catheters are passed up to the midpoint of the ureters and consecutive samples of urine obtained from each catheter, and 3 separate samples are necessary. Occasionally, there is a long delay in obtaining these specimens. The catheters are then withdrawn and the bladder urine, collected as a result of leakage round the catheters, is also sent to the laboratory. If the bladder urine is shown to be infected and the 6 ureteric samples are sterile, then a diagnosis of bladder infection is accepted. A diagnosis of upper urinary tract infection, unilateral or bilateral, is based on the demonstration of a 100-fold difference in bacterial counts in ureteric urine as compared with the washed bladder urine (Cattell et al., 1973).

Management

Patients with indwelling catheters, whether nephrostomy or urethral, will almost invariably develop bacteriuria. Chemotherapy is to be discouraged, since it is purely suppressive and withdrawal of the drug is followed by recurrence of the bacteriuria. Repeated courses of antibiotics lead to a changing bowel flora and so eventually only those organisms resistant to the drugs used will survive, and are the infecting bacteria in the urine. However, if the patient develops a systemic illness (with pyelonephritis or epididymo-orchitis), the appropriate antibiotic should be prescribed and a plain x-ray is necessary to exclude the development of stones which, if removed, may eliminate further bouts of septicaemia. In addition, considerable exudate and debris in the urine may result, caused by the catheter acting as a physical irritant to the urinary mucosa and by an infection, and this leads to blockage of the catheter. Bladder washouts should be undertaken with a weak antiseptic solution, and in these circumstances an appropriate course of antibiotic is often helpful in (temporarily) getting the urine free of debris.

In a small number of patients with grossly distended upper tracts, or large atonic bladders or diverticula, it is extremely difficult to eradicate asymptomatic bacteriuria. Although draining the urinary tract and giving very large parenteral doses of the appropriate antibiotic, followed by long-term chemotherapy, does sometimes produce a sterile urine, the bacteriuria often recurs after some weeks or months. It does seem that, in this selected small group of patients, the inherent defence mechanisms are poorly developed, and that, in the absence of symptoms, one must be prepared to accept the situation of a persistently unsterile urine.

References

Cattel W.R., Charlton C.A.C., McSherry A., Kelsey Fry I., O'Grady F.W. (1973). The localization of urinary tract infection and its relationship to relapse, reinfection and treatment. In *Urinary Tract Infection*, ed. (Brumfitt W., Asscher A.W., eds), p. 206. London: Oxford University Press.

Meares E.M.Jr., Stamey T.A. (1968). Bacteriologic localization patterns in bacterial prostatitis and urethritis. *Invest. Urol*; **5**:492–518.

O'Grady F.W., Richards B., McSherry A., O'Farrell S.M., Cattell, W.R. (1970). Introital enterobacteria, urinary infection and the urethral syndrome. *Lancet*; **2**:1208–10.

Smellie J.M., Normand I.C.S. (1968). Experience of follow-up of children with urinary tract infection. In *Urinary Tract Infection* (O'Grady F.W., Brumfitt W., eds.) p. 123. London: Oxford University Press.

Stamey T.A., Fair W.R., Timothy M.M., Chung H.K. (1968). The antibacterial activity of prostatic fluid. In *Urinary Tract Infection*, ed. (O'Grady F.W., Brumfitt W., eds.) p. 38. London: Oxford University Press.

Stamey T.A., Govan D.E., Palmer J.M. (1965). The localization and treatment of urinary tract infections. The role of bactericidal urine levels as opposed to serum levels. *Medicine*; **44**:1–36.

21

Obstruction

DAVID TOLLEY

The site of obstruction to the urinary tract may be divided conveniently into the upper and outflow tracts, the former consisting of the kidney and ureter, the latter from the bladder neck, through the urethra to the external urethral meatus. The majority of patients will present with lower urinary tract obstruction and its management forms a large part of modern urological practice.

Outflow tract

Anatomically, the outflow tract comprises the bladder neck and proximal and distal urethra, but not every case of outflow obstruction is due to an abnormality arising in these structures and neurological abnormalities must be borne in mind when assessing patients. The commonest cause of obstruction is benign prostatic hyperplasia; prostatic cancer and urethral stricture being relatively rare. Occasionally stenosis of the external meatus or phimosis may give rise to symptoms. Lower urinary tract obstruction in the female is unusual, and is mainly seen in association with other conditions such as infection, the menopause or following pelvic surgery.

Benign prostatic hyperplasia

One in ten males over the age of 65 will require prostatectomy for bladder outflow obstruction. The pros-

tate increases in size from the age of 40, but no definite aetiological factors have been identified, although eunuchs do not develop prostatic enlargement provided that they are castrated before puberty. Enlargement of the prostate is the result of hyperplasia of periurethral glandular tissue forming adenomas in the central zone (Fig 21.1; Blacklock, 1982). The developing adenomas form characteristic lateral and middle lobes which are readily recognisable at cystoscopy.

The outer zone of normal prostatic tissue is gradually compressed to form the 'surgical capsule' which surrounds the adenomas and the whole is further surrounded by a tough fibrous capsule, through which it receives its blood supply. The adenomatous tissue and the fibromuscular stroma have differing growth rates which accounts for the different characteristics noted when the prostate gland is examined. Thus adenomatous preponderance produces large discrete nodular hyperplasia with prostates often weighing more than

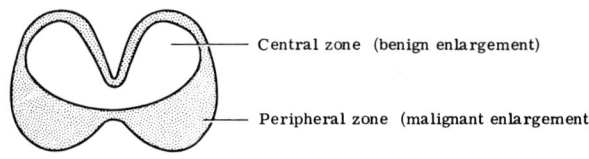

Central zone (benign enlargement)

Peripheral zone (malignant enlargement)

Fig 21.1 Anatomy of the prostate: cross section through the gland.

100 g. In the presence of previous infection, or fibro-muscular hyperplasia, the gland is usually small and firm. The gland may become infected and occasionally a prostatic abscess may form. Infarcts may occur and the subsequent oedema may cause transient enlargement of the gland sufficient to cause urethral obstruction.

As the adenoma enlarges, the urethra becomes obstructed as the lumen narrows. Initially, the bladder is able to compensate for the urethral obstruction and detrusor hypertrophy takes place in order to increase the voiding pressure and maintain the same flow. This is the stage of compensated outflow obstruction. If the obstruction is unrelieved, further muscular hypertrophy occurs, and the bladder appears coarsely trabeculated. Gaps occur between the trabecular folds and mucosal herniations may occur, initially as saccules, which eventually progress to diverticula.

Continuing chronic outflow obstruction in some cases leads to the replacement of muscle fibres with collagen; ultimately, the bladder may become little more than an atonic sac which is able to empty by changes in intra-abdominal pressure only.

As the bladder decompensates, the detrusor muscle becomes less efficient and the bladder fails to empty completely. The presence of residual urine carries a risk of urinary infection and stone formation. A large residual urine, e.g., greater than 1000 ml, may lead to progressive upper tract obstruction. Dilatation of the ureters and pelvicaliceal system occurs, resulting in obstructive renal failure due to atrophy of nephrons caused by raised intrarenal pressure which may in turn produce metabolic problems.

Clinical features

Prostatism is widely used as a term to indicate symptoms of bladder outflow obstruction. This is a rather imprecise word implying that the classical symptoms of outflow obstruction are present: namely, delay in initiating micturition, a poor stream followed by dribbling and increased frequency of voiding. Most patients with these symptoms will have an enlarged prostate, but this is by no means universal, particularly in the elderly. A careful history is required when one of the above symptoms is the only complaint.

As benign prostatic enlargement is a gradual process, many symptoms are of slow onset. There are often periods when patients are relatively free of symptoms. For this reason many men do not notice the deterioration in their stream and it is more common for patients to present complaining of hesitancy and dribbling due to relatively inefficient bladder emptying.

Urinary frequency seen in association with outflow obstruction is due to a reduction in the functional bladder capacity caused by an increasing residual urine. In the presence of urgency or urge incontinence, frequency of urine is due to bladder instability and provided that obstructive symptoms coexist, this symptom will usually be relieved by prostatectomy. However, in the absence of objective evidence of obstruction, patients complaining of urgency, incontinence and urinary frequency will be made worse by operation and should be offered treatment for their bladder instability. The sudden onset of urinary frequency in the absence of other symptoms may be due to polyuria (e.g. secondary to diabetes mellitus). Many elderly men develop symptoms of nocturia due to the inability of their kidneys to concentrate urine at night due to nephrosclerosis.

Urgency may be associated with cerebrovascular disease. Often patients will state that urinary frequency coincided with a stroke and it is virtually impossible to decide on clinical grounds whether the hemiplegia has compromised voiding by increasing the degree of outflow obstruction, or whether symptoms are due to bladder instability in association with a spastic hemiplegia. Further urodynamic evaluation is necessary in these patients.

Dribbling incontinence is often due to chronic retention of urine with overflow and in such patients the diagnosis is usually obvious. Sudden unexplained loss of continence may be due to loss of cortical inhibition and further direct questioning of the patient and observation of his behaviour will lead to clarification of the clinical picture.

Elderly patients frequently have other medical conditions for which they are receiving drug therapy and in these men symptoms of outflow obstruction may be drug induced. Many drugs provoke obstructive symptoms either by their effect on detrusor contractility or by increasing bladder outflow resistance (Fig 21.2), especially when normal voiding is already compromised by coexisting mild urethral obstruction.

Acute retention of urine is a common presenting feature and is often precipitated by urinary infection, excessive drinking – particularly alcohol – and cold weather. Provided that there is a good history of previous obstruction and the physical signs are compatible, it may be assumed that an enlarged prostate is the cause for this. Occasionally, patients will present with acute retention due to vertebral collapse, prolapsed intervertebral disc or a spinal tumour and the clinician must always be aware of this possibility. Retention may also be provoked by diuretic therapy, various drugs and constipation. Acute on chronic retention of urine may occur in the presence of pre-existing chronic retention of urine.

Physical examination of the patient often shows little in the way of physical signs. A man with uraemia secondary to chronic retention may appear sallow and exhibit features of uraemia. The patient's mental state

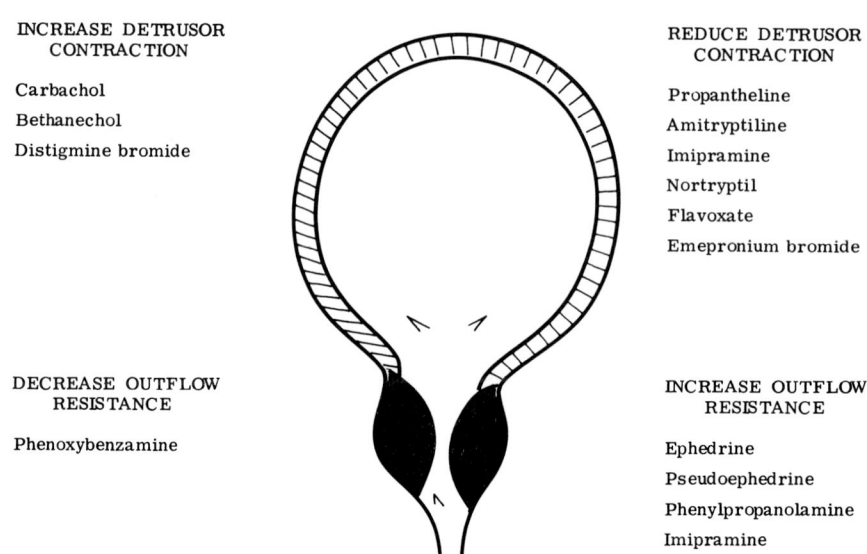

INCREASE DETRUSOR
CONTRACTION

Carbachol

Bethanechol

Distigmine bromide

REDUCE DETRUSOR
CONTRACTION

Propantheline

Amitryptiline

Imipramine

Nortryptil

Flavoxate

Emepronium bromide

DECREASE OUTFLOW
RESISTANCE

Phenoxybenzamine

INCREASE OUTFLOW
RESISTANCE

Ephedrine

Pseudoephedrine

Phenylpropanolamine

Imipramine

Fig 21.2 Effect of drugs on the lower urinary tract and bladder emptying.

should always be assessed. Abdominal examination may show evidence of incomplete bladder emptying, and this may be more obvious if a bimanual examination is performed (Fig 21.3).

Rectal examination will demonstrate enlargement of the prostate which is symmetrical, smooth and rubbery in consistency. Prostatic size should not be taken as an indication of the degree of obstruction: the patient with a small fibrous gland may have a severe degree of obstruction, whereas the man with a massive adenoma may be unobstructed. Although many irregular prostates are due to benign nodular hyperplasia, any gland which feels abnormally firm or asymetrical should be regarded as suspicious of malignancy.

All patients must have a basic assessment of renal function – blood urea, creatinine, electrolytes and haemoglobin estimation. The presence of urinary infection should be excluded by examination of a midstream specimen by culture and microscopy. An objective assessment of the degree of obstruction should be carried out by estimation of urine flow rate and intravenous urography.

Estimation of urine flow rate with the aid of a flow meter provides a simple non-invasive, objective assessment of the presence of bladder outflow obstruction. The finding of a low flow rate in an adequate volume of voided urine signifies the presence of some form of bladder outflow obstruction. A normal flow rate usually excludes obstruction, but this result should be interpreted in association with the intravenous urogram since patients with compensated obstruction may have

a normal flow rate. Ball *et al.* (1981) have shown that outflow tract symptoms in many men may change very little over a 5-year period and they have shown how valuable a urinary flow rate can be to sort out the significance of obstructive symptoms.

There has been much discussion of the place of the intravenous urogram in the assessment of outflow obstruction in recent years, but the short or limited IVU undoubtedly provides valuable information about the state of the lower urinary tract. Stones or a thick-

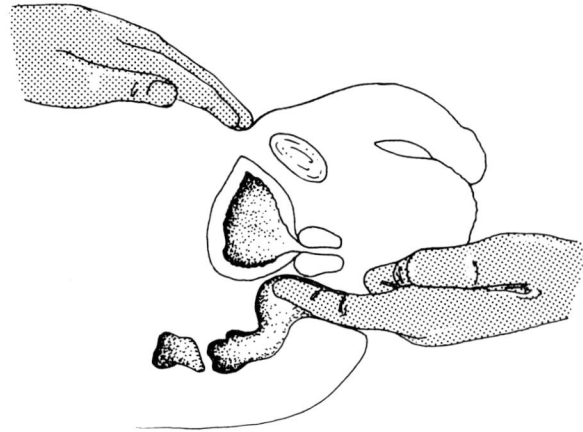

Fig 21.3 Bimanual examination of the bladder and prostate.

walled bladder may be noted on the control film and examination of the full bladder gives valuable information about the degree of trabeculation and the presence of saccules and diverticula from which an assessment of the *degree* of obstruction can be made (Marshall *et al.*, 1974).

Limited value should be placed on the presence of a residual urine on the postvoiding film in the assessment of outflow obstruction. A trabeculated bladder which empties completely may be a reflection of compensated obstruction and the presence of a large residual urine may be due to inhibition of normal micturition by a harassed patient, or delay in taking the film after voiding in a busy department (Fig 21.4).

The use of high dose urography with tomograms may provide valuable preoperative information in patients with obstructive uropathy and although the intravenous urogram should be performed in all patients with outflow obstruction, there should be no reason to delay operation in patients with acute retention simply because it is not possible to obtain the x-ray before operating.

Treatment

The only cure for patients with an enlarged prostate is prostatectomy. There is no acceptable drug treatment which reduces the size of the gland. Symptomatic urinary infection should be treated with an appropriate antibiotic before surgery.

There are four groups of patients whose management requires a different approach.

1 **The symptomatic healthy man**. Assessment is influenced by the patient's age, degree of social inconvenience caused by the symptoms, and the rate of progression of the disease. Although all patients with objective evidence of outflow obstruction should be offered surgery, the younger patient with severe symptoms will require more urgent treatment than the 75-year-old with mild obstruction. All these patients can be recommended to undergo prostatectomy. In most urological units this will be performed transurethrally and only the largest glands are removed by open operation.

Transurethral resection of the prostate (TUR) has become the preferred method of treatment in the last decade, because of advances in instrument design, improved fibre optics and lens systems and the introduction of solid state surgical diathermy machines. The disadvantage of a lengthy apprenticeship in acquiring the skills of endoscopic urology is greatly outweighed by the safety of TUR, short hospitalisation (5–7 days) and high patient acceptance. However, when performed by the inexpert surgeon, endoscopic prostatectomy is extremely hazardous (Mitchell, 1981).

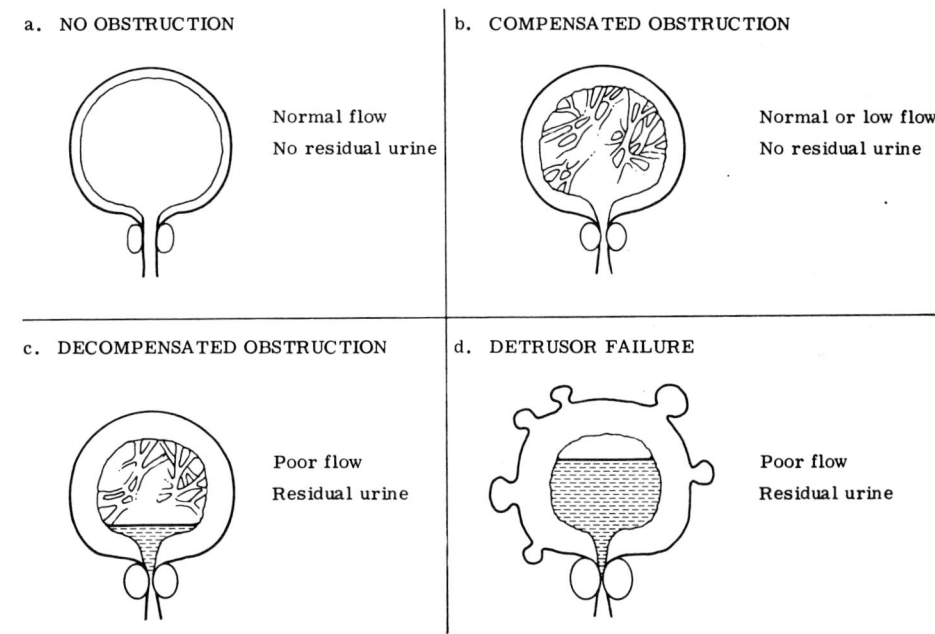

a. NO OBSTRUCTION

Normal flow
No residual urine

b. COMPENSATED OBSTRUCTION

Normal or low flow
No residual urine

c. DECOMPENSATED OBSTRUCTION

Poor flow
Residual urine

d. DETRUSOR FAILURE

Poor flow
Residual urine

Fig 21.4 The significance of residual urine in patients with bladder outflow obstruction.

For the large gland (> 100 g) and especially for the surgeon lacking in experience of transurethral prostatectomy, open prostatectomy remains the method of choice, but it has a number of disadvantages when compared with transurethral prostatectomy. Apart from a lower abdominal wound, and longer hospitalisation, bleeding is usually greater and enucleation of small adenomas or those containing carcinoma, may damage the external sphincter mechanism, resulting in urinary incontinence.

Transvesical prostatectomy was the simplest method of removing the obstructing adenoma, but carried a higher risk of bleeding and postoperative incontinence. In the retropubic approach described by Millin (1947) the adenoma is enucleated through a transverse incision in the capsule and this allows much better control of bleeding and a lower risk of incontinence.

Postoperatively, the bladder must be drained by a urethral catheter to allow free drainage, while the prostatic bed begins to heal and bleeding stops. After TUR or retropubic prostatectomy, this catheter can be removed as soon as the urine is clear but, if a transvesical operation is performed, it should be left in place for 7 days until the wound has healed.

Haemorrhage is the main postoperative hazard and is usually less of a problem after TUR than open operation because of more precise intraoperative control of bleeding. The risk of clot retention may be minimised by inducing diuresis with frusemide or by utilising continuous flow irrigation with a three-way catheter. Infection should be treated with a course of the appropriate antibiotic.

2 **The symptomatic patient with coexisting medical problems.** A patient's physical condition should rarely be an indication to refuse prostatectomy. With careful preoperative assessment, a skilled anaesthetist and help from physicians, patients with severe bronchitis, emphysema and myocardial problems may all benefit from relief of obstructive symptoms by transurethral prostatectomy. Intensive preoperative physiotherapy, antibiotics, and diuretic therapy if necessary, enable most patients to undergo transurethral prostatectomy under spinal anaesthesia.

Apart from the obvious advantages of the lack of a painful incision and the low risk of chest infection because of the avoidance of a general anaesthetic, transurethral resection and spinal anaesthesia enables rapid postoperative mobilisation, which is especially important in the elderly male.

In patients with a recent history of myocardial infarction or stroke, prostatectomy should be delayed for 6 months to allow full recovery to take place. Although a past history of myocardial infarction is no contraindication to operation, past history of cerebral vascular accident should lead to further careful preoperative evaluation of the patient with a full urodynamic assessment to exclude primary detrusor instability as the cause for the symptoms.

The demented patient with 'cerebral incontinence' should not be operated upon as even a perfect prostatectomy will not permit full return to continence.

3 **Acute retention of urine.** Patients presenting with a previous history of prostatism should be admitted to hospital and catheterised. A small self-retaining (Foley) catheter should be passed *per urethram* using an aseptic technique. Should this prove impossible, then a suprapubic catheter may be inserted percutaneously under local anaesthetic. Antibiotics should only be prescribed if there is microbiological evidence of infection. The patient should be operated upon as soon as possible after routine preoperative investigations have been performed. An intravenous urogram should be carried out at some time during the hospital admission, but it is not necessary to delay operation while waiting for the IVU.

In those patients who do not give a clear history of prostatism, a further history should be taken and appropriate investigations performed to clarify the diagnosis. This is particularly important in the elderly where constipation or concurrent medication is responsible for precipitating acute retention. Frequently, treatment of constipation or halting drug therapy is sufficient to establish normal micturition. Acute postoperative retention of urine may be relieved by catheterisation and when there is no pre-existing history suggestive of obstruction, the catheter should be removed as soon as the patient becomes mobile.

In the younger man, acute retention of urine in the absence of prostatic symptoms may indicate a neurological disorder such as tumour or prolapsed disc and a careful examination is required to exclude such conditions.

4 **Chronic retention of urine.** It is essential to determine whether or not there is any evidence of an obstructive uropathy at the first consultation, since any patient with obstructive renal failure should be admitted as an emergency. Other patients with chronic retention do not require immediate admission to the ward, but should be admitted at the earliest opportunity.

Assessment of renal function is made by checking blood urea, creatinine and electrolytes and an intravenous urogram should be obtained using double dose of contrast and tomography if necessary. The upper tracts may be dilated, but this does not necessarily imply impaired renal function. If renal function is normal and the patient is well, there is no indication for preliminary bladder drainage and prostatectomy may be planned electively.

In the presence of renal failure with associated

biochemical abnormalities, careful preoperative assessment is required. Dehydration and hyperkalaemia or other electrolyte disturbances should be corrected with appropriate intravenous fluids. A catheter is passed and prostatectomy carried out as soon as the patient is fit. While it is unnecessary to wait until the blood urea is normal (it may fail to fall); it is wise to wait a few days after catheterisation until the biochemical changes which occur after relief of obstruction and decompression of the urinary tract have stabilised. The relief of chronic obstruction is usually followed by an osmotic diuresis and increased sodium excretion due to tubular damage and, therefore, careful monitoring of urine output and fluid intake together with frequent estimations of blood urea and electrolytes is required (Chisholm, 1982). Occasionally the diuresis may be so severe that intravenous fluid replacement is necessary.

Exceptionally, a patient is unfit for surgery, and should be managed with a permanent indwelling silicone-coated catheter.

Sometimes, patients with chronic obstruction are unable to void when the catheter is removed postoperatively and this may be due to damage to the detrusor muscle caused by long-standing obstruction. In such cases it may be necessary to leave the catheter in the bladder for several weeks to allow bladder tone to return, and this may be aided by parasympathomimetic drugs such as Bethanecol. The patient should then be readmitted to hospital for a further trial without catheter about 6 weeks after the initial prostatectomy.

Bladder neck obstruction

In the elderly male severe outflow obstruction is sometimes due to bladder neck hypertrophy and this may be relieved by bladder neck resection. It is not clear whether this is a sequel to the condition of bladder neck dyssynergia, a condition typically seen in a younger man, often in his early forties, who complains of symptoms of outflow obstruction, associated with inability to void in public lavatories and a lifelong history of a 'non-competitive' stream. Flow rate is often dramatically reduced with a variable peak flow and, at cystoscopy, the bladder neck appears enlarged and there is a fine trabeculated appearance to the bladder. Synchronous pressure flow studies show inappropriately high voiding pressures and incoordination of the bladder neck causing functional obstruction. The symptoms are often dramatically cured by endoscopic bladder neck incision. Phenoxybenzamine 10 mg b.d. may also relieve symptoms and a trial of this may be used to diagnose the condition (Caine *et al.*, 1976, 1981).

Urethral obstruction

Urethral lesions causing obstruction are relatively uncommon. Prompt treatment of gonococcal venereal infection with antibiotics and the low incidence of tuberculosis has reduced the frequency of urethral strictures.

Pathology

Lesions may be congenital or acquired, the latter of infective, inflammatory, traumatic or neoplastic type.

Congenital posterior urethral valves occur only in boys and lie at the level of the verumontanum. Severe outflow obstruction and associated upper tract abnormalities occur.

Rarely a diverticulum may develop in the anterior urethra and give rise to obstructive symptoms. This condition is uncommon in men and even rarer in women.

Urethral injuries are described elsewhere, but stricture is an almost invariable late result of trauma to the urethra including inexpert catheterisation.

Gonococcal infections occur in the periurethral glands of the bulbous urethra and when treatment is inadequate, inflammation and subsequent fibrosis results in stricture formation. In the female, infection of periurethral glands may become chronic and urethral stenosis occur. Occasionally, distal urethral stenosis may be associated with infection in a urethral diverticulum.

Many problems may also arise with the foreskin and in patients whose personal hygiene is poor, the resulting balanitis may cause scarring and phimosis. Chronic infection or inflammation may scar the external meatus causing distal obstruction. This condition is also seen in children who have been circumcised while still wearing nappies and is due to an ammoniacal dermatitis.

A stone lodged in the fossa navicularis or in the bulb of the urethra is occasionally a cause of obstruction. Such stones rarely form in the lower urinary tract but arise in the kidney and then stick in the narrow part of the urethra.

Urethral tumours (usually transitional cell) are rarely seen in isolation and are related to primary bladder carcinoma. Squamous cell carcinoma may occasionally cause obstruction of the external meatus of the glans penis.

Symptoms and signs

The symptoms described by patients with urethral obstruction are often indistinguishable from those of prostatic enlargement. A previous history of venereal disease, tuberculosis, urethral instrumentation or trauma is suggestive of urethral stricture and patients with suspected outflow obstruction should be questioned directly about these features since urethral stricture is often a late event. A history of urethral bleeding may be elicited in those rare cases of tumour.

In males, the external genitalia should be examined carefully and the foreskin fully retracted to examine the external meatus. Rarely a stone may be palpated in the penile urethra. Abdominal examination may reveal the presence of a palpable bladder.

Examination of the vulva and introitus in the female may show features of atrophic vaginitis, but the female urethra is more easily examined under anaesthesia by palpation against the cystoscope.

Investigations

Renal function should be assessed with blood urea, creatinine and electrolyte estimation and the upper urinary tract assessed with an IVU. Urethrography in the form of an ascending urethrogram combined with voiding cystourethrography will help identify urethral strictures, but care should be taken not to confuse spasm of the distal sphincter with stricture of the membranous urethra. The best way of assessing a urethral lesion is at cystourethroscopy and it is often possible to perform definitive treatment at the same time.

Treatment

Posterior urethral valves may be treated endoscopically and destroyed by diathermy. Management of the associated upper urinary tract problems may be extremely difficult and infants with such problems are best dealt with in a special centre.

Phimosis is easily rectified by circumcision, although this operation may prove difficult in those men with balanitis xerotica obliterans, because of adhesions occurring between prepuce and glans penis. When circumcision is performed in a young boy, a meatal stricture may result due to ammoniacal dermatitis, but it can be controlled by meatal dilatation and often settles once the child comes out of nappies.

Meatal stricture in adult males is either secondary to balanitis, infection or trauma. When it is secondary to infection, it is best treated by a simple meatoplasty in which a flap of skin on the ventral aspect of the penis is turned into the urethra and sutured in place producing a mild degree of coronal hypospadias. A meatal or submeatal stricture occurring after instrumentation frequently responds to initial dilatation under local anaesthesia followed by regular self-dilatation with a spigot for a period of one or two months. In many cases the stricture could have been avoided initially by use of a smaller cystoscope or a simple meatotomy at the time of instrumentation.

Operations for urethral stricture fall into three types.

The time-honoured method of urethral dilatation under local anaesthetic with gum elastic bougies or metal sounds, occasionally supplemented by use of the Otis urethrotome to convert a tortuous stricture into a straight one, is being superseded in many urological units by the operation of optical urethrotomy. Urethral dilatation carries with it a high risk of bacteraemia and in many patients benefit is short-lived, since dilatation of the stricture frequently produces more scarring. Optical urethrotomy offers a precise method of incising a stricture under direct vision with the minimum amount of trauma. This procedure may be carried out quite safely on out-patients under general anaesthesia and a urethral catheter may be left in place for a variable length of time. Prophylactic antibiotics are unnecessary. Short strictures respond best to optical urethrotomy and if a stricture is greater than 2 cm or has been present for a number of years, several urethrotomies may be necessary (Desmond *et al.*, 1981). When difficulty is experienced in controlling the stricture or the patient is young, definitive treatment by urethroplasty should be considered. Frequently this may be a one-stage operation using an island patch of scrotal or penile skin, particularly when the stricture is a result of trauma, but in those patients with a long inflammatory stricture a two-stage operation is performed. The urethra is first laid open and the inflammation allowed to resolve. This is followed 6 months later by closure of the urethra with scrotal skin. Most urethroplasties can be accomplished through a perineal incision, but for the occasional dense stricture in the membranous urethra a transpubic approach is necessary (Waterhouse, 1977).

Recurrent urethritis in the female is frequently difficult to treat. Prevention by strict personal hygiene, avoiding foam baths and emptying the bladder immediately after intercourse, is often the most effective treatment. For those women who suffer with recurrent episodes of frequency and dysuria, a short course of a broad spectrum antibiotic as soon as the symptoms start and a copious fluid intake often averts a severe attack. Urethral dilatation may be necessary in patients who do not respond to conservative treatment or in women who develop evidence of urethral obstruction due to chronic inflammation.

A urethral diverticulum in the female is best dealt with transvaginally and, after excision, the defect in the urethra may be repaired with catgut.

Upper urinary tract

In terms of obstruction the upper urinary tract should be regarded as a tubular structure comprising the pelvicaliceal system and ureter. Obstruction is, therefore, caused by extrinsic compression, congenital and acquired intrinsic pathology or an intraluminal abnormality.

In the kidney the main causes are stones and tumours within the collecting system and pelvi-ureteric junction (PUJ) obstruction. In the adult, ureteric obstruction is most commonly due to intraluminal obstruction by stones, but may be the result of acquired intrinsic intramural abnormalities such as transitional cell carcinoma and specific infections (tuberculosis, bilharzia). Congenital abnormalities such as ureterocele, ectopic ureter, vesicoureteric reflux and primary megaureter, while common presenting features in the child, are rare causes of obstruction in the adult. Obstruction due to extrinsic compression of the ureter is usually bilateral and occurs secondary to retroperitoneal fibrosis, the presence of enlarged lymph nodes and malignant pelvic tumours. Occasionally, carcinoma of the colon or pancreas may cause unilateral obstruction of the ureter by direct invasion.

When dealing with a patient with suspected upper urinary tract obstruction, it is essential to confirm that the system is obstructed and that the appearances are not due to atonicity (*see* chapter on Investigation). This is particularly important in the management of children with a wide ureter and adults with congenital abnormalities.

Urinary tract stones

Pathology

Stones are initially formed in the kidney and are of two main types – metabolic (which is the more common) and infective. The two kinds of stone are easily distinguishable from each other on macroscopic examination.

A *metabolic* stone of calcium oxalate is hard and has an irregular dark surface, those containing uric acid appear light in colour and are radiolucent. Rarely the stone may have a waxy feel and is yellow, being composed entirely of cystine due to the congenital metabolic disorder of cystinuria. A number of aetiological factors have been identified and it is likely that several abnormalities occur together or in sequence for stone formation. Excess excretion of calcium in the urine (hypercalciuria) and high urinary oxalate urate levels may be associated with low urine volume and alteration in pH. The level of naturally occurring mucopolysaccharides which inhibit crystallisation of salts in the urine may also be reduced.

Infected stones are white, chalky and crumbly. They are composed mainly of calcium, ammonium and magnesium phosphates and usually occur in the presence of stasis or infection. There is often some underlying anatomical abnormality such as a diverticulum, pelvi-ureteric junction obstruction or ureteric reflux.

Obstruction and infection may recur in the presence of any type of stone, although the latter is more usually associated with infective stones. A combination of infection and obstruction causes severe damage to the kidney. Interstitial nephritis with subsequent scarring may occur and an acutely obstructed kidney containing infected urine may lead to the rapid development of pyonephrosis and septicaemia. Unrelieved obstruction will result in distal tubular atrophy with subsequent loss of renal function; an enlarging stone will also obstruct the urinary tract.

Symptoms and signs

The stone which causes acute obstruction to the upper urinary tract will often give rise to classical renal or ureteric colic. The patient develops severe colicky pain in the loin which causes him to roll around in an effort to obtain relief. It is frequently described as the worst pain known to man and is often severe enough to induce vomiting. As the stone passes down the ureter the pain alters in position, being felt in the iliac fossa, groins and occasionally in the scrotum or labia. Pain caused by a stone obstructing the ureteric orifice is often associated with urinary frequency or even strangury. Ureteric colic may be accompanied by frank, or more usually, microscopic haematuria.

The obstructed kidney often causes a dull ache in the renal angle, which persists after the colic has settled and which may be present on its own when the obstruction is of a more chronic nature. This pain may be worsened by a high fluid intake and is rarely, if ever, relieved by changes in posture. Symptoms of infection with a fever may occur occasionally, but if infection and obstruction coexist, the patient is frequently severely ill with a high fever, rigors, pain and a tense tender kidney.

Occasionally, patients with stones will have no symptoms and this is more likely to occur with staghorn calculi or stones which are wedged in the neck of a calix.

Clinical examination may demonstrate signs of uraemia due to renal failure and sometimes an obstructed kidney may be palpable. There may be an obvious anatomical or neurological abnormality such as spina bifida. In the presence of infection, or during an attack of ureteric colic some tenderness may be elicited in the renal angle, but usually examination of the patient is negative.

Investigation

This is dealt with in chapter 17.

Management

The clinical decision to be made is whether to adopt an expectant attitude or to remove a stone surgically. Two-thirds of all stones will pass spontaneously; only a third will need an operation (Williams, 1963).

A stone less than 5 mm diameter is likely to pass spontaneously, but if it becomes fixed causing a hydro-ureter and hydronephrosis, it must be removed, especially if the urine becomes infected. Stones between 5 and 10 mm diameter are less likely to pass and if they do not move for 12 weeks or cause obstruction, should be dealt with surgically. A stone greater than 1 cm is likely to stick in the ureter and cause obstruction. Therefore, if there is no medical contraindication, surgical removal should usually be advised. In all cases of ureteric stones, the decision about operation will be affected by the patient's symptoms. Hence a patient with a small stone with frequent attacks of colic causing absence from work will require operation sooner than the symptomless patient with a medium-sized stone and an unobstructed kidney.

Stones in the upper and middle third of the ureter must be removed by a formal ureterolithotomy. Under ideal conditions stones in the lower one-third of the ureter (i.e. below the pelvic brim) may be gently coaxed out endoscopically with the stone basket. There are a number of conditions which must be satisfied before this is done since ill-judged use of the instrument is dangerous. The stone should be small (less than 0.5 cm diameter) and should have been present in the ureter for a short time only and there should be no evidence of hydroureter. All attempted endoscopic stone extractions should be performed under image intensification and an ascending ureterogram should be performed after extraction to check that the ureter has not been damaged. Repeated manipulation should be avoided. If stone basket extraction is not successful, formal ureterolithotomy should be delayed for several days to allow oedema at the ureteric orifice, caused by repeated attempts at extraction, to settle.

Stones which cause obstruction to the PUJ are frequently larger in size than those causing ureteric obstruction and therefore removal by pyelolithotomy is common. In the presence of multiple stones or staghorn calculi more extensive surgery is required. In all elective cases a radioisotope scintiscan should be performed and if the affected kidney contributes more than 10% to overall renal function, attempts should be made to save it.

Before operating on the kidney an up-to-date IVU and a plain abdominal x-ray should be obtained. Preoperative CT scanning has been recommended for the difficult staghorn calculus (Wickham *et al.*, 1980), but in the majority of patients this is neither practical nor necessary. Intravenous fluids should be started on the evening before operation; the ensuing diuresis ensures that the kidney is tense and well-perfused so minimising renal damage caused by small emboli occurring during handling. In the presence of infected stones, antibiotic prophylaxis with a broad spectrum non-nephrotoxic antibiotic, (e.g. a cephalosporin) should be commenced with the premedication. For anything other than an uncomplicated pyelolithotomy, the kidney should be approached through a supracostal incision along the upper border of the 11th rib. This not only gives superior exposure, but allows for a quicker and easier approach to the renal pedicle especially in patients undergoing surgery for recurrent stone.

Removal of the stone from the renal pelvis (pyelolithotomy) should be an uncomplicated procedure and, other than the precautions outlined above, no special efforts are required to preserve renal function. Staghorn calculi which extend into the calices or occupy most of the pelvicaliceal system may require more extensive surgery to remove them and incisions may be made through the renal cortex directly onto stone fragments (nephrolithotomy). Alternatively, an incision in the renal pelvis may require extension into the infundibulum of the calix (Gil-Vernet approach). Under such circumstances it may be necessary to clamp the renal artery in order to obtain a bloodless operating field. The kidney should be cooled to 15°C by using cooling coils or an injection of Inosine may be given intravenously (Fitzpatrick *et al.*, 1981) prior to clamping the renal artery; the blood flow can then be interrupted for up to 60 min.

Removal of all stone fragments and correction of anatomical abnormalities is essential in order to minimise the chances of stone recurrence. The inside of the calices may be examined with a nephroscope and small stones removed with forceps and the kidney may also be irrigated with saline under pressure to remove multiple small fragments; contact x-rays should be taken to ensure that all these have been removed.

If the lower pole of the kidney is scarred due to recurrent infection and there is little remaining cortex, then removal of stones may be combined with amputation of the lower pole, although partial nephrectomy for stones does not decrease the incidence of recurrence.

Multiple stones within the pelvis and calices can be removed by trapping them in a coagulum of fibrinogen and thrombin injected through a small incision in the renal pelvis. After allowing the whole to coalesce, the incision is enlarged, the coagulum containing the stones is removed with forceps and the inside of the kidney washed out with saline.

Endoscopic extraction of stones from the upper urinary tract is a recent development. A small nephrostomy catheter is inserted percutaneously with the aid of image intensification and the tract thus formed is enlarged with dilators passed over a guide wire. The nephroscope is then introduced and the stone extracted under direct vision using specially designed forceps. If the stone is too large, ultrasonic or electro-hydraulic lithotripsy may be employed to fragment it. Some ureteric stones can also be extracted endoscopically with a ureteroscope. Percutaneous renal surgery is a rapidly expanding area of urology, at present the armamentarium is constantly changing and a fuller account of these procedures is described by Wickham and Miller, 1983.

A new non-invasive method of disintegrating kidney stones by means of shock waves has been developed by the Dornier Company of West Germany. Increasing experience has shown it to be a safe and efficient method of treating small/medium sized kidney stones.

Pelviureteric junction (PUJ) obstruction (idiopathic hydronephrosis)

Pathology

Dilatation of the renal pelvis and calices associated with a normal ureter is termed idiopathic or congenital hydronephrosis. Its exact cause remains obscure, but it is due to some obstructing lesion in the pelviureteric segment of the ureter.

Three theories have been advanced for PUJ obstruction. In 1923 Quimby suggested that an aberrant polar vessel acted as a window through which the distended renal pelvis could prolapse during diuresis. Murnaghan (1959) demonstrated a predominance of longitudinal muscle fibres in the PUJ, the relative absence of spiral fibres making it impossible for the affected pelviureteric segment to propel the contents downwards during peristalsis. A study of the electron microscopic characteristics of the pelviureteric junction by Notley (1968) demonstrated normal musculature and normal innervation, but a considerable increase in the amount of fibrous tissue in the wall of the ureter. It is thought that the excess collagen prevents distension of the pelviureteric junction by urine, resulting in obstruction. No theory, however, has satisfactorily explained why these abnormal situations arise. A high insertion of the pelviureteric junction or filmy adhesions around the junction are probably secondary to obstruction and infection and are not primary abnormalities. Unrelieved obstruction results in distension atrophy with gradual loss of renal function.

Symptoms and signs

The symptoms produced by a PUJ obstruction depend largely on its degree and the amount of functioning residual renal parenchyma. In its grossest form idiopathic hydronephrosis may be the cause of a symptomless mass discovered during routine physical examination. More usually, a moderately hydronephrotic kidney with ample renal cortex causes an ill-defined backache localised to one loin in a young person, which may be exacerbated by drinking large amounts of fluid of any kind. The acutely obstructed PUJ may give rise to symptoms indistinguishable from ureteric colic; these symptoms may also be initiated by alcohol. Frequently, no abnormality is found on physical examination and no abnormality is detected in the urine.

Investigation

When PUJ obstruction is suspected from the history, the initial investigation is IVU. In cases where the kidney is not visualised during conventional radiography, high doses of contrast, immediate tomography and delayed films provide sufficient information for diagnosis in most cases. In patients with repeated attacks of loin pain and a persistently normal IVU, x-rays taken during an attack of pain may demonstrate PUJ obstruction as the cause. Alternatively, the kidney may be stressed by administering a dose of frusemide intravenously during urography. In cases of equivocal PUJ obstruction, radioisotope scintigraphy, with diuretic stress if necessary, or pressure flow measurements through a percutaneous nephrostomy (Whitaker test) may provide the answer. Renal scintigraphy is also useful in determining which kidneys should be conserved and which should be removed.

Treatment

Patients with proven symptomatic PUJ obstruction require nephrectomy or surgery to relieve the obstruction. The decision to perform a nephrectomy will be made from the radiological appearances, supplemented if necessary by scintigraphy. Kidneys which consist of a gross hydronephrotic sac should be removed, but if function of the contralateral kidney is also impaired, even a poorly functioning kidney should be preserved.

Conservative operations are designed to relieve the obstruction and refashion the PUJ in such a way that there is free drainage of the renal pelvis into the ureter. This may be achieved in one of two ways. In the United Kingdom the most widely practised operation is the Hynes-Anderson pyeloplasty (Fig 21.5). This is a dismemberment pyeloplasty in which the obstructing segment is removed, together with a portion of the redundant renal pelvis, and a new PUJ is constructed. In the United States of America a flap of renal pelvis is rotated to widen the PUJ as in the Culp-Scardino pyeloplasty. Both operations are equally successful, but the Hynes-Anderson pyeloplasty is particularly useful

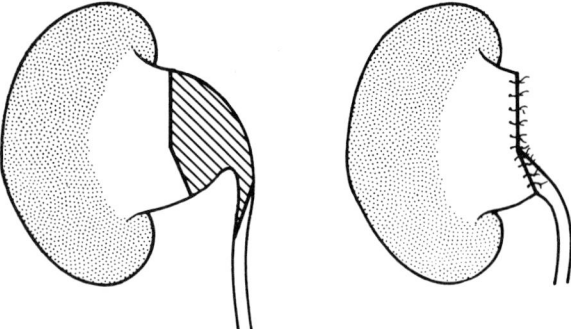

Fig 21.5 Hynes Anderson pyeloplasty for idopathic PUJ obstruction. The shaded area is excised and a new pelviureteric junction reconstructed with continuous 3/0 plain catgut.

when an aberrant lower polar vessel crosses the PUJ and is thought to be contributing to obstruction.

Retroperitoneal fibrosis

Bilateral ureteric obstruction is commonly due to fibrosis of the retroperitoneal tissues. The fibrosis encircles the ureters and causes hydronephrosis and hydroureter. There are three possible causes.

The most common condition is idiopathic retroperitoneal fibrosis. As its name implies the cause is unknown although there is an association with taking methysergide, methyldopa, analgesic abuse and beta blockers. Coexisting Dupuytren's contracture, mediastinal fibrosis or Riedel's thyroiditis may be present. An area of fibrotic tissue, which is microscopically devoid of cells, lies at the pelvic brim (most commonly over the fifth lumbar vertebra) and encases the ureters, drawing them medially. A mixture of acute and chronic inflammatory change may be present and this form of the disease usually follows a benign course.

Reactive retroperitoneal fibrosis may occur following radiotherapy or any surgical procedure to pelvic organs or retroperitoneal tissue. It is seen following extravasion of sclerosants after phenol sympathectomy or leakage of blood from an aortic aneurysm.

Malignant retroperitoneal fibrosis occurs in association with a primary retroperitoneal tumour, for example lymphosarcoma, or else it represents a metastatic process from various primary sites including the breast. Unlike the idiopathic variety, any part of the ureter may be affected (Thomas and Chisholm, 1973).

Symptoms and signs

Patients with benign retroperitoneal fibrosis may present with non-specific features of backache, loin pain, malaise and weight loss. If the ureters become acutely obstructed there may be severe oliguria or even anuria. Rarely, there is no preceding history and they present as an emergency with acute renal failure due to bilateral ureteric obstruction. Patients with reactive or malignant fibrosis usually give a history of previous treatment or disease, but sometimes bilateral ureteric obstruction will be the presenting feature of malignant disease.

On clinical examination, features suspicious of malignancy may be present such as weight loss, cachexia and an abdominal or breast mass, but there are frequently no physical signs other than those of fluid overload.

Investigation

In addition to tests of renal function, the initial assessment will consist of an IVU or ultrasound if the patient presents with renal failure (*see* chapter on Investigation). The classical radiological appearances of retroperitoneal fibrosis are bilateral hydronephrosis and hydroureter with medial displacement of the ureters, but frequently x-rays show ill-defined bilateral obstruction and ascending ureterography is required to delineate the site and nature of obstruction. It is rarely necessary to pass a ureteric catheter up to the kidney, but a classic feature of retroperitoneal fibrosis is the ease with which the catheter may be passed in the presence of seemingly total obstruction. A very high erythrocyte sedimentation rate (ESR) is a common finding in all types of retroperitoneal fibrosis and is a useful feature in assessing the course of the disease during treatment (Abercrombie and Vinnicombe, 1980).

Management

This depends on the initial cause of the retroperitoneal fibrosis and a histological diagnosis should be obtained. Patients with malignant RPF should be given symptomatic treatment only; there is little point in performing radical surgery. Where there is doubt as to the aetiology, initial management should be aimed at temporary relief of the obstruction and correction of the metabolic abnormalities pending definitive diagnosis. Preliminary ultrasound followed by bilateral percutaneous nephrostomy under local anaesthetic enables correction of electrolyte imbalance and reduction of fluid overload before proceeding to ureteric exploration, ureterolysis and biopsy. In centres where percutaneous nephrostomy is not available, bilateral ureteric catheterisation or peritoneal dialysis will achieve the same result. Ureterolysis, combined with wrapping the ureter in omentum to prevent recurrence is probably the best treatment (Osborn *et al.*, 1981). The administration of high doses of steroids may have a part to play in the initial management of the patient with the acute form of the disease.

In patients presenting with a more chronic picture, exploration of the ureter is the first choice. Steroid therapy may be of benefit in controlling development of further fibrosis once the diagnosis has been confirmed.

Transitional cell carcinoma (*see* chapter 22)

Tumours arising in the ureter are both rare causes of obstruction and rare forms of transitional cell carcinoma. The incidence of these tumours is approximately one for every 48 bladder cancers. Pathologically they behave like any other transitional cell carcinoma, but because the ureter is thin-walled, local extension occurs early and prognosis is relatively poor. Fifty per cent of patients have signs of urothelial dysplasia or second tumours in the ureter and 30% of patients will go on to develop bladder tumours (Cameron, 1969). Patients may present with renal pain due to obstruction or clot colic; haematuria is a late feature. Occasionally a mass may be palpable due to an obstructed kidney.

Treatment is considered in chapter 22 but usually nephroureterectomy is the treatment of choice.

Congenital ureteric obstruction

A variety of congenital abnormalities of the ureter and ureteric orifices may cause obstruction or give the appearance of the condition (Williams and Johnston, 1982).

Specific infection

Tuberculosis

This condition is uncommon in the United Kingdom. Progressive involvement of the ureter by this disease leads to stricture formation and occasionally complete obstruction. Urinary tract tuberculosis is frequently symptomless, but patients may present with urinary frequency or unexplained pyuria. The intense fibrosis associated with healing often causes worsening of the stricture and, therefore, prednisolone is frequently given at the same time as antituberculous therapy in order to avoid this complication. When strictures occur reimplantation of the ureter is necessary.

Bilharzia

Five per cent of the world's population suffers with this condition, which is due to infestation with a sexually differentiated trematode. The principal site of involvement is the bladder, but the whole urinary tract may be affected. The ureters are often involved, especially in the lower third as the organisms reach the site via veins associated with the vesical plexus. The middle third is less frequently affected and strictures in the upper part of the ureter and pelviureteric junction are rare.

Diagnosis depends upon the demonstration of ova in the urine or biopsy of the typical sandy patches which occur in the bladder. Effective treatment of the acute infection with niridazole may be obtained, but where ureteric obstruction is present various procedures may be necessary, including ureteric reimplantation or replacement of the ureter with a segment of ileum. The extent of surgery will be governed by the degree of renal involvement and the amount of renal damage.

References

Abercrombie G.F., Vinnicombe J. (1980). Retroperitoneal fibrosis: practical problems in management. *Brit. J. Urol*; **52**:443–5.

Ball A.J., Feneley R.C.L., Abrams P.H. (1981). The natural history of untreated 'prostatism'. *Brit. J. Urol*; **53**:613–16.

Blacklock N.J. (1982). Surgical anatomy of the prostate. In *Scientific Foundations of Urology*, 2nd edn. (Chisholm G.D., Williams D.I., eds.). London: Heinemann Medical.

Caine M., Perlberg S., Shapiro A. (1981). Phenoxybenzamine for benign prostatic obstruction. Review of 200 cases. *Urology*; **17**:542–6.

Caine M., Pfau A., Perlberg S. (1976). Use of alpha-adrenergic blockers in benign prostatic obstruction. *Brit. J. Urol*; **48**:255–63.

Cameron K.M. (1969). Ureteric tumours. *Proc. Roy. Soc. Med*; **62**:96–7.

Chisholm G.D. (1982). Pathophysiology of obstructive uropathy. In *Scientific Foundations of Urology*, 2nd edn. (Chisholm G.D., Williams D.I. eds.). London: Heinemann Medical.

Desmond A.D., Evans C.M., Jameson R.M., Woolfenden K.A., Gibbon N.O.K. (1981). Critical evaluation of direct vision urethrotomy by urine flow measurement. *Brit. J. Urol*; **53**:630–3.

Fitzpatrick J.M., Wallace D.M.A., Whitfield H.N., Watkinson L.E., Fernando A.R., Wickham J.E.A. (1981). Inosine in ischaemic renal surgery: long-term follow-up. *Brit. J. Urol*; **53**:524–7.

Marshall V., Singh M., Blandy J.P. (1974). Is urography necessary for patients with acute retention of urine before prostatectomy? *Brit. J. Urol*; **46**:73–6.

Millin T. (1947). *Retropubic Urinary Surgery*. Edinburgh: Churchill Livingstone.

Mitchell J.P. (1981). *Endoscopic Operative Urology*. Bristol, London, Boston: Wright.

Murnaghan G.F. (1959). Mechanism of congenital hydronephrosis with reference to factors influencing surgical treatment. *Ann. Roy. Cell. Surg.* Engl; **23**:25–32.

Notley R.G. (1968). Electron microscopy of the upper ureter and the pelvi-ureteric junction. *Birt. J. Urol*; **40**:37–41.

Osborn D.E., Rao P.N., Barnard R.J., Ackrill P., Ralston A.J., Best J.J.K. (1981). Surgical management of idiopathic retroperitoneal fibrosis. *Brit. J. Urol*; **53**:292–6.

Quimby W.C. (1923). Hydroenphrosis. *J. Urol*; **10**:45–8.

Thomas M.H., Chisholm G.D. (1973). Retroperitoneal fibrosis associated with malignant disease. *Brit. J. Cancer*; **28**:453–8.

Waterhouse R.K. (1977). Transpubic repair of membranous urethral strictures. In *Genitourinary Trauma. Urologic Clinics of North America*; **4**: pp.105–10.

Whitaker R.H. (1973). Diagnosis of obstruction in dilated ureters. *Ann. Roy. Coll. Surg. Eng*; **53**:153–66.

Wickham J.E.A., Fry I.K., Wallace D.M.A. (1980). Computerised tomography localisation of intrarenal calculi prior to nephrolithotomy. *Brit. J. Urol*; **52**:422–5.

Wickham J.E.A., Miller R.A. (1983) *Percutaneous Stone Surgery*. Edinburgh: Churchill Livingstone.

Williams R.E. (1963). Long-term survey of 538 patients with upper urinary tract stone. *Brit. J. Urol*; **35**:416–37.

Williams D.I., Johnston J.H. (1982). *Paediatric Urology*. London: Butterworth Scientific.

22

Malignancy

DAVID TOLLEY

Accurate histological diagnosis and staging of tumours is the basis of rational treatment of urogenital malignancies. Cooperation between surgeon, radiotherapist and chemotherapist has produced striking advances in the prognosis of patients with testicular tumours and a multidisciplinary approach to treatment has resulted in advances in some other areas of urological oncology.

Renal carcinoma

This is the commonest malignant tumour of the kidney and is responsible for some 1500 deaths per year in the United Kingdom. It occurs three times more frequently in men than women and most patients are over 40 years of age at presentation. It is a particularly fascinating tumour to the urologist because of the many different ways in which it may present and because it is a relatively slow-growing tumour.

Aetiology

While no causal factors have been demonstrated in man, renal tumours have been induced in experimental animals by the injection of viruses and prolonged oestrogen administration. Many different carcinogens induce tumours of the kidney in the laboratory animal; they include benzylpyrine, cholanthrene and nitrosamines. The latter substance is found in tobacco

smoke and Bennington and Laubscher (1968) found that more patients with renal carcinoma smoked than in a comparable control group.

Pathology

There is usually an obvious mass which may occur in any part of the kidney which, when cut, appears soft and homogeneous although there may be areas of haemorrhage and necrosis. Microscopically, renal carcinomas may consist of the more common clear cells or the rarer granular cell types. There is either a solid or tubular growth pattern, but many tumours will contain both cell types and exhibit a wide variety of differentiation.

Direct spread beyond the capsule is common and tumours may spread into the renal pelvis resulting in haematuria. The tumours metastasise to the para-aortic lymph nodes and invasion of the renal vein, often with extension into the inferior vena cava, occurs early.

Staging

The method of staging described by Flocks and Kadesky (1958) has the advantage that it is simple and correlates well with prognosis (Fig 22.1). The TNM classification revised in 1978 consists of both a pretreatment clinical classification and a postsurgical

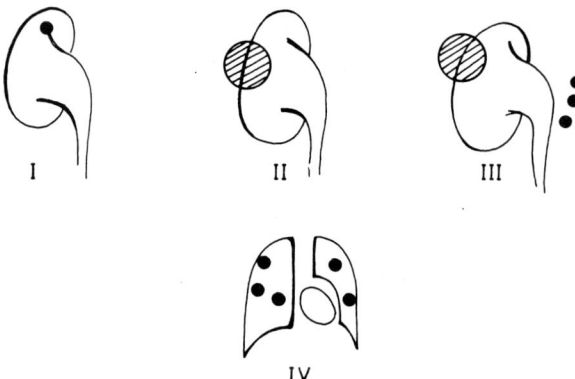

Fig 22.1 Staging for renal carcinoma (After Flocks and Kadesky, 1958).

histopathological classification. It has the advantage of being more comprehensive than the Flocks staging and also includes a histopathological grading. There is good correlation between grade of tumour and prognosis, but a lack of uniformity of opinion as to the most important histological features.

Clinical features

The classic triad of pain, haematuria and a mass in the loin only occurs in 15% of patients. Renal carcinoma is a great imitator and presents with many vague symptoms such as anorexia, malaise, weight loss and unexplained pyrexia. Alternatively, there may be a specific clinical condition such as hypertension, erythraemia or hypercalcaemia due to excess intrinsic or ectopic hormone production by the tumour. Hepatic dysfunction is common and may occur in up to 40% of patients with the disease (Utz *et al.*, 1970). This abnormality may be reversible after removal of the primary tumour and does not necessarily imply the presence of metastatic disease. The wide variety of presenting features are described as paraneoplastic syndromes and may be categorised into those producing non-specific effects and cases where the effect is produced by excess hormone production. Rarely, a tumour may present with evidence of metastatic disease causing bone pain or pathological fracture and occasionally tumours may be found following the discovery of the classical cannon ball metastases on a chest x-ray.

Investigation

The investigation of renal tumours usually begins as the investigation of a space-occupying lesion discovered in the renal parenchyma during intravenous urography (IVU). The main differential diagnosis lies between simple cyst and carcinoma. It is not possible to differentiate between the two on the IVU with certainty and, therefore, a simple diagnostic pathway should be followed in order to arrive at a firm diagnosis (*see* Chap. 16). The diagnosis is usually made with the aid of ultrasound, cyst puncture or angiography, but renal scintigraphy may also be used in the differentiation of renal masses. Cyst puncture is not always necessary to confirm the diagnosis of a simple cyst in elderly men with symptomless cysts (discovered during routine urography, or by ultrasound, during the assessment of bladder outflow obstruction); but in all other cases the diagnosis should be confirmed by cyst puncture since there is a small, but significant, incidence of tumours in these patients.

Should a renal carcinoma be confirmed by arteriography, then further information about the renal vein may be obtained by films in the venous phase of the examination. An inferior vena cavagram will provide additional knowledge of the extent of spread of the tumour if the renal vein is not clearly seen on the arteriogram.

A full haematological and biochemical profile including liver function tests should be performed preoperatively in order to determine the presence of a paraneoplastic syndrome, since the recurrence of such a syndrome after the tumour has been removed may provide early warning of recurrence. Further investigations should be performed to complete the clinical staging before deciding on treatment and these should include bone scan, chest x-ray and whole lung tomography. In centres where computed tomography (CT scanning) is available, further valuable information may be obtained about the extent of spread of the tumour and the presence of lymph node metastases.

Treatment

In patients with no evidence of metastatic disease and with a contralateral normal kidney, radical nephrectomy is the treatment of choice. Several approaches to the kidney are available. Many urologists choose the standard loin approach. However, this approach may be difficult with a large bulky tumour. A thoracoabdominal approach provides greater exposure, but some mobilisation of the kidney is required before the renal vessels can be identified. The theoretical advantage of the transabdominal approach with immediate ligation of the renal vein has not been translated into clinical practice. However, an anterior approach does offer a number of advantages; it provides excellent exposure, venous extensions of the tumour into the vena cava can be removed without difficulty and the kidney, perirenal fascia and involved regional lymph nodes can be removed en-bloc. The value of routine ipsilateral para-aortic node dissection is debatable: small tumours (<6.5 cm) rarely have node involvement while with larger tumours, the spread may not be in continuity.

Preoperative embolisation of the renal artery with a variety of substances including gel foam and Gianturco coils may be used to reduce the vascularity of the tumour. This may be done either immediately prior to surgery or nephrectomy may be delayed for 4–7 days. Delayed surgery following renal artery embolisation has the disadvantage of producing severe loin pain often associated with a high fever and malaise due to the extensive tumour necrosis which occurs. However it has been suggested that embolisation may have a therapeutic effect by alteration of the host immune response. Wallace *et al.* (1981) gave some clinical support to this possibility by demonstrating improved survival rates and objective regression following embolisation/ nephrectomy in patients with metastatic disease. Subsequent studies have not shown evidence of an immunological (T cell) response to embolisation and various clinical studies including further data from Wallace have been disappointing. Because of the unpredictable nature of renal carcinoma, any result attributed to treatment must be evaluated by controlled clinical trials before firm conclusions can be drawn.

While there is little doubt that a primary tumour which is causing symptoms should be removed in the presence of metastatic disease, there is a considerable lack of uniformity of opinion regarding the removal of the symptomless primary tumour with metastases. In these patients the operative mortality is higher (5–6%), very few patients survive for two years and threequarters will be dead within the first year. In patients with a solitary bony metastasis, removal of both primary tumour and metastasis may have limited value. There is no place for postoperative radiotherapy unless there has been incomplete removal of the tumour; some workers have suggested that radiotherapy appears to decrease the patient's chance of five-year survival. Palliative treatment of painful bony metastases, however, may be of value.

Despite the inhibition of growth of transplanted tumours in the hamster by a combination of orchiectomy, steroids and progesterone therapy, the use of medroxy-progesterone acetate (Provera) is of no value in the adjuvant treatment of renal carcinoma. To date no effective cytotoxic chemotherapeutic agent has been identified as having any activity against renal carcinoma (Spiers, 1982).

Prostatic cancer

Carcinoma of the prostate is the commonest cancer arising in the male genitourinary tract and the fourth most common type of cancer in men in England and Wales. There has been little improvement in a patient's chances of survival since the discovery by Huggins and Hodges in 1941 that many prostatic cancers are hormone responsive. This is despite increased understanding of factors influencing growth and better pretreatment staging.

Aetiology

The incidence of prostatic cancer increases with age and there has been a disturbing increase in the incidence of the disease especially in Scandinavia and in American negroes. This implies that environmental and dietary factors may be responsible. Epidemiological studies of black populations in North America and West Africa have shown a significant positive association between prostatic carcinoma and a sedentary occupation, sexual activity and venereal disease in both groups. There is now evidence of a relationship between sexual activity and venereal transmission in patients with prostatic cancer. Genital herpes virus (type 2) has been demonstrated in prostatic cells of patients with carcinoma of the prostate and an increase in antibody titre for both this virus and cytomegalovirus has been demonstrated in patients with prostatic cancer.

Pathology

More than 90% of tumours arise from the glandular tissue, but there are less common forms such as ductal tumours and mucinous and carcinoid tumours which are important as they can be difficult to diagnose and treat. The prostate may occasionally be infiltrated by urothelial carcinoma.

Prostatic carcinoma arises in the peripheral part of the gland and may appear to be solid, homogeneous and slightly granular. Microscopically the tumour is an adenocarcinoma though there is considerable variation in the degree of tumour differentiation even within the same tumour. There is good evidence that prognosis is better with well-differentiated than with poorly differentiated tumours and there is a high incidence of lymph node metastasis in patients with high grade tumours.

Clinical features

Most patients will present with symptoms of bladder outflow obstruction (*see* chapter 21). At least 45% of patients will have metastases at the time of diagnosis and while the vast majority of these are symptomless, some patients will be seen by orthopaedic surgeons with bone pain or pathological fractures.

In many cases the diagnosis may be first suspected on rectal examination which will reveal a hard craggy irregular prostate with loss of the median sulcus indicating locally advanced disease. However, in some cases where the tumour is less advanced, the prostate will feel firm or hard (T2) or there may be a localised nodule (T1). In some cases the diagnosis will only be made on histological examination of resected prostate and these findings are classed as incidental carcinoma (T0). Occasionally late disease will present as a fixed mass in the pelvis (T4) (Fig 22.2).

Investigations

All patients with suspected prostatic cancer should undergo histological confirmation of the diagnosis since the condition may be confused clinically with granulomatous prostatitis and occasionally with benign nodular hyperplasia. The only exception to this rule can be the elderly bedridden man with bone pain, a craggy mass on rectal examination, a high acid phosphatase and radiological evidence of sclerotic bony metastases in whom one wishes to give palliative oestrogen therapy. Prostatic tissue for histological examination may be obtained by needle biopsy of the prostate with a Trucut biopsy needle. This may be performed through the perineum, or transrectally, provided that the risk of bacteraemia is reduced by the administration of a broad-spectrum antibiotic. Material may also be obtained by transurethral resection of the prostate, but tissue from the outer zone of the prostate should be sent for examination, otherwise an erroneous diagnosis

of benign hyperplasia may be made in some cases of early cancer. Careful staging under anaesthesia is required to assess the T category, although imaging techniques such as transrectal ultrasound (Peeling *et al.*, 1979) provide for more precise definition of the local extent of the disease.

Estimation of serum acid phosphatase which is produced by the prostatic tumour should be performed routinely and should be repeated during treatment as a means of assessing the response to therapy and the way of predicting escape of the tumour from hormonal control (*see* below).

Assessment of lymph node involvement may be made by lymphography, but in most series the accuracy of prediction of pelvic lymph node involvement is only 75% (O'Donoghue *et al.*, 1976). For this reason lymphography is not widely practised in the UK except in the detection of para-aortic lymph nodes in patients who are likely to receive radiotherapy as a primary method of treatment. Assessment of regional lymph nodes by prostatic lymphoscintigraphy using Technetium labelled antimony are still being evaluated, but do not appear to be sufficiently accurate for routine use (Stone *et al.*, 1979). Pelvic lymph node biopsy or dissection certainly allows more accurate staging, but is not justified unless the primary treatment is radical prostatectomy or an iodine-125 implant, since the extra knowledge obtained is irrelevant when the primary treatment is to be hormonal.

The minimum requirements for assessing metastases – the M category in the TNM classification are: clinical examination, radiography, skeletal studies and relevant biochemical tests. The most important biochemical test is the serum acid phosphatase.

In practice, radioisotope bone scanning with Tech-

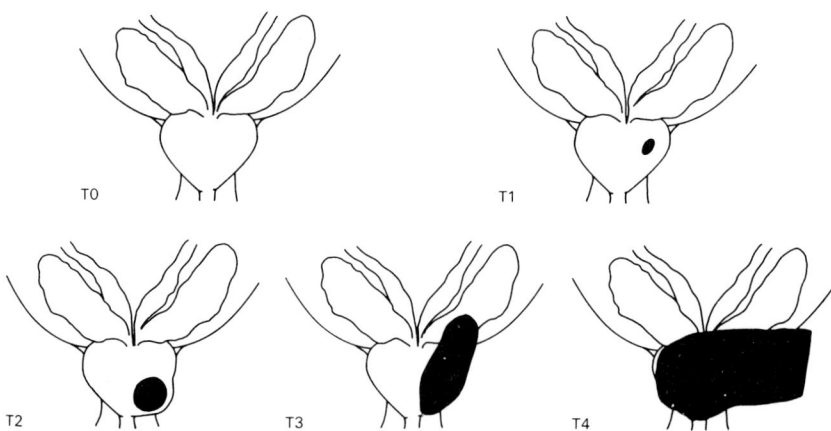

Fig 22.2 T category for carcinoma of prostate (From *Tutorials in Postgraduate Medicine: Urology* p. 227 by courtesy of Professor G.D. Chisholm and the publishers, William Heinemann Medical Books.)

netium ^{99m} methylene diphosphonate combined with x-rays of any areas showing increased uptake provides the most accurate method of assessing the presence of bony metastases. The bone scan will be positive in 20% of those patients with carcinoma of the prostate who have negative skeletal x-ray surveys (Chisholm, 1980) and the bone scan may also be used as a reliable tumour marker as it often provides evidence of progression of metastases before any other index (Fitzpatrick *et al.*, 1978).

Treatment

The incidentally diagnosed lesion (T0)

The finding of an unsuspected focus of carcinoma during prostatectomy accounts for about 10–15% of those patients diagnosed as having prostatic cancer. Most urologists adopt a 'watch and wait' policy if the tumour is only a focus, on the grounds that prostatectomy is in itself a form of radical treatment. However, further staging procedures should be carried out as occasionally these patients will have metastases.

If the tumour appears more diffuse and the pathologist is unable to say confidently that all malignant tissue has been resected, there is a strong case to be made for further transurethral resection to determine the completeness of removal of the tumour. Since a proportion of patients will develop metastatic disease, the protagonists of radical treatment (radiotherapy or radical prostatectomy) make a strong case for more aggressive initial management. To date there is no convincing evidence that radical treatment is any more effective than conservative treatment.

Locally advanced disease confined to the pelvis (T2, T3, T4, NXMO)

Those patients with negative bone scans and lymphography can be assumed to have disease confined to the pelvis and, following relief of obstructive symptoms by transurethral resection, should be offered radiotherapy as there is considerable evidence in the literature that the 10-year survival figures are superior to endocrine treatment alone (Harisiadis *et al.*, 1978). Radical prostatectomy has not become an accepted method of treatment for clinically localised (T1, T2) prostatic cancer in the UK, because of the higher mean age of patients at presentation, the high morbidity following operation (incontinence and impotence), and the lack of convincing evidence that this form of treatment is superior to a more conservative approach.

Symptomless metastatic disease (M1)

Since the discovery by Huggins and Hodges (1941) that an elevated level of acid phosphatase in patients with advanced prostatic cancer could be reduced, often to a normal level, by castration or by the administration of oestrogens, the primary treatment for patients with this disease has centred around control of androgenic hormones. Hormonal manipulation produces a symptomatic improvement in some 60–70% of patients with metastatic prostatic cancer. This largely subjective response is characterised by relief of bone pain, improvement of obstructive urinary symptoms, weight gain and a general feeling of well-being. Occasionally, there may be objective evidence of tumour regression, by a decrease in prostatic size or radiological improvement of bony metastases and reduction in acid phosphatase. Against this improvement must be balanced the high number of side-effects associated with oestrogen administration, namely fluid retention, gynaecomastia, impotence and the cardiovascular risks which are particularly prominent in men over the age of 75. Many of these side-effects may be eliminated if orchiectomy is used as the means of controlling androgen production, and indeed the only significant side-effect is that of impotence which is by no means universal.

Although androgen suppression is undoubtedly an excellent way of palliating symptoms, there is no evidence that hormonal therapy has any ultimate effect on survival. The Veterans Administration Co-operative Urological Research Group (VACURG) showed that the overall survival rates for patients with locally extensive disease with metastases who receive placebo treatment fared no worse than those in other endocrine treatment groups. They also suggested that the effect of oestrogens or castration is maximal when first applied and it does seem, therefore, that the timing of endocrine therapy must remain a matter for the individual clinician.

Symptomatic metastatic disease (M1)

Undoubtedly patients with prostatic cancer and generalised bone pain should undergo hormonal manipulation as the first choice of treatment. Since the side-effects following orchiectomy are less than those following stilboestrol, the former method of androgen control is to be preferred and, provided that histological confirmation of the diagnosis has been obtained either by previous Tru-cut needle biopsy or by frozen section, castration in the form of subcapsular orchiectomy can be performed at the time of the resection for relief of obstructive symptoms. Painful metastases showing evidence of gross bony destruction may also be treated with palliative radiotherapy.

Non-responders

Patients with prostatic cancer should be monitored regularly in the follow-up clinic and in addition to estimating and recording size of the primary tumour, estimation of serum acid phosphatase and serial bone scanning should be performed. If these show evidence of progression of the disease, the main choice lies between symptomatic treatment and an attempt to control the tumour with cytotoxic agents. There is no documented evidence that either increasing the dose of stilboestrol, switching to another oestrogen or castration offers more than a very temporary effect.

Symptomatic treatment may take the form of analgesics including drugs with an antiprostaglandin activity such as flurbiprofen, local palliative radiotherapy and further transurethral resection for obstructive symptoms.

A few non-hormonal cytotoxic agents have been shown to have some activity in prostatic carcinoma namely 5-fluoro-uracil, cyclophosphamide, nitrogen mustard, razoxane, but other agents have been either ineffective or too toxic (Torti and Carter, 1982). The effectiveness of other hormones such as cyproterone acetate, medroxyprogesterone, bromocriptine or glucocorticoids have yet to be assessed by controlled clinical trials. The combination of nor-nitrogen estamustine oestradiol-17 phosphate (Estracyt), when used as secondary treatment, produces a subjective response in 20–30% of patients and objective response in about 15% (Chisholm *et al.*, 1977).

Urothelial tumours

The urinary tract is lined with transitional cell epithelium which extends from the renal papillae to the external urethral meatus. This concept of a single lining, the urothelium, is of great importance when dealing with a urothelial tumour, because the whole of the urothelium is at risk of undergoing malignant change. Therefore in patients presenting with this type of tumour, the urinary tract should be considered as a whole and not just in isolation.

Some 8000 new cases of bladder cancer are diagnosed in the United Kingdom each year and the incidence is increasing. In contrast, tumours arising from the upper urinary tract urothelium are relatively rare. Deaths from bladder cancer in the United Kingdom are among the highest in the world (7.6 per 100 000 population) and men are four times as likely to be affected as women.

Aetiology

The rising incidence of the disease and its prevalence in males may be due to increasing exposure to exogenous carcinogens. Many chemicals have been identified as being carcinogenic; aniline dyes were first identified in Germany in the late 19th century and the higher incidence of bladder cancer in workers in the chemical and rubber industries led to a number of epidemiological studies by Case in the 1950s, as a result of which beta-naphthylamine and benzidine were identified as potent carcinogens. There is also evidence of a higher incidence of bladder cancer in other occupations such as tailors and hairdressers, but so far no definite carcinogen has been identified. Smoking and analgesic abuse has also been linked with bladder cancer. There appears to be increasing evidence of a link with cyclophosphamide. Rarely, squamous cell carcinoma may occur in the UK as a result of prolonged urothelial irritation by infection or stones. Chronic inflammation due to schistosomal infections also produces a high incidence of squamous cell cancer especially in the Middle East.

Any part of the urothelium is susceptible to malignant change. Tumours occur most frequently in the bladder which, acting as a reservoir, remains in contact with carcinogens for much longer than the upper urinary tract. Bladder tumours are almost 30 times more common than tumours in the upper urinary tract, but tumours may occur simultaneously in both sites and the whole urothelium must be regarded as being unstable in patients with bladder cancer.

Pathology

Although 98% of tumours seen in the UK are transitional cell carcinomas, in the Middle East squamous cell carcinomas are far more common and may be associated with chronic inflammation, urinary infection and stone formation. Adenocarcinoma occurs rarely in a urachal remnant in the dome of the bladder.

Most bladder tumours have a papillary growth pattern although some may contain solid areas and others may be entirely solid. The grade of malignancy varies from well-differentiated (G1) through intermediate grades (G2) to anaplasia (G3). These grades have been defined by the World Health Organisation.

There is good correlation between the morphological and histological characteristic of a tumour and the degree of invasion and survival. Well-differentiated (G1) papillary tumours are unlikely to be invasive whereas anaplastic solid tumours are almost invariably invading muscle at the time of presentation (Fig 22.3).

Carcinoma *in situ* is characterised by a thickened mucosa which may be widespread or patchy and may be associated with frank tumours or seen in isolation. Although the histological diagnosis rests with an evaluation of specific features, namely hyperplastic mucosa, increased cellularity, loss of polarity, pleo-

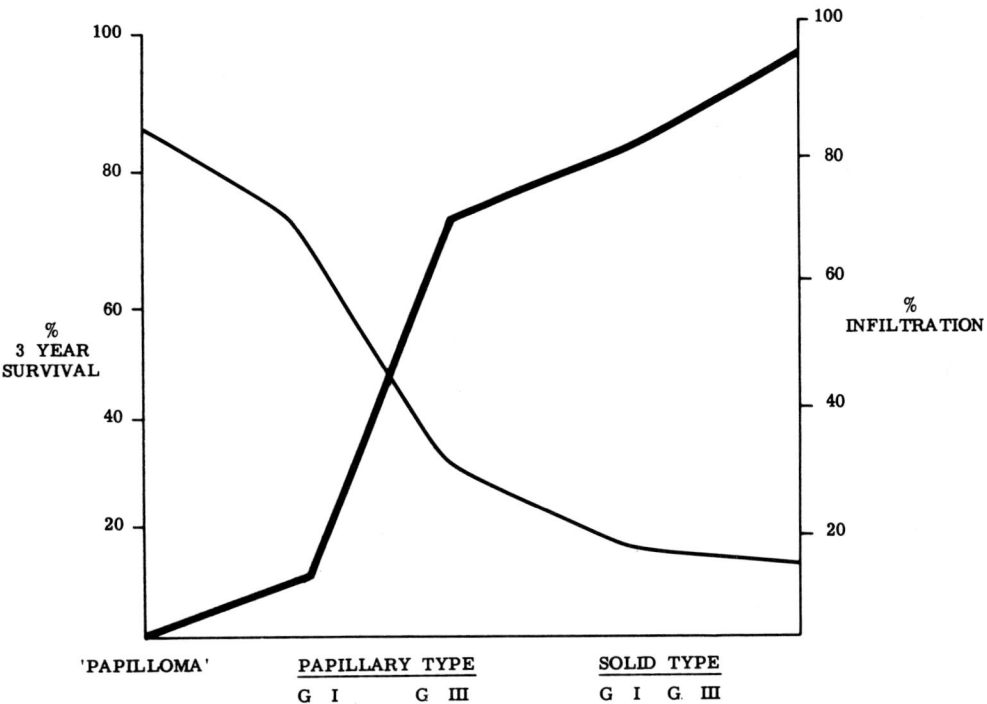

Fig 22.3 Relationship between tumour type, infiltration and survival. (After Wallace, 1959.)

morphism, nuclear hyperchromicity and lack of cohesion of superficial cell layers, in practice the diagnosis may be extremely difficult to make and certain non-neoplastic conditions must be excluded, in particular cyclophosphamide therapy, previous irradiation and urinary tract stone disease.

Clinical features

The vast majority of patients will present with painless haematuria and even the briefest episode of bleeding is in itself an indication for urgent full evaluation of the urinary tract, since delay in diagnosis and treatment significantly worsens the prognosis. For this reason many urological departments now hold special haematuria clinics providing immediate access for patients.

Other lower urinary tract symptoms, such as urinary frequency or pain on passing urine, may also be present due to the presence of carcinoma *in situ* or an infiltrating bladder tumour, and it is important that any patients with sudden unexplained onset of these symptoms be investigated to exclude the presence of malignant disease. Urothelial tumours occurring in the upper urinary tract may present with haematuria, clot colic or with pain due to obstruction (*see* chapter 21).

Physical examination is generally unhelpful, although general features suggestive of malignancy such as cachexia, weight loss or anaemia may be present. A tumour obstructing the ureter may result in a palpable hydronephrotic kidney and rectal examination may demonstrate a fixed bladder tumour.

Investigations

All patients with suspected urothelial tumours should have the urine examined microscopically for the presence of red cells and, wherever possible, cytological examination of a freshly voided sample of urine should also be performed. After IVU, with tomograms if necessary, cystourethroscopy under general anaesthesia should be performed and the whole of the lower urinary tract including the anterior urethra examined. In cases where there is an equivocal abnormality in the upper urinary tract, ascending ureterography should be performed in the theatre and in these cases cytological examination of specimens obtained from the upper ureter or renal pelvis with a special cytology brush may be of help in arriving at a diagnosis.

If a tumour is seen in the bladder at cystoscopy, biopsy should be obtained from both the superficial part of the lesion and its base. The place of random biopsies of apparently normal mucosa has yet to be fully defined (Wallace, *et al.*, 1979); these biopsies may show a variety of pathological abnormality, even carcinoma *in situ*. A careful, thorough, bimanual examination under general anaesthetic is essential for accurate clinical classification of tumours and subsequent rational treatment.

The TNM classification for bladder tumours (UICC, 1978) is now widely used throughout the United Kingdom and although it has shortcomings, has gained widespread acceptance (Fig 22.4). Patients with tumours which are thought to be invasive at the initial assessment require further staging procedures before radical treatment is instituted. Forty per cent of invasive lesions have lymph node involvement at the time of diagnosis and lymphography may be used to define the presence and extent of such metastases. Lymphography has been criticised because of the high incidence of false negative results in the pelvic nodes, but the detection of lymph node metastases in the para-aortic or high iliac nodes carries a drastic worsening of prognosis and militates against subjecting the patient to inappropriate radical therapy. Although distant metastases are rarely seen on presentation, further staging with chest x-ray, liver and bone scan should be performed in all patients being considered for radical treatment.

CT scanning in the initial assessment of the tumour is at least as accurate as clinical staging and may be of value in the assessment of para-aortic lymphadenopathy, although pelvic nodal involvement is poorly shown.

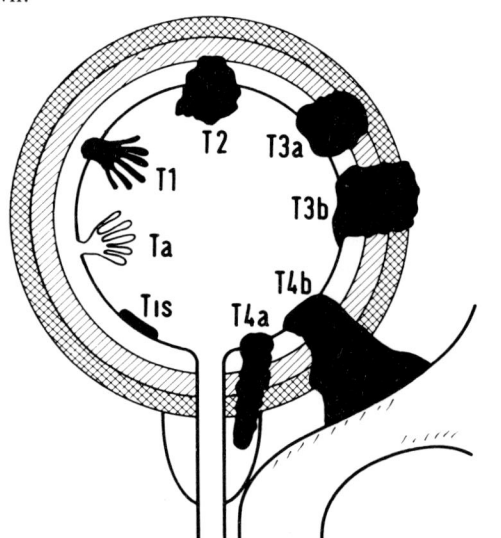

Fig 22.4 T category for carcinoma of bladder. (From *Tutorials in Postgraduate Medicine: Urology* p. 167 by courtesy of Professor G.D. Chisholm and the publishers, William Heinemann Medical Books.)

Treatment

Tumour occurring in the upper urinary tract should be treated by nephroureterectomy provided the contralateral kidney and ureter are normal. Regular follow-up with cystoscopy and IVU is essential as many patients will go on to develop recurrence in the bladder. In those cases where tumour occurs in a solitary kidney, or there is a solitary lesion in the patient considered unfit for radical surgery, segmental resection may be the treatment of choice. In those rare patients with synchronously occurring bilateral tumours, a combination of segmental resection, bench surgery with autotransplantation of the kidney and cytotoxic therapy is indicated.

Prognosis of tumours in the upper urinary tract is directly related to the histological grading and there is a marked reduction in survival in those patients in whom the tumour shows invasion of muscle.

Superficial tumours (Ta, T1)

Solitary bladder tumours with no evidence of abnormality in random biopsies are adequately treated by transurethral resection and regular cystoscopic follow-up. Well-differentiated multiple lesions may be treated initially by resection and diathermy and provided that they are easy to control, may not require any further treatment.

However, many patients with superficial tumours will develop multiple recurrences which may be difficult to control endoscopically and in these cases adjuvant intravesical chemotherapy has an important part to play in their management. These drugs act either by preventing or delaying the appearance of recurrences or by destroying active tumours.

Thiotepa has been used for 20 years with considerable success (Jones and Swinney, 1961). Forty per cent of patients with superficial tumours are cleared, but there is some risk of absorption and fatal bone marrow depression when a high dose of the drug is used. More recently England *et al.* (1980) reported a 75% decrease in the rate of new tumour-formation using a much smaller dose of thiotepa. Tumours which fail to respond may have a greater malignant potential and this may be of value in selecting patients for more radical therapy.

Riddle and Wallace (1971) reported the use of intravesical Epodyl and demonstrated a 50% response rate. This drug has the advantage that it is not absorbed and there are, therefore, no systemic side-effects. Non-response to Epodyl is also an indication for more radical therapy (Fitzpatrick, *et al.*, 1979).

Intravesical adriamycin produces a similar reponse with superficial tumours but the drug is expensive and is probably only advantageous in patients with carcinoma *in situ* (Edsmyr, 1980). Mitomycin C is also expensive but the early results indicate that this may be the best of the intravesical agents.

Over-distension of the bladder with the Helmstein balloon may be useful in arresting bleeding from superficial bladder tumours, but should not be used routinely in their treatment as there are a few reports of metastatic deposits occurring after treatment of superficial tumours in this manner.

Invasive tumours (T2, T3a, T3b)

Since these tumours have invaded muscle, local treatment is no longer adequate and the choice lies between radical radiotherapy, cystectomy or a combination of the two. Careful pretreatment staging is required to avoid submitting patients with incurable disease to a course of radical treatment.

Endoscopic resection of most T2 bladder tumours is inadequate and such patients should receive radiotherapy. Fifty per cent of patients may be expected to survive five years.

Radical radiotherapy for deeply infiltrating tumours is favoured by many urologists, mainly because this form of therapy preserves the bladder. Five-year survival is poor, being at best 30%. In addition to problems produced by irradiation cystitis and proctitis, the main disadvantage of radiotherapy is that failure of treatment leads to local recurrence. Under these circumstances salvage cystectomy is often difficult and is associated with a higher morbidity and mortality.

Radical cystectomy alone is unlikely to produce more than a 35% five-year survival rate and is associated with significant mortality. However, there is increasing evidence to show that planned preoperative radiotherapy (4000 rad in 4 weeks) followed by cystectomy 4 weeks later, produces significantly better survival rates at 5 years (Bloom *et al.*, 1982). Furthermore, patients whose tumours are 'down-staged' by preoperative radiotherapy fare significantly better than those whose tumours do not respond. Superior results obtained by this form of therapy may be explained by a much lower than expected incidence of pelvic lymph node involvement in those patients receiving preoperative radiotherapy.

Most patients with invasive bladder cancer die from distant metastases and it is clear that neither radiotherapy nor radical surgery provides adequate treatment in the majority. Adjuvant chemotherapy has not been used routinely in the treatment of bladder cancer and the evaluation of cytotoxic drugs has been limited to patients with advanced metastatic disease. A number of agents have now been identified as showing some activity against bladder cancer and a combination of these agents appears to be even more active. Cisplatinum, cyclophosphamide and adriamycin when given in combination show an objective response rate of 50% (Yagoda, 1982) and, in the future, the addition of chemotherapy to preoperative radiotherapy and cystectomy may provide more long-term survivors.

Tumours (T4)

The prognosis is extremely poor. Most patients are dead within 12 months of diagnosis and palliative radiotherapy for pain or bleeding is the only possible treatment.

Carcinoma *in situ*

The initial treatment of choice in these patients should be intravesical chemotherapy combined with careful and regular follow-up with cystoscopy and cytological examination of the urine. Sixty per cent of patients will progress to infiltrating carcinoma and if the lesion is widespread at presentation or progression occurs, cystourethrectomy is the treatment of choice since radiotherapy gives rather poor results.

Testicular tumours

Testicular tumours account for between 1–2% of all malignant neoplasms in man – an annual incidence of 2–3 per 100 000. A high incidence of clinical suspicion leading to early diagnosis, combined with advances in radiotherapy and cytotoxic chemotherapy enable many men with testicular tumours to be completely cured.

Aetiology

Testicular tumours are usually found in fit young men and are rare in negroes. There is a considerable difference in the peak age for occurrence of germinal cell tumours, teratomas tending to occur about a decade earlier than seminomas, which may continue to occur well into middle-age. Testicular tumours may be familial: there are a number of case reports of tumours occurring in twins and brothers. Men with undescended testes have approximately 30 times the risk of developing a testicular tumour than those with both testes descended. This is due to the high incidence of dysgenesis in the undescended testis and in approximately 10% of men who have both maldescent and a testicular tumour, there is evidence of carcinoma *in situ* in the contralateral testis. A considerable proportion of patients with testicular tumours give a history of injury to the testicle and on occasion there is a history of inflammatory disease.

Pathology

There are a few rare benign testicular tumours. Leydig cell tumours account for about 1%; they are almost all benign and production of hormones by the tumour causes precocious puberty in the prepubertal male and later, gynaecomastia. Sertoli cell tumours are also benign, the production of large amounts of oestrogen may also cause gynaecomastia. Very rarely, the testis may be infiltrated with malignant lymphoma which is more often a manifestation of widespread disease and bilateral testicular involvement is common.

The majority of tumours arising from the testis are of germ cell origin. Approximately 50% of these tumours will be seminomas which are characterised macroscopically by a firm, pinkish, rounded tumour divided by fibrous bands. In 75% of patients the tumour is confined to the testis at the time of diagnosis. Seminomas arise from the germinal epithelium of the seminiferous tubules and it has been suggested that the tumours may arise from any part of the spermatocytic element depending on the response of the cells to carcinogenic stimulus. Pure seminoma tends to metastasise first to the retroperitoneal lymph nodes, then to the mediastinum and supraclavicular lymph nodes. Haematogenous spread is rare.

The remaining types of non-seminomatous testicular tumours are embryonal carcinoma, choriocarcinoma, teratoma and terato carcinoma and these tumours can occur either alone or in combination. Genesis of these tumours is from primordial germ cells, embryonal carcinoma represents the results of early differentiation of tumour cells before the development of trophoblastic elements. Complete somatic differentiation results in the formation of teratoma whereas complete trophoblastic differentiation produces choriocarcinoma. Teratomas have been further subdivided reprsenting varying degrees of malignancy (Pugh, 1976). Choriocarcinoma and terato carcinoma usually metastasise to retroperitoneal nodes first, but haematogenous spread is common and is almost universal in cases of choriocarcinoma. Unlike seminomas, only 30–40% of non-seminomatous tumours are localised to the testis at diagnosis.

Clinical features

Most patients present with a history of a painless lump in the testis or a slowly enlarging painless testis. In many there is a definite history of trauma and patients may occasionally present with a painful swollen testis and a history suggestive of epididymo-orchitis. In all cases a high index of clinical suspicion is required and every scrotal mass should be considered malignant until proved otherwise. Usually there will be no doubt as to the nature of the scrotal swelling, but the diagnosis can be extremely difficult in patients who present with epididymo-orchitis. Following an acute inflammatory episode it is difficult to be certain whether a persisting lump in the testis is postinflammatory or is due to a testicular tumour, and then it is safer to explore the testis early through a groin incision and risk removing an inflammatory mass, than it is to watch a potentially curable testicular tumour grow over a number of months.

The physical signs will be those of a hard painless lump in the testis which may vary in size from a small 1 cm discrete nodule which is barely palpable, to an enlarged hard mass totally replacing the normal testis. Very rarely abdominal palpation will reveal evidence of retroperitoneal lymph node involvement.

Preoperative estimation of α-feto-protein and β-HCG (human chorionic gonadotrophin) is now an essential part of the management of all patients with testicular tumours. These tumour markers have been found to be elevated in non-seminomatous tumours of the testis and may be used as a guide to determining whether elements of embryonal cell carcinoma coexist with seminoma, whether the tumour has recurred or persisted and the efficacy of the therapy.

Clinical diagnosis of a testicular tumour should lead to the immediate admission of the patient and exploration of the testis through a groin incision on the next available operating list. Orchiectomy is performed through the groin and before the testis is mobilised, the cord is occluded to prevent haematogenous spread of the tumour caused by manipulation. When there is no doubt about the diagnosis, the spermatic cord and vessels should be ligated as high as possible in the inguinal canal, but in cases where there is some doubt as to the exact nature of the swelling, it is permissible to place a soft occluding clamp on the cord before delivering the testis for inspection. It is safer to risk removing a testis containing an inflammatory lump than to leave the tumour behind.

Further staging procedures should be carried out in the postoperative period. α-feto protein and βHCG levels should be sent 7 days after orchiectomy and at varying intervals during the follow-up period. Bilateral pedal lymphography should be carried out. In the UK this is reckoned to be an accurate assessment of the presence of malignant disease in the lymph nodes, with reported accuracy rates as high as 87% (Borksi, 1973). In the USA, however, retroperitoneal lymph node dissection is carried out routinely as a staging procedure. The operation carries a low mortality and morbidity, but impotence is almost universal after this procedure. CT scanning is of value in confirming the presence of retroperitoneal disease and is of value in the follow-up of these patients. Chest x-ray and whole lung tomography is also required for full staging of these tumours (Fig 22.5).

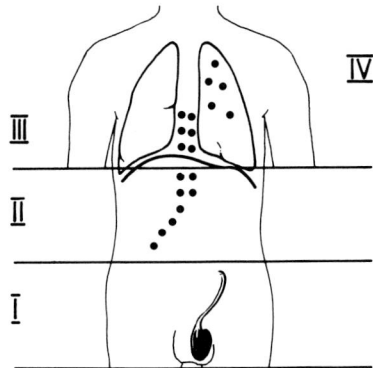

Stage I Tumour confined to testis. No lymph node involvement

II Involvement of sub-diaphragmatic lymph nodes

III Involvement of supra-diaphragmatic lymph nodes

IV Extra lymphatic metastases

Fig 22.5 Staging for testicular tumours (Stages II–IV have three subgroups according to size and number of metastases).

Treatment of testicular seminoma

A combination of surgical excision of the primary testicular tumour and radiotherapy to the nodal metastases is successful in over 90% of cases of seminoma (Calman *et al.*, 1979). Radiotherapy is based on the assumption that the disease is one step ahead of the point where it has been positively identified. Thus stage I tumours are routinely treated by radiotherapy to the para-aortic and ipsilateral pelvic nodes and patients with stage II disease also receive radiotherapy to the mediastinal and supraclavicular nodes. Patients with stage III and stage IV disease will also receive chemotherapy in addition to radiotherapy. Many different cytotoxic agents have been used including cyclophosphamide, but recently a combination of cis-platinum, vinblastine and bleomycin (PVB) has been used with dramatic success (Einhorn and Donoghue, 1977, Einhorn and Williams, 1982). In North America, retroperitoneal lymph node dissection is combined with radiotherapy. A review of the world literature carried out by Smith in 1979 indicates that the survival of patients with stage I disease is over 90% and patients with stage II disease survival approaches 70%. The overall survival rate for patients with stages III and IV is 22% (Smith *et al.*, 1979).

Non-seminomatous testicular tumours

In the UK patients with early non-seminomatous testicular tumours (stages I and II) have been treated by radical orchiectomy and radiotherapy, whereas in North America the standard treatment has been orchiectomy followed by radical node dissection. Comparison of just over 150 patients treated by orchiectomy and radiotherapy at the Royal Marsden Hospital and the collective American experience of just over 600 cases treated by orchiectomy and retroperitoneal lymph node dissection shows virtually identical survival figures at 3 years (Table 1). It would appear that the American policy of lymphadenectomy is unnecessary as a routine in these *early* cases.

Table 1

	Stage	n	% Survival
UK	I	111	81
	II	45	51
US	I	373	82.6
	II	257	49.4

Comparison of survival of patients with early testicular tumours treated by orchiectomy and radiotherapy (UK) and orchiectomy and radical node dissection (US).
(After Hendry, 1980).

In patients with more advanced disease in the para-aortic nodes, combination therapy is given starting with chemotherapy (PVB) and followed some weeks later by irradiation of the para-aortic and pelvic lymph nodes. It is possible that laparotomy and excision of residual bulk disease may be beneficial in selected patients (Hendry *et al.*, 1980), but this concept requires further evaluation.

The precise timing of the various treatment options is still to be assessed in the management of this condition, but it is clear that the use of combined treatment regimes has transformed the prognosis for patients with testicular tumours. The use of tumour markers provides early warning of the presence of recurrent disease and enables the presence of unsuspected non-seminomatous elements to be detected in patients who are thought to have pure seminoma.

Penile cancer

Penile cancer is rare in developed countries and is almost never seen in the circumcised male. The development of carcinoma of the penis has long been associated with poor hygiene and exposure to still-undefined carcinogens in the smegma. The tumour usually presents in the sixth and seventh decades and up to 50% of patients will have clinically palpable inguinal lymph nodes on initial presentation, although only 50% of these will contain tumour.

Pathology

Macroscopically the tumour will appear as an ulcerating papilliferous growth which on occasion is confined to the foreskin, but more usually arises on the glans penis and may be infiltrating one or both corpora cavernosa. Macroscopically the tumour may be confused with gross condylomata acuminata (Buschke-Lowenstein) tumour.

Microscopically the tumour is of squamous cell type and there may be varying degrees of differentiation. Distant metastases are rare, but involvement of inguinal lymph nodes is common. A simple clinical staging is used (Fig 22.6) according to the degree of penile involvement and the presence or absence of lymph node metastases. Stage I tumours are confined to the glans penis or prepuce, and the five-year survival rate of patients in this group approaches 95% (De Kernion and Persky, 1978). Stage II tumours include those that invade the shaft of the penis or corpora, but in whom there is no clinical evidence of lymphatic or distant metastases. The estimated five-year survival is approximately 70% (Williams, 1975). Inguinal lymph node metastases are evident in patients with stage III tumours. Stage IV tumours are locally invasive from the penile shaft or accompanied by unresectable lymph nodes or distant metastases. Even with extensive radiotherapy and chemotherapy five-year survival in these patients is extremely poor.

Clinical presentation

Patients are often elderly and showing signs of self-neglect. They may present with symptoms of a bloody discharge from the tip of an uncircumcised penis. The tumour may be discovered incidentally during routine clinical examination for some other reason, as many patients try to hide their disease.

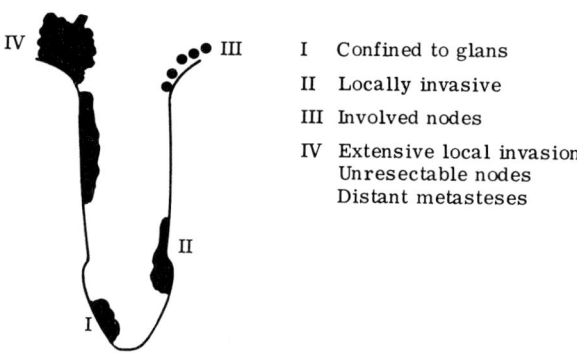

I	Confined to glans
II	Locally invasive
III	Involved nodes
IV	Extensive local invasion Unresectable nodes Distant metasteses

Fig 22.6   Staging for carcinoma of the penis.

Although frequently the diagnosis is not in doubt, a biopsy of the tumour must be obtained before definitive therapy is undertaken, as occasionally the tumour may be confused with giant condylomata acuminata. Due to the associated presence of infection about half the patients will have evidence of inguinal lymphadenopathy at presentation, but their presence must not be assumed to be due to tumour as many nodes disappear once infection has been treated.

Management

Careful examination under anaesthetic with palpation of the shaft of the penis to stage the disease is required. This should be combined with the creation of a dorsal slit in the foreskin and biopsy of the suspected tumour. Thorough cleansing of the lesion and the penis can be carried out at the same time. Culture swabs are taken and the patient is given a broad spectrum antibiotic. Once the infection is under control at least 50% of enlarged lymph nodes will become smaller and disappear.

In patients with a superficial lesion confined to the foreskin, simple circumcision is the most appropriate management. Other patients with stage I and early stage II lesions may be treated with radiotherapy, but patients with more advanced lesions are best treated by partial penectomy.

In all cases, the lymph nodes should be managed expectantly for at least 6 weeks after removal of the primary tumour, as much lymphadenopathy is due to the presence of infection. Overall only 20% of patients will present with metastases and it is, therefore, extremely difficult to justify block dissection in all patients who present with enlarged lymph nodes. Furthermore, there is no evidence that there is any deterioration in prognosis if lymphadenectomy is delayed (Grabstaldt, 1979). In patients with persisting clinically palpable lymph nodes, inguinal lymphadenectomy should be performed. If lymph nodes become palpable they should be removed.

References

Bennington J.L., Laubscher F.A. (1968). Epidemiological studies on carcinoma of the kidney: Association of renal adenocarcinoma with smoking. *Cancer*; **21**:1069–71.
Bloom H.J.G., Hendry W.F., Wallace D.M., Skeet R.G. (1982). Treatment of T3 bladder cancer: controlled trial of pre-operative radiotherapy and radical cystectomy versus radical radiotherapy. Second report and review (for the Clinical Trial Group, Institute of Urology). *Brit. J. Urol*; **54**:136–51.
Borski A.A. (1973). Diagnosis, staging and natural history testis tumours. *Cancer*; **42**:1202–11.

Calman F.M.B., Peckman M.J., Hendry W.F. (1979). The pattern of spread and treatment of metastases in testicular seminoma. *Brit. J. Urol*; **51**:154–60.

Chisholm G.D. (1980). Urological malignancy: prostate. In *Tutorials in Postgraduate Medicine: Urology* (Chisholm G.D., ed.) pp. 223–46. London: Heinemann Medical.

Chisholm G.D., O'Donoghue E.P.N., Kennedy C.L. (1977). Treatment of oestrogen escaped carcinoma of the prostate with estramustine phosphate. *Brit. J. Urol*; **49**:717–20.

De Kernion J.B., Persky L. (1978). Neoplastic lesions of the penis. In *Genioto-urinary Cancer* (Skinner D.C., De Kernion J.B., eds.) ch. 28. Philadelphia: Saunders.

Edsmyr F. (1980). Intravesical therapy with adriamycin in patients with superficial bladder tumours. In *Bladder Cancer: Progress in Combination Therapy* (Oliver R.T.D., Hendry W.F., Bloom H.J.G., eds.). London: Butterworth.

Einhorn L.H., Donoghue J.P. (1977). Improved chemotherapy in disseminated testicular cancer. *J. Urol*; **117**:65–9.

Einhorn L.J., Williams S.D. (1982). Chemotherapy of testicular cancer. In *Chemotherapy and Urological Malignancy* (Spiers A.S.D., ed.) ch. 10. Berlin: Springer-Verlag.

England H.R., Paris A.M., Blandy J.P. (1980). Intravesical thiotepa as adjuvant to cytodiathermy in multiple recurrent superficial bladder tumours. In *Bladder Cancer: Progress in Combination Therapy* (Oliver R.T.D., Hendry W.F., Bloom H.J.G., eds.). London: Butterworth.

Fitzpatrick J.M., Constable A.R., Sherwood T., Stephenson J.J., Chisholm G.D., O'Donoghue E.P.N. (1978). Serial bone scanning in the assessment of treatment response in carcinoma of the prostate. *Brit. J. Urol*; **50**:555–61.

Fitzpatrick J.M., Khan O., Oliver R.T.D., Riddle P.R. (1979). Long-term follow-up in patients with superficial bladder tumours treated with intravesical epodyl. *Brit. J. Urol*; **51**:542–8.

Flocks R.H., Kadesky M.C. (1958). Malignant neoplasms of the kidney: an analysis of 353 patients followed 5 years or more. *J. Urol*; **79**:196–201.

Grabstaldt H. (1979). Cancer of the penis. *J. Contin. Educ. Orol*; **18**:15–17.

Harisiadis L., Veenema R.J., Senyszn J.J. (1978). Carcinoma of the prostate: treatment with external radiotherapy. *Cancer*; **41**:2131–40.

Hendry W.F., Barrett A., McElwain T.J., Wallace D.M., Peckham M.J. (1980). The role of surgery in combined management of metastasis from malignant teratomas of testis. *Brit. J. Urol*; **52**:38–44.

Huggins C., Hodges C.V. (1941). Studies on prostatic cancer. I. Effect of castration of oestrogen and of androgen injec-

tion of serum phosphatases in metastatic carcinoma of the prostate. *Cancer Research*; **1**:293–7.

Jones H.B., Swinney J. (1961). Thiotepa in the treatment of tumours of the bladder. *Lancet*; **ii**:645–8.

O'Donoghue E.P.N., Shreidhar P., Sherwood T., Williams J.P., Chisholm G.D. (1976). Lymphography and pelvic lymphadenectomy in carcinoma of the prostate. *Brit. J. Urol*; **48**:689–96.

Peeling W.B., Griffifths G.J., Evans K.T., Roberts E.E. (1979). Diagnosis and staging of prostatic cancer by transrectal ultrasonography. A preliminary study. *Brit. J. Urol*; **51**:565–9.

Pugh R.C.B. (1976). Testicular tumours introduction. In *Pathology of the Testis* (Pugh R.C.B., ed.) pp. 139–59. Oxford: Blackwell.

Riddle P.R., Wallace D.M. (1971). Intracavity chemotherapy for multiple non-invasive bladder tumours. *Brit. J. Urol*; **43**:181–184.

Smith R.B., Skinner D.G., De Kernion J.B. (1979). Management of advanced testicular seminoma. *J. Urol*; **121**:420–31.

Spiers A.S.D. (1982). Cytotoxic drugs and hormonal manipulations in the management of carcinoma of the kidney. In *Chemotherapy and Urological Malignancy* (Spiers A.S.D., ed.) ch. 2. Berlin: Springer-Verlag.

Stone A.R., Merrick M.V., Chisholm G.D. (1979). Prostatic lymphoscintigraphy. *Brit. J. Urol*; **51**:556–60.

Torti F.M., Carter S.K. (1982). Chemotherapy of cancer of the prostate. In *Chemotherapy and Urological Malignancy* (Spiers A.S.D., ed.) ch. 7. Berlin: Springer-Verlag.

UICC (1978). *TNM Classification of Malignant Tumours*, 3rd edn. Geneva: UICC.

Utz D.C., Warren M.M., Gregg J.A., Ludwig J., Kelalis P.P. (1970). Reversible hepatic dysfunction associated with hypernephroma. *Mayo Clin. Proc*; **45**:161–9.

Wallace D.M.A., Hindmarsh J.R., Webb J.N., Busuttil A., Hargreave T.B., Newsam J.E., Chisholm G.D. (1979). The role of multiple mucosal biopsies in the management of patients with bladder cancer. *Brit. J. Urol*; **51**:535–40.

Wallace S., Chuang V.P., Swanson D., Bracken B., Hersh E.M., Ayala A., Johnson D. (1981). Embolisation of renal carcinoma: experience with 100 patients. *Radiology*; **138**:563–70.

Williams J.L. (1975). Surgical treatment of carcinoma of the penis. *Proc. Roy. Soc. Med*; **68**:781–3.

Yagoda A. (1982). The chemotherapy of advanced carcinoma of the urothelial tract. In *Chemotherapy and Urological Malignancy* (Spiers A.S.D., ed.) ch. 6. Berlin: Springer-Verlag.

23

Trauma

GEOFFREY D. CHISHOLM

Though most of the urinary tract is deeply placed, it does not escape its share of injury. The principles of care of the injured patient are discussed elsewhere (Chapter 44). It is important to keep an open mind as to the likely extent of any injury: an apparently minor injury to the loin in a child can result in kidney fragmentation: the multiplicity of injuries that can occur in a major road accident can easily divert attention away from the damage to the bladder/urethra often associated with a fractured pelvis.

Because of the nature of most injuries, the urological surgeon is unlikely to be the *first* doctor to attend these patients and it is the casualty officer/trauma surgeon who will have noted an abnormality of the flank, or blood at the external meatus or contusion of the perineum. Much of the controversy about the optimum treatment of some injuries of the urinary tract is derived from the assumption that a urologist, experienced in trauma, is always available to carry out the ideal urological treatment. The distinction must be made between the ideal and what is the most likely course of events.

In this context, the role of urethral catheterisation must be clarified. The measurement of urine output in the severely shocked and/or comatose patient is essential for fluid balance calculations. If there is no evidence of pelvic injury, then the aseptic, gentle passage of a 16F Foley catheter may be helpful to check that the patient is producing urine; the catheter does not need to be left *in situ* if the patient can void spontaneously and has a residual volume of 30 ml or less. If, however, there is a pelvic injury and/or blood at the meatus, then urethral damage should be assumed and a catheter should not be passed unless the situation has been further clarified (*see* p. 380). If the patient has had a pelvic injury and voids blood-stained urine, it is still better to act as if there is an injury and to investigate accordingly.

Kidney trauma

Aetiology

Open injuries

The kidney or renal pedicle may be injured either by a gunshot wound (GSW) or by stabbing. A percutaneous needle biopsy can, occasionally, damage an intrarenal vessel and cause severe bleeding: this may be a rare cause of an arteriovenous fistula. Open injuries are usually associated with other abdominal injuries.

Closed injuries

These are of two types:

Direct, blunt injury as when a child slips and falls against the edge of a bath or, as in sports injuries, where there is a punch or kick in the loin. If the injury seemed relatively trivial then it may be that the kidney was already abnormal (e.g. hydronephrotic.) There may also be fractured ribs with either a splenic or liver injury.

Deceleration injuries as in RTA or aircraft accident may injure the pedicle, for this is the only fixed part of the kidney. The usual damage is an intimal tear with spasm and thrombosis as a possible sequel.

The late effects of renal trauma include a perirenal collection of urine (urinoma) which is at risk of becoming infected, scarring of the kidney or renal artery stenosis causing hypertension. Hydronephrosis may be either an early or late complication.

Clinical features and management

Injuries to the kidney are classified in four groups (Fig 23.1): (a) contusions; (b) lacerations; (c) fragmentation; (d) renal pedicle injuries.

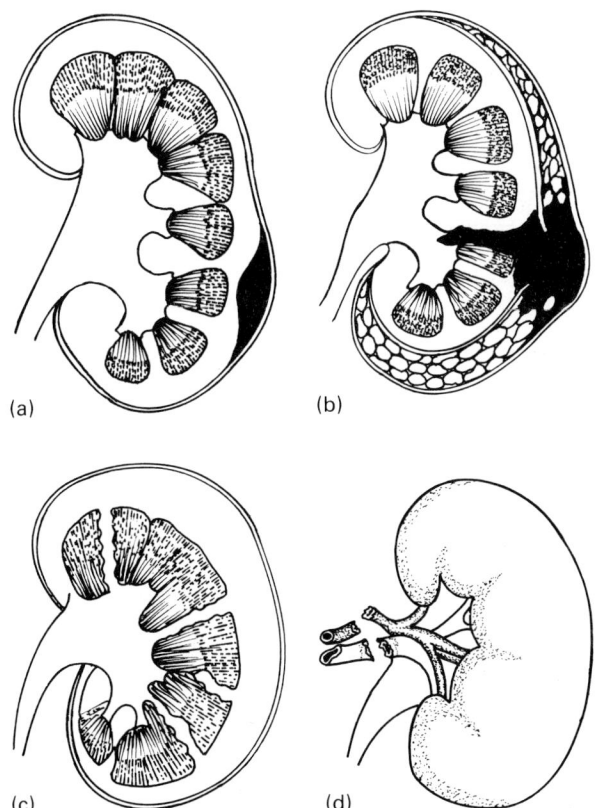

(a)

(b)

(c)

(d)

Fig 23.1   Injuries to kidney (a) contusion; (b) laceration; (c) fragmentation; (d) pedicle injury.

Contusions

These are the most common injuries and range from a subcapsular haematoma to minor cortical lacerations, but not involving the calices. Haematuria is present, but usually lasts for only a very few days. An IVU may show some irregularity of the renal outline but nothing else. No further investigations are needed. Treatment consists of bed rest, routine monitoring of pulse and BP and serial examination of the urine.

Lacerations

These extend deep into the collecting system. An IVU may show a wedge-shaped defect and there is likely to be a deformed outline due to haematoma. Extravasation is best seen on later x-rays. There may be clot in the collecting system causing obstruction. A laceration, if part of an open injury, needs exploring to determine the overall extent of the trauma. The majority of lacerations with a closed injury can be treated conservatively; the decision to explore a laceration early will be made if the clinical condition of the patient deteriorates and/or the loin swelling increases in size (Peters and Bright, 1977). Late exploration may be considered if haematuria is heavy and persistent (*see* Fig 23.2, Lang, 1975).

Fragmentation

Severe lacerations will result in fragmentation of the kidney and this injury almost always needs to be explored (Fowler *et al.*, 1982). The IVU may show gross extravasation or non-function of a part of the kidney. Ultrasound can be helpful, but angiography is essential to establish the severity of damage. A retrograde ureteropyelogram will add little to the diagnostic information and is not advised. The extent of the surgical procedure depends on the severity of the lacerations, but preservation of some of the kidney should be the aim.

Pedicle injuries

Sudden deceleration injuries may lead to an arterial intimal tear (with subsequent thrombosis) or the pedicle injury may be combined with severe lacerations and fragmentation. As soon as suspicion of a major renal injury is raised, an IVU is carried out: there may be no excretion by the kidney and even doubt as to the presence of the kidney. Ultrasound can be helpful, but there should be no delay in proceeding to an angiogram (Williams, 1976). Early operation offers a fair chance of saving the kidney, but if the delay is more than 24–26 h, then the kidney will be beyond salvage.

The place of angiography in the management of a patient with renal injury is shown in Fig 23.2.

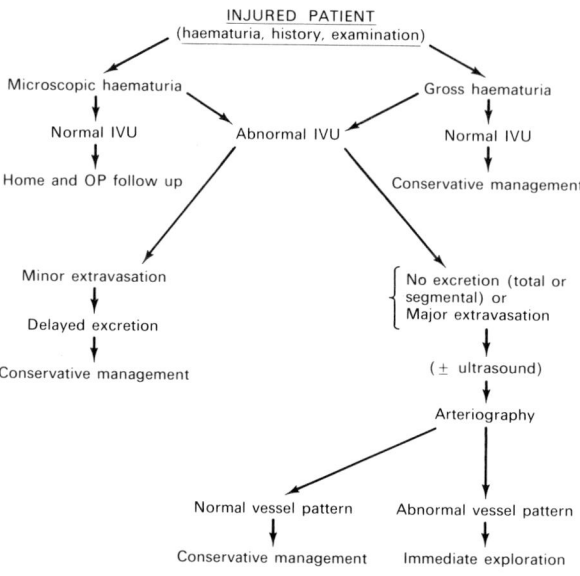

Fig 23.2 Flow chart for investigation of renal injury.

Ureteric trauma

The problems of ureteric injury concern not only the urologist but the general surgeon and gynaecologist (Yeates, 1980). Although the majority of these injuries are iatrogenic, a distinction should be made between those that occur as part of an operative procedure, those that occur accidentally, but are recognised, and those that are not recognised, thereby presenting as a complication of damage to the ureter (Newsam and Buist, 1980).

Aetiology

Ureteric injuries may be either closed or open.

Closed injuries

These are rare. The ureter is occasionally involved in major accidents such as 'run-over' injuries; children are prone to a rupture at the pelvi-ureteric junction with closed injuries. The ureter may be avulsed by the stone basket in an attempt to extract a ureteric stone (Riberio and Quartey, 1976).

Open injuries

These are almost always in association with other injuries and chance may include the ureter in a stab wound or, more commonly, a gunshot wound (GSW) (Peterson and Pitts, 1981). The main causes of injury to the ureter are operations involving the colon, rectum, bladder, major abdominal vessels or most commonly of all, operations on the uterus. The anatomical relationship of the ureters to these organs makes it inevitable that a variety of pathological conditions will affect the ureter e.g. retroperitoneal fibrosis, carcinoma of the large bowel, carcinoma of the prostate etc. The urologist may damage the ureter during an endoscopic basket extraction of a stone. The radiotherapist may cause either early or late (fibrotic) damage to the ureter in the course of treatment.

Clinical features and management

Ureteric resection planned at operation

In such a situation, the ureter will have been deliberately included in a surgical procedure, usually an extensive dissection for malignancy. Less commonly, a urologist may decide to carry out a local excision of a ureteric tumour, rather than a nephroureterectomy. In the confident expectation of a successful primary anastomosis 2–3 cm of a ureter can be excised spatulating the ends of the ureter and closing with continuous 4/0 CCG (Fig 23.3).

If a large piece of ureter has been removed, and especially if the overall prognosis of the patient is not good, then it is best to remove the kidney and not to burden the patient with tubes or 'ostomies.

If the ureteric excision is within the pelvis, then reimplantation into the bladder may be the simplest choice. If the gap between the ureter and bladder is too great for implantation, a Boari flap or psoas hitch may be considered; however, it may be expedient to place a catheter in the proximal end of the ureter and then review the situation at a later date.

If the ureter is unsuited for primary repair, then it should not be tied off (it will almost certainly leak or become infected). A ureterostomy should not be done, for it will cause endless problems unless the ureter was already dilated. It is better to put either a T-tube or a catheter into the ureter and review at a later date.

Accidental injury recognised at operation

Provided that the ureter is healthy, there is no reason why a careful anastomosis should not be successful and trouble-free (Fig 23.3); there is no need for splinting or a T-tube.

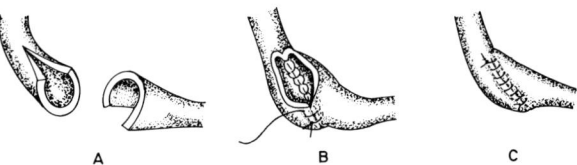

Fig 23.3 Ureteric anastomosis, (a) ureter is cut transversly and opposite border is cut back for 1.0–1.5 cm; (b) anastomosis with continuous 4/0 chromic catgut; (c) anastomosis complete.

If the damage is deep in the pelvis and technically awkward, the ureter may best be implanted into the dome of the bladder, ideally with a submucosal tunnel but this is not essential (Fig 23.4).

If the ureter is unhealthy e.g. from previous irradiation or from enmeshment in retroperitoneal fibrosis, then repair across a T-tube may be necessary. A urologist may prefer to swing the healthy upper ureter across to the other ureter – a transuretero-ureterostomy, but this should not be used for patients with either stones or tumours. An ileal loop replacement of the ureter may be preferred.

Accidental injury, not recognised at operation

The injury to the ureter may be either a cut, crush, excision, ligation or ischaemic necrosis (from a suture or forceps injury). Thus the sequelae may be either

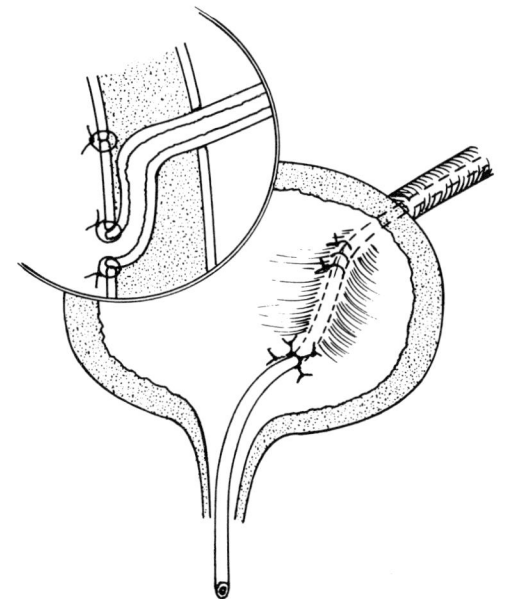

Fig 23.4 Ureteric reimplantation into bladder (Leadbetter–Politano technique).

complete or partial obstruction with subsequent hydronephrosis, or a urinary fistula. The fistula may occur immediately if the damage is not recognised at operation or later if the injury caused ureteric necrosis. The urine may leak to the skin (cutaneous fistula) or form a urinoma, or leak through the vagina after a gynaecological operation (ureterovaginal fistula).

The patient may complain of renal pain after an operation but, surprisingly, a completely obstructed kidney may cause few symptoms. However, if infection should occur in an obstructed kidney, then the patient soon becomes ill with pain, fever and rigors (Mendez and McGinty, 1978). An excessively 'watery' discharge from a wound is highly suspicious of a urinary fistula. The fistula may cause little or no upset to the patient unless superadded infection occurs. A rapid way to determine that a watery discharge is either urine or serum is to measure the concentration of urea in this fluid. Alternatively, an IVU will show the side of the damage: whether the ureter is cut or injured, there is always some hold-up of contrast on the affected side. This differs from the urogram in a patient with vesicovaginal fistula where the upper tract is normal. If there is still uncertainty as to whether a vaginal leak is from the ureter or bladder, then discolouration of a vaginal swab after intravesical methylene blue will confirm that the leak is from the bladder.

If the leak occurs late i.e. after 10–14 days, then a minimal partial injury may be suspected: a ureteric catheter may be passed endoscopically and left for 10–14 days to allow the area to heal. In general, early exploration is advised to avoid the hazard of operating in inflamed-infected tissues. If the procedure is carried out early enough, it may be possible to carry out a primary repair of the ureter. Usually the damaged ureter is best reimplanted into the bladder (Fig 23.4). If the ureter cannot be reimplanted comfortably without tension, then some method must be used to bring the bladder to the ureter (Boari flap or psoas hitch) (Turner Warwick and Worth, 1969). If the ureter is very short, then an ileal ureter may be fashioned or a transuretero-ureterostomy may be preferred. However, if there is severe infection or the patient has a limited prognosis from the primary disease, it may be safer to remove the kidney.

Emergency management of penetrating injuries

A clean incision from a stab wound may allow for careful primary suture. With a GSW, the devitalised tissue may be excised (for 2–3 cm) and the ureter anastamosed over a splint (either T-tube or a Cummings nephrostomy tube). If the gap is larger, then temporary ureteric tube drainage should be used.

Bladder trauma

Although bladder and urethral injuries will be described separately, it must be remembered that both structures may be damaged in severe trauma. In a series of lower urinary tract injuries in Bristol, the anterior urethra was ruptured in 21, the posterior urethra in 63 and the bladder in 34 cases: double injuries occurred in 10% (Mitchell, 1973). Serious injury to the bladder/urethra occurs in 10% of all closed pelvic fracture-dislocations, so that the index of suspicion of urinary tract injuries should be high in these patients. The severity of the trauma is evident from the fact that 80% sustain other severe injuries (of head, chest, bowel or limbs) while up to 20% die of their multiple injuries (Coffield and Weems, 1977).

Aetiology

Injuries to the bladder may be either open or closed.

Open injuries

Penetrating injuries to the bladder are now most commonly due to GSW or some other war injury; these are usually multivisceral, associated with severe soft tissue damage and are heavily contaminated. Penetrating injuries can also occur when a person becomes impaled as on a fence; the urethra and rectum are also likely to be involved.

The bladder may be injured in the course of extensive cancer operations in the pelvis; it may be damaged because unrecognised in a large inguinal hernia. Any of these events may be followed by a wound fistula, or vesicovaginal fistula or vesicocolic fistula. (The latter may also occur as a complication of diverticulitis, Crohn's disease or carcinoma of colon.)

Closed injuries

Two types of bladder injury can occur from quite different mechanisms:

Intraperitoneal. Typically, the person has been drinking (alcohol), has a full bladder, is then assaulted and kicked in the abdomen; the dome of the bladder ruptures and urine extravasates into the peritoneum (Fig 23.5a).

Extraperitoneal. These injuries are almost entirely due to high-speed road traffic accidents in which the pelvis is fractured (Fig 23.5b). Urologists may also cause a closed extraperitoneal leak in the course of resecting either the prostate or the bladder; provided

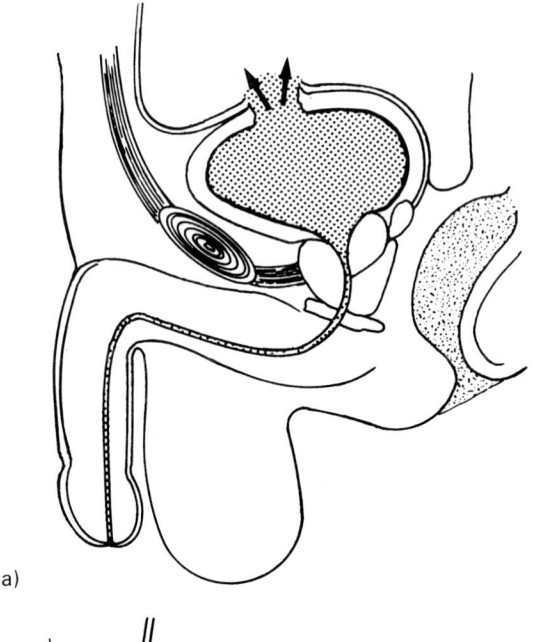

(a)

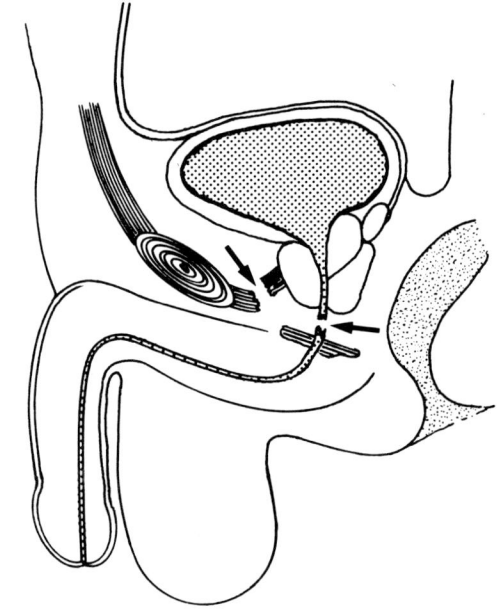

(b)

Fig 23.5 (a) intraperitoneal bladder rupture; (b) extraperitoneal, intrapelvic posterior urethral rupture.

that there is good bladder drainage per urethram, these rarely cause any clinical problems.

A vesicovaginal fistula (VVF) is a form of extraperitoneal injury to the bladder, seen mainly in less affluent countries as a complication of obstructed labour. A very prolonged second stage of labour can lead to pressure necrosis of the tissues between the inferior margins of the pubic bones and the head of the baby. The ensuing defect may vary from a very small fistula low down at the bladder neck to an extensive defect that includes the urethra, trigone and posterior bladder wall.

Clinical features and management

In general, the aetiology will indicate the most likely type of injury.

Penetrating injuries

Penetrating injuries, especially from war and terrorist violence, require immediate blood replacement, resuscitation and early exploration of the area. Diversion of the urine and/or bowel, together with debridement and drainage are usually necessary.

An intraperitoneal rupture

This may cause little evidence of the seriousness of the injury at first, but within hours there is ileus and distension (Fig 23.5a). If inebriated, there may be an even longer delay before the abdomen is examined and the history of a blow on the abdomen may be vague or even forgotten. A history of anuria is an important clue. A soft urethral catheter is passed and confirmation of a bladder rupture obtained by a cystogram. At laparotomy, the ruptured bladder is oversewn, urethral catheter drainage is established and other abdominal injuries excluded.

An extraperitoneal rupture

An extraperitoneal rupture that occurs as part of a major accident with a pelvic fracture may be difficult to distinguish from an intrapelvic rupture of the posterior urethra (Fig 23.5b). If there is blood at the external urinary meatus, the patient is unable to void and there is suprapubic pain, a urethrogram must be carried out. If the urethra is intact, then the bladder rupture should be explored and closed, with urethral and paravesical drainage established.

An extraperitoneal injury associated with a surgical procedure usually manifests as a wound fistula or vaginal fistula. Urethral catheter drainage is the first procedure, to see if the fistula dries up; a suprapubic drain is rarely needed. It may be necessary to distinguish between a ureterovaginal and vesicovaginal fistula (*see* p. 377). Urinary leakage following a difficult labour, due to a VVF, may vary from a tiny leak only, while the patient is standing, to gross incontinence – according to the size of the fistula. Gynaecologists and

urologists differ in their surgical approach to these problems, but both must use a careful multilayer closure of the fistula to avoid the risk of break-down and recurrence of the leak (Lawson and Hudson, 1980).

Urethral trauma

Aetiology

Open

Penetrating injuries especially GSW or from shrapnel, may involve either the anterior or posterior urethra.

Closed

Injuries may also involve either the anterior or posterior urethra and each may be either a complete or partial rupture.

Anterior urethral injuries typically occur by falling astride a rigid edge e.g. a fence or wall. A kick on the perineum can cause a similar injury. A difficult labour may result in a urethral fistula.

Posterior urethral injuries occur only with major trauma such as a road traffic accident. For such an injury to damage the urethra, a fracture of either the pubis or a fracture-dislocation of the pelvis must occur. Injury to the posterior urethra may also be iatrogenic due to inexpert instrumentation or even catheterisation which tears the mucosa and may cause a false passage, and later, a urethral stricture.

Clinical features and management

Open injuries

Since open injuries are usually part of a GSW, they will require debridement and, usually, proximal urinary diversion with a suprapubic catheter. It is unlikely that any formal repair can be done, since such injuries are contaminated. The area should be allowed to heal completely before reconstructive surgery is done.

Anterior urethral injuries

These are usually contusions located on the bulb of the urethra (Fig 23.6). Examination will reveal a haematoma. If the patient has passed urine, no further steps need be taken. A large haematoma with or

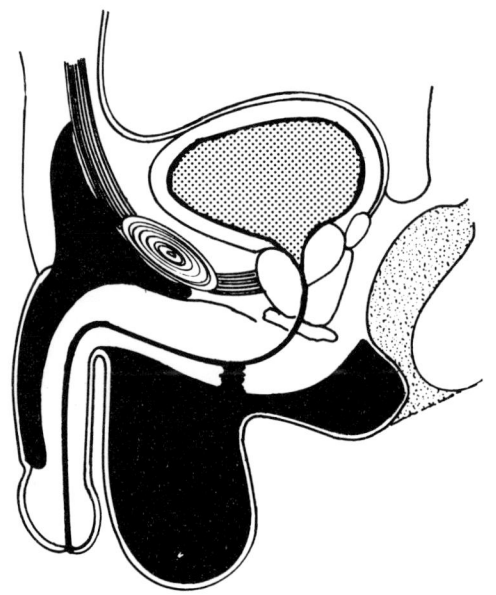

Fig 23.6   Bulbar urethral rupture, showing extent of urinary extravasation.

without extravasation of urine will need to be drained, the urethra examined and a rupture repaired; the bladder is drained by a urethral or suprapubic catheter.

If, however, there is blood at the meatus or the patient has passed blood-stained urine, then a diagnostic urethrogram using water soluble contrast material may demonstrate the extent of the damage. If the damage appears minimal, a silastic urethral catheter is inserted to act as a splint and to drain the bladder. If the injury is more severe, or catheterisation has been attempted and failed, then a suprapubic cystostomy, evacuation of haematoma and open repair of the partial or complete rupture is necessary. Antibiotic cover is essential; close follow-up with regular dilatation and/or urethrotomy under vision should avoid the need for a urethroplasty.

Posterior urethral injuries

These are often presented as an area of conflicting medical views and much confusion surrounds the management of these injuries (Morehouse and MacKinnon, 1977; DeWeerd, 1977). It is essential to recognise that there is a high risk of urethral injury in a road traffic accident victim who has a fractured pelvis. As with other injuries of the urethra (and ureter), they may be complete or partial ruptures or only contusions. The fear that routine urethral catheterisation will convert a partial to a complete rupture or a contusion to a partial rupture is justified. There is also a risk of introducing

infection. In addition, the information gained by the catheterisation may be confusing – if there is no urine, is it because the bladder is empty, or the bladder has ruptured or is the catheter coiled outside the bladder?

For these reasons a diagnostic retrograde urethrogram is recommended in all cases where there is blood at the external urethral meatus, and/or the bladder is distended and the patient unable to pass urine (Newsam and Buist, 1980).

If blood-stained urine has been passed, a urethrogram is still a useful procedure to demonstrate the state of the lower urinary tract. It is, however, true that the radiological distinction between an extraperitoneal bladder rupture and a rupture of the membranus urethra may be difficult.

If the urethrogram shows a partial rupture, but continuity of the urethra, a suprapubic cystostomy only is done and this is left for 3 months before the state of the urethra is reviewed.

If the urethra is ruptured and bladder separated, then the choice of procedure depends on the experience of the surgeon and the state of the patient. It is quite acceptable to carry out a suprapubic cystostomy, as with a partial injury, and to wait until the pelvic tissues settle and heal (Mitchell, 1975). Alternatively, the surgeon may open the bladder and rail-road a catheter across the disrupted urethra in order to replace the 'floating' prostate and realign the urethra in the hope of minimising the severity of the stricture that follows such an injury; this is also dependent on realignment of the pelvic fracture (Glass *et al.*, 1978). Attempts to suture the damaged urethra are usually prevented by the general state of the patient and by the damage to the urethral tissues. Evacuation of clot, drainage of the area and a suprapubic cystostomy are essential to hasten the early healing in the pelvis.

Urethral trauma is a major cause of stricture formation. Strictures due to a gonococcal urethritis are now much less common due to better and earlier antibiotic treatment. Although urethrotomy under vision (optical urethrotomy) is very successful for the simpler strictures of the penile and bulbar urethra, some are well managed by gentle regular urethral dilatation. Posttraumatic posterior urethral strictures remain a major urological challenge and most will eventually require urethroplasty (Waterhouse *et al.*, 1980).

Genital trauma

Injuries to the penis, scrotum, testes and spermatic cord can arise from diverse causes that range from circumcision to auto-amputation of the penis to scrotal avulsion to GSW.

The principles of management comprise the control of haemorrhage, conservative debridement and early repair. Extensive injuries and especially skin loss to the penis require a preliminary suprapubic cystostomy. Although the need for secondary reconstruction of the genital area is not common, a range of skin graft and flap techniques have been described (Horton *et al.*, 1977).

Injury to the testis may lead to a tear in the tunica albuginea and an haematocele which must be evacuated and the bleeding points diathermised. Early exploration results in more surgical repairs and fewer orchiectomies (Schuster, 1982). Scrotal avulsion or debridement may leave healthy but exposed testes: these can be placed temporarily under nearby thigh or abdominal skin.

Fracture of the penis follows trauma to the erect penis, usually with intercourse. The fracture is a rupture of the tunica albuginea (Buck's fascia). Most will heal spontaneously; a few require evacuation of haematoma and suture of the tunica. Fibrosis, deformity and impotence may be sequelae (Pryor *et al*, 1981).

References

Coffield K.S., Weems W.L. (1977). Experience with management of posterior urethral injury associated with pelvic fracture. *J Urol*; **117**:722–4.

DeWeerd J.H. (1977). Immediate realignment of posterior urethral injury. *Urol. Clin. N. Amer*; **4**:75–80.

Fowler J.W., Smith M.F., Buist T.A.S. (1982). The assessment and management of severe renal trauma. *Brit J. Urol*; **54**:329–33.

Glass R.E., Flynn J.T., King J.B., Blandy J.P. (1978). Urethral injury and fractured pelvis. *Brit. J. Urol*; **50**:578–82.

Horton C.E., McCraw J.B., Devine C.J., Jr., Devine P.C. (1977). Secondary reconstruction of the genital area. *Urol. Clin. N. Amer*; **4**:133–41.

Lang E.K. (1975). Arteriography into assessment of renal trauma. *J. Trauma*; **15**:553–66.

Lawson J.B., Hudson C.N. (1980). The management of vesicovaginal and urethral fistulae. In *Surgery of Female Incontinence*; (Stanton S.L., Tanagho E.A. eds.) ch. 14. Heidelberg: Springer-Verlag.

Mendez R., McGinty D.M. (1978). The management of delayed recognised urethral injuries. *J. Urol*; **119**:192–3.

Mitchell J. P. (1973). Trauma to the urinary tract. *New Eng. J. Med*; **288**:90–2.

Mitchell J.P. (1975). Trauma to the urethra. *Injury*; **7**:84–8.

Morehouse D.D., MacKinnon K.J. (1977). Posterior urethral injury: etiology, diagnosis, initial management. *Urol. Clin. N. Amer*; **4**:69–74.

Newsam J.E., Buist T.A.S. (1980). Trauma. In *Tutorials in Postgraduate Medicine: Urology*. (Chisholm G.D., ed.) Ch. 23. London: Heinemann Medical.

Peters P.C., Bright T.C. (1977). Blunt renal injuries. *Urol. Clin. N. Amer*; **4**:17–28.

Peterson N.E., Pitts J.C. (1981). Penetrating injuries of the ureter. *J. Urol*; **126**:581–90.

Pryor J.P., Hill J.T., Packham D.A., Yates-Bell A.J. (1981). Penile injuries with particular reference to injury to the erectile tissue. *Brit. J. Urol.*; **53**:42–6.

Ribeiro B.F., Quartey J.K.M. (1976). Traumatic avulsion of the ureter with obstruction, pseudocyst formation and hypertension. *Brit. J. Urol*; **48**:107–10.

Schuster G. (1982). Traumatic rupture of the testicle and review of the literature. *J. Urol*; **127**:1194–6.

Turner-Warwick R., Worth P.H.L. (1969). The psoas bladder hitch procedure for the replacement of the lower third of the ureter. *Brit. J. Urol*; **41**:701–9.

Williams J.E. (1976). Renal trauma – the place of arteriography. *Brit. J. Radiol*; **49**:743–4.

Waterhouse K., Laungani G., Patil, U. (1980). The surgical repair of membranous urethral strictures, experience with 105 consecutive cases. *J. Urol*; **123**:500–5.

Yeates W.K. (1980). Ureterovaginal fistulae. Chapter 15. In *Surgery of Female Incontinence*. (Stanton, S.C., Tanagho, E.A., eds.). Ch. 15. Heidelberg: Springer-Verlag.

24

Penis and scrotum

GEOFFREY D. CHISHOLM

Penis

Penile infections

Infection that involves the glans penis and prepuce may lead to problems requiring surgical intervention.

Balanitis and balanoposthitis

Bacterial infection developing under the prepuce is liable to occur in any male, but especially if the prepuce does not retract completely and prevents adequate washing of the glans. Secretions retained under the prepuce may become infected and lead to local inflammatory changes of the glans (balanitis) or glans and prepuce (balanoposthitis). If a chronic infection is neglected then the risk of developing a squamous carcinoma of the penis is increased (Chapter 22). The treatment of an acute infection is a dorsal slit of the prepuce to allow drainage and cleansing of the area, and systemic antibiotics. A circumcision can be advised for a later date.

Balanitis xerotica obliterans

This disease whose aetiology is still unknown, has been defined as a local manifestation of *lichen sclerosus et atrophicus*. It may involve the prepuce, glans, coronal sulcus and sometimes the fossa navicularis

(Kherzi *et al.*, 1979). Involvement of the prepuce is best treated by circumcision. Meatal involvement may lead to stenosis which responds to meatal dilatation, although of severe meatoplasty may be needed. Topical steroids may help in mild cases.

Condylomata acuminata

These warty growths may be either single or multiple on the glans penis, the prepuce and sometimes within the terminal few millimetres of the urethra. The warts are viral in origin and are also called venereal warts because they may be transmitted from sexual partners. A long standing and effective treatment is topical 20% podophyllin in tincture of benzoin, but diathermy and cryosurgery have also been used. It is important to recognise that the incorrect use of any of these methods may lead to a meatal stricture. Several topical chemotherapeutic agents have also been used with success (e.g. 5-fluorouracil, thio-tepa, bleomycin).

Veneral diseases

Syphilis and chancroid may produce ulcerative lesions on the penis, gonorrhoea affects primarily the urethra and paraurethral glands. The differential diagnosis between these conditions and other inflammatory or malignant diseases may ultimately require a biopsy if microbiological texts do not establish the diagnosis.

Phimosis and paraphimosis

The prepuce is normally non-retractile in the first few months of life. By the end of the first year it will retract fully in most, but not completely for three or four years in some boys. Ammoniacal balanitis (due to urea-splitting organisms) may occur and if the reaction is severe then there is scarring and constriction of the preputial orifice, preventing its retraction i.e. phimosis. A similar sequence may occur with infection in the adult and lead to difficulty in micturition; chronic infection may also involve the external meatus. Phimosis may be dealt with either by a dorsal slit or circumcision. Meatal narrowing will require a meatoplasty.

Paraphimosis is a complication of phimosis. In this condition, the narrowed prepuce retracts, but with difficulty. If there should be difficulty in returning the prepuce to its normal position, the constriction at the level of the coronal sulcus leads to severe swelling of the glans, even necrosis. This painful condition is a surgical emergency and if the prepuce cannot be manipulated forwards then the constricting band of the prepuce is slit under a general anaesthetic.

Circumcision

Circumcision in the adult may be necessary as a result of the inflammatory processes described above. It may be required in the male whose prepuce has never retracted, but in whom a bloody discharge develops, in order to see the state of the glans penis. Young adults may find that the frenulum of the glans is painful on erection and especially with intercourse; examination may show that the frenulum is both prominent and appears to draw the glans ventrally. Simple division may suffice, but circumcision may be preferred.

Reluctance to deal with a phimosis by circumcision in earlier years may lead to considerable problems for the urologist later should the patient require either cystocopy or urethral catheterisation.

Disorders of erection

Priapism

In this uncommon condition there is a maintained erection unassociated with sexual desire. In most patients the cause is unknown although the increasing use of psychotropic drugs as well as anti-hypertensive drugs and anti-coagulants may be associated. There is a significant incidence in patients on renal dialysis. Sickle cell disease, leukaemia and metastases to the corpora are known to cause priapism (Wasmer *et al.*, 1981). The mechanism of the erection is believed to be due to sludging of venous blood in the sinuses of the corpora cavernosa; the corpus spongiosum and glans remain unaffected.

A variety of non-operative methods have been used to relieve the congestion e.g. spinal anaesthesia, heparinisation or sedation. These are all ineffective and only delay the chances of success by other more interventional methods. Aspiration of a corpus cavernosum and heparin irrigation may be successful, but usually is not. The technique of creating a fistula between the glans penis and corpora cavernosa using a biopsy needle has met with considerable success (Winter, 1980), but should this fail then a venous anastomosis between either a corpus cavernosum to corpus spongiosum or a saphenous vein shunt to the corpus cavernosum should be made. The earlier the procedure (i.e. within 6 to 12 h) the better the chances of the patient achieving normal erections subsequently. If treatment is delayed or ineffective, the erectile tissue is damaged, becomes fibrosed and the patient will be impotent. Such patients may be candidates for a penile-prosthesis – *see* later.

Peyronie's disease

This condition is characterised by the development of a hard fibrous plaque (or plaques) in the wall of the corpora cavernosa and these may or may not lead to a lateral curvature of the penis. It is most commonly seen in the 5th and 6th decade, though difficulties with intercourse due to a painful curvature will lead the younger man to seek advice more urgently!

Peyronie's disease is not a single entity and is associated with many aetiological factors including trauma and atherosclerosis. Histologically, the fibrous lumps are similar to keloid or Dupuytren's contracture, indeed a significant proportion of these patients also have a Dupuytren's contracture. The natural history of the condition is of slow progression and also of spontaneous remissions (Chesney, 1975). Thus a surgical approach to this problem has not generally been taken seriously, until recently. Most conservative measures, including cortisone injections, vitamins, irradiation or short wave diathermy, have relied more on the passage of time than the effect of treatment for the occasional apparent response. However, attempts to excise the nodules have not always been successful and some caution should be advised to those seeking surgical treatment. If the penile curvature is sufficient to prevent intromission or if the curvature is painful or if either of these lead to impotence, then surgery may be indicated. The plaque(s) may be either excised or the defect corrected with a dermal graft or an ellipse of tunica albuginea may be excised *opposite* to the maximum curvature. In some instances, straightening of the penis may be combined with insertion of a semi-solid rod-type penile prosthesis.

Impotence

Impotence may be psychogenic, organic or drug-induced. Although loss of libido may be due to a generalised illness or endocrine disease, the majority of patients who complain of impotence have a psychosexual disturbance which may require specific therapy (Tulloch *et al.*, 1982).

Psychogenic causes can be established from a careful history that includes details of sexual habits. However, it is always important to exclude organic causes so that the correct advice may be given.

Organic impotence may occur with diabetes mellitus, after priapism, with neurogenic disorders, after major pelvic injury or operations (e.g. total cystectomy, abdominoperineal resection) vascular disease of the pelvic vessels (e.g. Leriche syndrome) and Peyronie's disease. Most of these conditions cause irreversible impotence, but angiography may help to define a treatable abnormality of the arterial supply to the penis and procedures for revascularisation may now be considered in some circumstances. There is no drug treatment and the only other surgical approach that should be considered is to implant a pair of semi-solid rod-type penile prostheses (Fig 24.1).

Drug induced impotence occurs in patients receiving oestrogen treatment for prostatic cancer. In addition, a range of antihypertensive drugs may cause loss of erection or inability to ejaculate. Drugs such as barbiturate, benzodiazepan, corticosteroid, phenothiazine and spironolactone may all effect libido and lead to the complaint of impotence.

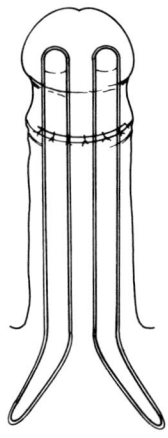

Fig 24.1 Penile prosthesis: showing two semirigid silicone rods in the corpora cavernosa (Small – Carrion type).

Scrotum

Scrotal skin infection

Infections of the scrotum are usually secondary to infections involving either the testis or its appendages or as a complication of severe urethral stricture with urinary infection which progresses to fistula formation. The latter may proceed to multiple fistulas – a 'watering-can' perineum. Initial treatment requires diversion of urine away from this area by means of a suprapubic cystostomy.

Scrotal gangrene may result from these infections, but may also be caused by mechanical, chemical or thermal injuries. The most dramatic form of gangrene of the scrotum and penis is associated with the name of Fournier and is also called necrotising gangrene of the scrotum. The aetiology of this is debatable, most cases are secondary to some infection, especially microaerophilic streptococci and *Staphylococcus aureus* but up to one-third are idiopathic, there being no apparent cause. Antibiotic therapy supplemented by antiseptic dressings may be sufficient, but the condition can progress rapidly with increasing toxicity and may even be fatal. These patients require radical debridement to remove the gangrenous tissue and ultimately skin grafts or flaps (Bejanga, 1979).

Skin changes accompanying scrotal oedema may occur in a wide variety of diseases: cardiac failure, ascites, renal disease. The scrotum may become enlarged in elephantiasis due to filariae (*Wucheria bancrofti*) and a reduction scrotoplasty may be required.

Epididymo-orchitis

Acute epididymo-orchitis is the preferred term to describe acute orchitis or acute epididymitis since both testis and epididymis are jointly involved in any acute inflammatory reaction. Also, the spermatic cord is often thickened from inflammation (funiculitis). The usual cause of epididymo-orchitis is bacterial, either from infected urine or gonococcal urethritis. The affected side of the scrotum is swollen and very tender. The skin becomes red and smooth and sometimes oedematous. In all cases the urine or urethral discharge must be cultured. Sometimes there is no evidence of an infective cause and a viral aetiology may be suspected, especially if the testis alone appears involved (as in mumps orchitis). The possibility of a testicular tumour must always be considered and excluded.

Treatment is with an antibiotic selected by the result of culture of the organism, bed rest and a scrotal support. If there is doubt about the diagnosis and especially if there has been no satisfactory response to treatment, the testis should be explored. An ultrasound study may be helpful in the diagnosis of tumour. Acute epididymo-orchitis in a teenager is so unusual that the first diagnosis to consider is torsion of the testis (*see* later). If antibiotic treatment is delayed, or ineffective, an abscess may form and require incision and drainage.

After an infection has subsided, the epididymis alone may remain thickened and irregular so that chronic epididymitis may be diagnosed. A late sequel to a gonococcal infection is thickening of the tail of the epididymis which, if bilateral, causes infertility (obstructive azoospermia). A later effect of tuberculosis is a hard and craggy epididymis. Syphilis can mimic these conditions, but is now very rarely seen while a gumma of the testis is to be found only in museum specimens.

Torsion of testis (spermatic cord)

Torsion of the testis is a surgical emergency *see* chapter 13: if the twist in the spermatic cord is not corrected within 6–12 h, there is a high risk of infarction and subsequent atrophy of the testis (Johnston, 1982). The most common form of torsion is due to an abnormality of the visceral layer of the tunica vaginalis which normally completely covers the testis to the level of the upper part of the epididymis. In cases of torsion, part of spermatic cord is also covered by the visceral tunica so that the testis is suspended within the parietal layer (bell-clapper deformity, Fig 24.2) and the cord can twist. Thus a torsion of the testis is, more correctly, a torsion of the spermatic cord. A far less common type of torsion can occur in neonates. The abnormality is extravaginal and appears to be due to failure of the epididymis to become attached to the posterolateral wall of the scrotum.

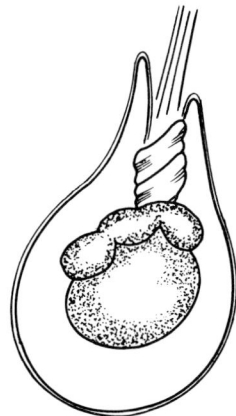

Fig 24.2 Torsion of the testis: showing the abnormality of the visceral layer of the tunica vaginalis that allows the spermatic cord to twist.

The characteristic history of torsion is of a teenager who suddenly develops an acutely swollen tender testis. There may be a history of minor trauma or previous episodes of pain in the testis due to partial temporary torsion. If the patient is seen soon after the onset, it may be possible to palpate the abnormality, but usually the hemiscrotum is red, swollen and too tender to palpate. The pain may be referred to the lower abdomen and there may be nausea and vomiting.

The differential diagnosis is mainly between torsion and acute epididymo-orchitis. The history and physical signs may help, but because of the serious risks of infarction of the testis any doubt must favour immediate exploration. Doppler studies of blood flow in the testis and radioisotope scintiscan to study perfusion have been described, but unless easily available a clinical decision on management should not be delayed.

Manipulation of a torsion has been successful (rotating the testis outwards), but preferably the testis should be explored as soon as possible through a scrotal incision (Lord, 1980). The cord is untwisted and the testis observed for evidence of restored circulation by pulsation and colour. Unless it is obviously gangrenous, it is best to leave the testis *in situ* and to fix it to the parietal tunica with chromic catgut sutures. The tunica should be left open to ensure good adherence of the layers. Since the underlying abnormality of the tunica is bilateral, the other testis must be similarly fixed at the same time to avoid the disaster of bilateral damage and infertility.

Torsion of the *testicular appendages*, usually the appendix testis, should be considered in a differential diagnosis. The pain is usually not so severe and the tenderness is localised to the upper pole of the testis. The need for certainty in the diagnosis makes the urgency of action the same as above and at operation the twisted appendage is excised.

Hydrocele

The collection of fluid in the tunica vaginalis producing a painless swelling of the scrotum is a common condition.

The cause of most hydroceles is unknown (idopathic). The fluid is a straw coloured protein-rich transudate. Rarely, and almost always in children, there is a patent processus vaginalis allowing the hydrocele to vary in size. In others, the hydrocele develops as a sequel to epididymo-orchitis, or rarely, but more sinister, it may develop with a malignant testis the so-called secondary hydrocele.

On examination of the scrotum, there is a tense, smooth oval swelling, above which a normal spermatic cord can be palpated and there is no cough impulse. The fluid around the testis transilluminates though in a chronic hydrocele this may be difficult because of fibrosis and thickening of the tunica. It may be possible to palpate the testis and confirm that it is normal, but this is unusual. Most idiopathic hydroceles occur in elderly men; in a younger man an underlying malignancy must be excluded and it is advisable to aspirate the fluid by needle and syringe in order to palpate the testis fully. If there is still doubt about the testis, ultrasound and/or urgent exploration is indicated.

A large scrotum that looks like a hydrocele but does not transilluminate may be due either to an *haematocele* or a tumour. A history of injury should clarify the diagnosis. A small haematocele will usually settle without specific treatment. If there is a recent history of trauma and the mass is large and/or painful, the scrotum should be explored and the haematoma evacuated. There may be a tear in the tunica of the testis and this should be sutured.

The surgical management of a hydrocele is preferred, especially since the mass has usually presented either because of its size or discomfort. Aspiration may have been done to exclude testicular pathology, but the tunica will refill with fluid within a few months. A few urologists favour repeated aspiration combined with the injection of a sclerosing solution especially if there is a contra indication to operation. Infection is the main risk of repeated needling.

There is a choice of several operative procedures. The tunica may be incised and evaginated and the cut margins sutured behind the epididymis. The tunica may be exposed through a small anterior scrotal incision and plicated (Fig 24.3) (Lord, 1964). Neither of these is suitable if the tunica is thick from chronic inflammation and excision of the parietal tunica is then necessary. Postoperative scrotal drains are to be avoided because of the risks of infection; compression dressings and good scrotal support are preferred.

Cysts of epididymis

Small cysts in the epididymis are a common finding in the older male. Their origin is thought to be from diverticula of the vasa efferentia. If a solitary cyst enlarges, it may have a remarkable resemblance to a testis: usually there are multiple cysts so that the surface of the mass feels irregular. Epididymal cysts transilluminate easily

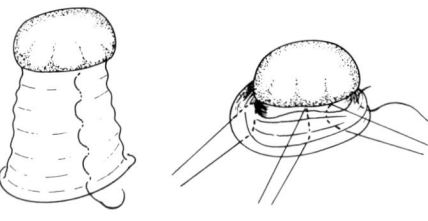

Fig 24.3 Hydrocele operation: demonstrating the plication of the parietal tunica vaginalis (Lord, 1980).

and, because of their characteristic position above and behind the testis, there should be no confusion with a hydrocele. The cysts contain fluid that is clear and watery, but sometimes the fluid is opalescent due to an abundance of sperms (*spermatocele*).

It is better to leave these cysts alone unless increasing size warrants excision. The operation requires careful dissection to remove the cysts completely; often there are several other little cysts which, if not removed, will increase in size and produce a so-called recurrence. Any operation on these cysts will almost certainly result in obstruction to the vasa efferentia and because a bilateral operation could result in sterility, the patient must be advised accordingly.

References

Bejanga B.I. (1979). Fournier's gangrene. *Brit. J. Urol*; **51**:312–16.

Chesney J. (1975). Peyronie's disease. *Brit. J. Urol*; **47**:209–18.

Johnston J.H. (1982). Acquired lesions of the penis, the scrotum and the testes. In *Paediatric Urology* (Williams, D.I., Johnson, J.H., eds.) Ch. 38. London: Butterworths.

Kherzi A.A., Dounis A., Dunn M. (1979). Balanitis xerotica obliterans. *Brit. J. Urol*; **51**:229–31.

Lord P.H. (1964) A bloodless operation for the radical cure of idiopathic hydrocele. *Brit. J. Surg*; **51**:814–916.

Lord P.H. (1980). Testis and epididymis. In *Tutorials in Postgraduate Medicine: Urology*. (Chisholm G.D., ed.) Ch. 29. London: Heinemann Medical.

Tulloch A.G.S., Keogh E.J., Csillag E.R., Dunn J.C., Brown D.S., Morlet A. (1982). Impotence – the team approach to investigation and surgical treatment. *Brit. J. Urol*; **54**:755–8.

Wasmer J.M., Carrion H.M., Mekras G., Politano V.A. (1981). Evaluation and treatment of priapism. *J. Urol*; **125**:204–07.

Winter C.C. (1980). Priapism. *Current Urologic Therapy* (Kaufman J.J., ed.), pp. 338–40. Philadelphia: Saunders.

25

Incontinence

J.R. HINDMARSH

Incontinence of urine is a symptom of bladder and or urethral dysfunction, often associated with frequency, urgency and nocturia. Under normal circumstances urine is stored in the bladder at low pressure, continence being maintained by the high closure pressure of the bladder neck and urethra. Incontinence is due either to active contraction of the bladder muscle when not desired (unstable bladder) or to relaxation of the urethra (unstable urethra). Structural damage to the sphincter mechanisms will also produce passive or stress incontinence.

A simple classification is:

1　Disturbances of neuromuscular or psychological control
　　a　functional
　　b　neuropathic
2　Structural abnormalities (ICS, 1981)

Some confusion surrounds the pathophysiology of incontinence despite an increased knowledge of the morphology and function of the bladder and urethra and their nervous control.

Embryology

The detrusor is of endodermal origin and is supplied by the parasympathetic (S2,3,4,): the superficial trigone and urethra are of mesodermal origin primarily supplied by the sympathetic nervous system. Fusion occurs along the lateral and cranial borders of the superficial trigone, deep trigone and bladder neck. Distal to the bladder neck a ring of striated muscle develops but is not in continuity with the pelvic floor muscles.

Anatomy

The detrusor muscle is a smooth muscular meshwork in layers that are more or less at right angles to adjacent ones, but none enters the urethral wall, superficial trigone or prostatic urethra. The superficial trigone is unimportant as far as trigono-urethral function is concerned. However, the deep trigone is densely packed smooth muscle contributing bundles to the proximal part of the urethra (Woodbine, 1960). In the male the preprostatic sphincter is a complete collar merging with the prostatic capsule, but separate from the detrusor muscle, its function being primarily sexual as none occurs in the female. In the male the distal urethral sphincter is a powerful muscle situated below the verumontanum whereas in the female a horse-shoe shaped striated muscle is present throughout the length of the urethra, mainly around the mid-point.

Physiology

The bladder and urethra act synergistically to perform two functions (Fig 25.1), storage and expulsion.

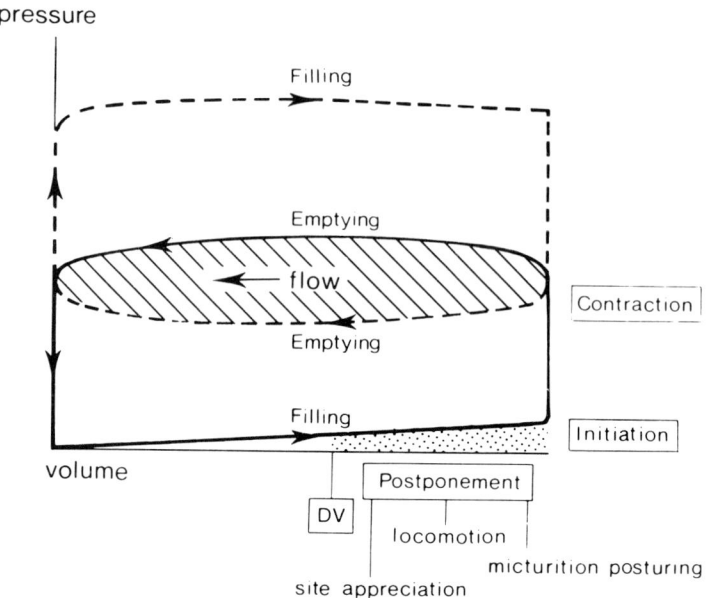

Fig 25.1 Diagram showing main features of normal bladder function. Continuous lines indicate bladder pressures, interrupted lines urethral pressures. Arrows to right indicate filling; arrows to left indicate emptying. Shaded area indicates flow. (From *Tutorials in Postgraduate Medicine: Urology*, p. 297, by courtesy of Prof. G.D. Chisholm and the publishers, William Heinemann Medical Books.)

During storage the detrusor muscle is inactive and urine accumulates slowly at low pressure. The urethral closure pressure is higher than bladder pressure at all times due to basal sphincter tone of the smooth and striated muscle, elastic tissue, and the submucosal vascular plexus. The proximal urethra is intra-abdominal, so when the pressure rises it is equally distributed to the bladder and urethra. During exercise additional closure is provided by the striated muscle of the distal sphincter and pelvic floor. When the desire to void is felt, postponement is achieved by voluntary increase in sphincter pressure. When appropriate, the voiding sequence is initiated by voluntary pelvic floor relaxation followed by detrusor contraction, thus overcoming urethral resistance. Continued detrusor contraction is aided by nervous control stimulated by urinary flow. When the bladder is empty, the sphincters contract until the next voiding cycle.

Peripheral motor innervation

The parasympathetic S2, 3, 4 innervates the detrusor muscle via the pelvic nerves and is only active during voiding. During bladder filling there is no neurally mediated detrusor activity, the rise in bladder pressure being produced by the resistance to stretch of the bladder wall. The smooth muscle of the urethra is innervated by the sympathetic (T10 to L2) via the hypogas-tric and pelvic plexuses. The alpha-adrenergic receptor sites, which are predominantly on the smooth muscles of the bladder base, produce contraction of the bladder neck and urethra during bladder filling. In the male their primary function is probably to prevent reflux of ejaculate. The urethral striated muscle is supplied by somatic efferent fibres via the pelvic plexus (Gosling *et al.*, 1977) and pudendal nerves.

Central innervation

The afferent receptors in the bladder and urethra have not been identified; the sensation of fullness is probably produced by stimulation of posterior urethral receptors by increased bladder volume and bladder wall tension. These impulses travel via the pelvic plexus to the posterior columns and spinothalamic tracts to the sensory cortex. Afferent impulses from the bladder muscle itself are probably stimulated by tension in the collagenous elements and travel via the pelvic nerves and spinoreticular tract to the pontine mesencephalic nucleus, detrusor motor centre (Uerema *et al.*, 1973). The integrity of this pathway, the nucleus and the descending motor pathways is essential for a coordinated sequence of filling and voiding in the human. There are many higher areas of the brain that influence the pontine centre both excitatory and inhibitory (Nathan, 1976). The periurethral muscle afferents pass via the pudendal nerve to the sacral cord and pons where they inhibit the detrusor motor centre playing an important part in the postponement phase of bladder filling. Detrusor motor neurones in the conus medullaris can act as a primitive voiding reflex centre in spinal injuries.

Pathophysiology

Any consideration of the pathophysiology of the lower urinary tract must take three factors into account (Table 1):

1   The range of symptoms produced.
2   Pathological conditions that can produce similar symptoms.
3   The anatomical differences between male and female urethral closure.

In the male, the distal urethral sphincter is a powerful muscle capable of producing very high pressures in the neurologically normal and compromised patients; the female urethra is shorter and has a weaker distal sphincter mechanism.

Functional abnormalities

Childhood

Learning bladder control can be dificult for some children. Poor reception of bladder filling can result in activation of the reflex at inappropriate times and

Table 1
CAUSES OF OVERACTIVITY OF DETRUSOR REFLEXES

Bladder Urethra	Mucosal afferents	Inflammation Stones Interstitial cystitis Infection Carcinoma *in situ* Urethral syndrome
	Muscle	Hypertrophy Idiopathic Dyssynergia Obstruction
Cord	Trauma Tumours Osteophytes Discs	
Cerebrum	Multiple sclerosis Cerebral vascular accident Parkinson's disease Cerebral degeneration Anxiety	

secondary hypertrophy of the bladder. Uncoordinated voiding similarly encourages detrusor muscle hypertrophy. Interruption of the stream by pelvic floor and distal sphincter contraction will act as a physiological obstruction in males. Subsequently unstable bladder contractions produce symptoms of urgency, urge incontinence, nocturia and nocturnal enuresis. Early re-education encouraging sphincter relaxation during voiding is essential, otherwise longterm damage is done to the bladder and urethra. A patient who was enuretic as a child will often have lifelong frequency and urgency. Some children develop nocturnal enuresis after attaining bladder control. In this group an emotional cause is normally found (Rutter *et al.*, 1973).

Adult females

Adult females with motor urge incontinence can be cured by bladder retraining. Symptoms often date back to childbirth or hysterectomy and social pressures exacerbate it. It is tempting to suggest sensory and motor nerve damage during surgery, or pressure necrosis during childbirth, as the cause. Intensive physiotherapy, bladder drill and a clear description of the function of the bladder and urethra to the patient will cure 80% (Jarvis and Millar 1980). A number of females have both stress and urge incontinence which require a combined approach of bladder training and surgery.

Adult males

Adult males rarely develop idiopathic detrusor instability spontaneously. Symptoms of urgency with incontinence are more likely to be secondary to mechanical obstruction, or neurogenic, or occasionally psychiatric in origin.

Neuropathic abnormalities

Traumatic

The response to the bladder and urethra following spinal damage is dependent on the level of the injury, its completeness and viability of the distal cord. A simple classification is difficult as the urethral sphincter mechanism is innervated by both sympathetic and somatic nerves with outflow at different levels (Table 2).

Injuries involving the cauda equina or conus medullaris result in bladder insensitivity and paralysis with sparing of the sympathetically innervated urethral smooth muscle. Damage between the sympathetic outflow between T10 and L2 and the conus produces many different pictures. However, damage above the sympathetic outflow with a viable distal cord allows

Table 2

1   Detrusor hyperreflexia
        Coordinated sphincter
        Striated sphincter dyssynergia
        Smooth muscle sphincter dyssynergia
2   Detrusor areflexia
        Coordinated sphincter
        Non-relaxing striated sphincter
        Denervated striated sphincter
        Non-relaxing smooth muscle sphincter

reflex micturition to occur. In the early stages of spinal shock, aseptic intermittent catheterisation is performed until the patient becomes neurologically stable, usually after 80 days (Rossier, 1974). If spontaneous voiding occurs a careful monitoring of residual urine, infection and the state of the upper urinary tracts must be maintained. If deterioration occurs, sphincter balancing or destruction should be performed with drainage into an external appliance. In the female, a urinary diversion may be required to spare the upper urinary tracts at an early stage. Renal failure due to infection and obstruction still remain a major cause of mortality.

Non-traumatic

Loss of sensation of bladder filling due to demyelination occurs in diabetes mellitus and subacute degeneration of the cord, resulting in a large acontractile bladder. A mixed picture is seen in multiple sclerosis and Parkinson's disease. The principles of management are essentially the same as for traumatic lesions. Damage to the brain centre involved in controlling bladder function usually results in failure of inhibition of the detrusor with urgency and incontinence. Old people with mild cerebral atrophy frequently suffer from urgency and incontinence partly because they cannot inhibit detrusor contractions and partly because they cannot wait long enough to get to the toilet.

Structural abnormalities

Stress incontinence

The female urethral closure mechanism is subjected to a variety of injuries, the most severe of which is childbirth. Direct pressure can produce anatomical weakness or atrophy so that the effective closure pressure is reduced. Prolapse of the urethra through the pelvic floor results in loss of intra-abdominal closure pressure so that coughing with a partially full bladder results in leakage. Repositioning of the urethra above the pelvic floor by colpo-suspension is effective (Stanton *et al.*, 1976). Female patients must be assessed by simple cystometry as operation will exacerbate urge incontinence

if this is the major component. Few male patients have stress incontinence. Usually it is produced by prostatic carcinomatous infiltration of the sphincter, inadvertent damage to the distal sphincter during prostatectomy and high pressure chronic retention with overflow. Sphincter implants are appropriate in patients with sphincter damage not due to cancer.

Fistula

Congenital absence of the lower abdominal and anterior bladder wall, *ectopia vesicae*, results in total incontinence. Ectopic ureters can also produce continuous leakage of urine if the distal end is in the vagina or distal urethra. In adult females fistulas can occur after obstetric trauma, carcinoma of the cervix and iatrogenic injury and cause incontinence.

Clinical

Symptoms

The symptoms relating to disordered bladder function are few and may be due to a number of conditions. Occasionally two factors contribute to the symptoms, e.g. prostatic obstruction and multiple sclerosis.

1   Detrusor motor overactivity produces a group of symptoms that can be identified: frequency, urgency, urge incontinence, nocturia or nocturnal enuresis.
2   Stress incontinence is produced on coughing, lifting or sneezing when the bladder is partially full.
3   Continuous incontinence is symptomatic of a fistula between the vagina and ureter or bladder or total urethral sphincter damage.
4   Unconscious incontinence when sitting or asleep is typical of high pressure chronic retention with overflow associated with increasing abdominal girth and poor flow.
5   Reflex incontinence is associated with spinal injury or neurovascular damage.

Examination

1   *Abdominal examination* may reveal a large bladder. However, most chronically distended bladders are difficult to feel, particularly in fat patients.
2   *The nervous system* must be carefully examined from the waist down and comparing the two sides. Perianal sensation, anal tone and ability to grip the examining finger must be noted. The

bulbo-cavernosus and ano-anal reflexes reveal the integrity of the sacral reflex arcs. The bulbo-cavernosus reflex is present in about 80% of females (Blaivis *et al.*, 1981).

3 *The external genitalia* may reveal prolapse or urethral stenosis and coughing will induce urinary leakage in females with stress incontinence. In males the patient should be standing.

4 *Locomotor systems.* Older patients may be immobilised by disease of the knees and hips.

Investigations

Urine

In all cases the urine is examined to exclude glycosuria and an MSU is sent to the laboratory for culture and sensitivity. Urinary tract infection superimposed on the overactive bladder makes the symptoms more severe.

The presence of blood in the urine demands urography and cystoscopy to exclude urinary tract neoplasia.

Urodynamic investigations

All patients with lower urinary tract dysfunction should have some form of urodynamic studies performed, preferably in a fully equipped laboratory. Initial screening is performed by free flow rate recorded with a flow meter and residual urine checks by ultrasound or catheter drainage.

1 Simple filling cystometry is performed in female patients with genuine stress incontinence to confirm the diagnosis and exclude gross bladder instability.

2 More complicated systems combining video cystography with synchronous filling and voiding pressures are required for most functional disorders (Bates *et al.*, 1970).

3 EMG of the pelvic floor is used in addition to the above for a neuropathic bladder. Measuring mean transit times through spinal reflex arcs may be used in cases of cauda equina lesions (Siroky *et al.*, 1979).

4 Male patients with sphincter weakness require both cystometry and urethral closure pressure profile measurements to assess peak closure pressures. Some patients with suspected urethral muscular dysfunction are investigated by continuous urethral pressure monitoring during bladder filling.

Cystoscopy

Most incontinent patients are cystoscoped under anaesthesia to assess sphincter mechanisms and capacity. The trigone and bladder mucosa are examined and a bimanual examination performed. Bladder neoplasia and interstitial cystitis can then be excluded.

Urography

Upper urinary tract radiology does not contribute to the final diagnosis. However, a plain film of the kidneys, ureters and bladder should be performed to exclude upper urinary tract calculi.

Management

Due to the diversity of conditions that can present with urinary incontinence, it is not possible to detail specific types of treatment. However there are several principles which should be borne in mind (Yeates, 1980).

1 Relieve excessive bladder distension.
2 Remove the primary cause of the dysfunction.
3 If (2) is not possible, balance expulsive forces with outlet resistance.
4 Where (3) is not possible, substitute bladder function by (a) apparatus or pads, (b) catheter drainage, (c) urinary diversion.

The broad outlines of some specific treatments are presented in Table 3.

Table 3
MANAGEMENT

	Non-operative	Operative
Female stress incontinence		Colposuspension
Male stress incontinence	Collecting device Clamp Catheter	Sphincter prosthesis Urinary diversion
Motor urge incontinence	Bladder drill Anticholinergics	Overdistension Bladder transection Caecocystoplasty Diversion
Chronic retension with overflow		Releave obstruction Urethrotomy Prostatectomy
Neuropathy	Catheterisation Anticholinergics Collecting devices	Sphincterotomy Diversion

References

Bates C.P., Whiteside C.G., Turner-Warwick R.T. (1970). Synchronous cine/pressure/flow cysto-urethrography with special reference to stress and urge incontinence. *Brit. J. Urol*; **52**:714–22.

Blaivis J.G., Zayed A.A.H., Labib K.B. (1981). Bulbocavernosus reflex in urology: prospective study of 299 patients. *J. Urol*; **126**:197–99.

Gosling J.A., Dixon T.S., Lendron R.G. (1977). The anatomic innervation of the human male and female bladder neck and urethra. *J. Urol*; **118**:302–5.

International Continence Society (1981). Fourth report on the standardisation of terminology of lower urinary tract function. *Brit. J. Urol*; **53**:333–35.

Jarvis G.J., Millar D.R. (1980). Controlled trial of bladder drill for detrusor instability. *Brit. Med. J*; **281**:1322–3.

Nathan P.W. (1976). The central nervous connections of the bladder. In *Scientific Foundations of Urology*, 1st edn., vol. 2. (Williams D.I., Chisholm G.D., eds.) pp. 51–58. London: Heinemann Medical.

Rossier A.B. (1974). Neurogenic bladder in spinal cord injury. *Urol. Clin. N. Amer*; **1**:125.

Rutter M., Yule W., Graham P. (1973). Enuresis and behavioral deviance. In *Bladder Control and Enuresis. Clinics in Developmental Medicine No. 48/49*. (Kolvin I., MacKeith R.C., Meadows S.R., eds.) pp. 137–47. London: Heinemann Medical.

Siroky M.B., Sax D.S., Krane R.J. (1979). Sacral signal tracing: the electrophysiology of the bulbocavernosus reflex. *J. Urol*; **122**:661–4.

Stanton S.L., Williams J.E., Ritchie D. (1976). The colposuspension operation for urinary incontinence. *Brit. J. Obstet. Gynaec*; **83**:890–5.

Uerema E., Fletcher T.F., Bradley W.E. (1973). Distribution of sacral afferent axons in cat urinary bladder. *Amer. J. Anat*; **136**:305–11.

Woodbine R.T. (1960). Structure and function of the urinary bladder. *J. Urol*; **84**:79–85.

Yeates W.K. (1980). Incontinence. In *Tutorials in Postgraduate Medicine: Urology* (Chisholm G.D., ed.) pp. 296–316. London: Heinemann Medical.

Further reading

Abrams P., Feneley R., Torrens M. (1983). *Urodynamics*. In *Clinical Practice in Urology*. Heidelberg: Springer Verlag.

Bors E., Commar A.E. (1971). *Neurological Urology*. Basel: S. Karger.

Denny Brown D., Robertson E.G. (1933). On the psychology of micturition. *Brain*; **56**:149–90.

Gosling J.A. (1982). *Functional Anatomy of the Urinary Tract*. Edinburgh: Churchill Livingstone.

Iggo A. (1955). Tension receptors in the stomach and urinary bladder. *J. Physiol*; **128**:593–607.

Kolvin I., MacKeith R.C., Meadows S.R., eds. (1973). *Bladder Control and Enuresis. Clinics in Developmental Medicine No. 48/49*. London: Heinemann Medical.

Krane R.J., Siroky M.B. (1979). Classification of neurourological disorders. In *Clinical Neuro-urology* (Krane R.J., Siroky M.B., eds.) pp. 143–158. Boston: Little, Brown and Company.

Kuru M. (1965). Nervous control of micturition. *Physiol. Rev*; **45**:425–495.

Ruch T.C. (1965). The urinary bladder. In *Physiology and Biophysics* (Ruch T.C., Patton H.D. eds.) pp. 000–000. Philadelphia: Saunders and Co.

Sunder G.S., Parsons K.F., Gibbon N.O.K. (1978). Outflow obstruction in neuropathic bladder dysfunction. The neuropathic urethra. *Brit. J. Urol*; **50**:190–9.

26

Infertility, fertility and sexual dysfunction

T.B. HARGREAVE

Infertility

Fertility has been of great concern to the human race since the earliest written records. It has been estimated that the incidence of involuntary infertility is 1 in 15 marriages (Macleod, 1971).

The couple should, where possible be investigated together. In those centres where the man is still investigated in isolation by the surgeon, efforts should be made to run joint clinics with gynaecologists. The first reason for this is that in one-third of couples there are problems requiring treatment in both partners. The second reason is that it is now possible to diagnose accurately conditions for which there is no treatment other than artificial insemination by donor and this type of help is best managed by a joint clinic.

At the initial interview a general history should be taken from both partners. In most cases it is appropriate to begin further investigations immediately. In cases where the wife is under 25 and the couple have been trying to have a child for only a short time it is reasonable to wait for 2 years before full investigation. It is also worth remembering that there is often a period of relative infertility in the wife for about 1 year after stopping oral contraception.

Investigation of the male

It is usual to investigate the man first because most of the tests are simple and safe (Fig 26.1). The following investigations are carried out: history, examination, seminal analysis, follicle stimulating hormone (FSH) estimation and antisperm antibody testing.

History

The main features to be elicited by history taking are shown in Table 1. A questionnaire is very helpful in obtaining a general history from both partners prior to their clinic attendance. This leaves more time to discuss difficult subjects such as past history of sexually transmitted diseases. It is better to enquire about previous children by another partner and sexually transmitted diseases when the wife is not present. This is most conveniently done when the man is examined in a separate room (Hargreave, 1983).

Physical examination

During physical examination note is made of the general physique and body hair distribution, since this

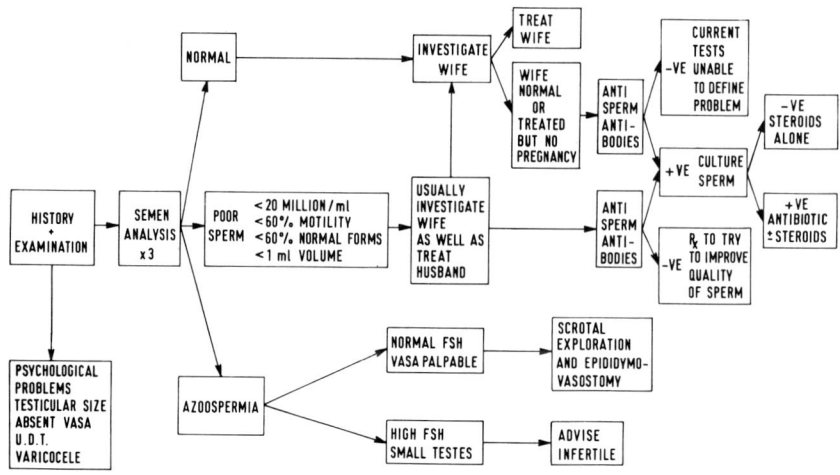

Fig 26.1 Flow diagram to illustrate sequence of investigation of the male partner of an infertile marriage.

Table 1
POINTS TO NOTE ON HISTORY TAKING

Years married

Years trying for a child

A. SEXUAL HISTORY
1. Voluntary abstinence
   religious proscriptions
2. Involuntary abstinence
   Impotence
   illness
   drugs (antihypertensives)
   ageing
   penile deformity
   psychiatric (premature ejaculation)
   Illness
   either husband or wife
   organic, psychiatric
   Unavoidable temporary separation
   e.g. husband on North Sea oil rig
3. Coital frequency. This is not the important factor that many think. Extremes of coital frequency usually affect the delay to conception of a fertile couple by a maximum of 6 months.

B. FACTORS INFLUENCING FERTILITY
1. Husband's biological fertility
   previous children
   occupation (pesticide worker, lead worker)
   previous venereal disease, genital infection or inflammation, *e.g.* mumps orchitis
   previous genital trauma or operation
   testicular descent
2. Wife's biological fertility
   previous children, pregnancy, miscarriage or abortion
   previous veneral disease or pelvic inflammatory disease
   menstrual history
3. Use of contraception
4. Previous voluntary sterilisation *e.g.* vasectomy

may be a guide to hormonal or chromosomal problems. Thus a tall man with scanty body hair and a history of delayed puberty could have a pituitary disorder. A man with breast enlargement and complaining of impotence may have hyperprolactinaemia. These specific endocrinological disorders are, however, very rare. Congenital deformities are sometimes associated with chromosomal abnormality.

The external genitalia should be examined. It is rare to find abnormality of the penis but note should be made of any phimosis, hypospadias or epispadias. The contents of the scrotum should also be examined carefully. The size and consistency of the testes are judged. Small, soft testes are usually associated with grossly deranged spermatogenesis. Normally the epididymis is soft on palpation, but occasionally engorged cystic areas are felt and in some cases this will be consequent on previous epididymitis resulting in obstruction which is amenable to surgery. Bilateral absence of the vas deferens is found in approximately 5% of cases of azoospermia. A unilateral absence of the vas is much rarer and is usually associated with absence of the kidney on that side. It is easier to examine for varicocele with the patient standing: distended veins may be felt above the testicle, usually on the left side, and the testicular size is sometimes reduced on that side. Rectal examination with prostatic massage should be performed on patients with a past history of sexually transmitted disease, with a poor semen volume or with pus cells in the semen sample. If in these cases the sample produced after prostatic massage shows numerous pus cells, antibiotic treatment may be appropriate.

Semen analysis

There is a natural variation in semen from day-to-day, from month-to-month and as the patient gets older. It is unreliable to base any confident prediction on one sample, because of these biological variables. It is also worth realising that the examination is imprecise, with laboratory errors of up to 40%. The minimum routine semen examination includes an estimation of seminal volume, of sperm motility, and of the numbers of sperm in millions per ml. A normal sample has a volume greater than 1 ml, a motility of more than 60% within the first 3 h after production (Hafez, 1977) and a sperm density greater than 20 million per ml. In some centres additional examinations are made of the viscosity and chemical constituents of seminal plasma and the morphology and vitality of sperm. Occasionally, samples are encountered where the seminal plasma is hyperviscid and there appears to be incomplete liquefaction. In such cases artificial insemination techniques using the husband's sperm have been helpful.

The finding of semen measurements that are below the accepted normal values does not necessarily mean sterility, but rather that the chances of fertility are reduced. Whether or not the husband is the true father in every case is impossible to say, but it is unwise to counsel a man as infertile as long as some sperm are present.

Follicle stimulating hormone estimation

The normal hormonal control of the testes is illustrated in Fig 26.2. Follicle stimulating hormone drives spermatogenesis and there is negative feedback from this. If there is damage to spermatogenesis, this negative feedback is reduced and the pituitary compensates by increasing FSH output to drive the failing testes harder. Thus FSH levels accurately reflect testicular damage and will in some cases obviate the need for testicular biopsy.

Antisperm antibodies

These were shown to be clinically important by Rumpke *et al.* (1974) who found that high titres were associated with diminished fertility in a large number of patients followed up for 10 years. These antibodies may either immobilise or agglutinate sperm and can be detected in the blood, seminal plasma, cervical mucus, or attached to the sperm. Their presence may be indicated by a high degree of autoagglutination noted during routine semen analysis, but in many cases there is no indication from history, physical examination or semen analysis. The way in which antisperm antibodies interfere with fertility has not yet been defined accurately. In cases with significantly high titres the move-

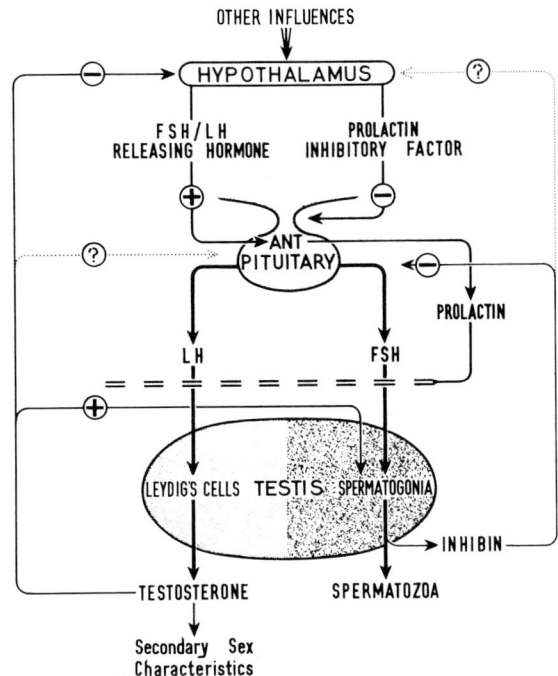

Fig 26.2   Hormonal control of the testis.

ment of sperm through mid-cycle cervical mucus is converted from progressive movement through the mucus to a non-progressive shaking movement. There is also evidence that some antibody coated sperm may not be able to penetrate the ovum.

Results from investigation

As a result of the above investigations certain problems are commonly seen.

1. No sperm present in the ejaculate – azoospermia.
2. Generally poor measurements on semen analysis, either low sperm density or poor motility or both – oligozoospermia.
3. Positive antisperm antibodies.
4. Psychological problems.
5. Poor seminal volume – retrograde ejaculation.
6. Other more complex problems, *e.g.* a very high sperm density with poor motility.
7. Chromosome abnormalities.
8. No obvious problem detected in the man.

Azoospermia

The two main causes of azoospermia are severe testicular damage or a block between the seminiferous tubule and the external urinary meatus. Testicular damage is not usually amenable to treatment, whilst a block can in some cases be corrected by surgery. The distinction is usually easy to make, since cases secondary to testicular damage will have small testes which are soft and a high FSH level. Cases with blockage will normally have good-sized testes and often an engorged epididymis is felt. Congenital absence of both vasa is rare and should be recognised at the initial physical examination. This is not usually amenable to surgery because of the length of the missing vas.

Oligozoospermia

There is no generally agreed lower limit of normal sperm density and it may be misleading to pay too much attention to this measurement in seminal analysis. It is, however, true to say that when sperm density is consistently below 10 million/ml an increasing number of patients will have testicular damage which can be detected on biopsy and is indicated by increased FSH levels. The chances of these men starting a pregnancy are reduced, and become less as the sperm density falls; however, it is almost certain that it is not the numbers alone that determine these chances; the poor numbers also reflect poor fertilising ability. In centres with facilities for accurate estimation of sperm morphology, the morphology of samples from men with a very low semen density is often bizarre, with a high percentage of abnormal forms. In addition, motility is often poor.

In most cases damage to the germinal epithelium can be surmised from the FSH level and the findings on semen analysis, and it is not usually necessary to perform a testicular biopsy. Sometimes, there is a history of previous undescended testis to account for this damage, but usually there is no obvious factor. Some occupations have been associated with infertility: for example, 50% of the work force of a pesticide factory in California were found to have azoospermia or oligozoospermia with high FSH levels. Impaired fertility has also been reported in lead workers.

Men with a poor semen analysis are usually offered treatment with hormones such as sublingual testosterone, mesterolone or clomiphene, or drugs such as bromocriptine or arginine. There is, however, little evidence that any of these preparations work and those with potentially serious side effects should be used with caution.

Treatment of antisperm antibodies

A 40% pregnancy rate using a regime of intermittent methyl prednisolone at high dosage has been reported by Shulman (1976), but this has not yet been confirmed elsewhere. Another approach is intrauterine insemination, using the husband's sperm in an attempt to bypass the cervical mucus barrier. There is still much need for basic research into the exact nature of antisperm antibodies and their treatment. There is a risk of aseptic hip necrosis when high dose steroid treatment is used.

Psychological problems

It is rare for infertility to be the presenting symptom of a psychological problem. It is true, however, to say that the infertile couple is often put under much stress by not having a family. A man with a psychosexual problem may be unable to provide a semen sample for analysis, but may give a history of nocturnal semen emissions at other times. Occasionally on examination of the wife, the marriage is found to be unconsummated. Impotence or premature ejaculation in the young man may also indicate psychological problems.

It should be remembered that many men feel threatened by infertility investigations and the opportunity should not be lost to explain that the male hormones, libido, genital size and maleness are all perfectly normal, when indeed they are so.

Low semen volume (Fig 26.3)

A small proportion of men attending the clinic are unable to produce a sample for examination. Androgen lack (hypogonadotrophic eunuchoidism) can have this effect; such patients lack male secondary sex characteristics and usually present to the endocrinologist because of delayed puberty. Neurological damage may result in failure of ejaculation, but is usually associated with other neurological signs and symptoms. Diabetes is often associated with autonomic neuropathy and this

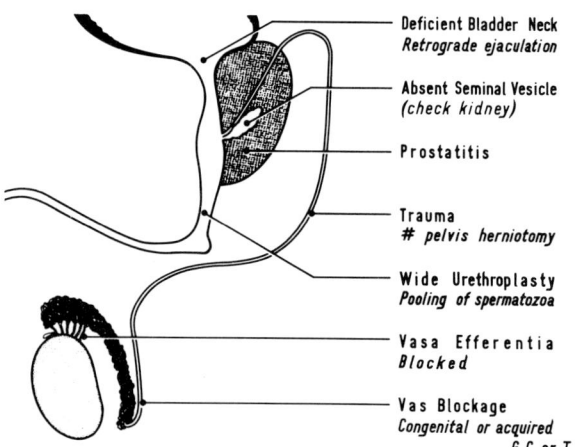

Deficient Bladder Neck
Retrograde ejaculation

Absent Seminal Vesicle
(check kidney)

Prostatitis

Trauma
 # pelvis herniotomy

Wide Urethroplasty
Pooling of spermatozoa

Vasa Efferentia
Blocked

Vas Blockage
Congenital or acquired
G.C. or T.B.

Fig 26.3 The mechanical causes of aspermia and azoospermia and low semen volume.

may cause disorganisation of ejaculation, with reflux of semen into the bladder. In many cases of retrograde ejaculation, no obvious neurological or structural abnormality can be detected. In such cases treatment is unsatisfactory, although some pregnancies have been reported following artificial insemination using the husband's sperm recovered from alkalinised urine. There may be obstruction to the seminal fluid at prostatic level after gonococcal or tuberculous prostatitis or because of urethral stricture following pelvic injury. In the latter case, there is usually a history of a poor urinary stream. Urethroplasty may result in a flaccid urethra and pooling of semen at that point with failure of ejaculation. This can also occur after hypospadias reconstruction. After both open and transurethral prostatectomy approximately one-third of potent men will continue to have some ejaculation; thus prostatectomy is not a sure method of contraception.

Other problems

Occasionally patients are encountered who appear to have good numbers of sperm, but very poor motility and in such cases, if electron microscopy is available, deficiencies in the make-up of the sperm tail are sometimes identified. In Kartagener's syndrome there are missing microtubules in the sperm tail and also in cilia throughout the body, resulting in clinical sinusitis, bronchiectasis and infertility, all associated with *situs inversus*. Abnormalities of the cilia causing infertility and chest problems, but not associated with *situs inversus* have been called the immotile cilia syndrome.

Sometimes when the seminal sample is examined, there is evidence of chronic infection, denoted by the presence of pus cells or organisms. Such cases may show dramatic improvement in semen quality following antibiotic treatment. Another obscure group comprises patients who are found to have an extremely high sperm density often associated with poor motility, and there is some evidence that this may be associated with seminal plasma prostaglandin deficiency.

Chromosome abnormality

There is an increase in the incidence of chromosomal abnormalities amongst men attending an infertility clinic (Fig 26.4), but this probably does not justify routine chromosome analysis in all cases. Exceptions are men with azoospermia or where there are clinical indications, *e.g.* congenital deformity, abnormal stature or delayed maturity. Klinefelter's syndrome XXY is the commonest chromosomal abnormality presenting with azoospermia. These men usually have a degree of androgen lack and small, soft testes. Medical follow-up may be necessary because of associated cardiac abnormalities. In some cases androgen therapy helps secondary sex characteristics to develop and may help libido.

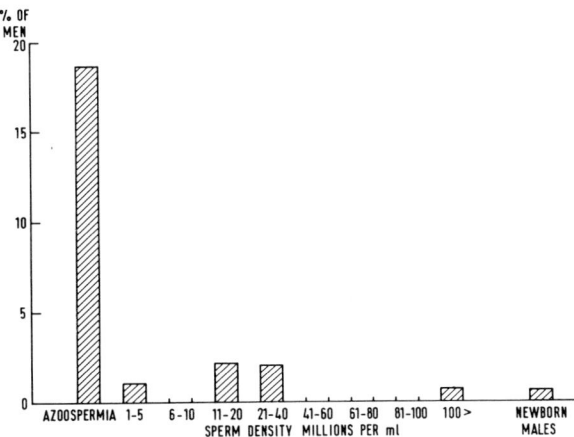

Fig 26.4   Chromosome abnormalities and sperm density in 683 men with infertile marriages (Redrawn from data by Chandley *et al.*, 1975). *Note:* The incidence of chromosomal abnormality in men with some sperm present does not usually justify routine chromosomal analysis.

No obvious problem detected in the man

In cases where all of the husband's investigations are normal, a problem may be found when the wife is investigated. She should undergo tests to determine whether the fallopian tubes are patent and whether regular ovulation is occurring, except in cases where the husband is azoospermic or has a very severe impairment of semen. Even then, it will often be necessary to investigate the wife should the couple subsequently request artificial insemination by donor. In a small number of couples all tests on both partners appear to show normal fertility. In these cases current tests are unable to define the problem.

Surgery of infertility

Orchiopexy

Normally the testicles have descended fully and lie in the scrotum by one year of age. The seminal tubules begin to elongate between the fifth and ninth year and spermatogenesis commences between the ninth and fifteenth year, probably at about 11½ years of age (Short, 1976). In order to preserve fertility, orchiopexy is ideally performed before the age of 6. There is also evidence that the risk of malignancy is reduced if orchiopexy is performed before this age.

There are three main types of maldescent to be considered:

1 **Retractile testes.** The testes should lie in the scrotum shortly after birth, but as the cremasteric reflexes develop each retracts to the external inguinal ring. This reflex is most marked in 5 to 6-year-olds. It is difficult at this age to distinguish between true maldescent and retractile testes and, unfortunately, this is the time when many children are examined at school.

2 **Ectopic testes.** Ectopic testes are those which become diverted from the normal path of descent. It is thought that inappropriate fibrous tissue may encroach on the gubernaculum, causing a mechanical barrier to descend. The commonest type of ectopic testes lie in the superficial inguinal pouch. More rarely they are found in the perineum or at other sites such as the femoral canal, pubic region or opposite sides of the scrotum.

3 **Incomplete descent.** The testes may arrest at any point on the normal pathway of descent between the posterior abdominal wall and the external inguinal ring. Such testes are usually impalpable when they are intra-canalicular or intra-abdominal. The incidence of impalpable testes is approximately 20% of the undescended testes population. Anorchism is very rare, but can be distinguished by hormone measurements and a challenge with chorionic gonadotrophin (Levitt *et al.*, 1978). The aetiology of arrested descent is probably different from that of the fibrous bands described above. In some cases there may be a failure of the proper hormonal milieu during the latter months of pregnancy. In other cases the testicular tissue may be abnormal and it is possible that only this group is more liable to malignant change.

Orchiopexy should, if possible, be performed before the age of 6. Often, however, the maldescent is not discovered until a later age, in which case orchiopexy should be attempted as early as possible before puberty. The adult with unilateral maldescent can have an orchiopexy if the testis is easily placed in the scrotum. If not, orchiectomy with placement of a testicular prosthesis is probably the treatment of choice. If there is bilateral maldescent, then orchiopexy should be attempted for psychological reasons and to place the testicles in a position where they can be easily examined. It should be remembered in adult cases that testosterone production will often be normal despite the maldescent and thus bilateral orchiectomy is not usually justified.

Varicocele ligation

Tulloch (1952) described a case of azoospermia associated with bilateral varicoceles. A biopsy taken before operation confirmed lack of spermatogenesis. Following varicocele ligation, spermatogenesis

returned and a second biopsy confirmed this. Subsequently this man fathered children. Following this classic description many centres have reported favourable results from varicocele ligation. Some doubt, however, has been cast on the significance of a varicocele in causing infertility by the observation that many fertile men attending for vasectomy have large varicoceles. In a controlled trial Nilsson *et al.* (1979) showed no benefit from varicocele ligation. In spite of the conflicting evidence, the weight of clinical experience still indicates that varicocele ligation is reasonable and probably effective treatment for some cases of male infertility.

It seems possible that it is not the size of the varicocele but the type of blood flow that is significant. If a Doppler is used to study varicoceles in some there is a continuous reflux of blood, whereas in others it is only intermittent (Fig 26.5).

Three different surgical approaches have been used: lower abdominal (Pallamo), inguinal and scrotal. The scrotal approach has now been abandoned because of a number of cases of testicular atrophy following inadvertent ligation of branches of the testicular artery. When the higher approaches are used the vessels are more easily defined (Fig 26.6). In many cases varicoceles can now be treated by embolisation using a catheter introduced into the testicular vein under x-ray control.

PREOPERATIVE

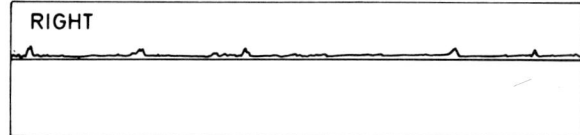

RIGHT

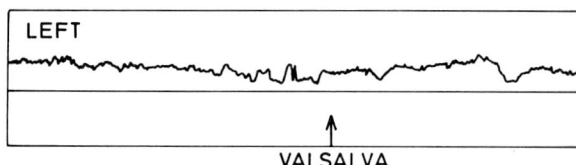

LEFT

↑
VALSALVA

POSTOPERATIVE

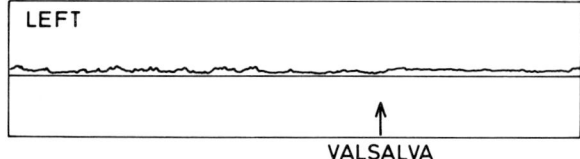

LEFT

↑
VALSALVA

Fig 26.5 The Doppler findings in a man with a clinical left-sided varicocele before and after operation. *Note* the continuous reflux of blood on the left side in the preoperative graft which is abolished by varicocele ligation.

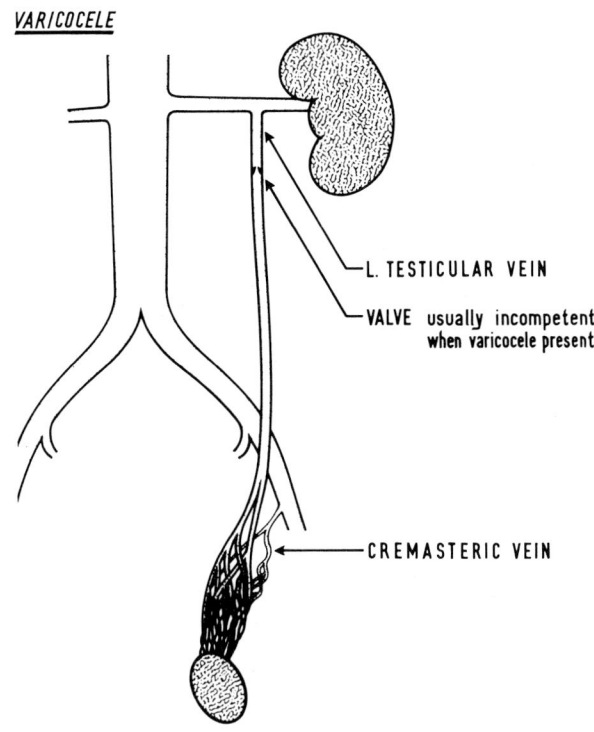

VARICOCELE

L. TESTICULAR VEIN

VALVE usually incompetent
when varicocele present

CREMASTERIC VEIN

Fig 26.6 Diagram to show dilated testicular veins secondary to an incompetent valve. Often cremasteric veins become varicose as well.

Epididymovasostomy

When there is a block to sperm passage in the tail of the epididymis or in the vas near the testes, the operation of epididymovasostomy may be used to bypass the blockage. Approximately 40% of men presenting with azoospermia have evidence of normal spermatogenesis on testicular biopsy and it is this group that would seem suitable for this type of management. Reported results range from an 80% success rate with a good pregnancy rate to 10% or even less. It seems probable that the reason for this discrepancy is differing aetiology of obstruction. In some reports, a past history of sexually transmitted disease or smallpox is obtained and presumably epididymal scarring causes a mechanical obstruction. In contrast in other reports, the incidence of sexually transmitted disease is low and it seems that azoospermia is due to a different aetiology. In some cases there may be a failure of sperm conduction rather than a mechanical block. Cases favourable for epididymovasostomy can be recognised during clinical examination, since obvious cystic lesions are felt in the head of the epididymis.

When a man has azoospermia, a palpable vas and normal FSH, then testicular biopsy is not indicated as a separate procedure. It is best to carry out a scrotal exploration, when the whole testis and vas are examined carefully, a vasogram is performed to check the proximal vas patency and a small testicular biopsy can be taken to confirm spermatogenesis. The operation consists of a careful anastomosis between the nearest patent portion of vas and the head of the epididymis (Fig 26.7). If there is a cystic lesion in the head of the epididymis, it is possible to take a small sample of seminal fluid and use this for artificial insemination, provided the wife is at the right time of her menstrual cycle. This idea has been developed and pieces of saphenous vein have been used in an attempt to create sperm reservoirs attached to the epididymis which could be aspirated through the scrotum. Despite the ingenuity of this technique, there has been a lack of success in terms of pregnancy.

Surgery for fertility

Vasectomy

Bilateral vasectomy for contraceptive purposes is now one of the most frequently performed minor operations in the United Kingdom. This has in part resulted from disquiet over long-term oral contraceptives for women and also because of the lack of other aesthetically acceptable methods. The perfect vasectomy would be 100% effective in a very short time, have no complications or side effects and be easily reversible. There are various methods but none is perfect. The technique described in Fig 26.8 is simple and the incidence of complications using this technique is low (Table 2). Nevertheless, it is worth noting that complications do occur and it is unwise with any type of operation to give absolute guarantees that recanalisation can never happen.

Clearance of sperm

In the majority of cases azoospermia will be achieved 3 months after vasectomy. Dodds (1972) found 10.5% of 1600 cases still had positive analyses 3 months after operation. One patient in his series continued to produce sperm until 17 months after vasectomy. In some cases these long delays seem to be related to infrequent ejaculation; coital frequency of less than once per week in men aged over 40 is associated with significantly prolonged periods before azoospermia is achieved, only 54% of men aged 50 becoming azoospermic at 12 months. Whether these non-motile sperms can fertilise is not known. Dodds (1972) stated that if sperm were dead on vital staining and the numbers were not

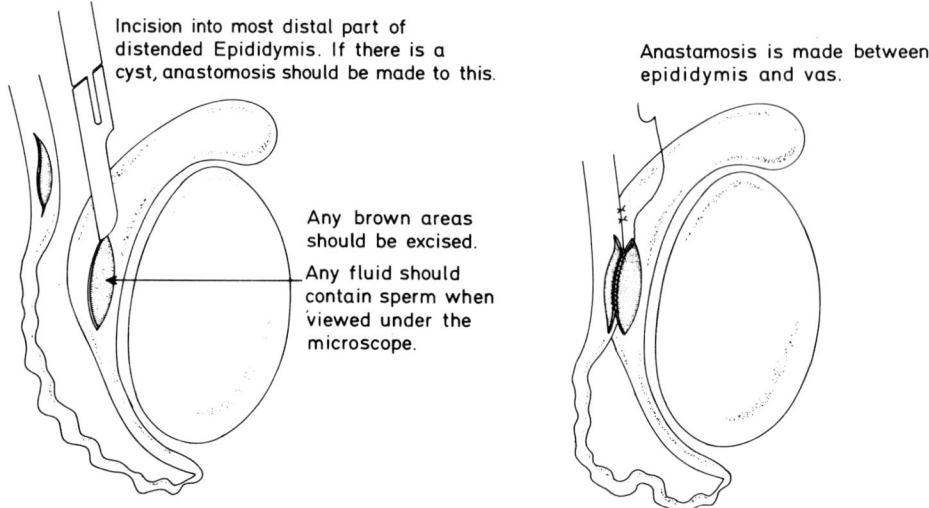

Incision into most distal part of distended Epididymis. If there is a cyst, anastomosis should be made to this.

Anastamosis is made between epididymis and vas.

Any brown areas should be excised.

Any fluid should contain sperm when viewed under the microscope.

Fig 26.7 Epididymovasostomy: operative technique.

increasing, then assurance of sterility could be given. Unfortunately, the occasional pregnancy is reported, and although this is likely to be due to a temporary recanalisation this cannot be proved. It is thus worth noting that 'two negative sperm counts (with a week between each sample) taken 3 months after operation are acceptable evidence of sterility'.

Complications

The immediate complication of serious concern to the patient is scrotal haematoma. Minor degrees of bruising are common and patients should be warned about this. If a haematoma larger than 2 cm develops, this is best managed by admission to hospital and evacuation of the haematoma with scrotal drainage under general anaesthesia. However, the incidence is low – approximately 0.5% (Table 2).

Table 2
COMPLICATIONS OF VASECTOMY

2343 Vasectomies between 1970–1976

5 Re-operation because of persistent positive sperm count		0.2%
10 Haematoma	Requiring medical advice	0.4%
4 Bleeding from skin edges		0.17%
4 Infection	Requiring medical advice	0.17%
3 Epididymitis		0.12%
2 Sperm granuloma	Requiring re-operation	0.08%
1 Impotence		0.04%
2 Pregnancy		0.08%
Total complications 31 = 1.3%		

(Two patients reported pregnancy following vasectomy. Sperm counts in both were negative, but one had had intercourse without contraception soon after vasectomy.)

Infection is also a risk following vasectomy and can in some cases develop into the dangerous Fournier's gangrene. In our series, using a strict aseptic technique and absorbable sutures, the rate of minor infection was 0.3%.

A later complication is the development of painful granulomas at the site of vasectomy. Extravasation of sperm from the vas gives rise to a characteristic foreign body giant cell reaction. These granulomas may appear up to 6 years after operation. Uusually they settle down with conservative measures, e.g. hot baths and a scrotal support. If symptoms persist, religation is sometimes necessary; in such cases, it is usually better to divide the vas or the tail of the epididymis at a site distal to the granuloma.

Recanalisation. In most cases this occurs within the first 3 months after operation. There is often a history of scrotal haematoma or sperm granuloma into which epithelial channels grow and then unite. The presence of motile sperm in the ejaculate at 3 months should make one suspect this complication. Another explanation for persisting motile sperm is the failure to ligate a duplicate vas at the original operation, but this is extremely rare.

Antisperm antibodies. Fifty per cent of patients following vasectomy appear to develop circulating antisperm antibodies. The presence of these antibodies may be related to the testicular granulomas which are known to develop as a consequence of vasectomy in various animals, *e.g.* guinea pigs and also in man. These antibodies are not known to have any harmful

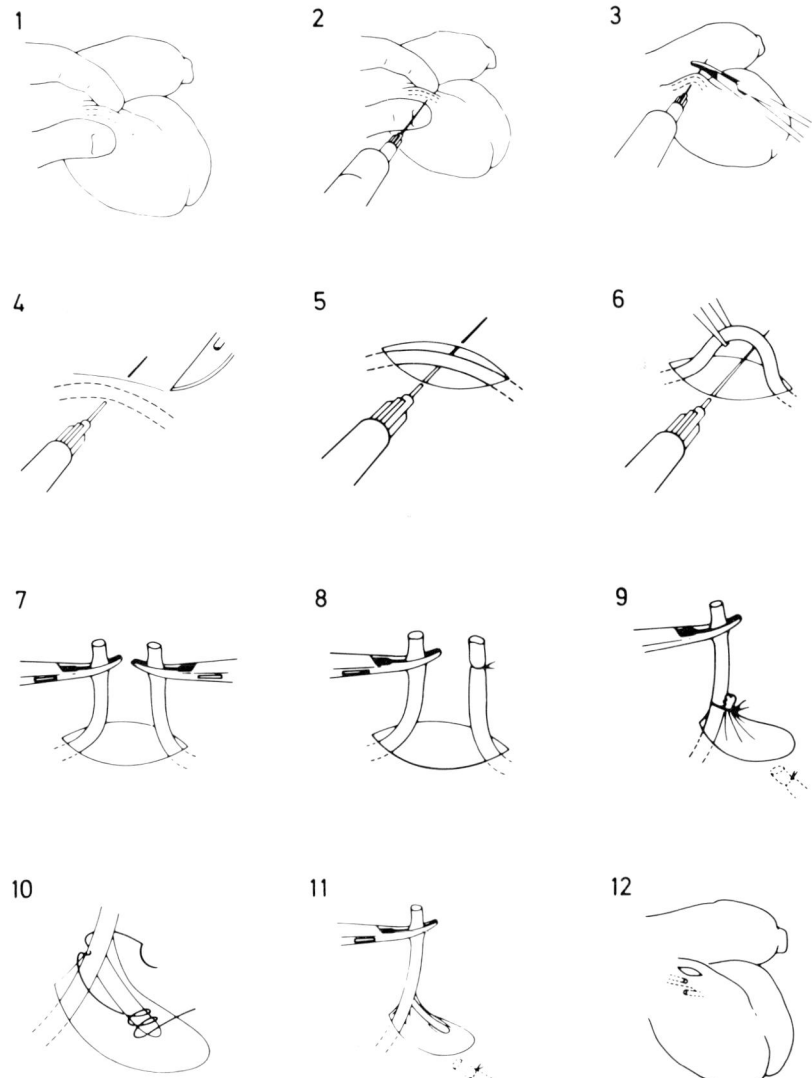

Fig 26.8 A method of vasectomy ideally suited to a local anaesthetic.

effects in man, although several long-term studies are being conducted. It is worth noting that Alexander and Clarkson (1978) reported that vasectomy increases the severity of diet-induced atherosclerosis in cynomolgus monkeys. The presence of these antibodies may affect the chances of fertility if a vasectomy reversal operation is required, but precise evidence about this is not yet available.

Psychiatric aspects. After vasectomy there is a tendency for the man to adopt a more masculine role. This does not seem to cause harm or marital break-up.

If, however, the patient is psychologically unstable, then vasectomy can precipitate psychiatric illness. For this reason pre-operative counselling should not be neglected.

Contraindications

There are few contraindications to vasectomy. It is unwise to perform the operation if the wife is pregnant in case the child is still-born or deformed. It is also unwise to recommend vasectomy if the marriage is unstable, the man psychiatrically unstable or if the wife is about to have a hysterectomy.

Vasectomy reversal

Whether a vasectomy can be reversed or not depends on the type of operation originally performed and how much time has elapsed since the operation. The operation shown in Fig. 26.8 is the minimum required to ensure success and can more easily be reversed. A nylon splint placed in the lumen of the vas helps the anastomosis, but is not essential. In such cases about 50% of the wives subsequently become pregnant and 80% of men have sperm in the ejaculate. The chances of subsequent success, however, appear to depend on the lapse of time since the original vasectomy and are much better if the reversal is attempted within 2 years of the original operation.

Surgery of sexual (erectile) dysfunction

Circumcision

In general, circumcision is not indicated in young babies except for reasons of religion or tradition. Some adults do, however, develop scarring of the foreskin, resulting in phimosis which interferes with sexual function. Such cases are best managed by circumcision.

Impotence

Penile splintage may be indicated in cases of impotence to enhance sexual function. A small proportion of men in their late thirties and forties develop impotence which does not yield to medical or psychiatric treatment and the prognosis after 3 years' duration is poor. Another indication is impotence associated with spinal cord injury.

Two types of artificial splintage are commonly used. The Small-Carrion penile prosthesis is a solid silicone elastamer rod which is implanted on each side into the corpora cavernosa. The Scott-Bradley prosthesis is an inflatable prosthesis implanted into the corpora with a reservoir in the scrotum. The advantage of the Small-Carrion device is simplicity of operative technique, but there is the disadvantage of continuous partial erection; with the Scott-Bradley device mechanical failure can be a problem. In general, older patients, patients with Peyronie's disease and paraplegics in wheel chairs who have condom catheter drainage are more suited to the Small-Carrion device, whereas young patients who participate in athletic activities should be considered for the Scott-Bradley implant. It is important that there is full counselling of both partners if this type of surgery is to be a success.

Peyronie's disease

This condition usually affects men between 40 and 60 years of age. Fibrous plaques develop, causing distortion of the penis which is particularly evident during erection. The condition is rather similar to Dupuytren's contracture of the hand and is indeed associated with this condition. The full extent of the plaque is often difficult to assess, but can be demonstrated by injecting contrast medium into the corpora cavernosa and taking x-ray pictures under the image intensifier.

Treatment is unsatisfactory. Radiotherapy, vitamin E, hyperpyrexia, oestrogens, the alkylating agent procarbazine, hyalase injections, systemic steroid therapy, dermo-injection of dexamethasone, ultrasound therapy, anticoagulants and pyschotherapy are some of the many therapies that have been tried without success. Medical treatment with para-aminobenzo-acidic potassium (POTABA) taken orally for several months may limit progression of the fibrosis, but it is doubtful if existing fibrosis resolves. The disorder tends to be self-limiting and this makes it difficult to evaluate any treatment. Surgical treatment is to excise the plaque and repair the area with a graft or to insert a penile prosthesis.

Penile deformity

Scarring of the glans and external meatus may follow phimosis with attacks of balanitis, although this is not usually associated with the failure of erection or difficulty in having intercourse. The congenital abnormality, hypospadias, is nearly always associated with chordee. This fibrosis causes gross penile bending during erection to such an extent that intercourse may be impossible; unfortunately, plastic repairs to reconstruct the urethra do not always satisfactorily deal with the chordee. The extent of any deformity should be assessed by saline injection into the corpora at operation so that correction can be attempted. It is also helpful to ask the patient or his partner to take polaroid photos of the erect penis from at least two different planes. Often this will mean the length to be constructed is extended and it may be necessary to obtain extra skin cover with a scrotal flap.

References

Alexander N.J., Clarkson T.B. (1978). Vasectomy increases the severity of diet-induced atherosclerosis in Macaca fascicularis. *Science*; **201**:538.

Chandley A.C., Edmond P., Christie S., Gowans L., Fletcher J., Frackiewicy A., Newton M. (1975). Cytogenetics and infertility in man. I. Karyotype and seminal analysis. *Ann. Human Genetics*; **39**:231.

Dodds D.J. (1972). Reanastomosis of the vas deferens. *J. Amer. Med. Ass*; **220**:1498.

Hafez E.S.E. (1977). Human reproductive medicine. In *Techniques of Human Andrology* (Hafez E.S.E., ed.). Netherlands: Elsevier.

Hargreave T.B. (1983). Questionnaire for assessing infertility. In *Male Infertility* (Hargreave T.B., ed.) pp. 28–45. Berlin: Springer Verlag.

Levitt S.B., Kogan S.J., Engal R.M., Weiss R.M., Martin D.C., Ehrlich R.M. (1978). The impalpable testes, a rational approach to management. *J. Urol*; **120**:515.

MacLeod J. (1971). Human male infertility. *Obstet. Gynec. Surv*; **26**:335.

Nilsson S., Edvinsson A., Nilsson B. (1979). Improvement of semen and pregnancy rate after ligation and division of the internal spermatic vein. Fact or fiction? *Brit. J. Urol*; **51**:591.

Rumpke P., Van Amstel N., Messer E.N., Bezemer P.D. (1974). Prognosis of fertility of men with sperm-agglutinins in the serum. *Fertil. Steril*; **25**:393.

Short R.V. (1976). The evolution of human reproduction. *Proc. Roy. Soc. B*; **195**:3.

Shulman S. (1976). Treatment of immune male infertility with methyl-prednisolone. *Lancet;* **ii**:1243.

Tulloch W.S. (1952). Consideration of sterility. Subfertility in the male. *Edinb. Med. J*; **59**:29.

27

Transplantation

P.R.F. BELL and R.F.M. WOOD

Techniques for organ transplantation were developed in the early years of this century but it took the dramatic development of immunology in the 1940s and 50s to make clinical transplantation a possibility. An understanding of the immune response involved in the rejection of organ grafts led to research into drugs capable of suppressing the response. During the last 15 years, transplantation has become an established part of clinical practice particularly in the treatment of renal failure and, in a few specialised centres, liver and heart transplant programmes have continued with increasing success. Practical solutions to the technical problems of whole organ pancreatic transplantation have emerged and cellular grafts of bone marrow and isolated pancreatic islets have also met with some success.

This chapter outlines the immune response to allografted organs, methods of immunosuppression and organ preservation. In addition, the techniques and results of transplantation of specific organs are presented. There has been some disappointment that despite so much research effort, clinical transplantation has not progressed more rapidly. However, there have recently been a number of encouraging advances in tissue typing, chemical immunosuppression and modification of recipient immunity. The significance of these new developments is considered in the final section of the chapter on future prospects for transplantation.

Transplant rejection

The mechanism of rejection

In many early reports of organ grafts using experimental animals, although the histological features of acute rejection were accurately described, the appearances were thought to be due to infection. However, in the early years of this century, geneticists and immunologists had established the basis of 'individuality' and with hindsight it is perhaps surprising that the process of rejection was not elucidated at an earlier stage. Schöne (1908) had found that while rat skin could be successfully autotransplanted, allotransplants were always unsuccessful. He concluded that the intensity of rejection was inversely proportional to the degree of affinity between the donor and recipient. Although this fundamental study had explained the probable reason for rejection, it was another 25 years before the mechanism was discovered. In 1942, Gibson and Medawar recorded in detail the rejection of human skin grafts. A 22-year-old woman with severe burns was grafted with skin from her brother. An initial set of pinch grafts were taken from the brother's thigh and applied to the granulation tissue in the burnt area. However, an extensive raw surface remained and 15 days after the first grafting a second set of pinch grafts of the brother's skin were applied. By serial histological examination of both sets of grafts, Gibson and Medawar established that there was rapid degeneration of the second set and they formulated the hypothesis that this was due to acquired immunity on the part of the recipient. Medawar then embarked on a series of animal experiments which confirmed the hypothesis. The fact that the immunity was basically cellular in origin was then proved by Mitchison (1954) who demonstrated that transplant immunity could be passively transferred by means of the lymphoid cells of sensitised donors.

An organ graft acts as a major antigenic challenge to the immune system. The potential effect of this stimulation on cellular and humoral immunity is illustrated in Fig 27.1. The major component of the immune system is the lymphocyte. Two subpopulations of lymphocytes are recognised – T cells and B cells – both thought to originate from a common stem cell in haemopoietic tissue. The T or thymus derived lymphocytes mature after passage through the thymus and are found in large numbers in the paracortical areas of lymph nodes. These cells respond to challenge by enlarging and dividing into blast cells specifically sensitised to the stimulating antigen. Humoral immunity, resulting in antibody production, is mediated by B lymphocytes. The B stands for Bursa as, in avian species, the lymphocytes responsible for antibody production originate from the Bursa of Fabricius. In mammals, there is no direct equivalent of the Bursa and B lymphocytes may come from the bone marrow or gut lymphoid tissue.

The classic acute rejection reaction is due to an activation of cell mediated immunity in response to graft antigen. Antigenic fragments may be washed out into the recipient circulation at the time of transplantation and, after phagocytosis by macrophages, are presented to the host immune system. This recognition phase results in the production of a population of T lymphocytes sensitised against the graft. In addition T lymphocytes may migrate to the transplant and undergo blast cell transformation within the organ itself. These cells have considerable cytotoxic potential and their activity is mediated by the release of soluble factors known as lymphokines.

In addition to cytotoxic factors, the lymphocytes release lymphokines capable of recruiting macrophages and polymorphs to cause further destruction of the graft. In any organ transplant, episodes of acute rejection are commonest in the first two to three months after surgery. Following this time fulminating rejection crises are rare and the recipient appears to develop an almost symbiotic relationship with the graft. The reasons why rejection is less common after the first few months are still not fully understood, but have been attributed to the immunological phenomenon of 'enhancement'. This is the suppression of host responses by protective antibodies or 'suppressor cells'. Biopsy studies show that even in well functioning renal transplants, antibodies can be demonstrated in the glomerular capillaries by using fluorescent techniques. It may be that this antibody, rather than damaging the graft, is coating the vascular endothelium and protecting it from further cellular attack. 'Suppressor cells' (Fig 27.2) are a subset of the T lymphocyte population which can be shown to suppress the cytotoxic

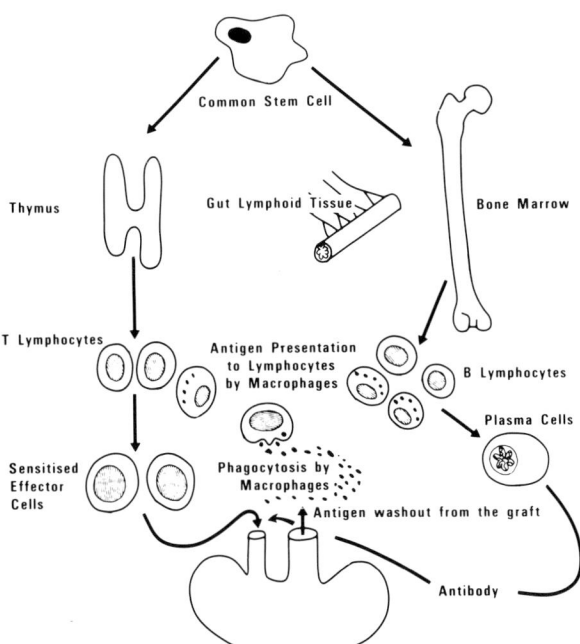

Fig 27.1 Lymphocyte subpopulations and the response to antigen challenge.

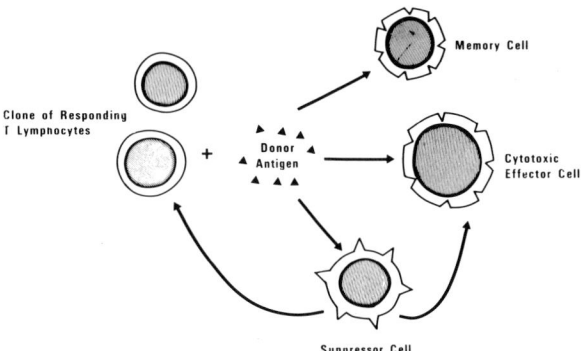

Fig 27.2 T lymphocyte response to donor antigen.

potential of the remaining lymphocytes. The exact role of these two mechanisms *in vivo* is still poorly understood.

It is now clear that in addition to the cell mediated immune response, humoral mechanisms are also important in transplantation. Potential transplant recipients may have generated circulating antibody as the result of pregnancy, a previous failed transplant or blood transfusion. If these antibodies are cytotoxic to donor cells, then transplantation will be followed by an accelerated or 'hyperacute' rejection. When the organ is revascularised these antibodies rapidly become fixed to endothelial surfaces and cause activation of the complement cascade. Platelets become attached to the damaged endothelium and there is rapid coagulation in the microcirculation. Although cell mediated immune responses can be controlled by immunosuppression, hyperacute rejection has so far proved to be an irreversible process despite attempts at treatment with anticoagulants and antiplatelet agents.

Apart from their proven role in hyperacute rejection, antibodies were thought to play little part in acute rejection which has traditionally been regarded as a purely cell mediated immune phenomenon. However, it would be surprising if such a large antigenic challenge as an organ graft did not produce a significant antibody response. Circulating antibodies to the transplant have been difficult to demonstrate in patients with a graft *in situ* but it has been noted that following removal of a rejected transplant, antibodies could be detected readily in the serum. The failure to detect circulating antibody is, therefore, due largely to the ability of the transplant to fix the vast majority of antibody produced. The potential importance of antibody in acute rejection is implied by the reported successes of plasma exchange in reversing rejection which has failed to respond to conventional therapy.

Antibodies have also been implicated in the process of 'chronic' rejection which is characterised by slowly progressive failure of the transplant, usually associated with histological features of ischaemia. It may be difficult to distinguish chronic rejection from the previous cause of organ failure. In the liver, the graft becomes cirrhotic with portal fibrosis and biliary stasis. In the heart, there is interstitial fibrosis with areas of infarction. A biopsy from a chronically rejecting kidney may show features indistinguishable from end stage glomerulonephritis. There are arterial changes with intimal thickening and reduplication of the internal elastic lamina. The glomeruli become sclerosed and the damage to the basement membrane commonly results in increasing proteinuria.

In human transplantation it has so far proved impossible to prevent the recognition phase of the immune response and rejection, therefore, remains a constant threat to any organ graft.

Prevention of rejection: donor-recipient matching

Blood groups

Compatibility is an essential for successful transplantation. There is a tendency, however, to use O kidneys in patients of all blood groups, thereby creating a shortage of organs for patients of blood group O. This is unfortunate, particularly as results indicate that recipients with blood group O receiving O kidneys do best in the long-term.

Tissue typing

The major histocompatibility complex in the human is situated on chromosome 6 (Lamm *et al.*, 1974) and has been shown to be largely responsible for the rejection of allografts (Solheim *et al.*, 1977). The antigens responsible in man are situated at four loci designated A, B, C and D (Fig 27.3).

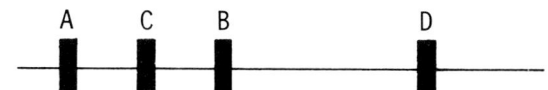

Fig 27.3 Arrangement of the human HLA area on chromosome 6.

HLA – A,B,C

Human leucocyte antigen (HLA) typing is a serological technique using antisera to A, B and C locus antigens to test against separated lymphocytes. At present, 20 antigens are recognised at the A locus, 33 at the B locus and 6 at the C locus, though there are probably more to be discovered. There is considerable controversy about the importance of matching at the A, B and C loci and some reports claim that typing is of little importance. However, there is evidence to show that survival of the graft can depend on the degree of match. There are two alleles at each locus and individuals, therefore, have a total of four antigens at the A and B loci. Because of the large number of antigenic determinants, the chances of achieving an identical match between donor and recipient are very small. This problem is overcome by centralising tissue typing information and organising the despatch of an appropriate donor kidney to a well matched recipient. A and B locus matching is of proven value in patients in whom all four antigens are compatible; these patients have an excellent graft survival rate. In addition, those patients who have had a previous transplant and have cytotoxic antibodies in their serum have poor graft survival with a second transplant unless there is a good A and B match. For first cadaver grafts there is relatively little difference in overall survival rates between groups of recipients with 1, 2 or 3 A and B locus antigens in common with the donor.

HLA – D

Until recently the D locus could only be typed by means of the mixed lymphocyte culture reaction (MLC). This has been known to provide accurate indication of the outcome of live donor transplants (Opelz and Terasaki, 1977). However, the test takes 5 days to complete and is of no use in cadaver transplantation. Recently, D locus determinants have been discovered on a number of cells including B lymphocytes. By harvesting B lymphocytes, it is now possible to type serologically for the D region – DR typing. Since there are only two alleles at the DR locus and only ten antigens have so far been described, the chances of an identical match between recipient and donor are much better than with A and B locus typing. Early results suggest a graft survival in excess of 80% at one year in patients matched for both DR antigens. Even when there is only one DR antigen in common, graft survival at a year is well over 60%, with relatively poor results in patients who share no DR identities.

Antibodies

Because of the possible presence of preformed antibodies, it is mandatory to perform a direct cross match between the recipient's serum and donor lymphocytes prior to transplantation. The presence of cytotoxic antibodies has been regarded as a complete contraindication to transplantation. However, it is now clear that a positive cross match is not necessarily an indication of the presence of broadly reactive antibodies. Some patients have been shown to have auto-reactive lymphocyte antibodies which will not cause hyperacute rejection. In addition antibody specificity can be ascertained by subdividing recipient lymphocytes into T and B cell populations. Transplantation is possible despite a positive B cell cross match and long-term graft survival is equivalent to patients with a completely negative cross match (Ting, 1982).

Recipient selection

There is evidence to suggest that selection of patients for transplantation on the basis of their immune response may be important. Recent evidence has suggested that patients with a strong immune response while on dialysis have poorer graft survival rates than those who have a weak response. This has led to the suggestion that each patient should have his immune response tested prior to being accepted for transplantation and, in the event of a normal response, should perhaps be refused a transplant. It is too early to say whether this approach is correct, but where facilities permit, patients waiting for transplantation should have their immune response tested using one of the available techniques such as the DNCB skin test (Watson et al., 1979) which provides an estimate of cell mediated immunity.

Immunosuppression

The two most frequently used drugs are Azathioprine (Imuran) and steroids. These agents were not particularly successful when originally used in animals, but were more effective when applied to man (Calne, 1960). In the early years of transplantation, Actinomycin C was used as an additional treatment, but has since been abandoned. Other drugs, such as Cyclophosphamide have been used in patients who have shown an intolerance to Azathioprine (Starzl et al., 1971). More recently, Cyclosporin A has been evaluated as a potentially more specific antirejection agent. In the biological area, antilymphocyte globulins have been tested and used extensively, mainly in North America. Monoclonal antibodies to lymphocyte subsets are now commercially available and provide the prospect of immunosuppresive therapy directed specifically at the T cell.

'Conventional' immunosuppression

Since 1960 when Azathioprine and Prednisolone were found to be useful in preventing rejection in dogs, these agents have been used as standard immunosuppression for renal transplantation in man. The general principles are to give the patient a large loading dose of Azathioprine (3–5 mg per kg body weight) at the time of operation and then to adjust the dose on the basis of a daily white cell count in order to maintain a level of between 4000 and 7000. Eventually, the dose of Azathioprine can be stabilised and white cell counts need only be obtained infrequently. Steroids act synergistically with Azathioprine to suppress the immune response and are initially given at a dose varying from 100 mg to 200 mg of either Prednisolone or Methylprednisolone. The dose is reduced slowly over the next few weeks to a maintenance level of 10 to 15 mg per day by the third month after transplantation. As most of the complications that occur following transplantation are due to steroids, some centres give these drugs on an alternate day basis, as this appears to reduce the incidence of side effects. Some centres also give the patient 1 g of Methylprednisolone at the time of re-vascularisation as this has been shown to kill T lympho-cytes. After 3 months the aim should be to have the patient on a daily dose of Azathioprine consistent with a white cell count of 5000–6000 mm^3 and a dose of Prednisolone of 20 mg on alternate days.

Low dose steroid therapy

A regimen of low dose steroid therapy from the time of transplantation has been popularised by McGeown from Belfast (1981). Initial steroid treatment is given in the form of intravenous hydrocortisone (total dose 800 mg), patients are then treated with 20 mg of oral Pred-nisolone per day and no bolus doses of intravenous Methylprednisolone are used. Rejection is treated by increasing oral Prednisolone to 200 mg per day and then rapidly tapering the dose over a period of 5 to 7 days. Results from the Belfast group show excellent long-term graft survival with low morbidity from steroid side effects.

Antilymphocyte globulin (ALG)

Antilymphocyte globulin is produced by the injection of lymphocytes into a different species, thereby causing immunisation against the injected cells. The serum is collected at a defined interval, refined and the globulin fraction (ALG) injected into the recipient. This ma-terial was first shown to be a potent inhibitor of graft rejection in animals by Woodruff and Anderson (1963). Antilymphocyte globulin has a marked effect on T lymphocytes and has been used since 1967 in clinical transplantation, but controlled clinical trials have been difficult to evaluate until relatively recently. ALG as a biological product cannot be standardised easily and may produce a severe reaction in recipients who have had multiple injections. High potency ALG can pre-vent rejection in man and if access to an active, safe preparation is available, it is a useful addition to stan-dard immunosuppression provided that precautions are taken and it is given for short periods of time.

Monoclonal antibodies

Monoclonal antibodies are produced by isolating individual antibody secreting cells in tissue culture and using hybridisation with a mouse myeloma cell line to create a new population of cells which will manufacture pure antibody in large quantities (McMichael and Fabre, 1982). Reagents are now available with reactivity against determinants on lymphocyte sub-populations and these monoclonals have been used to study the ratio of T helper to T suppressor/cytotoxic lymphocytes in the peripheral blood of transplant recipients. Preliminary clinical trials have been carried

out where pan T cell monoclonals have been used to treat acute rejection. The antibodies employed, OKT3 and anti-T12, have been shown to be effective in reversing rejection although the development of anti-bodies to mouse immunoglobulins precludes their use on a long-term basis.

Cyclosporin A

Cyclosporin A (CyA) is produced as a metabolite by a fungal organism *Tolypocladium inflatum* grains. The immunosuppressive activity of CyA has been under investigation for the past 10 years and animal experi-ments demonstrated its ability to prolong the survival of all types of organ allografts in a wide variety of species. CyA does not appear to affect antigen binding to T cells but acts by interfering with the transmission of the antigen derived signal to the synthetic machinery of the cell. If given at the time of transplantation it will therefore prevent the development of a population of sensitised effector cells.

Initial clinical trials of CyA were carried out in Cam-bridge (Calne *et al.*, 1979). Although CyA was clearly extremely successful in preventing rejection there were worrying problems with both hepatotoxicity and nephrotoxicity. In addition there was a 10% incidence of lymphomas. The lymphomas appear to have been caused by oversuppression when CyA was combined with large doses of other immunosuppressive agents. In subsequent clinical trials the frequency of malignant lesions has been the same as in patients on other forms of immunosuppression. Results from a European multicentre trial of CyA in 232 patients have shown encouraging results. The patients treated with CyA had a significant improvement in one-year graft survival at 73% compared to the 53% one-year graft survival in the control grup treated with conventional immuno-suppression (European Multicentre Trial, 1982). Nephrotoxicity remains a problem and there is concern that this may affect long-term survival. Therefore the concept of using CyA at the time of transplantation with subsequent conversion to Azathioprine and Pred-nisolone is attractive and clinical trials in Oxford have shown this to be an effective policy (Morris *et al.*, 1983). CyA can be given alone although impressive results have been reported when it is combined with low dose oral steroids (Starzl *et al.*, 1982). Initially the drug is given in a dosage of from 12.5–17 mg/kg/day reducing to maintenance levels of around 5 mg/kg/day. The drug is poorly absorbed after intramuscular injection and should be given either orally or intra-venously.

Radiation therapy

In the early years of transplantation, total body irra-diation was used to prevent rejection. This treatment was abandoned because of the morbidity and high mortality it produced. Later, local irradiation was often practised in order to reduce the numbers of active cells in the graft during a rejection episode. Opinion varies as to its usefulness but a small dose of about 250 rads to a swollen rejecting kidney in association with other antirejection therapy appears to shrink the graft.

Another method of using radiotherapy may provide good results in the future. Total lymphoid irradiation (TLI), often practised in the treatment of Hodgkin's disease, has been shown to produce indefinite graft survival if donor bone marrow is given over the period of lymphoid irradiation (usually lasting several weeks). After this, the recipient will accept an organ from the same donor and keep it in the long-term. This technique may be useful in live donor transplants and, perhaps in the long-term, with cadaver transplants.

Donor pretreatment

It was shown experimentally that the most important way in which the recipient became sensitised to a graft was through cells transferred with the transplanted tissue. These cells have been called 'passenger leucocytes' and have been shown to be powerful instigators of the immune response; if these cells are destroyed, graft survival can be enhanced without any other therapy. In view of this finding, some centres advocated a policy of donor pretreatment where the donor was infused with huge quantities of Cyclophosphamide and steroids in order to destroy as many lymphocytes as possible. This added a significant work load to the preparation of a donor and has not become universally accepted.

Manipulation of the immune response

Experimentally, many attempts have been made to produce specific immunosuppression by preventing the recognition of antigen by the host, thereby avoiding the need to use drugs which are relatively non-specific and may be dangerous. It is known from tumour immunology that one of the reasons for cell growth is the probable existence of weak antibodies in the serum which form antigen-antibody complexes with tumour tissue and in some way block the immune system enhancing tumour growth. This model has been used in experimental organ transplantation to enhance and protect organ grafts, particularly in rodents. This can often be achieved by injecting donor lymphocytes into a recipient strain animal over a period of weeks. The serum is then harvested and injected into the recipient at the time of organ transplantation. This weak serum has the ability to protect the graft completely if given for a short period over the first few days after grafting. The animal retains the ability to reject other organs from other donors and to resist normally any infection. The mechanism is uncertain, but may be that antibody given to the recipient either attaches itself to the graft, thus masking the sites normally exposed to T lymphocyte recognition or by centrally attaching itself to T lymphocytes and thus immobilising them. The method does not work well in species other than rodents. The use of enhancement in human cadaver transplantation is probably impossible for logistic reasons but it has been used in live donor transplants where the serum has been raised in one of the parents (French and Batchelor, 1969). So far it has not been very sucessful, but may well be useful in the future if enhancement can be better defined and large quantities of specific serum made available.

Blood transfusion

Prior to 1970, blood transfusions were given frequently to patients on dialysis because of their tendency to become anaemic. As a result, a number of them developed cytotoxic antibodies which made transplantation impossible. Because of this problem, most units changed to a no-transfusion policy, or transfusion with frozen red cells or leucocyte-poor blood. In addition, improvements in dialysis techniques meant that less blood was needed anyway. In contrast to this general policy of avoiding transfusion, some authors suggested that blood transfusions were not necessarily harmful and could possibly induce enhancement due to the formation of weak antibodies to the leucocytes in the transfused blood (Opelz *et al.*, 1973). Since these observations, several studies in monkeys and in man have shown that patients who receive a blood transfusion fare better than those who have not. The difference in graft survival can be as high as 50%. The reason for the effect remains to be determined. It may be that patients who need a blood transfusion have a poor immune response and produce weak antibodies which protect the graft. Those who have a strong immune response may well react normally by producing a large number of cytotoxic antibodies which excludes them from transplantation. Another possibility is that blood transfusion does actively 'switch on' the subpopulation of cells called suppressor T cells which protect the transplant. Although no-one is certain about the mechanism of the transfusion effect, most centres now give blood prospectively to all their patients. It would seem that one unit of blood is all that is required, provided it is given while the patient is on dialysis and approximately 2 months before transplantation. However, it has also been suggested that one unit given at the time of transplantation is equally effective.

Complications of immunosuppressive therapy

Because chemical agents suppress the immune response in a non-specific fashion, most of the complications that occur are related to infection or directly to the use of steroids. In the early postoperative period when the dose of immunosuppressive drugs is high, infection is a particular problem, and during this period the patient ought to be barrier-nursed for at least 48 h. Many units use a single parenteral dose of a broad spectrum antibiotic immediately before transplantation. However, prolonged administration of prophylactic antibiotics is dangerous and encourages the growth of more exotic organisms. Bacterial infection of the lungs, urine and wound can easily occur and regular screening cultures are essential. Any evidence of bacterial infection should be dealt with by specific antibiotic therapy.

More difficult problems are seen when infections with other organisms occur. Viruses, for example, cytomegalovirus, Herpes simplex or influenza virus, can all cause serious problems, often necessitating the cessation of immunosuppression and loss of the graft. Fungal infections are also seen, particularly if antibiotics are used excessively. The commonest is monilia, but other fungal infections affecting mainly the upper respiratory tract, can occur. Should there be any suggestion of a continuing infection, sputum or tracheal specimens should be taken for culture, if necessary by aspiration.

When an infection is first discovered and the cause determined, specific therapy should be given. In the case of bacteria, appropriate antibiotics are often effective. Infections with viruses such as cytomegalovirus, Herpes simplex, or influenza are difficult to treat. Some, in fact, accentuate the rejection process, leading to loss of the organ. Most viral diseases are, however, self-limiting provided that the immunosuppression is reduced. Should the condition of the patient deteriorate, the possibility of using some of the newer methods of treatment such as Interferon or Adenosine – Arabinoside should be considered. Fungal infection with aspergillosis, candidiasis, toxoplasmosis, and cryptococcus, are best dealt with by stopping all antibiotic treatment and giving specific chemotherapy. Flagyl is useful in the treatment of moniliasis and 5-Flurocytosine in systemic infections with candida. Amphotericin B can be used in other severe fungal infections, but it is nephrotoxic and its use should be controlled carefully to keep the total dose below 3 g. If the patient suffers from a protozoal infection such as pneumocystis carinii, pentamidine isothionate or cotrimoxazole is useful. These infections are unusual, but if the condition of the patient fails to resolve, then the immunosuppression should be stopped and the kidney removed if necessary.

Once the early postoperative phase has been passed, the long-term complications of immunosuppression are due mainly to steroids. Avascular necrosis of bone can occur in as many as 10 to 15% of patients, producing a severe disability in otherwise fit patients with good renal function. Recourse to alternate day treatment with steroids may help to alleviate this problem.

The other difficulty with long-term immunosuppression is the increased incidence of malignancy. It has now been shown that tumours, particularly lymphomas, are more common in patients who have been immunosuppressed for a long period of time. Lymphomas are one hundred times more common than in the general population, but tumours of almost every other variety have been discovered in various surveys. Apart from lymphomas, the commonest appear to be in the skin, lip, uterus and cervix (Penn, 1977). It seems that although patients are statistically more liable to develop cancer this does not override the benefits of transplantation. Those who are likely to be at risk should, wherever possible, be screened regularly and treatment started early.

The detection of rejection

General principles

Rejection is essentially an inflammatory reaction and as such it may present with systemic features such as pyrexia and general malaise. Although it is an immunological process its clinical significance lies in the degree of functional impairment it can cause to the grafted organ. There are three main techniques for detecting rejection:

1 Immunological monitoring to pick up alterations in the recipients cellular and humoral immunity.
2 Measurement of the normal biochemical and physiological parameters reflecting the function of the particular organ.
3 Biopsy of the graft.

A great deal of research effort has been undertaken in an attempt to make an early diagnosis of rejection based on immunological tests. However, there have been no clinical trials to establish whether early treatment has any long-term effect on graft function. All current transplant programmes rely mainly on standard methods of assessment of organ function to diagnose rejection.

Immunological monitoring

Ideally immunological monitoring should attempt to detect a response in the recipient specifically directed against the donor. Therefore, the majority of studies have concentrated on cellular and humoral immunity to either donor cells or donor antigen preparations. These investigations have been carried out almost exclusively in renal transplant recipients.

Donor directed cell-mediated immunity. Three tests reflecting lymphokine production have been used and all three have been shown to be capable of predicting rejection. The leucocyte migration test (Wood *et al.*, 1978) is now usually referred to as the LIF test after the soluble mediator involved – leucocyte inhibition factor. This technique measures the ability of LIF to prevent the migration of recipient leucocytes from a capillary tube into a well containing donor antigen. The leucocyte aggregation test (LAT), developed by Kahan *et al.* (1974) demonstrates a cell mediated response when recipient leucocytes clump around viable donor cells maintained in a monolayer culture. Finally, the tanned erythrocyte electrophoretic mobility (TEEM) test (Shenton *et al.*, 1977) investigates the effect of recipient lymphokine on slowing the movement of tanned sheep erythrocytes in an electromagnetic field.

Mixed lymphocyte culture (MLC) reactivity has been monitored after transplantation in the hope that it might provide a sensitive index of alterations in donor/recipient reactivity preceding rejection. Miller *et al.* (1978) have shown that there is a fall in MLC responsiveness which frequently heralds graft rejection. They have identified MLC reactive cells within the graft and postulate that the fall in MLC response is due to trapping of these cells within the graft. An MLC test takes at least 3 days to complete and although the results are interesting, they are of no predictive value. Direct cytotoxicity of recipient lymphocytes for donor cells can be assessed in the lymphocyte mediated cytotoxicity (LMC) test. Several studies have shown excellent correlation with rejection, but in most cases positive test results coincide with biochemical evidence of rejection.

Donor directed humoral immunity. There are four tests for antibody in current use: complement dependent cytotoxicity (CDC), complement dependent cytotoxicity to B lymphocytes (CDC-B), erythrocyte-antibody inhibition (EAI) and antibody dependent cell mediated cytotoxicity (ADCC).

The development of cytotoxic antibody formed after transplantation can be tested using the same CDC technique as the standard pretransplant crossmatch. The development of a positive CDC response after transplantation has shown a strong correlation with rejection. However, the test is of little value in predicting graft outcome and CDC often remains positive long after a rejection episode is over (Stiller *et al.*, 1978). Transplantation in the presence of positive B cell antibody has already been discussed and the evidence suggests that preformed anti-B cell antibody is not a

contraindication to transplantation. However, the development of B cell antibody *de novo* after transplantation has a significant association with rejection. The EAI test detects the presence of antibody to Fc receptors on B lymphocytes. The test utilises ox red blood cells coated with a rabbit anti-ox IgG. In the controls, rosettes of the IgG coated ox red cells form around B lymphocytes. In the test, if antibodies present in the recipient's serum are directed against donor B cell Fc receptors, the receptor sites will be blocked and there will be a reduction in the number of rosettes formed. Positive EAI results may provide a better correlation with rejection than CDC to B lymphocytes. In some situations, although antibody directed against the donor develops, it is unable to produce cell killing on its own and requires the assistance of a population of non-sensitised effector cells (K or killer cells). In the ADCC, chromium (^{51}Cr) labelled donor lymphocytes are primed with recipient serum and then incubated with third party effector cells. The published studies of ADCC in renal transplantation show a mixture of results with some demonstrating a clear correlation with rejection while others report few positive results.

Non-specific immunological tests. A number of non-specific techniques have been used in transplantation, including the rosette inhibition test (RIT) and lymphoblast transformation to mitogens such as phytohaemagglutinin. These techniques have generally been replaced by the donor specific assays mentioned above. Estimates of the numbers of T and B cells in the peripheral blood are of relatively little value in detecting rejection, but have been widely used in patients on antilymphocyte globulin to regulate the dosage schedule (Thomas *et al.*, 1978).

There has been renewed interest recently in antibodies to vascular endothelium after transplantation. The original non-specific test using vascular endothelium from umbilical cord vessels as the target has been developed by Claas *et al.* (1980) using small biopsies of donor kidney removed prior to transplantation. Thin kidney slices are incubated with recipient serum and then labelled with a fluorescent immunoglobulin preparation. They have found that the development of antibody to the endothelium in the peritubular capillaries showed a high correlation with rejection. The antibody is not absorbed by red cells, platelets or granulocytes, but is absorbed by glass adherent monocytes. It is, therefore, possible to screen for the presence of this antibody after transplantation by testing recipient's sera against panel monocytes.

T lymphocyte subpopulations can now be monitored using fluorescein conjugated monoclonal antibodies. The cells can be counted either by using immunofluorescence microscopy or by employing a fluorescence activated cell sorter. Reagents are now available which will recognise T helper cells (Leu-3a, OKT4) and T suppressor/cytotoxic cells (Leu-2a, OKT8). A number of studies have now been reported in which the ratio of T helper to T suppressor/cytotoxic cells (T_h/T_s ratio) has been measured in the peripheral blood of renal transplant patients. It has been suggested that increases in T_h/T_s ratio may be predictive of acute rejection. However, a careful longitudinal study where samples were analysed on a daily basis has failed to demonstrate an increase in the T_h/T_s ratio either before or at the time of rejection (Carter et al., 1983). The normal T_h/T_s ratio is 1.9–2.0 and there is evidence of a correlation between low T_h/T_s ratios (<1.0) and viral infection in transplant patients. The majority of reported cases have had Cytomegalovirus infection (Chatenoud et al., 1983). In general, patients with a ratio of less than 1.3 are unlikely to experience rejection. However, if rejection does occur it is much more likely to result in graft loss than in patients with higher ratios.

Techniques for the assessment of graft function

In kidney transplantation, rejection is still diagnosed by routine estimation of renal function and reliable biochemistry is essential for patient management. Rejection is accompanied by an increase in the serum creatinine and a fall in the creatinine clearance. In liver transplantation, rejection is associated with jaundice and deranged liver function tests. Monitoring for rejection in cardiac transplantation involves daily electrocardiograms. The tracing during rejection typically shows an overall reduction in the voltage. In whole organ transplantation of the pancreas, rejection is accompanied by deterioration in the control of blood sugar.

Biopsy. Histological studies of transplanted livers and kidneys can readily be undertaken by performing needle biopsies of the graft. This is not possible in cardiac transplantation, but the development of endomyocardial biopsy by threading a catheter through the venous system and into the right side of the heart has proved beneficial in the management of cardiac transplant recipients.

The classical feature of acute rejection is mononuclear cell infiltration of the graft. In severe reactions, other inflammatory cells are also involved with prominent numbers of polymorphonuclear leucocytes and plasma cells. This is often accompanied by interstitial oedema and haemorrhage. There is damage to specialised structures with liver cell necrosis in hepatic transplants, tubular disruption in the kidney and destruction of myocardial fibres in the heart. There may also be evidence of arteriolar damage with fibrinoid necrosis of the vessel walls.

Fine needle aspiration cytology

Fine needle aspiration biopsy (FNAB) with subsequent cytological examination of the infiltrating cells was originally proposed as a monitoring technique in the 1960s. It has been revived by Hayry and von Willebrand (1981) and they have described a number of patterns of cellular infiltration. Early reversible rejection tends to be dominated by the presence of lymphoblasts. Progressive rejection is accompanied by increasing numbers of monocytes and macrophages. The presence of significant numbers of large tissue macrophages is an ominous sign usually indicating irreversible rejection. The tubular cells of the kidney can also be identified by FNAB and it has been claimed that the technique is of value in assessing cyclosporin A nephrotoxicity (von Willebrand and Hayry, 1983). Monoclonal antibodies with immunoperoxidase staining can be used to provide precise identification of lymphocyte subpopulations (Wood et al., 1982). The focal nature of the cellular infiltrate in acute rejection may affect results and the value of FNAB in clinical management is still undecided.

Reversal of rejection

In spite of the precautions outlined above and even in patients who are apparently identically matched with their donors, rejection episodes will occur and result in loss of the graft unless the patient is, of course, an identical twin. Most rejection episodes are relatively minor and may or may not continue to graft destruction, but when treated will often reverse. For therapeutic reasons, rejection is best divided into acute and chronic. Acute, by definition, is that type of reaction which occurs within 3 months of transplantation; the chronic type occurs at a later date and usually results in the loss of the graft.

Treatment of acute rejection

Once this has been diagnosed, whether clinically or by biochemical means, it can be dealt with in a number of ways. The most common method is to give the adult patient 1 g (0.5 g in the case of a child), of methylprednisolone (Solumedrone) i.v. over a period of about 1 h. This has been shown to be effective in reversing experimental and clinical rejection (Bell et al., 1971) although recent evidence suggests that this type of therapy may not be necessary and that a simple elevation of the oral steroid dose can also be effective. If no response occurs after giving a gram of methylprednisolone the dose should be repeated on three further occasions. If renal function fails to respond, it is unlikely that any other method will be effective

(Fig 27.4). Large doses of intravenous steroid given in this way over a limited period are rapidly excreted and appear to have no serious side effects. Other methods of reversing rejection including the use of antilymphocyte globulin, Cyclosporin A and Azathioprine, have been tried, with limited success. Actinomycin C is occasionally worth trying if other attempts to reverse rejection fail. If rejection does not reverse quickly, it is best

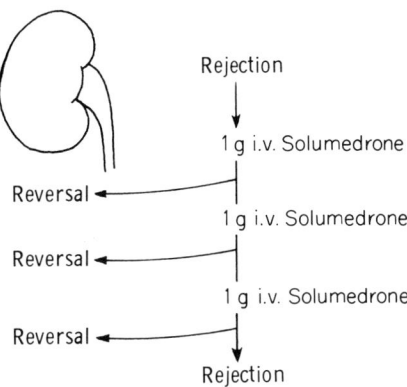

Alternatively oral steroids can be used

Fig 27.4 Treatment of rejection.

to stop trying, otherwise the patient can be put at serious risk of death from infection with little chance of regaining useful renal function. Recently, plasmapheresis has been used in otherwise irreversible rejection episodes. Removal of antibodies by plasmapheresis in some patients has led to dramatic improvements in their condition and maintenance of long-term renal function. However, the results of controlled trials of plasmapheresis have been disappointing.

Chronic rejection

This is an ill understood process characterised by gradually decreasing renal function with each biopsy showing progressive thickening of arterioles and fibrosis. In some cases, the process is accompanied by proteinuria which reflects glomerular rather than tubular damage. No effective method has as yet been found of preventing the progression of chronic rejection. One or two courses of therapy with intravenous methylprednisolone may be worthwhile, but will only serve to defer the time of complete organ destruction. At best, the patient survives with impaired renal function, and at some stage a decision needs to be taken to abandon therapy, remove the kidney and return the patient to dialysis.

The retrieval of organs for transplantation and organ preservation

General principles

The cells of vascularised organs undergo rapid degeneration at body temperature when they are deprived of a blood supply – warm ischaemic damage. Intracellular metabolism can be slowed down dramatically by cooling the organ to 4°C and prolonged storage at this temperature is possible. However, it is impossible to reverse the damage from an initial period of warm ischaemia. It is to minimise this problem that organs are now almost always removed from 'heart beating cadavers' where brain death has been diagnosed using established criteria (for full details *see Brit. Med. J.*, 1976, 2, 1187–8 and *Brit. Med. J.*, 1979, 1, 3320). Immediate function is essential in heart transplantation and of critical importance in liver grafts. In renal transplantation warm ischaemic damage may lead to tubular necrosis which, although it will usually recover, means a period of continued dialysis after transplantation. This may also cause difficulty in diagnosing rejection. Suitable donors for transplantation are patients in intensive care units maintained on intermittent positive pressure ventilation in whom a diagnosis of brain death has been made. The patient should be under the age of 60 and for heart transplants, ideally under the age of 30. There should be no evidence of systemic infection or malignancy (apart from primary brain tumour). It is important to ensure that there is no history of damage or disease to the organ to be transplanted. Once the relatives and other appropriate authorities have given permission for transplantation, blood samples should be sent for tissue typing and arrangements made for organ removal.

During this time it is important to maintain the donor blood pressure and urine output at satisfactory levels. In addition to adequate hydration, it may be necessary to give Mannitol and Dopamine to maintain the donor in a stable condition. The help of an anaesthetist is essential to maintain adequate ventilation and oxygenation throughout the operation. Muscle relaxation with Curare is of considerable benefit in removing abdominal organs. The operation should always be carried out in a properly equipped operating theatre with strict asepsis throughout the whole period of removal and preservation.

Organ preservation

Infusion and ice storage

In kidney, heart and liver transplantation the standard form of preservation consists of an initial cold flush with a preservation solution in order to clear the organ of blood and to reduce rapidly the core temperature to 4°C. Organs removed from heart beating donors with short warm ischaemic times can then be stored in ice for several hours. This allows time for transport to the recipient centre and preparation of the patient. In heart transplantation this 'cold ischaemic time' should be kept as short as possible and ideally not more than 3–4 h. Liver grafts can be satisfactorily preserved in this way for up to 10 h and kidneys stored in ice for over 24 h.

A number of preservation solutions are in current use, all attempting to prevent further deterioration of the organ during cold storage. Collins solution (Collins *et al.*, 1969) mimics intracellular fluid and is rich in potassium and magnesium. It was formulated to prevent potassium loss from the organ which results in oedema from an influx of sodium and water. Research into solutions capable of preserving organs for several days demonstrated the importance of osmolality: thus increasing the osmolality from 300 to over 400 mosmol/kg by the addition of Mannitol to an electrolyte solution. This is basically similar to Collins, allowing an increase in total storage time of up to 72 h. Good results have also been reported with the use of a hypertonic citrate solution and in general a hyperosmolar composition appears to provide more efficient preservation in organs which have suffered a degree of warm ischaemic damage (Ross *et al.*, 1976).

Machine perfusion

The maintenance of the circulation through an isolated organ in the period prior to transplantation is an attractive concept offering the possibility of long-term storage. Practical techniques for organ perfusion were developed by Belzer *et al.* (1967) and led to the development of portable machines for continuous hypothermic perfusion. Using colloid solutions such as cryo-precipitated plasma, experimental studies demonstrated that kidneys can be successfully transplanted after perfusion for 7 days. In clinical practice preservation machines have been used almost exclusively in renal transplantation. They provide an excellent method of assessing organs with warm ischaemic damage. Kidneys which have suffered irreversible ischaemia tend to have poor perfusion characteristics with a high level of lactate in the perfusate. However, at the present time the availability of kidneys with minimal warm ischaemic damage has reduced the necessity for machine preservation. Research in this field is continuing and if the preservation time could be extended by a further 7 to 14 days, then there would be a realistic possibility of effecting immune modification of the recipient before transplantation.

Cryo-preservation

Single cell suspensions can be successfully frozen and stored in liquid nitrogen. In transplantation this has proved extremely useful by providing viable cells from the donor which can be used in postoperative immunological tests. The technique may also prove valuable in storing isolated pancreatic islets for transplantation. Despite much research effort, it has so far proved impossible to freeze whole organs. An even rate of cooling cannot be maintained and the resultant intracellular formation of ice crystals leads to cell disruption on thawing.

Renal transplantation

The first successful renal autograft was performed by Ullman (1902) in the dog but it was Alexis Carrel who really established the technique of renal transplantation. Using the technique of excising a patch of donor aorta around the renal artery to allow subsequent anastomosis to the recipient aorta. Carrel (1908) performed 14 renal transplants in cats; 9 of the animals survived and considering the many advances in surgery and anaesthesia since Carrel's time, this success rate is truely remarkable. In 1911 Carrel reported the results of an orthotopic renal autograft and contralateral nephrectomy in a dog, in which the animal had survived for 2.5 years. The dog died of an intestinal obstruction, but at postmortem the renal artery and vein were of normal calibre and the ureter and pelvis were also normal. Carrel concluded 'that from a purely surgical stand point, the grafting of organs is a real possibility.'

In human transplantation, most centres now use a technique where the kidney is placed in an extraperitoneal pouch in either iliac fossa, anastomosing the renal artery and vein to the internal iliac vessels of the recipient. This method was first described by Küss *et al.* (1951) after experiments in cadavers had convinced them that the internal iliac could be mobilised sufficiently to provide a blood supply for the transplanted kidney. The technique was then modified and developed by the Boston transplant group, Merrill *et al.* (1956).

Surgical techniques

Cadaver nephrectomy

In removing kidneys from donors maintained on intermittent positive pressure ventilation during operation, it is best to attempt to isolate the aorta and vena cava above and below the renal vessels. A wide subcostal incision is made and the kidneys identified by dividing the overlying peritoneum. On the left side the renal vein is identified and its adrenal and gonadal branches divided. In mobilising the renal arteries, it is important to make a careful search for polar vessels. A lower pole renal artery usually supplies the ureter and if this is not revascularised at the time of transplantation, then there is a high risk of ureteric necrosis. In mobilising the aorta above the renal arteries, it is usually a help to divide the attachments of the diaphragm to free a sufficient length of the vessel for cross clamping. This also allows access to divide and ligate the superior mesenteric artery and the coeliac axis. The ureter is identified and dissected out as far distally as possible taking care not to strip off the connective tissue surrounding it, as this contains most of the blood supply. Once complete mobilisation of the vessels, kidneys and ureters has been achieved, the donor should be given an intravenous injection of 10 000 i.u. of heparin and the ventilator switched off. The aorta and vena cava can now be clamped and the kidneys removed with a cuff of both inferior vena cava and aorta. The aortic patch should be large enough to include any polar vessels (Fig 27.5). An alternative approach is to perfuse the kidneys *in situ* with Ringer's lactate solution containing Mannitol and Heparin. The aorta is clamped proximal and distal to the renal vessels and the inferior vena cava is also clamped distally. A large perfusion catheter is introduced into the aorta and the kidneys cooled, allowing the perfusate to circulate back into the proximal inferior vena cava. The kidneys and ureters can then be excised en bloc with a segment of aorta and vena cava. Following removal using either of these techniques the kidneys should be flushed immediately with preservation solution at 4°C and then placed on ice in two sealed sterile plastic bags.

Live donor nephrectomy

In considering a patient as a live donor, it is essential to proceed from matching tests to an evaluation of renal function and anatomy. Even if the intravenous urogram is normal, an angiogram is required to ensure that the kidney has a single artery. The right kidney may be removed in order to avoid problems with adrenal and gonadal branches of the left renal vein. The patient should receive a preoperative fluid load and a diuresis should be stimulated by the administration of intravenous Mannitol during the operation. The kidney is usually approached through a standard loin incision excising the twelfth rib. It is important to avoid damaging the hilum in mobilising the kidney. Once the renal artery and renal vein have been mobilised, the ureter should be carefully dissected to the level of the pelvic brim. As in cadaver nephrectomy it is essential to preserve the periureteric fat and connective tissue. Once the ureter has been divided and ligated, the renal vessels can be clamped and the kidney removed. To obtain a sufficient length of renal vein it may be necessary to place a vascular clamp on the inferior vena cava and oversew the renal vein stump with monofilament nylon.

The recipient operation can be started as soon as the donor kidney has been mobilised and it has been confirmed that there are no anatomical problems. The kidney is, therefore, transplanted with minimal warm and cold ischaemia and should function immediately it is revascularised.

The transplant operation

The iliac vessels are approached by a curved incision above the inguinal ligament dividing the external oblique aponeurosis and the internal oblique muscle. The peritoneum is swept upwards from the floor of the iliac fossa to allow dissection of the iliac vessels. An important technical detail is the careful ligation of lymphatics running along the vessels – if these are damaged and not ligated a lymphocele may form around the graft. The kidney is transplanted so that the vessels lie posteriorly with the ureter anteriorly. This means that the left kidney is transplanted into the right side and *vice versa*. The renal vein is anastomosed end-to-side to the external iliac vein and for a kidney with a single renal artery the ideal anastomosis is end-to-end with the internal iliac artery (Fig 27.6). In recipients with diseased internal iliac vessels or if there are multiple renal vessels on an aortic patch, then an end-to-side anastomosis is made with the external iliac artery.

Various methods of ureteric anastomosis are described, but most surgeons favour either a modification of the technique of implantation through a submucosal tunnel or an extravesical tunnel technique. A simple technique of implantation of the ureter in to the dome of the bladder is favoured by some units. In this method it is common practice to splint the anastomosis with a ureteric catheter brought out through a separate incision in the bladder.

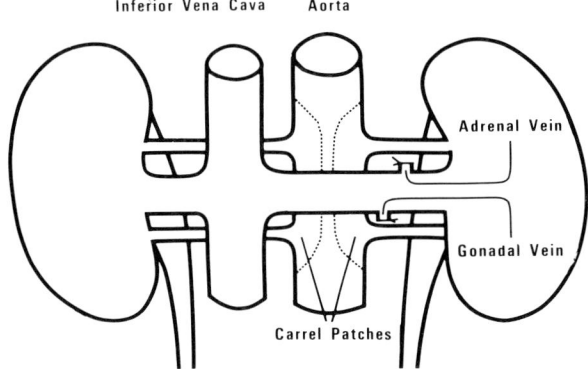

Fig 27.5 En-bloc technique for removing kidneys with multiple arteries.

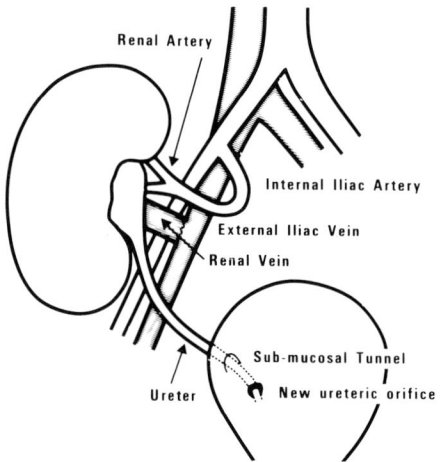

Fig 27.6 Renal transplantation – vascular and ureteric anastomoses.

Postoperative management

Patients are usually nursed in isolation for the first 48 h after operation and careful bacteriological surveillance is essential. Kidneys with a short warm ischaemic time usually function immediately after transplantation. In this situation, biochemical estimations are the mainstay of the diagnosis of rejection. The serum creatinine, creatinine clearance and blood urea should be estimated daily. Of these the serum creatinine is the most reliable index of rejection. Confirmatory clinical signs are often present. These include graft swelling and tenderness, a reduction in urine volume, pyrexia, unexplained weight gain or a rise in blood pressure.

There has been considerable research effort to find methods of detecting rejection before deterioration in graft function, in the hope of preventing the rejection episode or at least reducing the amount of damage to the graft. A large number of immunological techniques have been used and these have already been referred to. In addition, isotope techniques such as gamma camera scinti-scanning, the uptake of ^{125}I fibrinogen and the injection of indium labelled autologous platelets have all been used to give early warning of rejection. The urine may also be tested for the presence of cells, fibrin/fibrinogen degradation products and specific urinary enzymes such as N-acetyl glucosaminidase.

One of the most difficult problems in the postoperative management of renal transplant patients is the presence of anuria. This is frequently due to acute tubular necrosis and may last for several days or even weeks. However, the anuria may also be due to rejection or to a vascular accident (renal artery or renal vein thrombosis). Scinti-scanning techniques can be used to

demonstrate whether the graft has a blood supply and in anuric patients with features suggesting rejection then a renal biopsy is indicated.

Long-term follow-up

Patients with satisfactory renal function can usually be discharged from hospital 2 to 3 weeks after the operation. Regular monitoring on a daily or alternate day basis is essential during the first month after operation. The interval between outpatient visits can then be gradually extended with patients who have a well functioning graft at a year being followed up on a monthly basis.

Results of renal transplantation

Despite an undoubted improvement in the quality of kidneys transplanted, the overall results of transplantation have not significantly improved during the last 10 years. The collected statistics for Great Britain published by the 'UK Transplant' organisation show a 1-year graft survival rate for cadaver transplants of almost exactly 50% with the 2-year survival at just over 40% (Fig 27.7). The effect of blood transfusion and tissue matching on transplant results has already been discussed. It may well be that the introduction of DR typing will prove an important factor in improving the rate of graft survival.

A live donor transplant offers a much greater chance of success than a cadaver graft. Excellent results can be expected in the rare cases of transplantation between identical twins. However, with a kidney from an HLA identical sibling the 1-year graft survival in most centres is over 90%. In sibling transplants without complete

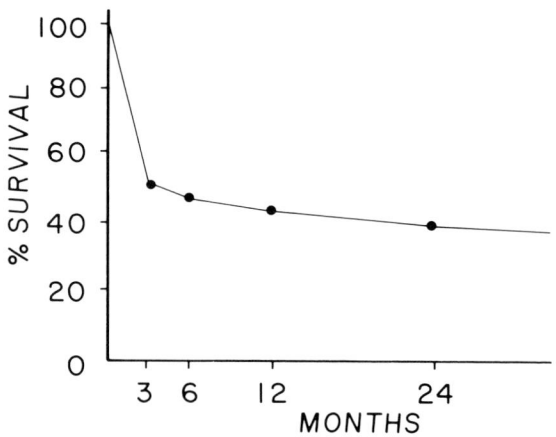

Fig 27.7 Survival of first cadaver grafts

HLA identity and in parent to child operations, the levels of graft survival are lower, but still around 75% at 1 year. Preoperative donor specific blood transfusion can be used to improve results of mis-matched live donor transplants. Salvatierra *et al.*, (1983) have reported a one-year graft survival rate of 94% in 101 patients transplanted with a one-haplotype matched kidney after donor specific transfusion.

An increasing awareness of the potentially lethal effects of immunosuppression has led to a gradual reduction in the morbidity and mortality of transplantation. The complications of immunosuppressive therapy have already been discussed and most units have now adopted a 'low dose' steroid policy.

An interesting statistic to emerge from nationally collected figures is the wide variation in results between the different centres. This 'centre effect' is partly due to the skill of medical and surgical teams and the extent of their back-up facilities. However, there are undoubtedly other factors of which patient selection may be the most important. The general failure to improve overall results may reflect a willingness to offer transplantation to a wider group of patients with chronic renal failure. This includes individuals over 45 and patients with systemic diseases such as diabetes – both risk factors associated with poorer long term survival.

Transplantation of the pancreas

Transplantation of the pancreas remains a goal for all who wish to prevent the complications of diabetes. Experimental evidence has shown that diabetic rats, dogs and monkeys, with the complications of diabetes, can be helped by transplantation of pancreatic tissue. Progress in this area has tended to be in the transplantation of whole or part of the organ (Jonasson, 1979) or in the use of isolated islet cells (Kretschner *et al.*, 1977). It is probable in future that both of these methods will be useful depending on the type of diabetes encountered. Juvenile diabetics with severe uncontrolled disease associated with renal failure often respond to transplantation of the pancreas at the same time as renal transplantation. In the mature onset diabetic, however, where control is less of a problem, it seems unlikely that a serious procedure, such as transplantation of part of the pancreas, will be acceptable even if immunosuppression becomes readily and simply available. It seems more likely in this situation that transplantation of islet cells would be more acceptable.

Transplantation of the whole pancreas

Initial attempts to transplant the whole organ usually met with failure, because of the difficulty of dealing with the exocrine secretion which inevitably led to severe complications such as digestion of tissue and death of the patient. This type of transplant has, therefore, been abandoned and instead the tail of the organ based on the splenic artery and vein has been used in recent years. The problems remain the same, however; although the endocrine function is acceptable, leakage from the duct has posed a problem. Attempts to overcome this have been made in a variety of ingenious ways. First, ligation of the duct at the time of transplantation was thought to be the answer. However, in spite of giving steroids to reduce inflammation and glucagon to reduce pancreatic secretion, severe pancreatitis has occurred, and this method has largely been abandoned. Najarian and his colleagues (1979) recently suggested that leaving the duct open to drain freely into the peritoneal cavity was safe. Provided that the pancreatic juices do not come into contact with the GI tract, they remain inactive and as such are non-digestive. This method does, however, cause problems, and has not been uniformly successful. Implantation of the duct into the ureter or the intestine has also caused problems and is no longer used in many centres. The most useful method has been the suppression of exocrine secretion by the injection of Neoprine or latex rubber into the duct system without any other treatment (Traeger *et al.*, 1979). This method appears to have successfully prevented the complications seen with other techniques of duct management and has now been used in several units with success.

Islet cell transplantation

Removal of the islets from the pancreas by mincing and collagenase digestion prior to injection into the liver has proved a useful method of reversing diabetes in animal models. This method has also been used successfully in patients given their own pancreatic tissue following pancreatectomy for pancreatitis, establishing that these cells can produce insulin and control diabetes (Najarian *et al.*, 1979). The reasons for using isolated islet cells have been twofold. Firstly, so that the cells could be injected directly into a favoured site, such as the spleen or liver, without the need for a major operation, and secondly, because endocrine cells may be less of an immunological stimulus than whole organ grafts. Although it has now been shown that cells will survive and work well in the liver or the spleen, they are certainly not less immunogenic. A major problem has been that these cells are more rapidly destroyed, possibly because of their particulate nature. Recent work has suggested that antimacrophage agents may prevent this from occurring (Nash and Bell, 1979). Another problem is that of obtaining sufficient cells to reverse diabetes successfully. Although research continues, the difficulties in this area remain those of preventing rejection and getting enough islet cells into the patient.

Clinical heart transplantation

In heart transplantation, as in liver transplantation, failure of the graft will result in the death of the patient and the operation can only be considered in patients whose ultimate prognosis is measured in weeks rather than months. Patients suitable for cardiac transplantion are individuals under the age of 50 with severe myocardial ischaemia in whom coronary artery bypass surgery is not possible. The other major group of patients in whom cardiac transplantation can be considered is those with cardiomyopathies with severe cardiac failure. Transplantation can also be considered in patients with valvular disease of the heart where previous cardiac surgery has failed or is not possible.

Following the first cardiac transplant by Barnard in 1967, a number of heart transplants were carried out in Cardiothoracic units throughout the world. In general the results of these operations were poor with few patients surviving for a year or more. Shumway in California, backed by an extensive research programme, has continued with cardiac transplantation and has demonstrated that it is now an effective form of treatment for a small group of patients with end-stage cardiac failure. Between 1968 and 1983 Shumway's group carried out more than 250 cardiac allografts. There has been a progressive improvement in survival figures and for the period 1974 to 1980 65% of patients were alive at one year and the projected five-year survival was between 45 and 50% (Jamieson *et al.*, 1982).

The technique of orthotopic heart grafting was developed by Lower and Shumway (1960) after extensive research in experimental animals. The recipient heart is removed leaving a cuff of both the left and right atria and stumps of the aorta and pulmonary artery to anastomose to the donor heart. The donor heart must be removed from a brain dead patient maintained on intermittent positive pressure ventilation and, after flushing, the heart must be transplanted within two to three hours to guarantee that it will function satisfactorily. The transplant operation involves anastomosis of the donor atria to the cuff of atrial tissue left in the recipient and then end-to-end anastomoses between the donor and recipient aorta and pulmonary artery.

The patient is maintained on the same form of immunosuppression as for renal transplantation with the addition of antilymphocyte globulin. The diagnosis of rejection is made on the basis of the ECG supplemented by transvenous endomyocardial biopsy.

Liver transplantation

Transplantation of the liver is technically the most difficult of the various operative procedures in the field of transplantation. This large organ, in order to be successfully implanted, requires the anastomosis of several major vessels, plus the difficulty of arranging biliary drainage, something which is difficult enough to do even in patients who have not had a transplant. Several hundred liver transplants have now been performed, and although the results are gradually improving, many difficulties remain. One of the problems has been the lack of an hepatic support system to make the patients fit for surgery and to tide them over rejection episodes. The result has been that patients are often presented for transplantation at a time when they are extremely ill, usually terminal, and really not fit for an operative procedure. This problem led to a trial of heterotopic transplantation, which is the term used for the insertion of an additional liver. Removal of a diseased organ and its replacement in the same position by another is termed orthotopic transplantation (Fig 27.8).

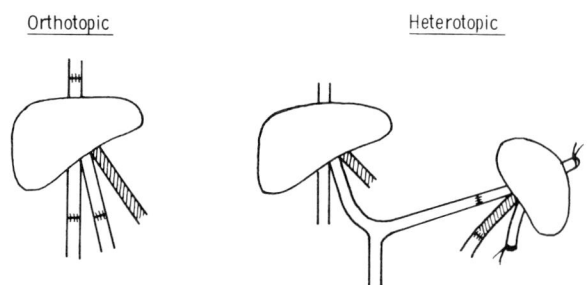

Orthotopic   Heterotopic

Fig 27.8   Liver transplantation.

Heterotopic liver transplantation

This type of transplant has proved to be relatively unsuccessful. Although it has the attraction of preserving what function remains in the patient's own liver, the obvious problem of providing enough space is such that the patient often cannot breathe properly following the insertion of a second, usually smaller organ. Secondly, and perhaps unexpectedly, the heterotopic liver often fails to function adequately and usually atrophies after a few weeks. This was shown to be due, among other things, to a lack of insulin in the blood supply to the liver. Because of these problems, heterotopic transplantation of the liver has not been clinically successful and is now used in relatively few cases.

Orthotopic transplantation

The results of this procedure have improved over the last 5–10 years and the long-term survivors of over 5–6 years are not, by any means, uncommon (Starzl *et al.*, 1979). The indications for the operation include biliary atresia in children, end-stage cirrhotic disease in adults, and primary biliary cancer. Because of the lack of adequate hepatic support facilities and relatively poor methods of hepatic preservation, it is vital that a well-preserved organ from a heart-beating donor is used. The patient's liver is removed and the recipient liver is inserted completing anastomoses between the vena cava, portal vein and the hepatic artery of the donor and recipient. During this period, the patient is usually very ill and anaesthesia is difficult. The provision of a shunt to pump blood from the lower trunk to the heart is beneficial and helps to maintain the blood pressure during the procedure. Once the liver is inserted, and provided that it is not damaged, the patient's circulation recovers rapidly and coagulation, which is otherwise a problem, will become stabilised.

One of the main difficulties in liver transplantation over the years has been the arrangement of biliary drainage. There are various ways of doing this, including anastomosis of the gallbladder to the intestine, the bile duct directly to the intestine, and bile duct to bile duct, all of which have caused problems (Fig 27.9). Many patients may lose their liver from ascending cholangitis due to thick biliary sludge, rather than to rejection. The problem can be reduced by perfusing the biliary tree during preservation to remove sludge and bile residue, and secondly organising bile drainage to avoid complications. This is done by using the gallbladder to bridge the gap between the donor and recipient bile ducts (Calne, 1976) (Fig 27.9).

Encouraging results have been obtained with the use of Cyclosporin A and in a review of cases transplanted between 1980 and 1982 Calne (1983) reported a 75% one-year graft survival rate.

Future developments

Rejection remains the major problem preventing the wider application of transplantation in clinical medi-

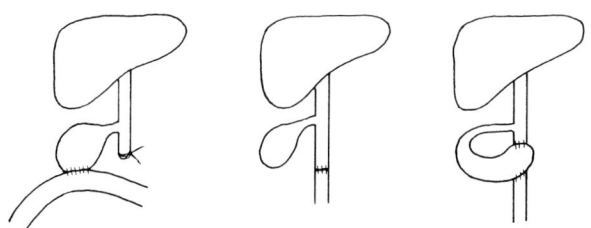

Fig 27.9 Liver transplantation – bile drainage.

cine. If completely reliable means of preventing rejection can be developed, then transplantation could be introduced on a much wider scale. For example, it would be possible to offer pancreatic transplantation either in the form of whole organ grafts or isolated islet grafts to all insulin dependent diabetics. Lung transplantation, which has currently been abandoned, could be reintroduced offering hope to patients with end-stage respiratory failure. In addition it would be possible to consider transplanting bowel in patients who have had massive small intestinal resections. This expansion of transplantation depends on the following developments in the current fields of research:

1   Tissue typing

The major histocompatibility system is an extremely complex structure and even with the introduction of new techniques, such as DR typing, it seems unlikely that tissue matching alone will have a significant effect in reducing the incidence of rejection.

2   Immunosuppression

Transplantation has suffered from a failure to develop more specific and effective immunosuppressive drugs. The only really effective new agent is Cyclosporin A and like many potent drugs it appears to have a number of side effects which can be hazardous. However, the development of this drug gives hope that clinical immunosuppressive agents will be developed with more specific effects on the components of the immune response involved in transplantation.

3   Manipulation of the immune response

Manipulation of the recipient immune response to induce a state of unresponsiveness to the graft seems to offer the best possibility for combating rejection. Work in experimental animals has clearly demonstrated that antisera with 'enhancing' properties can be developed. These antisera when given to the animal at the time of transplantation can completely abrogate rejection with long-term survival of the graft (French and Batchelor 1969). Unfortunately, it has not been found possible to develop reliable means of inducing enhancement in man. However, the observation that blood transfusion improves the results of renal allografting indicates that enhancing phenomena do occur in human transplantation. Research is now concentrating on the development of 'monoclonal' antibody of high specificity. It is possible that using such techniques enhancing antisera may be developed for use in human transplantation.

Another practical means of achieving a state of unresponsiveness is by the use of a total lymphoid irradiation and bone marrow reconstitution. This technique
has been developed for the treatment of leukaemic
patients but offers a potential method of grafting
organs into tolerant hosts. Using fractionated doses of
radiation to the lymphoid areas and shielding structures
subject to radiation damage, such as the bowel, sufficient suppression can be induced to allow bone marrow grafts to be accepted with minimal reaction.

Conclusion

Transplantation now has an important role in the
management of many disease processes. The continued
application of experimental discoveries in immunology
to clinical practice will inevitably lead to more precise
methods of controlling the immune response. It, therefore, seems likely that in the next few years there will
be a much wider application of transplant techniques.

References

Barnard C.N. (1967). A human cardiac transplant, an interim
report. *S. Afr. Med. J*; **41**:1271–4.
Bell P.R.F., Briggs J.D., Wood R.F.M., Calman K.C., Paton
A.M., McPherson S.G., Kyle K. (1971). Reversal of clinical
and experimental organ rejection using large doses of
intravenous prednisolone. *Lancet*; **i**:876–80.
Belzer F.O., Ashby B.S., Dunphy J.E. (1967). 24-hour and
72-hour preservation of canine kidneys. *Lancet*; **ii**:536–9.
Calne R.Y. (1960). The rejection of renal homografts inhibition in dogs by 6-mercapto purine. *Lancet*; **i**:417–18.
Calne R.Y. (1976). A new technique for biliary drainage in
orthotopic liver transplantation utilising the gallbladder as a
pedicle graft conduit between the donor and recipient common bile ducts. *Ann. Surg*; **184**:605–9.
Calne R.Y. (1983). Recent advances in clinical transplantation
of the liver and pancreas. *Transplant. Proc*; **15**:1263–8.
Calne R.Y., Rolles K., Thiru S., McMaster P., Craddock
G.N., Aziz S., White D.J.G., Evans D.B., Dunn D.C.,
Henderson R.G., Lewis P. (1979). Cyclosporin A. Initially
as the only immunosuppressant in 34 recipients of cadaveric
organs: 32 kidneys, 2 pancreases and 2 livers. *Lancet*;
ii:1033–6.
Carrel A. (1908). Transplantation in mass of the kidneys. *J.
Exp. Med*; **10**:98–140.
Carrel A. (1911). The ultimate result of a double nephrectomy
and the replantation of one kidney. *J. Exp. Med*; **14**:124–5.
Carter N.P., Cullen P.R., Thompson J.F., Bewick A.L.T.,
Wood R.F.M., Morris P.J. (1983). Monitoring lymphocyte
subpopulations in renal allograft recipients. *Transplant.
Proc*; **15**:1157–9.
Chatenoud L., Chkoff N., Kreis H., Bach J.F. (1983). Cor-
relation between immunoregulatory T-cell imbalances and
renal allograft outcome. *Transplant. Proc*; **15**:1184–5.
Claas F.H.J., Paul L.C., van Es La, van Rood J.J. (1980).
Antibodies against donor antigens on endothelial cells and
monocytes in eluates of rejected kidney allografts. *Tissue
Antigens*; **15**:19–24.
Collins G.M., Bravo- Shugarman M., Terasaki P.I. (1969).
Kidney preservation for transportation. *Lancet*; **ii**:1219–22.

European Multicentre Trial (1982). Cyclosporin A as sole
immunosuppressive agent in recipients of kidney allografts
from cadaver donors. *Lancet*; **ii**:57–60.
French M.E., Batchelor J.R. (1969). Immunological enhance-
ment of rat kidney grafts. *Lancet*; **ii**:1103–6.
Gibson T., Medawar P.B. (1942). The fate of skin homografts
in man. *J. Anat*; **77**:299–310.
Hayry P., von Willebrand E. (1981). Monitoring of human
renal allograft rejection with fine-needle aspiration cytol-
ogy. *Scand. J. Immunol*; **13**:87–97.
Jamieson S.W., Stinson E.B., Shumway N.E. (1982). In
Tissue Transplantation, (Morris, P.J. ed.) Edinburgh:
Churchill Livingstone.
Jonasson O. (1979). Transplantation of the pancreas 1978.
Transplant Proc; **11**:325–30.
Kahan B.D., Tom B.H., Mittal K.K., Bergan J.J. (1974).
Immunodiagnostic test for transplant rejection. *Lancet*;
i:37–42.
Kretschner G.J., Sutherland D.E.R., Matas A.J., Cani T.L.,
Najarian J.S. (1977). Autotransplantation of pancreatic
islets without separation of exocrine and endocrine tissue in
totally pancreatectomised dogs. *Surgery*; **82**:74–81.
Küss R., Teinturier J., Milliez P. (1951). Quelques essais de
greffe de rein chez l'homme. *Mémoires de l'Académié de
Chirurgie*; **71**:755–64.
Lamm L.U., Friedrich U., Petersen C.B., Jorgensen J.,
Nielsen J., Therkelsen A.J., Kissameyer-Neilsen F. (1974).
Assignment of the major histocompatability complex to
chromosome No. 6 in a family with a pericentric inversion.
Hum Hered; **24**:273–84.
Lower R.R., Shumway N.E. (1960). Studies on orthotopic
homotransplantation of the canine heart. *Surg. Forum*;
11:18–19.
McGeown M.G. (1981). Clinical renal transplantation and
immunosuppression. In *Immunosuppressive Therapy*. (Sala-
man, J.R., ed.) Lancaster: MTP Press.
McMichael A.J., Fabre, J.W. (1982). *Monoclonal Antibodies
in Clinical Medicine*. London: Academic Press.
Merrill J.P., Murray J.E., Harrison J.H., Guild W.R. (1956).
Successful homotransplantation of the human kidney
between identical twins. *J. Amer. Med. Ass*; **160**:277–
82.
Miller J., Lifton J., Wilcox C. (1978). The use of second-
generation assays in pre- and post-transplant monitoring:
the primed or second-degree MLC. *Transplant Proc*;
10:573–8.
Mitchison N.A. (1954). Passive transfer of transplantation
immunity. *Proc. Roy. Soc. Lon*; **142** series B:72–87.
Morris P.J., French M.E., Dunnill M.S., Hunnisett A.G.W.,
Ting A., Thompson J.F., Wood R.F.M. (1983). A controlled trial of Cyclosporin A in renal transplantation with conversion to Azathioprine and Prednisolone after 3 months.
Transplantation; (in press).
Najarian J.S., Sutherland D.E.R., Matas A.J., Gotz F.C.
(1979). Human islet auto-transplantation following pac-
reatectomy. *Transplant Proc*; **11**:336–40.
Nash J.R., Bell P.R.F. (1979). Effect of macrophage suppres-
sion on the survival of islet allografts. *Transplant Proc*;
11:986–98.
Opelz G., Sengar D.P.S., Mickey M.R., Terasaki P.I. (1973).
Effect of blood transfusion on subsequent kidney transplants. *Transplant Proc*; **5**:253–9.
Opelz G., Terasaki P.I. (1977). Significance of mixed leucocyte culture testing in cadaver kidney transplantation.
Transplant; **23**:375–80.
Penn I. (1977). Development of cancer as a complication of
clinical transplantation. *Transplant Proc*; **9**:1121–7.
Ross H., Marshall V.C., Escott M.L. (1976). 72-hour canine
kidney preservation without continuous perfusion. *Transplantation* **21**:498–501.

Salvatierra O., Vincenti F., Amend W., Garovoy M., Iwaki Y., Terasaki P., Potter D., Duca R., Hopper S., Slemmer T., Feduska N. (1983). Four year experience with donor specific blood transfusions. *Transplant. Proc*; **15**:924–31.

Schöne G. (1908). Vergleichende Untersuchugen über die Transplantation von Geschwülsten und von normalen Geweben. *Bruns Beitre Klin. Chir*; **61**:1–49.

Shenton B.K., Jenssen H.L., Werner H., Field E.J. (1977). A comparison of the kinetics of the macrophage electrophoretic mobility (MEM) and the tanned sheep erythrocyte electrophorectic mobility (TEEM) tests. *J. Immunol. Methods*; **14**:123–39.

Solheim B.G., Engerbretsen T.E., Flatmark A., Jerrell J., Enger E., Thorsby E. (1977). The influence of HLA-A, -B, -C and -D matching on kidney graft survival. *Scand. J. Urol. Nephrol. Suppl*; **42**:28–31.

Starzl T.E., Halgrimson C.F., Penn I. (1971). Cyclophosphamide and human organ transplantation. *Lancet*; ii:70–4.

Starzl T.E., Koep L.J., Halgrimson J., Hood G.P., Schröter P.J., Porter K.A., Weil R. (1979). Liver transplantation 1978. *Transplant Proc*; **11**:240–6.

Starzl T.E., Hakala T.R., Iwatsuki S., Rosenthal T.J., Shaw B.W., Klintmalm G.B., Porter K.A. (1982). Cyclosporin A and steroid treatment in 104 cadaveric renal transplantations. In *Cyclosporin A*. pp. 364–77. (White, D.J.G. ed.) Amsterdam: Elsevier Biomedical Press.

Stiller C.R., Sinclair N.R., St C., McGirr D., Jevnikar A., Ulcen R.A. (1978). Diagnostic and prognostic value of donor specific post-transplant immune responses: clinical correlates and *in vitro* variables. *Transplant. Proc*; **10**:525–30.

Thomas F., Mendez-Picon G., Thomas J., Lee H.M., Lower R. (1978). Effective monitoring and modulation of recipient immune reactivity to prevent rejection in early post-transplant period. *Transplant Proc*; **10**:537–41.

Ting A. (1982). HLA and organ transplantation. In *Tissue Transplantation*. (Morris, P.J., ed.) Amsterdam: Churchill Livingstone.

Traeger J., Dubernard J.M., Touraine J.L., Neyra P., Malik M.C., Pelissard C., Ruitton A. (1979). Pancreatic transplantation in man: a new method of pancreas preparation and results of diabetes correction. *Transplant Proc*; **11**:331–5.

Ullman E. (1902). Experimentelle Nierentransplantation. *Wien Klin Wochenschr*; **15**:281–2.

Watson M.A., Briggs J.D., Diamandopoulos A.A., Hamilton D.N.H., Dick H.M. (1979). Endogenous cell mediated immunity, blood transfusion and outcome of renal transplantation. *Lancet*; ii:1323–6.

von Willebrand E., Hayry P. (1983). Cyclosporin A deposits in renal allografts. *Lancet*; **ii**:189–92.

Wood R.F.M., Gray A.C., Bell P.R.F. (1978). Daily immunologic tests in the prediction of renal transplant rejection. *Transplant Proc*; **10**:593–4.

Wood R.F.M., Bolton E.M., Thompson J.F., Morris, P.J. (1982) Monoclonal antibodies and fine needle aspiration cytology in detecting renal allograft rejection. *Lancet*; **ii**:278.

Woodruff M.F.A., Anderson N.A. (1963). Effect of lymphocyte depletion by thoracic duct fistula and administration of anti lymphocye serum on the survival of skin homografts in rats. *Nature*; **200**:702.

Heart, lungs and blood vessels

Introduction

Unlike every other structure to which the surgeon has access, the heart is of necessity in a state of continuous motion and with the individual at rest continues to pump about 5 litres per minute. For this reason, the heart was one of the last structures in the body to be amenable to precise, accurate, restorative surgery.

It was in 1953 that a real breakthrough occurred with the first clinical use of a machine designed to substitute the function of the heart and lungs in man. Thus it became possible to perform an operation upon the heart. Two years later, methods were developed for deliberately arresting the heart, so that not only was it functionless but also motionless, and this considerably increased the accuracy of attempts at surgical correction of defects. The next 25 years were occupied in refining the techniques of cardiopulmonary bypass, and of perfecting methods of myocardial protection when the heart was arrested and deprived temporarily of its blood supply. During this time also, there has been an increasing understanding of the pathophysiology and anatomy of congenital heart disease and of its surgical correction. Simultaneously, in order to deal with the problems created by acquired disease there has been a steady improvement in the design and manufacture of artificial heart valves.

In the last 10 years the surgery of coronary artery disease has become highly developed and its place in the treatment of angina pectoris and the surgical pathology resulting from myocardial infarction has become well established. The surgical treatment of certain rhythm disturbances is now on a sound basis, but the electrophysiological investigation and surgical management of a wider range of disturbances of rhythm is still in its infancy.

The surgical techniques of cardiac transplantation have been largely standardised, following extensive animal and human experience world wide. Despite the immense problems associated with rejection and its prevention, 5-year survivals of better than 50% are now being reported. However, the enormous cost of transplantation and the shortage of donor material continue to limit the availability of this method of treatment for the great bulk of sufferers from crippling heart disease. While the design of implantable artificial hearts continues to concern many investigators, mainly in the United States, the mechanical problems remain considerable and the difficulties of adequate power supplies have not yet been overcome. There is, as yet, no perfect artificial heart valve and the artificial ventricle is even less well developed. It would, however, be surprising if such devices were not available within a very few years.

H.H.B.

Heart, lungs and blood vessels

28

Acquired heart disease

H.H. BENTALL

Valve disease

Acquired valvar heart disease still constitutes an important part of the work of the cardiac surgeon. During the period 1950–1960, operations for rheumatic valve disease constituted the bulk of his work and were, predominantly, closed operations for mitral stenosis. In the decade ending in 1980, however, there has been a progressive reduction in the incidence and in the mortality and morbidity in the British Isles from rheumatic heart disease, and there is, therefore, a changing pattern of patients presenting for surgical treatment. Acquired valve disease, however, has other aetiologies, in addition to rheumatism, and may be either degenerative or the result of previous congenital deformity of the valve. As such lesions are, however, specific to particular valves, they will be dealt with in considering each individual site.

Valve lesions may be stenotic or regurgitant or a combination of both. Stenotic lesions are invariably chronic in nature, as are the combined lesions, but regurgitation may occur acutely, usually due to infective endocarditis; it may, however, be due to a degenerative condition or to ischaemic changes in association with coronary artery disease (*see* Ch. 29).

Haemodynamic effects of chronic valve disease

Stenosis

The chamber behind (upstream of) the narrowed valve becomes progressively hypertrophied, for example left atrial hypertrophy in mitral valve stenosis or left ventricular hypertrophy in aortic valve stenosis. This hypertrophy may be recognised clinically, and objectively by measurements obtained at cardiac catheterisation. A gradient can be recognised across a valve at the end of diastole in the case of an atrioventricular valve and in systole across a ventriculoarterial valve. Angiocardiography gives a clear demonstration of both stenosis and regurgitation but is an invasive method. Non-invasive techniques of echocardiography can frequently confirm the diagnosis of mitral or aortic stenosis for example, but it is essentially an inferential technique rather than a direct measurement. Similar methods can be applied to the tricuspid and pulmonary valves. Normal heart valves can handle flows in excess of five times the resting flow rate without difficulty and thus any valve must be seriously narrowed before physical signs and later symptoms develop. When a valve is so stenosed that it causes serious symptoms and threatens the health and the life of the patient, it is said to be critically stenosed.

Regurgitation

Incompetence of an atrioventricular valve produces effects both in the atrium and in the ventricle. Generally, the atrium dilates and the ventricle, initially at least, both dilates and hypertrophies. At first, the cardiac output at rest remains normal, but there is increased cardiac work due to the addition of the regurgitant flow to the forward flow: the stroke volume is increased.

Stenosis and regurgitation frequently coexist, although in practice one or other aspect is usually dominant.

Secondary effects of the valve lesions

As aortic valve stenosis becomes increasingly severe, secondary dilatation of the mitral valve annulus occurs producing mitral regurgitation and this, in turn, increases the left atrial pressure and, therefore, the pulmonary venous pressure. Secondary changes begin to occur in the lungs; the raised left atrial pressure is ultimately reflected in a rise in pulmonary arterial pressure and hence in right ventricular pressure, which results in dilatation of the tricuspid valve annulus as the right ventricle dilates. This train of events is delayed for some years in aortic valve stenosis and is made worse by the insufficient blood supply to the hypertrophied myocardium resulting from the aortic valve stenosis. A similar sequence occurs in mitral valve disease, but the course is more chronic and the pulmonary vascular disease more severe. Eventually, right ventricular dilatation and tricuspid regurgitation occur with the development of all the signs and symptoms of chronic congestive cardiac failure.

Chronic mitral valve disease

Only about one-third of patients with rheumatic heart disease give a history of previous rheumatic fever, but the pathological features of the rheumatic valve are remarkably constant.

Mitral stenosis

Initial fusion of the leaflets leads gradually to thickening and finally to calcification. On the ventricular side of the valve, the chordae tendinae progressively fuse and thicken and contract (Fig 28.1a,b).

As the left atrial pressure rises, dyspnoea on exertion and tiredness cause the patient to present for operation, even those who are in normal sinus rhythm. Such patients may have a valve diameter of approximately 1.5 cm (compared with the normal 3–4 cm). Symptoms may occur, however, with a valve of 2 cm or more if, as frequently happens, a patient should develop atrial fibrillation. In either case, mitral valvotomy may be recommended, but invariably permission is also obtained for valve replacement should it prove necessary. The onset of atrial fibrillation sometimes declares itself in another way. It may encourage thrombus to form in the auricle and on the atrial wall, which subsequently may be released as emboli to the brain, intestinal tract or limbs. Such an embolus may be the first sign, and when the diagnosis of mitral stenosis has been established, operation on the valve should seriously be considered after recovery from the embolus. In the earlier stages of the disease, before calcification has occurred, mitral valvotomy can give very useful palliation; it was formerly carried out as a closed procedure performed 'blind', using the Tubbs' or similar dilator through the transventricular route. In most centres throughout the world, mitral valvotomy is now carried out as an open operation using cardiopulmonary bypass. The commissures are carefully divided under direct vision, the chordae tendinae are separated where possible and the valve mobilised to the maximum possible without the production of regurgitation. In the later stages of the disease, when the valve is so thickened, contracted and calcified that it cannot be made into a useful structure, it is removed and replaced by one of a number of different prostheses.

Mitral regurgitation

Isolated rheumatic mitral regurgitation is very commonly seen in patients with the most severe attacks of rheumatic fever. It is this variety of disease which is most common in Mediterranean and tropical countries; the more slowly evolving mitral stenotic lesions are seen as the more common variety in Northern Europe. In pure mitral regurgitation, the valve is thickened, but the valve ring is widely dilated. The valve leaflets gradually prolapse with lengthening of the chordae tendinae (Fig 28.2). Calcification is uncommon. The left atrium becomes enormously dilated. The patient with rheumatic mitral regurgitation, in the earlier stages of disease, before gross valve prolapse and chordal lengthening, can have the valve made competent again by the use of a Carpentier ring (Carpentier *et al.*, 1974). This is a cloth-covered metal ring whose size is so arranged that, when sutured to the patient's valve ring

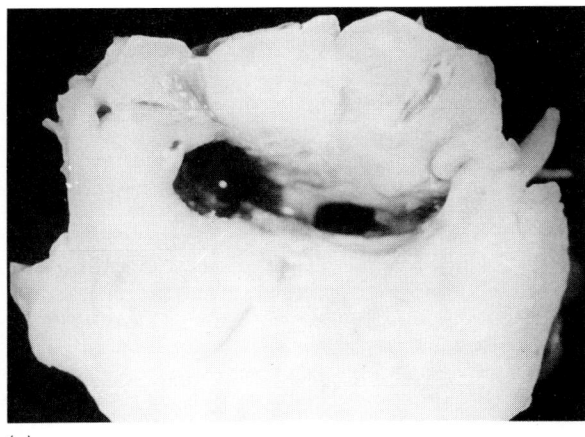

(a)

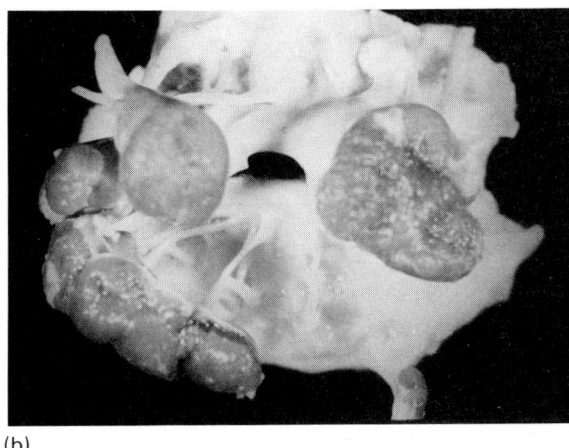

(b)

Fig 28.1 (a) Critical rheumatic mitral valve stenosis with calcification – left atrial aspect of surgical specimen; (b) The same valve – left ventricular view – fusion and shrinkage of chordae tendinae.

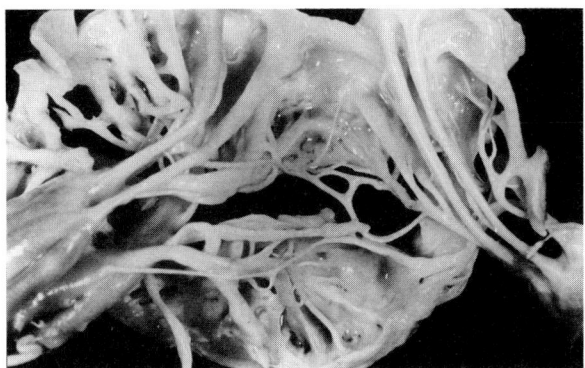

Fig 28.2 Rheumatic mitral regurgitation. The chordae tendinae are stretched and permit leaflet prolapse into left atrium.

by multiple interrupted sutures, the orifice is reduced to a normal size. Once gross changes have occurred, replacement is necessary.

The mortality and morbidity of operations for pure mitral valve disease are now very low, mortality being less than 5%. Modern techniques of intensive care have allowed this low mortality to extend to those with pulmonary hypertension. Once congestive cardiac failure has occurred, however, the risks of operation begin to rise and the morbidity increases. If, at the time of mitral valve replacement, tricuspid regurgitation is present, this should be treated at the same operation, usually by a plastic procedure such as the de Vega repair (de Vega, 1972; Boyd *et al.*, 1974) or a Carpentier ring (Carpentier, *et al.*, 1974). Where possible a tricuspid valve prosthesis is avoided, owing to a much higher risk of valve thrombosis than on the left side.

When chronic congestive failure has been present for months and even years with chronic hepatomegaly and liver failure, cardiac cachexia ensues and the risks of operation rise to prohibitive levels of 50% or more. Moreover, such patients are not candidates for transplantation.

The trend, therefore, is to earlier operation in rheumatic mitral valve disease, but such a course would be more readily advised were there more perfect mitral valve prostheses which combined both freedom from thromboembolic complications and longevity.

Results of operation

Very useful palliation is obtained in those patients who have a successful mitral valvotomy and while it is possible that the course of the disease in the leaflets is unaffected, recurrence of the stenosis is so slow that 15–20 years may elapse before further surgical treatment is needed, and in many patients it is never required. Mitral valve replacement in the absence of tricuspid disease also gives very satisfactory results, but long-term anticoagulation is required with prosthetic valves. Stent mounted heterograft valves require anticoagulants only for 3 months until the stent is incorporated, but valve failure due to wear and tear is inevitable after about 8–10 years on average, though occasionally it may occur earlier or later. The modern prosthetic valve is not subject to wear. Patients who have had valve replacement by whatever method are, however, subject to roughly 1% per annum risk of endocarditis and about the same of thromboembolism. The risks of thromboembolism are, however, appreciably less with the heterograft bioprosthesis but the risk of infective endocarditis is little different from that in the mechanical valve.

Acute mitral valve regurgitation

Rarely, sudden chordal rupture occurs in a patient with chronic rheumatic mitral valve disease, but much more commonly this lesion is part of a degenerative process in which the chordae tendinae become increasingly thin so that even the major chords are mere threads. Occasionally, a patient with chordal rupture will give a history of an acute pain at the time of some increased exertion such as straining at stool, but in most patients the onset of the rupture is apparently spontaneous. The consequent sudden rise in left atrial pressure produces acute dyspnoea. Chordal rupture may affect either the anterior or the posterior mitral leaflet. If several chordae have ruptured, the valve is so grossly flail that urgent surgical treatment is required. In less severe cases, the patient may not present for surgery until weeks or even months have passed since the event. The surgical treatment is by open operation. When one or two chordae only have ruptured, it may be possible to do a resection of that portion of the leaflet and restore competence. More often, however, valve replacement is required. Even severely disabled patients may be accepted for surgery as there is no underlying rheumatic carditis and the ventricle can respond well to the restoration of a competent mitral valve.

Acute papillary muscle rupture

This is a severe complication of myocardial infarction in which the base of the papillary muscle is infarcted and a large area of mitral valve becomes flail. The papillary muscle may even pass into the outflow tract in systole producing partial obstruction to aortic outflow. This is a very serious complication of chronic ischaemic heart disease. The only surgical treatment available is mitral valve replacement and the operative mortality is high. The long-term prognosis depends on the extent of the ischaemic heart disease and the severity of the infarction.

Aortic valve disease

Like the mitral valve, the aortic valve may be subject either to stenosis or regurgitation. The former may be part of the rheumatic process and be accompanied by mitral valve disease, but in an increasing proportion of patients (due to the reducing incidence of rheumatic heart disease) adult pure aortic stenosis is due to calcification of a congenitally deformed functionally bicuspid valve. In patients with rheumatic aortic stenosis, some regurgitation is common and calcification is less extensive as a rule. Pure aortic regurgitation due to

rheumatic heart disease is frequently seen both with and without coincident mitral valve disease. There is increasing evidence that when patients with aortic valve disease become symptomatic, they should be offered operation within a short period of time. The only operation possible is aortic valve replacement with either a mechanical valve or with a bioprosthesis. The same considerations apply as in the mitral valve with respect to choice of prostheses. The unmounted human allograft which was the subject of great interest in the 1960s has not proved a practical valve replacement on a wide scale due to a number of factors. It is difficult to get a close anatomical match with the patient's own aortic sinus, which in many cases is deformed by the disease. The operation is time-consuming and difficult and the supply of material is hard to come by. In enthusiastic hands, however, a fresh human allograft has much to offer, as it is free from thromboembolic complications and is usually functionally perfect initially. Late failure is, however, commonly seen between 5 and 10 years. There may, however, still be indications for its use. Irradiated allografts lose tensile strength, are subject to early calcification and are no longer used.

Indications for operation in the patient with aortic valve disease

A deteriorating electrocardiogram may indicate operation before any symptoms have occurred or while they are still trivial. All symptomatic patients with aortic valve disease should be considered for operation unless there are other factors which make it impossible. In patients with calcific aortic stenosis based on a congenitally deformed valve, presentation may be very late, even into the 7th and 8th decades possibly due to late onset of disease. The myocardium has not been affected by the ravages of rheumatic disease and advanced age is no barrier, of itself, to successful valve replacement.

All patients over the age of 50 who are having either mitral or aortic valve replacements should have coronary arteriography and younger patients who have angina or risk factors for coronary artery disease, in addition to their valve lesions, should be similarly investigated. Coronary artery disease should be treated by coronary artery bypass graft coincidentally with the valve replacements.

Aortic root aneurysm occurs with aortic valve regurgitation in patients who have Marfan's disease and more rarely in syphilis and in yaws. These patients are treated by aortic valve replacement, with a special prosthesis having a dacron tube already attached, which is used to graft the ascending aorta. The ostia of the coronary arteries are anastomosed to holes appropriately cut in the wall of the cloth graft. Fortunately, in most patients, the ascending aneurysm stops just below the innominate artery and a successful result can be achieved, or at least good palliation for many years in a high proportion of cases (Singh and Bentall, 1972).

Acute aortic valve regurgitation

This is almost invariably the result of infective endocarditis. In a patient with a previously normal aortic valve, its destruction by endocarditis produces a catastrophic acute left ventricular failure, the left atrial pressure rises and pulmonary oedema develops. Immediate operation is indicated on diagnosis without waiting for identification of infecting organism or its control by antibiotics. No patient should be considered too ill for valve replacement as death in these patients occurs within hours of admission to hospital unless there is surgical intervention. About two-thirds of these patients can be rescued by timely surgery.

Infection occurring in a patient who is already suffering a chronic valve lesion does not deteriorate so rapidly, as a damaged valve is less likely to become completely regurgitant or, if already regurgitant, has ventricular hypertrophy which protects against the catastrophic decline.

Acute tricuspid valve regurgitation

This occurs most commonly in drug addicts, as a result of the self administration of infected intravenous injections. Infective endocarditis affects the tricuspid valve in these patients. Regurgitation is usually severe and may be accompanied by infective emboli in the lungs. While valve replacement after sterilisation of the blood stream by antibiotics might seem to be the treatment of choice, these patients so often relapse that excision of the valve has been recommended without replacement. Treatment thus has to be directed at the whole patient as the outlook is exceedingly poor with or without surgery.

Pulmonary valve disease

This is invariably primarily congenital in origin, although it may increase in severity even to complete obstruction after a successful pulmonary to systemic shunt used to treat the tetralogy of Fallot. Chronic pulmonary regurgitation is a complication of severe pulmonary arterial hypertension which may be seen in some patients with chronic rheumatic mitral valve disease, but more commonly in patients with pulmonary hypertension due to congenital heart disease. There is no merit in surgical treatment directed at the pulmonary valve in these patients. Chronic pulmonary regurgitation is also seen as the result of surgical treatment of the tetralogy of Fallot, especially when an outflow tract patch has been placed across the pulmonary valve ring. Such regurgitation should not be regarded as a benign event, but it is compatible with long-term survival without symptoms. Replacement of the pulmonary valve usually with a bioprosthesis may, however, be required in some patients.

The complications of valve replacement

Anticoagulant-related complications

All patients with either mechanical or bioprosthetic valves are liable to thromboembolic complications maximal during the first 3 months after surgery. During this period, the cloth skirt of the valve, through which sutures secure it to the patient, becomes gradually incorporated into the patient's valve ring and covered, for the most part, with neointima. Patients with a mechanical valve continue with anticoagulant treatment for life and usually require estimation of prothrombin activity at monthly intervals with readjustment of the dose of anticoagulants during any intercurrent illness or infection. Patients with bioprostheses, on the other hand, do not require long-term anticoagulants once the valve has healed in place.

Should surgery be required in a patient who is receiving anticoagulant treatment, the prothrombin level should be investigated and the patient brought to operation with a prothrombin level at the upper end of the therapeutic range. The risks of thromboembolism caused by the sudden cessation of anticoagulants are, in most cases, greater than the risks of haemorrhage during careful surgery. A possible exception to this rule, perhaps, will be in patients who need liver surgery, where the risks of haemorrhage are very great. Cholecystectomy, however, has not proved a problem in these patients in the author's experience. Similarly, anticoagulants are not stopped should a patient require reoperation for his heart disease. Anticoagulants are restarted after such an operation as soon as the drains are removed. A patient with mitral valve disease or mitral valve prosthesis may present to the general surgeon requiring urgent embolectomy. It is particularly important that anticoagulants are continued in these patients.

Haemorrhagic complications of anticoagulant treatment

Gastrointestinal haemorrhage is particularly likely to occur in patients receiving long-term anticoagulants if they have a concomitant duodenal ulcer, which is not uncommon. It is the author's practice, if at all possible, to recommend definitive treatment of the duodenal ulcer before embarking on valve surgery. In a few patients in whom it was appropriate on gastroenterological grounds, a highly selective vagotomy was performed at the time of valve surgery. Massive gastrointestinal haemorrhage, however, due to acute erosion may occur during the stress of the postoperative period after cardiac surgery, or it may occur as a late complication due to lack of effective control of anticoagulant therapy. This massive haemorrhage may be lethal and, therefore, is an important consideration in deciding which valve is the most appropriate for any individual patient.

Prosthetic valves

The introduction by Starr of a ball valve prosthesis which could be implanted into the natural site of an excised, diseased valve was a major watershed in the development of cardiac surgery (Starr *et al.*, 1962). For the first time stenotic or regurgitant valves could be operated on with the knowledge that if conservative surgery was impossible an alternative treatment was immediately available. This gave great impetus to valve design and many surgeons worked in close relationship with manufacturers to produce improved designs of replacement valves. Two examples are illustrated here, Starr-Edwards (Figs 28.3a,b), perhaps the most widely used and best evaluated ball valve, and Björk-Shiley

(Figs 28.4a,b), a well tried tilting disc valve. These two valves remain the yardsticks by which other valves are assessed.

The Starr-Edwards prosthesis has a dacron sewing ring, a Stellite metal cage and a silicone rubber ball. The Björk-Shiley valve has a similar sewing ring, a 'Stellite' cage and a pyrolytic carbon disc (the disc was originally of 'Delrin', a polyamide similar to nylon). The majority of other types make use of similar materials.

Bioprosthesis is the name now used to describe a valve manufactured from animal materials combined with metals and/or plastics to form a valve, in which the proteins are fixed by an agent such as glutaraldehyde (Fig 28.5). These valves are non-antigenic and can be implanted by the same techniques as are used for the mechanical valves. They are, however, subject to failure by fracture of the cusps within a period of 5–10 years and, therefore, replacement is likely to be necessary at least every 10 years. Most bioprostheses are made from pig aortic valves though human dura mater and pig and calf pericardium have also been used for the cusps.

In general terms, it can be argued that the trileaflet valve pattern found in the ventriculoarterial position in nature is probably less suitable for use in the atrioventricular position in man: the results of valve replacement bear this out. The ideal valve replacement has yet to be made.

A comparison of valves may conveniently be made with some accuracy after 10 years and the following factors considered:

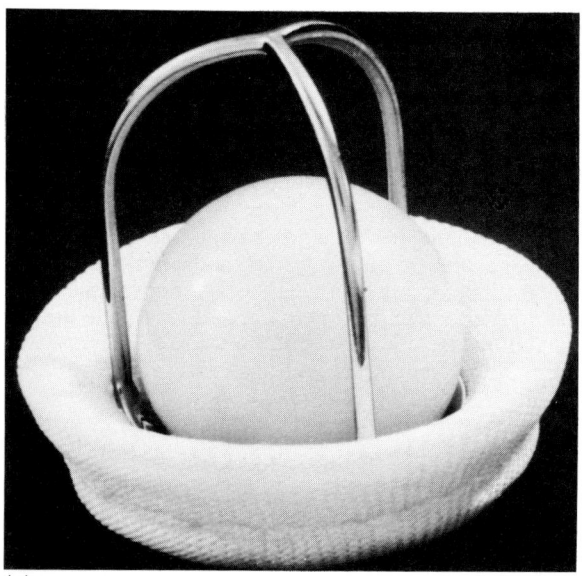

(a)

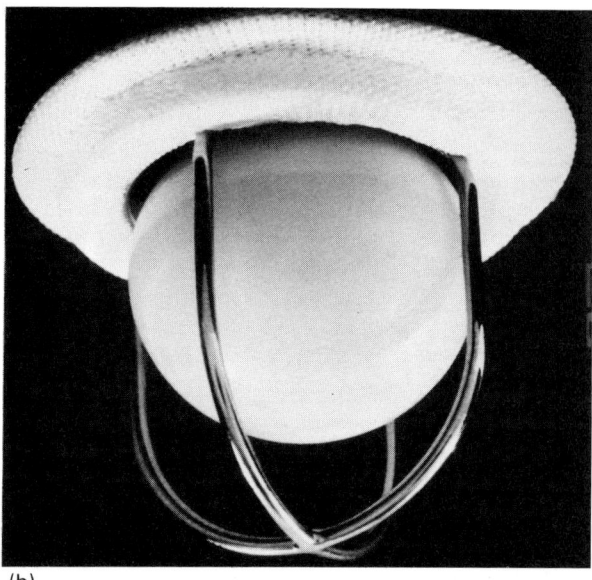

(b)

Fig 28.3 Starr-Edwards silicone-rubber ball valves. (a) aortic valve prostheses. (b) mitral valve prostheses.

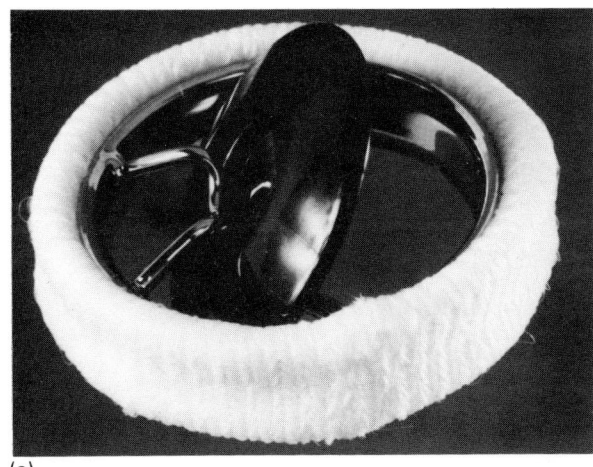

(a)

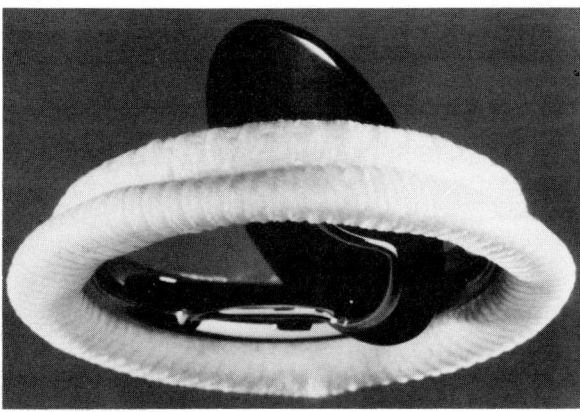

(b)

Fig 28.4   Björk-Shiley tilting disc valves. (a) aortic valve prostheses. (b) mitral valve prostheses.

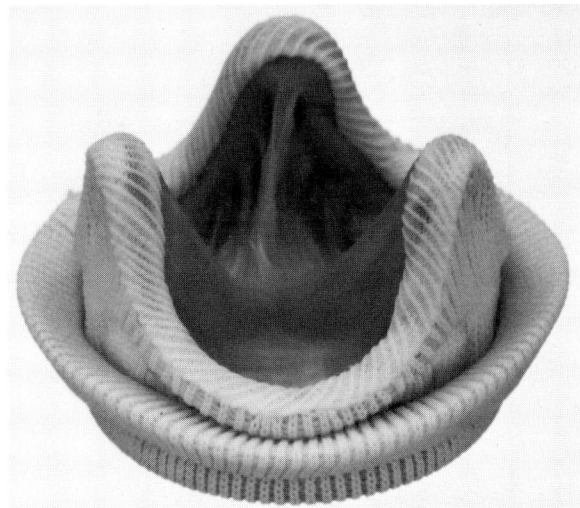

Fig 28.5   Stent mounted porcine xenograft aortic valve (Hancock Laboratories Inc.)

Patient survival

In Fig 28.6 (Starr *et al.*, 1976; Björk and Henze, 1979) a comparison of the 10-year follow-up is shown comparing the Starr-Edwards with the Björk-Shiley aortic valve prosthesis with respect to survival. Figure 28.7 depicts the same comparison for the mitral valve (Starr *et al.*, 1975; Björk and Henze, 1979).

Valve related complications

Thromboembolism

Table 1 gives the incidence of embolism expressed as a percentage figure per year; this is equated with the

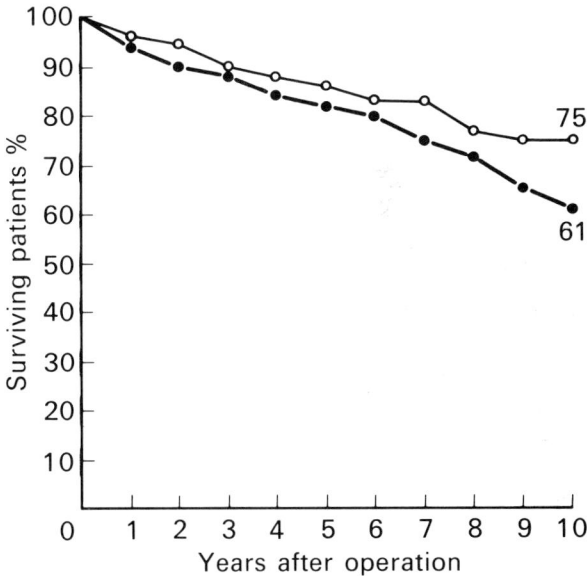

• Starr-Edwards silicone rubber ballvalve
  (type 1260)
○ Björk-Shiley tilting disc valve
  (type – standard)

Fig 28.6 Survival rates for aortic valve prostheses of Starr-Edwards and Björk-Shiley.

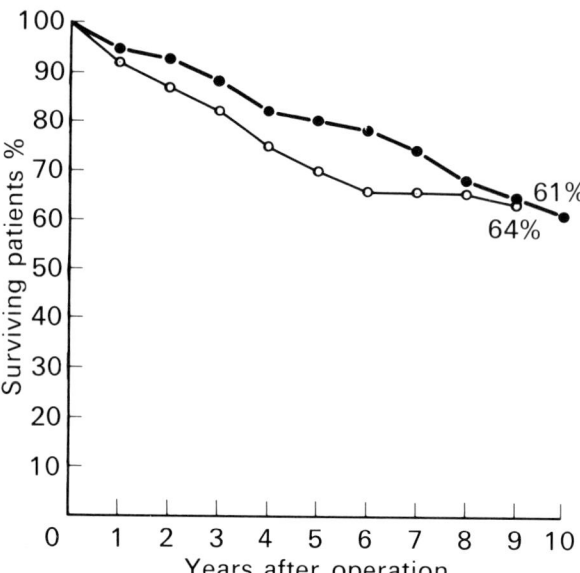

• Starr-Edwards silicone rubber ballvalve
  (type 6120)
○ Björk-Shiley tilting disc (type – standard)

Fig 28.7 Survival rates for mitral valve prostheses of Starr-Edwards and Björk-Shiley.

quoted rate per hundred patient years in the case of the Björk-Shiley valve.

Haemorrhage

Haemorrhagic complications due to anticoagulant treatment are rarely fatal in western countries at the present time, but non-fatal bleeding from this cause is relatively common. Starr gives an incidence of 1.4% per year for serious bleeds and a further 1.3% per year for minor bleeds, a total of 2.7% haemorrhagic com-

Table 1
INCIDENCE OF THROMBOEMBOLISM IN PATIENTS RECEIVING ANTICOAGULANTS

Aortic valve	
Starr-Edwards (Type 1260)	Björk-Shiley (Type – standard)
5.2% per year	0.7% per year

Mitral valve	
Starr-Edwards* (Type 6120)	Björk-Shiley† (Type – standard)
6.0% per year	4.1 per year

* Includes 'transient ischaemic attacks' and 'significant emboli'.
† Includes fatal and all non-fatal emboli.

plications per year. This risk is possibly continued throughout life, but is probably influenced by personal factors related to management both by the doctor and the patient of his anticoagulant regime and the reliability of the laboratory.

Infection

The incidence of infection is discussed under the heading of endocarditis (p. 433).

Thrombotic stenosis

A creeping pannus of organised clot gradually imprisons the valve ball or disc and prevents it from moving. Severe stenosis (and slight regurgitation) are produced. Urgent operation is required to relieve the obstruction. This may take the form of simple removal of the thrombus, but more usually excision and replacement of the valve is required. The incidence of this complication is shown in Table 2.

Table 2
INCIDENCE OF THROMBOTIC OBSTRUCTION IN PATIENTS RECEIVING ANTICOAGULANTS

Aortic valve	
Starr-Edwards (Type 1260)	Björk-Shiley (Type – standard)
None	0.3% per year

Mitral valve	
Starr-Edwards (Type 6120)	Björk-Shiley (Type – standard)
0.38% per year	1.3% per year

Sudden death

Unidentified causes of sudden death should be assumed to be thromboembolic though a patient with a valve prosthesis is not immune from all the other cardiac and non-cardiac causes. Autopsy is rarely obtained when the patient is at home and all series contain a number of deaths which are not certainly attributable to valve complications. The overall figures given include deaths from all causes.

Summary

At the present time, valve replacement is a relatively safe routine procedure. The patient lives a useful life with considerable or complete relief of symptoms. The dangers and nuisance of anticoagulant treatment have to be balanced against the certain necessity of replacing a bioprosthesis when it fails. Valve development continues: the foregoing account indicates the nature and extent of improvements in valve design which are required.

The surgical aspects of infective endocarditis

Infective endocarditis occurs as a spontaneous disease classically in a subacute form and due to infection with a streptococcus viridans originating in the patient's own mouth flora. This infection is more likely to attack previously damaged heart valves (rheumatic or congenitally deformed) (Fig 28.8) and can also attack a prosthetic valve. This well recognised infection is usually easily controlled by a penicillin and surgical treatment is rarely required. A much greater spectrum of organisms are now being found in infective endocarditis (Table 3) (Bentall, 1979) and not all are satisfactorily controlled by antibiotics, or valve damage may be so severe that haemodynamic causes necessitate surgical intervention. Infection of a prosthetic valve is a serious and potentially lethal complication. The commonest organism is a *Staphylococcus epidermidis* or a *Staphylococcus aureus*. (Table 4) (Bentall, 1979).

Prosthetic valve endocarditis may be early (within 2 months of operation) and is then due to infection at operation or associated with it. Late infection occurs at any time after this at a steady rate of approximately 0.5% per year. In nearly 10 000 valve replacements collected from the world literature there were 71 early cases of whom 53 died and 91 late of whom 34 died (Rossiter *et al.*, 1978). The death rate in early prosthetic valve endocarditis is thus 75% and of the late cases 37%.

Table 3
BACTERIAL ENDOCARDITIS – ORGANISMS

	Non-prosthetic valves	Prosthetic valve endocarditis
Strep. viridans	12	2
Strep. faecalis	3	0
Streptococcus, ∝-haemolytic	2	0
Streptococcus, anaerobic	3	0
Strep. pneumoniae	1	0
Staph. epidermidis	3	5
Staph. aureus	2	3
Micrococcus	1	
Diphtheroid	1	1
Corynebacterium	1	0
Pseudomonas	1	0
E. coli	2	0
Klebsiella	0	2
Candida albicans	0	1
Negative cultures	8	3

Hammersmith Hospital, 1968–1976. (From *Proceedings of the VIII World Congress of Cardiology*, Tokyo, Sept. 1978. International Congress Series No. 470. By courtesy of the Editors, S. Hayase and S. Murao and the publishers, Excerpta Medica, Amsterdam, Oxford and Princeton.)

Table 4
PROSTHETIC VALVE ENDOCARDITIS – BACTERIOLOGY

	All cases	Early cases
Staph. epidermidis	5	2
Staph. aureus	3	1
Strep. viridans	2	1
Klebsiella	2	
Diphtheroids	1	1
Candida	1	1
Negative cultures	3	2
	17	8

Hammersmith Hospital, 1968–1976. (From *Proceedings of the VIII World Congress of Cardiology*, Tokyo, Sept. 1978. International Congress Series No. 470. By courtesy of the Editors, S. Hayase and S. Murao and the publishers, Excerpta Medica, Amsterdam, Oxford and Princeton.)

The principle of treatment for all cases of infective endocarditis is primarily medical until the bloodstream is sterilised, then by excision of the valve and replacement if there is a haemodynamic fault (such as perivalvar leak). In a few patients operation is forced earlier by the impending death of the patient from haemodynamic deficit. These principles apply in both natural and prosthetic valve endocarditis (Westaby, 1983).

Ventricular aneurysm

The great majority of ventricular aneurysms arise in the anterior wall of the left ventricle and are a late

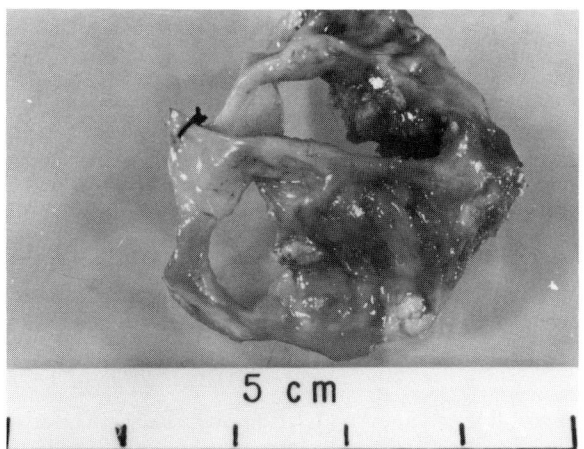

5 cm

Fig 28.8 Aortic valve destroyed by infection – congenitally bicuspid aortic valve with fenestrations and vegetations.

result of myocardial infarction due to coronary artery disease. Very rarely ventricular aneurysms may be found as a result of blunt trauma to the chest wall (Fox *et al.*, 1980) or at the site of previous ventriculotomy (Samarrai *et al.*, 1976).

Pathological features

Damaged cardiac muscle cannot regenerate, but is replaced by fibrous tissue. A fibrous scar anywhere has a tendency to stretch and, when it forms part of the wall of the heart, this tendency is frequently demonstrated by the formation of an aneurysm. Pressure in the left ventricle is four times that in the right and this coupled with the fact that the left anterior descending coronary artery is the most frequent site of a complete block, makes the territory of this artery the most frequently involved with aneurysm formation. The development of aneurysm is progressive as the tension in the wall increases directly with its diameter and with the reciprocal of the wall thickness. Cardiac aneurysms do eventually rupture, if death does not result from other causes, but these patients are not usually seen in hospital practice as rupture tends to occur outside the hospital environment and is almost invariably fatal. Saccular ventricular aneurysms tend to accumulate thrombus which may help to support the wall, but friable thrombus may be thrown off and form a cerebral or more peripheral embolus.

The less common posterior wall aneurysms lie in the territory of the circumflex coronary artery or its branches and may involve the posterior papillary muscle of the mitral valve, producing one form of mitral regurgitation. Aneurysms of the right ventricle are very much less common, but may be seen after incomplete operations for right ventricular outflow tract obstruction. In these patients the pressure in the right ventricle may be equal to or even greater than that in the left ventricle.

Diagnosis and treatment

The incidence of ventricular aneurysm following myocardial infarction is difficult to determine, but it has been found to be as high as 12–15% of myocardial infarctions in postmortem series (Abrams *et al.*, 1963). Early aneurysms may be completely asymptomatic initially and there has been an increasing tendency to treat these conservatively. The use of echocardiography is of great value in the diagnosis and follow-up of small aneurysms as unlike x-ray ventriculography, it is non-invasive and free from risk. Should the patient suffer from angina pectoris and coronary angiography is carried out and indicates the need for coronary artery

bypass grafting, then surgical excision of the aneurysm will be undertaken at the same time as the bypass surgery. Congestive cardiac failure occurs in the presence of a large aneurysm due either to the damping effect of the paradoxically enlarging aneurysmal chamber or to associated mitral valve regurgitation; in both these instances the reduction of the contractile mass of the left ventricle due to myocardial disease is obviously a contributory factor. These large aneurysms require excision and the mitral valve is readily replaced through the open left ventricle if required. Coronary artery bypass grafting to the remaining vessels is carried out as the coronary arteriogram indicates, at the same operation. Serious ventricular arrhythmias are frequently seen in association with ventricular aneurysm and are an indication for operation. Until recently, the operative mortality in this class of patient was exceedingly high (42% in one series) (Harken *et al.*, 1980) but modern methods of electrophysiological mapping of the heart at operation have made it possible to identify the area of myocardium from which the ventricular tachycardia arises, and the operation designed to interrupt the localised myocardial re-entry circuits involved. It has been found that a subendocardial incision in the apparently normal ventricular wall about 2 cm from the visible junction between the aneurysm and the surviving myocardium will abolish the arrhythmias in most patients. While it is possible to carry such an incision around the entire aneurysmal neck, most surgeons specialising in this work prefer to identify by mapping the site or sites of earliest activation of the ventricular muscle and perform a more localised incision. Such an approach has resulted in a dramatic improvement in the operative mortality and late results in these patients (7% hospital mortality in another series) (Harken *et al.*, 1980) which is approximately the same as for excision of aneurysm without arrhythmia.

Surgical techniques

The methods of treatment of ventricular aneurysm are now well standardised worldwide, apart from the more recent additions of surgery for rhythm disturbances.

The chest is opened through a median sternotomy and the pericardium opened in the same line. The aorta and right atrium are then prepared for cannulation, but no attempt is made at this stage to separate the pericardium over the bulk of the ventricular mass and the aneurysm. The aorta and right atrium are cannulated in the routine manner and cardiopulmonary bypass is started. The patient's temperature is lowered to approximately 27°C, the aorta is cross-clamped and the heart arrested with a cold cardioplegic solution. Only at this stage is the left ventricle and the aneurysm completely freed from the pericardial sac. In this way the danger of dislodgement of thrombus or rupture of the aneurysm is avoided. The aneurysm is then opened down its whole length and the contained thrombus carefully removed. The aneurysm is then excised leaving a fringe of aneurysmal wall of 1–2 cm around the entire periphery. The mitral valve and its papillary muscles are inspected and, if indicated, mitral valve replacement is carried out at this stage. The distal ends of any coronary grafts to be placed are then inserted. The left anterior descending coronary, in whose territory the aneurysm most often lies, is usually completely occluded and unsuitable for grafting. Heavy mattress sutures are then inserted through 'Teflon' felt strips placed on each side of the ventricular wound, and made to emerge in the normal-looking myocardium just beyond the junction with the aneurysm. The fibrous aneurysmal fringe is then sutured as a second layer with a continuous stitch from end-to-end to complete the haemostasis. The patient is rewarmed and, after evacuation of all air from the left side of the heart, the heart is restarted and bypass discontinued.

In patients with arrhythmias, a slight modification of this technique is required as mapping must be carried out before cooling and careful attention is paid to maintain the patient at 37°C or even higher until the electrophysiological study has been completed. The operation is then carried out as above, but with the addition of myocardial incision as indicated by the electrophysiological study. Remapping of the ventricles is then performed with the heart beating after the completion of the operation to confirm abolition of the arrhythmias.

The late results of operation

The long-term outlook for these patients, despite the severity of the operation and the myocardial disease, is surprisingly good. In one recent large series (Cosgrove *et al.*, 1978) of surgical patients, the survival rate at 7 years of those who underwent ventricular aneurysmectomy, together with coronary artery revascularisation, was 69% for patients with single vessel disease and 65% for those who had multiple vessel disease with complete revascularisation. This compares very closely with the results for coronary artery bypass grafting without aneurysmectomy (Ratcliffe *et al.*, 1983).

Cardiac tumours

The commonest primary benign tumour of the heart is the myxoma. It is at least ten times more frequent in the left atrium than in the right atrium. It is very rarely found in the right ventricle. It usually arises from the margin of the fossa ovalis by a narrow pedicle and slowly becomes a pedunculated mass. This mass may nearly fill the left atrium and causes symptoms by passing through the mitral valve. Typically, it causes intermittent obstruction of the mitral valve with physical signs which vary with posture, though not all patients exhibit this feature. Clinically, patients may present with a story suggestive of rapidly developing mitral stenosis with early onset of pulmonary hypertension, or, if the tumour is soft and friable, with peripheral embolus before any cardiac symptoms and it is these patients who present to the general surgeon. Patients with these soft tumours may also present with fever, raised sedimentation rate and even splinter haemorrhages suggestive of infective endocarditis. The blood cultures are negative and the true diagnosis may be missed if the possibility of myxoma is not considered.

Those patients with peripheral emboli are usually diagnosed by histological examination of the embolus and this should not be omitted in any patient who has an unusual or unexpected embolus – for example in a child.

The diagnosis of myxoma was formerly dependent on angiography, but is now rapidly and accurately made by echocardiography. There are difficulties only if there is such a large tumour that it fills the atrium and there is a limited blood-tumour interface.

Treatment is excision using cardiopulmonary bypass. The results are excellent and recurrence is exceedingly rare.

Malignant tumours of the heart are more commonly secondary to lung, breast or lymphoma of the mediastinum than the primary angiosarcoma of the heart.

Presentation is often as a result of bloodstained pericardial effusion although, rarely, there is a sessile relatively circumscribed tumour growing in right or left atrium or ventricle which may present like a myxoma or give rise to cardiac arrhythmia. Thoracotomy or even cardiotomy may be required for diagnosis. Surgical excision is rarely possible and never curative.

Radiotherapy or cytotoxic drugs may be used, but give poor palliation.

Surgery of cardiac arrhythmias

A supraventricular tachycardia occurring in otherwise healthy young adults originally described by Wolff *et al.*, in 1930 has become amenable to surgical treatment since the discovery of its physiological basis: that it is a tachycardia usually initiated in the atrium in which an aberrant conduction pathway permits the ventricle to reactivate the atrium and thus establish a closed loop autonomous re-entry circuit. The anatomical basis of these re-entry circuits is accessory conducting tissue around left or right atrioventricular grooves which have been described since Kent first reported them in 1893, but for which no function was found for nearly one hundred years! Some of these patients are controllable by drugs, but for others surgical ablation of the aberrant conducting tissue is required. This is carried out using cardiopulmonary bypass and, as the pathways are invisible, requires an electrophysiological study in the operating theatre for the identification of their location. The tissue is then either divided surgically or ablated with a cryothermic technique. The results are excellent and permanent in most cases.

Similar techniques are used in certain patients with atrial fibrillation and an abnormal pathway, although here ablation of the atrioventricular node and insertion of a ventricular pacemaker may be a more appropriate treatment.

Recurrent unifocal ventricular tachycardias may be due to small, even microscopic, re-entry circuits near a ventricular aneurysm. These are now within the ambit of surgical treatment using the same kind of approach.

In all these three groups of patients, life threatening tachycardias can be successfully controlled at low risk, thus eliminating the necessity for lifelong drug treatment.

Surgery of the pericardium

The pericardium may be involved in any acute generalised infection. It may be viral, for example Coxsackie virus or the influenza virus. Viral pericarditis may be associated with myocarditis. Both conditions require differentiation from bacterial pericarditis, notably that due to tuberculosis. Initially, while the inflammation is fibrinous, a pericardial rub may be heard, but when fluid develops, the rub disappears. The pericardial fluid is readily detected by echocardiography which has rendered angiocardiography less important in its diagnosis. Aspiration of fluid or pus is valuable diagnostically. It should always be cultured for tubercle bacilli, even if it is heavily bloodstained. Whilst tuberculous pericarditis is much less common now in the indigenous population of the British Isles, it should be kept firmly in mind in the immigrant population. Early antituberculous treatment may result in complete resolution of the condition, but in some patients it proceeds to constrictive pericarditis which will require surgical treatment. Chronic tuberculous pericarditis may progress eventually to calcification. Pericarditis in rheumatoid disease may also cause constriction, but without calcification. Pericardectomy is usually successful in the relief of the constriction and gives excellent clinical results in both conditions.

Haemopericardium

Haemopericardium may occur in response to trauma, either blunt or penetrating, or may be one method of presentation of subacute rupture of an aneurysm of the aortic root or it may be of insidious onset in uraemia, in spontaneous haemorrhage in patients who are in receipt of anticoagulants, or due to ill-conducted attempts at pericardiocentesis. Haemopericardium may also be a manifestation of a malignant tumour, either spreading from lung or mediastinum or as a primary tumour of the pericardium; this may be mesothelioma or some form of sarcoma. If the cause of haemopericardium is obscure, cytology should always be done on the aspirate.

Pericardial tamponade may present in the early postoperative course following cardiac operations. It is heralded by a rise in pulse rate followed by the so-called pulsus paradoxus in which inspiration transiently reduces the volume of the peripheral pulse (Friedman *et al.*, 1980). For this sign to be useful, however, there must be an adequate cardiac output, thus in severe tamponade or even in slight tamponade in patients with a low cardiac output for other reasons, the diagnosis may easily be missed. Even if the embarrassment in cardiac filling is due to blood clot and the bleeding has already ceased, removal is always beneficial.

Chronic pericardial effusion

This occurs as a relatively common complication in patients receiving long-term renal dialysis. Repeated pericardiocentesis is not often necessary. Very rarely it may be so severe as to warrant open biopsy and pleural drainage.

Endomyocardial fibrosis

This rare disease first described in Uganda in 1948 is occasionally a surgical problem. The aetiology is unknown. It is characterised by a spreading layer of fibrous tissue over the endocardium and frequently involves the papillary muscles of the mitral valve. Mural thrombi occur and may embolise. Occasionally the right ventricle may also be involved. The fibrosis restricts left ventricular wall movement and by involvement of the papillary muscles, causes atrioventricular valvar regurgitation. Surgical treatment consists in removal of the fibrous layer from the inside of the left ventricle with or without excision of the mitral valve and mitral valve replacement. It is usually a disease of young Africans; the long-term outlook is uncertain.

Cardiac transplantation

This technique, developed since the first human transplant in 1967 by Christiaan Barnard, can offer significant palliation to a small number of individuals who would otherwise die from cardiac failure. There is an absolute limitation of numbers enforced by the limited supply of suitable hearts for transplantation. It is estimated in the British Isles to be a maximum of about 1000 hearts per year. In practice very few of these are, in fact, available for transplantation. Deaths from atherosclerotic heart disease are about 50 000 per year. Recipients have been mostly patients suffering from advanced coronary artery disease due to this cause. It is important that recipients are stable, phlegmatic individuals without disease in other organs and of sufficient intelligence and determination to collaborate with the exacting schedule of continued immunosuppression combined with transvenous cardiac biopsy when rejection episodes occur. Careful recipient selection is, therefore, of the utmost importance.

In the UK the 'donor' heart is derived from individuals declared dead according to the criteria of the Code of Practice of the Joint Royal Colleges (1979). The heart is removed after arrest with cold cardioplegic solution and immersed in normal saline at 4°C. It may then be transported at a temperature of 6°–8°C and implanted in the recipient. Cold storage time has been as long as 3 h with successful survival.

The techniques of implantation are essentially those of Lower and Shumway devised for the dog in 1960. Shumway and his associates (Baumgartner *et al.*, 1979) at Stanford University have been responsible for the majority of the cardiac transplants performed worldwide during the first decade of cardiac transplantation. Survival after transplantation is given by Shumway as 56% ± 4.4 at one year and 31% ± 5.2 at 5 years. Results were progressively worse the older the patient. Age over 50 is regarded as a contraindication to acceptance for transplantation.

The cardiac function of the transplanted heart is not normal in that it is, of course, denervated (British Medical Journal, 1980). Being free from vagal inhibition the rate is 90–100 per min and varies only with catecholamine drive. There is thus a slow response to exercise. The quality of life of these patients is undoubtedly improved and they and their families in general find the operation and its aftermath worthwhile.

Despite this remarkable progress in sophisticated surgical treatment, in the long-term the extension of facilities for cardiac transplantation is unlikely to make a noticeable overall contribution to the death rate and morbidity of cardiac disease (*see also* Ch. 27).

References

Abrams D.L., Edelist A., Luria M.H., Miller A.J. (1963). Ventricular aneurysm. A reappraisal based on a study of sixty-five consecutive autopsied cases. *Circulation*; **27**:164–9.

Baumgartner W.A., Reitz B.A., Oyer P.E., Stinson E.B., Shumway N.E. (1979). Cardiac homotransplantation. *Curr. Prob. Surg*; **XVI**:1–61.

Bentall H.H. (1979). The surgical aspects of bacterial endocarditis. In *Proceedings of the VIII World Congress of Cardiology*, Tokyo 17–23 September 1978 (Hayase S., Murao S., eds.) pp. 541–44. Amsterdam, Oxford, Princeton: Excerpta Medica.

Björk V.O., Henze N. (1979). Ten years' experience with the Björk-Shiley tilting disc valve. *J. Thorac. Cardiovasc. Surg*; **78**:331–42.

Boyd A.D., Engelman R.M., Isom O.W., Reed G.E., Spencer F.C. (1974). Tricuspid annuloplasty, five and one-half years' experience with 78 patients. *J. Thorac. Cardiovasc. Surg*; **68**:344–51.

British Medical Journal (1980). Function of the transplanted heart. *Brit. Med. J*; **281**:529.

Carpentier A., Deloche A., Hanania G., Forman J., Sellier P., Piwnica A., Dubost C. (1974). Surgical management of acquired tricuspid valve disease. *J. Thorac. Cardiovasc. Surg*; **67**:53–65.

Code of Practice, drawn up by a Working Party on behalf of the Health Departments of Great Britain and Northern Ireland (1979). The removal of cadaveric organs for transplantation. Appendix 5, *Diagnosis of Brain Death* and *Diagnosis of Death*, papers produced by the Conference of Royal Colleges and Faculties of the United Kingdom, pp. 32–6.

Cosgrove D.M., Loop F.D., Irarrazaval M.J., Groves L.K., Taylor P.C., Golding L.A. (1978). Determinants of long-term survival after ventricular aneurysmectomy. *Ann. Thorac. Surg*; **26**:357–63.

De Vega N.G. (1972). La anuloplastia selectiva, regulable y permenente: Una tecnica originale para el tratamiento de la insuficiencia tricuspide. *Rev. Esp. Cardiol*; **25**:555–6.

Fox K.M., Rowland E., Krikler D.M., Bentall H.H., Goodwin J.F. (1980). Electrophysiological manifestations of non-penetrating cardiac trauma. *Brit. Heart J*; **43**:458–62.

Friedman H.S., Sakurai H., Choe S.S., Lajam F., Celis A. (1980). Pulsus paradoxus: A manifestation of a marked reduction of left ventricular endiastolic volume in cardiac tamponade. *J. Thorac. Cardiovasc. Surg*; **79**:74–82.

Harken A.H., Horowitz L.N., Josephson M.E. (1980). Comparison of standard aneurysmectomy and aneurysmectomy with directed endocardial resection for the treatment of recurrent sustained ventricular tachycardia. *J. Thorac. Cardiovasc. Surg*; **80**:527–34.

Lower R.R., Shumway N.E. (1960). Studies on orthotopic homotransplantation of the canine heart. *Surg. Forum*; **11**:18–23.

Rossiter S.J., Stinson E.B., Oyer P.E., Miller D.C., Schapira J.N., Martin R.P., Shumway N.E. (1978). Prosthetic valve endocarditis. Comparison of heterograft tissue valves and mechanical valves. *J. Thorac. Cardiovasc. Surg*; **76**:795–803.

Samarrai A.A.R., McCloy R., Ablett M.B. (1976). Biloculate false aneurysm of the right ventricle after cardiac surgery. *Brit. Heart J*; **38**:297–300.

Singh M.P., Bentall H.H. (1972). Complete replacement of the ascending aorta and the aortic valve for the treatment of aortic aneurysm. *J. Thorac. Cardiovasc. Surg*; **63**:218–25.

Starr A., Edwards M.L., Griswold H.E. (1962). Mitral replacement: late results with a ball valve prosthesis. *Prog. Cardiovasc. Dis*; **5**:298–312.

Starr A., Grunkemeier G. L., Lambert L., Okies J.E., Thomas D. (1975). Mitral valve replacement. A 10-year follow-up of non-cloth-covered vs. cloth-covered caged-ball prostheses. *Cardiovasc. Surg* 1975, *Circ.* 1976; supp. **3 54**:111–47, 111–56.

Starr A., Grunkemeier G.L., Lambert L.E., Thomas D.R., Sugimura S., Lefrak E.A. (1976). Aortic valve replacement. A ten-year follow-up of non-cloth-covered vs. cloth-covered caged-ball prostheses. *Cardiovasc. Surg.* 1976, *Circ.* 1977; **supp.2 56**:11–133, 11–139.

Starr A., McCord C.W., Wood J., Herr R., Edwards M.L. (1964). Surgery for multiple valve disease. *Ann. Surg*; **160**:596–613.

Wolff L., Parkinson J., White P.D. (1930). Bundle branch block with short P-R interval in healthy young people prone to paroxysmal tachycardia. *Amer. Heari J*; **5**:685.

Further reading

Ratcliffe P.J., Oldershaw P.J., Dawkins K., Cotter L., Lennox S.C., Paneth M. (1983). Long-term survival following left ventricular aneurysmectomy. *J. Cardiovasc. Surg*; **24**:461–6.

Westaby S., Oakley Celia, Sapsford R.N., Bentall H.H. (1983). Surgical treatment of infective endocarditis with special reference to prosthetic valve endocarditis. *Brit. Med. J*; **287**:320–3.

Myocardial ischaemia

DONALD ROSS

Pathology and natural history

Myocardial ischaemia results from atherosclerotic degeneration of the coronary arteries. It should, therefore, be recognised clearly as a disease of the arteries and not primarily a disease of the myocardium. As such it is analogous to atherosclerosis occurring elsewhere in the body as in the legs and cerebral vessels. Characteristically, the disease affects all the blood vessels, but with its main incidence proximally in the larger arteries. It is segmental or localised in its distribution and often with its maximum incidence at vessel bifurcation.

As with the surgical treatment of atherosclerotic vessel disease at any site in the body, surgery is dependent first on establishing the exact anatomy by angiography. Secondly, the aim of treatment should be to relieve symptoms and to abort the progression of the disease before it reaches a stage where death or permanent injury to the area supplied by the diseased vessel occurs. This latter aim is best achieved in the case of the coronary vessels by bypassing the diseased vessel segment with some form of tubular graft, for example, a saphenous vein.

Where narrowing or blockage of the arteries results in occlusion and permanent ischaemia of the tissue, that segment of myocardium in the case of the coronary arteries, undergoes infarction and the resulting electrical instability may cause sudden death from ventricular arrhythmias. Alternatively, there may be localised destruction of the muscle and healing by scar tissue. This results in a permanent impairment of ventricular function.

Symptoms

Patients with a reduced blood flow in the coronary vessels, short of occlusion and tissue destruction, experience angina which is pain of a crushing nature felt beneath the sternum and radiating to neck, back and arms. It is relieved by rest or by trinitrin tablets. The estimated 5-year survival for patients with this symptom complex is in the range of 65 to 80% or there is an expected annual death rate of between 4 and 7%.

Where muscle dysfunction predominates (as a result of repeated infarcts) breathlessness is an important symptom and angina may be absent or minimal since only living and contracting muscle causes pain.

Indications for surgery

The commonly quoted indication for coronary artery surgery is angina which is resistant to medical therapy, but this implies that medical treatment is a valid alternative to surgery, whereas medical and surgical treatment are, or should be, regarded as complementary. A sensible approach, at least until radioisotope scanning techniques are more refined, is to base our surgical decisions on the angiographic appearance of the coronary arteries. This means we have first to decide on the type of case which should be studied in this way and the study must include an assessment of the functional integrity of the left ventricle.

Indications for coronary angiographic study include:

1 patients with severe angina particularly those resistant to medical therapy;
2 patients who have had a documented myocardial infarction;
3 patients over the age of 40 years prior to surgery on their valves;
4 patients with angina plus a strong family history of heart attack and those with diabetes and hyperlipidaemia.

Based on these criteria all patients with severe angina and with proven coronary artery disease are potential candidates for saphenous vein bypass grafting.

Most studies indicate that where only one coronary artery is diseased, the prognosis of life expectancy is the same for medically and surgically treated patients. With two and three vessel disease the odds favour surgical treatment and, in left main stem disease, the prognosis for life is considerably better with surgery.

It follows that surgery should be offered to all patients with angina where there is over 50% narrowing of two or three main coronary arteries and in left main stem disease. At the same time, in assessing the importance of a single vessel involvement, a lesion involving the proximal anterior descending left coronary artery is potentially more important than a similar lesion in a non-dominant right coronary. Particularly in the absence of obvious collateral vessels, an important proximal lesion in the left anterior descending coronary artery may be an indication for surgical treatment in the hope of avoiding a massive infarction of the antero-lateral wall and septum of the left ventricle.

An important consideration in deciding on surgical treatment is the state of the left ventricle as judged clinically by breathlessness and by evidence of increased heart size and pulmonary congestion on the chest x-ray. The efficiency of contraction of the ventricle can also be judged angiographically. Localised dysfunction of the ventricle has some adverse bearing on the results of surgery, but a diffusely impaired poorly contracting left ventricle increases mortality and militates against a good result and may even be considered a contraindication to surgery.

Surgical anatomy

Coronary angiography has brought us into contact with the detailed anatomy of the coronary arteries and has afforded us a much clearer understanding of them than can be learnt from standard textbooks of anatomy.

There are two major arteries, the right and left, although from the surgeon and cardiologist's point of view there are three major sources of blood supply to the myocardium, since the main left coronary artery has a short stem which, in fact, may be absent with the left coronary arising as two separate arteries – circumflex and anterior descending.

The right coronary artery is a large vessel which arises from the anteriorly placed right aortic sinus and runs in the fatty groove between the right atrium and the right ventricle (Fig 29.1). It supplies branches to the front of the right ventricle and a large marginal bunch which runs along the acute margin of the heart. It then crosses the diaphragmatic surface of the heart towards the left atrioventricular groove. When it reaches the interventricular sulcus posteriorly, it gives off the posterior descending coronary artery which gives branches to the posterior surface of the left ventricle. In 10% of people, the posterior descending territory is supplied exclusively by the left coronary artery (left dominance) and in a further 10%, the supply to this area is balanced between left and right coronary arteries.

The right coronary is, therefore, an important vessel supplying the right atrium and a large part of the right

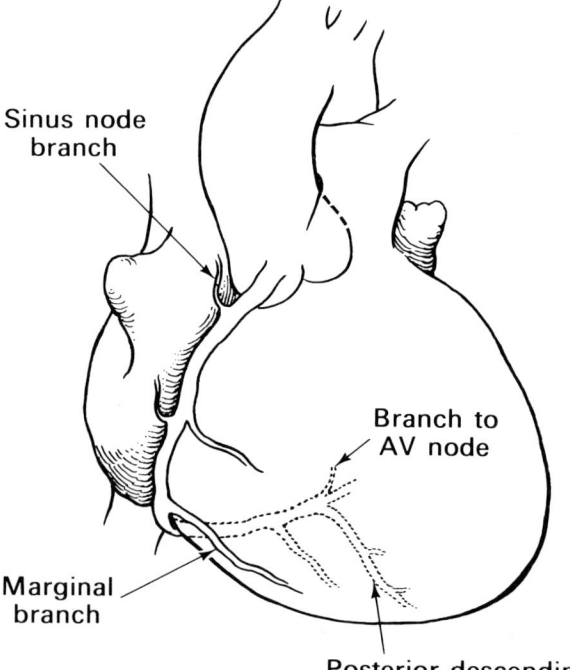

Fig 29.1 The anatomy of the right coronary artery and its branches.

ventricle and also a great deal of the posterior surface of the left ventricle through its posterior descending branches. It also gives branches to the sinus node and the atrioventricular node. Consequently, a lesion of this vessel may well be responsible for dysrhythmias or heart block and also an infarct or dysfunction of the posterior wall of the left ventricle.

The left main stem artery arises from the left coronary sinus and runs for a variable course behind the pulmonary artery before dividing into a circumflex branch and an anterior descending branch (Fig 29.2).

The circumflex artery runs posteriorly in the left atrioventricular groove close to the base of the left atrial appendage to join up with the right coronary running in corresponding right atrioventricular groove between the right atrium and right ventricle (Fig 29.3).

As it runs posteriorly along the upper margin of the left ventricle it gives off a variable number of marginal arteries (29.1–29.4) which come off more or less at a right angle and supply the postero-lateral wall of the left ventricle. The circumflex artery may be a dominant vessel taking over the territory of the right coronary artery as shown in Fig 29.4.

The left anterior descending coronary artery usually arises as the left main coronary appears behind the lateral margin of the pulmonary artery. It runs to the apex in the interventricular groove between the right and left ventricles correspondingly with the posterior

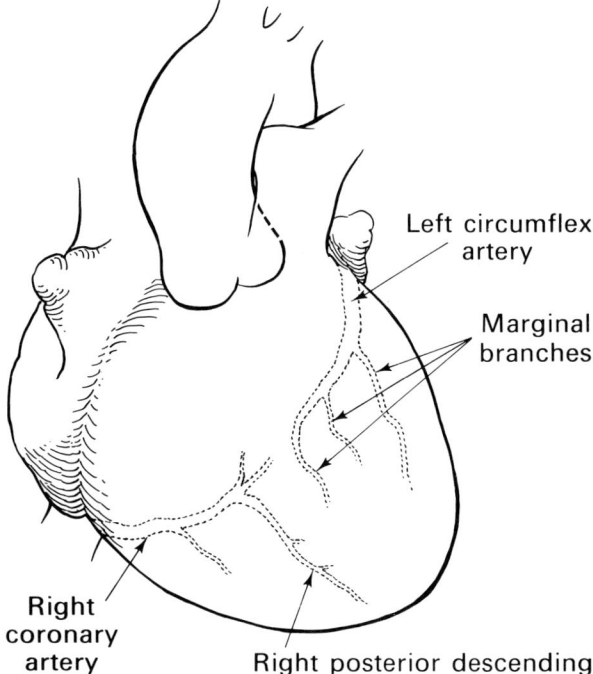

Fig 29.3   Distribution of circumflex and right coronary arteries (right dominance).

descending branch of the right coronary, but is a much bigger vessel. Its important branches are the septal branches, which supply most of the interventricular septum with blood of which the first septal is the largest vessel. It also gives off one or two diagonal arteries to the lateral wall of the left ventricle (Fig 29.2).

It is sometimes difficult to differentiate between branches of the circumflex artery and left anterior descending angiographically, but the left anterior descending runs characteristically to the apex and its septal branches come off vertically like the teeth of a comb. Also, being in the relatively immobile septum, the left anterior descending artery and its branches show less movement with ventricular contractions than the circumflex arteries which are in the contractile left ventricular wall.

The saphenous vein bypass operation

A length of saphenous vein is either removed first or synchronously with the opening of the chest. The lower leg vein is preferred, since it is less disproportionate in diameter and healing is less likely to be associated with

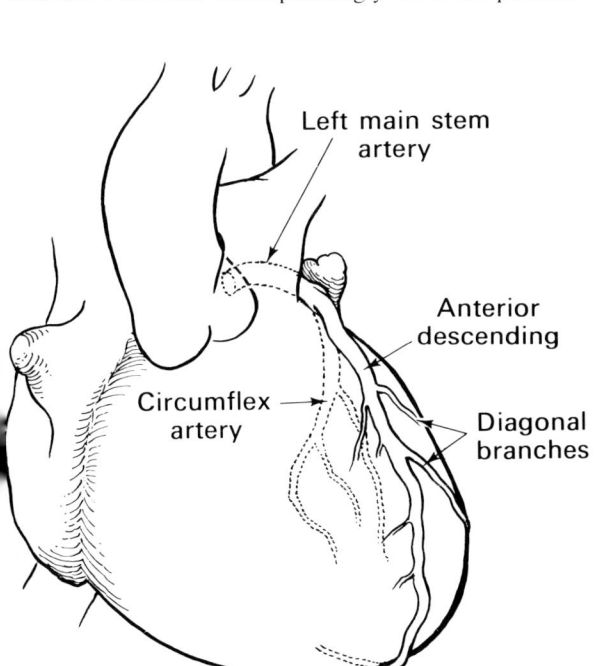

Fig 29.2   The distribution of branches from the left main stem artery.

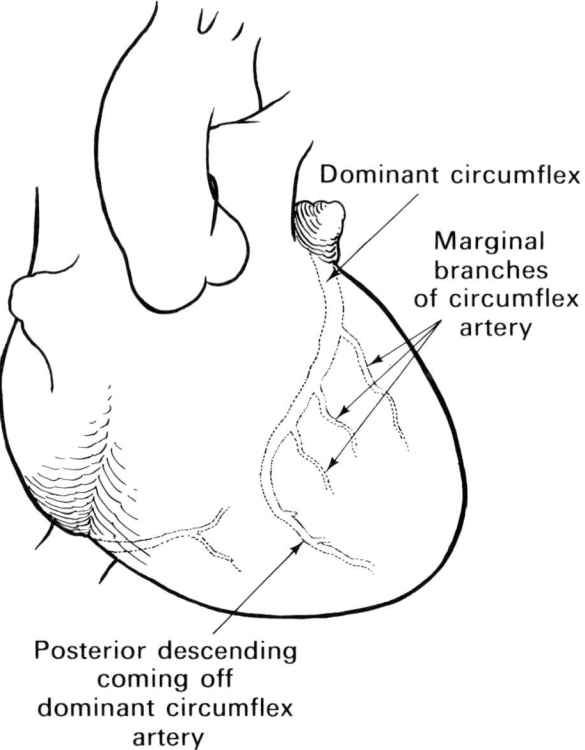

Fig 29.4 Distribution of circumflex in left dominance.

haematoma than in the thigh. Nevertheless, it is usual to extend the incision above the level of the knee in removing the vein. Where the leg veins have already been removed or are varicose, the short saphenous or arm veins can be used.

Immediately the vein has been removed, it is distended, preferably with heparinised blood and any patent side branches are ligated or oversewn. Cardiopulmonary bypass is then instituted and it is usual to cool the body temperature to between 20–30°C. The heart is then excluded from the circulation by cross-clamping the aorta and it is necessary to arrest and protect the ischaemic myocardium further by an infusion of cold blood or other cardioplegic solution directly into the aortic root.

For access to the marginal branches of the circumflex artery the operating table is tipped towards the surgeon and the apex of the heart held over towards the surgeon by an assistant. Access to the anterior descending and right coronary arteries is much simpler.

Without preliminary dissection or trauma to the vessels, an incision is made through the epicardium into the vessel at the chosen site, with progressively deeper linear sweeps of the knife till the lumen is entered. The

incision is then enlarged with Potts angled scissors. (Fig 29.5e,f).

Where an atheromatous plaque is encountered, it is better to extend the incision beyond the plaque after which a flexible probe is run along the lumen of the vessel proximally and distally to establish the patency and diameter of the lumen (Fig 29.5g).

A length of vein is prepared by cutting it at an angle and then splitting it longitudinally (Fig 29.5a–d). A suitable suture is of 6/0 Prolene on an 8 mm needle, but there are a number of options available in relation to the type of suture and suture material. Some surgeons routinely employ magnifying spectacles to improve the field of vision.

A convenient suture technique is to start at the distal end of the arterial incision with a single knot and then fix the vein with a whip stitch, (Fig 29.5g,h,i) proximally for half the length of the incision. The vein is then flipped over and the suture continues. This technique has a double advantage in that it enables one to enlarge the size of the vein or artery incision as the need arises and the upper angle is automatically retracted and kept open.

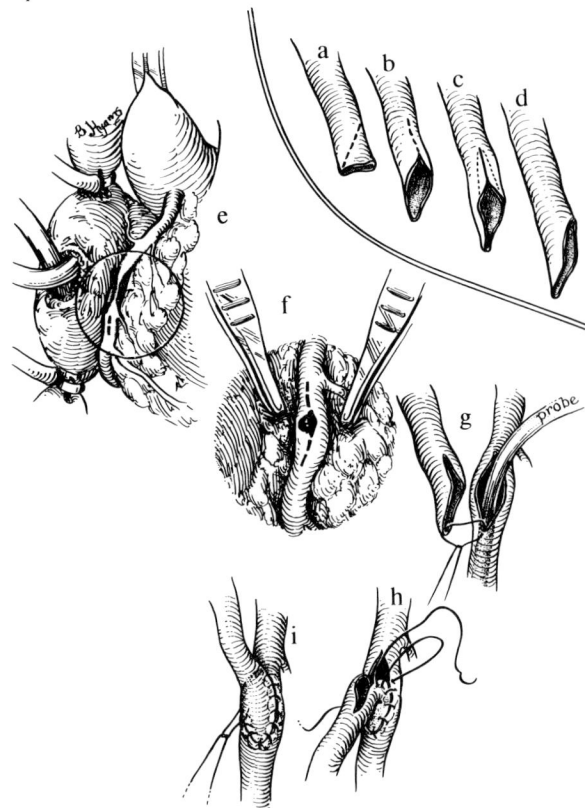

Fig 29.5 The technique of saphenous vein anastomoses to the coronary arteries.

On completion of the anastomosis, it can be tested by an injection of blood and the vein should then be temporarily clamped distally and distended so as to assess its length under pressure conditions.

A suitable site is chosen on the ascending aortic root. This is cleared of adventitia before being side-clamped and incised. It is advisable to punch out a disc of aorta with a punch or bone forceps. The proximal anastomosis is completed again with a 6/0 Prolene suture (Fig 29.6a–d). In practice, it is usual to complete all the distal anastomoses first, then re-establish the coronary circulation, defibrillate and rewarm the heart while the proximal anastomoses are completed.

Where it is desirable or convenient to anastomose the same vessel to more than one artery, like the 2nd and 3rd marginal circumflex vessels, a jump or snake graft is achieved by making small incisions in the vein and corresponding artery, where the distended vein crosses the artery (Fig 29.7). Again a continuous suture anastomosis is used.

Alternatively, two grafts may be joined as a 'Y' graft depending on the anatomical circumstances or the preference of the surgeon (Fig 29.8).

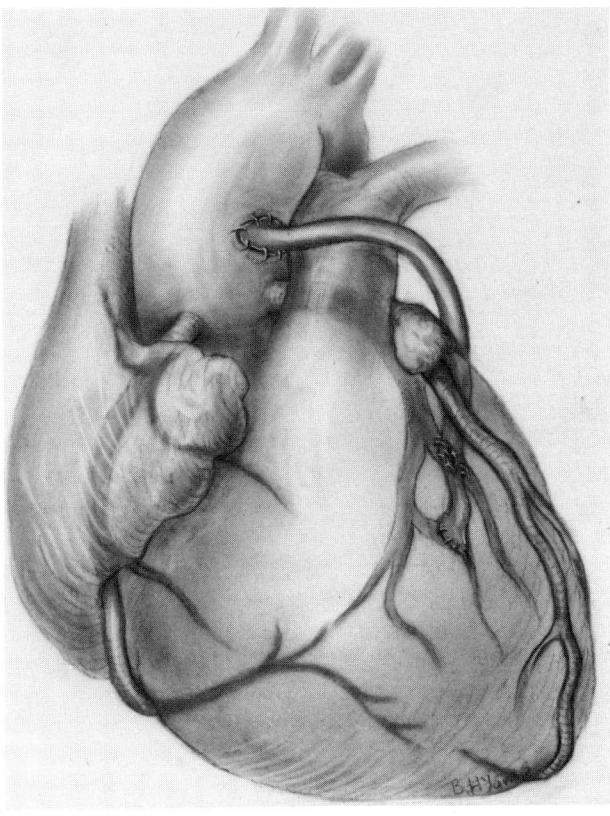

(A)

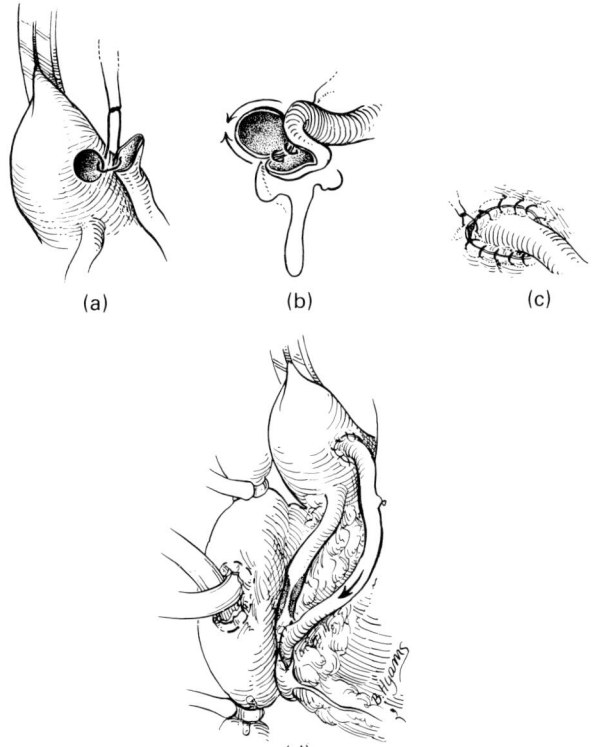

(a)   (b)   (c)

(d)

Fig 29.6 Anastomoses of saphenous vein graft to root of aorta.

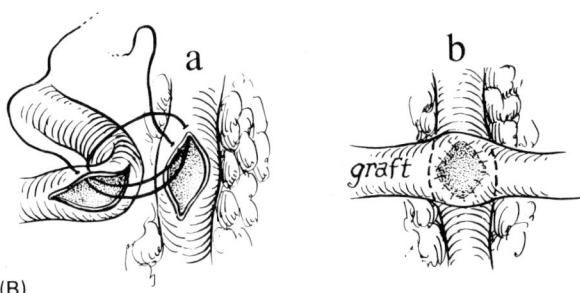

(B)

Fig 29.7 A. Two marginal circumflex arteries anastomosed to one vein graft. B. Diamond shaped orifice created on side-to-side anastomosis of jump graft.

When the arterial lumen is filled with atheroma, this can be extracted after careful freeing in the correct tissue plane by means of blunt dissection or suitable probes. Some surgeons distend and develop the plane of cleavage with CO_2 gas to facilitate the endarterectomy.

It is essential that the vessels be cored out cleanly distally including all the branches. Proximally, the

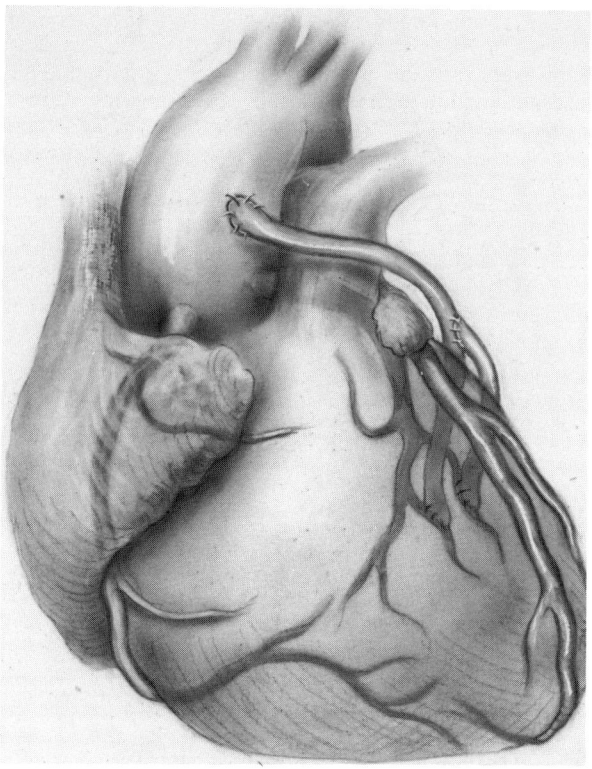

Fig 29.8 Y graft anastomosed to two marginal circumflex arteries.

removal of the atheroma should be limited and cut off
sharply with scissors.

The left internal mammary artery can be used as a
source of blood, particularly for the left anterior
descending and diagonal arteries. The advantage of the
method is that the long-term patency rate for this vessel
is even higher than for vein grafts, but the dissection is
somewhat time-consuming and the volume of blood
carried by the artery is sometimes disappointingly
small. A reasonable compromise is to graft the internal
mammary onto the diagonal and a vein graft into the
anterior descending artery.

The results

The surgical treatment of angina by saphenous vein
bypass grafting is certainly able to relieve the pain of
angina in medically resistant cases. From all centres
there is general agreement that there will be relief of
this symptom in 80–90% of survivors and the relief of
pain is long-lasting.

Furthermore, the mortality for the operation is surprisingly low being in the region of 1–3% in uncomplicated cases.

The experience of the operating team and the number of cases being handled has an important bearing on
results, but a more important determinant is the presence of associated lesions like aneurysm, infarcts, septal defects, aortic and mitral valve disease and poor
ventricular function. The best results and lowest mortality are achieved in patients with good ventricular
function and isolated coronary artery disease.

An additional satisfactory feature relates to graft
patency. At least 70–75% of grafts remain patent 3
years after operation, and an even higher patency rate
is recorded where the internal mammary artery has
been used as a graft.

More controversy surrounds the other claims and
counterclaims relating to the effectiveness of the operation. These include the possibility of increasing life
expectancy and preventing further infarcts as well as
improving ventricular function.

Of these, an increased life expectancy is probably the
least controversial and accumulating experience tends
to support the view that patients with disease of the left
main stem artery and disease of all three coronary vessels have a better life expectancy with surgical than with
medical therapy.

The evidence for improvement in ventricular function and the effectiveness of the operation in preventing further infarcts is currently the subject of a great
deal of clinical and experimental study, but there is at
present not enough evidence to support these claims.

On the other hand the chances of damaging the ventricle have receded with the introduction of more
sophisticated techniques of myocardial protection and
the claims for an acceleration of the disease in the natural coronary arteries have not been convincingly substantiated.

In summary, saphenous vein bypass grafting is certainly effective in relieving the pain of angina pectoris
in a significant number of cases resistant to medical
therapy. The mortality of the operation is low and the
long-term prospects for graft patency are high.

The patient's long-term prognosis with regard to
improved life expectancy are definitely improved with
surgery in cases with left main stem disease and three
vessel disease and probably also in cases with two vessel
disease. Results correlate better with the state of the
left ventricular damage or dysfunction preoperatively
and the best functional results can be expected in cases
with good or reasonable left ventricular function
preoperatively. This raises the question as to whether
the operation improves ventricular function and while
it is reasonable to expect that this is the case, proof is at
present lacking. What is less controversial is the fact
that the operation cannot be expected to improve

prognosis in patients with poor left ventricular function who have diffuse left ventricular disease, no angina and evidence of congestive cardiac failure.

There is no evidence at present available on the efficiency of the operation in preventing further infarcts. Certainly the operation does nothing to halt the progress of the underlying atherosclerotic process and the prevention and treatment of this process should remain our primary aim.

Transluminal angioplasty

Despite the outstanding success of coronary artery bypass grafting, it was inevitable that methods of treating coronary artery stenosis without operation should be developed. In 1979, Grüntzig and his colleagues introduced percutaneous transluminal coronary angioplasty (PTCA) as a non-operative technique for the treatment of certain types of coronary stenosis. The method involves the passage of a guiding catheter into a peripheral artery until it is engaged in the coronary ostium. A fine balloon catheter is passed into the coronary artery and through the stenosis. The balloon is then distended with radio-opaque contrast medium to dilate the stenosis; angiograms are performed before and after dilatation. This technique is applicable to discrete, non-calcific, subtotal, proximal stenosis of a major vessel. It is not suitable for left main stem disease, nor for diffuse narrowing. This technique has now been employed by many centres and its place in the treatment of coronary artery disease is being defined. Recent developments have allowed the method to be applied even in total stenosis though with less success than in incomplete obstruction.

Meier, Grüntzig and their colleagues (1983) have now reported the longer term results of this treatment at a mean follow-up interval of 29 months and they have shown that successful revascularisation approximately doubled the work capacity of their patients whether achieved by PTCA or by PTCA plus subsequent coronary artery bypass grafting. They concluded that failed PTCA (21%) does not compromise subsequent grafting either as an emergency or as an elective procedure. They noted that recurrence rates were the same in each of the above groups and all occurred within the first 9 months after the procedures. It is noteworthy that there were no deaths in either group of patients. Their results are similar to those obtained with coronary artery bypass grafting. While these early results are good, it is considered that a period of 10 years must still elapse before the place of these closed techniques can be properly evaluated.

Further reading

Braunwald E. (1978). Evaluation of the efficacy of coronary bypass surgery. II. *Amer. J. Cardiol*; **42**:161.

Conley M.J., Wechsler A.S., Anderson R.W., Oldham H.N., Sabiston D.C., Rosati R.A. (1977). The relationship of patient selection to prognosis following aortocoronary bypass. *Circulation*; **55**:158.

Dervan J.P., Baim D.S., Charniles J., Grossman W. (1983). Transluminal angioplasty of occluded coronary arteries: use of a movable guide wire system. *Circulation*; **68**:776–84.

European Coronary Surgery Study Group (1979). Coronary artery bypass surgery in stable angina pectoris: survival at two years. *Lancet*; **i**:889.

European Coronary Surgery Study Group (1980). Prospective randomised study of coronary artery bypass surgery in stable angina pectoris. Second interim report. *Lancet*; **ii**:491.

Grüntzig A.R., Senning A., Siegenthaler W.E. (1979). Non-operative dilatation of coronary artery stenosis: percutaneous transluminal coronary angioplasty. *N. Engl. J. Med*; **301**:61–8.

Hultgren H.N., Takaro T., Detre K.M., Murphy W.L. (1978). Evaluation of the efficacy of coronary bypass surgery. I. *Amer. J. Cardiol*; **42**:157.

Kloster F.E., Kremkau E.L., Rahimtoola S.H. *et al.* (1977). Prospective randomized study of coronary bypass surgery for chronic stable angina. *Cardiovasc. Clin*; **8**:145.

Loop F.D., Proudfit W.L., Sheldon W.C. (1978). Coronary bypass surgery weighed in the balance. *Amer. J. Cardiol*; **42**:154.

Meier B., Grüntzig R., Siegenthaler W.E., Schlumpf Maria. (1983). Long-term exercise performance after percutaneous transluminal coronary angioplasty and coronary artery bypass grafting. *Circulation*; **68**:796–802.

Tecklenberg P.L., Alderman E.L., Miller D.C., Shumway N.E., Harrison D.C. (1975). Changes in survival and symptom relief in a longitudinal study of patients after bypass surgery. *Circulation*; **52** suppl.1: 1–98.

30

Congenital heart disease

CHRISTOPHER LINCOLN and G. CRUPI

The application by Gibbon of a mechanical heart and lung apparatus to provide an extracorporeal circuit for cardiac surgery in 1953 saw the beginning of corrective intracardiac surgery, following which, at the present time, there are few congenital heart defects, either complex or simple in which correction cannot now be attempted.

Current concepts

Patients with heart disease can either undergo correction of their congenital anomaly, or palliation with a view to total correction in the future.

Simple defects such as patent ductus arteriosus or coarctation of the aorta can be totally corrected in infancy and early childhood. Complete intracardiac correction of congenital heart defects in early infancy may not always be possible because of the size of the patient, or the complexity of the lesion.

There are compelling sociological, psychological, economic and surgical arguments for one-stage total correction of simple and complex congenital heart disease, when the patient first requires surgical help. However, if such a policy is to be pursued, one-stage total correction must have a morbidity and mortality which is equal to palliation followed by correction at a later date.

With ever-increasing improvement of surgical and anaesthetic techniques, together with a better understanding of myocardial preservation, there has been a move towards early one-stage total correction in the last ten years with an acceptable mortality and morbidity in many instances.

Principles of cardiopulmonary bypass

Success in the surgery of congenital heart disease is dependent upon accurate preoperative diagnosis, perfect operative conditions, preservation of the myocardium and all the vital organs, and maintenance of total body function in the postoperative period.

Congenital cardiac anomalies, which in part are extracardiac, can be surgically treated without resorting to the use of cardiopulmonary bypass machinery, since the anomaly lies outside the main chambers of the heart and does not require interruption of flow of the blood to the vital structures – e.g. patent ductus arteriosus and coarctation of the aorta.

In order to carry out corrective surgery within the heart, a heart-lung machine must be used. This entails using apparatus by which the pumping action of the heart and gas transfer of the lungs is substituted by mechanical, artificial and physiological devices. By means of this apparatus, it is possible to exclude the heart from the circulation, when the body is connected to the heart-lung machine, allowing intracardiac surgery to be performed. The limitations of such apparatus is that the pump (artificial heart) is usually non-pulsatile, and the artificial lung is usually of the type which allows blood and gas to mix, thereby causing damage to the blood constituents. More recent developments of pulsatile pumps and membrane oxygenators have allowed great improvement in the application of cardiopulmonary bypass techniques. The addition of hypothermia, haemodilution and isolated cardiac ischaemia using cardioplegic drugs, increases the facility of cardiopulmonary techniques, reduces the time on the bypass machine, and thereby facilitates the cardiac surgery.

Hypothermia reduces oxygen consumption and metabolism, thereby aiding survival of tissues during the period of cardiopulmonary bypass perfusion. Oxygen consumption falls with the temperature 0°C. It is known that the oxygen consumption per kilogram body weight of tissue and perfusion of blood per unit mass of tissue is twice as much in children as that in adults; therefore, if hypothermia is in use during surgery, perfusion and oxygen requirements are reduced even more significantly in children than in adults.

Cardiopulmonary bypass techniques are usually incorporated with either (a) profound hypothermia when the body is cooled to 15°C or (b) moderate hypothermia when the body is cooled to 28°C.

In patients below the weight of 5 kg, previous surface cooling by ice bags applied to the surface of the body reduces the patient's body temperature to 28°C. This has the advantage of slowing the heart rate, and facilitates the surgery to connect the heart to the cardiopulmonary bypass perfusion apparatus. In addition, the previous surface cooling reduces the time spent on bypass to achieve the cooling, be it moderate or profound hypothermia.

At 15°C circulation can be arrested for an arbitary period of 60 min, during which intracardiac surgery can be performed. This gives an ideal operating field and is particularly applicable to patients under the weight of 5 kg.

Preservation of the myocardium with good long-term function must be achieved, in addition to the preservation of all other vital organs. Use of hypothermic biochemical perfusates within the coronary arterial circulation and topically applied hypothermic solutions to the surface of the heart, has improved the preservation of the myocardium. Immediate satisfactory cardiac function does not necessarily mean that there will be good long-term cardiac function.

Monitoring of brain activity is an important part of the overall monitoring which is carried out during cardiac surgery, particularly when using hypothermic techniques.

Monitoring during and after cardiac surgery

Since the circulation is being manipulated artificially during the period of cardiopulmonary bypass perfusion, it is important to be able to monitor various physiological parameters, in particular the central venous pressure (right atrial pressure) and left atrial pressure together with systemic arterial pressure and urine output. Frequent estimations of acid-base status and oxygenation must be performed. Cardiac rhythm is monitored by means of electrocardiogram, and during hypothermia it is important to know the rectal and nasopharyngeal temperatures.

Following cardiac surgery, all patients are returned to an intensive care unit, staffed by those specially trained in this area of care. In the postoperative period the physiological parameters are monitored as during cardiac surgery. These are recorded every 15 min. Blood loss via the chest drains is measured and replaced accordingly. The routine measurement of cardiac output in the postoperative period, although ideal, is not widely practised, nor in the majority of patients is it necessary.

Management and ventilation

It is customary for most patients to return to the intensive care unit ventilated and sedated. During the transition from the operation room to the intensive care unit, it is vital that the patient is sedated, and that there is control over the airway.

In children under the age of 5 years a nasoendotracheal tube is preferable to an oral endotracheal tube. They are more easily held in place, and may require to be in place for several days.

When all the vital systems of the patient are stable following return to the intensive care unit, and when the patient is fully awake, but sedated, he is transferred from mechanical artificial ventilation to continuous positive pressure breathing. This allows the patient to breathe spontaneously, but permits accurate monitoring of the inspired gas concentration and allows, in addition, for an expiratory resistance to be included with the ventilatory circuit, assisting the prevention of microatelectasis which is a not uncommon complication following cardiopulmonary bypass surgery. Only when the patient has shown that he can breathe spontaneously at normal inspiratory pressure with normal inspired gas concentrations is he extubated, if all the other vital signs are normal.

Palliative operations

Patients with congenital heart disease can in many instances be well palliated by extracardiac procedures.

Palliation can be performed for patients who have diminished pulmonary blood flow, inadequate mixing within the heart, or excessive pulmonary blood flow; the first two cause cyanosis and the third causes pulmonary plethora with congestive cardiac failure.

Decreased pulmonary flow

In patients with an obstructed flow of blood to the lungs, and a right to left shunt in the heart a systemic pulmonary artery anastomosis can be constructed to allow an increase in the flow of blood to the pulmonary arteries. This can be carried out by:

1 anastomosing one or other subclavian artery to the right or left pulmonary artery (Blalock);
2 anastomosing the right pulmonary artery to the back of the descending aorta (Waterston);
3 anastomosing the left pulmonary artery to the front of the first part of the descending aorta (Potts);
4 using an artificial tube prosthesis connecting the aorta or subclavian artery to one or other of the pulmonary arteries.

The systemic artery/pulmonary artery anastomosis of choice is still that of Blalock, the first palliative operation performed for patients with restricted pulmonary blood flow. This anastomosis allows the correct amount of blood to pass into the pulmonary arteries, thereby precluding the complications of pulmonary vascular disease which are sometimes seen in the other forms of anastomosis (Fig 30.1).

In patients with transposition of the great arteries with an intact atrial and ventricular septum, there is complete separation of the systemic and pulmonary circulations except through a patent ductus arteriosus. The situation is incompatible with life as soon as the ductus closes. Urgent opening of a connection between the left and right sides of the circulation is achieved in the first few days of life by the balloon atrial septostomy (Rashkind procedure) which has now supplanted surgical attempts to the same ends by the Blalock-Hanlon procedure of closed atrial septostomy. The complete mixing of the circulation allows survival of these infants until a subsequent more radical open correction.

Excessive pulmonary flow

In patients with anomalies which allow excessive flow of blood to the lungs, restriction of blood flow to the lungs can be performed by banding or narrowing the main pulmonary artery. This can be carried out by means of a constricting tape, so that the distal pulmonary artery pressure is reduced to 30% of the proximal

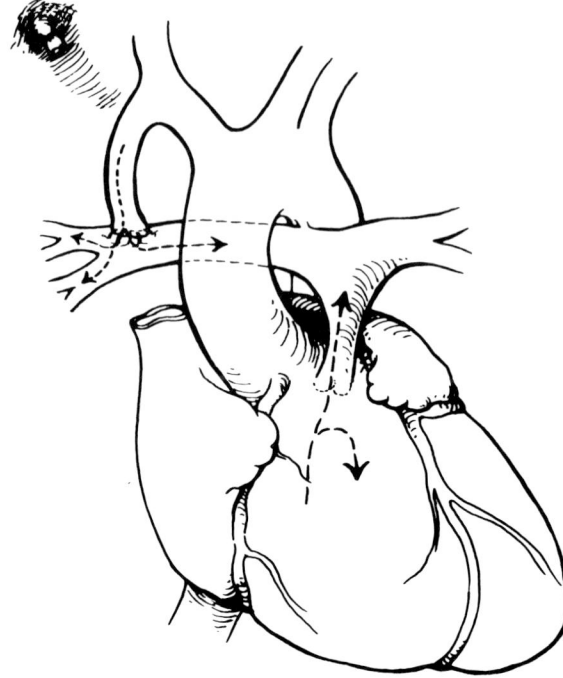

Fig 30.1 The classical Blalock-Taussig shunt in a patient with restricted pulmonary blood flow.

pulmonary artery pressure, thereby causing a gradient across the narrowed area (Fig 30.2).

Patent ductus arteriosus

Patients with this condition have signs of a high pulmonary blood flow due to a left-to-right shunt between the aorta and the patent ductus arteriosus. The patent ductus arteriosus usually closes spontaneously within 48 h of birth, but when it remains patent a communication exists between the first part of the descending thoracic aorta and the left pulmonary artery.

Treatment

Patent ductus arteriosus is an external cardiac anomaly which should be closed either by ligation or transection (Fig 30.3). The operation can be performed at any age or weight.

Results

The hospital mortality for this condition is 0–3%.

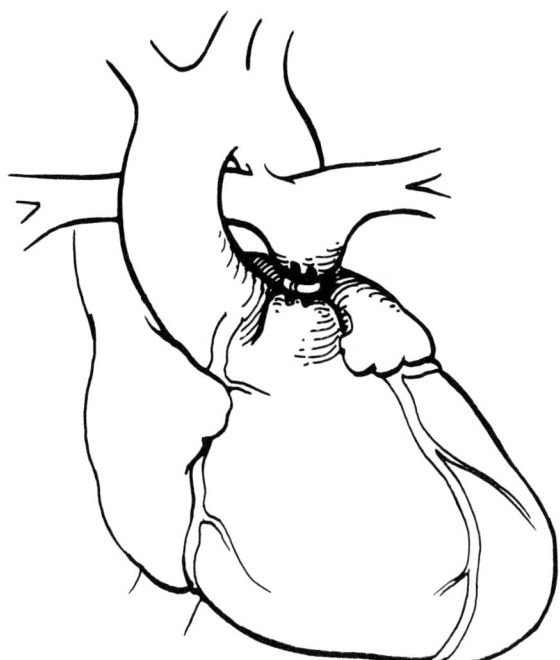

Fig 30.2 Banding of the pulmonary artery in a patient with increased pulmonary blood flow.

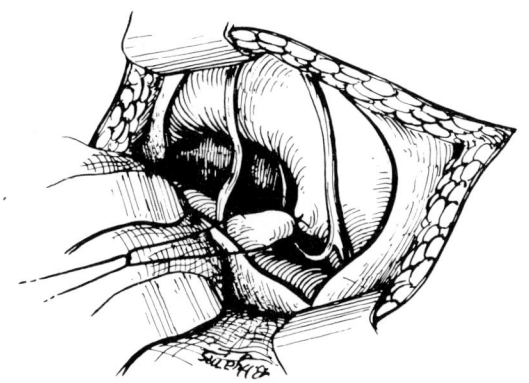

Fig 30.3 Ligation of patent ductus arteriosus.

Aorticopulmonary window

This is a rare anomaly in which there is a large communication between the main pulmonary artery and the ascending aorta. This situation is analogous to a patent ductus arteriosus, but the shunt is much larger as a rule and the patient may be symptomatic. Treatment is by open operation and primary colosure of the defect by a patch.

The hospital mortality of this condition is 0–5%.

Coarctation of the aorta

Coarctation of the aorta consists of a narrowing of the descending thoracic aorta. Early repair of this anomaly is indicated in those children with congestive heart failure who fail to respond to medical treatment. Elective repair should be performed before the age of 10 years to avoid the risk of residual hypertension.

Coarctation of the aorta can be divided according to its relationship to the ductus arteriosus into:

1 Preductal
2 Juxtaductal

A high incidence of associated intracardiac defects has been noted in infants with this anomaly.

Treatment

Aortoplasty using the left subclavian artery to widen the narrowed area is the treatment of choice in infancy. This technique is effective in preventing the incidence of restenosis at the site of repair. Resection of the coarctation and end-to-end anastomosis is commonly used in older children. The use of a dacron tube prosthesis is necessary in those instances in which the presence of a long hypoplastic segment precludes an end-to-end anastomosis (Fig 30.4).

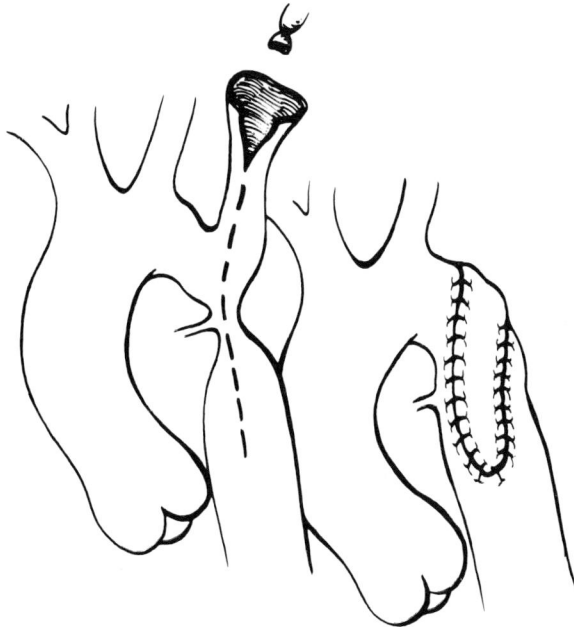

Fig 30.4 Stages in the reconstruction of coarctation of the aorta using the subclavian artery.

In older children and in adults, coarctation is best treated by a plastic widening of the aorta at the site of the coarctation using a diamond-shaped Dacron gusset.

Interrupted aortic arch

Three types of aortic arch interruption can be encountered and these are interruption between:

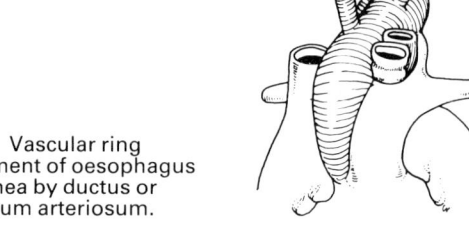

Fig 30.5 Vascular ring encirclement of oesophagus and trachea by ductus or ligamentum arteriosum.

1. the innominate artery and the left common carotid artery;
2. the left common carotid and the left subclavian;
3. the left subclavian and the distal descending aorta.

In these patients the descending aorta is perfused by means of a large persistent ductus arteriosus. A ventricular septal defect must be present in order to support life.

Treatment

Success of treatment of this critical anomaly depends on the reconstruction of the arch of the aorta. This can be performed by means of an interposition graft using the ductus arteriosus as an autologous tube graft. The condition remains one of the most challenging encountered in all surgery of congenital heart disease.

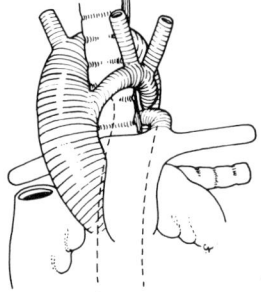

Fig 30.6 Vascular ring: double aortic arch.

Results

This anomaly is so rare as to preclude a meaningful figure for the results of surgical treatment.

Vascular ring

Treatment

In all these anomalies the underlying object of the treatment is to relieve the constricting ring compressing the trachea and the oesophagus. All anomalies can be treated through a left thoracotomy.

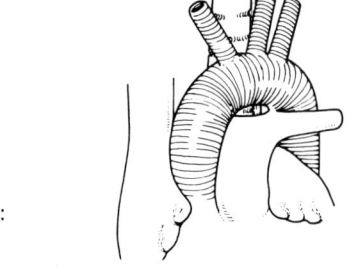

Fig 30.7 Vascular ring: abnormal position of innominate artery.

1. Right aortic arch with left ligamentum arteriosus or patent ductus arteriosus (Fig 30.5).
2. Double aortic arch (Fig 30.6).
3. Abnormal position of the innominate artery (Fig 30.7).
4. Anomalous right subclavian artery (Fig 30.8).
5. Anomalous left pulmonary artery arising from the right side of the main pulmonary artery.

In (1) it is only necessary to divide the patent ductus arteriosus or ligamentum arteriosum, breaking the constricting ring. In (2) there is a minor and major arch; the major arch usually gives rise to the head vessels.

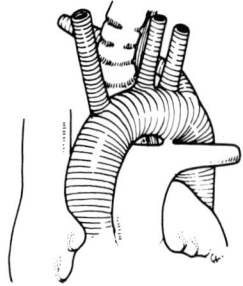

Fig 30.8 Vascular ring: aberrant right subclavian artery.

The division of the minor arch does not compromise the vital structures. (3) The innominate artery crosses the front of the trachea compressing it when present in infancy because the vessel arises abnormally to the left of the midline. In this abnormality, the innominate artery is suspended from the back of the sternum, thereby lifting it off the trachea. (4) Anomalous right subclavian artery is rarely symptomatic, although it can cause symptoms in later life. Division of the subclavian artery as it arises from the first part of the descending thoracic aorta relieves the constriction and pressure on the back of the oesophagus. (5) Anomalous left pulmonary artery is treated by detachment of this vessel from the right side of the pulmonary artery and reanastomosing it to the left side of the main pulmonary artery.

Results

There should be no hospital mortality.

Atrial septal defect (secundum)

This anomaly is characterised by absence of part of the atrial septum. Patients with this defect are usually asymptomatic in childhood and the indication for operation is the presence of a large left–right shunt which, if left untreated, can cause pulmonary vascular obstructive disease. Closure of this defect is usually carried out before school age, even if the patient is asymptomatic.

Atrial septal defects are divided according to their position in the atrial septum.

1   Secundum defects in which there is deficiency of the septum secundum (Fig 30.9; lower defect).
2   Sinus venosus defects in which there is abnormal drainage of the right pulmonary veins such that they drain into the right atrium (Fig 30.9; upper defect).

Intracardiac repair is performed through a right atriotomy. With secundum atrial septal defects it is often possible to close the defect by direct suture. In sinus venosus defects the atrial incision extends into the right lateral aspect of the superior vena cava and a baffle is placed to divert blood from the anomalously positioned right pulmonary veins into the left atrium.

Results

The operative mortality for all types of atrial septal defects is less than 2%.

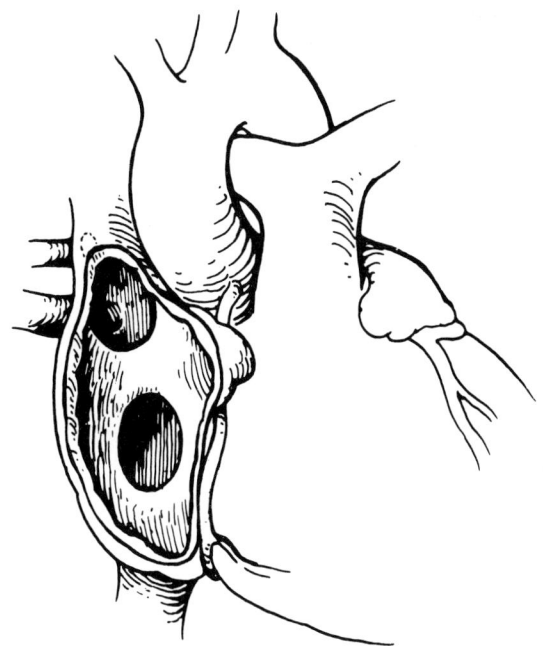

Fig 30.9 Atrial septal defects; right atrium opened. Sinus venosus defect at upper end of atrium; ostium secundum defect in middle of atrium.

Ventricular septal defect

Patients with this anomaly are symptomatic because of excessive pulmonary blood flow due to a large left-to-right shunt. Patients can undergo palliation or primary correction of this defect. In patients with a single ventricular septal defect a primary repair is performed at all ages. In those patients with multiple ventricular septal defects, when seen in early infancy, pulmonary artery banding is appropriate.

Treatment

Palliation, banding of the main pulmonary artery reduces the blood flow to the lungs and is reserved for small patients with multiple ventricular septal defects.

In infancy, isolated ventricular septal defects can usually be closed via the right atrium and tricuspid valve, thereby avoiding an incision in the right ventricle and the possible sequel of right ventricular failure. The defect must be closed by means of a patch, since there is an absolute deficiency in the ventricular septum and it is not possible to close the defect by direct suture.

The hospital mortality for this condition is 0–5%.

Tetralogy of Fallot

Patients with this condition are symptomatic because of cyanosis and polycythaemia, secondary to obstruction of flow of blood to the lungs from the right ventricle and the shunting of blood from right to left of the heart.

Young age, body surface area, high haematocrit and the need to enlarge the pulmonary valve annulus are risk factors to be considered when planning total repair.

The anatomical features of Fallot's tetralogy are a large ventricular septal defect, anterior displacement of the infundibular septum of the right ventricle, hypertrophy of the muscle bands of the right ventricle, pulmonary valve stenosis and rightward shift of the root of the aorta.

Treatment

Patients with tetralogy of Fallot can be palliated by means of a systemic artery/pulmonary artery shunt or can undergo one-stage total correction. Total correction in infancy is dependent upon the anatomy of the main right and left pulmonary arteries.

Successful intracardiac repair of tetralogy of Fallot must fulfil the following criteria:

1 The ventricular septal defect or defects must be securely closed.
2 Right ventricular outflow tract obstruction must be relieved at ventricular pulmonary valve and pulmonary artery level; and
3 The myocardium must be preserved from prolonged ischaemia or damage to the coronary arteries.

Because of the extreme variation in the anatomy of the main pulmonary artery and the pulmonary valve ring, it is sometimes necessary to enlarge this vessel by means of a gusset. In addition, it is not always possible to resect anteriorly and so relieve the obstruction to the outflow of blood from the right ventricle into the pulmonary artery. A gusset can also be placed in the right ventriculotomy to overcome this obstruction. The ventricular septal defect is closed by means of a patch of dacron. Since the placement of this patch is in the region of atrioventricular conducting tissue, knowledge of the conducting tissue is obligatory for surgical closure, as damage can result in heart block. A satisfactory early and late postoperative course is associated with a right ventricular/left ventricular peak systolic pressure ratio below 0.75 after correction.

In 2% of patients the anterior descending coronary artery is supplied by a large branch from the right coronary artery, which crosses the right ventricular outflow tract. In this case, obstruction to outflow from the right ventricle into the pulmonary artery must be relieved by means of an external tube conduit, since division of this anomalous artery would cause fatal ischaemia of the left ventricle (Fig 30.10).

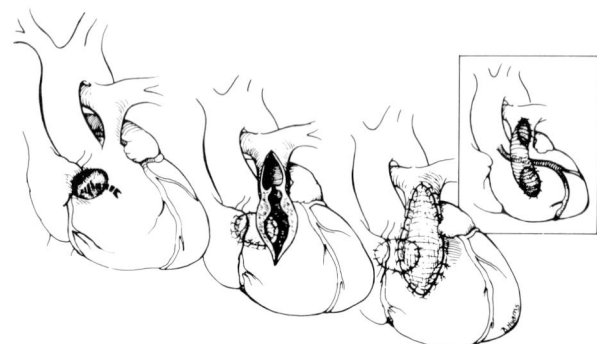

Fig 30.10   Tetralogy of Fallot; stages in correction. Patch closure of interventricular defect and patch enlargement of right ventricular outflow tract. *Inset* shows alternative management of outflow tract by external conduit in presence of abnormal coronary artery.

Results

Corrective treatment in this condition carries up to 8% mortality in children and around 20% in infants.

Pulmonary atresia with ventricular septal defect

Patients with this condition have symptoms similar to those with tetralogy of Fallot. This defect can be considered an extreme form of tetralogy of Fallot.

In this defect there may be hypoplastic right and left pulmonary arteries and there is usually discontinuity between the right ventricle and the main pulmonary artery according to the degree of severity of the condition.

Treatment

A palliative systemic artery/pulmonary artery shunt allows relief of symptoms and encourages growth of the hypoplastic pulmonary arteries. Palliation is performed early in life, correction being possible around the age of 5–8 years. Total correction is carried out along the same principle as in tetralogy of Fallot. Since there is right ventricular pulmonary artery discontinuity, it is nearly always necessary to reconnect them, using an external valved conduit. There are frequently very large systemic artery/pulmonary artery collateral vessels present, which must be ligated before corrective surgery is performed. Failure to ligate these very large vessels can result in high output cardiac failure, which increases the postoperative morbidity.

Results

The hospital mortality for the treatment of this complex form of heart disease is 25%.

Double outlet right ventricle

In this condition, in which both great arteries arise from the morphological right ventricle, a ventricular septal defect must be present for survival of the patient.

Patients with double outlet ventricle may be symptomatic early in life, because of increased pulmonary blood flow in which banding of the main pulmonary artery can be carried out, as a palliative procedure, or decreased pulmonary blood flow, in which case a systemic artery/pulmonary artery anastomosis can be performed. Total correction is performed at a later date before the age of 4 years.

Results

The hospital mortality for this condition ranges from 10–30%.

Transposition of the great arteries

In *classical* transposition of the great arteries the anomaly causes cyanosis which leads to the patients becoming symptomatic. In classical complete transposition of the great arteries, the atria and ventricles are normally connected, atrioventricular concordance, but the aorta arises from the right ventricle and the pulmonary artery from the left ventricle. There may or may not be an intra-atrial communication.

Treatment

Most patients are seen in early infancy when they are usually successfully palliated by means of a balloon atrial septostomy allowing interatrial mixing of the blood.

Operative correction can be accomplished by using either the Mustard operation or the Senning operation. Intracardiac repair in both consists of rerouting the systemic and pulmonary venous return at atrial level by means of a baffle, so that the systemic venous blood empties into the left ventricle via the mitral valve and thence to the pulmonary artery, and the pulmonary venous blood exits into the right ventricle via the tricuspid valve and thence into the aorta. The two circulations are then separate. In Mustard's operation pericardium or synthetic material is used for the baffle, but in the Senning operation it is not necessary (Fig 30.11).

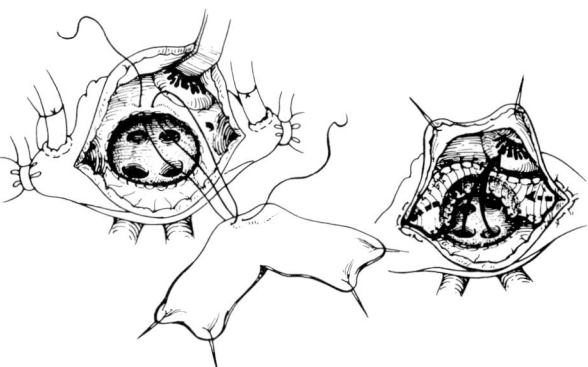

Fig 30.11 Classical complete transposition; right atrium opened. Stages in Mustard procedure. *Left:* attachment of pericardial patch. *Right:* patch completed. Pulmonary venous blood arrowed to tricuspid valve.

Results

The hospital mortality for this condition is 2–5%.

Transposition with ventricular septal defect

Early surgical repair is indicated in these patients to avoid the risk of pulmonary vascular obstructive disease. These patients are usually not cyanosed because there is mixing and an increased flow of blood to the lungs.

Intracardiac repair is carried out by using either the Mustard or Senning operation and closing the ventricular septal defect via the tricuspid valve.

An alternative procedure is the anatomical correction whereby the great arteries are switched with reimplantation of the coronary arteries as described by Jatene. So far this procedure has only been successful when applied to patients in whom the left ventricle has been pumping at systemic pressures (Fig 30.12).

Results

The hospital mortality for this condition ranges from 5–20%. With the repositioning of the great arteries the mortality is around 30%.

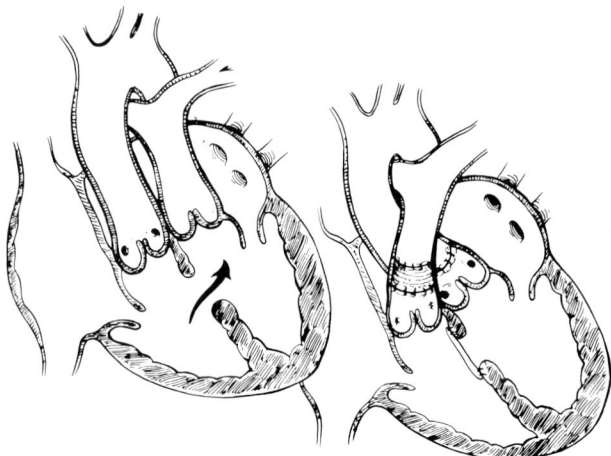

Fig 30.12 Transposition of the great arteries with ventricular septal defect. Jatene procedure for arterial switch and closure of ventricular septal defect.

Transposition with ventricular septal defect and pulmonary stenosis

These patients are symptomatic because of cyanosis. The pulmonary stenosis is usually subvalvar. Pulmonary valve stenosis is rare in this condition.

Treatment

Radical operation is not performed below the age of 5 years and patients are palliated when seen early in life by means of systemic artery/pulmonary artery shunt. Intracardiac repair is accomplished by closure of the ventricular septal defect in such a way as to connect the aorta to the left ventricle. The pulmonary artery is closed off at pulmonary valve level and the right ventricle is reconnected to the distal main pulmonary artery by means of an external valve tube conduit incorporated in the original right ventriculotomy.

Results

The mortality for this condition is 15–25%.

Congenitally corrected transposition of the great arteries

The anatomy of this anomaly is characterised by atrioventricular discordance whereby the normally placed right atrium is connected to a right-sided morphologically left ventricle which gives rise to the pulmonary artery, and the left atrium empties into a left-sided morphological right ventricle which gives rise to the aorta. If there are no intracardiac septal defects, these patients may live a normal lifespan without any symptoms. The anatomical arrangement of the intracardiac conducting system is abnormal and complete heart block may occur at any age. If there is a ventricular septal defect with or without pulmonary valvar or subvalvar stenosis, these patients may be symptomatic: a restriction of pulmonary blood flow causes cyanosis, or excessive pulmonary blood flow causes pulmonary congestion.

Treatment

This entails closure of the ventricular septal defect by means of a patch placed on the left side of the septum in order to avoid the abnormally placed conducting tissue. Pulmonary stenosis must be relieved by means of an external tube conduit since resection of subvalvar pulmonary stenosis will damage the conducting tissue.

Results

The hospital mortality of this condition is 10–20%.

Atrioventricular defect

This spectrum of anomalies is due to a deficiency of the atrioventricular septum and is variable in degree. The partial form is characterised by an interatrial communication and a cleft due to abnormal alignment between the anterior and the septal mitral valve leaflets. This cleft causes regurgitation in about 30% of individuals. The complete form of the defect has a ventricular septal defect as well and the mitral and tricuspid valves may be incompletely separated, so that a common atrioventricular orifice is present.

Treatment

In partial atrioventricular defects, palliation is inappropriate and one-stage corrective surgery is performed when operation is necessary, regardless of age. Closure of the cleft in the mitral valve may not be required if the mitral valve is competent. Attempts at complete closure of this cleft may produce either mitral stenosis or, by drawing together the anterior leaflet, may produce more mitral regurgitation than the patient already has. Experience with this condition is crucial in determining the extent of the closure of this cleft. The septal defect is closed with a patch, and mitral valve replacement is avoided in these patients whenever possible (Fig 30.13).

In the complete atrioventricular defect, palliation is also unsatisfactory and the malformation of the mitral

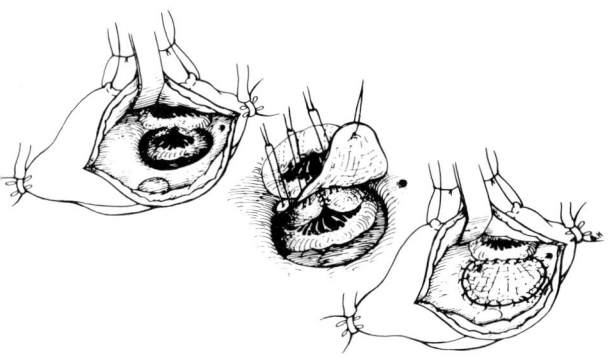

Fig 30.13 Atrioventricular defect (partial); right atrium opened. Left-to-right closure of cleft and reconstruction of interatrial defect with patch.

and tricuspid valves may be so severe that curative treatment is difficult and sometimes impossible. The mitral and tricuspid valves must be refashioned from the common valve tissue and the atrioventricular septum reconstructed in such a way as to leave the mitral valve completely on the left of the septum and the tricuspid valve completely on the right, with attachment of these valves to the new septum. Right ventricular outflow tract obstruction is not uncommon in the complete form of the defect, especially in Downs syndrome. Left ventricular outflow tract obstruction may also be present and require treatment.

Results

Hospital mortality of this complex form of congenital heart disease varies from 15–40%.

Pulmonary and aortic valve stenosis

Critical stenosis of one or other of these valves can occur in infancy requiring emergency valvotomy. Frequently the valve tissues are grossly myxomatous and malformed, and can be bicuspid or quadricuspid. Surgery of this defect in early infancy is unrewarding.

Valve stenoses in childhood and thereafter are more easily treated with a greater degree of success. It is unusual for patients to require valve replacement.

Results

The hospital mortality for this condition in childhood is 0–6%, but in infants ranges from 20–40%.

Total anomalous pulmonary venous connexion

Patients with this anomaly are typically seen in early infancy and are usually critically ill due to pulmonary plethora. In this defect the pulmonary veins do not enter into the left atrium and there may be pulmonary venous obstruction or excessive blood flow to the right heart. Palliation is not appropriate with this anomaly.

There are three anatomical types:

1   Intracardiac type of TAPVC

In this the pulmonary veins drain into the right atrium, usually by way of the coronary sinus.

Treatment

The coronary sinus is opened by cutting back its superior wall, thereby opening into the atrial septal defect which may or may not be present. An intra-atrial baffle is placed to incorporate the ostium of the coronary sinus into the atrial septal defect, thereby directing the pulmonary venous blood into the left atrium.

2   Supracardiac type of TAPVC

In this type the horizontal collecting vein is placed retropericardially and is immediately posterior to the posterior surface of the wall of the left atrium, but not connected to the left atrium. The horizontal collecting vein drains into the persistent left superior vena cava which, in turn, drains directly to the innominate vein and thence to the right superior vena cava.

Treatment

An incision in the anterior surface of the horizontal collecting vein and the posterior surface of the wall of the left atrium is made and these two are anastomosed, thus allowing free communication between the collecting vein and the left atrial chamber.

3   Infracardiac type of TAPVC

The common collecting vein is retropericardial, but in the vertical plane.

Treatment

As in the supracardiac type, an anastomosis is constructed between the front of the vertical collecting vein and the back of the left atrium.

Results

The hospital mortality of the treatment of these conditions is from 20–50%.

Tricuspid atresia

Cyanosis with poor exercise tolerance is the common presentation in patients with this form of congenital heart disease.

The anatomical abnormality of absence of the right atrioventricular valve with underdevelopment of the right ventricular cavity is such that both a ventricular septal defect and an atrial septal defect must be present to allow survival.

Treatment

When diagnosis is made early in life, following cardiac catheterisation, palliation is performed by constructing a systemic artery/pulmonary artery anastomosis to allow an increase in blood flow to the lungs.

Corrective surgery can be achieved by anastomosing the right atrial appendage to the main pulmonary artery by means of an external valved conduit, at the same time closing the atrial septal defect. In carefully selected patients with ideal haemodynamics this operation can achieve a great improvement in the patient's condition (Fig 30.14).

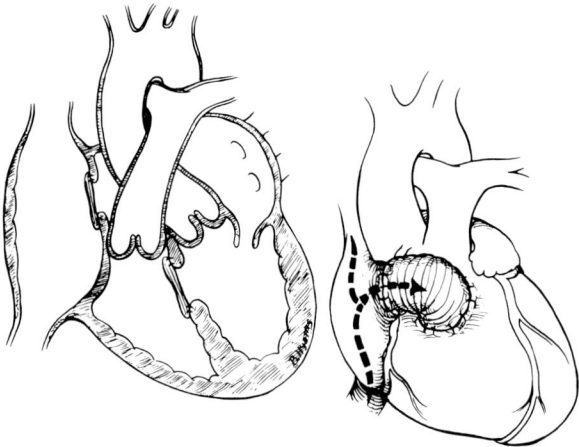

Fig 30.14   Tricuspid artesia. *Left*: patch closure of interatrial and interventricular defects. *Note* atretic tricuspid valve. *Right*: right auricle joined to right ventricular outflow tract by external conduit (Fontan procedure).

Results

The hospital mortality for this operation is between 5–10%.

Truncus arteriosus

The anatomy of this condition is such that there is a common arterial trunk as opposed to discrete pulmonary artery and aorta. The pulmonary arteries arise from the back of the common arterial trunk.

Treatment

This depends upon the detaching of the pulmonary artery or arteries from the back of the common arterial trunk, the reanastomosing of the right ventricle to the confluence of the pulmonary arteries, and the closing of the ventricular septal defect. The continuity between the right ventricle and pulmonary artery is achieved by means of an external valved tube conduit (Fig 30.15).

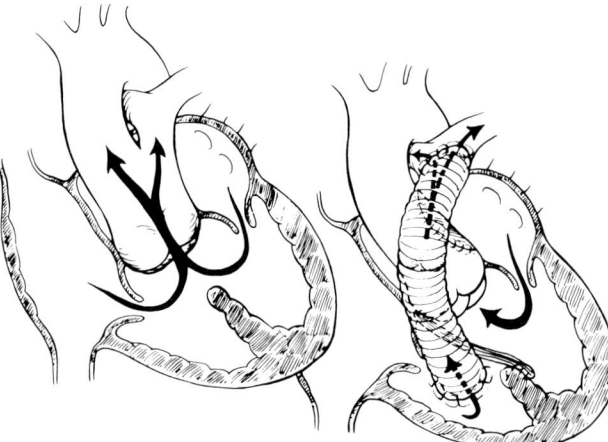

Fig 30.15   Truncus arteriosus. Closure of interventricular defect and external valved conduit from right ventricle to main pulmonary artery. Origin of pulmonary artery from common trunk closed by a patch.

Results

The hospital mortality for this condition is 20–30%.

Ebstein's malformation

A wide range of anatomic variation of right ventricle and tricuspid valve can be encountered in this malformation. Most have a displaced and hypoplastic septal and posterior leaflet of the tricuspid valve, and an enlarged anterolateral leaflet. 'Atrialised' segments of the right ventricle, deficiency of the anterior leaflet of the tricuspid valve, and abnormal papillary muscle and chordae can also occur. It is also commonly seen as part of congenitally corrected transposition in which there is atrioventricular discordance.

Treatment

The aim in the surgical correction is to obtain a competent tricuspid valve, allowing forward flow of blood from the right ventricle to the pulmonary artery without damage to the conducting tissue. Surgical treatment aims at annuloplastic repair of the tricuspid valve, with excision of redundant right atrial tissue. Valve replacement is avoided where possible.

Results

The results of surgery for this condition are poor. Complications of surgery include rhythm disturbances due to accessory atrioventricular conducting pathways, damage to the atrioventricular conducting tissue, and residual tricuspid valve incompetence. The hospital mortality for this condition is 20–30%.

Further reading

Anderson R.H., Arnold R., Wilkinson J.L. (1973). The conducting system in congenitally corrected transposition. *Lancet*; **i**:1286–8.

Becker A.E., Becker M.J., Edwards J.E. (1970). Anomalies associated with coarctation of aorta. Particular reference to infancy. *Circulation*; **41**:1067–75.

Burnell R.H., Ghadiali P.E., Joseph M.C., Paneth M. (1970). Management of critical valvular outflow obstruction in neonates. *Thorax*; **25**:116–19.

Clarke D., deLeval M., Pincott J., Stark J. (1976). Correction of total anomalous pulmonary venous drainage in infancy. *Brit. Heart J*; **38**:879.

Fontan F., Baudet E. (1971). Surgical repair of tricuspid atresia. *Thorax*; **26**:240–8.

Hamilton D.I., Di Eusanio G., Sandrasagra F.A., Donnelly R.J. (1978). Early and late results of aortoplasty with a left subclavian flap for coarctation of the aorta in infancy. *J. Thorac. Cardiovasc. Surg*; **75**:699–704.

Kirklin J., Applebaum A., Bargeron L.M. (1976). Primary repair versus banding for ventricular septal defects in infants. In *The Child with Congenital Heart Disease after Surgery* (Kidd B.S.L., Rowe R.D., eds.). Mount Kisco, New York: Futura Publishing Co Inc: 3–9.

Kirklin J.W., Karp R.B. (1970). *The Tetralogy of Fallot from a Surgical Viewpoint*. Philadelphia: WB Saunders.

Kirklin J.W., Pacifico A.D., Hannah H., Allarde R.R. (1973). Primary definitive intracardiac operations in infants: intraoperative support techniques. In *Advances in Cardiovascular Surgery* (Kirklin J.W., ed.), pp. 85–99. New York: Grune and Stratton.

Lincoln J.C.R., Deverall P.B., Stark J., Aberdeen E., Waterston D.J. (1969). Vascular anomalies compressing the oesophagus and trachea. *Thorax*; **24**:295–306.

Lincoln J.C.R., Jamieson S., Joseph M., Sinebourne E.A., Anderson R.H. (1977). Transatrial repair of ventricular septal defects in relation to their anatomic classification. *J. Thorac. Cardiovasc. Surg*; **74**:183–90.

Lincoln J.C.R., McKay R., Miller G.A.H., Joseph M.C., Sinebourne E.A. (1978). Surgical correction of complete atrioventricular canal in infants and children. *Brit. Heart J*; **40**:451–2.

Marcelletti C., Mair D.D., McGoon D.D., Wallace R.B., Danielson G.K. (1976). The Rastelli operation for transposition of the great arteries. Early and late results. *J. Thorac. Cardiovasc. Surg*; **72**:427–34.

Pennington D.G., Liberthson R.R., Jacobs M., Scully H., Goldblatt A., Daggett W.M. (1979). Critical review of experience with surgical repair of coarctation of the aorta. *J. Thorac. Cardiovasc. Surg*; **77**:217–29.

Stewart R.W., Kirklin J.W., Pacifico A.D., Blackstone E.H., Bargeron L.M. (1979). Repair of double outlet right ventricle. *J. Thorac. Cardiovasc. Surg*; **78**:502–14.

Ullal R.R., Anderson R.H., Lincoln J.C.R. (1979). Mustard's operation modified to avoid disrhythmias and pulmonary and systemic venous obstruction. *J. Thorac. Cardiovasc. Surg*; **78**:431–9.

Wright J.S., Newman D.C. (1978). Ligation of the patent ductus. Technical considerations at different ages. *J. Thorac. Cardiovasc. Surg*; **75**:695–8.

Lungs and trachea

M. PANETH

Bronchial carcinoma

This is the commonest cause of death from cancer in the United Kingdom. In recent years 40% of all cancer deaths in men and 13% in women were due to malignant disease of the respiratory tract. The steady increase in the early part of this century is tending to level off among men, but among older men and among women there is still a steady rise.

There is a strong association with smoking and 90% of lung cancers in men are due to this. The risk of developing the disease increases 25-fold if the consumption of cigarettes reaches 25 per day and there is also an increase in town – as compared with country-populations. Occupational hazards include working with pitchblende, uranium, asbestos, nickel, haematite and contact with gas retorts.

Tumours arise from the bronchial epithelium and consist of four main histological types: *squamous cell carcinomas* account for approximately 50%, are generally fairly well differentiated and comparatively slow growing; *adenocarcinomas* are frequently peripheral in position and probably not related to smoking; *large cell anaplastic* growths are fairly fast growing, but the most aggressive tumour is the *oat cell carcinoma*.

Indications for operation

It is simpler to list the contraindications to operation and it should be remembered that more than 50% of intrathoracic radiological abnormalities which have defied diagnosis before operation are malignant when removed.

Factors not primarily related to the carcinoma

Inadequate cardiac and respiratory reserve

The best and simplest test of combined cardio-respiratory reserve is to walk the patient up a flight of stairs at a normal pace. If he is no more dyspnoeic than his surgeon, then he will probably tolerate a pulmonary resection. In addition, the forced expiratory volume at 1 s (FEV_1) may be estimated as a percentage of his forced vital capacity (FVC). As a good rule an FEV_1 of 1.5 l or more allows the surgeon to resect the whole of one lung provided the patient is of average build.

Advanced cerebral deterioration

Pre- and postoperative physiotherapy requires the willing and active cooperation of the patient. However, actual age is unimportant, the physiological state of the patient being decisive.

Factors directly relating to the presence of the tumour

Local extension

Invasion of the oesophagus. The oesophagus may be directly invaded by the tumour or may be involved secondarily by enlarged mediastinal lymph nodes. Clinically progressive dysphagia suggests inoperability. Direct invasion of the oesophagus by the tumour or by involved lymph nodes as shown by barium examination is a strong contraindication to surgical removal.

Superior caval obstruction may be the first manifestation and is an absolute contraindication to thoracotomy and/or mediastinoscopy by the suprasternal route. Its development is an indication for urgent radiotherapy, usually coupled with heparinisation even in the absence of a positive histological diagnosis. Biopsy is obtained when the caval obstruction has been relived.

Bronchoscopy. 1½ to 2 cm of normal bronchial mucosa above the upper limit of the tumour is allowed on bronchoscopy so as to be clear of the zone of upward infiltration. If in doubt, a number of mucosal biopsies from the proposed line of resection may be taken and their histology awaited before proceeding to thoracotomy.

Invasion of the pericardium may occur. Increases in, or an abnormal shape of, the cardiac silhouette should be investigated by pericardial aspiration. A blood-stained effusion is highly suggestive of invasion, but mere involvement of the pericardium may be treated by wide excision.

Direct invasion of the heart may manifest itself as bouts of supraventricular tachycardia culminating in established atrial fibrillation. Though only a guarded prognosis with regard to resection must be given, it is possible in some patients to resect portions of involved atrial wall.

Pleural effusions should be aspirated and analysed for cells. Pleural effusions are not a contraindication, but a bloodstained effusion should raise suspicion of widespread pleural seeding.

A high ipsilateral diaphragm, confirmed on screening to be due to phrenic nerve paralysis, is an absolute contraindication in the presence of upper lobe tumours. Lower lobe tumours may involve the phrenic nerve as it lies on the pericardium, but resection, taking a wide sweep of the pericardium, will still be possible.

Paralysis of the left recurrent laryngeal nerve, as it passes around the ligamentum arteriosum, is an absolute contraindication since neither the left bronchus nor the left main pulmonary artery will be safely accessible for resection.

Involvement of the brachial plexus (superior sulcus or Pancoast tumour). Pain along the distribution of the first and second thoracic dermatomes together with evidence of involvement of the cervical sympathetic chain giving a Horner's syndrome is due to perineural invasion. These tumours are usually slow growing and, by the time they give rise to pain, have extended too far to be successfully resected. Pain is probably best relieved by tractotomy.

Distant extension

Brain, bony skeleton and liver. The brain, the bony skeleton and the liver are the commonest sites for secondary deposits; x-rays and CAT scanning aid diagnosis. Changes in behaviour pattern and biochemical alteration of liver enzymes may arouse suspicion. Fixed bone pain, even without radiological evidence, is suggestive of involvement. Isotope uptake may indicate more widespread bony involvement.

Adrenal deposits are common, but evidence of adrenal insufficiency is difficult to obtain. Inappropriate hormone secretion may interfere with potassium and water balance, *see* chapter on adrenal surgery.

Direct invasion

Direct invasion of the chest wall is not a contraindication to thoracotomy since a wide excision of the ribs together with their intercostal muscles and neurovascular bundles is possible, especially if the resulting defect of the chest wall will be covered by the scapula, as is often the case. Similarly, enlarged and involved paratracheal nodes can be excised en bloc, provided they are not fixed.

There are a number of non-metastatic extrathoracic manifestations which are not, by themselves, contraindications to operation. They may be listed thus:

Finger clubbing, also seen in empyema.

Hypertrophic pulmonary osteoarthropathy which may be painful, especially at night and is dramatically relieved by removal of the primary tumour.

Inappropriate vasopressor, ectopic ACTH and parathyroid hormone secretion which are rare. Gynaecomastia, thyrotoxicosis and hypoglycaemia can also occur.

Dementia, peripheral neuropathy, myopathy, myasthenia and cerebellar ataxia which are not necessarily due to direct central nervous system involvement.

Radiotherapy

The place of radiotherapy in the treatment of carcinoma of the bronchus is not yet fully defined, response to this treatment depending on cell type. Adenocarcinomas are virtually radioresistant, the oat cell type highly sensitive, while the squamous variety occupy a position between these.

On the whole, radiotherapy should be reserved for palliation of symptoms such as pain from bony deposits, superior caval obstruction, intracranial deposits, haemoptyses and obstruction to main bronchi or trachea. Reports of five-year recurrence-free survival following radiation are so few that this form of treatment should not be advised as an alternative to resection, but its place as palliative treatment is well established. Radiotherapy does not prolong life, but can improve its quality.

Although it was hoped that preoperative radiotherapy would improve survival after resection, this has not been shown to be true; and against its use is the higher incidence of postoperative complications, especially bronchopleural fistula, which undoubtedly offsets any potential benefit. The same arguments apply to its routine use postoperatively, except in patients where the line of bronchial division has shown microscopic submucosal or peribronchial infiltration and there is no evidence of distant metastases. Local high dose exposure to the region of the bronchial stump is then indicated.

The question of whether radiotherapy should be given to patients in whom involved lobar, hilar and/or mediastinal lymph nodes have been excised, cannot be answered, since properly conducted trials have not been carried out.

Preoperative radiotherapy is indicated in the rare case where the origin of the tumour is too close to the highest possible line of resection, but the tumour is still almost entirely intrabronchial. Radical x-ray treatment, especially for the squamous variety, will quite often reduce the tumour to such an extent that a clear bronchial division often coupled with a 'sleeve' resection, can be performed.

Chemotherapy

What has been said for radiotherapy applies even more to chemotherapy since the side-effects are severe and present a definite risk to life.

Preoperative investigations and preparation

Radiography

The routine PA and lateral x-rays of the chest should be supported by tomograms which clearly define any opacity in the lungs and indicate whether it is solitary or associated with others – possibly hidden behind the cardiac shadow. Tomography can analyse the composite shadows which make up the mediastinum and may have to be taken in two planes. Bronchography is rarely indicated, but may occasionally be necessary to outline the bronchi in relation to a pulmonary opacity which has resisted all other forms of diagnosis.

CAT and other scans are not yet used routinely.

Sputum cytology

This should be used routinely analysing three consecutive early morning samples of sputum. An accuracy of 80% is claimed by some units.

Cytology of secretions aspirated from the appropriate bronchus at the time of bronchoscopy will also frequently give positive results.

Bronchoscopy

It is axiomatic that no operation on the respiratory system should be undertaken until this investigation has been performed. Preferably the surgeon performing the thoracotomy should also do the bronchoscopy, but some bronchoscopy clinics are staffed by chest physicians. The popularity of fibreoptic instruments has given added scope, since this instrument is passed under local anaesthesia, whereas general anaesthesia is the rule for conventional bronchoscopy.

The advantages of the fibreoptic system are that it can be more easily used and that the bronchial tree can be inspected beyond its secondary divisions and therefore provides biopsies from peripheral tumours. On the other hand, the rigid instrument provides vital information as to the mobility of the bronchial tree at the proposed line of resection; fixity at this level means that there is extensive peribronchial infiltration.

Aspiration needle biopsy

This is also being used with increasing frequency and confidence, since the theoretical danger of implanting malignant cells along the needle track has not been found to exist in practice.

The investigation is performed under x-ray screen control and the aspirate is obtained with a wide-bore needle under local anaesthesia, is immediately transferred to a slide and fixed by the histologist. Positive results are helpful, but a negative result should not be taken as an indication that thoracotomy is not necessary since, even in skilled hands, the aspirate may not have been obtained from the peripheral tumour, but from the lung immediately adjacent to it.

Mediastinoscopy/mediastinotomy

This investigation is performed to obtain diagnostic tissue from the superior mediastinum on either side (Figs 31.1; 31.2a,b,c). In some centres it is used routinely to assess operability and thoracotomy is not undertaken if the ipsilateral paratracheal lymph nodes show malignant infiltration. This investigation is not used by the author to assess operability, since good tomography of the mediastinum will demonstrate enlarged lymph nodes. In his experience there is still a worthwhile, albeit small, chance of recurrence-free survival, even if these nodes are involved, provided they are removed by block dissection.

Either route of exploration is applicable, but by excising the appropriate 2nd or 3rd costal cartilage the exposure is better and the procedure is safer than by the suprasternal route.

Pleural aspiration and biopsy

Pleural effusions may be due to (a) pleural involvement by a peripheral tumour, or (b) collapse/consolidation of a part of the lung distal to a central tumour.

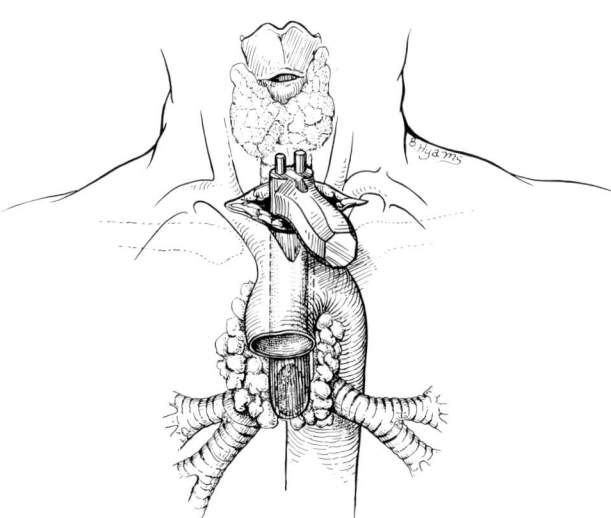

Fig 31.1 Mediastinoscopy. This shows the relationship of the mediastinoscope to the aorta and its branches, and the extent of the lymphatic region which can be reached for biopsy.

Pleural involvement by growth should be suspected if the effusion is large, uniformly blood-stained and reaccumulates rapidly, even if malignant cells are not found in it. When in doubt, thoracoscopy or even a small, limited thoracotomy may provide evidence of involvement of the parietal pleura.

Pleuropneumonectomy gives disappointing results; and this operation is not advised. If the effusion causes cardiorespiratory embarrassment, pleurodesis may be effected by the instillation of talc or nitrogen mustard and temporary intercostal underwater seal drainage with suction.

Lymph node biopsy

Lymphatic metastatic spread from the lung and pleura ultimately reaches the scalene nodes, most commonly on the right. If such nodes are palpably enlarged they should be excised, preferably under general anaesthesia, and their involvement is an absolute contraindication to thoracotomy since the malignant process has now extended beyond the hemithorax. The same applies to subcutaneous nodules.

Axillary lymph nodes will only become involved when the tumour has invaded the chest wall; they can be removed en-bloc at the time of operation together with the involved portion of the thoracic cage, the invading tumour and its lobe of origin.

General preoperative preparation

The patient should be prepared for the operation both mentally and physically. Attention should be paid to hydration, renal and hepatic function and correction of anaemia.

Physiotherapy must be initiated preoperatively since many patients are unable to breathe effectively. Postoperative breathing exercises are vital to an uneventful recovery and instruction in their performance must precede the operation including diaphragmatic breathing, coughing and leg exercises. Broad spectrum antibiotic cover using two antibiotics simultaneously for a period of 6 days, starting 12 h before operation is routine.

Finally, particular attention should be paid to any loose teeth which are at risk during bronchoscopy and intubation.

Operative technique

After intubation, a central venous line for rapid fluid and blood replacement is inserted and after the ECG skin electrodes have been attached, the patient is turned onto his side with the involved hemithorax uppermost. Pelvic and anterior chest supports with a pelvic strap stabilise the position. The upper arm is

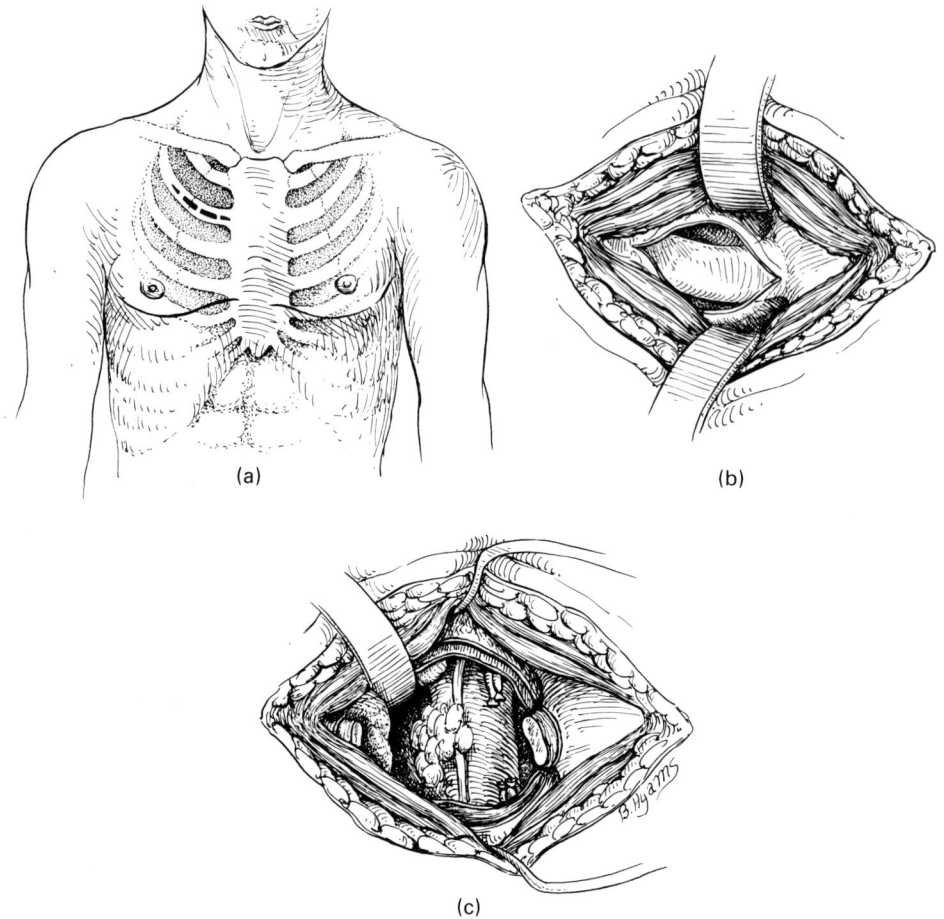

Fig 31.2 Anterior mediastinotomy. (a) The skin incision based on the right (or left) 2nd costal cartilage. (b) Excision of the 2nd costal cartilage. (c) The internal mammary pedicle has been divided, the pleura reflected laterally and the lymph nodes biopsied.

pulled forwards and upwards and strapped in position. This will pull the scapula forwards and upwards and allow more space for the incision.

Anteriorly, the 5th costo-chondral junction marks the anterior limit of the incision and is identified by counting the ribs from below upwards.

For a lower thoracotomy (6th or 7th rib) the skin incision is simply placed an appropriate rib space lower in front and extends a few centimetres lower at the back.

For lesser procedures, such as pleurodesis or lung biopsy, a small incision, parallel to the ribs in the ausculatory triangle may be used with minimal division of the muscles; or for anterior mediastinal exposure, a submammary incision extending posteriorly to the anterior border of the latissimus dorsi and dividing the

pectoralis major with splitting of the fibres of the 5th digitation of the serratus magnus gives a very satisfactory exposure.

For a satisfactory resection of malignant tumours of the bronchi it is important to have an understanding of the lymphatic drainage of the lung, because en-bloc dissection is still considered to be the best procedure.

Each lung has a lymphatic sump into which the lobar lymph nodes drain. The lymphatic sump of the right lung consists of a group of nodes situated below and behind the right upper lobe bronchus and also surrounding the intermediate bronchus below this level, but above the origin of the apical lower segmental bronchus and middle lobe bronchus. All three lobes of the right lung drain into this sump, but the right upper lobe does not drain below this level, whereas the right middle and lower lobes may drain higher up than the sump level. Tumours of the right side will spread to the right superior tracheobronchial group of nodes and from there to the paratracheal nodes and, finally, to the right scalene nodes.

On the left side the lymphatic sump lies in the greater fissure and consists of nodes lying between the upper and lower lobe bronchi as well as those situated behind the pulmonary artery just before it enters the greater fissure. From this sump spread will occur equally frequently to the subcarinal and paratracheal nodes on the right as on the left side. Lower lobe carcinomas on either side may involve the nodes in the pulmonary ligament and the paraoesophageal group.

Figures 31.3 and 31.4 indicate the extent of block dissection of the superior mediastinum on the right and left sides respectively. On the right side, the azygos arch is divided: the anterior limit is the line of the phrenic nerve unless this is deliberately sacrificed because of extension anterior to it; superiorly the thoracic inlet is exposed containing the origin of the right subclavian

artery and posteriorly the oesophagus forms the boundary.

On the left, the arch of the aorta forms the posterior and superior limits of the dissection and the phrenic nerve is again the anterior limit. In front of the arch and above it one may expose the left innominate vein in an extended high dissection if this is indicated for the removal of lymph nodes along the phrenic nerve.

Once the chest has been entered and the rib spreader opened, resectability should be further assessed by visual inspection of the major surrounding viscera and by palpation of the hilum. As a first step, it is good practice to secure the venous pedicle, since manipulation of the tumour-bearing area may result in haematogenous spread. The pericardium is opened longitudinally, usually behind the phrenic nerve and the pulmonary vein(s) is/are ligated in continuity. In the case of the right upper lobe, the superior pulmonary vein, exclusive of its middle lobe tributary, is secured outside the pericardium. Intrapericardial dissection of the venous pedicles is easier, safer and quicker. If the

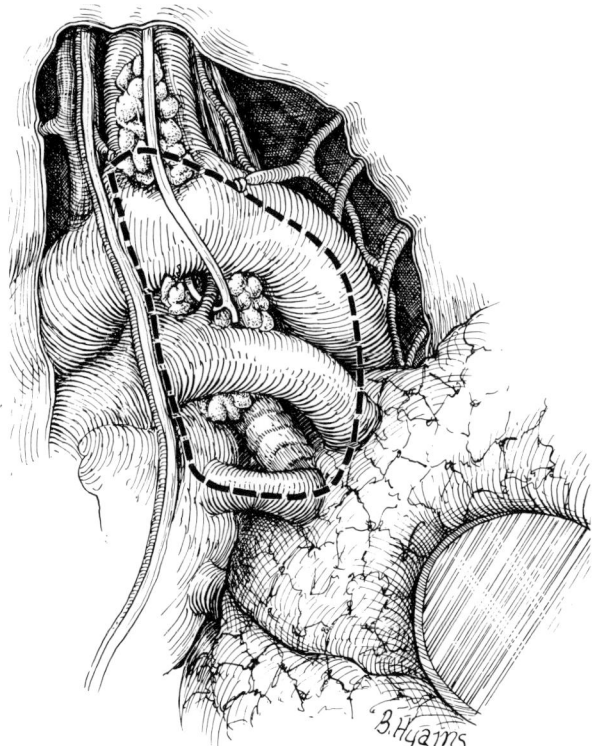

Fig 31.3 Right block dissection. The extent of the superior mediastinal block dissection on the right is indicated. *Note* that the azygos arch has been divided and that the right recurrent laryngeal nerve is frequently identified superiorly.

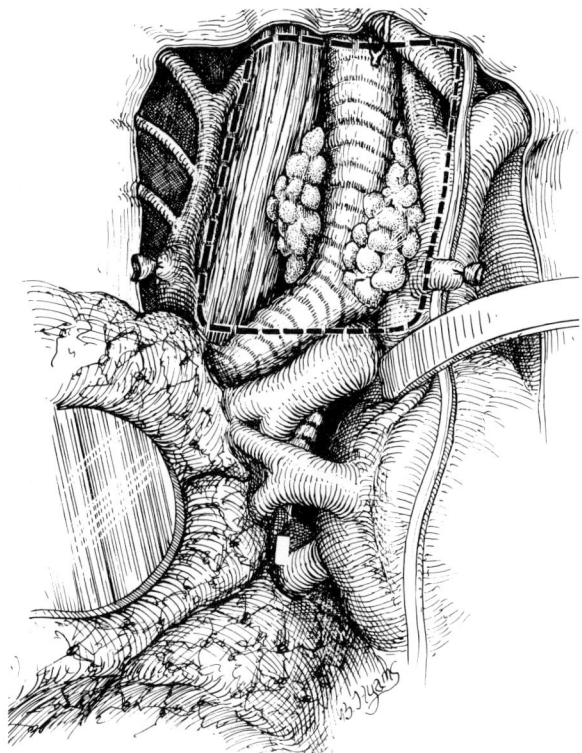

Fig 31.4 Left block dissection. The extent of the superior mediastinal block dissection on the left is indicated. *Note* that the left recurrent laryngeal nerve is always exposed and that superiorly the dissection extends to the origin of the head vessels and left innominate vein (not shown).

histological diagnosis has not been made pre-operatively, a frozen section biopsy of any suspicious areas is next obtained.

The technique of pneumonectomy and lobectomy is best conveyed in Figs 31.5 to 31.10.

Results

About 50% of patients presenting for treatment are inoperable from the outset; at exploratory thoracotomy a further 50% are found to have a lesion too extensive for 'curative' resection. Thus of the original group only 25% have resection with hope of cure; of these only about one-third are alive at 5 years. Thus in a large series only 8–10% of those originally presenting are 5-year survivors.

Involvement of lymphnodes reduces survival rate. Oat cell and anaplastic tumours have a very poor operative survival and some authors prefer radio-therapy for these. Small, solitary peripheral lesions have the best prognosis with a 5-year survival of about 50%.

(*continued* on p. 470)

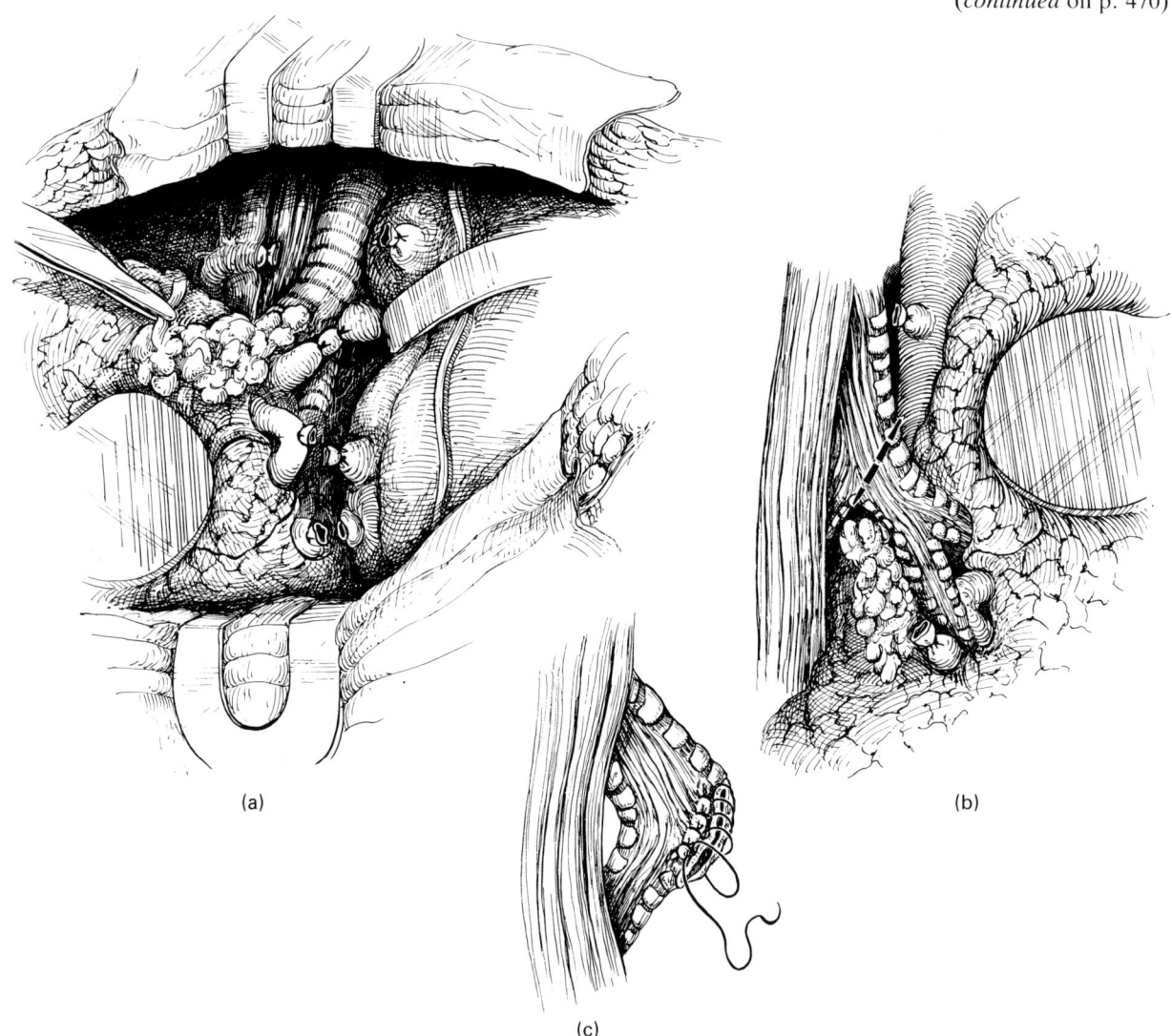

(a)

(b)

(c)

Fig 31.5 Right pneumonectomy. (a) The superior mediastinal block dissection has been completed and the right pulmonary artery is doubly tied and transfixed prior to its division. (b) The origin of the right main bronchus and its line of division. (c) Technique of bronchial closure by vertical mattress sutures and a covering over-and-over running suture.

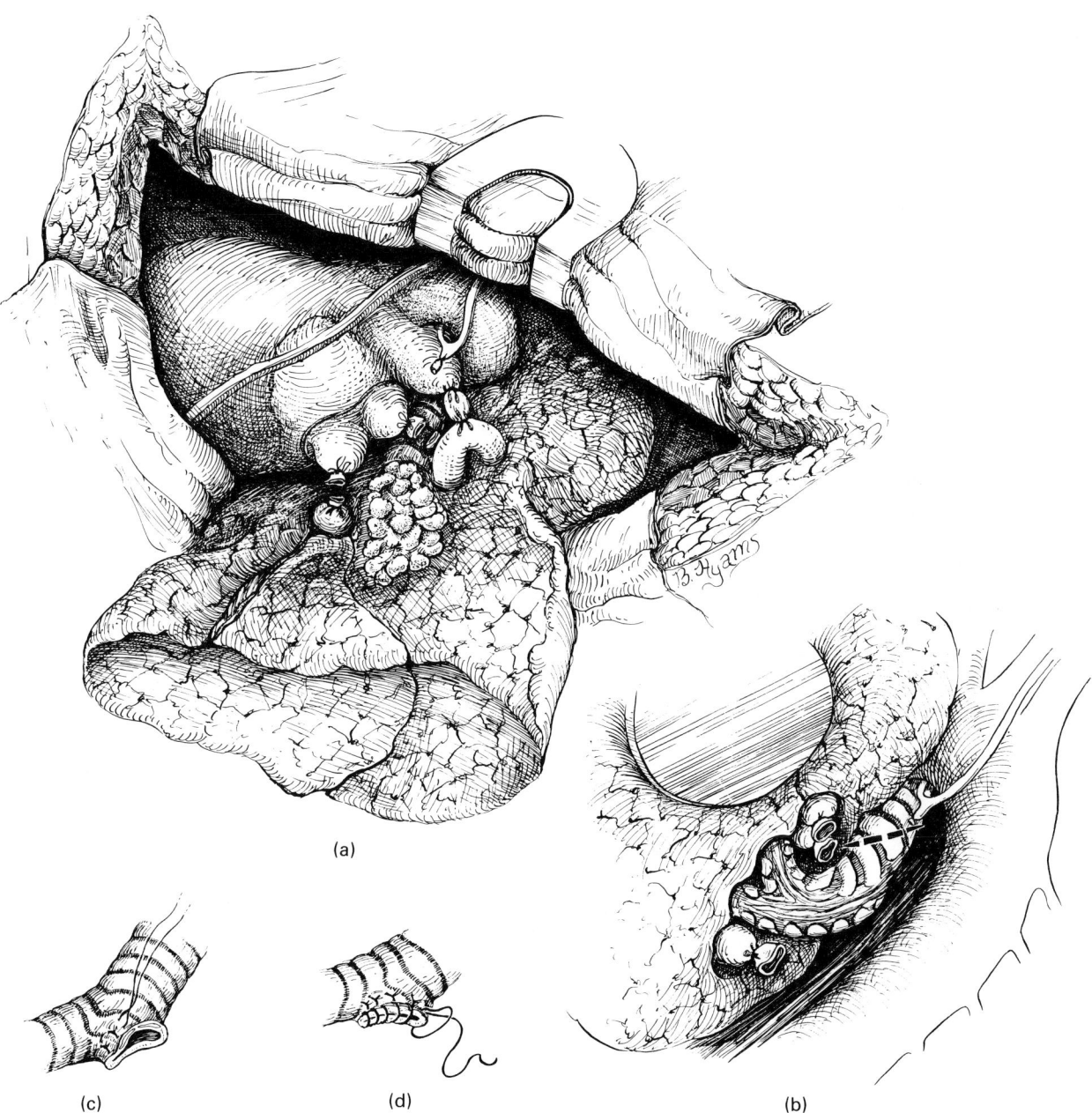

(a)

(c)   (d)   (b)

Fig 31.6   Left pneumonectomy. (a) The superior mediastinal block dissection has been completed, the left pulmonary veins divided inside the pericardium and the left main pulmonary artery has been doubly ligated and transfixed prior to its division. (b) Exposure of origin of the left main bronchus and its line of division. (c) Technique of closure of left main bronchus with interrupted vertical mattress sutures (d) covered by a continuous over-and-over suture.

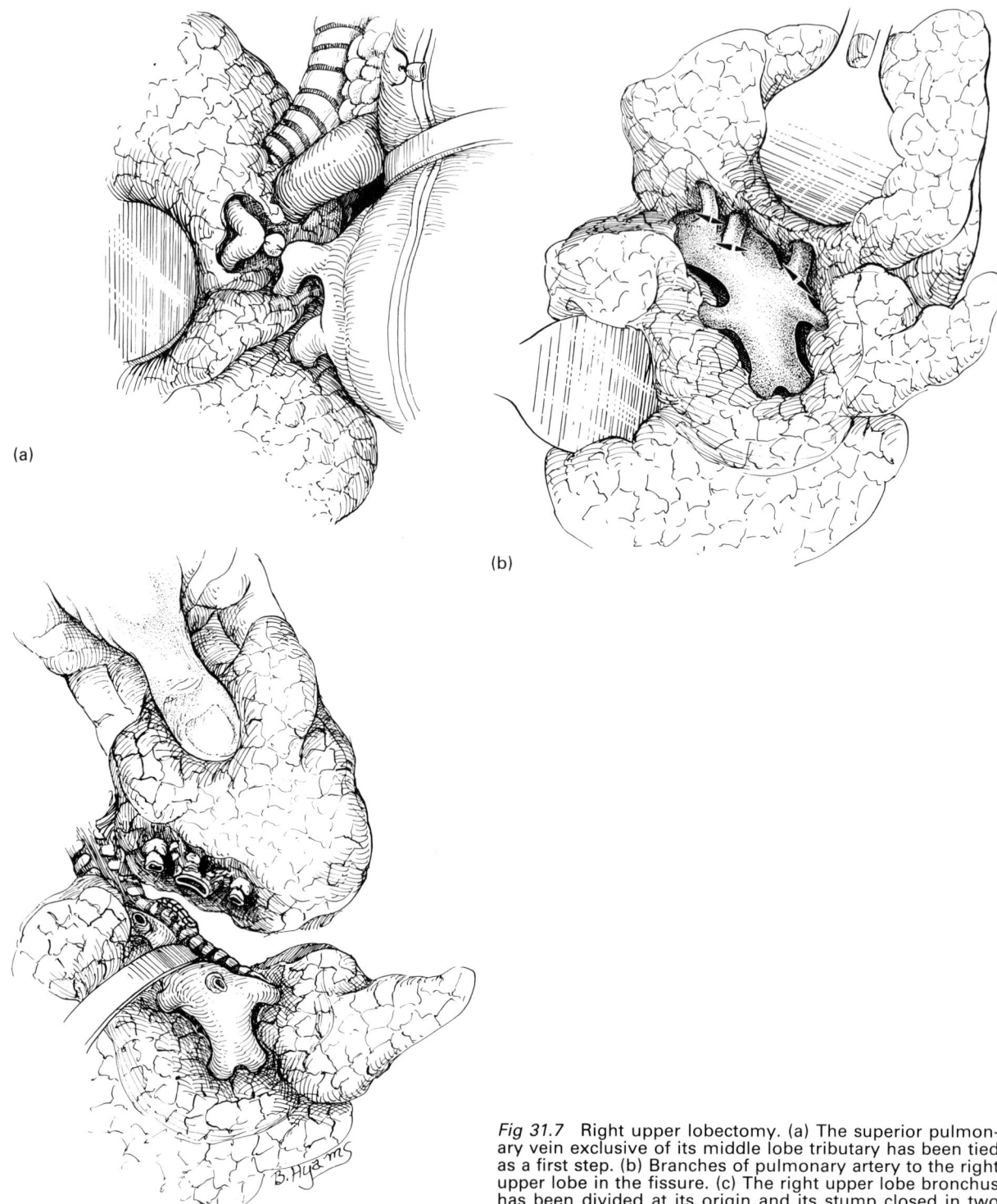

(a)

(b)

(c)

Fig 31.7 Right upper lobectomy. (a) The superior pulmonary vein exclusive of its middle lobe tributary has been tied as a first step. (b) Branches of pulmonary artery to the right upper lobe in the fissure. (c) The right upper lobe bronchus has been divided at its origin and its stump closed in two layers.

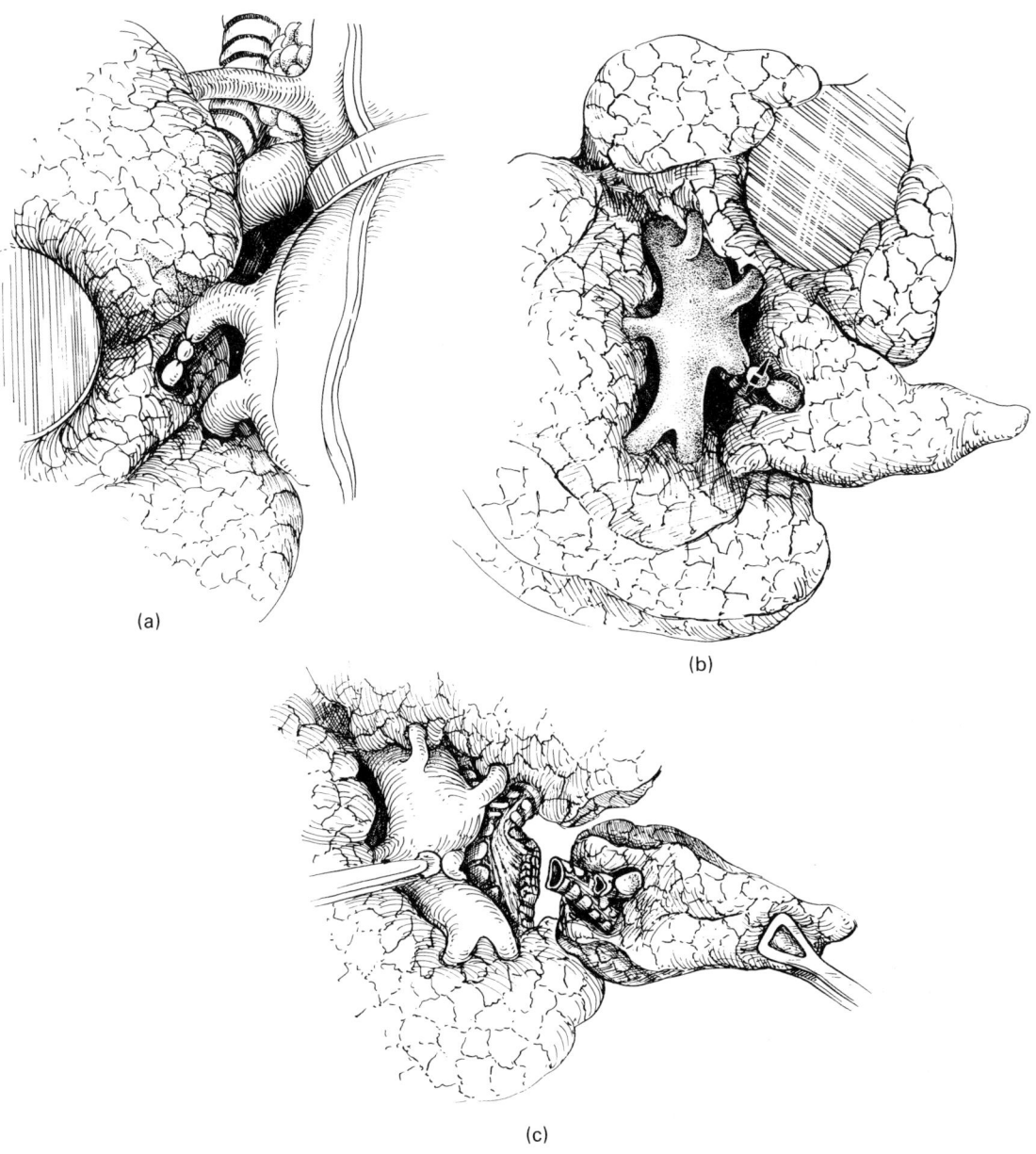

(a)

(b)

(c)

Fig 31.8 Right middle lobectomy. (a) The middle lobe vein has been ligated outside the pericardium where it ends in the superior pulmonary vein. (b) The fissures have been developed and the middle lobe artery(ies) has been divided between ligatures. (c) The pulmonary artery in the fissure is retracted to expose the origin of the middle lobe bronchus, which can then be divided and its stump closed in two layers.

(a)

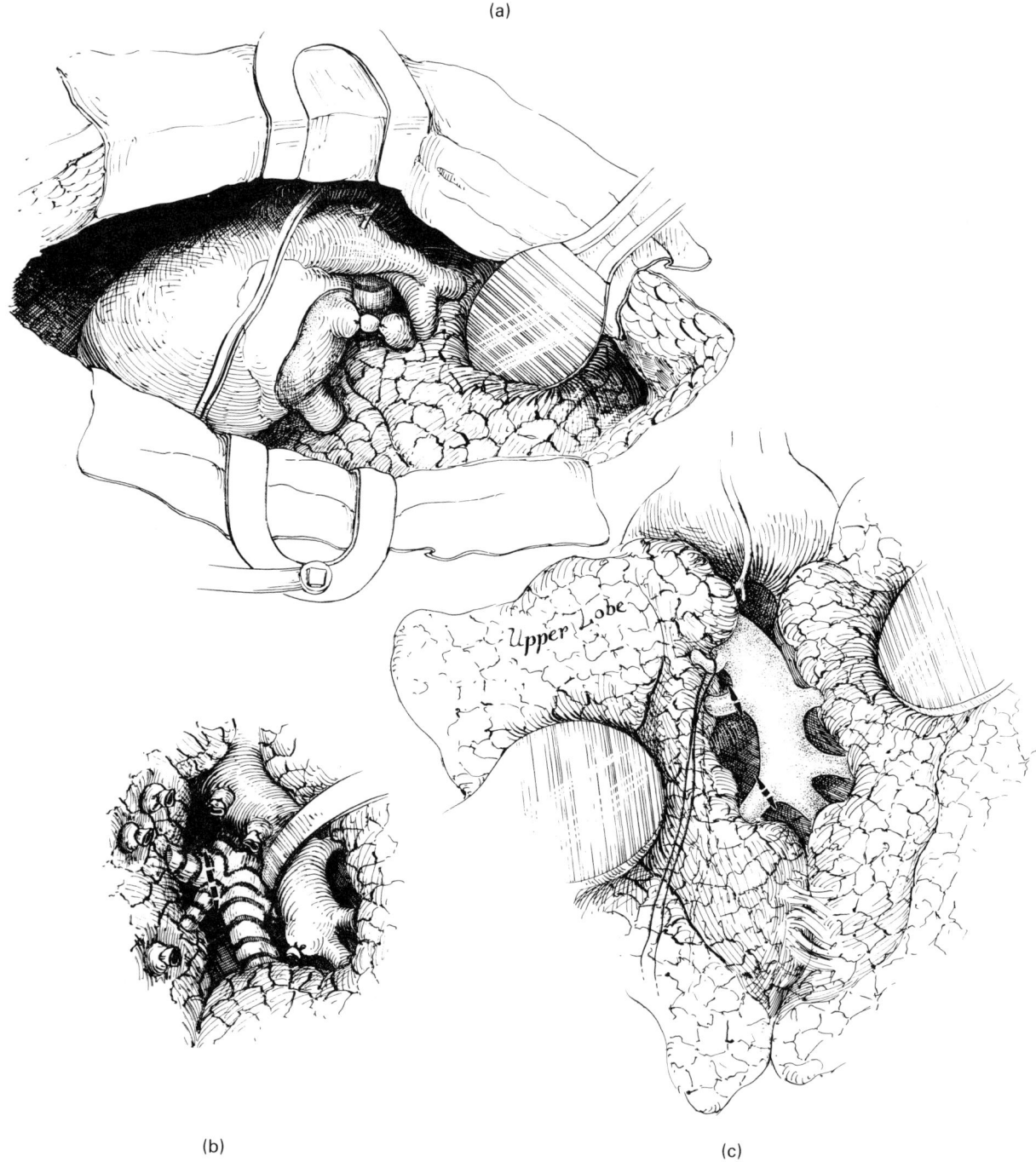

(b)

(c)

Fig 31.9 Left upper lobectomy. (a) The branches of the pulmonary artery to the upper lobe in the fissure are exposed. (b) The left superior pulmonary vein has been ligated as a first step. (c) The left upper lobe bronchus is exposed by retracting the pulmonary artery in the fissure posteriorly. The line of division is indicated.

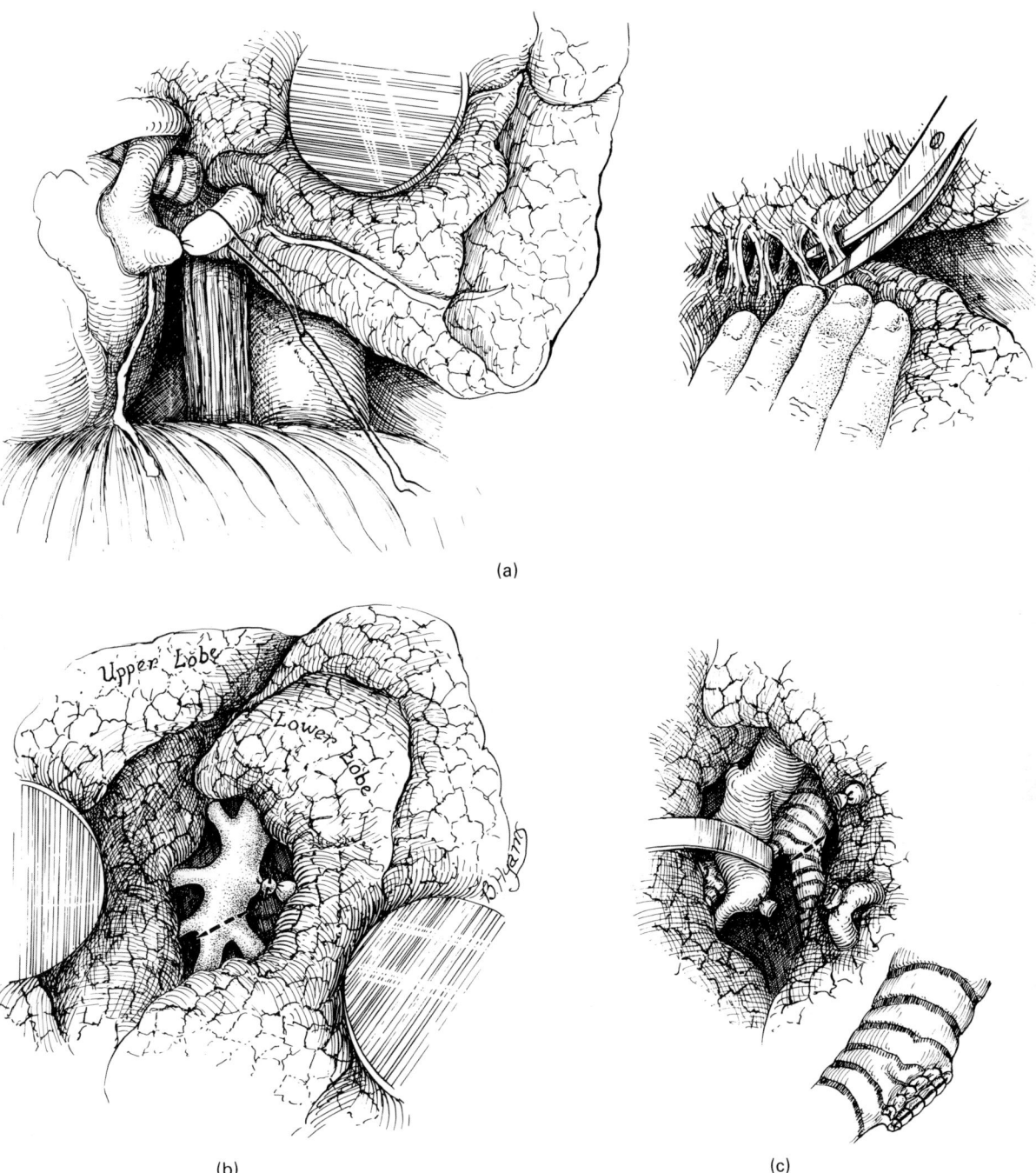

(a)

(b)

(c)

Fig 31.10 Left lower lobectomy. (a) The left inferior pulmonary vein has been tied inside the pericardium as a first step. (b) The branches of the pulmonary artery to the lower lobe are identified in the fissure, the apical lower branch being tied separately. (c) The line of division of the lower lobe bronchus is indicated.

The Pancoast tumour

This carcinoma results in a characteristic clinical picture and requires special treatment. It was described by Pancoast in 1932 as a tumour of the superior pulmonary sulcus 'characterised by pain, Horner's syndrome, destruction of bone and atrophy of hand muscles'. Originally thought to be extrapulmonary in origin, it is now generally agreed that it is of bronchogenic origin, either squamous or adeno-carcinoma, arising by metaplasia in the periphery of the lung, with direct extension into the adjacent extrapulmonary structures.

Commonly these tumours are of low grade malignancy and metastasise late, but invade the lymphatics of the endothoracic fascia, aided by apical pleural adhesions and quickly involve the lower roots of the brachial plexus, the intercostal nerves, stellate ganglion, the sympathetic trunk, the posterior ends of the first few ribs, the transverse processes and, finally, also the adjoining vertebral bodies.

Initially, there is localised pain in the shoulder or deep to the scapula high up; but later it extends down the ulnar side of the arm in the T1 and C8 dermatomes, and weakness, with atrophy of the small muscles of the hand, becomes evident. Horner's syndrome is also found due to destruction of the sympathetic chain. Pulmonary symptoms are conspicuous by their absence and positive bronchoscopic findings and sputum cytology are unusual.

Complete extirpation of the tumour is not possible when it has extended along the perineural lymphatics to produce a full Pancoast syndrome; a bad prognostic sign is destruction of the transverse processes of the vertebrae and the adjoining parts of ribs.

Since the tumours initially are rather like flat, pleural plaques, their radiological detection before they give rise to pain is not practicable and one could justifiably conclude that by the time the patient complains of the characteristic referred pain down the arm, the situation does not warrant extensive surgery. In the past, operative treatment has, therefore, been disappointing, but the combination of incomplete resection either preceded or followed by irradiation has produced relief of pain with long-term survival. American authors favour preoperative irradiation delivering a dose of 3000 rads over a 2 week period. Radical resection is then performed 3–4 weeks later. The aim is to remove the involved upper lobe and portion of invaded chest wall en-bloc.

The resulting defect in the chest wall will be covered when the scapula is replaced in its normal position and, although resection is extensive, it is usually well tolerated and leads to very little disability. On occasion, it may be necessary deliberately to sacrifice the lowest contribution of the brachial plexus and the patient should be warned of this possibility and its consequences.

Tumours invading the chest wall, other than the apex, may be resected by a similar technique, but if the defect in the chest wall is not going to be covered by the scapula, it should be reinforced by a sheet of Marlex mesh or Tantalum wire gauze sewn tautly to the edges of the defect to prevent postoperative paradoxical movement.

Benign tumours

These tumours are uncommon representing less than 10% of all solitary pulmonary lesions found on routine chest x-ray. In general, they may be divided into those in the lung parenchyma and those with primary bronchotracheal origin.

The commonest is the hamartoma in its various histological forms. Characteristically, these appear as asymptomatic intrapulmonary shadows with clearcut edges, slightly lobulated in outline and only rarely containing radio-opaque flecks of calcification in their substance. They are usually solitary and at thoracotomy appear to be very mobile within the lung substance. They are easily removed by incising the overlying lung when they will virtually 'shell out'. Their cut surface presents a characteristic whorled appearance. The residual cavity in the lung is obliterated by interrupted absorbable sutures.

The commonest intrabronchial benign tumour is the adenoma which has a variety of histological appearances. Bronchial adenomas give rise to symptoms because they obstruct the lung distal to them. If a ball-valve-like action results, there will be obstructive emphysema, but if the bronchus becomes totally occluded then collapse/consolidation will occur. The symptomatology may superficially resemble that of carcinoma, but the history is usually much longer and symptoms may occur intermittently.

Although the final diagnosis can only be made by histology, the bronchoscopic appearances of a round, cherry red, smooth tumour covered by intact mucosa, which may move with respiration, is highly suggestive of a benign lesion. Biopsy of the red adenoma may lead to troublesome haemorrhage and is best avoided, but biopsy of its paler variety is quite safe.

The carcinoid variety contain Kulchitsky cells which explains the occasional carcinoid syndrome due to the secretion of serotonin. They invade the bronchial wall and spread to adjacent lymph nodes by direct extension and this finding worsens the prognosis. When a carcinoid tumour arises at the origin of an upper lobe bronchus, lobectomy alone will not clear the tumour, and this is equally true of an early carcinoma in this position. It is necessary, therefore, to resect more of the bronchus by performing a sleeve resection of the main bronchus in association with a lobectomy.

Tracheal tumours

The most important tracheal tumour is the cylindroma or adenocystic tumour which affects the lower trachea or its bifurcation. This tumour has a slow but relentless progression, is extremely difficult to eradicate surgically because it may have a multicentric origin and is almost completely resistant to radio- and chemotherapy.

Macroscopically the tumour appears to be widely based with extensive submucosal infiltration of the upper bronchi and lower trachea. Treatment of these tumours has varied from the repeated endoscopic piecemeal removal to radical resection and insertion of plastic tracheal prosthesis combined with radiotherapy. Adequate primary excision of the early growth is probably still the best form of treatment.

Mediastinal tumours

The commonest extrapulmonary tumour in the posterior mediastinum is neurogenic and includes neurilemmoma, neurofibroma, neurosarcoma, ganglion-neuroma, sympatheticoblastoma, paraganglioma and phaeochromocytoma. Precise determination, even after their removal, is difficult and, on the whole, in adults they tend to be benign, but in children there is a greater tendency towards malignancy. Typically the neural tumours are situated in the paravertebral sulcus, are clearly delineated and commonly arise from an intercostal nerve or its sheath or the sympathetic chain. The neurilemmoma may be dumb-bell in shape, a portion of it passing through the intervertebral foramen and then expanding again in the spinal canal. This may be indicated by widening of the involved intervertebral foramen and their complete removal may require the attendance of a neurosurgeon at the time of thoracotomy. Symptoms of spinal compression before operation are rare.

Neurofibromas of the mediastinum may occur as part of a generalised neurofibromatosis or these isolated tumours may precede the onset of the generalised disease. The neuroblastoma is a highly malignant tumour of the sympathetic chain and requires radical surgical excision combined with chemotherapy and irradiation.

Tumours of the middle mediastinum are most commonly teratomas and may be solid and cystic in parts. They frequently contain teeth and hair and, histologically, all three germinal layers are represented in varying degrees. Untreated, they may enlarge and may rupture into the lung or pleural space when their removal becomes more difficult because of secondary infection.

Tumours of the anterior mediastinum usually originate in the thymus and a thymoma may be associated with myasthenia gravis. Histologically it may be difficult to determine the malignancy of a thymic tumour and this will then depend on the findings at operation

such as invasion of pleura and lung or the presence of discrete secondary nodules.

Lymphomas, though they may occur as part of a generalised disease, may start as an isolated lesion in the anterior mediastinum; they include Hodgkin's disease, reticulum cell sarcoma and lymphoblastoma.

Surgical treatment

The posterior and middle mediastinal tumours are best approached by a posterolateral thoracotomy. For tumours of the anterior mediastinum, anterolateral thoracotomy may be made if radiological investigation suggests that the lesion is still unilateral. If a wide exposure of the anterior mediastinum is deemed necessary for complete extirpation of the thymus, in Hodgkin's disease for instance, or when the tumour has extended to both sides of the midline, a vertical median sternotomy gives the best exposure.

Tumours of the pleura

Tumours of the pleura, by definition, arise from the cellular elements of the pleura and therefore any malignancy originating in the lung, mediastinum or in other organs with secondary seeding or involvement of the pleura is excluded. The elements which compose the tumours are derived from either the mesothelial cells or the underlying connective tissue. But when the pleural cavity is diffusely involved by neoplastic tissue, it may be very difficult to decide whether this is a true primary growth. The confusion continues because mesothelial cells may form tubular structures histologically which resemble adenocarcinomas with pleural involvement.

It is now recognised that asbestos is a definite aetiological factor in the development of the malignant mesothelioma and asbestos bodies may be found within the tumour tissue. The patient's exposure to asbestos may have occurred a few decades ago and need not necessarily have been prolonged. Asbestos bodies are not usually found in the 'benign fibroma' of the pleura.

The fibroma, initially solitary, will usually be found on routine chest x-rays, but may give rise to pressure symptoms simply from its size. These tumours at thoracotomy may be lying almost free within the pleural space, with only very tenuous attachment to either pleura. They are usually associated with gross clubbing and hypertrophic pulmonary osteoarthropathy and are very easily removed with rapid relief of the symptoms. The sessile variety may require excision of the affected pleura. Although regarded as benign for many years, it is now clear that they tend to recur as multiple nodules or as fibrosarcomas.

The diffuse mesothelioma of the pleura will produce

refractory effusions and a fixed type chest pain of increasing severity. The diagnosis can be made by cytology of the fluid, but more often requires an open pleural biopsy. When this condition is suspected on clinical grounds the diagnosis may be confirmed at operation, when the parietal pleura is stripped out in an attempt to obtain a pleurodesis and so prevent the continuous accumulation of the fluid which causes respiratory embarrassment. Although chemotherapy has been tried, treatment is primarily directed towards the prevention of the reaccumulation of the effusion and to the relief of the intractable pain which is such a prominent distressing feature of the later stages of the disease.

Suppurative pulmonary disease

The most important of these is pulmonary tuberculosis. It is the purpose of this section to concentrate on surgical management. Operative intervention is only indicated when the infection has been eradicated by chemotherapy and the patient is, therefore, only suffering from the complications of the original infection. In these cases resection of the affected segments, lobes or lung is indicated. The lobectomies, usually upper, are performed by an extrapleural technique without gland clearance. Since pulmonary tuberculosis causes extensive peribronchial fibrosis, care must be taken in the hilar dissection. After a pneumonectomy, which may involve an extrapleural mobilisation of the lung, it is advisable to follow the resection after a suitable interval by a space-reducing thoracoplasty.

If only one or two segments of an upper lobe are involved together with the apex of the ipsilateral lower lobe, then it is advisable to perform segmental resection.

Resections for bronchiectasis rarely involve the upper lobes, since sputum drains readily from them. Bronchiectasis should only be treated surgically when antibiotic treatment and physiotherapy carried out properly and over a long period have failed. In the great majority of patients the disease is bilateral and this responds poorly to resection. Unilateral disease may be resected, especially if there is crowding of the diseased bronchial segments due to destruction of the lung tissue served by them. Lower and middle lobectomy on the right, and lower lobectomy with resection of the lingula on the left are the commonest procedures. In unilateral bronchiectasis limited to the basal segments of the lower lobe, no attempt to preserve the unaffected apical segment of the lower lobe should be made. If left behind, this segment is very likely to swing down into the space created by the segmental resection. Its bronchus then kinks and the segment too quite quickly becomes infected and bronchiectatic. In general, surgical opinion has swung from the aggressive to the conservative over the last three decades.

The other most important suppurative condition which may demand surgical intervention is fungus infection of the 'sterile' (tuberculous) cavity. *Aspergillus fumigatus, flavus, niger, nidulans* and *clavatus*, in that order, are the offending organisms and when a fungus ball in the cavity with its surrounding diagnostic halo of air is present, the patient may suffer from the effects of chronic pulmonary sepsis on the one hand, and, on the other, may have massive and life-threatening haemorrhages. The latter are caused by a combination of pressure from the enlarging fungus ball on the branches of the pulmonary artery which traverse the cavity and also lie in its wall together with secondary infection which always accompanies the presence of a fungus ball within the cavity. An erosion occurs in the wall of the artery which is not severed and, therefore, does not retract and the haemorrhage is severe and prolonged. The patient may succumb from a combination of blood loss and suffocation as the blood spills into the healthy regions of his lungs. At times, emergency resection is necessary to save life. These operations, usually upper lobectomies since the fungus multiplies in the sterilised tuberculous cavity, can be technically the most difficult ones the thoracic surgeon is asked to perform because of the intense fibrosis which accompanies first the chronic pulmonary tuberculosis and then the superadded fungus infection. It is advisable to mobilise the lobe extrapleurally so as to minimise the risk of spillage of fungus material from the cavity into the pleural space. Should a postoperative 'pleural' space persist at the apex of the hemithorax for any length of of time, the risk of reinfection with a fungus becomes increased if the cavity has been accidentally entered during the resection.

If resection is not possible because of poor respiratory reserve or bilateral aspergillomas of considerable size, then cavernostomy must be carried out. Through an appropriately sited skin incision a segment of the lowest rib overlying the cavity is resected and the cavity is entered directly by removing a 2 cm square portion of its wall, which will consist of the greatly thickened and fused pleural layers and destroyed lung. The fungus ball is removed entirely and the incision is closed with through-and-through vertical figure-of-eight mattress sutures with a drainage tube. Appropriate antifungal agents may be instilled locally into the cavity until all evidence of fungus infection has been eradicated and the tube may then be removed and its track covered with a firm dressing. These cavities have multiple bronchiolar openings into them and, therefore, can never be expected to heal, but they can be sterilised by this relatively simple and safe manoeuvre. However, there is always the risk that they will eventually become reinfected.

Pulmonary actinomycosis should be recognised and preferably not treated by resection.

Parasitic infections

Amoebic infections are usually secondary to hepatic abscesses. These abscesses generally occur in the right lobe of the liver and may rupture through the diaphragm, often without formation of a subphrenic abscess, directly to enter the lower lobe. Amoebic pus (anchovy paste) and bile will be coughed up by the patient and these are highly irritative to the bronchial mucosa, the bile particularly giving rise to characteristic yellow bronchorrhoea which allows the patient very little rest. Occasionally, the abscess may rupture into the pericardial sac. The acute phase of the disease is treated by specific antiamoebic chemotherapy. If the amoebae are not identifiable then a diagnositic course of emetine, chloroquine or metronidazole may confirm the clinical suspicion (*see* Chapter 14). Only rarely will operative intervention be indicated and then only to drain residual abscesses below the diaphragm, in the pleura (empyema) and to decorticate or resect involved portions of the lung.

Hydatid disease is caused by the *Taenia echinococcus* which divides its parasitic life between sheep and dogs. In this cycle, man may inadvertently take the place of the sheep. The parasitic larvae burrow through the gastric mucosa and enter the liver via the portal system where most of them are filtered out to form hepatic hydatids, but some escape into the lungs where they may form one or more hydatid cysts. These may grow slowly or quickly without necessarily causing symptoms unless, by their sheer size, they may produce respiratory symptoms or those due to pressure on neighbouring viscera. On the other hand, they may also rupture into the adjacent bronchus or into the pleura. In the former instance, the cyst with its contents will be coughed up, in the latter the pleura becomes heavily infested with daughter cysts. Occasionally hypersensitivity reactions to the contents of the cyst cause severe symptoms and rarely death. In any event a ruptured cyst becomes infected, the daughter cysts and scolices die in this case, and the situation then resembles a lung abscess. Radiologically, the pathognomic 'water lily sign' is due to the true endocyst falling away from the layer of compressed lung which forms the pericyst.

Extirpation of the cyst is advised because of these likely complications. Two techniques are described, the extrusion method and the extraction method. In the former, the pericyst is carefully incised until the white, laminated endocyst is uncovered. At this stage the anaesthetist vigorously and progressively inflates the lung and causes the cyst to be extruded. It is caught in a spoon or basin unruptured. In the other method, the cyst is located and the wound edges are packed off with large swabs soaked in 1% formalin. The contents of the cyst are then partially aspirated with a syringe also containing 1% formalin and this syringe is then emptied into the cyst. The pericyst is incised and the cyst and its contents can be extracted. The cavity in the lung resulting from the removal of the cyst is obliterated as it has a number of open bronchioles in its wall.

Pyogenic infections

Lung abscesses, other than those arising from conditions already mentioned, have become rare with the advent of new antibiotics. Brock emphasised the segmental localisation and explained their 'axillary' predilection by gravitation of infectious material from the oropharynx into these dependent segments of the lung. The administration of the appropriate antibiotics remains the first line of treatment. At times, it may be necessary to resect a segment or more for a chronic lung abscess.

The multiple thin-walled staphylococcal lung abscesses occurring in infancy present a frightening clinical and radiological picture and are due to an uncontrolled septicaemia. With vigorous antibiotic therapy the surgeon will only be required to deal with the occasional spontaneous pyopneumothorax which occurs when an abscess ruptures into the pleura. A fine intercostal catheter for underwater seal drainage is all that is required and, in some cases, repeated pleural aspirations will suffice.

Pleural infections

These are always secondary to infection of the underlying lung or more rarely the chest wall or infection may be inadvertently introduced with a needle. In the simplest example, a spontaneous pneumothorax, if it becomes infected, will give rise to an empyema, but more commonly an empyema results from infection of the pleural effusion overlying an unresolved pneumonia. These empyemas are usually based posterolaterally since the patient will have been lying in bed.

The diagnosis is made by aspirating the pus from the pleural space. By this time the aetiology will have been established and as much as possible should be aspirated and a broad spectrum antibiotic instilled until the bacteriological culture and sensitivity studies of the causative organism are available.

Repeated thoracocenteses will demonstrate that the pus becomes thicker and that aspiration becomes more difficult because of the development of fibrin masses. If the patient's general condition has improved sufficiently, decortication should be undertaken without delay before contraction of the chest wall has taken place.

A posterolateral thoracotomy is performed, but at first the pleura is not entered, as it is often thickened by the cortex. Instead, an extrapleural plane is developed, at first with the finger and then with a dissecting swab until normal pleura is reached, usually at the upper limit of the empyema. The parietal aspect of the empyema is then progressively mobilised by blunt and sharp dissection, care being taken not to injure the diaphragm inferiorly and the phrenic and vagus nerves medially; but it is most unusual for the fibrous process to involve the mediastinal aspect.

Eventually, for complete excision of the whole abscess, it may have to be opened, its contents sucked out and its walls excised piecemeal from within its cavity. Provided the underlying lung has returned to normal and the cortex covering the visceral pleura has been completely removed, the previously encased and compressed lung will easily expand to fill the empyema space. The incision is then closed routinely with two fenestrated drainage tubes. If irreparably damaged lung underlies the empyema, then it should be resected at the same time.

In children, early excision of the empyema is now advised since their powers of recovery after removal of the abscess are very great and they develop chest wall contraction with accompanying scoliosis early.

It is clear that though decortication removes the affected parietal pleura, the visceral pleura is left in place. If it is not technically possible to decorticate the visceral pleura adequately, then this area should be cross-hatched by incisions into it down to the level of the pleura.

Decortication is a major operation and should not be performed in the old and debilitated patient in whom 'silent' empyema has led to amyloid disease. In these patients, rib resection and tube drainage is indicated. It must be emphasised that intercostal tube drainage alone can never result in adequate drainage.

It is important to identify the most dependent point of the empyema by instilling heavy, radio-opaque liquid into the abscess cavity and then taking postero-anterior and lateral x-ray films to show the lowest ribs. Counting from below upwards, the rib to be resected is identified and also the appropriate part of it is localised. The resection can best be done with the patient sitting upright on the operating table. One should never resect any rib lower than the 9th, since after drainage of the empyema the diaphragm will usually rise to this level and drainage lower down will thereby be closed off. At least 3.5 cm of rib is removed. The wall of the empyema and the floor of the rib bed is then excised (and sent for section) creating a generous stoma. The contents of the cavity are sucked out and the cavity is then inspected with a light on a stalk. After thorough cleansing of its walls, a large drainage tube is placed in the most dependent part of the cavity and fixed to the skin. The incision is loosely closed with vertical figure-of-eight through-and-through mattress sutures.

For the first few days the drainage tube is connected to an underwater seal, pleurograms are then obtained by instilling radio-opaque fluid and the tube shortened as necessary. Appropriate antibiotics are given until the volume of drainage has diminished sufficiently to be absorbed comfortably by a large gauze pad dressing.

Spontaneous pneumothorax and emphysema

A spontaneous pneumothorax occurs because of leakage of air through a breach in the visceral pleura. It occurs more commonly in males than in females and the rupture of the visceral pleura occurs at weak areas such as over a pleural bleb or bulla. A subpleural tuberculous focus may sometimes cause it, trauma may be the aetiological agent, but in many instances the pneumothorax occurs without any identifiable cause.

Sudden chest pain and dyspnoea of varying degree are the commonest symptoms. The severity of the dyspnoea will depend on the size of the pneumothorax and may become severe if tension develops in the pleural space, because of a valvular effect at the point of pleural rupture. Since bullas are commonly bilateral, a patient occasionally sustains a pneumothorax on both sides.

Pleural adhesions may limit the pneumothorax and it is thought that adhesions may keep the leak open. Rupture of an adhesion may result in the development of a haemothorax.

If a chest x-ray demonstrates fluid in the presence of a pneumothorax, then diagnostic aspiration of the fluid should be undertaken. If the fluid is found to be blood, urgent thoracotomy, evacuation of the haemothorax, suture ligation of the bleeding point and pleurodesis should be undertaken.

In the absence of intrapleural bleeding, an asymptomatic, spontaneous pneumothorax, occurring for the first time, requires no active intervention since it will be absorbed over a matter of days. At most, aspiration of air on one occasion may be performed.

Thoracocentesis with syringe and needle may be all that is necessary to relieve dyspnoea and tension, but on the whole a large pneumothorax, with or without tension, is best treated by the insertion of an intercostal tube into the second anterior intercostal space. The underwater seal drainage is connected to a suction pump to maintain a constant negative pressure in the hemithorax so that the lung is allowed to expand, thereby closing the leak. The intercostal drain may be removed 48 h after it has ceased to function and there has been no swing in it when taken off suction with the patient breathing deeply.

More aggressive treatment is indicated when the pneumothorax is recurrent, when there is respiratory insufficiency, when simple tube drainage and suction for 5–6 days has failed to produce complete expansion and when there is obvious bullous formation. In these cases, an open pleurodesis is advocated using a limited anterolateral thoracotomy.

Patients suffering from cystic fibrosis of the lungs present rather a special problem. The incidence of recurrent spontaneous pneuomothorax is high in this group, but surgical intervention should only be undertaken after prolonged and repeated tube drainage with suction has failed. Only the minimum compatible with achieving a pleurodesis should be performed, as these patients invariably have stiff lungs, grossly impaired respiratory function and any substantial interference with chest wall movement will necessitate the institution of artificial ventilation. This, in turn, interferes with clearance of highly infected and copious bronchial secretions.

The forms of emphysema for which surgery may be advocated are congenital lobar emphysema and bullous emphysema causing lung compression.

In congenital lobar emphysema the upper lobes are most commonly affected and with equal frequency, the middle lobe sometimes, but the lower lobes very rarely. Symptoms occur soon after birth consisting of, often extreme, respiratory distress with tachypnoea, wheezing and cyanosis. Hyperresonance is noted on the affected side with contralateral mediastinal shift and marked radiolucency on the affected side. Excision of the grossly over-expanded lobe is the treatment of choice. In about 40% of cases a deficiency in the amount of supporting bronchial cartilages will be found.

Bullous emphysema

Considering the frequency of incidence of this degenerative condition, patients in whom removal of these cysts will significantly improve respiratory function are relatively rare. Although sophisticated tests have been devised to demonstrate that healthy lung will come into normal use if allowed, a good plain radiograph in conjunction with tomograms will give just as much information.

Congenital vascular disorders of the lung

The pulmonary arteriovenous fistula is a cavernous vascular malformation and may be associated with hereditary haemorrhagic telangiectasis. There may be one or more sizeable communication between a pulmonary artery and vein which may result in cyanosis. The lesions consist of multiple thin-walled saccular channels. Usually they are discovered as shadows on a routine chest x-ray unless cyanosis and dyspnoea on exertion are already obvious. The fistulas do not give rise to murmurs or cardiomegaly. Polycythaemia, if severe, may give rise to cerebral thrombosis. The fistula produces a characteristic shadow on x-ray of a convoluted shape with clear outline. Vascular shadows are seen radiating from it on tomography.

Eradication of the malformation may require lobectomy, but isolated lesions may be treated by excision. Multiple ligation of vessels is not satisfactory.

Lobar sequestration is a congenital abnormality in which a part of the lung retains an abnormal systemic blood supply and fails to gain a pulmonary arterial supply. These lesions may involve the whole of one lobe or only part of it and occur most commonly in the lower lobes. Bronchial connection is only established secondarily due to retained secretions in the cystic, sequestered part, and then will give rise to symptoms of cough, sputum and attacks of infection in the involved lung tissue. During the operation for excision of the lobe care must be taken to identify and secure the aberrant systemic artery, which may often be subdiaphragmatic in origin and can be most easily dissected out as it passes into the lung between the pleural folds which make up the inferior pulmonary ligament.

Congenital abnormalities of the trachea

The commonest abnormality is the tracheo-oesophageal fistula, and the chapter on paediatric surgery (ch. 13, pp. 255–83) should be consulted for more details.

Congenital tracheal stenosis presents in many forms. Web-like structures are seen in the neonate and there are also three main types: in generalised hypoplasia the trachea is of normal diameter at its origin and then becomes severely narrowed to just above the carina; in the funnel type stenosis, the narrowing is progressive over the whole length of the trachea, and in segmental narrowing, the affected part may occur at any point in the trachea. In these cases the bronchi are usually of normal calibre. Segmental narrowing may be associated with vascular rings, the division of which may bring relief of respiratory difficulty.

Because of the difficulty of maintaining an adequate airway after operation on the new born trachea, conservative management for as long as possible is favoured. It may be wise in the first instance to perform a tracheostomy below the level of obstruction to allow the infant to grow to a more easily managed size, before definitive tracheal resection is undertaken.

Tracheal surgery

The commonest forms of traumatic lesions of the trachea are those following prolonged tracheostomy and intubation with an inflatable cuff, when either a tracheo-oesophageal fistula develops or a stricture. Blunt trauma to the front of the neck as in steering wheel accidents may cause complete rupture of the trachea without initially showing any evidence of serious respiratory embarrassment.

In the diagnosis of lesions of the trachea, plain x-rays and tomograms of the neck are important and should always be performed except in cases of suspected rupture where rapid intubation may be necessary, or emergency tracheostomy to save the life of the patient.

In the case of resectable tumours, tracheal reconstruction will be necessary and every effort should be made to complete the reconstruction in such a way that the patient can breathe on his own at the end of the procedure, since prolonged postoperative intubation and ventilation greatly increases the risk of suture line dehiscence.

Lesions of the upper half of the trachea can be approached through a collar incision in the neck to which may be added a short vertical incision dividing the manubrium. The lower half, or entire intrathoracic trachea is best exposed through a 4th rib right postero-lateral incision. Only rarely will it be necessary to combine these two types of approach.

The addition of cardiopulmonary bypass is only justified in those cases where resection and reconstitution of both bronchial origins and the carina is indicated to ensure complete resection of a tumour.

Up to 4.5 cm of trachea can be removed if the head is flexed while the anastomotic sutures are tied, but in some cases the carina may require mobilisation via an incision extended laterally into the right chest, or the larynx can be mobilised by dividing the thyrohyoid muscles, the thyrohyoid membrane and the superior horns of the thyroid cartilage. Care should be taken not to injure the superior laryngeal nerves.

For lower tracheal resection and reconstruction via a posterolateral thoracotomy, the intrathoracic trachea is mobilised, resected and anastomosed. Additional mobilisation may be obtained by freeing the hilum of

the right lung. Distal intubation and ventilation is also performed and the tube may have to be passed temporarily into the left main bronchus, resulting in one lung anaesthesia, if the lesion to be resected is so low as to leave an inadequate length of cuff above the carina. In patients with poor respiratory reserve, two endotracheal tubes (right and left) may be required, connected to two anaesthetic machines until tracheal continuity has been established.

Carinal resection and reconstruction involves implanting the right main bronchus end-to-end to the cut end of the trachea and then anastomosing the left main bronchus end-to-side to the medial aspect of the right main bronchus just below the level of the origin of the right upper lobe bronchus. Alternatively, the left main bronchus may reach the trachea above the anastomosis of the right main bronchus. The reverse anastomotic procedure may be necessary.

Further reading

Arrigoni M.G., Woolmer L.B., Bernatz P.E., Miller W.E., Fontana R.S. (1970). Benign Tumours of the lung: a ten year surgical experience. *J. Thorac. Cardiovasc. Surg*; **60**:589.

British Thoracic and Tuberculosis Association (1970). Aspergilloma and residual tuberculous cavities – the results of a re-survey. *Tubercle*; **51**:227.

Dines D.E., Arms R.A., Bernata P.E., Gomes M.R. (1974). Pulmonary arterio venous fistulae. *Mayo Clin. Proc*; **49**:460.

Grillo H.C. (1973). Reconstruction of the trachea. Experience in 100 consecutive cases. *Thorax*; **28**:667.

Grillo H.C., Greenberg J.J., Wilkins E.W. (1966). Resection of bronchogenic carcinoma involving the thoracic wall. *J. Thorac. Cardiovasc. Surg*; **51**:417.

Kirsch M.M., Rotman H., Argenta L., Bove E., Cimmio V., Tashian J., Ferguson P., Sloan H. (1976). Carcinoma of the lung: results of treatment over 10 years. *Ann. Thorac. Surg*; **21**:371.

Knudson R.J., Gaensler E.A. (1965). Surgery for emphysema: collective review. *Ann. Thorac. Surg*; **1**:332.

Lichter I. (1972). Surgery of pulmonary hydatid cyst – the Barrett technique. *Thorax*; **27**:529.

Pancoast H.K. (1932). Superior pulmonary sulcus tumor. *JAMA*; **99**:1391.

Paulson D. (1973). Selection of patients for surgery for bronchogenic carcinoma. *Ann. Surg*; **39**:1.

Pearson F.G. (1968). An evaluation of mediastinoscopy in the management of presumably operable bronchial carcinoma. *J. Thorac. Cardiovasc. Surg*; **55**:617.

Shields T., Higgins G., Keelin R. (1972). Factors influencing survival after resection for bronchogenic carcinoma. *J. Thorac. Cardiovasc. Surg*; **64**:391.

Arterial surgery

L.T. COTTON

There has been a remarkable increase in atherosclerotic vascular disease since the Second World War and it is now the greatest killer disease in the developed world. With the increase in vascular disease there has been an impressive development in the field of reconstructive arterial surgery. Perhaps the biggest stimulus to this development was the Korean War in which it was found possible to fly a soldier with an arterial wound to a base hospital within an hour or so, where the full facilities for arterial repair could be made available. This development in acute ischaemia has later been applied to the much larger problem of chronic ischaemia with which vascular surgery is mainly concerned.

Chronic ischaemia of the legs

Most chronic ischaemia is due to atherosclerosis and the larger part affects the legs. Rarer causes are thromboangeitis, cystic degeneration and entrapment of the popliteal artery (p. 487). Diseases commonly associated with atherosclerosis are diabetes mellitus and hypertension. Heavy smoking must be a causative factor for 94% of patients with chronic ischaemia of the legs are heavy smokers as compared with 40% in the general population. In addition, the chances of failure after arterial reconstruction are five times greater if patients continue to smoke. A high level of haemoglobin is another risk factor, possibly in the causation of the disease and its effect on the chances of successful surgery. It is known that thrombotic incidents are very common in polycythemia rubra vera and it is known that success or failure after arterial surgery can be related to the haemoglobin level. Smoking can cause a physiological polycythemia. Interlinked with a high level of haemoglobin can be a raised blood viscosity that may be associated with causation of symptoms and possibly related to failure after surgery (Greenhalgh, 1978).

Clinical presentation

The symptoms of chronic ischaemia are exercise pain (intermittent claudication) and rest pain. The signs are those of poor tissue blood perfusion leading to signs of deficient nutrition of the extremity from coldness and changing colour to the signs of pregangrene or established gangrene. Intermittent claudication is the commonest presenting symptom and is evidence of stenosis or occlusion of a major artery which can be compensated by the collateral circulation at rest, but not during exercise when there is a need for increase in blood flow to satisfy the leg muscles by a factor of five. What it is that causes the pain is unknown; it is thought to be the accumulation of metabolites and perhaps kinins that stimulate pain nerve endings in the muscles.

It is important to appreciate that intermittent claudication is a benign symptom that often remits spontaneously. It can be said that of 100 cases, 40 will improve spontaneously, 40 will stay the same and only 20 will require an operation (Taylor and Calo, 1962). Only 8 will come to amputation and usually these present with rest pain in addition to claudication. Spontaneous improvement may continue for up to two years from the onset of symptoms.

Rest pain is much more unpleasant and potentially dangerous. Claudication occurs in the muscles of the calf, thigh or buttock, rest pain in the toes and foot. Rest pain is evidence that tissue perfusion is inadequate even at rest. Typically, it is worse in the early hours of the morning due to a depression of cardiac output, pulse rate and blood pressure during sleep. Patients with rest pain learn to avoid sleeping deeply by sleeping in a chair or even on the floor. In this 'twilight sleep', they learn to wake at the slightest sensation of rest pain and walk about to raise their vital functions. Some find benefit by hanging their legs down out of bed, which helps to relieve pain by assisting blood flow by gravity. Rest pain, pregangrene and gangrene are all indications for immediate admission to hospital. In diabetic patients gangrene may be painless if there is an associated neuropathy. Indeed, there may be signs of an 'autosympathectomy', a warm dry foot and dilated veins and yet gangrenous toes due to a neuropathic degeneration of sympathetic nerves.

The important features of physical examination are first to assess any nutritional changes in the feet or legs and secondly to identify arterial pulses. Pulses are best felt synchronously in both limbs to detect differences between the two sides. Absent pedal and popliteal pulses are the most common finding when superficial femoral artery occlusion is the cause of the symptoms. Normal pulses in the presence of vascular disease would indicate small vessel disease. Occasionally an aneurysm may be detected. Weak pedal pulses may be felt when there is aortoiliac disease and misleadingly suggest the absence of any vascular obstruction. If the arterial circulation is very proximal and very well developed, the collateral circulation may allow pedal pulses to be felt. The femoral pulses should be felt synchronously to detect differences in amplitude. Bruits heard over the femoral arteries indicate more proximally sited disease and are accentuated by exercise.

Vascular examination should include abdominal palpation for an aneurysm, auscultation of the heart for evidence of disease and measurement of brachial blood pressure which is so often raised. The radial pulses should be felt synchronously for evidence of weakness or absence due to subclavian artery obstruction; the neck should be auscultated immediately above the clavicles for bruits that indicate subclavian artery disease and near the angle of the mandible for bruits indicating carotid artery disease. The urine should be examined to diagnose diabetes mellitus.

From the history and physical examination the surgeon should have a fair idea of the site of vascular occlusion or narrowing and the degree of treatment.

Vascular laboratory

Before the wide use of ultrasound in medicine the next step after clinical assessment could only be the invasive test of angiography. Ultrasound examination now provides an objective test for a disease which is often predominantly subjective in its symptomatic presentation. Ultrasound can be used to measure blood pressure to analyse the pulse wave form, to measure the pulse wave velocity and most recently to image vessels. During the last 5 years many centres have established vascular laboratories to obtain an objective assessment of the degree of severity of chronic ischaemia.

With ultrasound it is very simple to measure blood pressure at the ankle (Yao, 1970). Normally the blood pressure at the ankle is equal to or greater than the brachial pressure and after exercise the pressure is either unchanged or rises transiently above the brachial level. If there is a vascular occlusion, then the resting blood pressure at the ankle is less than the brachial. Exercise is usually simulated by walking on a treadmill. Most patients find personal estimation of their walking distance quite impossible (Fig 32.1). If their estimated walking distance is plotted against their actual walking distance on the treadmill, there is no correlation except that most people think they can walk 100 metres (Thomas and Quick, 1976).

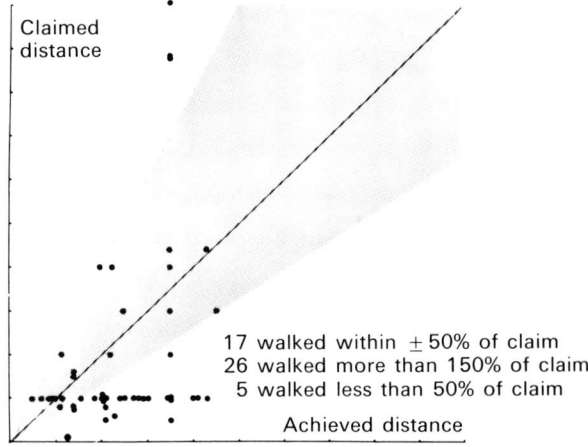

Fig 32.1 Patients' claimed distance plotted against distance achieved on treadmill.

The fall of pressure after walking is most significant (Lewis *et al.*, 1972). A fall to zero indicates a severe degree of ischaemia. A fall to less than zero implies a lesser degree of ischaemia and so to the surgeon a lesser degree of urgency or the great possibility of spontaneous recovery (Fig 32.2). The time taken for the pressure to return to the patient's baseline pressure may extend from 2–20 min and is an index of the adequacy of the collateral circulation. Serial measurements over a period of months are useful in showing patients their spontaneous improvement as the collateral circulation opens up and compensates for the haemodynamic defect.

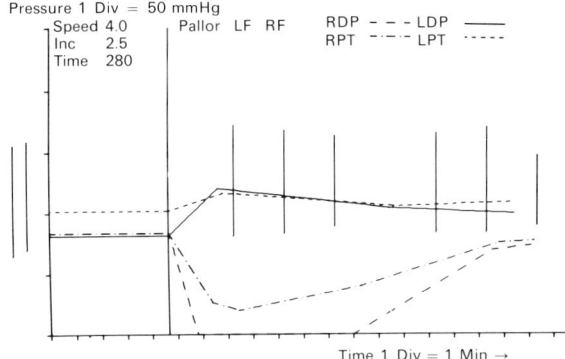

Fig 32.2 Postexercise pressure response curves.

Simple measurements such as this are invaluable in clarifying the diagnosis. Many patients complain of exercise pain who have no vascular disease and are suffering from such entities as nerve root compression as in intermittent claudication of the cauda equina. Others have a prolapsed intervertebral disc, spinal stenosis, osteoarthritis of the spine, or even osteoarthritis of the hip (Blau and Logue, 1961). Another less common presentation is a peripheral neuritis or part of a polyneuritis. Normal ankle pressures before and after exercise indicate the absence of a haemodynamically significant arterial occlusion or stenosis. Difficulty is met in those cases where there is evidence of both arterial disease and nerve root compression or other non-vascular disease. Usually in these cases the vascular element is the less important.

The form of the pulse wave can be analysed and displayed to demonstrate the many different blood streams in a vessel moving at innumerable different velocities. The beam of ultrasound directed into an artery is reflected from the circulating red cells. The signal detected can be displayed as a flow wave form composed of a number of dots reflecting the velocity profile in the arteries (Fig 32.3). Inspection of this analysed flow wave form can demonstrate where the block lies in the arterial circulation and can distinguish between the

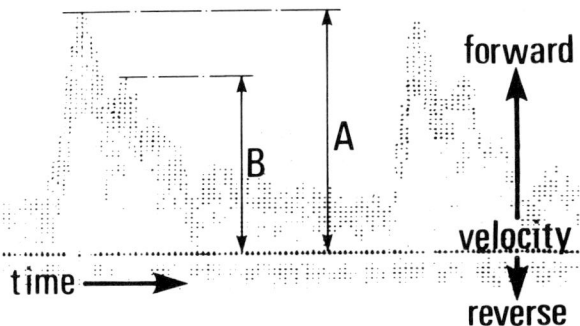

Fig. 32.3 Sonogram of a normal arterial pulse. Each dot represents a different red cell velocity.

up stream and down stream components of obstruction (Gosling and King, 1975).

Vascular laboratory tests demonstrate first if there is vascular disease, secondly how severe it is and thirdly where it is (Roberts and Cotton, 1979).

Techniques of visualisation of arteries

Angiography is still an important investigation in arterial disease. Its importance is to establish the site of blockage, the inflow pattern and the 'runoff'. The examination most commonly used has been aortography either by the translumbar or percutaneous transfemoral routes.

Angiography has its complications and should be avoided if possible. It usually necessitates general anaesthesia for a person who has generalised arterial disease and may well have disease of the heart. Vascular laboratory tests have already reduced the need for angiography by half. An absent femoral pulse in a patient with ischaemic disease of the leg who has a normally nourished foot indicates an adequate run off even if the superficial femoral artery is occluded, and in such a case an angiogram is usually unnecessary. It is now already obvious that many patients can be offered operations such as an aortofemoral bypass without any need for angiography, if vascular laboratory testing has been performed, thus saving time, expense and discomfort to the patient.

It appears that we are coming full circle in the need for vascular angiography. Historically, femoral angiography was first undertaken, but experience suggested that unsuspected aortofemoral disease could only be detected by translumbar angiography, so all patients were given translumbar angiograms. Ultrasound examination should detect aortoiliac disease and the need today is for angiography mainly to demonstrate the run off, especially where the disease is mainly below the inguinal ligament. Ultrasound scanning of the abdominal aorta can exclude or identify an aneurysm.

Techniques of radionuclide angiography may replace some of the more complicated techniques of angiography. In this method technetium-99^m is injected intravenously in a bolus and a picture of the arteries of the leg is built up by the use of a gamma scanner (Hurlow and Strachan, 1978). The full development of this method is yet unknown. Imaging of peripheral arteries by ultrasound is at present only of use where arteries are fairly superficial, for example at the carotid and femoral bifurcations. This method is in its infancy. Unlike nuclide imaging it is exceedingly expensive.

Treatment

It is important to stress that no treatment is necessary for the majority of those who have vascular disease apart from remedying the risk factors that may have contributed to the disease such as diabetes and hypertension. An absolute ban on smoking is stressed, but is very difficult to enforce. Many patients will swear they have given up smoking and yet their high blood carboxy-haemoglobin levels reveal the truth (Clyne *et al.*, 1982). Many patients openly state they would prefer an operation to stopping smoking and even a threat of loss of limb is no deterrent. There is much controversy over dietary restriction for atherosclerosis, so most surgeons encourage a low animal fat and low carbohydrate diet more with the idea of keeping weight down than in the hope of slowing down progress of the disease. It is doubtful if a high cholesterol level in the blood is a risk factor, nor are the lipid and triglyceride levels significant except in the relatively rare cases of hyperlipidaemia. Attempts to lower cholesterol and fibrinogen by such drugs as clofibrate have not proved to be effective in the control of atherosclerosis and, indeed, have their own harmful side effects such as an increased incidence of gallstones and in mortality. There is an enormous investment being made by the pharmaceutical industry into finding antiplatelet drugs that might prevent the thrombotic sequelae of atherosclerotic plaques so that the disease itself might be arrested or slowed down.

Non-surgical treatment

Only one in five claudicants require surgery (Taylor and Calo, 1962). The others can be assured they have a nearly 50–50 chance of spontaneous improvement that can happen over a period of up to two years so long as they stop smoking and slow down, that is accept the 'shop window disease'. So long as the subject can walk

more than 100 metres on the treadmill and the ankle pressure after exercise does not fall to zero, improvement can be confidently predicted in most patients.

Correction of anaemia may improve ischaemic signs and symptoms. It is very important to control diabetes. The level of haemoglobin is important because polycythaemia is associated with thrombosis and a high level of haemoglobin is associated with increased viscosity. Haemodilution produced by venesection may improve claudication in selected subjects and improve wound healing in some diabetics (Bailey *et al.*, 1979).

Most patients with peripheral vascular disease are given vasodilator drugs. At any one time there are between 20 and 30 vasodilator drugs in use, but there is no evidence as to their value. Because of the natural history of claudication many patients and their doctors become convinced that this is an effective method of treatment. Lastly, it should be stressed that good hygiene and chiropody are essential and patients who have vascular disease in their legs should avoid the physical extremes of heat, cold or exposure to the elements.

Those who have rest pain, pregangrene or gangrene need urgent hospitalisation and usually surgical treatment. Occasionally, however, bed rest and chemotherapy for cellulitis and perhaps releasing pus from under a nail may allow relief of rest pain and some healing. The history of the medical treatment of peripheral vascular disease has shown many different approaches in relation to drugs, such as Vitamin E, or quaint procedures such as the intermuscular implantation of amniotic membrane. However, few have stood up to the rigours of a double blind clinical trial.

Surgical treatment

The surgical procedures available for the treatment of peripheral arterial disease can be grouped under four headings, sympathetic denervation, arterial reconstruction, balloon dilatation and amputation. Operations to reconstruct arteries differ as to whether the aortoiliac or femoropopliteal segments are affected.

Lumbar sympathectomy

Sympathetic denervation is less often performed than earlier because of the increased number of arterial reconstructions that are now feasible. It took a long time for it to be appreciated that lumbar sympathectomy rarely benefitted intermittent claudication beyond its placebo effect. Occasionally it is useful for the claudicant with excessively cold feet by warming them up. Its main role is in the relief of rest pain when arterial reconstruction is not feasible or the general condition is poor. More and more surgeons are using chemical sympathectomy for rest pain and pregangrene (Walker *et al.*, 1978). Many arteriosclerotic patients are old and in a poor condition for surgery. In addition, operative lumbar sympathectomy benefits less than 50% of those suffering with rest pain. A paravertebral lumbar sympathectomy produced by the injection of 8% phenol in glycerine alongside the sympathetic chain is, in skilled hands, extremely effective and almost free of side effects. Occasionally there is irritation of the lumbar nerves producing an unpleasant pain and paraesthesia in the thigh which, however, always remits. Chemical sympathectomy can be performed as day case surgery, or even as an outpatient procedure, so little does it disturb the patient. Operative sympathectomy need only be offered to selected patients, for example younger people with Buerger's Disease.

Reconstructive operations for aortoiliac disease

Arterial reconstruction of the aorta and iliac arteries is performed either by rebore or bypass. Thromboendarterectomy or rebore is not often feasible because the disease is usually too extensive. Rebore is frequently possible if the disease is localised to the infrarenal aorta and the common iliac arteries. Disobliteration of the external iliac artery is difficult and potentially dangerous. Thromboendarterectomy depends on the surgeon's finding a plane of cleavage about one-third into the depth of the media. In the external iliac artery this leaves too diaphanous a vessel which is easily torn, especially where the artery goes deep to the inguinal ligament.

In chronic ischaemia the usual operation is an aortofemoral bypass using a plastic prosthesis joined end-to-side or end-to-end of the infrarenal aorta, end-to-side of the common femoral artery and extending into the proximal part of the deep femoral artery to bypass the posterior plaque that so often narrows the origin of the deep femoral artery (Fig 32.4).

These operations are standardised nowadays, but because they are major operations in people who are often old and less than fit, the mortality is about 5%. Three years after operation only 75% of these grafts are patent (Taylor, 1973). The reasons for failure are first the fact that the prostheses available are still far from perfect and, secondly the operation is only a bypass and does nothing to arrest the progress of the disease, especially distal to the graft, i.e. in the run-off. Complications of the operation include cardiac and respiratory failure, bleeding problems and sepsis. Sepsis is particularly dangerous because of the large buried foreign body the prosthesis represents (Charlesworth, 1980). The groin wounds are particularly prone to infection, because there may be organisms present in the lymph nodes and lymphatics which are disturbed by the dissection of the groin, especially if there is infec-

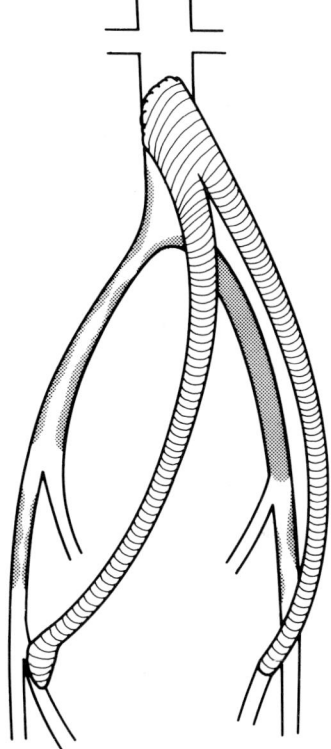

Fig 32.4 Aortofemoral bypass.

tion in the leg such as gangrene. Also, healing of the groin may be impaired by undercutting of the skin and deprivation of its blood supply. Collections of lymph in the groin also provide a medium for the growth of organisms. These groin infections pose great problems for the surgeon and are a hazard to the life and limb of the patient. Often there is a need for a rerouting operation as described on p. 483. There is some evidence that the use of antibiotics during the time of operation may be effective in reducing septic complication, especially if given by bolus injection (Charlesworth, 1980).

Reconstructive operations for femoropopliteal disease

It has become obvious that the larger the artery involved by disease the more satisfactory are the results of surgery. The critical vessel diameter seems to be about 5 mm. Below this diameter the resistance to blood flow mounts dramatically and hence the chance of early and late failure is that much increased. For this reason operations for disease below the level of the inguinal ligament should only be performed for crippling claudication or for fear of loss of limb, where there is rest pain, pregangrene or gangrene. There is no greater disaster than for a patient to lose a limb for a symptom like intermittent claudication which can be relieved by sitting down or walking slowly. The reconstructive operations commonly performed for infrainguinal disease are extended deep femoral angioplasty, femoropopliteal bypass and femorotibial bypass.

Extensive deep femoral angioplasty (Fig 32.5) is indicated for crippling claudication rest pain, pregangrene and minimal digital gangrene (Cotton and Roberts, 1975). The inflow from the aortoiliac segment must be proven to be unimpaired by angiography and ultrasonography. The theoretical reason for success of the operation is the presence of a critical stenosis at the origin of the deep femoral artery (Berguer and Huwang,

1974). In most cases of infrainguinal atherosclerotic disease the superficial femoral artery is occluded, presenting therefore a 50% stenosis. The presence of atheroma in the deep femoral artery increases the stenosis to 67% if the atheroma measures 0.5 mm and 83% if it is 1 mm thick (Fig 32.5).

Normally in the branching arterial system, at each bifurcation the joint surface area of the cross sections of the arterial branches is greater than the main stem by a factor of 1.1 (Berguer *et al.*, 1975). Simply doubling the diameter of the deep femoral artery by a dacron patch will largely abolish the degree of stenosis. How far to extend the patch will depend on the extent of the disease in the deep femoral arteries. It should always extend to a bifurcation and its length will vary from 3–16 cm. Early failures are common in patients with diabetes and where the run-off is poor. Success is most likely for rest pain and minimal digital gangrene, about 50% of claudicants benefit.

Follow-up for up to 7 years has shown satisfactory progress to be maintained so long as the inflow or run-off does not deteriorate. The operation is simple and relatively free of complications. Limb swelling is not a feature as it is after bypass grafting. It is also an operation that can be carried out after failure of a bypass graft.

Femoropopliteal autogenous reversed vein bypass has now been performed for at least 25 years. The patient's own long saphenous vein is removed, its branches sealed off and the vein is reversed so as to nullify the effects of its contained valves. The vessel is joined end-to-side above to the common femoral artery and below to the popliteal artery, preferably above the level of the knee joint. The anastomosis should be as wide as possible, greater than 2 cm in diameter and spout-shaped to allow minimal disturbance of the blood flow (Fig 32.6, p. 484). The operation has also been done with the vein *in situ* with the valves being excised or destroyed by a vein stripper. However, there does not appear to be any advantage to this procedure and it is more difficult to perform.

The operation is well standardised and complications are few (Grimley *et al.*, 1979). Sepsis is not a great problem because there is no foreign body left in the leg. Chronic limb swelling is a feature, probably due to lymphatic disturbance. The main problem is the size of the vein graft. Veins less than 5 mm in diameter are prone to close by thrombosis either early or late in the postoperative period. Early closure may prove disastrous, especially if the operation has been performed for gangrene. Late closure, however, may bring back claudication, but more often than not does not precipitate gangrene. Obviously the process of collateral formation is not inhibited by the presence of an open graft, which is surprising.

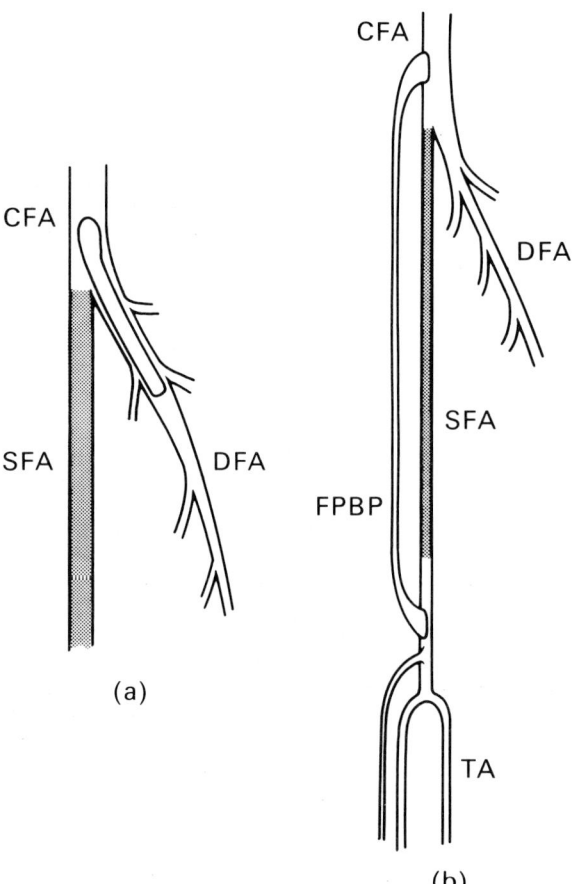

Fig 32.5 (a) Extended deep femoral angioplasty. (b) Femoropopliteal bypass. CFA = common; DFA = deep; SFA = superficial femoral arteries; TA = tibial arteries; FPBP = reversed autogenous long saphenous femoropopliteal venous bypass.

If there is no vein because it has been removed in a stripping operation or if the vein is too small to be a useful graft, other graft materials may be used, but the chances of success are less. Dacron and expanded polytetrafluoroethylene (Goretex) graft materials are used, but, though published results are conflicting, there is no doubt they are inferior to natural grafts such as autogenous long saphenous vein. Recently denatured homologous umbilical vein grafts have become available and seem promising, though they are very expensive (Dardik and Dardik, 1976).

Femorotibial grafting is particularly indicated when the trifurcation of the popliteal artery is involved by disease and a long vein bypass can be achieved by joining the vein below to a tibial artery, usually the posterior tibial, down as far as the ankle. These operations are more difficult to perform because of the small size of the distal artery. Good results have been claimed using both autogenous vein grafts and umbilical vein grafts (Reichle and Tyson, 1975).

Rerouting operations have been devised to divert arterial blood flow from a good to a bad limb either because of failure of one of the standard methods of arterial reconstruction or the poor condition of the patient. These are usually less traumatic operations and can even be performed under local or regional anaesthesia.

1. Cross-over femorofemoral graft. This is a simple relatively small operation in which arterial blood is piped from one femoral artery to another (Ayvazian *et al.*, 1972). It may be the operation of choice when only one iliac artery appears occluded and the aorta and the other iliac artery appears relatively free of disease. In some cases it can also be used when a single limb of an arterial prosthesis has become occluded. The theoretical disadvantage of stealing blood from a normal leg is not realised because the flow down the normal iliac artery is usually doubled when the extra graft is inserted.

2. Axillofemoral and bifemoral graft. In this operation the graft is taken from one axillary artery and placed deep to the pectoral muscles and then subcutaneously joined to the common and deep femoral arteries in one or both groins (Moore *et al.*, 1971).

This operation is for poor risk patients who would not tolerate a more major procedure such as aortofemoral bypass. It is also used when an aortic prosthesis has become infected and must be removed.

3. Obturator canal bypass graft. If there is sepsis in the groin either due to an infected wound, a mycotic aneurysm or an infected prosthesis it may be possible to bypass the site of infection by taking a straight tube graft through the obturator foramen, burrowing it through the muscles of the thigh and joining it to the femoral artery where it is clear of infection (Spiro and Cotton, 1970).

Balloon dilatation

Balloon dilatation of localised strictures and short (less than 10 cm) occlusion of arteries can be very effective in relieving symptoms. The collapsed balloon is precisely located radiologically at the site of the lesion and then rapidly inflated to compress the artherosclerotic tissue against the arterial wall to restore the lumen.

Amputation

Amputation is unfortunately still the only procedure available in some cases of peripheral vascular disease, either because of the extent of arterial disease rendering impossible the feasibility of arterial reconstruction, or because of the poor condition of the patient. Not all arterial operations are successful and failure may indicate amputation. Even after a successful arterial reconstruction, dead tissue may have to be removed by amputation, particularly when toes are involved. Formal flap amputations are to be avoided; it is better to fillet' out the bones from the healthy tissues proximal to the gangrene. The wounds need not be sutured, but merely approximated by surgical tapes. Penicillin must be given against the possibility of gas gangrene.

The commonest major amputations are below knee and above knee, more limited amputations such as the Syme's or transmetatarsal are rarely indicated. One great advance in amputation has been the realisation that wound healing is far better so long as the flaps are constructed of skin, subcutaneous tissue and muscle without separating the skin from the muscle and so reducing the blood supply to the skin. This and suction drainage have been the two major advances in amputation in recent years (Fig 32.6).

The most often used method of below knee amputation utilises the long posterior flap (Thompson, 1978). In this the skin, subcutaneous tissue and calf muscles are tailored to cover the lower edge of the amputation and sutured to the skin over the end of the tibia. This must be cut very obliquely to avoid painful protrusion of bone under the end of the skin. It is still difficult to be sure that a below knee amputation will heal with certainty. A pressure at the ankle measured with ultrasound of less than 40 mmHg makes success very unlikely. A pressure over 100 mmHg is a good prognostic sign (Yao, 1978), but in diabetics pressure at the ankle may be misleadingly high, because diabetics have stiffer, even calcified, arteries as in Mönckeberg's degeneration.

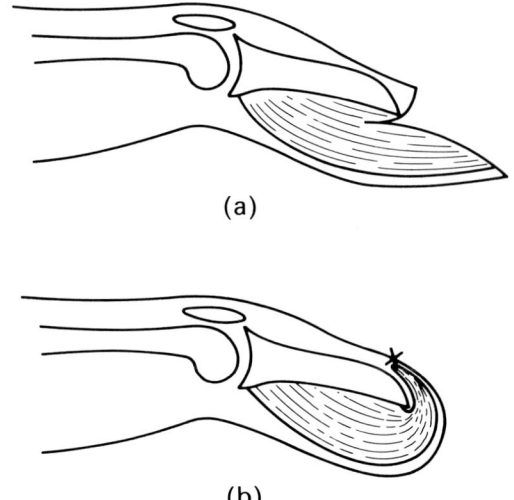

Fig 32.6 Long posterior flap below knee amputation. (a) flaps (b) after suture.

Through-knee amputations and Gritti-Stokes amputations have proved to be less needed because so many patients can have a successful below knee amputation. Above knee amputations are certainly best favoured by the limb fitters, rather than the through-knee amputations. A major advance in below-knee amputation has been the suction prosthesis which enables the patient to walk with a normal gait and without cumbersome buckets and belts.

There is still a need for a pylon to be worn for about 3 months to obtain an optimal shape for the stump which should be conical, free of oedema and free of pain. Good walking training and firm bandaging are essential during this period, under the expert supervision of an experienced physiotherapist.

Graft and suture material

The ideal graft is the autogenous graft, but so often a vessel of appropriate size is not available. Homologous arterial grafts taken from cadavers thrombose or become aneurysmal, usually within a period of a year, but occasionally one may remain patent for many years. Homologous vein grafts suffer the same fate. Presumably anything other than autogenous vascular tissue is antigenic and provokes a rejection reaction by the host. The recent introduction of the denatured umbilical vein graft has probably overcome the rejection phenomenon.

Artificial prostheses have been in use for the last 20 years or more. Those most commonly in use today are made of dacron or Teflon. Different weaves are employed and broadly the grafts are either woven or knitted. More recently velour materials are being used. The choice of plastic material such as dacron or Teflon derives from their almost total lack of reactivity with the host tissues. These plastic materials invoke no inflammatory reaction (Charlesworth, 1980).

When a prosthesis is inserted into the vascular system the suture line becomes covered by endothelium which extends from the host vessel to a variable distance along the graft from either end. Fibrin and blood cells line the rest of the graft with a pseudointima which is, however, poorly attached and likely to dissect and cause thrombosis. In an attempt to procure attachment, the knitted materials are used which have larger interstices through which fibroblasts and macrophages can pass to anchor the intima. Such grafts must be preclotted with the patient's own blood so that fibrin fills the porous material and stops leakage of blood. Velour materials have a weave that allows better entrapment of cells and fibrin from the blood on the inner surface and allows free passage of reparative cells and hence allows greater incorporation.

However, despite all these efforts about 25% of aortic grafts fail within 3 years after insertion, partly due to graft failure and partly to progress of the disease. At the present time there are large numbers of new types of plastic prostheses being produced, but it is extremely difficult to know whether any of them is better than the existing woven and knitted dacron and Teflon materials. Probably improvement of the results of the aortofemoral grafting will only be made by measures which are taken to slow down the progress of the disease, but how to do this is as yet unknown apart from ceasing smoking (Myers *et al.*, 1978).

Upper limb ischaemia

The commonest cause of ischaemia of the upper limb today is, unfortunately, damage sustained at the time of catheterisation of the brachial artery by the cardiologist for coronary angiography. The brachial artery is very sensitive to trauma and is easily sent into spasm. Damage may result in complete or partial severance of the artery, pulsating haematoma and arteriovenous fistula. Careful documentation must be made of the pulses before and after catheterisation. The physician must treat the procedure as a surgical operation and call for surgical help wherever damage is suspected. Immediate surgical reconstruction should then be attempted with patch grafting after patency has been restored by balloon catheterisation. Occasionally, late occlusion occurs and patients present with claudication of the upper arm. Most of these settle spontaneously because of the well-developed collateral circulation in the upper limb. In a few an upper dorsal sympathectomy may give relief from pain.

Apart from iatrogenic trauma, the brachial artery is particularly prone to damage in children who have suffered a supracondylar fracture of the humerus. In these patients it is imperative to record the presence or absence of pulses before and after the reduction of the fracture. If the pulse is absent even after reduction, an expert opinion must be sought. The first move is a fasciotomy to decompress the antecubital fossa. If the artery is in spasm, manoeuvres such as distending it with lignocaine may restore the circulation. The fear is that the widespread spasm may lead to infarction of the forearm muscles, followed by ischaemic contracture of the hand (Volkmann's) and often ischaemic nerve palsies. The artery may be contused with an intimal tear, or even severed by the bone ends. In such cases repair must be attempted by vein graft. Other causes of acute ischaemia in the arm are trauma and embolism, which are considered below.

Cervical ribs rarely cause vascular symptoms and signs unless the artery has been damaged by the rib so as to produce an aneurysm distal to the rib (post-stenotic aneurysm) or an ulcerated plaque where the artery is hooked up by the rib. In both instances ischaemic symptoms such as pain, and signs such as Raynaud's phenomenon, or even digital gangrene may arise because of embolism of thrombus from the aneurysm, or platelets and cholesterol from the plaque (p. 493). Neurogenic symptoms may present in the C.5, 6 or C.8, T.1 dermatomes. The treatment is to remove the rib, resect the aneurysm, if that is possible, or repair the plaque and perform an upper dorsal sympathectomy.

Costoclavicular compression is even rarer and arises when the gap between the clavicle and the first rib is so narrow that the neurovascular bundle becomes nipped between them, causing pain in the arm. Tests for this syndrome are unsatisfactory. Little reliance can be placed upon the obliteration of pulses by elevation of the arm, or bracing the shoulders back because this may happen in normal people. The diagnosis is to be made by exclusion and nowadays, fewer cases are diagnosed now that the syndromes of cervical spondylosis and carpal tunnel syndrome have become so well defined. The treatment is resection of the inner part of the first rib allowing the neurovascular bundle to sink back into the chest, an operation of some difficulty and magnitude.

Intermittent claudication of the arm, Raynaud's phenomenon and even gangrene may be caused by stenosis or thrombosis of the first part of the subclavian artery or in some part of the innominate artery as a manifestation of atherosclerosis or arteritis. In addition, there may be symptoms of subclavian steal (p. 492). A weak radial pulse, lower blood pressure in one arm and a

bruit low down in the neck all suggest the diagnosis. More rarely, the axillary artery may be involved, perhaps from damage by long-term use of an axillary crutch and very rarely after irradiation e.g. for cancer of the breast.

Severe ischaemic symptoms and signs are usually the indication for surgical reconstruction after angiography. Most operations can be performed through the neck, though sometimes the exploration must be carried into the mediastinum through a sternal splitting incision.

Peripheral acute ischaemia

Acute ischaemia of the limbs is most usually due to embolism or trauma and may affect both legs and arms. The symptoms are coldness of the extremity, with or without pain or numbness in the fingers and toes. Loss of sensation indicates a very severe degree of ischaemia. The signs include pallor going on to blotchiness, discolouration and gangrene. Absence of pulsation is an indication of the site of arterial blockage.

Arterial embolism

Atrial fibrillation is by far the commonest cause of arterial embolism due to the breaking off of part of a thrombus in the left atrial appendage. Sudden onset of pulse irregularity may precipitate the liberation of an embolus. A second cause is embolism from a mural thrombosis where thrombus has accumulated at the site of a coronary infarct in the left ventricle about 10 to 20 days after the event. Other causes are the breaking off of thrombus from laminated clot in an aneurysm, or from the surface of an atherosclerotic ulcerating plaque at the carotid bifurcation, or from the abdominal aorta. If no obvious cause can be found atrial myxoma should be sought. Rarely, no primary cause can be found, so-called pseudoembolism. In recent years cardiologists have looked at the possibility of emboli coming from abnormal heart valves, for example in mitral regurgitation. Twenty-four hour tape recordings are useful in picking up intermittent dysrhythmias. Acute ischaemic signs and symptoms present not only in the limbs but in the cerebral circulation, causing stroke, and in the visceral circulation, causing ischaemia of the gut (p. 496), spleen or kidneys.

Many emboli cause only transient episodes of ischaemia, presumably because the thrombus breaks up or slips down an arterial branch where it does no harm. In the upper limb, because of the better collateral circulation, spontaneous relief is common. A saddle embolus blocking the aortic bifurcation may cause ischaemia of both legs, but one may recover if the embolus slips down the other leg. Emboli lodge at bifurcations, in the leg either at the bifurcation of the common femoral artery or at the bifurcation of the popliteal artery. Loss of sensation indicates a severe degree of ischaemia, so severe as to produce ischaemia of the peripheral nerves and merits urgent surgical treatment.

Arterial embolism treated early and before loss of sensation can be treated urgently by intravenous injection of heparin with the idea of preventing the propagating thrombus that spreads distal to the embolus. If this does not produce improvement within an hour or two then embolectomy should be performed by the passage of a Fogarty balloon catheter via an arteriotomy sited immediately above the site of lodgement of the embolus. Where saddle embolus is diagnosed, it can be removed by retrograde balloon catheterisation from the groin on either side. Patients with arterial embolism are often very unfit and in them the operation can be performed under local analgesia.

Operations for arterial embolism are most likely to succeed if performed within 12 h of the onset of symptoms, but many cases have been dealt with successfully up to several days, or even weeks, from the onset. The catheter must be passed down to the tibial or radial arteries until no more clot can be retrieved and a good backflow of blood is obtained. The catheter should also be passed retrogradely to ensure as good a forward flow as possible. The application of a tourniquet is also useful in squeezing the clot out from the periphery towards the arteriotomy.

After operation careful consideration should be given to long-term anticoagulation therapy with Warfarin. In suitable cases cardiac surgery to deal with the mitral valve lesion and the atrial thrombus may be indicated. Recurrence of the embolism is common and mortality is high because of associated cardiac failure, and in the aged, atherosclerosis and poor respiratory reserve. Many patients come to amputation because of a long delay in making the diagnosis, often due to the slowness of the development of symptoms in such cases and the age and poor condition of the patient.

Trauma

Apart from iatrogenic injury to arteries and fractures, direct injury from stabbing or gunshot wounds is becoming more of a commonplace than hitherto. The signs may be very obvious because of the signs and symptoms of acute ischaemia. In other cases a history of profuse blood loss at the time of injury is very suggestive. A torn artery as in an avulsion injury may bleed less than a clean division. In the tear the intima tends to rupture first and the adventitia curls round and plugs the vessel in nature's attempt to arrest haemor-

rhage. Usually the diagnosis is simple, but if there is any doubt about the continuity of the vessel, Doppler examination to reveal arterial patency, or blood pressure at the wrist or ankle may be invaluable. It may also reveal evidence of an arterio-venous communication (p. 495). The rule is that wherever arterial trauma is suspected the wound must be explored and both the artery and the vein repaired if possible. It is very important to repair the vein as well as the artery as cases have been described where arterial reconstruction has been successful, but amputation has followed because of venous obstruction. Arterial damage may only become obvious later, for example a pulsating haematoma may appear days or weeks after injury, so too may the signs of arterio-venous fistula (p. 495). Similarly, a pulsating haematoma may arise days or weeks after femoral puncture for the purpose of angiography. It cannot be stressed too much that in any case of suspected arterial trauma the vessels should be explored and if necessary repaired urgently.

Trauma to the intrathoracic aorta is a feature of major injuries occurring in car crashes. For a patient who has suffered severe injuries, x-rays showing widening of the aortic shadow with signs of cardiac tamponade or cardiac failure indicate the possibility of aortic trauma. The aorta must be exposed, clamped and repaired during cardiac bypass. Even complete transections can be repaired successfully.

Less common aspects of arterial disease

The vast majority of patients affected by arterial disease suffer from the effects of atherosclerosis. It is important, however, to recognise the rarer causes of arterial disease which are amenable to treatment.

Diabetics

Diabetics are prone to arterial disease. Atherosclerosis presents earlier in diabetics than in non-diabetics. The distribution of disease in diabetes is atypical in that additional to major vessel occlusion or stenoses, smaller vessels are typically affected. Because of this many vascular surgeons view diabetic vascular disease as an entity different from atherosclerocis in non-diabetics but the results of reconstructive arterial surgery in diabetics are not generally worse than in non-diabetics. Peripheral neuritis, or diabetic neuropathy, and the increased susceptibility of diabetics to infection increase the chances of developing peripheral gangrene, often with a spreading cellulitis. It is difficult to know why, but local amputations are often more likely to be successful in diabetics even where there is an ischaemic element, especially if they are not polycythaemic (Bailey *et al.*, 1979). Chronic infection in the bones of the foot is best dealt with by 'filleting' operations. It is vital that the diabetic condition is urgently controlled, otherwise the vicious circle of infection leading to the instability of the diabetes and ketosis allows the spread of infection. The appropriate antibiotics must be given. It is common for diabetics to present for the first time with symptoms of ischaemia or infection in the foot. Always a careful assessment of the three elements of 'diabetic gangrene' must be made – arterial disease, neuropathy and infection.

Thromboangiitis obliterans

This is a rare arterial disease that affects younger people. Most vascular surgeons believe that this is a true entity and perhaps an example of extreme hypersensitivity to smoking. Angiographically, the disease mainly affects smaller vessels, for example from the mid-tibial level downwards. Proximally the arteries are smooth and free of atherosclerotic plaques. Histologically the internal elastic lamina is well preserved and in early cases there may be seen an acute inflammatory infiltrate involving arteries, nerves and veins in the neurovascular bundle. The erythrocyte sedimentation rate is often raised and there may be abnormalities in the spectrum of serum proteins. The course of the disease may be prolonged over many years with long periods of remission. In other cases there is a relentless continuous progress of the disease.

The clinical presentation is of severe ischaemia of the skin at the periphery. Rest pain, colour changes and gangrene of the toes are the commonest presentation, but the disease may occur in the fingers and even the tips of the ears and nose may be affected. Amputation, either major or minor, of the limbs may be forced. Because the smaller arteries are involved, arterial reconstruction is not usually feasible. Lumbar or upper dorsal sympathectomy is usually beneficial in relieving rest pain and possibly improving the healing of amputation wounds. Coronary thrombosis and visceral arterial thrombosis are likely to occur and on the whole the outlook is poor. In the past there have been claims that steroid administration and adrenalectomy are beneficial, but there is no scientific evidence that these methods are of any use.

Cystic degeneration and entrapment (Whelan and Bergan, 1977) particularly affect the popliteal artery. They are very rare conditions, but should be thought of in cases of leg ischaemia, particularly in young people.

Cystic degeneration

In cystic degeneration a gelatinous material accumulates in the media, most often in the popliteal artery behind the knee joint. Angiographically the appearance is typical of a filling defect either partially or completely obstructing the artery. At operation the appearance is similar to a ganglion and simply evacuating its contents is often curative, but sometimes the wall is so damaged that it must be resected or bypassed.

Entrapment of the popliteal artery

This is due to an anomalous congenital origin of the popliteus muscle that causes repeated compression of the artery during movement and eventually causes damage to the arterial wall to the extent of resulting in thrombosis. If it can be detected early, it can be cured by dividing the muscle. The angiographic appearance is a typical lateral displacement of the popliteal artery. Once occlusion has occurred it can only be treated like any other cause of chronic ischaemia of the leg.

Aneurysm

Usually arterial aneurysms are due to atherosclerosis and most are sited in the infrarenal part of the abdominal aorta (Gordon-Smith *et al.*, 1978). In most cases atherosclerosis is an intimal disease, resulting in stenosis followed by thrombosis. For some unknown reason the main impact of the disease may be upon the media. In this 'dilating disease' the elastin fibres of the media that make up its larger part become degenerate. The repeated force of the arterial pulsation seems only to be withstood by the integrity of the elastin. The smooth muscle and collagen fibres become fibrosed and stretched. The eventual result is an aneurysm.

Abdominal aneurysms usually lie distal to the renal arteries. They may extend into the common iliac and external iliac arteries. The next common site for aneurysm is in the popliteal artery. Such aneurysms are often bilateral. Other sites are the common femoral, tibial, brachial and rarely the carotid arteries. The natural history of aneurysms is that they may remain unchanged, but more often they thrombose or rupture. Abdominal aortic aneurysms are held to rupture in 60% of cases within 2 years of their recognition. Popliteal and femoral aneurysms are more likely to thrombose than to rupture. In some patients multiple aneurysms appear in a number of sites in the arterial system, as if there had been a generalised breakdown of the structures in the arterial wall. Most aneurysms are asymptomatic. Symptoms and signs are due to increase in size when veins and nerves may be compressed, or from complications such as thrombosis leading to ischaemia, or the signs and symptoms of impending or complete rupture.

Another cause of aneurysm is trauma. Injury to the arterial wall may lead to leakage of blood resisted by the surrounding tissues. Two or three weeks after an injury a pulsating swelling may appear in the limb, a so-called pulsating haematoma. In other cases injury may cause a true aneurysm, usually in a smaller artery such as the radial artery. A mycotic aneurysm arises in cases of septicaemia or pyaemia where infection lodges in the arterial wall, or after injury to an artery. Dissecting aneurysms occur where a split in the intima allows dissection by blood in a plane that runs through the media, usually the site of cystic degeneration. A generation ago the aetiology of aneurysm was reversed inasmuch as syphilis was the major cause and atherosclerosis the lesser. Syphilitic aneurysms nowadays are mostly found in the arch of the aorta.

Abdominal aortic aneurysms

Symptomless abdominal aortic aneurysms are usually detected when the abdomen is being palpated for a routine examination or in cases of abdomindal pain. Occasionally the patient has noted a swelling or abnormal pulsation, or it is found where peripheral ischaemia has been diagnosed in cases of claudication, rest pain or, rarely, gangrene. Another presentation is in a routine abdominal x-ray where calcification in the wall of the aneurysm is discovered.

The pulsation of an aneurysm is expansile rather than transmitted. Small aneurysms may be difficult to distinguish from normal pulsation in a thin person with a thin abdominal wall, especially if there is an element of hypertension. In such patients a plain x-ray of the abdomen may be very helpful because most aneurysms show a thin zone of calcification which outlines the extent of the aneurysm. It may be even better seen in a lateral view. Examination with ultrasound is also very useful in gauging the size of the abdominal aorta and may readily depict an aneurysm. Rarely angiography is needed to define the size of the aneurysm and its relation to the renal arteries. CAT scanning can identify an aneurysm, its relation to the renal arteries and the thickness of its wall.

Abnormal pulsation in the abdomen is usually found to the left of the mid-line because the abdominal aorta tends to lengthen to the left side as it dilates. If the upper limit of pulsation is easily defined, then it can be assumed with reasonable certainty that the aneurysm lies below the renal arteries. It is in those cases in which the upper limit of pulsation cannot be defined clear of the costal margin that angiography is indicated. Angiography may be misleading because a large part of the aneurysmal sac is filled by laminated thrombus and so the apparent aortic dilatation is much less than would be expected from the size of the aneurysm felt by the fingers.

There is no doubt that the majority of aortic abdominal aneurysms should be resected because they eventually rupture and may cause death (Gordon-Smith *et al.*, 1978). The operation is a major abdominal operation often in poor risk patients, but life expectancy charts have clearly shown that the patient whose abdominal aneurysm is treated surgically lives longer than if it is left *in situ* (MacVaugh and Roberts, 1961). In the operation the neck of the aneurysm is isolated and divided, the sac of the aneurysm is opened and evacuated of thrombus. Any bleeding lumbar arteries are closed by sutures from within the sac. If the aneurysm is confined to the aorta it can be replaced with a straight tube of dacron. If the iliac arteries are involved, then a bifurcation graft is inserted, usually down to the common iliac bifurcation. The mortality of the operation is usually between 3 and 5%.

An aneurysm may cause pain if rupture is threatening. The aneurysm may be tender to touch. The presentation may be very varied. Biliary and renal colic may be simulated, as may diseases of the large bowel such as carcinoma and diverticulitis. Indeed, the finding of an aneurysm that causes symptoms must indicate a careful examination of the entire abdominal viscera because there may be so many other causes that may have produced pain. The rule is that aneurysm plus pain indicates immediate and urgent laparotomy. A rupturing aneurysm is a very dangerous condition and carries a high mortality, up to 25% of patients being likely to die. Ruptured abdominal aortic aneurysm is highly fatal and may be a cause of sudden death. Some patients present with a generalised peritonitis. There may be signs to help in the diagnosis, such as pallor and the signs of intraperitoneal bleeding and shock. A pulsating swelling may be felt in the abdomen. Haemorrhagic staining in the perineum and flanks is usually late in appearance. Oliguria and anuria are very serious prognostic signs, as most patients who die after operation die from renal failure.

Urgent operation is indicated and anaesthesia should be induced in the operating theatre because muscular relaxation may allow total rupture of the aneurysm to occur, in which case rapid laparotomy should be undertaken to control the aorta by digital pressure and then by clamping. Once the bleeding is controlled then the aneurysm can be replaced by a prosthesis. Often massive blood replacement is necessary, but not until the aortic leak has been controlled. The operation is usually not difficult, but the problems come later in the immediate and intermediate postoperative phase, which should be carried out in the Intensive Care Unit. The problems then are cardiorespiratory, shock and renal failure and, if recovery is prolonged, local infection and septicaemia. A high proportion of ruptured abdominal aneurysms grow organisms on culture and so appropriate chemotherapy should be instituted, both during the operation and immediately afterwards. The results overall are not good, for some 60–75% of patients succumb after rupture of an aortic abdominal aneurysm (Butler *et al.*, 1978).

Popliteal aneurysm

Popliteal aneurysms are often found accidentally during a routine examination. Often they are bilateral, commonly they are found to be thrombosed on presentation. The diagnosis is easy, the swelling lies behind the knee joint, the pulsation is expansile and the swelling is superficial. Typically, the swelling disappears on flexion of the knee joint. There may be aneurysmal disease elsewhere, such as in the abdominal aorta, femoral artery or brachial artery. Without symptoms, they can be left alone and observed at 3 or 6 monthly intervals.

Thrombosis of a popliteal aneurysm may produce acute or chronic signs and symptoms of ischaemia, or may produce no symptoms at all. Pressure signs on the popliteal vein or adjacent nerves are rare. A solid oval swelling is felt behind the knee; often a symptomless aneurysm is felt behind the opposite knee as well. Acute ischaemia may merit urgent operation in which the aneurysm is bypassed by the insertion of an autogenous vein or, if that is lacking, then less preferably by a plastic prosthesis. In some, the presentation is intermittent claudication, which may remit spontaneously. If not, and if there is in addition rest pain, a bypass operation may be needed.

Rupture of a popliteal aneurysm is a rare event and indicates an urgent operation to arrest haemorrhage and repair by arterial reconstruction if that is possible. It may be that the bypass graft must be extended down to a tibial or peroneal artery if the trifurcation is involved. Occasionally the condition cannot be repaired, when amputation is inevitable.

Other arterial aneurysms

Atherosclerotic aneurysms may arise in any artery; common sites are in the common femoral, brachial and carotid. Similarly aneurysms also occur in other arteries such as the renal and branches of the coeliac. Usually the presenting signs and symptoms are of thrombosis or rupture of the aneurysm. Common femoral aneurysms may require treatment from their size alone. Carotid artery aneurysms may also demand treatment from their size and potential for liberating emboli and causing strokes or transient ischaemic episodes. Where indicated the treatment is resection and arterial reconstruction.

In Marfan's syndrome an aortic aneurysm may present in the thoracic or abdominal aorta. If the aortic arch is involved, dilatation of the aortic valvular ring may cause aortic valvular incompetence and in some cases left ventricular failure. Valve replacement may be necessary. The diagnosis may be made from the patient's spidery fingers, high arched palate and dislocated ocular lenses.

Traumatic aneurysms

Aneurysms due to trauma may be true, false or arteriovenous aneurysms. An example of a true aneurysm is an aneurysm of the radial or ulnar arteries in a young person, or in a person without evidence of atherosclerosis, and which presumably arise from trauma, isolated or repeated. These small, tense painful aneurysms often simulate ganglia and may cause considerable surprise when they are explored. The appropriate feeding artery is tied, the sac removed and cure results.

A false aneurysm, or pulsating haematoma, is due to incomplete division of an artery allowing a leak into the surrounding tissues which limit the spread and size of the aneurysm. An example is damage to a palmar artery from a tool such as a chisel. A tender swelling is felt in the palm which may compress branches of the median nerve and cause numbness and tingling in the fingers. Another example is a stab wound in the thigh that 2 or 3 weeks later may give rise to a pulsating, tender swelling. If this is left, it may eventually rupture, or even become infected. False aneurysms may also follow angiography in the groin after percutaneous transfemoral angiography, and in the antecubital fossa after coronary angiography. The diagnosis may be difficult to make initially because the peripheral pulses are often well preserved.

Angiograms may be deceptively normal in appearance, or show only a small leakage into the surrounding tissue. Operative treatment entails proximal exposure of the feeding vessel to allow its temporary control. Then the sac of the false aneurysm is opened to evacuate clots and to expose the site of the damage. The artery can then be repaired, usually with a patch, but occasionally the damaged artery must be excised and replaced. In this situation a composite graft is useful. A part of the long saphenous vein is dissected, opened and then sutured to another part of the vein of equal length to provide a tube equivalent in diameter to the damaged artery. End-to-end suture is then carried out.

Arteriovenous aneurysms due to trauma may follow stab wounds when both artery and vein are incised. Operative trauma such as dealing with a prolapsed intervertebral disc may result in a major arteriovenous communication, between the aorta and the inferior vena cava.

Immediate exploration may reveal a communication, in which case careful repair of both artery and vein should be carried out, if necessary using a patch for both vessels. Late presentation of an arteriovenous communication may be serious because the load on the heart due to the left to right shunt may precipitate cardiac failure. The signs of a communication are a loud continuous or machinery murmur, dilated superficial veins and a considerably warmer limb. If the communication is large then gangrene of the periphery may appear. The use of an ultrasound probe is very helpful in locating an arteriovenous shunt, either in the early or late phase of its presentation. The treatment is operative repair of both the artery and vein, if that is possible. Occasionally there is a sac separating the vein from the artery. Dissection and division of the communication is curative. A major communication of the aorta and the vena cava is best controlled by passing a balloon catheter up the aorta from the common femoral artery and thus obstructing the site of communication, after which it can be displayed and repaired.

Mycotic aneurysm

Mycotic aneurysms are fortunately rare. Infection in the arterial wall may be a feature of pyaemia or septicaemia. In addition, there is often an injury to the artery that favours the lodgement of infection. This may happen if a pulsating haematoma becomes infected or most often it happens where the anastomosis of a prosthetic graft to a host artery is involved. This may happen soon after surgery or at an interval of months or years. Considerable ingenuity must be used to bypass the site of infection. Commonly, the infected aneurysm is in the groin. Bypass may be achieved either by the obturator femoral route, or by a crossover graft from the common femoral of the affected side. Intensive chemotherapy is essential. Once the bypass is achieved the aneurysm is opened and its infected contents evacuated so that the cavity can be treated with antibiotic and, if necessary, packed to control haemorrhage from any residual feeding vessels.

Dissecting aneurysm

The commonest cause of a dissecting aneurysm is a tear of the intima in the ascending aorta just distal to the sinuses of Valsalva. Commonly there is a cystic degeneration of the media and often hypertension is a feature. Blood enters the split and dissects the aorta and the peripheral arteries to a very variable extent. Dissection may be a cause of sudden death. Rarely, a spontaneous cure may result if the dissection ruptures back into the aorta well distal to its origin, in which case

the aorta has a double lumen that may be compatible with life for many years.

Patients with dissection are often admitted with symptoms indicating a coronary occlusion, although often the cardiogram is normal and the patient may recover and, indeed, be discharged from hospital. More often the dissection is diagnosed by the discovery of an aortic bruit that characteristically changes in intensity in time. Widening of the aortic shadow in a plain chest radiograph may indicate the diagnosis. Some patients may be precipitated into cardiac failure because of the dilatation of the aorta rendering the aortic valve incompetent.

If the dissection progresses down the limb arteries the patient may present with a cold, pulseless arm or leg and arterial embolism may be simulated. Dissection of the renal arteries may be followed by anuria and usually death.

Treatment of a dissecting aneurysm is usually undertaken in collaboration with a cardiac surgeon. As soon as it is safe to proceed, a percutaneous transfemoral angiogram is performed to define the extent of the dissection. Hypertension is controlled by appropriate drug therapy. Immediate surgery may be needed if cardiac failure is present. Surgery is delayed as long as possible to allow fibrosis to occur when the aorta may have to be transected or sutured to a prosthesis. The definitive operation to remove the dissection is the excision of the descending aorta during cardiopulmonary bypass and replacement of it with an aortic prosthesis. This is a serious condition and carries a high mortality (Vecht *et al.*, 1980).

Extracranial arterial disease

During the last 25 years it has become more and more appreciated that many attacks of neurological symptoms and signs are due to disease in the extracranial arteries supplying the brain. These so-called transient ischaemic attacks (TIAs) often progress to full or completed strokes, many of which can be prevented by appropriate surgery. In most cases TIAs are separated by intervals of complete normality. The intervals may vary from minutes to years. In some a partial neurological deficit persists.

Carotid artery stenosis

Typically, the lesion of carotid artery stenosis is an ulcerated plaque sited at the carotid bifurcation and extending variably up the internal and external carotid arteries. Variation in the degree of stenosis is present and can be measured in angiograms and expressed as anything up to a 95% stenosis. The disease is very typically confined to the three carotid arteries and centred within a centimetre or so of the bifurcation. Symptoms are thought to be due to the liberation of atherosclerotic material from the plaques, comprising cholesterol, fibrin and platelets. Confirmation of this theory has often been shown by the appearance of cholesterol crystals in the vessels of the retina easily observed by the ophthalmoscope.

Ischaemic attacks due to carotid artery stenosis lead to interference with the function of the ipsilateral cerebral hemisphere. For example, transient mono- or diplegias, with or without loss of sensation, are common on the opposite side to the affected hemisphere. Often one side of the face is affected. Speech disorders occur if the dominant hemisphere is affected. Ocular symptoms vary from partial to complete loss of vision and are restricted to the same side as the lesion. Total irreversible blindness is rare, but may occur if the central artery to the retina is blocked.

Sometimes stenosis of the carotid arteries is bilateral, in which case it may be difficult, from the symptoms and signs, to localise the side of the responsible stenosis. Localisation is helped by the hearing of a bruit over the side of the stenosis. Sometimes one internal carotid artery is stenosed and the other is thrombosed completely. Obviously a very important factor is the crossover circulation through the circle of Willis in determining the deficit that may occur after stenosis or thrombosis of one or both internal carotid arteries. Less often, the common carotid or innominate arteries are the site of the stenosis.

All these variables make the diagnosis and assessment of carotid artery stenosis very difficult and many attempts have been made first to diagnose the stenosis non-invasively before confirming it by angiography. Timing of the pulse wave arrival can be measured by oculoplethysmography (Kartchner *et al.*, 1973) in which the pulsation of the eyes is recorded by two little cups applied to the anaesthetised corneas connected to pressure transducers. A delay on one side would indicate a stenosis on that side. The pulse wave velocity can also be measured by ultrasound from the suprasternal notch to the supraorbital artery where it emerges from the supraorbital notch on the skull. The supraorbital artery is a terminal branch of the internal carotid artery. The time for transit of the pulse wave can be related to the degree of carotid artery stenosis. If the internal carotid artery is occluded then there may be reversal of blood flow in the supraorbital artery. Occlusion by pressure on the frontal artery, a terminal branch of the external carotid artery, may reduce or promote flow in the supraorbital artery depending on the degree of stenosis in the internal carotid. The main drawback to these methods occurs where there is bilateral disease and where there is a very good crossover flow through the circle of Willis (Horrocks *et al.*, 1979).

The most recent method of non-invasive measurement is by ultrasound imaging in which a picture of the bifurcation is built up and the actual blood flow through the stenosis can be measured (Mercier *et al.*, 1978). When the stenosis is confirmed, angiography can be performed, either by direct puncture of the common carotid arteries, or by arch angiography in which all four arteries supplying the brain are visualised. Ultrasonic imaging will eliminate the need for much angiography. At the present time the machinery for it is extremely expensive and not freely available.

The operation of carotid endarterectomy is carried out by exposure and mobilisation of the carotid bifurcation. Some surgeons anaesthetise the sinus nerves with local anaesthetic because of vasomotor instability both during and after the operation when there is a sensitive carotid sinus. The three carotid arteries are clamped and an incision made from the common carotid extending into the internal carotid just distal to the limit of thickening due to atherosclerosis. With gentle dissection a plane is found in the media which is smooth and allows the atheromatous material stenosing the internal carotid artery to be removed completely because it is so clearly limited to the bifurcation. The incision is closed with a fine continuous prolene suture without a patch.

The operation takes 10–15 min during which time the carotid arteries are clamped and there is fear of brain ischaemia. Brain protection may be achieved by insertion of a plastic shunt. Other methods have been tried and often rejected. Hypercarbia produced by carbon dioxide inhalation does dilate cerebral arteries, but probably not on the clamped side, so this method could actually be harmful by promoting a steal of blood from the clamped to the non-clamped side. Temporary clamping with the patient conscious is very unpleasant for the patient and is no longer used. Monitoring by the electroencephalogram is probably not worthwhile for the EEG is more sensitive to carbon dioxide accumulation than it is to hypoxia. Stump pressure measurement, that is measurement of the pressure in the clamped carotid, is said to be of help. If the pressure is over 50 mmHg some hold that the carotid can be safely clamped. Anticoagulation with heparin either locally or systemically is used by many surgeons and is probably the best method of protection.

Some vascular surgeons take no precautions and claim as good results as those who do. Unfortunately, there is no satisfactory test before the operation of the capacity of the cerebral circulation to withstand a period of carotid clamping. The question of brain protection during carotid surgery is much discussed, but proof of efficiency of any one method is hard to come by.

Many large series have now been published showing excellent short- and long-term results (Thompson and Talkington, 1976). The mortality of the operation is about 2% and the morbidity about 6%. Morbidity includes both transient and permanent strokes after surgery. Risk factors are hypertension, bilateral disease and evidence of peripheral vascular disease. The mortality and morbidity are directly related to the number of risk factors present (Bouchier-Hayes *et al.*, 1979) and have made neurologists more cautious in referring patients for surgery.

Another problem that exercises the vascular surgeon is what should be done after the detection of a symptomless bruit in the neck. Some workers have claimed that approximately 25% of patients with symptomless bruits eventually do go on to develop carotid artery stenosis and permanent strokes. There is great reluctance by many surgeons to operate on such patients and the general view is that symptomless bruits should not be treated, but merely observed over a period of time. Perhaps with the more modern non-invasive methods of treatment this problem may be solved by the detection of the degree of stenosis associated non-invasively.

Operations for patients who have a neurological deficit following an ischaemic attack do not fare so well as patients who have fully recovered after a TIA. Emergency operations for strokes on the whole have not proved to be satisfactory. Surgeons have opened the carotid artery system and sucked out clots, but the tendency to rethrombosis is very high. Also, there is always a possibility that if the blood flow is restored to the brain after a period of ischaemia a serious, if not fatal, cerebral haemorrhage may result because of local brain softening not being able to withstand blood flow even at normal pressure.

Subclavian steal

If a stenosis or occlusion arises in either the subclavian or innominate arteries that is proximal to the site or origin of the vertebral artery then a reversal of blood flow may occur in that artery. This is because the obstruction produces a low pressure in the affected arm vessels which is aggravated by exercise because of peripheral vasodilatation. Arterial blood will then flow from the opposite vertebral artery over the basilar artery. Effectively this is a form of steal and deprives the structures of blood at the base of the brain or in the posterior fossa. The cause is usually atherosclerosis or an arteritis.

Symptoms of vertebrobasilar disease include giddiness, unsteadiness and 'drop attacks'. Less often there is intermittent claudication in the arm following exercise even so trivial as combing the hair. The situation is complicated when there is also disease at the carotid bifurcation when there may also be symptoms of cerebral hemisphere deficiency.

The syndrome is easy to diagnose. A radial pulse

may be diminished in amplitude or even absent. Systolic bruits are heard over one or both subclavian arteries immediately above the clavicles. It is possible with ultrasound to detect flow in the vertebral arteries in the neck and its direction. If reverse flow is found it can be changed to the normal direction by inflation of a sphygmomanometer cuff around the upper arm. This is good confirmatory evidence of a steal.

Arch angiography, preferably with separate catheterisation of the four extracerebral cranial arteries is carried out where possible. There are a variety of operations to reverse a subclavian steal either by direct exposure and local endarterectomy through a sternal splitting incision, or by some form of bypass, for example subclavian-subclavian, axillo-axillary or carotid-suclavian. When there is carotid disease as well, correction of this may improve the blood supply to the brain to such a degree as to vitiate the effects of the steal. In any event, subclavian steal is not so dangerous as carotid artery disease for there is no fear of stroke or death.

Raynaud's phenomenon

There is a continuing debate about the terminology of Raynaud's phenomenon or disease. Maurice Raynaud in 1862 described cases of ischaemia of the periphery which we would probably not call by his name today. He did, however, think that there was an underlying vasomotor instability with which we would now agree. The Raynaud phenomenon is best defined clinically as an abnormal sensitivity to cold in which colour changes in the digits are manifest. There may be episodes of acute onset of pallor, or there may be chronic cyanosis. After pallor hyperaemia may cause a startling redness. Warming the extremities may produce a marked and painful cyanosis.

Many conditions are associated with Raynaud's phenomenon and they are listed in Table 1. Most are rare, but must be identified in the process of investigation. Diseases such as systemic sclerosis may present with

Table 1
RAYNAUD'S PHENOMENON

Arterial disease, Atherosclerosis, Thromboangeitis

Thoracic inlet syndrome, Cervical rib, Costoclavicular pressure

Disease of CNS, Syringomyelia, Poliomyelitis

'**C**ollagen disease', Scleroderma, Dermatomyositis, Cryo and macro globulinaemia, Disseminated Lupus erythematosis

Drugs, Ergotism, B-blocking agents

Trauma, Frostbite, Immersion foot, Occupation, Vibratory tools, Polyvinyl industry

Idiopathic, (the majority)

Raynaud's phenomenon and only years later does the underlying process become evident. Systemic sclerosis must always be suspected when fingers are swollen and stiff and where there are necrotic changes, ulceration and gangrene. Subcutaneous calcinosis may also be a feature simulating pus under the skin, or even gout. Occasionally the fingers are atrophied, tapering and glossy. Radiographs of the hand may reveal the typical deposits of calcinosis and atrophic changes in the terminal phalanges. Wider manifestations are dysphagia due to sclerosis of the oesophagus drawing the stomach into the chest and producing a hiatus hernia. Pulmonary fibrosis causes dyspnoea and even right sided cardiac failure. Telangiectases in the skin are common. The facial appearance is typical in that the angles of the mouth are drawn down and the lips appear thin. There may also be patches of sclerosis of the skin, particularly over the chest. Occasionally, if the gut is involved, there may be diarrhoea and a malabsorption syndrome.

Unilateral Raynaud's phenomenon suggests a local vascular disease or a thoracic inlet syndrome. Any vascular disease from atherosclerosis to thromboangeitis obliterans may present with skin colour changes. Thoracic inlet syndromes include cervical ribs, very rarely cervical bands and very, very rarely costoclavicular compression. A cervical rib usually causes pain in the neck due to its hooking up the lower cords of the brachial plexus thus rendering them more superficial than usual and thus more exposed to touch and trauma. Pain round the shoulder and pain in the hand results. Vascular symptoms are rare and usually due either to a traumatic ulcer in the intima or a poststenotic subclavian aneurysm. From these lesions emboli made up of platelet aggregates and fibrin are likely to be sent to the periphery and cause ischaemic symptoms. Presumably the ulcer in the artery is due to its being elevated abnormally by the rib. Poststenotic dilatation is a well known sequel to a stenotic lesion in an artery.

In costoclavicular compression the gap between the clavicle and the first rib is very narrow and decreased by movement of the shoulder girdle. It is rarely diagnosed now that the frequency of cervical spondylosis and carpal tunnel syndrome have been recognised. A rare cause of costoclavicular compression is following a dislocation or fracture of the medial end of the clavicle when the instability of the fracture imposes repeated trauma on the subclavian artery.

Plain radiographs will reveal cervical ribs or some abnormality such as a prominent transverse process pointing to a cervical band. Pulses may disappear on bracing back the shoulder and elevating the arms. This is a normal finding in quite a number of people. Systolic bruits may be heard over the subclavian arteries. Cervical ribs may be removed if they are troublesome; usually only one side causes symptoms. If the surgeon is convinced of costoclavicular compression then the medial end of the first rib is removed, a difficult and rarely performed operation.

Raynaud's phenomenon caused by vibration is very common. Probably a third of workers using vibrating tools develop Raynaud's type syndromes, but only a few complain. The coarser the vibration the worse are the symptoms. Interestingly, the thumb is rarely involved. In some cases the worker must change his job and the condition is now accepted for industrial compensation.

Ergotism is known to cause digital artery spasm and even gangrene. Bread made from grain infested by 'rust' has been known for centuries to cause madness and digital ischaemia (St Antony's Fire). Ergotamine and its derivatives are used for migraine and every now and again a patient will become sensitive to it and present with a crisis of digital and even brachial ischaemia. This passes off spontaneously or with the assistance of a sympathetic paravertical block. Workers with polyvinyl alcohol have also been known to develop Raynaud's syndrome with digital necrosis and even bone necrosis and gangrene.

Neurological disorders must be excluded, particularly syringomyelia which may present with Raynaud's symptoms. Damage to the sympathetic nerve supply, for example in poliomyelitis, may also produce Raynaud's symptoms in a wasted limb.

As in so many medical conditions the list of potential causes for a syndrome is long, but the cause of the majority of cases is unknown. What the surgeon sees is usually a young woman who has trouble with her hands on exposure to cold. This may be so extreme as to happen merely on change of temperature even in a warm environment. Amongst this group over a period of years a significant number go on to show signs and symptoms of systemic sclerosis with nutritional changes in the digits.

Investigations

After a detailed history and careful physical examination, radiographs of the thoracic inlet and thorax are taken. Haematological examination includes blood count and sedimentation rate. Measurement of IgM and IgG paraproteins is requested. Tests for autoimmune complexes include C1Q binding capacity. In some laboratories blood viscosity and the red cell deformability are measured.

Digital angiography is relatively difficult to perform and has its dangers. The need for it has been eliminated by ultrasound non-invasive investigation with a Doppler probe of each digital artery. With a Doppler probe each digital artery can easily be insonated and its patency revealed. Digital artery occlusion in Raynaud's phenomenon is segmentally arranged and the segments correspond to the phalanges. Two digital arteries and three phalanges make up the six potential arterial segments for each finger. In the thumb there are only two phalanges so there are only four segmental arteries. Each normal hand then has 28 digital artery segments. Mapping of the fingers produces a pattern which correlates well with angiograms (O'Reilly *et al.*, 1979). The digital artery patency can then be expressed as a percentage (28' = 100%).

Preferably the patient should be examined in a temperature controlled room (21°C). The hand should be examined after immersion in water baths 'cold' at 15°C, 'warm' at 21°C and 'hot' at 45°C. 15°C may not seem very cold, but below this temperature the hands may exhibit the 'hunting phenomenon' described by Sir Thomas Lewis in which the digital arteries open and close capriciously. At 45°C the digital arteries open completely in most patients, even when there are necrotic ulcers or terminal gangrene. Examination at 15°C and 21°C suffices particularly for diagnosis and also to follow the course of treatment (Fig 32.7).

Digital artery pressure can also be measured on either side of the finger using small sphygmomanometer cuffs and a Doppler probe. Pressure measurements can be shown to follow precisely the pattern of digital artery patency. By screening patients with Raynaud's phenomenon 80% show some degree of digital occlusion, especially at 15°C. In the other 20% a further cause must be sought. Perhaps in some the test is not sensitive enough or perhaps the site of the occlusion is in the arterioles.

Pathology

It has always been assumed that digital artery occlusion is due to thrombosis or fibrosis, but the evidence for this has been mostly derived from amputation specimens. Dynamic testing with ultrasound before and after thermal stressing shows that almost all occluded digital arteries can be opened at high temperatures. Recent work has shown that in Raynaud's phenomenon the blood is more viscous than normal at low and high shear rates and when the ambient temperature is low. In addition, red cell deformability is less in patients with Raynaud's phenomenon, that is red cells are stiffer than normal. Normally the red cells size 7–8 microns must negotiate the capillary circulation where the vessel diameter averages 5 microns. To flow smoothly the red cells must be flexible. Basically the method of measurement of red cell deformability is the assessment of the capacity of the cells to pass through a filter with 5 micron pores.

Platelet activity is also increased in the blood of patients with Raynaud's phenomenon. The platelets show increased aggregation when exposed to ADP. Most recently platelet activity is assessed by measurement of β thromboglobulin in the plasma which demonstrates an increase in platelet enzyme activity in Raynaud's phenomenon.

Treatment

If a local cause can be found such as thoracic inlet compression, or the effects of vibration disease, or a drug toxicity, or exposure to a toxic chemical agent, these can be dealt with logically.

These factors, however, only account for a small proportion of patients. For the majority the first advice is to avoid cold by wearing sensible gloves and avoiding the immersion of the hands in cold water. There is no evidence that vasodilator drugs have any effect, although many are prescribed. Upper dorsal sympathectomy in which the second and third dorsal sympathetic ganglia are removed improves only about half the patients, and even where relief is gained it is often shortlived. The reason for this is probably that complete denervation of the upper limb is extremely difficult to achieve. It is well known that autonomic nerves

SEGMENTAL

DIGITAL ARTERY PATENCY

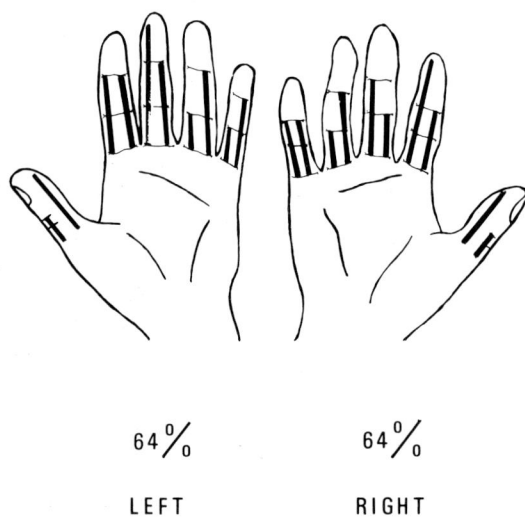

64 %   64 %

LEFT   RIGHT

Fig 32.7 Digital artery patency, recorded by ultrasound. Patency is expressed as the number of arterial segments open as a percentage of the normal 100% = 28 segments.

have a tremendous capacity for regeneration unless they are totally sectioned. The nerves regenerate by collateral sprouting and in this regeneration they may well travel into other nerves both somatic and autonomic. One of the complications of sympathectomy is postgustatory sweating, where newly sprouting nerves become re-routed via the gustatory mechanism to sweat glands of the face.

A promising treatment is plasma exchange (O'Reilly *et al.*, 1979). In this blood is removed from one arm and passed through a centrifuge to remove the plasma. The plasma is replaced by purified protein fraction and gelatin solutions. Up to 3 l of plasma can be removed at one time as an outpatient procedure. How plasma exchange works is as yet unknown. The evidence would suggest that an unknown plasma factor is removed which must reform very slowly, because improvement can last up to two years after a course of plasma exchange. Usually four exchanges are given at weekly intervals. The treatment is expensive, but satisfying in that digital patency is improved and necrotic lesions heal. Tests show that the blood viscosity is improved for at least 6 months after completion of treatment. For less severe cases electrically heated gloves are very helpful in cold weather. Injection of prostaglandin (PGI_2) intravenously is also claimed to help.

Congenital arteriovenous fistulas

Most arteriovenous malformations occur in the limbs and usually only one limb is affected. In the legs the presentation may be only an extensive naevus obvious from birth involving a variable part of the limb or trunk, but often of the whole limb down to the toes. It does not cross the mid-line. As the child grows the cutaneous naevus usually fades and leaves a pale brown pigmentation. The parents may notice that one limb is bigger than the other, or simply find difficulty in fitting shoes. There may well be an endocrine factor in the opening up of arteriovenous malformations, because in a number of patients complications present round about puberty.

Rarely, the appearance is of a gross arteriovenous shunt with gigantism of the limb, a hot limb and the presence of continuous bruits and 'machinery murmurs' over the limb arteries. In such patients left ventricular hypertrophy may be obvious in chest x-rays or in the electrocardiogram. The cardiac output and total blood volume may be grossly increased, but left ventricular failure is rare. Arterial ulcers may appear at the ankle, with patches of gangrene in the base of which are spurting arteries. In some cases there is a marked lymphatic abnormality as well, adding to the gigantism of the limbs.

Purely venous malformations are more common in which varicose veins arise at an early age and lead to the usual venous complications in later life, swelling, pigmentation and ulceration. Unusual veins appear, especially on the lateral side of the leg. In some, phlebograms show total absence of venous valves.

In between these two extremes are cases with both an arterial and a venous element. Ultrasound is useful in such patients because it is the most delicate method of detection of arteriovenous shunts (Sabri and Cotton, 1971). Hearing a continuous noise with ultrasound both in systole and diastole, indicates some degree of arteriovenous shunting. The extent of arteriovenous shunting can be mapped out by scanning the legs.

In most patients no treatment is needed. A yearly examination is made to watch for increased growth in a limb. Careful fitting of shoes is indicated. If the limb grows too much, consideration of epiphyseodesis that is operative fusion of the epiphyses should be undertaken at about 11 years of age to arrest the growth of the limb at the knee. Venous malformations are treated just like varicose veins, preferably by stripping and avulsion of varicose tributaries.

Very rarely, when the shunt is very large as shown by Branham's sign (compression of the artery proximal to the fistula causing a fall in pulse rate and blood pressure), or where there arc signs of left ventricular strain, or increase in blood volume, operative measures must be undertaken. In the Malan operation the main stem vessels are denuded of their branches over very extensive segments. This may be followed by healing of gangrenous ulcers. Embolisation is now widely practised, first by localising the site of shunting by angiography and then by injecting various substances intra-arterially to block off the abnormal circulation. The substance most commonly used is gelatin sponge, but more recently acrylic plastics have been employed. One of the problems of embolisation is the very great capacity for shunts to open up adjacent to the site of blockage. Recurrence, therefore, can be troublesome.

Malformations can occur almost anywhere in the arterial circulation. In most cases they can be safely left, but occasionally they grow almost like malignant tumours and heroic procedures must be devised for their correction and control including deep x-ray therapy to fibrose the microcirculation. Occasionally, if the malformations are small, for example in the digits or on the scalp, they may be excised in their entirety, preferably under hypotensive anaesthesia.

Renovascular hypertension

It has for long been known that stenosis of a renal artery can produce hypertension by activation of the renin-angiotensin system. In a few cases of hypertension, correction of the stenosis can result in prolonged relief. The problem is one of selection of patients because the process of identification of suitable cases is time consuming and expensive, and not without hazard. Pessimists point to poor long-term results after operations to correct renal artery stenosis.

Promising candidates are the young in whom endocrine causes have been excluded such as a phaeochromocytoma, Cushing's syndrome and Conn's syndrome. A urogram that shows a contracted kidney with increased contrast indicates the need for angiography. Selective renal angiography may show a stenosis that may be congenital or atherosclerotic. Some show evidence of fibromuscular hyperplasia.

Operations to bypass the obstruction use either the splenic artery, a vein graft or a plastic prosthesis. Recently strictures have been convincingly dilated by balloon catheterisation. The vascular surgeon also sees renal artery stenosis associated with atherosclerosis of the abdominal aorta and in cases of aneurysm where the atherosclerotic disease has spread from the aorta to involve one or both renal arteries. In such patients the renal arteries can be divided and anastomosed to a prosthesis. This, however, means making the kidney ischaemic. Twenty minutes of ischaemia is recoverable, but if the operative procedure takes longer, then some measure must be undertaken to protect the kidney. The kidney may be cooled locally, but this method is cumbersome and occasionally the freezing coil becomes adherent to the kidney. More recently it has been found that intra-arterial infusion can allow ischaemia of the kidney for up to an hour.

Intestinal ischaemia

Mesenteric infarction from either thrombosis or embolism is fatal in more than 90% of cases. It is to be expected in a patient with arteriopathy who shows evidence of an abdominal catastrophe. Intestinal obstruction and peritonitis are evident. There may be rectal bleeding. If external hernia is excluded and there have been no previous operations to cause adhesions, then mesenteric infarction is one of the likely conditions to be present, especially if there is evidence of coronary disease, peripheral vascular disease or hypertension.

At operation, varying lengths of the mid-gut are found infarcted and dead. Embolectomy or thrombectomy is rarely feasible. Gut resection is usually the only procedure possible. The length of gut removed is irrelevant – what matters is the length left behind. As long as 50 cm of small bowel can be preserved, it is possible for long-term life to be worthwhile, so long as the appropriate vitamin supplements including vitamin B12 and folic acid and a high protein and carbohydrate diet is given.

Chronic intestinal ischaemia is difficult to diagnose

and usually made by exclusion of other causes. It may be more obvious as a cause if there is already evidence of aortoiliac disease. Angiography may show dilatation of the inferior mesenteric artery as the major collateral. For mesenteric ischaemia to occur, more than one intestinal artery must be narrowed or occluded. Evidence such as this calls for lateral angiography to show the origin of the coeliac axis and the origins of the superior and inferior mesenteric arteries.

A bruit heard in the epigastrium may suggest coeliac axis compression and cases have been demonstrated where the coeliac axis is compressed by fibrous bands or the origins of the crura of the diaphragm. Relief of this compression has been claimed to be of great benefit, but there are doubts about its efficacy. Abdominal bruits are not uncommon in normal people and are not necessarily related to intestinal ischaemia.

However, there are a few examples of unexplained abdominal pain where narrowing of at least two intestinal arteries can be demonstrated radiologically. Some people lose weight, and suffer pain but steatorrhea is surprisingly rare. Bypass of the obstruction by a prosthetic graft from the aorta to an intestinal artery, or from one intestinal artery to another distal to the site of obstruction, may be dramatically successful (Marston, 1977). This is a field of great confusion and each possible case must be examined in the greatest detail before a reconstructive procedure is advocated.

The future

It must be clearly understood that vascular surgery for atherosclerosis treats only symptoms while the disease pursues its course over months or years. Arterial reconstructions may fail because of progress of the disease, either proximal or distal to the reconstruction. Risk factors such as smoking, hypertension or diabetes must be taken into account. The medical treatment for arterial disease is only now becoming evident. Measures to correct high blood viscosity and decrease red cell deformability are coming to the fore. Dietary factors are still a matter of debate. Exercise may well be crucial to success. The use of prostaglandins, prostacyclin, and the search for other antiplatelet drugs may well contribute to this field in the near future.

References

Ayvazian V.H., Auer A.I., Hershey F.B. (1972). Limb salvage by extended femorofemoral bypass. *Surg. Gynae. Obstet*; **135:**737–41.

Bailey M.J., Johnston C.L.W., Yates C.J.P., Somerville P.G., Dormandy J.A. (1979). Preoperative haemoglobin as a predictor of outcome of diabetic amputation. *Brit. Med. J*; **1:**168–70.

Berguer R., Huwang N.H.C. (1974). Critical arterial stenosis: a theoretical and experimental solution. *Ann. Surg*; **180**:39–50.

Berguer R., Higgins R.F., Cotton L.T. (1975). Geometry, blood flow and reconstruction of the deep femoral artery. *Amer. J. Surg*; **130**:68–??.

Blau J.N., Logue V. (1961). Intermittent claudication of the cauda equina. *Lancet*; **i**:1081.

Bouchier-Hayes D., De Costa A., Macgowan W.A.L. (1979). The morbidity of carotid endarterectomy. *Brit. J. Surg*; **66**:433–7.

Butler M.J., Vhant A.D.B., Webster H.H. (1978). Ruptured abdominal aortio aneurysm. *Brit. J. Surg*; **65**:839–41.

Charlesworth D. (1980). Arterial replacements. In *Recent Advances in Surgery* (Taylor S.F., ed), pp. 93–111. London: Churchill Livingstone.

Clyne C.A.C., Arch P.J., Carpenter D., Webster J.H.H., Chant A.D.B. (1982). Smoking ignorance and peripheral vascular disease. *Arch. Surg.*; **117**:1062–5.

Cotton L.T., Roberts V.C. (1975). Extended deep femoral angioplasty: an alternative to femoropopliteal bypass. *Brit. J. Surg*; **62**:340–3.

Dardik H., Dardik L.L. (1976). Successful arterial substitution with modified human umbilical vein. *Ann. Surg*; **183**:252–8.

Gordon-Smith I.C. *et al.* (1978). Management of abdominal aortic aneurysm. *Brit. J. Surg*; **65**:834–8.

Gosling R.G., King D.H. (1975). *Ultrasonic Angiology. Arteries and Veins*. Edinburgh: Churchill Livingstone.

Greenhalgh R.M. (1978). Biochemical abnormalities and smoking in arterial ischaemia, in gangrene and severe ischaemia of the lower extremities (Bergan J., Yao J.S.T., eds) pp. 39–60. New York: Grune & Stratton.

Grimley R.P., Obeid M.L., Ahston F., Stanley G. (1979). Long term results of autogenous vein bypass grafts in femoropopliteal arterial occlusion. *Brit. J. Surg*; **66**:723–6.

Horrocks M., Roberts V.C., Cotton L.T. (1979). Doppler ultrasound in the evaluation of carotid artery stenosis – a comparative study in progress in stroke research (Greenhalgh R.M., Rose F.C., eds) pp. 287–97. Tunbridge Wells: Pitman Medical.

Hurlow R.A., Strachan C.J.L. (1978). Clinical scope and potential of isotope angiology. *Brit. J. Surg*; **65**:688–90.

Kartchner M.M., McRae L.P., Morrison F.D. (1973). Non-invasive detection and evaluation of carotid occlusive disease. *Arch. Surg*; **106**:528–35.

Lewis J.D., Yao S.T., Eastcott H.H.G. (1973). *Blood Flow and Pressure in Peripheral Vascular Disease in Blood Flow Measurement* (Roberts V.C., ed) pp. 69–73. London: Sector Publishing Ltd.

MacVaugh H., Roberts B. (1961). Results of resection of abdominal aortic aneurysm. *Surg. Gynae. Obstet*; **113**:17–23.

Marston A. (1977). *Intestinal Ischaemia*. London: Edward Arnold.

Mercier L.A. *et al.* (1978). *High-resolution Ultrasound Arteriography: a Comparison with Carotid Angiography in Non-invasive diagnostic Techniques* (Bernstein E.F., eds) pp. 231–43. Saint Louis: C.V. Mosby.

Moore W.S., Hall A.D., Blaisdell F.W. (1971). Late results of axillary-femoral bypass grafting. *Amer. J. Surg*; **122**: 148–54.

Myers K.A., King R.B., Scott D.F., Morris P.J. (1978). The effects of smoking on the late patency of arterial reconstructions in the legs. *Brit. J. Surg*; **65**:267–71.

O'Reilly M.J.G., Talpos G., Roberts V.C., Cotton L.T. (1979). Assessment of treatment in Raynaud's phenomenon by Doppler ultrasonic velocimetry. *Brit. J. Surg*; **66**:365.

Reichle R., Tyson R. (1975). Comparison of long term results of 364 femoropopliteal or gemorotibial bypasses for revascularisation of severely ischaemic lower extremities. *Ann. Surg*; **182**:449–55.

Roberts V.C., Cotton L.T. (1979). *The Clinical Vascular Laboratory – its Role in the Management of Vascular Disease in Haemodynamics of the Limbs* (Puel P., Bocelaon A., Engalbert A., eds) pp. 519–27. Toulouse, France: S.E.P.E.S.C.

Sabri S., Cotton L.T. (1971). New test for the detection of peripheral arteriovenous fistulae. *Brit. Med. J*; **3**:761–2.

Spiro M., Cotton L.T. (1970). The obturator canal as a route for iliofemoral bypass. *Brit. J. Surg*; **57**:168–72.

Taylor G.W. (1973). Chronic arterial occlusion. In *Peripheral Vascular Surgery* (Birnstingl M., ed) pp. 211–34. London: Heinemann Medical.

Taylor G.W., Calo A.R. (1962). Atherosclerosis of arteries of lower limb. *Brit. Med. J*; **1**:507–10.

Thomas M., Quick C.R.G. (1976). Letter. Intermittent claudication. *Brit. Med. J*; **1**:1531.

Thompson J.E., Talkington C.M. (1976). Carotid endarterectomy. *Ann. Surg*; **184**:1–15.

Thompson R.S. (1978). Performance of major amputation for severe ischaemia in gangrene and severe ischaemia of the lower extremities (Bergan J.J., Yao S.T.T., cds) pp. 407–17. New York: Grune & Stratton.

Vecht R.J., Beesterman E.M.M., Bromley L.L., Eastcott H.H.G., Kenyon J.R. (1980). Acute dissection of the aorta: long term review and management. *Lancet*; **i**:109–11.

Walker P.M., Kay J.H., MacKay I.M., Johnston K.W. (1978). Phenol sympathectomy for vascular occlusive disease. *Surg. Gynae. Obstet*; **146**:741–4.

Whelan T.J., Bergan J.J. (1977). Popliteal artery entrapment and adventitial cystic disease of the popliteal artery. In *Vascular Surgery* (Rutherford R.B., ed) pp. 563–76. Philadelphia: W.B. Saunders.

Yao, J.S. (1970). Haemodynamic studies in peripheral arterial disease. *Brit. J. Surg*; **57**:761.

Yao J.S. (1978). Surgical use of pressure studies in peripheral arterial disease. In *Noninvasive Diagnostic Techniques* Bernstein E.F., ed) pp. 288–303. Saint Louis: C.V. Mosby.

33

Veins

ANDREW NICOLAIDES

Varicose veins

Aetiology and prevalence

Although minor grades of varicosities are very common, the incidence of symptomatic prominent varicose veins has been found to be 6% in adults between 40 and 70 years (Hobbs, 197?).

In the lower extremity varicose veins may be primary or secondary. Primary varicose veins develop in the absence of any demonstrable obstruction. Secondary varicose veins are due to venous obstruction or damage to valves, commonly from deep vein thrombosis and less frequently from extramural compression. Although recanalisation often occurs, the valves remain incompetent. The transmission of high pressure from the deep veins of the leg to the superficial veins through communicating veins whose valves have become incompetent, results in the dilatation and tortuosity of the superficial veins.

Although the aetiology of primary varicose veins is unknown, there are certain well recognised predisposing factors: age, sex and heredity. Age has been found to be the most important predisposing factor. The second most important predisposing factor is sex. Varicose veins are from twice to five times more prevalent in women than in men. The incidence of varicose veins increases if one parent is affected and when both parents are affected this is even higher. Even the frequently reported low prevalence in coloured races may be due to the different life expectancy between African tribes and the Western population. Although men are more rarely affected than women, the relatives of male patients, especially their fathers and brothers have a higher incidence than relatives of affected women.

Pathology

The main features which characterise varicose veins are elongation and tortuosity, loss of elasticity, dilatation, thickening of intima, hypertrophy or atrophy of the muscular layer, disappearance or atrophy of valves, spontaneous thrombosis and enlargement of collaterals with occasional calcification. In a large number of patients with primary varicose veins the only site of incompetence is the saphenofemoral or saphenopopliteal junction without evidence of incompetent communicating veins in the calf. It is not known what causes incompetent valves in these patients. In secondary varicose veins the destruction of valves and the occlusion of deep veins is responsible for the high pressure and dilatation and explains the presence of the incompetent communicating veins.

Three types of varicose veins are recognised:

1 'Spider veins' are small intradermal venules which may first appear when major hormonal changes

are taking place such as puberty, pregnancy and the menopause. They are rarely seen in association with gross varicose veins and postphlebitic limbs. The patients seek medical advice for cosmetic reasons only.

2   Visible subcutaneous veins which are tributaries of the long and short saphenous.

3   Dilated main trunks and main tributaries of long and short saphenous systems with marked valvular incompetence, sometimes associated with symptoms.

In well developed varicose veins with incompetent valves in the saphenous trunks there is no flow when the patient is standing still. During walking the flow is directed distally and blood passes from superficial veins to the deep via communicating veins in the lower calf; flow through the communicating veins is inward in the 'foot lifting' phase (diastole) and outward in the 'foot on ground' phase (systole), but the resultant mean flow is inward from superficial to deep veins. In the presence of deep venous incompetence the flow in the saphenous main trunk during walking may be a back-and-forth movement, a retrograde flow as in saphenofemoral incompetence, or a propulsive flow towards the heart.

The complications of varicose veins are oedema of the ankle and foot, dermatitis, pigmentation of skin, superficial thrombophlebitis, haemorrhage usually after minor trauma and ulceration, although this is rare if the deep veins are patent with competent valves.

Presentation

Patients seek medical advice because of cosmetic reasons, skin changes, irritation, aching or pain on standing, haemorrhage which is either spontaneous or follows minor trauma, muscle cramps, swelling or ulceration. These symptoms may or may not be the result of varicose veins and this must be established before the correct therapy can be decided. Effective treatment depends on correct diagnosis and determining whether the symptoms are really caused by the varicose veins. The history taking should include a careful inquiry about previous deep vein thrombosis, injury or fracture of a limb or abdominal operation with subsequent swelling, attacks of superficial thrombophlebitis, diabetes and anaemias and, finally, inquiry about family history and pregnancies, particularly in relation to the onset of varicose veins.

Examination

For rational treatment it is necessary to determine the extent and severity of the varicose veins, but particularly to determine the presence or absence of incompetence of:

1   saphenofemoral junction
2   saphenopopliteal junction
3   calf communicating veins
4   mid-thigh communicating veins
5   deep veins

The distribution of the affected veins is noted with the patient standing and it is decided whether the long or the short saphenous vein is chiefly affected. Nutritional changes are observed. Varicose oedema is usually local and minimal; substantial oedema should raise the suspicion of old or recent deep vein thrombosis. If a cough impulse is transmitted to the dilated veins, it may be concluded that there is no organic venous occlusion, and that there are no competent valves above that point.

The Trendelenburg test is then performed. The patient lies down and the leg is elevated; if the varices empty immediately, there is no organic venous obstruction. Digital pressure is then applied to the saphenous vein just below the fossa ovalis, and the patient stands; if the great saphenous vein remains empty for as long as the digital pressure is maintained, there is a valvular defect at the termination of the great saphenous vein, the communicating veins which perforate the deep fascia are open and competent, and the circulation in the communicating veins is in the proper direction, from without inwards. The compressing finger is now released; if the vein fills immediately, the incompetence of the highest saphenous valve is confirmed, and the extent of subsequent dilatation shows the area over which valvular incompetence extends.

If the varices fill quickly, in spite of digital compression at the saphenous opening, the communicating (perforating) veins between superficial fascia and deep spaces are incompetent, and the flow in them is reversed. Even if this effect is obtained, the removal of the compressing finger will occasion an immediate and appreciable increase in the venous dilatation if the saphenous valve is also incompetent.

Perthes' test is complementary to the Trendelenburg test. Instead of digital pressure, a tourniquet is applied high in the thigh sufficiently tight to occlude the superficial veins, but no tighter. Ochsner and Mahorner refined this test: three tourniquets are tied sufficiently tightly to occlude the superficial veins, one as high as possible in the thigh, one in the lower third and one just below the knee. The incompetent communicating vein or veins may be presumed to lie in that third of the lower extremity in which the superficial veins fill in spite of tourniquet compression. When the veins are distended, the downward transmission of fluctuation by the column of blood in them indicates over what extent the valves are defective.

These tests are not applicable to the short saphenous vein which drains by a narrow channel through the fibrous roof of the popliteal fossa to join the popliteal vein which is provided with several valves at higher levels. The short saphenous vein always refills slowly, even when varicose.

If the varicose veins in the calf are not controlled by a below knee tourniquet, the presence of incompetent communicating veins is suspected. The fascial orifices in the region of the perforating veins are then detected and marked with a skin pencil on the elevated relaxed leg. Each site is then compressed by fingers and the patient is asked to stand. The fingers are withdrawn one by one and the filling of the varicose veins by blood from the deep venous system is observed. Thus, the 'points of control' are determined where incompetent communicators join the superficial veins.

Performing and interpreting all the above tests is a time consuming procedure for a busy clinic. Moreover, the reliability of the tourniquet tests has been questioned. Because the accurate determination of the sites of incompetence is essential for the correct management of varicose veins, simpler methods have been sought in recent years. Directional Doppler ultrasound is not only accurate, but also quick in determining the presence or absence of saphenofemoral and saphenopopliteal incompetence. The patient is examined standing and the direction of the flow at these sites on thigh and calf compression and release is noted. In the presence of incompetence, there is marked retrograde flow. Directional Doppler ultrasound can also determine the patency of the popliteal, femoral and iliac veins (Nicolaides and Yao, 1981) and the presence or absence of popliteal reflux. This confirmation, obtained quickly, is very useful when confronted with a swollen limb.

The presence of a suspected mid-thigh incompetent communicating vein can be demonstrated by the triple tourniquet test and confirmed by venography. Ascending deep to superficial venography is the best method of determining the site of thigh and calf incompetent communicating veins, especially with stereoscopic views, but this is usually reserved for special complicated cases. The main indication for venography is to confirm the presence of suspected femoral or iliofemoral occlusion in patients with venous claudication and a postphlebitic limb. Ambulatory venous pressure is an invasive method requiring the insertion of a needle in a vein on the foot. Ambulatory foot and calf volumetry (Fernandes *et al.*, 1979) are promising new non-invasive methods.

Treatment

The available methods for the treatment of varicose veins are the injection of sclerosing solutions, ligation and excision or stripping. These have been used separately or in combination.

In 1950, Fegan popularised sclerosant therapy using small volume injections of sodium tetradecyl sulphate into an empty vein followed by local compression. Fegan had a two-fold rationale, that varicose veins were due to incompetence of calf communicating veins and that the obliteration of distal sites of incompetence would diminish the abnormally high flow in the superficial system. In spite of the striking short-term symptomatic and cosmetic success with even the grossest of varices, neither premise has been shown to be true. Up to 3 years after treatment the technique has been found to compare more than favourably with surgery. However, 65% of patients treated by sclerotherapy were classed as failures after 6 years by comparison with 22% of those matched individuals managed by surgical means. Further analysis shows that trivial superficial varices without manifest deep-to-superficial incompetence respond well to sclerotherapy and poorly to surgery. Injection also controls incompetence of communicating veins in the calf. By contrast, varicose veins in the presence of saphenofemoral and saphenopopliteal incompetence, have a high 6-year failure rate.

These results suggest that compression sclerotherapy should be used only after ligation of incompetent saphenofemoral and saphenopopliteal junctions. Because compression is difficult to maintain in the upper two-thirds of the thigh, incompetent communicating veins should also be ligated before sclerotherapy. This means that in an average clinic, about 75% of patients will need some form of surgery prior to sclerotherapy, the remainder can obtain lasting relief from sclerotherapy alone (Nicolaides and Yao, 1981).

Technique of compression sclerotherapy

The treatment of varicose veins by injection and compression requires much practice and is better performed in a specially equipped clinic devoted exclusively to it, an excellent description of the technique is given by Fegan (1967).

'Having decided on the advisability of injection and selected the exact points at which injection should be placed, the usual procedures for i.v. injection are observed.

'A 2 ml syringe loaded with 1 ml of 3% sodium tetradecyl sulphate and a 25 gauge disposable needle is used. The patient sits vertically on a waist-high couch with the legs horizontal. In this position the vein contains sufficient blood for venepuncture. Holding the syringe in the right hand, the vein is punctured at the exact site. A drop of blood is aspirated and 0.1 ml of sodium tetradecyl sulphate is injected to clear the needle. The syringe is now clamped to the patient's leg with the left hand in order to prevent movement between the syringe and vein. It is not necessary to hurry over this procedure because the needle contains sclerosant and will not block. The patient now lies quietly and the leg is elevated and time allowed for the blood to drain out of it. The syringe is taken in the right hand and the ring and index fingers of the left hand are placed along the course of the vein on either side of the puncture site with firm compression. The middle finger rests gently over the point of the needle in order to detect extravascular injection.

'Sclerosant (0.5–1 ml) is injected into the now isolated and emptied segment of vein. The syringe is withdrawn by the right hand and the left hand is maintained in position, holding the sodium tetradecyl sulphate in the isolated segment of vein.

'The bandage is taken in the free hand and applied on either side of the compressing fingers. The left hand is removed, a further turn of the bandage is applied and a bevelled sorbo rubber pad placed directly over the site of venepuncture. The bandaging of this segment is completed and secured. It is advisable to start at the most distal chosen site for injection, but this may produce spasm of the proximal veins, making injection of a more important site more difficult.

'A full length two-way stretch elastic stocking is fitted over the completely injected and bandaged leg and held in place by a suspender belt from the waist. It is wise to make the patient walk around an average room between the application of the bandages and the fitting of the stocking. The application of the stocking holds the bandages in position, especially in bed at night when bandages are inclined to loosen or roll into cords. The stocking, therefore, must be worn throughout the 24 h.

'The compression is of three types. The sorbo rubber pad effects specific compression upon the vein at the site of injection. The cotton crepe bandages without rubber fibre will hold the leg firmly and exert an isometric compression and the elastic stocking will keep the bandages in position following reduction of swelling.

'The importance of walking for 1 h immediately and thereafter for 3 miles each day with avoidance of standing is emphasised. If the bandages loosen, the patients are told to lie down immediately and to have them reapplied with the leg raised.

'Patients are given an explanatory leaflet in the waiting room before entering the clinic and are asked whether they have read it and fully comprehended what the treatment entails. If they are not prepared meticulously to carry out instructions treatment is not given.

'After 2–3 weeks the patient is re-examined and any remaining sites of retrograde filling are dealt with in an identical manner. The use of multiple injections at the first visit greatly reduces the number of attendances required and yields superior results. If successful in dealing with all the sites of retrograde filling at the first visit, the results are extremely gratifying. In the author's experience there are usually not more than three or four such sites and it is worthwhile making a great effort to find them all at the first treatment. Compression is maintained for 6 weeks after the final injection.'

Complications of compression sclerotherapy. Pigmentation of the skin occurs over the sclerosed cords particularly if insufficient compression is applied after the injection. Skin necrosis can occur with an extravascular injection which can be avoided by using a correct technique. Deep vein thrombosis and pulmonary embolism are rare, but have been reported; they are minimised if the patient obeys the instructions of full ambulation. Injection in the region of the post tibial artery is avoided for fear of gangrene.

Contraindications to compression sclerotherapy. Patients not fully ambulant, venous obstruction by extramural compression or recent deep vein thrombosis, severe cardiac disease and arterial disease are contraindications. Previous allergic reaction to the sclerosant is a contraindication, but is very rare.

Technique of saphenous ligation

Aird's (1957) description still remains the best. There are three fundamental principles in the operation:

1 The ligature must be placed close up to the femoral vein so that all subcutaneous tributaries are included, a duplication of the vein is not overlooked, and a pouch of saphenous vein does not remain above the ligature to dilate later.
2 The vein must be doubly ligated and divided, for if it is ligated in continuity, recanalisation is almost certain.
3 All branches of the terminal 5 cm of the vein must be ligated, for if any, either above or below the ligature, remain untied, they may serve as collateral channels for the filling of the potential space in the thick-walled, rigid, saphenous trunk.

Under local or general anaesthesia the fossa ovalis is identified 1.5 cm below and 2.5 cm lateral to the pubic tubercle. An incision 5 cm long is then made over the fossa ovalis in the skin line of the thigh, which curves medially and downwards. The fossa ovalis is identified with the great saphenous vein disappearing under its firm border. Several branches are cleared by dissection and divided between ligatures:

1 A lateral superficial femoral vein curving away laterally and downwards
2 Several superficial veins
3 The superficial circumflex iliac vein
4 The superficial epigastric vein or veins
5 The superficial external pudendal vein

Certain of these, particularly the superficial epigastric and superficial circumflex iliac, may join the saphenous vein in the superficial tissues, but sometimes they pierce the cribriform fascia of the fossa ovalis independently to join the saphenous vein at a deeper level or to enter the femoral vein at a rather higher level than does the saphenous. The cribriform fascia must, therefore, be divided and the vein followed to its termination in the femoral. After division of its tributaries the saphenous vein is doubly tied and divided. The upper ligature is further reinforced by a transfixion ligature as a safeguard against blow-out. If one of these ligatures slips, great care should be taken in controlling haemorrhage. The femoral artery may be traumatised by a clamp applied to the stump of a saphenous vein. Even if the artery is not damaged, the common femoral vein may be obliterated. This should not produce untoward symptoms, and repair of the femoral vein may indeed be necessary if it is lacerated. Occasionally femoral vein ligation produces massive venous thrombosis with loss of arterial pulses and even gangrene. A lateral defect in the femoral vein is best closed by suture. The patient should stay in bed overnight, sometimes if she walks home the upper ligature comes away with production of a considerable haematoma.

In about 2% of legs there are significant variations of the anatomy near the oval fossa. The superficial femoral artery may run extrafascially in the normal location of the long saphenous vein and may cross the oval fossa anterior to the saphenofemoral junction. Thus an incision long enough for complete exposure of the oval fossa is essential. Tortuous varicose veins in the upper two-thirds of the thigh are best excised. Very often the varicosities are tributaries of the long saphenous vein which may be normal, and stripping of it is unnecessary and not recommended. This vein may be useful in subsequent years for femoropopliteal reconstruction or for coronary vein grafts.

Deep vein thrombosis

Deep vein thrombosis (DVT) is used to describe the thrombosis which occurs in the deep veins of the lower limb and pulmonary embolism is migration of venous thrombi and their impaction into the pulmonary circulation. Although deep vein thrombosis and pulmonary embolism are manifestations of the same condition, their management is different and they are considered separately.

Pathogenesis

It is now realised that DVT has a multifactorial aetiology. Immediately after operation or tissue trauma, clotting factors are found circulating in the blood in an activated form. The production of thrombi depends mainly on the action of activated clotting factors in an area of stasis. Thrombosis is not produced by stasis alone, nor by activated factors alone, but by the combination of the two. Stasis in the soleal veins and valve pockets is considerable when the patient is supine with the legs immobile. This explains why the majority of thrombi start at these sites after operation. In addition, stasis stimulates white cells to migrate under the endothelium and damage it. Further information is given in chapter 53.

Factors such as low levels of antithrombin III in women on the contraceptive pill, high levels of urokinase inhibitor in patients with carcinoma, pregnancy and sickle cell disease may be significant. The ^{125}I-fibrinogen test has demonstrated that the incidence of deep vein thrombosis is much higher than previously thought. The majority of thrombi either lyse spontaneously or remain localised to the calf, while only 22% extend proximally to the popliteal or more proximal veins. Clinically detectable pulmonary emboli occur in patients of the latter group only. Certain clinical factors are associated with a high incidence of postoperative deep vein thrombosis viz age, severity of operation, immobility, history of previous deep vein thrombosis and pulmonary embolism, varicose veins, malignancy and obesity.

Clinical features

In the early stages of deep vein thrombosis, symptoms and signs may be absent and in 50% of patients they never become clinically manifest. In some patients thrombosis may be suspected by the occurrence of clinical pulmonary embolism, by a persistent low grade fever which fails to settle after operation, or by the occurrence of pain and swelling in the lower limbs. The patient experiences mild pain of gradual onset in the calf, with a sense of fullness, tightness or actual swelling. The severity of these symptoms depends on the extent of the thrombosis and whether the patient is ambulant or not. Extensive thrombosis involving the popliteal vein frequently produces ankle oedema, but thrombosis extending into the calf, popliteal and superficial femoral veins and terminating just below the sapheno-femoral junction without any oedema has been seen often in patients confined to bed. Swelling may be the only sign. Extensive iliofemoral thrombosis results in a typically swollen white leg (phlegmasia alba dolens). Massive iliofemoral thrombosis involving the collateral vessels results in a very tender, tense, dusky blue leg with distended veins (phlegmasia coerulea dolens).

Although the clinical signs are notoriously unreliable because they can be elicited in the presence of other conditions, the most useful are deep induration at the site of tenderness, and oedema proximal to the calf. An operation or a period of hypotension during the preceeding 3 days increase the probability of presence of thrombosis markedly. Homans' sign, i.e., calf pain produced by gentle dorsiflexion of the foot when the knee is flexed is unreliable because it is present whenever there is calf tenderness irrespective of cause. Ideally, therefore, the first step in the management of DVT is to confirm the diagnosis with an objective test. The relative value and place of venography, ^{125}I-fibrinogen test and other non-invasive tests is discussed below.

Ascending venography

Until recently this has been the method of choice. Contrast is injected in a vein on the dorsum of the foot and directed into the deep veins by an ankle tourniquet. Its ascent is slowed down by a second mid-thigh cuff or by having the patient in a semierect position. It is possible to demonstrate the deep veins consistently from the muscular veins in the calf up to the inferior vena cava, but not the internal iliac and profunda veins.

In a very small proportion of patients it is not possible to obtain good visualisation of the iliac veins and inferior vena cava with ascending venography and yet it is essential to do so. A good example is the patient with gross oedema and iliofemoral vein occlusion in whom anticoagulants are contraindicated and an interruption procedure of the inferior vena cava is contemplated. A cavogram through a percutaneous injection of contrast into the contralateral common femoral is indicated prior to caval interruption. Intraosseous venography has been used to study the venous collaterals in iliac vein obstruction, but is not used routinely because it requires a general anaesthetic and there is the possibility of osteomyelitis and fat embolism.

The criteria for the diagnosis of deep vein thrombosis were established by de Weese and Rogoff (1963) as:

1   The presence of well defined filling defects in opacified veins
2   The demonstration of these defects on at least two radiographs.

Non-visualisation of one or more calf veins was not considered diagnostic of thrombosis since, in normal extremities, these veins are frequently not all visualised. Non-visualisation of the femoral vein with good opacification of the proximal and distal veins and the presence of collaterals was considered evidence of thrombotic obstruction.

Loose thrombus appears as a cylindrical filling defect surrounded by a thin white line of contrast medium. Obliteration of the white line of contrast indicates adherence to the wall. The use of the image intensifier and obtaining several views of the same vein just before and after a Valsalva manoeuvre helps distinguish most artefacts from thrombosis. Fresh thrombus fills most of the venous lumen but is not adherent to the wall. Old thrombus is partly adherent to the wall and partly lysed so that it produces the appearance of a recanalised vein.

The complications of ascending venography are pain, extravasation of contrast and thrombosis. Pain may be prevented by giving the patient an analgesic and injecting the contrast slowly during the early part of the examination. Thrombosis due to the contrast medium is another serious complication. Minimal pain, tenderness or swelling on the day following the venogram has been observed in a small number of patients. These symptoms are rarely severe and clear within 3 days of heparin therapy. In 50% of patients who had venography for varicose veins associated with recurrent leg ulcers on the day before operation, thrombi were found not only in the superficial but also in the subfascial veins at operation. This was despite the routine flushing of the veins with heparinised saline. Since thrombosis may be caused by venography, it is now recommended that it should be done under full heparin cover administered for 24 h. Non-ionic contrast media, now available, should be used in order to minimise the above complications.

[125]I-fibrinogen test

This is now regarded as the most sensitive method for detecting the presence of developing thrombus, whether it is extending or lysing. The test is based on the demonstration that ^{125}I-fibrinogen injected into the circulation is incorporated into a forming thrombus as ^{125}I-fibrin which can be detected by an external scintillation counter. Venography performed in patients with a positive ^{125}I-fibrinogen scan has demonstrated the presence of thrombosis in 93%. However, the test is by no means specific. Any inflammatory condition such as superficial thrombophlebitis, haematoma, wounds, fractures, ulceration, cellulitis and arthritis will result in an increase in the radioactivity. Unless such causes are excluded by careful examination of the patient's legs the test will lead to false positive findings. The ^{125}I-fibrinogen test will not detect any thrombosis in the region of the groin and pelvis because of the high background radioactivity in the bladder.

There are three practical uses of this test. Firstly, it is a useful research tool. Secondly, with the increased awareness of the dangers of venography the ^{125}I-fibrinogen test is used more frequently in the diagnosis of established thrombosis in patients presenting with symptoms and signs. Finally, the ^{125}I-fibrinogen test is useful in the management of limited deep vein thrombosis detected in the calf of patients who are ambulant. If the patient's legs are scanned daily for 1 week and the increased radioactivity extends up to the popliteal fossa, then full anticoagulation therapy with heparin should be started and the patient confined to bed.

Non-invasive tests

Other objective tests such as Doppler ultrasound and impedance plethysmography are non-invasive and easy to perform. They will detect recent occlusion of veins proximal to and including the popliteal, although they may not detect isolated thrombi confined to the calf. When Doppler ultrasound is combined with impedance plethysmography, the diagnostic accuracy is almost the same as venography (Nicolaides and Yao, 1981).

Management

The management of DVT is directed towards the prevention of pulmonary embolism, limitation of local venous damage, the relief of symptoms and prevention of recurrence.

Thrombosis confined to the calf

It has been demonstrated that thrombi confined to the calf are responsible for small silent pulmonary emboli only and serious post-thrombotic sequelae, but not for large clinical pulmonary emboli. It is, therefore, advisable to treat extensive thrombosis in the calf i.e., thrombi longer than 10 cm involving two or more tibial veins with i.v. heparin for 48 h followed by oral anti-coagulants for 6 weeks. Thrombi which are smaller and isolated to the tibial or muscular veins of the calf tend to lyse spontaneously, particularly in patients who are ambulant, wear elastic stockings and are not allowed to keep their legs in a dependent immobile position. Anticoagulant therapy can be avoided in these patients. However, because 20% of thrombi in the calf extend proximally, the above policy is only safe if the ^{125}I-fibrinogen test is used. Patients who are not ambulant and have thrombi confined to the calf should be treated with conventional anticoagulant therapy because the risk of proximal extension in immobile limbs is very high.

Thrombosis proximal to the calf

When thrombosis involves the popliteal and more proximal veins, the risk of pulmonary embolism and post-thrombotic sequelae is high. When the pelvic veins are involved the incidence of clinical pulmonary embolism is 50%. Prompt treatment of these patients is therefore essential. The place of thrombectomy, thrombolytic therapy and anticoagulants in the management of proximal thrombosis is summarised below. The value of defibrinating agents has not yet been fully evaluated.

Thrombectomy. The use of Fogarty's embolectomy catheters allows better clearance of the proximal venous system, diminished risk of pulmonary embolism and less blood loss than the use of suction catheters. Radiological control during thrombectomy and the use of radio-opaque medium in the balloon of Fogarty's catheter have been advocated as aids to obtaining complete clearance. Passage of the Fogarty catheter distally in the leg destroys the valves and should be avoided. Distal thrombus can be expressed by elastic bandages and manual compression. By introducing a small catheter into the iliac segment, postoperative venography and the administration of heparin and fibrinolytic agents is possible. The best results are obtained if thrombectomy is done within 3 days from the onset of thrombosis. Complete clearance is difficult to achieve if the thrombus is more than 5 days old and further clotting is then common. Pulmonary embolism during thrombectomy has been reported but is uncommon. The technique of using two Fogarty balloon catheters reduces the risk, although most surgeons rely on a Valsalva manoeuvre performed during extraction of the iliac clot.

Despite meticulous technique and careful postoperative management, the incidence of recurrence is high, and it seems that thrombectomy neither reduces early morbidity nor prevents valvular damage and the post-thrombotic sequelae. Because of this, thrombectomy has not been generally accepted for patients with proximal thrombosis except in the presence of impending or established venous gangrene. Most patients with phlegmasia coerulea dolens will respond to conservative therapy provided the limbs are not so tense that the arterial supply is impaired; thrombectomy should be reserved for very oedematous tense limbs with impending or actual venous gangrene. Anticoagulant therapy and heparin for several days and subsequent oral anticoagulants for several months should follow thrombectomy.

Fibrinolytic and defibrinating agents. Urokinase and streptokinase stimulate the natural fibrinolytic mechanism in the body by converting the circulating plasminogen into plasmin which is the active substance that lyses thrombus. Complete lysis may require fibrinolytic therapy for several days and the high cost of urokinase makes streptokinase the drug of choice. Bleeding is the commonest complication and occurs at sites of previous venous and arterial punctures and at sites of operation. Other complications include rigors, fever, anaphylactic reactions and embolism.

The evidence available suggests that thrombolytic therapy will produce rapid clearance of the veins with preservation of valves in patients with recent deep vein thrombosis, but further studies are still required to confirm its therapeutic effects and define its exact place in the management of thrombosis.

Ancrod, extracted from Malayan viper venom, is a defibrinating agent which removes fibrinogen from the circulation so that thrombi cannot propagate and are, therefore, more susceptible to natural fibrinolysis. It is as effective as heparin and the incidence of bleeding is less. Its chief disadvantage is that its defibrinating effect can be established safely only after 4–6 h while the anticoagulant effect of heparin is immediate. Further clinical trials are required before this drug is fully assessed.

Heparin therapy. Soon after heparin was discovered it was found to be effective in the treatment of DVT and lifesaving after pulmonary embolism, but it is now realised that the beneficial clinical effect of heparin is not always accompanied by clearance of thrombi as determined by venography.

Heparin may be administered by intermittent i.v. injection, continuous i.v. infusion or subcutaneously. Intermittent i.v. injection allows blood levels of heparin to fluctuate from high to below the therapeutic range. Continuous i.v. infusion produces more constant blood levels, but the risk of bleeding is higher. The subcutaneous route produces more sustained blood levels, but may make neutralisation by protamine sulphate more difficult. It is the method of choice in treating patients outside the hospital.

The amount of heparin required to produce an adequate therapeutic level depends on the patient's weight and on the amount of circulating antiheparin substances which are extremely variable. Usually 30 000 to 60 000 u of i.v. heparin over 24 h are required to prolong the whole blood clotting time to between 2 and 3 times the normal, a level which is effective and safe. It is safer to start with a high dose and then reduce it, than to start with a low dose and gradually increase to the required level. Effective therapy during the early hours will arrest thrombosis and eliminate thromboembolic recurrences.

The optimum duration of heparin therapy has not been established. There is general agreement that a minimum period of 48 h is required, provided the administration of oral anticoagulants is commenced at the same time. This may be adequate for thrombi distal to the popliteal vein, but in patients with proximal thrombosis, heparin may be required for 8–10 days before oral anticoagulants are commenced. After this period most thrombi are firmly attached to the venous wall.

Supportive treatment. Bed rest with leg elevation during the first few days of anticoagulant therapy helps to reduce oedema and, theoretically, prevents dislodgement of thrombi which are not firmly adherent to the vessel. Analgesics may also be required during the same period, but salicylates should be avoided because of the risk of GI bleeding and the potentiation of oral anticoagulants. Active exercises are encouraged in bed and most patients are allowed up after they have been on anticoagulants for 1 week. The study of the fate of thrombi labelled with ^{125}I-fibrinogen suggests that active leg exercises and ambulation encourage early lysis. Elastic stockings with graded compression (decreasing proximally) should be used.

Venous interruption. In patients with DVT proximal to the knee, interruption of the vena cava is indicated when there is failure of anticoagulants to prevent embolism or when anticoagulants are contraindicated. The operative mortality from pulmonary embolism and from other complications after caval interruption is several times higher than that from embolic and haemorrhagic deaths during treatment with anticoagulants. Failure of anticoagulants is the commonest indication for surgical interruption of the vena cava.

The retroperitoneal route through a right-sided transverse incision at the level of the umbilicus is the approach to the inferior vena cava. A variety of techniques of interruption have been practised, including ligation, flattening of the cava to a lumen of 3 mm using stainless steel or Teflon clip, temporary ligation using catgut, plication using multiple sutures, a toothed plastic clip or a mechanical stapler. In recent years umbrella filters have been developed.

Oral anticoagulants. Oral anticoagulants act by inhibiting the production of Factors VII, IX, X and prothrombin by the liver (*see* chapter 53). Their action is antagonised and slowly reversed by the administration of vitamin K. Warfarin and phenindione have become the most popular because they are suitable for both short- and long-term therapy. Toxic and sensitivity reactions are relatively infrequent with warfarin and it is, therefore, the drug of choice. Laboratory control is essential for effective and safe therapy, *see* chapter 53.

Certain drugs are contraindicated during anticoagulation therapy. Salicylates, broad spectrum antibiotics, ACTH, quinidine, alcohol, phenylbutazone and clofibrate may cause haemorrhage. Barbiturates, aminophylline, chloral hydrate and certain tranquilisers such as diazepam antagonise the effect of therapy. Drug resistance is rare and is an indication for changing to a different anticoagulant. The contraindications to oral anticoagulants are the same as for heparin.

The duration of therapy with oral anticoagulants is controversial. In patients with thrombi extending to the veins proximal to the knee, oral anticoagulants are recommended for 6 weeks provided that the patient is ambulant and symptom-free. In patients with clinical pulmonary embolism, therapy for 3–6 months is recommended and in patients with thromboembolic pulmonary hypertension, therapy should be permanent. There is now some evidence that therapy for more than 6 weeks in patients with DVT might be beneficial although the optimum time is not known. It is, however, recommended that after venous thrombosis proximal to the knee, oral anticoagulants should be administered for 3–6 months and in patients with pulmonary embolism this period should be even longer.

Prophylaxis

Methods of preventing venous stasis

Specific attempts to reduce the incidence of DVT by preventing venous stasis have produced variable results. When leg elevation was used in combination with graded elastic stockings and frequent supervised active leg exercises, it was found to reduce the incidence of thrombosis by approximately 50% in patients over the age of 60 undergoing major operations, but this strains the resources of the departments of physical medicine and nursing in any hospital.

Active intermittent compression of the calf by enclosing the leg in a pneumatic bag during and after operation has prevented DVT but is not always effective in patients with malignant disease. The disadvantage of this method is the task of applying the bags, not only at operation but during the postoperative period.

Passive dorsiflexion of the foot during operation by motor driven pedals has reduced the incidence of DVT during the first three postoperative days, but is not effective during the subsequent postoperative period. Electrical stimulation of the calf muscle during operation can produce a reduction in the incidence of DVT but has not always been confirmed. Cinévenographic studies have shown that the soleus muscle and its veins act as a peripheral pump and by recording the changes in blood velocity in the femoral vein it was possible to determine the most effective electrical calf stimulus, which is once ever 4 s. When this stimulus was used in a controlled clinical trial in patients scanned with the ^{125}I-fibrinogen test during the first nine postoperative days, it produced a 92% reduction in the incidence of DVT.

Methods altering the composition of blood

Dextran. Experimental work with Dextran has demonstrated that it prevents thrombi in injured vessels. It is thought that Dextran-70 acts by coating the venous endothelium and the formed elements of the blood, interfering with the platelet adhesiveness and aggregation.

The results of clinical trials with Dextran-70 suggest that the incidence of DVT and pulmonary embolism is diminished but by no means abolished.

Antiplatelet agents other than Dextran. Hydroxychloroquine inhibits ADP-induced platelet aggregation in man and red cell 'sludging'. Aspirin inhibits ADP- and collagen-induced platelet aggregation. Their clinical value awaits further confirmation.

Anticoagulants. The most promising form of prophylaxis is the use of low doses of subcutaneous heparin. The results of an international multicentre trial suggested that subcutaneous heparin diminishes the incidence of postoperative pulmonary embolism, although it has not demonstrated a reduction in the mortality rate in the heparin group. Although we can now say that small-dose subcutaneous heparin can prevent DVT and pulmonary embolism in patients having general

and thoracic operations, many problems remain which are summarised below:

1 Ineffective prophylaxis. The small dose heparin regimen is of limited value in patients with hip fractures and those undergoing elective hip reconstruction. It is also ineffective in patients with an active thrombotic process.

2 Bleeding. In many trials there have been more haematomas in the heparin group and the combination of Dextran infusion with small-dose subcutaneous heparin has led to excessive bleeding and clearly such practice is dangerous. If the increased incidence of wound haematoma is to be prevented, the administration of heparin should be modified so as to avoid plasma heparin levels greater than 0.2 units per ml.

Pulmonary embolism

The incidence of fatal pulmonary embolism has been estimated as 5 per 1000 and of non-fatal pulmonary embolism as 20 per 1000 inpatients.

The diagnosis of pulmonary embolism is difficult because of the great variability of the clinical picture and the lack of a specific laboratory test. The introduction of the ventilation perfusion lung scan which can demonstrate high probability lesions and the measurement of pulmonary artery pressure and selective pulmonary angiography have also contributed towards more accurate diagnosis and better monitoring of therapy.

The effect of sudden obstruction to the pulmonary circulation depends on its size and the state of the cardiac and respiratory systems prior to embolism. In the presence of severe lung or heart disease a small embolus may have the same effect as a massive one in a patient with normal cardiac and respiratory function. By using perfusion lung scans, pulmonary artery pressure measurements and pulmonary angiography, it is possible to classify acute pulmonary embolism as major or minor.

Acute major pulmonary embolism

Clinical features and diagnosis

Although the clinical picture is very variable the commonest symptoms are dyspnoea, pleuritic pain, apprehension and cough. The commonest signs are raised central venous pressure, a loud pulmonary second sound S_3 or S_4 gallop sounds, cyanosis, tachypnoea and tachycardia. When more than 40% of the major pulmonary arteries become occluded the pulmonary embolus is defined as massive, causing marked reduction in cardiac output and right ventricular failure with the possibility of syncope or circulatory arrest. Central chest pain which mimics myocardial infarction may be the result of reduced coronary perfusion.

In the absence of sepsis, the white cell count is less than 15 000 and this may help differentiate major pulmonary embolism from pneumonia in which it is usually raised. Consolidation on the chest x-ray and a raised diaphragm are common and suggest a high probability of embolism. The ECG is a sensitive but not very specific test, many of the changes, which may be transient, reflecting acute right ventricular strain. However, it is very useful in excluding myocardial infarction.

Pulmonary perfusion scan is the most frequent investigation employed; it is a sensitive technique but lacks specificity. Tumours, bullae and areas of inflammation will alter blood flow in the pulmonary arterial tree and produce perfusion defects. However, if the perfusion scan is normal in all posterior, anterior and lateral views, the presence of pulmonary embolism is excluded. Perfusion defects are significant only if the corresponding area on the chest x-ray (or better on a ventilation scan) is normal. Such defects will become smaller or disappear within 4 days. The presence of a doubtful lesion on the pulmonary perfusion scan and the additional finding of vein occlusion in the lower limbs by a non-invasive test such as Doppler ultrasound or impedance plethysmography indicates a high probability (>90%) that pulmonary embolism is present.

Pulmonary angiography is the most specific diagnostic test of major pulmonary embolism and provides a means of demonstrating the anatomical extent of the emboli. At the time of angiography, measurements of the pulmonary artery, right ventricular and right atrial pressures reveal the severity of the haemodynamic disturbance, and a catheter left *in situ* provides effective monitoring. The greatest value of pulmonary angiography is in confirming the presence and extent of embolism in patients whose condition is deteriorating and are considered for pulmonary embolectomy, and excluding those with myocardial infarction.

Management

The initial management depends on the severity of the disturbance. The patient with circulatory arrest needs immediate resuscitation with external cardiac massage, DC shock in the small proportion of patients with ventricular fibrillation (most patients are in asystole), oxygen administration by endotracheal tube, correction of metabolic acidosis with sodium bicarbonate and improvement of right ventricular function with intravenous isoprenaline infusion. A single i.v. injection of heparin (15 000 units) may abolish bronchoconstriction and pulmonary vasoconstriction by blocking serotonin release from platelets on the embolus. External cardiac massage often causes fragmentation and distal propagation of the embolus in the main pulmonary artery, thus reducing the obstruction to overall pulmonary flow.

The patients who fail to respond to the above measures can only be saved with immediate pulmonary embolectomy. Without cardiopulmonary bypass, pulmonary embolectomy using outflow occlusion or inflow occlusion has a high mortality. Partial cardiopulmonary bypass after cannulating the common femoral artery and vein at the bedside enables the transfer of the patient to the operating theatre for establishment of full cardiopulmonary bypass and subsequent embolectomy with a lower, but still unacceptably high, mortality.

A number of patients with circulatory arrest will respond to the initial resuscitation, but remain critically ill. It is recommended that if after 1 h of maximal medical management, there is a systolic blood pressure of less than 90 mmHg, urinary output of less than 20 ml per hour or an arterial Po_2 of less than 60 mmHg, pulmonary embolectomy should be considered and the cardiac surgical team should be assembled urgently. The availability of a portable pump oxygenator as a means of partial cardiopulmonary bypass will provide support during pulmonary angiography and allow a definitive preoperative diagnosis to be made. In patients with a systolic pressure below 10 mmHg and occlusion of more than 70% of the pulmonary circulation there is a 70% chance of death or deterioration on streptokinase or heparin therapy. For them pulmonary embolectomy is indicated.

A direct comparison between the results of embolectomy or heparin in patients who have survived the initial impact of pulmonary embolism, but are critically ill, is not available, but in the majority the treatment of choice is adequate heparin as described for deep vein thrombosis for 7 to 10 days followed by oral anticoagulants for 6 months to a year; heparin, 60 000 units in the first 24 h, is the minimum. Thereafter, a smaller dose may be given, but it should be sufficient to keep the clotting time prolonged for at least twice the control level.

Supportive therapy for acute pulmonary embolism includes bed rest, sedation, aspiration of pleural effusions particularly in the presence of dyspnoea, the treatment of cardiac arrhythmias and oxygen therapy in severe cases. Isoprenaline is the drug of choice in hypotension because of its ionotropic effect. It should be given at a rate which maintains the systolic blood pressure at 100 mmHg (usually 2 μg/min).

Acute minor pulmonary embolism

Clinical features and diagnosis

The patient presents with pleuritic pain or haemoptysis because of the development of a pulmonary infarct. The ECG remains normal, but the chest x-ray may reveal an infarct shadow, pleural effusion, raised diaphragm or linear atelectasis. A pulmonary scan will show areas of reduced perfusion. The presence of one or more perfusion defects in areas which are normal on the x-ray or ventilation scan suggest pulmonary embolism. The improved perfusion when the scan is repeated 4 days later confirms the diagnosis.

Management

Heparin therapy by continuous i.v. infusion for 7 to 10 days followed by oral anticoagulants for 6 months to a year is the treatment of choice. If anticoagulant therapy is contraindicated, or if a second pulmonary embolism occurs during adequate heparin therapy, interruption of the vena cava is indicated. A minor pulmonary embolus should be diagnosed promptly and treated effectively because it often heralds a subsequent massive one.

Subclavian and axillary vein thrombosis

Pathogenesis

Subclavian and axillary vein thrombosis is less frequent than iliofemoral thrombosis. The aetiological factors are the same as for DVT in the lower limb, but trauma to the axillary vein wall as a result of the great mobility at the shoulder joint is the commonest mechanism. The subclavian vein wall is also susceptible to intermittent external compression, injury after fractures of the clavicle and compression by metastases from carcinoma, usually the breast. Thrombosis may be secondary to i.v. therapy, to surgical trauma or scar tissue, but often a cause is not found. Pulmonary embolism following subclavian and axillary vein thrombosis is uncommon and venous gangrene extremely rare.

Diagnosis

There is gradual swelling of the upper limb with symptoms of heaviness, fullness and a 'bursting sensation'. The hand becomes blue with distended veins which on arm elevation are slower to empty than normal. A history of doing gymnastics, lifting heavy weights or a forceful outstretched movement of the upper limb may be obtained. After several days, collateral veins appear over the shoulder, there is diffuse tenseness with some pitting oedema over the whole limb and a tender brachial vein may be palpable. All arterial pulses are normal. Examination by Doppler may reveal absent venous flow or when the collaterals are well developed, continuous flow not affected by respiration. Venography will demonstrate the extent of the lesion and differentiate between extravascular compressions and thrombosis.

Treatment

The initial treatment consists of heparin by continuous i.v. infusion as for DVT in the lower limb, with arm elevation for 1 week followed by oral anticoagulants. In the majority of patients these measures suffice, but a high proportion will have persistent oedema for weeks or months. Recanalisation can be hastened by a temporary ateriovenous fistula using the radial artery at the wrist. The fistula is usually closed 3 months later and the patient continues on oral anticoagulants for 6 months to a year. Thrombectomy is not recommended unless there is threatened gangrene and should always be done in association with a temporary arteriovenous fistula.

Superficial thrombophlebitis

This is a common condition of the superficial veins which consists of localised thrombosis with perivenous inflammation, redness of the skin and pain.

Pathology

Superficial thrombophlebitis is common in varicose veins, but may occur spontaneously in normal veins. It often involves the long saphenous system and its tributaries. It is common in varicose veins because of stasis and because they are more liable to trauma. Other predisposing factors are febrile illness, dehydration, long parturition, bed rest and oral contraceptives. Superficial thrombophlebitis does not give rise to pulmonary embolism, unless it extends into the deep veins through the saphenofemoral, saphenopopliteal junctions and communicating veins.

Thrombophlebitis migrans

This is the term used to describe multiple episodes of superficial thrombophlebitis which may also involve the deep veins. It may be associated with polycythaemia rubra vera, collagen vascular diseases and visceral carcinoma arising most commonly in the pancreas, stomach and lungs.

Infusion thrombophlebitis

This is the commonest cause of iatrogenic superficial thrombophlebitis in the upper limb associated with infusion therapy and injection of contrast media. Hypertonic solutions, low pH and length of infusion are the main factors responsible. It is more frequent on the dorsum of the hand than in the ante-cubital fossa following injection for induction of anaesthesia. It has been shown that neutralisation of low pH by phosphate buffer also reduces the incidence. For parenteral hyperalimentation, a superior vena cava cannula via a subclavian puncture is less likely to cause thrombophlebitis than one via the antecubital fossa.

Suppurative thrombophlebitis

This is a serious condition which may lead to septicaemia and death. Frequent changes of a peripheral cannula and full aseptic technique are good measures for preventing this.

Diagnosis

Superficial thrombophlebitis can usually be diagnosed from red tender globular enlargement of the vein which soon becomes a solid cord. The process may extend up the saphenofemoral junction or it may stop at any point. It may remain localised to a tributary of the long or short saphenous vein.

Superficial thrombophlebitis must be distinguished from lymphangitis by the absence of a clotted vein and lymphadenitis. When it involves the tributaries of the short saphenous, careful examination will avoid the mistake of diagnosing DVT because of calf tenderness and a positive Homans' sign.

Treatment

Firm compression bandages, analgesics and increased walking activity are the essential measures. If there is extensive involvement up to the sapheno femoral junction, then flush ligation of the latter will prevent pulmonary embolism and recurrence. Persistence of severe pain in a large tortuous varicose vein can be treated by evacuation through a stab wound or excision of the thrombosed vein. Bandages are worn for 2 weeks, by which time the tenderness and swelling have subsided and the patient is instructed to wear an elastic stocking for another 2 weeks. Treatment of the varicose veins is the best method to prevent a recurrence.

References and further reading

Aird I. (1957). *A Companion in Surgical Studies*, 2nd edn. Edinburgh: E and S Livingstone.

De Weese J.A., Rogoff S.M. (1963). Phlebographic patterns in acute deep venous thrombosis of leg. *Surgery*; **53**:99.

Dodd H., Cockett F.B. (1976). *The Pathology and Surgery of the Veins of the Lower Limb*, 2nd edn. Edinburgh, London and New York: Churchill Livingstone.

Fegan G. (1967). *Varicose Veins*. London: William Heinemann Medical Books.

Fernandes e Fernandes J., Horner J., Needham T., Nicolaides A. (1979). Ambulatory calf volume plethysmography in the assessment of venous insufficiency. *Brit. J. Surg*; **66**:327.

Hobbs J.T. (1977). *The Treatment of Venous Disorders*. Philadelphia and Toronto: J.B. Lippincott.

Kakkar V.V., Thomas D.P. (1976). *Heparin-Chemistry and Clinical Usage*. London, New York and San Francisco: Academic Press.

Kinmonth J.B. (1982). *The Lymphatics – Disease, Lymphography and Surgery*, 2nd edn. London: Edward Arnold.

Nicolaides A.N. (1975). Thromboembolism – aetiology. In *Advances in Prevention and Management*. Lancaster: Medical and Technical Publishing.

Nicolaides A.N., Hobbs J.T. (1978). Diagnosis of venous thrombosis by the ^{125}I-fibrinogen test. In *Venous Problems* (Bergan J.J., Yao J.S.T., eds.). Chicago and London: Year Book Medical Publishers.

Nicolaides A.N., Yao J.S.T. (1981). *Investigation of Vascular Disorders*. New York, Edinburgh, London, Melbourne: Churchill Livingstone.

Endocrine system

Introduction

Endocrine surgery like gut surgery has benefitted greatly in recent years from the setting up of joint clinics in which physicians and surgeons work side by side. Many countries have also seen the formation of societies for endocrine surgery and now there is, in addition, an International Association devoted exclusively to it. Meanwhile, endocrinology itself has expanded enormously with newer knowledge in many fields; hypothalamus, pituitary, thyroid, parathyroid, adrenal and especially those endocrine cells scattered throughout the gut which produce a variety of hormones and are occasionally the major constituents of tumours.

Thyroid disease and especially hyperthyroidism is more often treated by surgery in the United Kingdom than in most countries in the world today and many would aver that there is no place for the occasional thyroid surgeon. The identification of the C cells and their secretion calcitonin has led to a reappraisal of medullary carcinoma of the thyroid. The association of this tumour with multiple endocrine neoplasia has latterly revived interest in the operation of total thyroidectomy and its potential hazards.

Parathyroid disease was considered a great rarity until the introduction of automated biochemical analysis in the diagnostic laboratory and the rapid and regular production of accurate calcium analyses of blood. As a result, this now proves to be probably the commonest endocrine abnormality in the general population, because approximately one in a thousand are shown to have a raised calcium level, and by far the commonest cause of this is an adenoma of a parathyroid gland. It is true that many of these patients are asymptomatic, although it is also true that when the abnormality is corrected surgically, such patients often volunteer the information that they have been relieved of symptoms which previously they had accepted as normal. The knowledge of mechanisms which both raise and lower the calcium level in the blood, changes almost daily at the present time. The surgery of parathyroid disease can still be very challenging. It clearly adds a new dimension to the care of the patient with renal failure.

The adrenal glands received a great deal of attention when, for a while, adrenalectomy was widely used in the treatment of metastatic cancer, especially of the breast. Today diagnostic techniques both of hormones in the laboratory and the newer imaging processes have made the identification and localisation of adrenal tumours a precise science. The screening of patients suffering from hypertension has provided a considerable harvest of Conn's tumours and diagnosis of the MEN syndromes many phaeochromocytomas.

The pituitary gland, from the surgeon's point of view, is such a highly specialised area that it is not dealt with independently in this section of the book, but the reader is referred to the chapter on brain tumours.

S. T.

34

Thyroid

SELWYN TAYLOR

Development and abnormalities

The thyroid gland develops from the inner end of the first two pharyngeal pouches and the actual site of origin remains as the foramen caecum at the back of the tongue. The anlage of the gland migrates downwards and, traversing the area behind the hyoid bone, ends over the first two or three rings of the trachea dividing into lateral lobes which are then closely applied to it and to the thyroid cartilage. Occasionally remnants of its path remain as thyroglossal cysts or a thyroglossal duct and most rarely the whole of the thyroid remains buried in the posterior third of the tongue, the lingual thyroid gland. The pyramidal lobe of the thyroid gland, which is usually present, represents the lower part of the thyroglossal tract. Occasionally there is complete agenesis of one lobe of the thyroid.

The size of the thyroid gland varies from district to district according to the amount of iodine in the diet. The average weight in the United Kingdom is between 18 and 30 g; in Iceland where the diet is rich in iodine the gland may weigh as little as 10 g in normal health. A rare abnormality of development, but one of importance to the surgeon, is the sequestered or unfused nodule which is an area of normal thyroid tissue completely divorced from the main gland, but occasionally attached to it by a fine fibrous thread. It can readily be mistaken for a deposit of well differentiated thyroid carcinoma.

Vascular connections

A thorough knowledge of the blood supply is essential in surgery of the gland. The superior thyroid artery on each side of the neck arises from the external carotid and passes down the side of pharynx and larynx to break up into branches around the upper pole of the gland. The branches always appear very superficial and are more in evidence on the anterior than the posterior part of the gland, but they anastomose with branches of the inferior thyroid arteries and the gland is very vascular throughout. The inferior thyroid artery arises from the thyrocervical trunk which comes off the first part of the subclavian artery near to the inner border of the anterior scalene muscle. It passes upwards in front of the vertebral artery, behind the carotid sheath and is related to the sympathetic trunk. It is always tortuous and divides into two branches as it approaches the thyroid gland; the recurrent laryngeal nerve lies close to it at this point and the artery may be in front, behind or even embracing the nerve. For the most part the veins draining the thyroid accompany the arteries and this is especially so in the superior part of the gland. The middle thyroid vein and its various tributaries, short and broad, enter the jugular vein directly, while the inferior group usually run down towards the mediastinum often closely associated with the capsule of the thymus. Considering the fact that arteries and veins are usually tied together in operations on the gland, it is surprising that an arteriovenous connection does not more commonly form. However, frequently in hyperthyroidism or in patients who have been over-treated with antithyroid drugs, a loud bruit or machinery murmur is heard over the gland which could easily be mistaken for such a shunt, but it is almost always due to increased blood flow in individual vessels.

Lymphatic drainage

The drainage of lymph from the gland and the associated lymph nodes deserve mention because of the spread of papillary carcinoma by this route. Studies using dye and radio-active substances have shown that the main flow of lymph is towards the wall of the trachea but lymph also flows to a chain of lymph nodes which lie in the groove between the trachea and oesophagus and others drain downwards towards the mediastinum to nodes lying on the thymus gland. A group of lymph nodes lying at the isthmus and, therefore, in front of the larynx have been called the Delphian nodes because it used to be said that if they were palpable it was diagnostic of carcinoma, but this clinical sign is as misleading as was the oracle at Delphi whose name the lymph nodes have been given. Involved lymph nodes may also be found lying alongside the jugular vein or infolding its walls on each side of the neck. They may also be found on each side of the neck above the clavicles. Dense intrathyroidal lymphatics lead to metastases in the contralateral lobe.

The nerves

The recurrent laryngeal nerves are of great importance to the thyroid surgeon since damage to them leads to paralysis of the vocal cords. Severing one of the nerves leads to loss of abduction and the affected vocal cord then lies in the mid-line and the voice is hoarse and has little power. In addition sensory fibres run in these nerve trunks and, as a result, there is usually difficulty in swallowing liquids because they tend to cause choking attacks as some slips past the epiglottis and enters the trachea. When both recurrent nerves are damaged, the two vocal cords come together in the mid-line and this causes respiratory distress during effort so that it is then often necessary to perform a tracheostomy. On the right side, the recurrent nerve arises from the vagus at the root of the neck and passes in front of the first part of the subclavian artery, then ascends behind it in the groove between trachea and oesophagus. If there is an anomalous right subclavian artery arising from the left side of the aorta, the nerve passes directly from the vagus into the larynx and it is thus much more liable to injury at operation; this

abnormality may be associated with coarctation of the aorta. On the left side, the nerve arises in the thorax from the vagus and behind the arch to ascend in the groove between the trachea and oesophagus. In the neck both nerves are closely related to branches of the inferior thyroid artery and then on the posterior aspect of the thyroid gland at the level of the thyroid cartilage they pass under the inferior constrictor muscles into the larynx bending acutely in so doing. The nerve can often be identified more easily low down than near the thyroid gland and can then be rolled under the finger against the wall of the trachea. It has a very distinctive little blood vessel which runs up its anterior surface.

Injury to a recurrent nerve often results in only temporary loss of function and hoarseness, which may appear for the first time 24 or 48 h postoperatively. Recovery is often complete, occurring in 1 or 2 weeks. Such hoarseness should not be confused with that caused by tracheitis due to intubation during anaesthesia. For a correct diagnosis it is essential to perform indirect laryngoscopy both before operation and about 14 days after operation. Even when a cord is paralysed, the opposite vocal cord swings across to the other side to compensate for the loss. As a result, the voice improves greatly in 3 months and may sound normal until the patient is tired, i.e. at the end of the day.

The superior external laryngeal nerve on each side of the neck is principally sensory, but its motor part supplies the cricothyroid muscle. The nerve is at particular risk when the superior thyroid vessels are being ligated and, if it is damaged, the patient finds it impossible to shout explosively and is unable to sing in tune, the tone of the voice dropping quite characteristically. Most superior laryngeal nerve injuries recover in 3 months, but not always. It is possible to identify the nerve as it runs across the cricothyroid muscle in a horizontal direction.

Function

The thyroid gland synthesises, stores and secretes two hormones, thyroxine (T4) and tri-iodothyronine (T3) (de Visscher, 1980). Iodine in the diet is absorbed from the gut and actively concentrated in the cells of the follicles; it is oxidised and combined with thyroglobulin to form monoiodotyrosine (MIT) and di-iodotyrosine (DIT) that are then coupled to form the hormones T4 and T3 which are stored in the colloid in the space inside the follicles. T3 may also be formed by the loss of one iodine molecule from T4. T3 is some three times as active as T4 in stimulating metabolism and as it is not firmly bound to a globulin in the blood, it is readily available and acts much more swiftly.

There is a feedback mechanism and initially the hypothalamus produces a thyrotropin releasing hormone (TRH) which releases thyrotropin (TSH) and this, in turn, stimulates the thyroid gland. The colloid is hydrolysed, little droplets are engulfed and T4 and T3 is carried into the bloodstream.

A third hormone, calcitonin, is also largely manufactured in the thyroid gland, although it is produced to a lesser extent at other sites. It is secreted by the C cells, derived from the neuroectoderm, which are represented by the ultimobranchial body in birds and fishes. The role of calcitonin in calcium metabolism is discussed in the chapter on the parathyroid glands. The C cells lie between and beside the follicular cells and, though scarce, are scattered throughout the thyroid, the greatest number being found in the upper poles.

Tests of function

The patient usually presents to the doctor with a thyroid gland which is either large or too active or both. The history should be most thoroughly obtained because the diagnosis may often rest on this alone. Family history of thyroid disease is important, the area where the patient lives, the diet consumed – especially its content of iodine, the age, sex and race of the patient are all contributory factors.

The three commonest laboratory tests are radioimmunoassay of the serum T3, T4 and TSH (Table 1). The T3 resin uptake is measured *in vitro* and indirectly expresses the concentration of the unsaturated thyroxine binding globulin in the serum and is useful in assessing if the patient is toxic. The radioactive iodine uptake is most valuable when followed by thyroid scanning for the estimation of function in nodules. Radioactive technetium with its short half life and much lower radiation dosage has largely replaced iodine in this respect. ^{123}I is even more acceptable, but at the present time is much more costly.

A rare familial abnormality is the occurrence of a raised thyroid binding globulin (TBG) in the serum. Large family groups have been identified in both the UK and USA and on laboratory testing the T4 level is proportionately raised into the toxic range. The condition is harmless and the individuals so affected are euthyroid, as with all laboratory tests the clinical findings override the abnormal tests on the serum.

Simple goitre

In the endemic areas of the world (Stanbury and Hetzel, 1980) which are usually mountainous, the iodine content of the diet is low and the thyroid enlarges, becoming nodular with the passage of time. Other causes of simple enlargement are puberty and pregnancy and the presence of goitrogens in the diet, especially when the iodine intake is barely sufficient or subliminal. Dyshor-

monogenetic goitre due to an inborn error of iodine metabolism should be considered.

The symptoms are usually a mass in the neck which increases with age and becomes nodular and may press on the great veins, trachea and eventually oesophagus.

The diffuse or parenchymatous enlargement of puberty, or in the young adult before the development of nodules, responds well to treatment with thyroxine by mouth and if 0.2 mg a day is given for one or two years the gland becomes soft and may return to normal size. With the passage of time, if untreated, the gland becomes nodular and thereafter no amount of thyroxine will shrink the nodules, though it may diminish the size of the paranodular tissue. Likewise an adequate intake of iodine in infancy will prevent the development of such swellings, but iodine given after the gland has become nodular is only effective in shrinking the paranodular tissue. Thyroidectomy is the only certain way of removing nodules, or a massive goitre, and the indications for surgery are pressure on the structures in the neck, an unsightly mass or the suspicion that a carcinoma has arisen in the gland.

Treatment of non-toxic goitre

The treatment of non-toxic nodular goitre which is causing symptoms is by partial thyroidectomy followed by thyroxine replacement. The operation for multinodular goitre is best carried out through a long horizontal incision in one of the neck creases about halfway between the manubrium and the thyroid cartilages. Division of the strap muscles gives excellent access and allows identification of the recurrent nerves and parathyroid glands. The aim should be to leave approximately 10 g to 20 g of non-nodular thyroid tissue on each side of the trachea after removing much of the nodular tissue and the pyramidal lobe. If there is a large retrosternal extension two courses of action are open. The simpler is to incise the capsule of the gland and scoop out the contents with a spoon. If the mediastinal extension is very large, then the recurrent nerves must first be clearly defined. Then the manubrium and upper pieces of the sternum are divided vertically with a Lebsche chisel, Gigli wire or vibrating saw, after introducing a metal spatula behind them with finger dissection. The two bony halves are forced apart with a screw retractor such as a Price-Thomas and the nodular mass is carefully dissected away from the great vessels, fibrous tissue making the cleavage plane easily defined. Thyroid tissue is retained on each side of the trachea in the neck as before and the sternum reconstituted with nylon or steel wire. Suction drainage tubes should reach to the bottom of the cavity.

Thyroxine, 0.1 mg to 0.2 mg daily is ordered postoperatively for at least the first year—it is better

Table 1
THYROID TESTS

Test	Indications	Normal	Raised	Lowered
T4 Radioimmunoassay	Screening for hyperthyroidism	70–150 nmol/l	Hyperthyroidism Pregnancy Contraceptive pill Liver disease	Hypothyroidism Aspirin Sulphonamide Patient taking T3
T3 Radioimmunoassay	Screening for hyperthyroidism and T3 toxicosis	1.0–2.8 nmol/l	Hypothyroidism T3 toxicosis	Severe illness Ageing
TSH Radioimmunoassay	Screening for hypothyroidism	< 4 mu/l	Primary hypothyroidism, Established Hashimoto's disease	Hyperthyroidism Secondary (pituitary) hypothyroidism
T3 RU T3 resin uptake	Use in conjunction with T4 Hyperthyroidism in presence of abnormal serum proteins, TBG abnormalities	Laboratory provides its own normal range 92–117 (Thyopac-3 method)	Hyperthyroidism	Contraceptive pill Pregnancy
Free thyroxine index FTI	When complicating factors e.g. pregnancy or drug therapy may alter tests	56–135	Hyperthyroidism	Hypothyroidism
Isotope uptake radioiodine ^{131}I, ^{130}I, ^{132}I, ^{123}I, radio-technetium ^{99}Tc	Scanning for nodules Measure of iodide clearance	^{99}Tc scan at 20 min ^{131}I scan at 30 h	Hyperthyroidism	Hypothyroidism
TRH test	Sensitive test for hyperthyroidism	Rise in TSH level in 20 min	Hypothyroidism	No rise in hyperthyroidism

continued for life. A number of prospective surveys have now demonstrated that approximately 50% of patients develop hypothyroidism after partial thyroidectomy for non-toxic goitre and since follow-up and studies to make sure whether it is no longer necessary to continue it are difficult to arrange long-term, it is probably safer at the present time to advise the patient to take 0.1 mg thyroxine daily for life. When this is not ordered approximately 50% of patients regrow a significant goitre within 7 or 8 years.

The solitary thyroid nodule

Much of the thyroid surgeon's work is involved in dealing with nodules, especially in deciding whether the lesion is benign or malignant (Taylor, 1981). The differential diagnosis is between benign simple goitre, cysts, thyroiditis and a malignant tumour. Again a careful history is helpful, especially the duration of the swelling, recent growth and any localising signs such as a change of voice which is very suggestive of malignancy. More general symptoms stem from hyperthyroidism or hypothyroidism when these arise. A family history or history of radiation to the neck in youth is particularly important since ionising rays in infancy or childhood, even small doses used in diagnosis, are associated with an increased likelihood of thyroid cancer in later life. Unlike other malignant tumours, it is in the young patient that the thyroid nodule is more likely to be malignant than in the older age group, and the surgeon should be suspicious of the solitary hard mass in the thyroid gland of a male patient because the prognosis is not as good as in the female (Mazzaferri et al., 1977).

Investigation

The incidence of carcinoma in the solitary thyroid nodule varies between 10 and 25% in most parts of the world and very careful palpation may reveal fixation, hardness or other changes suggestive of malignancy, such as the presence of enlarged lymph nodes in the drainage area. Scanning the lesion with an isotope such as technetium or iodine 123 or 131 will show whether it is single or multiple, non-functioning or functioning. It is amongst the cold, non-functioning solitary nodules that carcinoma is most frequently encountered. Hot or overactive nodules are very rarely malignant. Fluorescent scanning, if available, is a very safe way of finding out the function of any area in the thyroid.

A radiograph of the neck and mediastinum can be informative, fine calcified stippling is regularly seen in the well differentiated papillary carcinoma and is quite different from the more massive calcification seen fol-

lowing haemorrhage into a simple goitre. Ultrasound with good quality gray scale apparatus will demonstrate cysts as small as 2 cm in diameter.

Where the expertise of the cytologist is available, aspiration biopsy cytology, (ABC), using a fine needle provides an immediate diagnosis (Taylor, 1981). The final arbiter is always a biopsy and other techniques; high speed drill, Tru-cut or open operation require the making of frozen or paraffin wax sections.

Treatment

The optimal treatment for the solitary nodule which is suspicious of malignancy is to excise the whole lobe in which it arises, together with the isthmus and pyramidal lobe and give the patient supplementary thyroxine for at least 2 years, and preferably in small doses for life. The lobe is subjected to histology when it will be discovered whether or not it contains carcinoma. The patient's neck is examined at annual intervals thereafter. The well differentiated carcinoma, papillary or follicular, seen in young patients if removed entire in this way practically never recurs. Further operation is only indicated if there is histological evidence that malignant tissue has been cut across in removal or when palpable lymph nodes are later discovered on palpating the neck.

Hyperthyroidism

This disease is seven or eight times commoner in women than men, affects certain families, and some races have a predisposition to it. When the gland is diffusely enlarged, the disease is often called after Graves or Basedow. The nodular form is sometimes called Plummer's disease and tends to occur in older patients. The onset may be insidious or quite suddenly following a shock and the cause remains unknown, although it is common in certain families. Current belief is that it is a derangement of the immune system and it has been labelled an autoimmune disease because of the presence of TSH receptor antibodies in most patients with Graves' disease.

The severity of hyperthyroidism waxes and wanes and the disease may undergo spontaneous remissions. In the few studies made of its natural history, about 25% tend to go into remission, 25% do not become more severe and, of the remainder, with the passage of time there is progressive cardiovascular damage and some 25% will die of congestive heart failure. Hyperthyroidism can occur with a normal level of T4 in the blood, but a raised T3, so called T3 toxicosis. Individuals who are debilitated or critically ill may show a raised level of T4, but a lowered T3, presumed to be due to difficulty in conversion of T4 to T3.

Symptoms and signs

The typical findings in hyperthyroidism are a fast pulse, moderately and diffusely enlarged thyroid gland, nervousness, tremor, increased sweating, easy fatiguability and loss of weight. In severe cases there is a bruit to be heard over the thyroid gland and there may be diarrhoea and in later stages atrial fibrillation and congestive failure. The eye signs are the thrusting forward of the whole eye and, in addition, retraction of both lids. The resulting exophthalmos gives the patient a distinctive stare and if the ocular changes are severe, there may be muscle weakness. The first eye movement to be lost is that of looking upwards and there may be further paresis of the extraocular muscles with severe limitation of eye movements. In its most severe form the eyes show marked chemosis, and the conjunctivitis and keratitis which accompanies it may even lead to perforation of the cornea and loss of sight. CAT scanning is a very accurate method of measuring the soft tissue changes in the orbit which greatly increase in volume in exophthalmos.

Tests

In most patients the clinical findings are proof enough, but a raised T4 and T3 are also diagnostic, although the TSH is normal or low; the most sensitive test for hyperthyroidism is the TRH (thyrotropin releasing hormone) test. 200 to 400 μgm of TRH injected i.v. cause a rise in the serum TSH at 20 min in all normal patients, but there is no response at all in those with hyperthyroidism. The test is particularly valuable in those with mild or occult hyperthyroidism, such as a small hot nodule may produce.

Differential diagnosis

The likeliest, in mild cases, is anxiety neurosis, but heart disease, all types of diarrhoea, tuberculosis, pregnancy and symptoms sometimes associated with the menopause may all cause confusion. In phaeochromocytoma there may be tachycardia and other symptoms of a raised metabolic rate which is also seen in acromegaly. The most difficult diagnostic tease is the patient who takes thyroxine surreptitiously by mouth; as a result, all the symptoms of hyperthyroidism are produced, but under these circumstances the thyroid gland is usually impalpable and the TRH test shows a rise in TSH.

Choice of treatment

Hyperthyroidism may be treated with antithyroid drugs, radioactive iodine or thyroidectomy and the treatment should be chosen carefully to suit the individual patient (Friesen, 1978). In brief, antithyroid drugs are most suitable for the young patient with mild disease and a diffuse goitre; this therapy is also very useful in preparing a patient both for radio-iodine and surgery. Radioactive iodine is one of the most convenient forms of treatment, but should never be given to children or pregnant women because of the risk of carcinogenesis in the thyroid and is not well suited to the large nodular toxic gland. The high incidence of hypothyroidism which follows this therapy means that follow-up must be continued for life. Surgery is primarily indicated in those patients with a large and especially nodular toxic goitre; in the presence of any suspicion of carcinoma and where it is important that the patient return rapidly to full work and where there are not good facilities for follow-up. It is also well suited to the pregnant patient and those who are incapable or unwilling to maintain long-term drug therapy.

Antithyroid drugs

The principal substance used in the UK is carbimazole (Neomercazole) which is given in 5–10 mg doses 8 hourly and inhibits organic binding of iodine and also prevents the synthesis of the hormones in the gland. The response is rapid and the dose should be reduced as the patient becomes less toxic, or there may be complete suppression of hormone synthesis with greatly increased TSH secretion and as a result a large vascular gland. If there is a good chance of remission in the patient who takes thyroxine surreptitiously by mouth; as tailing off the dose. Sensitivity may occur with rashes, joint pains and agranulocytosis which is rare, but patients should be warned to stop the drug and see their doctor if a sore throat or fever develops.

Radioiodine

The isotope used is ^{131}I with an 8 day half-life; it is safe and is not associated with increased incidence of malignant disease except when used in infants and children. Much smaller doses are now given than heretofore, usually around 3 millicuries as opposed to 7 previously, and the patient's hyperthyroidism is controlled using antithyroid drugs or propanolol for at least 3 months and often a year after the dose, since radiation therapy takes this long to have its full effect. The incidence of hypothyroidism increases by about 2% per year after treatment and it is essential to have an annual check because the onset of symptoms is insidious, and easily mistaken for the normal changes of ageing.

Surgery

The indications for surgery (Heimann, 1978) have been stated, but the patient must be properly prepared for operation and this preparation can take many forms. If antithyroid drugs have already been given, they should be continued up to the day of operation. If the gland is very vascular, iodide or Lugol's iodine should be given for 10 preoperative days at the rate of about 50 mg or 5 drops 8 hourly in milk. This causes the laying down of good quality colloid, shrinkage of the gland and decrease in vascularity. If there is urgency in preparing the patient for treatment for any reason, propanolol 40 mg 8 hourly is given for 3 or 4 days and will control all the symptoms of the disease though in no way lowering the level of hormone in the blood. The patient is quite safe to operate upon and so long as the propanolol is continued after operation for at least a week, there is no risk of thyroid storm.

Thyroid storm is rare nowadays, but used to be one of the hazards of operating on an unprepared toxic gland and may still be seen when a patient is operated upon for some other condition and has an undiscovered hyperthyroidism. The pulse rate rises to uncountable levels, there is hyperpyrexia, air hunger and the patient may die in heart failure. Treatment (Das and Krieger, 1969) is by giving i.v. fluids, cooling the body and infusing very slowly 1–5 mg propanolol which rapidly slows the heart and lowers the temperature. An electric fan on the bed table both cools and assists breathing.

Subtotal thyroidectomy

The operation of subtotal thyroidectomy carries a negligible mortality of less than 1 per 1000 and the other complications include haemorrhage after operation which is due to technical faults, recurrent laryngeal palsy which can be minimised by demonstrating both nerves at operation and avoiding them; the incidence should certainly not be above 2% and most of these paralyses are only temporary. External laryngeal palsy can also be avoided by seeing the superior laryngeal nerves at operation. In very longstanding large retrosternal goitres there is the occasional risk of the trachea collapsing after operation and in any thyroid operation tracheostomy should be performed if there is any anxiety about the airway.

Under intratracheal anaesthesia, and with the neck slightly extended by a small inflated pillow under the shoulders (Fig 34.1), a long incision is made half-way between manubrium and hyoid bone in a horizontal plane following a natural crease (Fig 34.2). The platysma is raised with the skin flaps both above and below

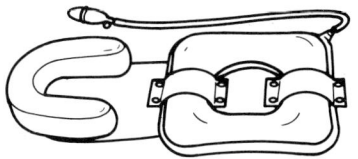

Fig 34.1   Head rest and inflatable shoulder rest.

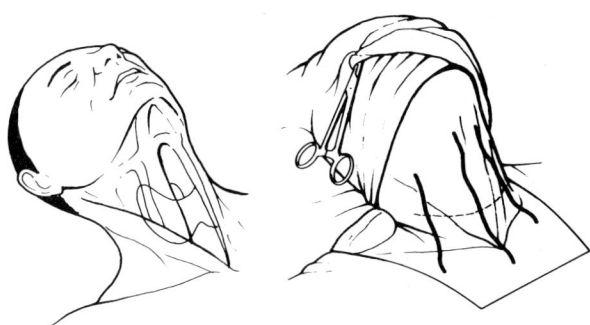

Fig 34.2   Incision.

(Fig 34.3); the sternothyroid and sternohyoid muscles are separated in the mid-line, secured with stay sutures and divided laterally so that the whole neck opens up like a book (Fig 34.4). The removal of the gland should follow a set plan, the superior thyroid vessels are doubly ligated and divided, the gland held forward with a transfixion stitch and the inferior thyroid artery defined and its relation to the recurrent nerve which should be sought at this time. If the parathyroid glands can be seen, this is an added advantage. The inferior thyroid artery is tied in continuity, but is not divided unless the gland is large. The leash of veins at the lower

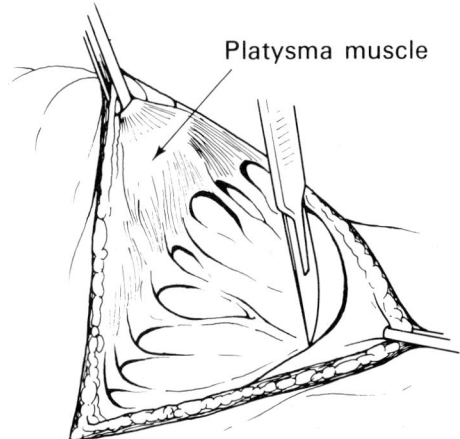

Platysma muscle

Fig 34.3   Separation of platysma from underlying tissues.

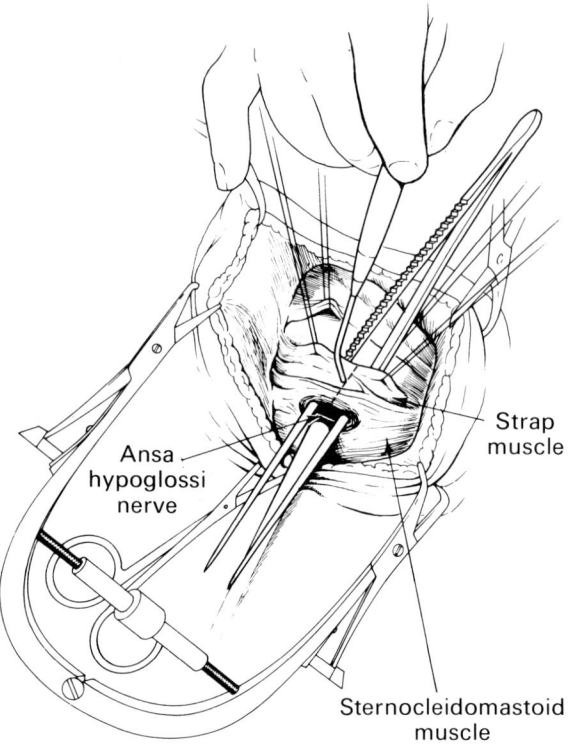

Fig 34.4   Division of strap muscles by diathermy.

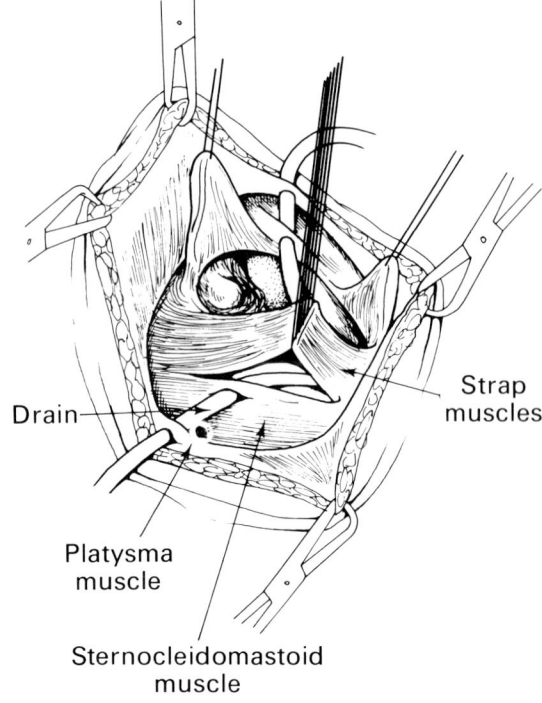

Fig 34.5   Wound closure; *note* drainage tube.

pole is then secured and divided. A similar procedure is carried out on the opposite side of the neck, a procedure which may be facilitated by working from the opposite side of the operating table. Then using fine Spencer Wells or haemostats the amount of gland which is to be retained is carefully marked by introducing the tips and closing the forceps at the level at which the tissue will be cut.

Eight to ten grams of healthy thyroid gland should be left in the neck without encroaching on the parathyroid glands, where they can be defined, and the recurrent nerves. The pyramidal lobe and isthmus is removed with the rest of the tissue and the cut surface of the gland on each side of the neck is oversewn or attached lightly to the adventitia of the trachea, to ensure haemostasis. Two fine rubber tubes are introduced into the neck using a Redon needle (Fig. 34.5) or are placed at the extremities of the wound which is then closed in layers, the skin with Kifa (Fig. 34.6) or Michel clips and a little negative pressure applied to the two drainage tubes. The patient should have a dressing which in no way restricts neck movement (Fig 34.7) and should be sitting up in bed as soon as this is possible and certainly getting out of bed at the end of 24 h. The drainage

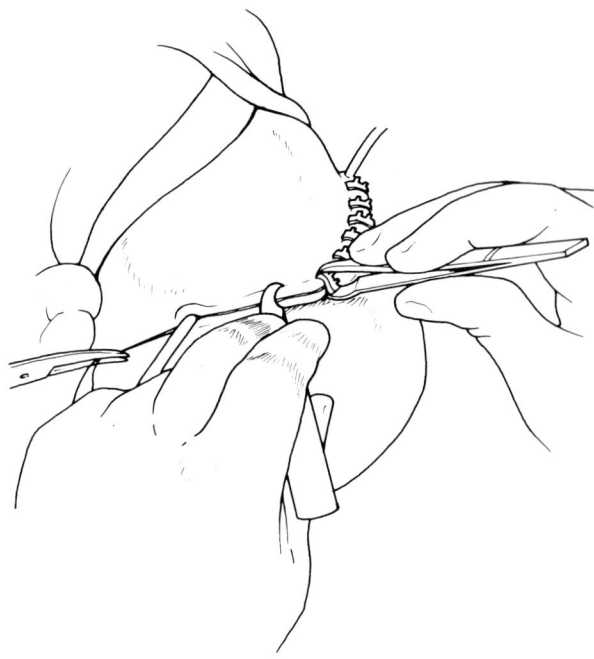

Fig 34.6   Skin closure with Kifa clips.

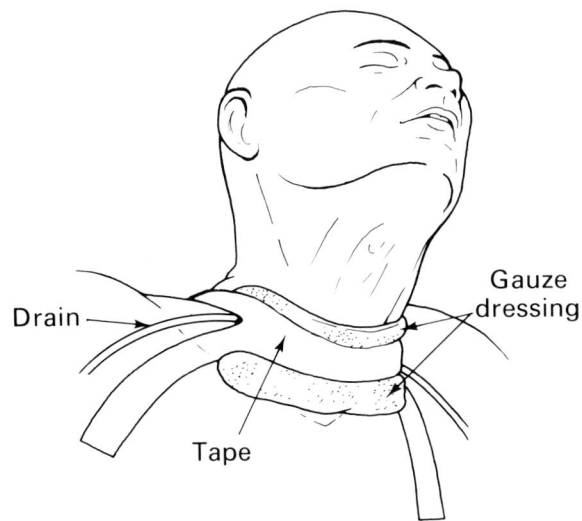

Drain

Gauze dressing

Tape

Fig 34.7 Dressing which does not restrict neck movement.

tubes are removed after 24 h and the clips on the third and fourth days, when the patient should be fit to return home.

Follow-up

All patients who have hyperthyroidism and are treated by any means are likely to develop hypothyroidism more often than the average population. The incidence is highest in those treated with radioiodine, less so after courses of antithyroid drugs. After surgery, there will be an immediate fall-off in the first year of about 10% who may show symptoms and signs of hypothyroidism but, after the first year, it is unusual for it to develop more frequently than in the rest of the population. This matter is still a controversial one and therefore all such patients must be followed-up annually by clinical examination by their practitioners and if there is the least doubt there should be an estimation of TSH and thyroid hormones. Thyroxine is then given when necessary.

Exophthalmos

Because the aetiology of exophthalmos is not known, the treatment has to be empirical but, fortunately, in most patients it is a self-limiting condition, the exophthalmos burning out.

If the symptoms are not severe, it is sufficient for the patient to wear spectacles which keep dust from blow-

ing into the rather sensitive and exposed conjunctiva and cornea and with large side pieces to the spectacles the safety is increased. If it is necessary to narrow the widened lid aperture, then drops of guanethidine 1% can be instilled and for a few hours has this effect. If the eye remains very exposed and unsightly, it is possible to stitch together the two eyelids at each external angle by the operation known as tarsorrhaphy and this can give an acceptable cosmetic result in many.

In that rare minority in whom the exophthalmos is progressive, treatment with steroids is essential and a brief course of very high dosage i.e. up to 60 mg prednisolone daily is better than a long course with lesser dosage. Finally, if the eyesight still remains threatened, the orbit should be decompressed and an approach through its floor via the maxillary antrum produces a very acceptable result and breaks the vicious circle of rising pressure which leads to so much trouble.

Malignant tumours of the thyroid

Thyroid cancer is rare, accounting for about 6 deaths per million of the population per year in most parts of the world (Duncan, 1980). There is a close relationship between irradiation of the neck or surrounding tissues in infancy or childhood and the development of thyroid carcinoma later in life, the interval can be anything from 10 to 30 years and the dose as low as 100 rads. Areas of endemic goitre appear to have a higher incidence of malignant change. When the iodine intake is high, papillary carcinoma is the usual form seen and this is also the commonest thyroid cancer overall, especially in young adults. Follicular carcinoma arises in a somewhat older age group and is the usual tumour seen in those countries where the iodine intake is low, as in endemic areas of the world. Undifferentiated or anaplastic carcinoma almost only appears after the age of 60 and is much commoner in women than men.

The C cells which secrete calcitonin and which migrate into the thyroid gland from neuroectodermal elements on the dorsum of the fetus give rise to medullary cell carcinoma and high levels of calcitonin in the blood. Since the thyroid is a vascular gland, secondary deposits may be seen from primary tumours occurring elsewhere in the body, the commonest is the renal carcinoma, followed by melanoma and tumours of the gastrointestinal tract. Carcinoma may also occur in the toxic thyroid.

Figure 34.8 shows the main types of malignant thyroid tumours and the cells from which they arise.

Papillary carcinoma

Papillary carcinoma (Mazzaferri *et al.*, 1977) accounts for almost 70% of thyroid tumours often

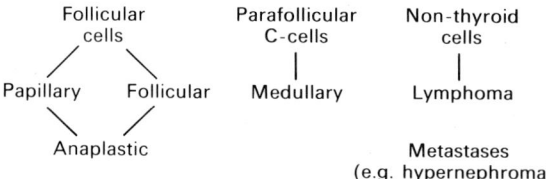

Fig 34.8   The cell origin of thyroid tumours.

appearing in late childhood or early adult life, growing rather slowly and spreading by the lymphatics both to the opposite lobe and to the lymph nodes along the jugular vein and in the lateral triangles of the neck. Later, it may spread by the bloodstream to the lungs and bones and the tumour is readily recognisable histologically being a mixture of papillary processes and small follicles with psammoma bodies scattered throughout the stroma, sometimes sufficiently numerous to give speckling on the x-ray.

The tumour is often discovered incidentally when a solitary thyroid nodule has been removed, when it is unnecessary to return and carry out further removal of thyroid tissue as long as the tumour was not transected. If, however, lymph nodes are enlarged, then these should be removed simultaneously by a modified neck dissection, it being unnecessary to remove the sternomastoid or intervening tissue planes. It will be found that that the involved nodes can be readily enucleated from the tissues and this is adequate removal. If it is known from previous node biopsy that carcinoma exists in the thyroid then it is desirable, whenever possible, to do a total thyroidectomy preserving the four parathyroids, recurrent nerves and surrounding structures. Where there is any difficulty in preserving them, a flake of thyroid tissue should be left behind, since this can be destroyed by radioactive iodine later although this is seldom necessary.

Prognosis

In children removal of the tumours, and nodes if they are present, is almost always followed by remission for life. In adults the factors which make the prognosis less good are tumours which are more than 2.5 cm in diameter, spread of the tumour to the lymph nodes in the neck and age over 40 years. Age is the single most important factor in determining prognosis. Males over 40 appear to do less well than females. In later life the tumour may become less differentiated and much more aggressive. The presence of involved lymph nodes does not necessarily presage a poor prognosis since they usually only occur in the younger patient in whom the tumour rarely kills. Undifferentiated or anaplastic carcinomas, however, with or without node involvement,

carry a uniformly bad prognosis. It is essential to give full replacement doses of thyroxine i.e. about 0.2 mg per day for the remainder of the patient's life and the neck must be checked at annual intervals to see if any further nodes develop. The chest should be x-rayed at less frequent intervals.

Follicular carcinoma

Follicular carcinoma (Taylor, 1981) is the second commonest malignant tumour in the thyroid, appearing a little later in life, peak age around 45 and the tumour is usually solitary and may grow to a large size and often feels rather springy on palpation. Unfortunately, more than 50% of the patients first seen with this tumour have already distant spread as their presenting feature. This commonly takes the form of a secondary deposit in a bone with a pathological fracture or metastasis in the lungs. It is possible histologically to subdivide these tumours into those completely enclosed within the capsule, the removal of which is curative, and those a little less differentiated which infiltrate not only the capsule, but the surrounding blood vessels, and as a result their prognosis is unpredictable.

The treatment is total removal of the tumour and, in addition, all normal thyroid tissue if this is surgically possible, or subtotal removal followed by ablation of the rest of the thyroid gland with radioactive iodine. Metastatic tissue may then be stimulated to take up radioiodine by an i.m. injection of 5 i.u. of TSH followed 24 h later by a tracer dose of 1 mCi of radioiodine and scanning of the whole body. If secondaries are present and take up a significant amount of the isotope, a treatment dose of radioiodine is next given, usually of the order of 80 mCi and the urine must be stored for a while because it is too radioactive to flush down the drain. After the isotope therapy the patient is put on fully suppressive doses of thyroxine by mouth and this should be checked at regular intervals by seeing if the TSH has been suppressed in the bloodstream. The patient is followed annually and repeated doses of radioactive iodine may be helpful. Not many tumours are so well differentiated that the metastases take up the isotope, but when this is the case, treatment can be highly successful.

Medullary carcinoma

Medullary carcinoma (Taylor, 1981) is rare, but has the distinctive histological feature of amyloid in a rather solid stroma; the tumour does not take up radioactive iodine. The cells secrete calcitonin which can be assayed and the tumour may occur in families, and when associated with bilateral phaeochromocytoma, and occasionally hyperparathyroidism, is known as Sipple's syndrome or multiple endocrine neoplasia type 2 (MEN II).

The sporadic tumour may arise apparently at any age and grow slowly and spreads by lymphatics especially to the anterior mediastinum. The familial variety may be present at birth and grows slowly in the early years of life, but may explode into activity later. The latter tumour is nearly always bilateral in the thyroid and may spread by lymphatics or bloodstream. The only successful treatment at the present time for medullary carcinoma is surgical excision and this means total thyroidectomy, but it may be impossible to achieve this by the time the patient presents for treatment, because of the very slow growth of the tumour. Radiotherapy may inhibit tumour growth and is a useful ancillary. Intra-arterial embolisation of liver metastases sometimes offers useful palliation. The success of the treatment is monitored by assaying calcitonin in the bloodstream both after operation and at annual intervals thereafter. Other members of the family should be investigated in case the disease is familial. A rare variant of this tumour which, however, is usually sporadic, is the occurrence of MEN II in a patient of Marfan type habitat with neuromas of the mucosal surfaces, especially the tongue and eyelids. The prognosis is poor because the patient usually dies, even though the primary tumours have been excised. It is sometimes designated MEN IIb.

Anaplastic carcinoma

The undifferentiated form of thyroid carcinoma (Duncan, 1980) which occurs much more commonly in women than men over the age of 60, often complicates an already existing well differentiated tumour which may not have been diagnosed for many years. The patient complains of a sudden increase in the size of the swelling in the neck with hoarseness, dysphagia and a feeling of being unwell. The diagnosis clinically is rarely in doubt, as the tumour becomes fixed to the neck tissues at an early stage and an aspiration needle biopsy confirms the diagnosis. Radiotherapy provides good palliation, but usually only for a limited period and many patients do not survive for more than 6 months. The only chemotherapy so far known to have significant effect is doxorubicin (Adriamycin) and cannot be recommended at the present time. If stridor occurs a tracheostomy must be performed and treatment with radiotherapy continued because of the risk of fungation of the tumour into the wound.

Lymphoma

Lymphoma of the thyroid is now a well recognised type of thyroid tumour and was probably, in the past, misdiagnosed as small-cell carcinoma of the thyroid. It typically affects women of 40–50 years, may grow slowly and is particularly sensitive to radiation therapy. Rarely a thyroid gland which is affected by Hashimoto's thyroiditis undergoes malignant change with rapid infiltrative growth and enormously high titres of thyroid antibodies in the blood. Radiation may offer palliation and a surgical operation, apart from tracheostomy, and confirming the diagnosis histologically, has not much to offer.

Thyroiditis

The term thyroiditis is used to describe all kinds of conditions in the thyroid gland including those due to inflammation.

Suppurative thyroiditis

This rare condition usually follows a sore throat and the patient has a sudden onset of severe pain in the neck made worse on swallowing, accompanied by dysphagia, high fever and often rigors. The inflammation, if untreated by antibiotics, may go on to suppuration and the organisms that have been incriminated are streptococci, staphylococci, coliforms and typhoid. If pus is produced, it must be evacuated as soon as possible or pressure on the trachea leads to severe dyspnoea.

Hashimoto's thyroiditis

This is the commonest thyroiditis and is seen in women especially in middle age when there is a moderate enlargement of thyroid, occasionally with tenderness although this is unusual, and there is the progressive development of hypothyroidism in most patients. There is often a family history of thyroiditis, myxoedema and pernicious anaemia, the latter with gastric cell antibodies. Occasionally, there is an initial period when the patient appears slightly hyperthyroid, but it is unusual to see the patient at this stage. The present theory is that this is an autoimmune disease in which the patient becomes sensitised to her own thyroid follicular cells and forms thyroid antibodies which may be identified with the colloid, microsomal parts of follicular cells, and other thyroid gland structures. Blood sent to the laboratory reveals a raised level of gamma globulin in the serum. Red cells coated with thyroglobulin provide a quantitative measurement by agglutination for the presence of antibodies.

There is a complement fixation test for microsomal antibodies and fine needle biopsy or removal of tissue from the thyroid gland provides good evidence of the diagnosis.

Treatment consists of giving replacement thyroxine and this usually provides the answer in that the gland becomes softer and smaller with the passage of time and the patient is maintained in a euthyroid state. However, there are some forms of Hashimoto thyroiditis which induce fibrous tissue formation and it is then necessary to remove the isthmus of the thyroid gland, not only to relieve pressure on the trachea, but at the same time to provide good histological evidence of the disease process which may mimic malignant disease.

de Quervain's thyroiditis

This condition is often called subacute or giant cell thyroiditis. It was first described by de Quervain in 1904 and is characterised by its sudden onset with pain in the neck which radiates to the ears, malaise, night sweats and a raised red cell sedimentation rate. The biopsy of the gland is diagnostic, with disruption and dissolution of the follicular cell walls so that the aggregation of their nuclei gives the appearance of multinucleated giant cells. Hence the old name for the disease, pseudo-tubercular thyroiditis. Slight enlargement of the thyroid gland in a patient, accompanied by pain which radiates to the ears and malaise of sudden onset should raise suspicion of this disease, and the high level of the ESR accompanied by complete suppression of radioiodine or technetium uptake in the gland should prove diagnostic. The disease is self-limiting and the treatment largely symptomatic. Aspirin by mouth, or in more severe cases cortisone, relieve the symptoms until the condition has burnt itself out, often in a few months.

Riedel's thyroiditis

This, the rarest of all the thyroiditis conditions, is seen as the involvement of the gland in a hard woody mass completely adherent to the other structures of the neck and only accompanied by a moderate diminution in thyroid function. The main complaint is of tracheal compression and the surgeon's responsibility is to free the trachea which can only be accomplished by dividing the isthmus, a difficult task when the fibrous tissue freely infiltrates all the surrounding tissue planes.

Riedel described how the condition might occasionally resolve completely, but this is by no means common. Occasionally, Riedel's thyroiditis is only one manifestation of a more generalised disease process and the author has seen it associated with retroperitoneal fibrosis with bilateral hydronephrosis, with biliary cirrhosis of the liver and obstructive jaundice, and with mediastinal fibrosis. These complications should be looked for if Riedel's thyroiditis is diagnosed, since they respond to high doses of prednisolone, 20–30 mg 8 hourly.

Acknowledgement

Figures 34.1–34.7 are redrawn from *Surgical Techniques Illustrated*, 1978, Vol 3, No 4 by courtesy of the Editors, Ronald A. Malt and Frank Robinson and the publishers Little, Brown & Co.

References and further reading

Andreoli M., Fabrizia M., Robbins J. eds (1982). *Advances in Thyroid Neoplasia*. Rome: Field Educational Italia.
Beaugié J.M. (1975). *Principles of Thyroid Surgery*. London: Pitman.
Das G., Krieger M. (1969). Treatment of thyrotoxic storm with intravenous propanolol. *Ann. Intern. Med*; **70**:935.
Duncan W. ed (1980). Thyroid cancer. In *Recent Results in Cancer Research*. Berlin: Springer-Verlag.
Friesen S.R. (1978). *Surgical Endocrinology*. Philadelphia: J.B. Lippincott.
Hall R., Evered D. eds (1979). Hypothyroidism and goitre. In *Clinics in Endocrinology and Metabolism*, Vol. 8. No. 1. London: WB Saunders.
Heimann P. (1978). Should hyperthyroidism be treated by surgery? *World. J. Surg*; **2**:281.
Kaplan E.L. (1983). *Surgery of the Thyroid and Parathyroid Glands*, London: Churchill Livingstone.
Mazzaferri E.L. *et al*. (1977). Papillary thyroid carcinoma: the impact of therapy in 576 patients. *Medicine*; **56**:171.
Montgomery D.A.D., Welbourn R.B. (1974). *Clinical Endocrinology for Physicians and Surgeons*. London: Arnold.
Stanbury J.B., Hetzel B.S. (1980). *Endemic Goitre and Endemic Cretinism*. New York: John Wiley.
Taylor S. (1979). The surgical treatment of thyroid disease in modern perspective. *Ann. Roy. Coll. Surg*; **61**:132–37.
Taylor S. (1981). Progress in the treatment of thyroid cancer. *World J. Surg*; **5**:1–84.
de Visscher M. ed (1980). The thyroid gland. In *Comprehensive Endocrinology*. New York: Raven Press.

35

Parathyroids

SELWYN TAYLOR

The parathyroid and calcium metabolism

Development

The parathyroid glands arise from the third and fourth branchial clefts and in more than 90% of people there are four glands, two on each side of the neck, which descend during development of the fetus, the fourth cleft glands usually being arrested posterior to the upper pole of the thyroid gland, but occasionally lying higher. The third cleft derivatives descend much further and although the commonest site is behind the lower pole of the thyroid, they may be arrested at any level or pass down to be found within the substance of the thymus gland or even descend as low as the arch of the aorta. Thus the development of the parathyroid glands determines the wide variety of sites in which these tumours may have to be sought, which can be from the base of the skull above to the arch of the aorta below and laterally as far as and including the sheaths of the carotid arteries (Fig 35.1).

In health the parathyroid glands are approximately 4–8 mm in length and diameter being oval in shape and of a distinctive tan or orange brown colour. Each gland weighs approximately 40 mg and is extremely vascular and usually lies enmeshed within the loose fibrous tissue which invests the thyroid gland on its posterolateral

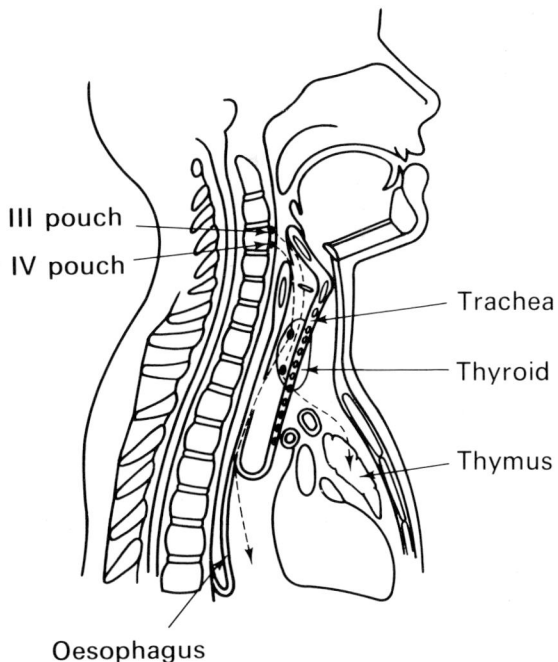

Fig 35.1 Parathyroid migration.

aspect. The glands are not only very vascular, but usually a small artery can be seen entering at a particular hilar point; this forms a sort of pedicle upon which it is usually possible to swing the gland when it is necessary to preserve it, but remove underlying tissue, as in total thyroidectomy (Fig 35.2).

Parathyroid hormone (PTH) and calcium metabolism

The three main hormones controlling calcium metabolism in the body are vitamin D, calcitonin and parathyroid hormone (PTH) (Taylor, 1976). The prime effect of parathyroid hormone is to mobilise calcium subperiosteally. The parathyroid glands secrete a very large prohormone which is broken down mainly in the bloodstream to much smaller and biologically more active fragments. The biologically active part of the PTH hormone is not the terminal part of the molecule which is usually labelled in the radioimmuno assay and this accounts for some of the lack of correlation between levels of parathyroid hormone and the diagnosis of the disease. Vitamin D is also metabolised in the body both in the liver and the kidney to its active form which is 25 dihydroxycholecalciferol and various commercial preparations of an active metabolite of vitamin D are available for use in patients. Vitamin D and its metabolites can be radioimmunoassayed in the blood. The role of calcitonin is still not entirely clear, but it is a potent inhibitor of subperiosteal calcium resorption and probably plays a major part in the modelling of bones. It also can be assayed in the serum.

When PTH is produced in excess, it not only increases subperiosteal resorption of calcium and, therefore, the secretion of calcium salts through the kidney, but leads to the deposition of calcium crystals in the renal tubules and thus, eventually, to renal damage and hypertension. In addition, it increases the absorption of calcium from the bowel, possibly because of its effect on vitamin D. The direct effect on the renal tubular cells is to decrease the resorption of phosphate and increase the resorption of calcium. If the levels are high enough and great enough, stone formation occurs in the kidneys, and then there may be deposition of calcium in the renal parenchyma causing nephrocalcinosis. The concurrent high levels of calcium in the bloodstream lead to mental changes and to constipation and the renal damage is accompanied by polyuria and polydipsia.

Pathology

The commonest abnormality is an adenoma occurring in one parathyroid gland and this accounts for approximately 90% of hyperparathyroidism (HPT). In patients who lose calcium abnormally, usually due to renal failure or losses from the gut, there may be secondary hyperplasia of all four parathyroid glands, which is referred to as secondary HPT. When severe and long continued, the four glands may pass through diffuse hyperplasia to nodular hyperplasia or what is apparently adenoma formation. Severe secondary hyperparathyroidism which exhibits some of the features of autonomy has been called tertiary HPT, but this remains a controversial term since most patients' serum calcium returns to normal after renal transplantation, if a *long* enough period can be allowed.

Parathyroid disease occurs as one feature of a number of endocrine syndromes, in particular multiple endocrine neoplasia, MEN both type I and type II, and it is, therefore, necessary when hyperparathyroidism has been diagnosed to exclude features of these syndromes before assuming that the diagnosis is one of uncomplicated primary HPT.

The commonest associated abnormality is an adenoma of the pituitary which can be revealed by radiology if it is large enough, since it then erodes the

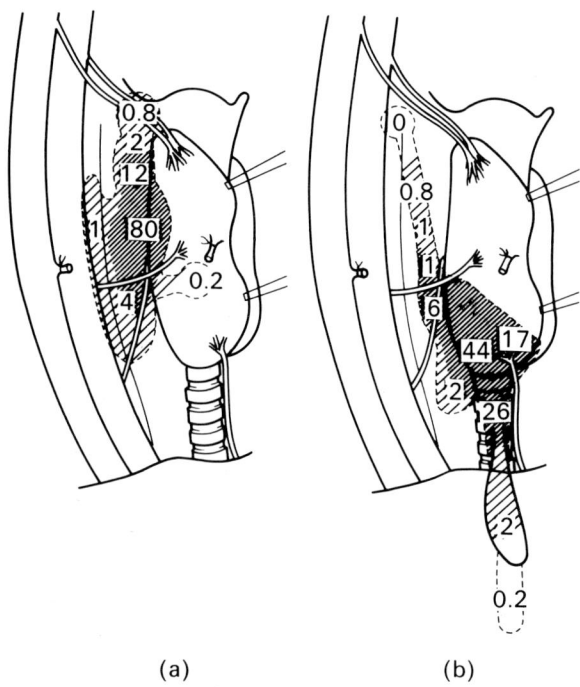

(a)   (b)

Fig 35.2 Localisation of (a) the superior and (b) the inferior parathyroid glands in 503 autopsies. (Redrawn from *The Parathyroids, Location and Histopathological Diagnosis*, 1981 by courtesy of the Editors, A. Grimelius *et al.* and the Institute of Pathology and Department of Surgery, University Hospital, Uppsala, Sweden.)

clinoid processes and expands the sella turcica. Other features of MEN I can be an elevated secretion of gastrin, insulin or adrenal cortical hormones or, more rarely, a combination of these, MEN II is characterised by an increase of calcitonin in the blood, the level of which is readily elevated before assay by an alcohol or pentagastrin stimulation test. Continued overproduction of PTH leads to subperiosteal removal of bone and the excess calcium is excreted by the kidneys; simultaneously the resorption of phosphate is impeded with hypophosphataemia. In longstanding cases the bone destruction may include cyst formation, a condition called osteitis fibrosa cystica.

There is a small group of patients who present with all the signs and symptoms of HPT, but have no parathyroid gland abnormality. This is due to the ectopic production of PTH or a PTH-like molecule by a malignant tumour. Such a tumour is usually large in size and may arise from bronchus, kidney, thymus or resemble a fibroma.

Diagnosis

HPT is much commoner than was previously thought and the routine examination of patients' blood attending clinics or hospital has revealed a significant hypercalcaemia in approximately 1 per 1000 of the population over 40 years of age (Heath et al., 1980). The commonest causes of hypercalcaemia are malignant disease and HPT, so there must be many patients with undiagnosed HPT and an unsolved problem at the present time is how many, and which, of these individuals should have operative treatment to lower the serum calcium.

The usual method of diagnosis today is finding a raised level of calcium when blood has been submitted to the autoanalyser for a chemical profile. However, a good case history can be very helpful, enquiring particularly about previous medical conditions, the possibility of increased thirst and urine formation and relatives may have noticed mental changes. Any history of renal colic is significant, peptic ulcer is particularly common in this group of patients and in the older patients the occurrence of gout. Bone pain is seen in those with severe disease and HPT may even present with pancreatitis when the calcium level is very high indeed.

Signs which may be looked for are band keratitis which is best demonstrated with a slit lamp. Hypertension is a common complication and it carries a poor prognosis since the blood pressure does not return to normal after correction of the HPT.

The laboratory tests are first and foremost calcium estimation which must be repeated on a number of occasions since there are natural fluctuations in its level. The measurement of ionised calcium is difficult and requires expensive apparatus, but undoubtedly correlates much better with the activity of the disease than does the total serum calcium which is the usual laboratory estimation. It is of particular value in the diagnosis of mild hyperparathyroidism. The calcium is normally bound to albumin and, therefore, anything which lowers this in the blood will give a relatively lower level of calcium. Thus the serum proteins should always be estimated and the use of a tourniquet should be avoided when taking blood samples, since in a short time this permits albumin molecules to pass through the capillary walls. If the serum proteins are low (e.g. 7.1), due allowance must be made for this in calculating the actual calcium level from the observed level, e.g:

$$\text{Calcium} \times \frac{7.8}{\text{total serum protein.}}$$

It is possible to have an overactive parathyroid gland in the presence of a normal level of calcium in the bloodstream if the binding capacity of albumin has been lowered or if there is severe hypovitaminosis D.

The other tests which are useful to do in HPT are estimation of the phosphate which should be low and the chloride and the alkaline phosphatase activity which may be considerably elevated when much bone is involved. Serum electrophoresis will exclude those with multiple myeloma and sarcoidosis, two other causes of raised calcium. Last, and perhaps of less value, the PTH assay should be done if a reliable method is available. A raised PTH undoubtedly indicates that there is increased parathyroid activity, but a normal or depressed level does not exclude the diagnosis of HPT in some patients.

The differential diagnosis (Edis et al., 1975) of a raised level of calcium in the bloodstream includes the presence of malignant disease almost anywhere in the body, but most commonly affecting a bronchus or breast; myeloma, renal disease, sarcoidosis, the intake of large quantities of alkali as is occasionally done by some dyspeptics and the intake of excess vitamin D usually as calciferol or in proprietary health products.

Familial hypercalcaemia or familial hypocalciuric hypercalcaemia is a benign form of hypercalcaemia that has now been reported from many countries (Paterson and Gunn, 1981; Foley et al., 1972). When symptoms occur, they are usually mild and difficult to assess, such as fatigue and impairment of memory. The skeleton is normally calcified and there is no predisposition to stone formation unlike primary hyperparathyroidism. Occasionally severe symptoms and signs of hyperparathyroidism occur in the newborn (Marx et al., 1982).

Among the special tests of great value is radiography. Good quality x-rays of the hand will demonstrate subperiosteal resorption on the radial side of the second phalanges even in early cases of HPT. A lateral view of the skull may show changes in the texture of the bone and an increased size of the pituitary fossa in MEN I. Soft tissue x-rays of the abdomen may show a stone in the urinary tract or nephrocalcinosis in the kidneys. A barium swallow will demonstrate in a small proportion of patients the presence of a parathyroid adenoma impinging on the oesophageal wall.

Bone biopsy (Becket *et al.*, 1973) is invasive and requires a trephine type of needle or a modified Vim-Silverman. It is difficult to interpret, but in skilled hands is a valuable adjunct especially when HPT is suspected in the absence of abnormal x-ray findings and a normal alkaline phosphatase.

Many tests have been devised to help in the diagnosis of this condition, but few have stood the test of time. It is still sometimes useful to use the hydrocortisone suppression test. Hydrocortisone given daily in a dose of 100 mg for 10 days will reduce the serum calcium concentration in most of those patients in whom the elevation is due to vitamin D intake or sarcoidosis, and also in many of those with carcinoma. HPT patients rarely show any depression of the calcium with this test.

The symptoms of HPT do not usually draw attention to the disease until the calcium level is well above the normal range of 2.1–2.6 mmol/1 or 8.5–10.5 mg/100 ml. Any history of renal tract calculus, e.g. an attack of colic should arouse suspicion. Increased thirst and polyuria occur early. Mental changes are common, but seldom helpful except in retrospect. Dyspepsia and peptic ulcer may reflect HPT or MEN I. There may be muscle weakness (Patten *et al.*, 1974) in severe hypercalcaemia, lethargy and drowsiness, all of which are reversible with lowering of calcium. Hypertension reflects renal damage and is rarely, if ever, improved by parathyroidectomy.

A 10-year prospective study of asymptomatic primary hyperparathyroidism (Scholz and Purnell, 1981) was reported by the Mayo Clinic in 1981 and failed to resolve the problem of predicting which patients will ultimately require parathyroid surgery. Recognised criteria for surgical treatment include:

1 Serum calcium 2.8 mmol/1 or 11 mg/dl
2 X-ray evidence of bone disease especially
   (a) Subperiosteal resorption of phalanges and clavicles
   (b) Thinning of distal phalangeal tufts
   (c) Cysts
   (d) Granular demineralisation of skull
   (e) Osteoporosis of vertebrae
3 Decreased renal function
4 Renal tract stones
5 Mental changes
6 Geographical remoteness
7 Peptic ulcer
8 Age of patient, e.g. if young.

Surgical treatment

Operative removal of the abnormal parathyroid tissue is the correct treatment for the majority of those with HPT. Since some 90% of patients will have a single adenoma, the removal of this is usually curative and it is wise to excise a small biopsy from what appears to be a normal gland as a check of the pathology and a frozen section diagnosis at the time of operation is of great help in this. If all four glands are involved in hyperplasia, then removal of 3½ glands leaving about 40 mg of normal-looking parathyroid tissue is one form of treatment which is successful in the short term. In most patients it is preferable to do a total parathyroidectomy and then implant 50 or 60 mg of the parathyroid tissue chopped up into little pieces into a muscle in the forearm, where, should there be a recurrence of the disease, it is easy to remove them under local anaesthesia.

After total parathyroidectomy and the grafting (Wells *et al.*, 1979) of tissue fragments into the forearm, there is a period of up to 3 months during which the patient requires to be treated for hypoparathyroidism, that is while the grafts are becoming vascularised. This can be achieved by giving one of the vitamin D metabolites and ensuring that the diet contains a more than adequate amount of calcium.

The commonest cause of failure to cure HPT by operation is a lack of knowledge of the anatomy of the glands on the part of the surgeon and, for success, the division of the strap muscles and middle thyroid vein is essential (Figs 35.3, 35.4), as is also the delivery of the thymus into the neck as it so often contains parathyroid

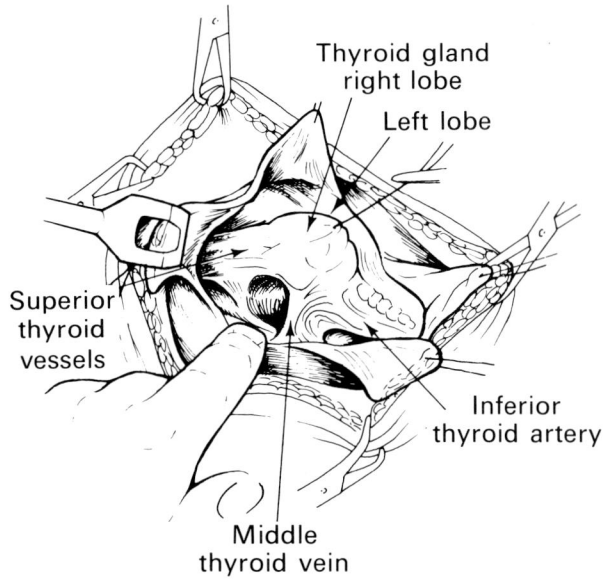

Fig 35.3 Exposure on right side.

Thyroid gland right lobe

Left lobe

Superior thyroid vessels

Inferior thyroid artery

Middle thyroid vein

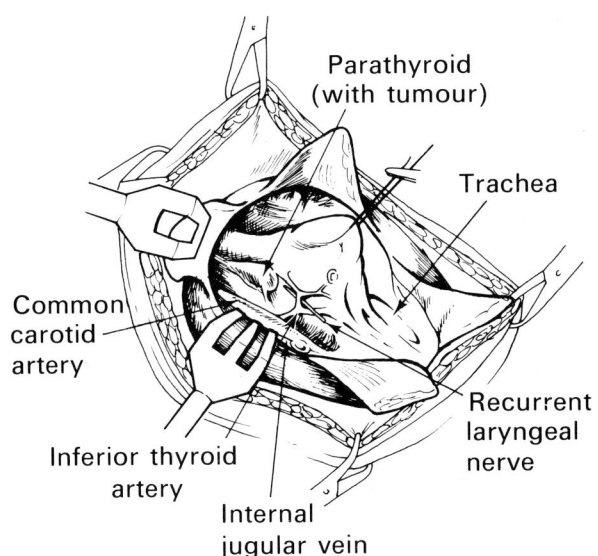

Fig 35.4   Relations of recurrent nerve, inferior thyroid artery and parathyroid.

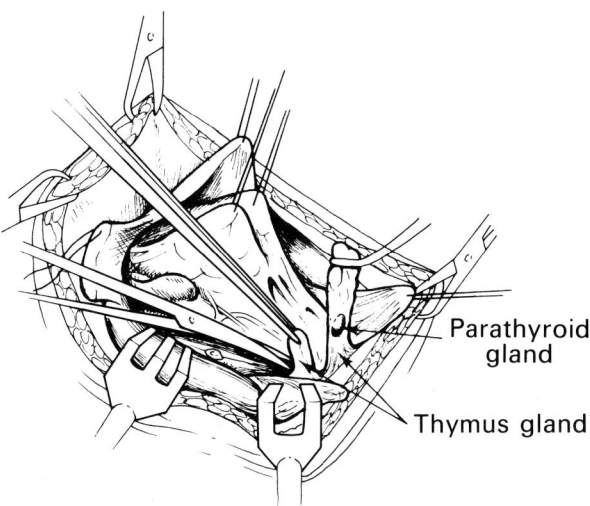

Fig 35.5   Exposure of thymus.

tissue (Fig 35.5). Other helpful aids are following branches of the inferior thyroid artery especially if they look abnormal or large, exploring behind the manubrium and in the region of the oesophagus. A very rare site is the carotid sheath. Intrathyroidal tumours (Spiegel *et al.*, 1975) only account for 2–3%.

Division of the sternum to permit removal of an adenoma from the mediastinum is only necessary in less than 1% of patients with HPT. If after a long, thorough and careful search in the neck and after examining the thymus, no tumour can be found, it is better to close the neck wound and then employ some of the localisation techniques described below before embarking on a sternal split. Under no circumstances should normal parathyroid tissue be removed, except a minute sliver for a frozen section biopsy for identification purposes.

Parathyroidectomy for secondary HPT (Arnaud and Bordier, 1979) can be of great value in patients on renal dialysis, especially those who may have to wait a long time for a renal graft. Some patients with renal failure gradually develop increasingly severe hyperplasia of all four glands and eventually decalcify the skeleton so severely that they have bone pain and spontaneous fractures. The level of serum calcium is usually slightly elevated. The preferred operation for these patients is total parathyroidectomy, a procedure made relatively easy by the enlargement of all four glands. About 60 mg is chopped into 10 or 20 morsels, each of which is transplanted into its individual muscle pocket in the fleshy part of brachioradialis, avoiding the arm that has the arteriovenous shunt which is used for dialysis. Post-

operatively, the calcium level is maintained by calcium by mouth and a vitamin D metabolite. In a few weeks or months the patient is weaned off this supportive therapy. Rarely, hyperplasia of the grafted material causes a return of the secondary HPT and some of the grafts have to be excised under local anaesthesia.

Localisation techniques

These are of especial value in patients with persistent or recurrent HPT which is usually due to one of two things; inadequate knowledge of the anatomy at the first operation, and MEN I.

Subtraction scanning using thallium-201 and technetium 99^m has produced the best results so far in the localisation of adenomas. (Ferlin *et al.*, 1981).

Imaging using ultrasound has not proved of much value in finding what are usually rather small adenomas although it will demonstrate the large ones but techniques improve steadily. CAT scanning is only of value for those lying behind the sternum, since in that situation the surrounding tissue is fat and the difference in density between the parathyroid tissue and fat is sufficient to give an image. Use of aortography, arteriography and selective arteriography is not now recommended since there is morbidity attached to all these techniques sufficient to outweigh their advantages. However, selective arteriography has been used successfully to embolise adenomas (Doppmann *et al.*, 1979) lying in the mediastinum. Selective venous catheterisation, however, has proved consistently useful in those patients in whom it is possible to pass a catheter into veins near the tumour, but the technique means that there will be an interval between this investigation and the operation for at least a week, while the samples of blood are assayed.

The technique is to introduce a catheter by the method of Seldinger in the left femoral vein in the x-ray department. The position of the catheter is checked by injecting small amounts of diodone and samples of blood are then aspirated from the IVC, SVC and neck veins, both left and right side, as far as the catheter can be manipulated. Each sample is carefully documented on a map of the neck. The only limiting factor is usually that many veins have been ligated at the previous exploratory operation and they are then impassable. The samples are cooled in ice and sent immediately for radioimmunoassay of PTH. The presence of an adenoma is revealed by a high titre in one of the samples.

Dyes have had much support recently, starting with orthotoluidene blue which proved to be toxic and caused heart irregularities, but this has been followed by the much safer methylene blue which, given during the 20 min before the neck incision, renders most parathyroid tissue a slatey blue colour and is favoured by some surgeons. Delivery of the thymus and careful exploration of it has already been mentioned. It is particularly helpful in those patients who have previously had an operation on the neck in which the thymus was not examined.

Finally the technique introduced of using flotation to determine what is pathological parathyroid tissue and what is normal or fat has proved valuable where a frozen section service is not available. Parathyroid tumour tissue will sink and normal parathyroid tissue will float if placed in a solution of specific gravity 1049–1069 which can conveniently be prepared using mannitol and placed in test tubes in a rack in the operating theatre.

An intrathyroid parathyroid adenoma is a considerable rarity and is usually due to the engulfment of the tumour by an enlarged or multinodular goitre.

Recurrent and persistent hyperparathyroidism

In some patients after an operation has successfully removed abnormal parathyroid tissue and the serum calcium has fallen to normal limits, there is a normocalcaemic interval of months or even years after which the patient is once more hypercalcaemic (Egdahl, 1977). The usual reason for this is that the patient has hyperplasia of all the parathyroid glands which may be sporadic, familial or one manifestation of MEN I.

In contradistinction the patient's calcium may not fall after operation (Brennan *et al.*, 1978) and the likely cause then is a failure to remove all the abnormal parathyroid tissue which may, indeed, be disease of a fifth

gland. Whatever the cause, the clinical problem is the same, that is a scarred neck and a high calcium. As a result of dealing with 21 such patients the author suggests the following plan:

1   Obtain an excellent case history with special note of unusual sex and age presentation, MEN I and II and familial hyperalcaemia and previous hospital records.
2   Obtain previously removed parathyroid tissue for further histology if possible.
3   X-ray pituitary fossa and skull, hands and vertebrae if not done.
4   If MEN I suspected, assay: gastrin, glucose, insulin, corticoids. If MEN II; assay calcitonin.
5   (a) Technetium-thallium subtraction scan, if available, or:
     (b) selective venous catheterisation with PTH assay.
6   Preoperatively infuse methylene blue if you prefer it.
7   Operate (Taylor, 1978) and identify all possible parathyroids with cryostat biopsy. Tag with silver clips and silk any 'normal' parathyroid left *in situ*. If MEN I or familial hyperplasia, remove all parathyroid tissue and implant 45 to 60 mg in forearm. Freeze remainder or leave tagged remnant.
8   Split sternum if adenoma suspected and not found. It may be under arch of aorta.

Carcinoma of the parathyroid

Carcinoma of the parathyroid (Schantz and Castleman, 1973) is rare, accounting for approximately 3% of all those patients seen with HPT. It is usually diagnosed by the surgeon at operation because the tumour infiltrates the surrounding tissues but, occasionally, this is not noticed at the time of the initial operation although the recurrence of the disease with an elevated calcium and new masses in the neck is diagnostic of malignancy. Even the most extensive operations frequently fail to cure these patients in a majority of cases. If carcinoma is recognised at operation, then a radical operation should be undertaken at that time removing all the surrounding tissue even although it may not appear to be affected to the naked eye. Recurrence is always local in the first place and is only rarely seen in the form of distant metastases at a late stage of the disease when the usual sites for secondaries are lung and bone.

Hypercalcaemic crisis

Patients in whom the diagnosis of HPT has been missed and in those with recurrent carcinoma of the parathyroid and occasionally those with a single adenoma which enters on a burst of cellular activity, present to the doctor with a hypercalcaemic crisis. The patient usually has mental blunting which is then followed by coma, there is numbness around the mouth and dehydration is always severe.

Treatment for hypercalcaemia is initially good hydration which means a rapid infusion of saline and then correction of the low level of potassium which almost always accompanies this condition. Hypomagnesaemia can also occur and muscle weakness may be profound. Most patients have a good response to hydration, but if the calcium level is still dangerously high then active methods should be used to lower it while the patient is being prepared to go to the operating theatre and have the parathyroid tumour excised. Calcitonin by infusion lowers the calcium for short periods as also does mithramycin, but the latter is a toxic substance. Neutral phosphate by infusion, though effective, has the disadvantage of causing deposition of calcium in the soft tissues and this is to be avoided in patients who are already suffering from this in greater or lesser degree. Most of these patients, though not all, have by this stage of the disease severe renal damage which makes the control of fluid and electrolyte balance extremely difficult. The assistance of a skilled nephrologist is enormously helpful with these problems.

Operative treatment should be carried out as an emergency and the response to the removal of the parathyroid tumour is often dramatic. Within hours the symptoms of hypocalcaemia can begin and rapidly become severe because of the 'hungry' bones, the skeleton having been so effectively drained of calcium.

Hypocalcaemia

The response of the patient to the treatment of HPT is a sudden lowering in the calcium and it is the extent of this lowering and the speed with which it occurs which causes symptoms of hypocalcaemia rather than any particular level. The symptoms and signs are tingling in the fingers and toes, numbness around the mouth followed by crampy pains in other muscle groups and finally painful spasms, which can even interrupt normal breathing. There are often marked mental changes, acute depression or sometimes a manic phase. Should the patient, due to anxiety, start to overbreathe then all the symptoms and signs will be exaggerated.

Treatment of hypocalcaemia is to give calcium when the patient is in pain or seriously disturbed. Ten to twenty ml of a 10% solution of calcium gluconate is added to a unit of saline run *slowly* into a vein; rapid infusion of calcium causes flushing and headache and may even lead to cardiac arrest. Oral calcium, especially in the form of effervescent tablets given twice or thrice daily, will help absorption and if this is not adequate then the addition of vitamin D in 50–100 000

units per day will rapidly increase absorption of calcium from the gut. In those patients who may have had normal parathyroid tissue removed at previous operations before finally having the tumour removed, the severe hypocalcaemia which results can be controlled by the use of dihydroxycholecalciferol in doses of 1 or 2 μg daily.

Acknowledgement

Figures 35.1, 35.3, 35.4 and 35.5 are redrawn from *Surgical Techniques Illustrated*, 1978, Vol 3, No 4 by courtesy of the Editors, Ronald A. Malt and Frank Robinson and the publishers Little, Brown & Co.

References

Arnaud C. D. Jr., Bordier P.J. (1979). *Management of Secondary Hyperparathyroidism in Endocrinology*, vol. 2 (de Groot *et al.* eds) New York: Grune and Stratton.

Becker F.O., Schwartz T.B., Economo S.G. (1973). Needle bone biopsy in primary hyperparathyroidism. *Arch. Int. Med*; **131:**650.

Brennan M.F., Doppman J.L. *et al.* (1978). Reoperative parathyroid surgery for persistent hyperparathyroidism. *Surgery*; **83:**669.

Doppman J.L., Brown E.M., Brennan M.F. *et al* (1979). Angiographic ablation of parathyroid adenomas. *Radiology*; **130:**577.

Edis A.J., Ayala L.A., Egdahl R.H. (1975). *Manual of Endocrine Surgery*. New York: Springer-Verlag.

Egdahl R.H. ed. (1977). Hyperparathyroidism: a surgical perspective. *World J. Surg*; **1:**689.

Ferlin G., Borsato N., Perelli R., Camerani M., Conte N., Mariente P., Giudice C. (1981). Technetium-thallium subtraction scan. A new method in the pre-operative localization of parathyroid enlargement. *Eur. J. Nucl. Med*; **6:**A12.

Foley T.P., Harrison H.L., Arnaud C.D., Harrison H.E. (1972). Familial benign hypercalcaemia. *J. Pediatr*; **81:**1060.

Heath H., Hodgson S.F., Kennedy M.A. (1980). Primary hyperparathyroidism; incidence, morbidity and potential economic impact in a community. *N. Engl. J. Med*; **302:**189.

Marx S.J., Attie M.F., Spiegel A.M., Levine M.A., Lasker R.D., Fox M. (1982). An association between neonatal hypercalcaemia in three kindreds. *N. Engl. J. Med*; **306:**257.

Patten B.M. *et al.* (1974). Neuromuscular disease in primary hyperparathyroidism. *Ann. Int. Med*; **80:**182.

Paterson C.R., Gunn A. (1981). Familial benign hypercalcaemia. *Lancet*; **ii:**61.

Schantz A., Castleman B. (1973). Parathyroid carcinoma. *Cancer*; **3:**601.

Scholz D.A., Purnell D.C. (1981). Asymptomatic primary hyperthyroidism: 10-year prospective study. *Mayo Clin. Proc*; **56:**473.

Spiegel A.M., Marx S.J. *et al.* (1975). Intrathyroidal parathyroid adenoma. *J. Amer. Med. Ass*; **234:**1029.

Taylor S. (1976). Hyperparathyroidism: retrospect and prospect. *Ann. Roy. Coll. Surg*; **58:**255.

Taylor S. (1978). Cervical parathyroidectomy. In *Surgical Techniques Illustrated*, vol. 3 No. 4. Boston: Little, Brown.

Wells S.A. Jr., Ross A.J., Dale J.K., Gray R.S. (1979). Transplantation of the parathyroid glands: current status. *Surg. Clin. N. Amer*; **59:**167.

36

Adrenal glands

R.B. WELBOURN

General features

Anatomy

The two adrenal glands, each weighing 4 to 5 g, lie retroperitoneally close to the upper poles of the kidneys. They bear important relationships to other structures (Fig 36.1), in particular the lower ribs and pleura on both sides, the vena cava and liver on the right and the spleen on the left (Harrison *et al.*, 1975; Montgomery and Welbourn, 1975; Friesen, 1978).

The arterial blood supply is provided by three small vessels on each side, which are rarely identified at operation. The venous drainage, however, is important surgically. A single vein emerges from the hilum of the gland and, on the right runs a short horizontal course directly into the posterolateral part of the inferior vena cava. Occasionally, there are two or even three veins on the right. The left adrenal vein is longer and runs caudally to join the left renal vein. Each gland has an outer cortex and an inner medulla, with different origins and separate functions.

Adrenal cortex

The adrenal cortex arises from coelomic epithelium, is orange-yellow in colour and is more compact in consistence than the surrounding fat. There are three histological zones, named glomerulosa (the outer), fascicu-

lata and reticularis (the inner). Ectopic nodules, a few millimetres in diameter, may be found retroperitoneally and are occasionally important clinically.

Adrenal medulla

The adrenal medulla is a specialised part of the sympathetic nervous system and arises from the neural

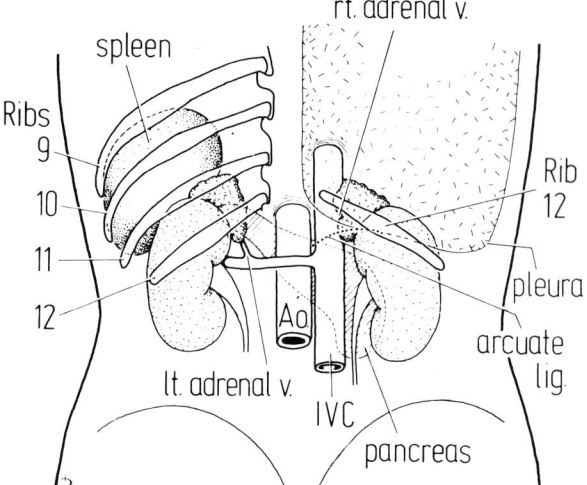

Fig 36.1 The adrenal glands and adjacent structures viewed from the back. Ao = aorta; IVC = inferior vena cava; lt. = left; rt. = right; v. = vein; lig. = ligament. (Welbourn, 1977.)

crest. It is reddish in colour and consists mainly of phaeochromocytes (chromaffin cells) together with a few ganglion cells. Both belong to the APUD series of cells (with a high **A**mine content and the capacity for amine **P**recursor **U**ptake and **D**ecarboxylation). The medulla is innervated by preganglionic fibres from the splanchnic nerves, which form synapses with the chromaffin and ganglion cells. Extra-adrenal collections of chromaffin cells, termed paraganglia, are usual alongside the spine from the neck to the pelvis in childhood, but normally disappear later. Those which persist are separate from ectopic cortical nodules.

Physiology

Adrenal cortex

The adrenal cortex secretes steroid hormones and is essential to life (Fig 36.2). Its main product is cortisol, which arises from the two inner zones and whose secretion is under the direct control of corticotrophin (ACTH) from the anterior pituitary (Fig 36.3). This, in turn, is stimulated by corticotrophin-releasing factor (CRF) from the hypothalamus. The normal feedback control ensures that a sufficiency of cortisol inhibits the further production of CRF and hence of ACTH and of cortisol itself. ACTH and cortisol (and presumably CRF) are secreted in a cyclical manner, their output and concentrations in the blood being normally lowest at night and highest early in the morning. Large amounts are secreted in response to stress, including that of trauma or a surgical operation.

Cortisol controls the intermediary metabolism of carbohydrate, protein and fat in many ways. In particular, it increases the synthesis and release of glucose by the liver and the catabolism of protein. It plays an important part in the control of electrolyte and water balance, and contributes to the maintenance of a normal blood pressure and the proper functioning of the nervous system.

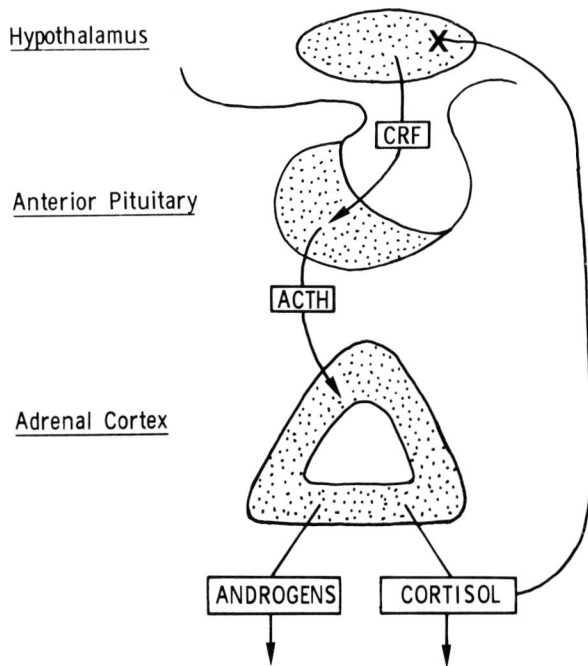

Fig 36.3 The normal hypothalamic-pituitary-adrenal axis. → = stimulates (when pointing to gland); X = inhibits; CRF = corticotrophin-releasing factor; ACTH = adreno-corticotrophic hormone = corticotrophin.

Adrenal androgens, which include testosterone, are secreted by the same two zones and are also under the control of CRF and ACTH. They do not influence the feedback control and their physiological role is uncertain. They are partly converted into oestrogens in the tissues.

Aldosterone, which is secreted by the zona glomerulosa, is important but not essential to life, and is concerned with electrolyte and water metabolism in the distal renal tubules, intestines and sweat glands. It promotes the reabsorption of sodium and the excretion of potassium and hydrogen ions, and these effects may be blocked by a specific antagonist, spironolactone.

The adrenal steroids are partly metabolised in the liver and other tissues and are excreted in the urine both unchanged and as metabolites.

Adrenal medulla

The adrenal medulla synthesises and secretes catecholamines in response to sympathetic nervous stimuli (Fig 36.4). The main product is adrenaline (epinephrine), which enters the blood and influences many metabolic processes including the heart rate and the pupils. It prepares the body for 'fight or flight'. Noradrenaline (norepinephrine), which is the principal

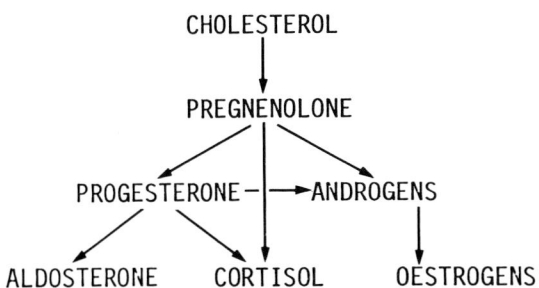

Fig 36.2 Biosynthesis of adrenal steroids (simplified).

adrenergic neurotransmitter, is synthesised at sympathetic nerve endings throughout the body. In the adrenal medulla, it is the precursor of adrenaline, whose synthesis requires the presence of cortisol. Some noradrenaline enters the blood. It constricts all blood vessels and is concerned with maintenance of the blood pressure.

Some actions of the catecholamines are stimulatory and some inhibitory and separate α and β receptors account for their different actions. The former are involved, for example, in peripheral vasoconstriction and the latter with stimulation of the myocardium. The receptors may be blocked therapeutically by specific α and β blocking agents.

The main metabolites of the catecholamines (Fig 36.4) are the 'metadrenalines' ('metanephrines') and vanilmandelic acid (VMA), which are excreted in the urine together with the catecholamines themselves. Small quantities of DOPA, dopamine, and homovanillic acid (HVA) are also excreted.

The nervous tissue of the adrenal medulla also synthesises a small amount of the vasoactive intestinal polypeptide (VIP), which may be a neurotransmitter.

Pathology

The cortex and the medulla may develop lesions which influence their function.

Adrenal cortex

Lesions causing *increased secretion* are: hyperplasia, adenoma and carcinoma.

Various clinical syndromes result, depending on the hormones which are secreted in excess, namely:

Cortisol	—	Cushing's syndrome
Aldosterone	—	Aldosteronism
		Primary (Conn's syndrome)
		Secondary
Androgens	—	Virilisation
Oestrogens	—	Feminisation

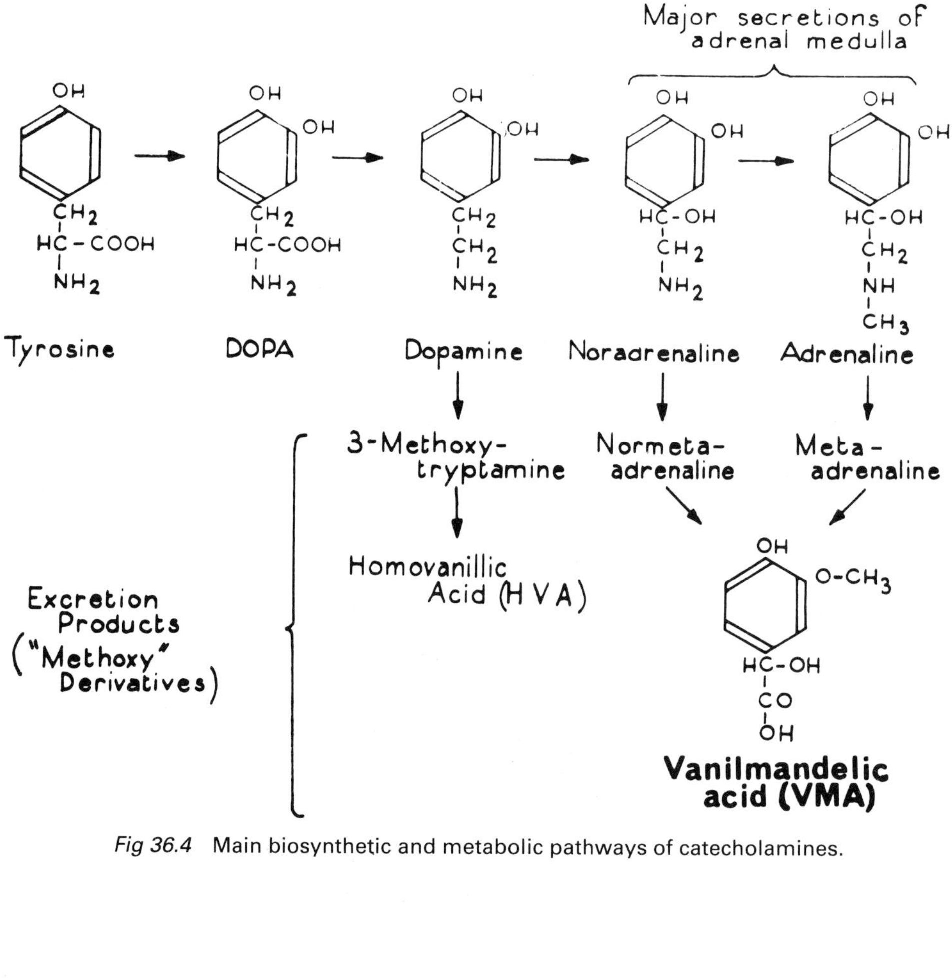

Fig 36.4 Main biosynthetic and metabolic pathways of catecholamines.

Benign lesions tend to cause pure syndromes, while carcinomas frequently secrete several steroids and consequently give rise to mixed syndromes.

Pathological adrenals are usually the same colour as normal ones. *Hyperplasia* is bilateral. The glands are larger than normal, sometimes very much so (over 20 g each), and often (in Cushing's syndrome) contain micronodules up to 2 or 3 mm in diameter.

Lesions causing *decreased secretion* may be primary, in which the adrenals themselves are at fault, or secondary, in which pituitary failure results in deficiency of ACTH. Primary lesions include autoimmune disease, haemorrhage, tuberculosis, infarction, metastatic cancer and bilateral adrenalectomy. Pituitary failure may arise in many ways and causes adrenal atrophy. Two causes which are important surgically are prolonged therapy with corticosteroids, which results in atrophy of both glands, and a cortisol-secreting adrenal tumour (benign or malignant), which leads to atrophy of the non-tumorous part of the gland in which it grows and the whole of the opposite one. Adrenal failure may be chronic, as in hypopituitarism or Addison's disease, or acute, as in an Addisonian crisis, which may be precipitated by a surgical operation.

Some lesions do not interfere with adrenal function. Non-functioning benign nodules may be bilateral and are sometimes found incidentally in life or at autopsy. Some carcinomas secrete steroids which are biologically inactive. Other rare tumours and cysts have no secretory activity.

Adrenal medulla

The only lesions which are important clinically are tumours, all of which belong to the general class of apudomas. They develop in the adrenals themselves or in extra-adrenal paraganglionic tissue. There are three main types, derived from different cells: (1) Phaeochromocytomas arise from chromaffin cells. Adrenal medullary hyperplasia may precede tumour formation in the syndrome of multiple endocrine neoplasia (adenopathy), MEN type II (MEN II)*; (2) Ganglioneuroma, which is benign, arises from sympathetic ganglion cells; (3) Neuroblastoma, which is malignant, is thought to arise from the primitive sympathogonia. Carotid body tumours, glomus tumours and retinoblastomas have similar cells of origin and are closely related. Nearly all phaeochromocytomas and varying

proportions of the other tumours secrete excessive amounts of catecholamines and sometimes of peptides, including VIP. These humoral agents cause characteristic syndromes.

Phaeochromocytomas develop in the abdomen in some 99% of cases and in the adrenals in about 80%. Occasionally there are several phaeochromocytomas in one gland. Tumours are bilateral (in the adrenals) in about 10% of adults, 40% of children and in almost 100% of patients with MEN II. Extra-adrenal tumours are found in the retroperitoneal tissues, including the bladder, and very rarely in the mediastinum or the neck.

The growths are round or ovoid and circumscribed, but rarely encapsulated. They are usually 2 to 10 cm in diameter and are homogeneous on section. Large ones may undergo central necrosis. The colour is grey or brownish and the cells stain dark brown with chromium salts (the chromaffin reaction).

Histologically the tumours resemble adrenal medullary tissue and about 90% are benign, even though many show histological characteristics usually associated with malignancy. Malignant tumours can be recognised as such only when they metastasise to lymph nodes, liver, lungs, bone and elsewhere, where chromaffin tissue is not normally found.

Ganglioneuromas and **neuroblastomas** develop in the adrenal medulla in about one-third of patients, elsewhere in the abdomen in one-third and in the thorax or neck in the remainder. Multiple primary tumours have been described. Although ganglioneuromas are benign and neuroblastomas malignant, many tumours reveal histological features of both. However, the presence of neuroblastoma elements implies that the tumour is malignant.

Ganglioneuromas develop in older children and adults. They are benign, firm, encapsulated tumours, which are occasionally associated with congenital deformities of the vertebrae and ribs. They grow slowly and may become very large. Rarely they penetrate the intervertebral foramina and compress the spinal cord. They are composed of mature ganglion cells, nerve fibres and fibrous tissue.

Neuroblastomas are among the commoner malignant tumours of young children and most of them appear between the ages of 6 months and 5 years. Thirty percent develop in the first year of life. The tumours are soft and fleshy, invade locally, and undergo necrosis and haemorrhage. They metastasise early and widely by the blood and by the lymphatics to liver, lungs, skeleton, lymph nodes and elsewhere. They are composed of small, round or oval cells, sometimes arranged in rosettes. They may contain nerve fibrils. About 5% of tumours, especially in the first year of life, regress

*MEN and MEA. The terminology of these syndromes remains a matter for debate, but as there is now preference for MEN (multiple endocrine neoplasia) this is used throughout this book. However Professor Welbourn rightly points out that MEA (multiple endocrine adenopathy, **not** adenomatosis) is a more accurate description because most of these patients have hyperplasia rather than neoplasia of the affected glands.

Eds.

completely. Others may mature slowly to form benign ganglioneuromas.

Investigation

Investigation of patients suspected of suffering from adrenal disease involves:

1 Determination of the nature and site of the underlying lesion, especially by radiological and related methods. These have much in common for all adrenal lesions and will be discussed together first.
2 Specific biochemical investigations, which involve measurements of steroids in the blood and urine for cortical lesions and similar estimations of catecholamines and their metabolites for medullary lesions. They will be described separately for each syndrome.
3 Non-specific investigations, which vary with the syndromes and will be described last.

Radiology and ultrasonography

A chest x-ray should always be taken, in particular to assess the state of the cardiovascular system (in hypertension), to show fractures of ribs or a primary bronchial tumour (in Cushing's syndrome) or to reveal secondary deposits from an adrenal carcinoma.

Several procedures are available for the localisation of tumours (Sutton, 1975). Medullary tumours are often bilateral or in extra-adrenal sites and special precautions are needed when invasive techniques, especially arteriography, are used. These involve preparation with an adrenergic α blocking drug, such as phenoxybenzamine, and careful monitoring of the blood pressure (and special measures if required) during the procedure. These are described under the measures required for operations.

The following methods are available for examination of the adrenals themselves:

A plain abdominal film may show downward displacement of the kidney by a large adrenal tumour and calcification may be seen in Addison's disease, in some malignant cortical and medullary tumours and in a few benign phaeochromocytomas.

Intravenous urography, especially when combined with tomography, reveals adrenal tumours and renal displacement in a higher proportion of cases.

Arteriography, performed selectively, is very helpful. Cortical adenomas are rather avascular but, if at least 2 to 3 cm in diameter, may show displacement of

vessels. Cortical carcinomas are usually very vascular, much larger and are readily seen (Fig 36.5). Most medullary tumours are revealed (Fig 36.6).

Venography is capable of displaying tumours under 1 cm in diameter, but is liable to cause haemorrhage and rupture of the gland, making subsequent operation difficult.

Selective venous sampling involves injection of just sufficient contrast into the adrenal or other veins to establish the positions of the catheters, so should not carry the same risks as venography. Samples of blood are withdrawn and the concentrations of hormones (cortisol, aldosterone, ACTH or catecholamines) are measured to determine the site or side of a secreting tumour. Samples are taken from blood in the vena cava below and above the adrenals, from a peripheral vein and from an artery at about the same time. In the case of extra-adrenal tumours secreting catecholamines or ACTH, samples may be taken from the neck to the pelvis.

Radioisotope scanning (Thrall *et al.*, 1978) with radiocholesterol (of which there are several forms) is a valuable non-invasive technique. The compound is

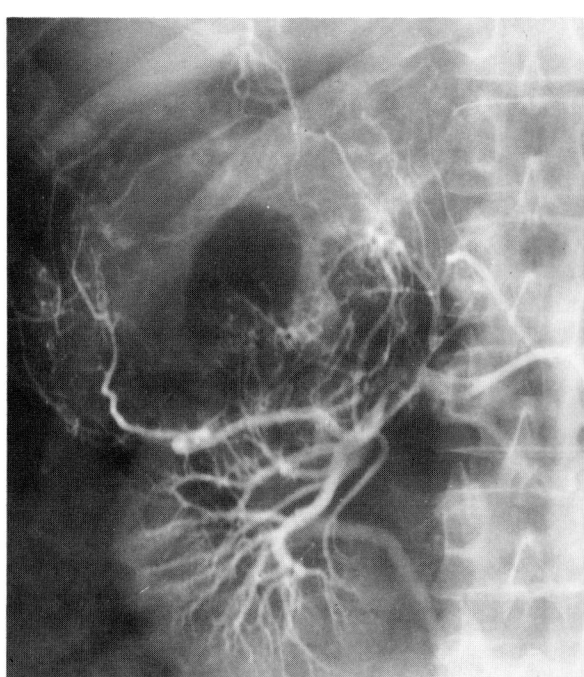

Fig 36.5 Selective renal arteriogram showing displacement of vessels and an abnormal circulation in an adrenocortical carcinoma above the right kidney. (By courtesy of Prof R.E. Steiner.)

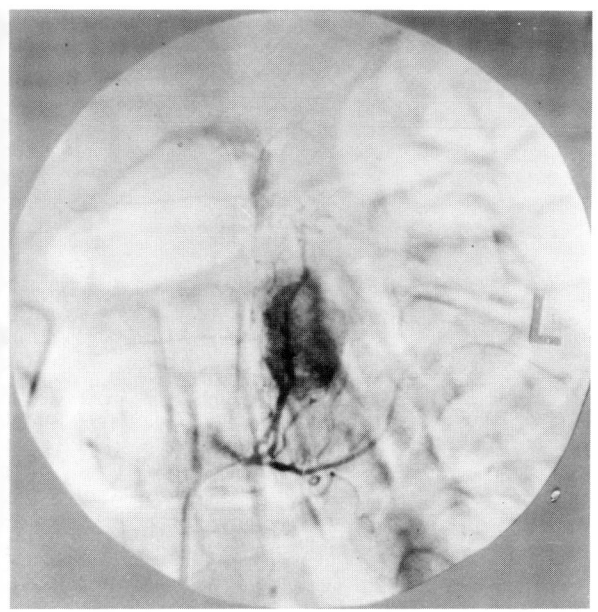

Fig 36.6 Selective adrenal arteriogram, with subtraction, showing abnormal tumour circulation in left-sided phaeochromocytoma. (By courtesy of Prof D.J. Allison.)

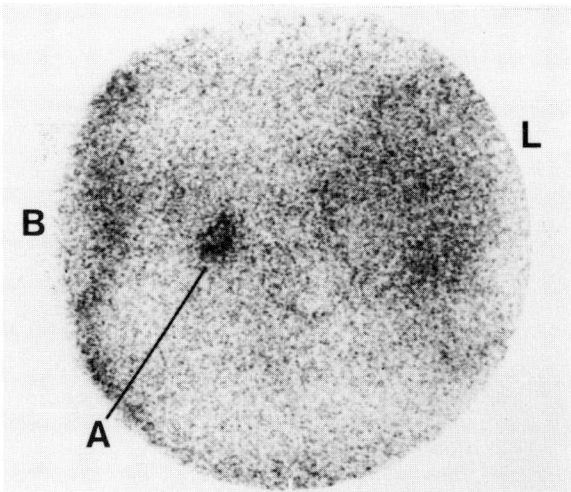

Fig 36.7 Adrenal scintigram in patient with left-sided aldosterone-secreting adenoma. 250 μCi of ^{75}Se cholesterol had been injected 7 days previously and the secretion of cortisol had been suppressed by dexamethasone (3 mg/day). The iodocholesterol has been incorporated in the aldosterone and shows as a hot spot (there is also some in the liver and in the bowel). A = lt. adrenal; L = liver; B = bowel. (By courtesy of Dr P. Lavender.)

taken up specifically by adrenocortical and gonadal tissue and 'hot spots' are recorded after some days by a gamma camera (Fig 36.7). The pattern varies with the nature of the pathological lesion and with the type of steroid secreted. Isotope scanning is being developed for adrenal medullary lesions also.

Ultrasonography is increasingly useful for detecting tumours of 2 to 3 cm or more in size and its value will probably increase (Fig 36.8).

CAT scanning is probably the best method for detection of tumours down to about 2 cm in diameter (Fig 36.9) and also reveals hyperplastic glands.

Cushing's syndrome

A syndrome originally named 'pituitary basophilism', was described by Harvey Cushing first in 1912 and more fully in 1932 (Harrison *et al.*, 1975; Montgomery and Welbourn, 1975; Friesen, 1978). In the naturally-occurring disease hypersecretion of cortisol by the adrenal cortex, which may arise in several different ways, causes the main metabolic and clinical features. An iatrogenic form results from exogenous administration of steroids or ACTH. Whatever the cause, however, the condition is now known as Cushing's syndrome. Some excessive secretion of androgens often accompanies that of cortisol, causing some virilisation in women, but this is less severe than that found in the pure virilising syndromes.

Causal lesions

The spontaneous syndrome arises in two main ways (Table 1). In the commoner variety bilateral adrenocortical hyperplasia is caused by an excess of ACTH, whose usual source is an anterior pituitary adenoma. In old terminology these tumours were described as basophil (hence 'basophilism') or sometimes chromophobe. Newer techniques, especially immunofluorescence and electronmicroscopy, show them to be corticotrophinomas. It is not yet known whether the primary disorder lies in the hypothalamus, which secretes an excess of CRF, or in the pituitary itself. Most of the tumours are benign, but a few are malignant, spreading and invading locally but not metastasising. The tumours are usually small and can only be recognised in life by elaborate investigations, needle biopsy or surgical operation. Some (about 10–15%) cause gross enlargement of the pituitary fossa. A few patients exhibit functional overactivity of the pituitary (and presumably of the hypothalamus) without any sign of tumour even at autopsy. The peak secretion of ACTH

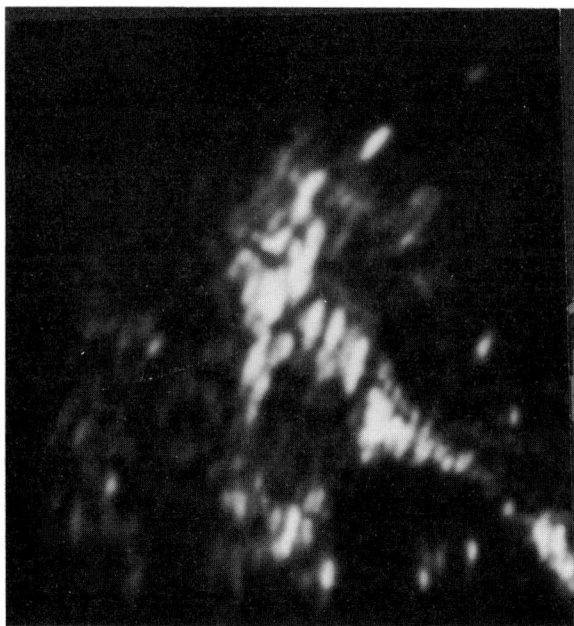

(a)

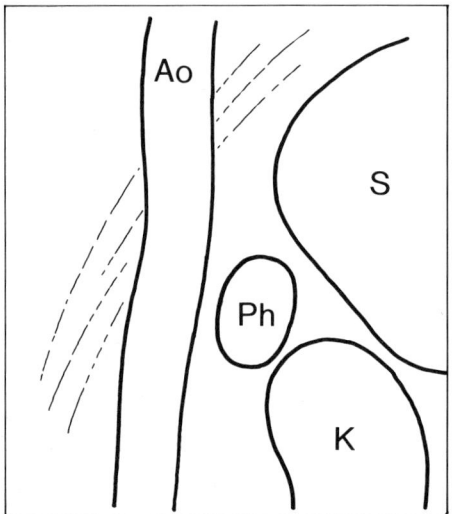

(b)

Fig 36.8 a. Ultrasonogram (coronal cut) in patient with left-sided phaeochromocytoma. (By courtesy of Dr N. Bowley.) b. Ph = phaeochromocytoma; A = aorta; S = spleen; K = kidney.

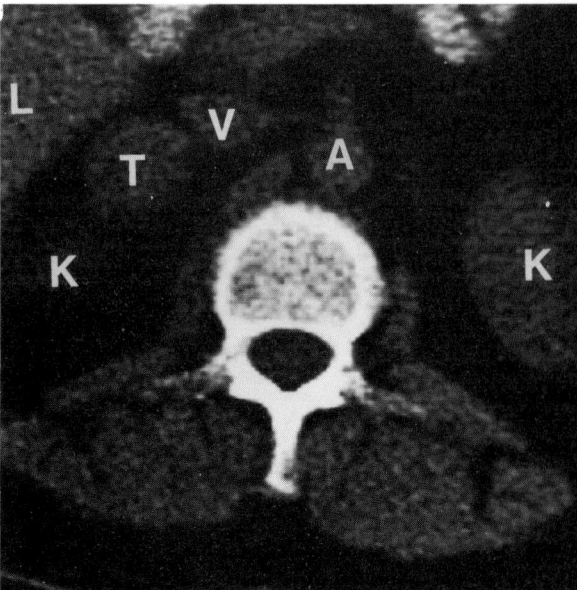

Fig 36.9 Computerised axial tomogram in patient with Cushing's syndrome, showing right-sided adrenal adenoma. T = tumour; L = liver; V = inferior vena cava; A = aorta; K & K = kidneys. (By courtesy of the BUPA Medical Centre.)

Table 1
CAUSAL LESIONS IN CUSHING'S SYNDROME

Bilateral adrenocortical hyperplasia	(ACTH +) 80%
Pituitary tumour	65%
Hypothalamic/pituitary hyperfunction	5%
Paraendocrine tumour	10%
Unilateral adrenocortical tumour	(ACTH −) 20%
Adenoma	10%
Carcinoma	10%

Percentages are approximate.

by the pituitary is often within the normal range or increased slightly, but the diurnal rhythm is absent so that the adrenals are stimulated continuously.

In some cases paraendocrine tumours elsewhere in the body secrete ACTH, usually in very large amounts, causing the *ectopic ACTH syndrome*. Most are malignant, the commonest being oat cell carcinoma of the bronchus, medullary carcinoma of the thyroid, islet cell tumour of the pancreas and thymic carcinoma. In these the Cushing's syndrome is usually an acute terminal event. A few are benign, the commonest being a bronchial carcinoid.

The second main cause of Cushing's syndrome is an adrenocortical tumour, which may be benign or malignant. Tumours secrete cortisol autonomously and inhibit the production of ACTH by the pituitary. Carcinomas often secrete significant quantities of androgens and other steroids in addition to cortisol, and cause mixed syndromes.

Metabolic and clinical features

Cushing's syndrome may develop at any time from infancy to old age, but is commonest between 20 and 50 years. It affects females two or three times as often as males. The length of history varies from a few weeks to many years, but is usually two to three years. The main symptoms are increase in weight, muscular weakness and impairment of sexual function. Patients are typically fat in the face and trunk, and have a florid complexion, thin limbs, hirsutism and striae (Fig 36.10). Most of the metabolic and clinical features result from the actions of excess cortisol on fat, protein and carbohydrate metabolism and electrolyte balance.

Fat is deposited excessively in the subcutaneous tissues of the face and trunk and within the abdomen.

Protein undergoes catabolism throughout the body. This causes wasting of muscles with general weakness and thinning of the limbs. Atrophy of the dermis reduces the thickness of the skin and causes livid striae

to develop on the trunk and proximal parts of the limbs in half the patients. The capillary walls are weakened and patients bruise easily, especially at the sites of venepuncture. Catabolism of protein in the bone matrix causes osteoporosis and kyphosis, and pathological fractures, especially in the ribs and lumbar spine, are very common (Fig 36.11). Loss of calcium from the skeleton may cause hypercalciuria and sometimes renal calculi.

Carbohydrate metabolism is altered in such a way that glucose tolerance is impaired and some patients develop frank diabetes.

Electrolyte metabolism is disturbed and potassium is excreted in excess in the urine. Intracellular base is depleted and some patients develop hypokalaemic alkalosis. Retention of sodium is less marked, but may contribute to ankle oedema, which is common.

Other features include hypertension, which is almost invariable and whose cause is not understood completely. It is often severe and is liable to all the complications of essential hypertension. Venous thrombosis

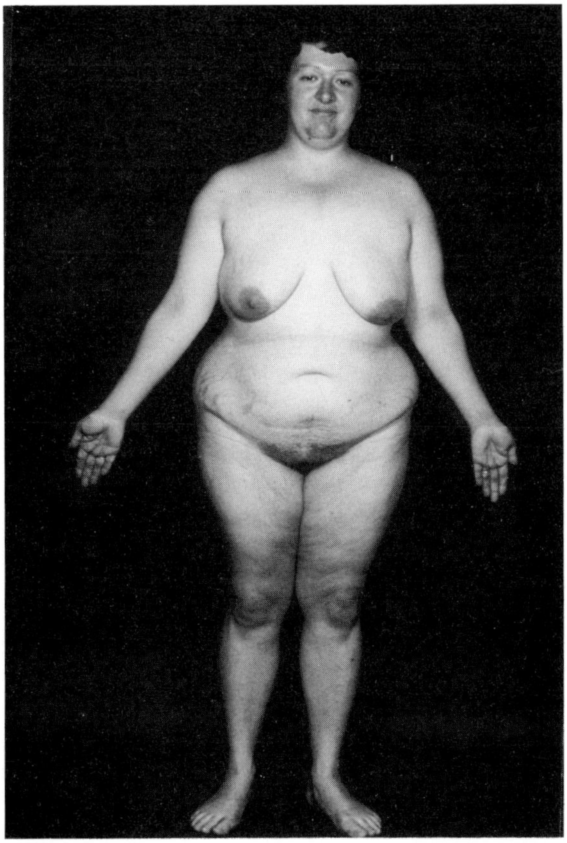

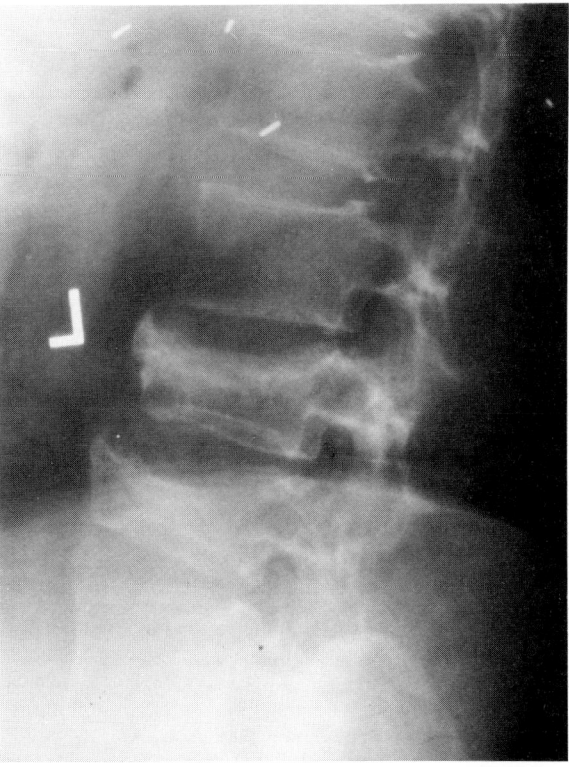

Fig 36.10 Female aged 28 with florid Cushing's syndrome.

Fig 36.11 Lateral x-ray of lumbar spine in patient with Cushing's syndrome, showing severe osteoporosis and pathological fractures. Clips had been inserted at an operation. (By courtesy of Prof R.E. Steiner.)

and embolism occur. Cortisol inhibits the secretion of gonadotrophins and sexual function is usually, but not always, impaired, women developing amenorrhoea, men impotence, and both sterility. Hirsutism and acne, as a result of androgen excess, are frequently seen. Some patients develop psychiatric symptoms, depression being most common, and a few become psychotic. Inflammatory reactions and healing are inhibited and chemosis is common. Cortisol inhibits the secretion of growth hormone, and growth is impaired seriously in children. Pituitary or other tumours secreting large amounts of ACTH may cause pigmentation. Very rarely the disease undergoes spontaneous remission, but in general the prognosis is bad and, without treatment, half the patients die within five years of the first symptom.

Investigation

These symptoms, signs and biochemical and radiological features may lead to a suspicion, and sometimes to a virtual certainty of Cushing's syndrome. However, two questions must be answered: Does the patient suffer from Cushing's syndrome? and, if so, what is the causal lesion?

The first depends on measurement of cortisol (with or without its metabolites) in the urine and/or blood (Table 2). In Cushing's syndrome the basal urinary free cortisol and 11-OHCS are raised and allow the diagnosis to be confirmed or refuted with confidence. Other groups of steroids are often raised also, but are less reliable.

Measurement of the plasma 11-OHCS is very helpful. The early morning (08.00 h) level is often raised, but may be normal. On the other hand, the midnight reading is almost always raised because of the lack of diurnal variation.

Plasma testosterone is variable, but tends to be similar in the two sexes when the adrenals are hyperplastic. It is relatively high in women, owing to adrenal stimulation, and relatively low in men as a result of testicular inhibition by cortisol. Testosterone levels tend to be highest in patients with adrenocortical carcinoma.

The pattern of the plasma ACTH is similar to that of the plasma 11-OHCS, when the corticotrophin originates in the pituitary. The level tends to be much higher when the source is ectopic and absent or very low in the presence of a cortisol-secreting adrenal tumour.

The nature of the causal lesion may be suggested by the metabolic and clinical features and by the measurements of steroids and ACTH which have been described (Table 3). It may be confirmed by functional tests and by x-rays and related investigations of the pituitary and of the adrenals.

The functional integrity of the hypothalamic-pituitary-adrenal axis (Fig 36.3) can be tested by stimulation with metyrapone and suppression by dexamethasone. The tests take from 1–4 days, depending on the methods employed. In normal subjects and in those with pituitary-dependent hyperplastic adrenal glands, metyrapone, by blocking to a great extent the synthesis of cortisol, removes its inhibitory effect on the hypothalamus and causes excessive secretion of ACTH. This results in increased production of the immediate precursor of cortisol, compound S (11-deoxy-cortisol) and of androgens, and these cause characteristic alterations in the urinary and blood steroids (Table 4). Dexamethasone, by suppressing the secretion of ACTH, reduces the production of cortisol, androgens and their metabolites.

Table 2
MAIN GROUPS OF STEROIDS MEASURED IN INVESTIGATION OF ADRENOCORTICAL DISEASE

Group of steroids	Abbreviated name	Significance
11-hydroxycorticosteroids*	11-OHCS	Relatively specific index of cortisol and its metabolites
17-oxogenic (ketogenic) steroids†	17-OGS	Less specific for cortisol and its metabolites
17-hydroxycorticosteroids*	17-OHCS	
17-oxosteroids (ketosteroids)†	17-OXOS	Mainly androgens and their metabolites

* Measured in blood and urine.
† Measured in urine only.

Table 3
CUSHING'S SYNDROME CLINICAL AND BIOCHEMICAL FEATURES IN RELATION TO CAUSAL LESIONS

Features	Lesion			
	Adrenal hyperplasia		Adrenal tumour	
	Pituitary lesion	Para endocrine tumour	Adenoma	Carcinoma
Sex	F >M	M>F	F>>M	F>M
Age	>10	>30	>20	<20&>40
Length of history	Years	Weeks	Years	Months
Hypokalaemia	±	++	±	±
Urinary free cortisol or 11-OHCS	+	+++	+	++
Plasma 11-OHCS	+	+++	+	++
Plasma ACTH	+	++	–	–
Stimulation and suppression	+	–	–	–

Table 4
INFLUENCE OF METYRAPONE AND DEXAMETHASONE ON URINARY AND BLOOD STEROIDS AND BLOOD ACTH WHEN THE HYPOTHALAMIC-PITUITARY-ADRENAL AXIS IS FUNCTIONALLY INTACT

	Urine		Blood	
	Increased	*Decreased*	*Increased*	*Decreased*
Metyrapone stimulation	17-OGS 17-OHCS 17-OXOS	Free cortisol 11-OHCS	Compound S 17-OHCS ACTH	11-OHCS
Dexamethasone suppression		Free cortisol 11-OHCS 17-OGS 17-OHCS 17-OXOS		11-OHCS 17-OHCS ACTH

In patients with adrenal tumours, which secrete cortisol and other steroids autonomously, the axis cannot be stimulated or suppressed (Table 3). Similarly, para-endocrine tumours secrete ACTH without hypothalamic control. Sometimes patients with adrenal carcinomas or the ectopic ACTH syndrome *appear* to show a response to metyrapone or dexamethasone. However, their excretion of steroids is usually very high and often varies greatly from day-to-day, so that such effects are probably illusory.

Plain x-rays of the pituitary fossa reveal only tumours greater than about 1 cm in diameter (Fig 36.12). More complex procedures, such as triaxial spiral tomography, CAT scanning and magnification carotid angiography, may reveal smaller ones. Most adrenal tumours can be demonstrated, as has been described. Ectopic ACTH-secreting tumours occur most often in the lungs, and the chest should be x-rayed first. If no tumour is seen, and if there are no other clues to the site of one, CAT scanning and selective venous sampling, with measurement of ACTH, are sometimes helpful.

Pituitary-dependent adrenal hyperplasia without obvious tumour

This is the commonest variety of Cushing's syndrome and requires no special additional description. The first regularly effective method of treatment was bilateral adrenalectomy, which became safe in about 1950, when cortisone was made available for replacement therapy. Since then many other procedures have been introduced. Emergency measures may be required to treat hypokalaemia, diabetes, heart failure, pathological fractures, infections, psychosis or other complications.

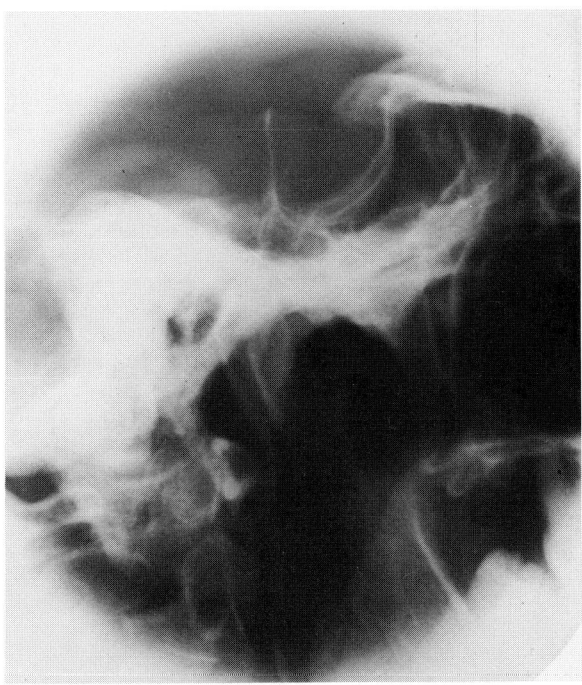

Fig 36.12 Lateral x-ray of pituitary fossa in patient with Cushing's syndrome due to a large pituitary adenoma, which subsequently became invasive. (By courtesy of Prof F.H. Doyle.)

Treatment

The present possibilities for definitive treatment are as follows:

Medical
Aminoglutethimide — inhibits synthesis of all adrenal steroids
Metyrapone — inhibits synthesis of cortisol
Mitotane — causes necrosis of adrenal cortex.

Radiotherapeutic
External — photons (conventional radiotherapy)
— protons
Internal — interstitial with seeds of radioactive material

Surgical
Bilateral adrenalectomy
Microsurgical excision of pituitary adenoma

These methods may be used alone or in combination. Several of them are effective in experienced hands and the method of choice in any particular patient depends on local expertise. No prospective controlled therapeutic trials have been reported.

Medical treatment

Of the medical measures metyrapone is probably the most effective as a temporary measure. In divided doses of 0.5 to 4 g per day it induces biochemical and clinical remission within a few weeks or months. The only reported side-effects are aggravation of hirsutism and acne, which may be severe in women. Metyrapone is of value in combination with other methods of treatment because it brings the disease under control rapidly and safely. If used alone, treatment must be permanent (Jeffcoate *et al.*, 1977)

Radiotherapy

External conventional radiotherapy of the pituitary, in a dose of 4500 to 5000 rads, causes remission in about 30% of patients, more often in adolescents than in adults. It has been used alone, but is probably best combined with metyrapone or adrenalectomy. With the former it may control the disease and allow the drug to be discontinued. With the latter it may reduce the risk of further tumour growth. Proton therapy is available in only two or three centres, but is reported to produce excellent results.

Interstitial irradiation of the pituitary with seeds of yttrium-90, together with needle biopsy of the gland, has been perfected in a very few centres, where it probably provides the best form of therapy available (Burke *et al.*, 1973). It is applicable to nearly all patients and its results are similar to those of bilateral adrenalectomy at least for 10 years or so. Replacement therapy is rarely needed. The further growth of small pituitary tumours is largely prevented.

Adrenalectomy

Bilateral adrenalectomy involves the total removal of both glands, followed by permanent steroid replacement (Welbourn *et al.*, 1971; Montgomery and Welbourn, 1978). Early attempts to restore normal adrenal function by subtotal adrenalectomy, or by the implantation of adrenal tissue in superficial muscles, were often followed by adrenal insufficiency or recurrence of the syndrome within a few years. The operative mortality was about 5% in experienced hands. Now, if patients are prepared with metyrapone, it is probably lower. Wound healing is impaired in Cushing's syndrome, but can be improved by vitamin A (50 000 iu per day by mouth for 1 week before operation, intramuscularly until the patient is eating, and then by mouth again until the wounds have healed). Venous thromboembolism is a serious problem and should be prevented, if possible, by intermittent pneumatic compression of the legs or by other methods.

The plasma ACTH usually rises after adrenalectomy, since its secretion is no longer inhibited by a high level of cortisol. Slight pigmentation, especially in the scars, is common. If a pituitary tumour continues to grow, the ACTH reaches very high levels and is accompanied by pigmentation (Nelson's syndrome).

Patients who survive operation undergo remission and require permanent replacement therapy. Very occasionally, probably owing to hypertrophy of ectopic cortical nodules, steroids are not required permanently and the syndrome may even recur. About 70% of patients survive for 10 to 15 years and about 50% for 20 years (Fig 36.13).

Remission

Effective treatment causes remission of the disease. After adrenalectomy the blood pressure falls, but remains labile, the skin often peels, particularly at the hair margins, until remission is complete, and the electrolyte balance returns to normal. Diabetes usually remits if it is mild, but tends to persist if it is severe. During the next few weeks to months the appearance (Fig 36.14), shape, strength, energy, mental state and sexual function all return towards normal. The cardiovascular system improves in most patients, but deteriorates in a few who suffer cardiovascular accidents. Later, after months to years, the blood pressure returns almost to normal in most patients and the cardiovascular system reaches a stable state. The bones regain their protein matrices, but do not recalcify (except in children). Deformities become stable and the bones no longer fracture. Hirsutism diminishes but does not disappear completely. Cutaneous striae become pale. Growth is restored in children, but lost height is rarely regained. Renal stones, if treated, do not reform. Fertility is restored.

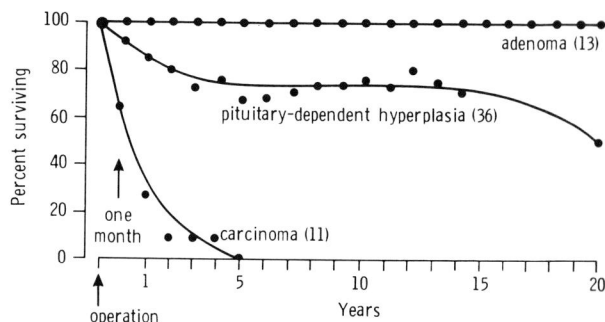

Fig 36.13 Survival after adrenalectomy for Cushing's syndrome (Welbourn, 1980). Figures in brackets indicate numbers of patients.

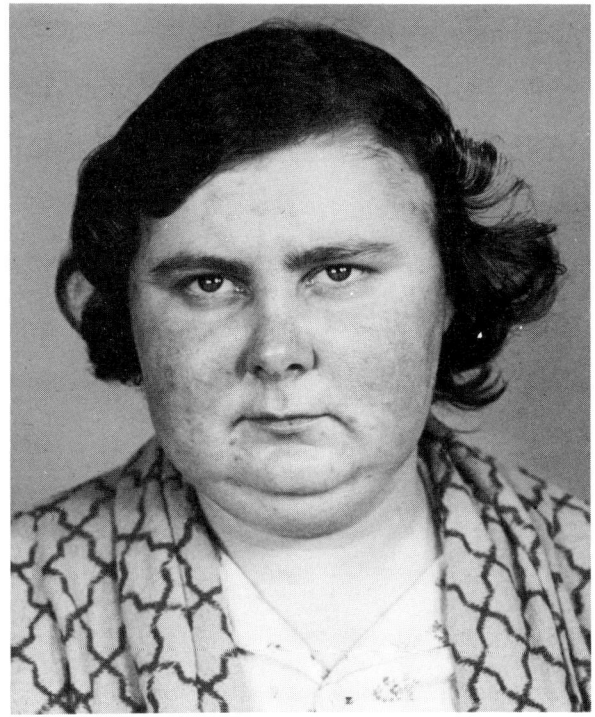

Fig 36.14a Cushing's syndrome in a girl aged 19.

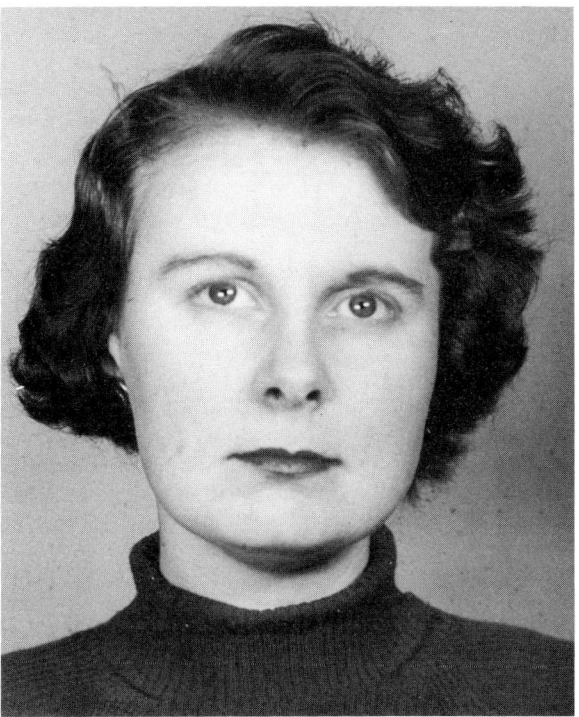

Fig 36.14b The same patient 3 years after bilateral adrenalectomy.

Pituitary operations

Microsurgical exploration of the pituitary fossa by the transsphenoidal route, without special preoperative methods for the detection of a tumour, is being practised in some centres (Wilson *et al.*, 1979). Any adenoma which is found is enucleated and the normal pituitary tissue is left *in situ*. If no tumour is discovered the whole gland is removed and a tumour may be found on serial section. Preliminary reports indicate that microadenomas are found in a high proportion of patients, that nearly all undergo satisfactory remission, and that few require replacement therapy. Those who fail to respond must be treated by another method. No long-term results are yet available.

Pituitary tumour

The more extensively patients are investigated radiologically, the more frequently are pituitary tumours diagnosed with confidence without needle biopsy or operation (Salassa *et al.*, 1978). The clinical features are not remarkable unless the tumour is large enough to cause local pressure effects. Very rarely a large and usually invasive tumour, secreting great amounts of ACTH, causes cutaneous pigmentation.

Although, as described, the majority of patients with Cushing's syndrome *may* be treated by measures directed primarily at the pituitary, this is only essential if a tumour is large enough to expand the fossa or to cause pressure effects or pigmentation. Surgical removal is the method of choice, and the transsphenoidal route may be used even when there is moderate suprasellar extension of the tumour. The transfrontal approach is required for gross intracranial expansion. The whole tumour and all normal pituitary tissue must be removed or destroyed by surgical excision combined with external or internal irradiation. Permanent replacement therapy is required. The prognosis for benign tumours is good, but invasive ones are incurable and cause death within two or three years.

Nelson's syndrome

In some 50% of patients who had no obvious pituitary tumour initially, small adenomas increase in size after adrenalectomy. The patient develops severe cutaneous pigmentation, the pituitary fossa usually enlarges greatly, the plasma ACTH rises to very high levels and, if the tumour is invasive, local pressure signs appear. The syndrome generally develops within a year or two of operation, but may not do so for many years. It is claimed that the incidence is reduced by irradiation of the fossa at the time of adrenalectomy, but the evidence is inconclusive (Moore *et al.*, 1976).

Paraendocrine (ectopic) ACTH-secreting tumours

Adult males are affected most frequently and, when the tumour is malignant, the onset is usually acute. Metabolic features, especially hypokalaemia, often develop within weeks before the patient shows outward signs of the disease. Very high levels of ACTH and cortisol are found in the blood and very large amounts of cortisol in the urine. In these circumstances Cushing's syndrome usually develops terminally and no active treatment is indicated. When the tumour is benign the syndrome is not usually so severe. If it can be located, it may be removed and the disease cured. This rarely happened in the past, but CAT scanning is now revealing more tumours at an early stage. If a tumour cannot be found or removed, the patient may be treated with metyrapone or bilateral adrenalectomy.

Adrenal adenoma

There are no special clinical features. The tumour is very rare in men. The plasma ACTH is undetectable and the tumours are independent of pituitary control. They can usually be localised without difficulty. Surgical removal of the tumour is highly effective and the results are better than those for any other variety of Cushing's syndrome (Fig 36.13). It is usually possible to wean the patient off steroid replacement, but the suppression of the other gland may be so profound that it takes many months, or even years, to do so, and occasionally permanent replacement is necessary.

Adrenal carcinoma

Most patients are less than 20 or more than 40 years of age and Cushing's syndrome in children under the age of 8 is nearly always due to adrenal carcinoma. The history is usually less than 1 year. Most carcinomas secrete several steroids in addition to cortisol. Androgens often cause virilism and aldosterone may cause severe hypokalaemia. The plasma ACTH is undetectable and blood and urinary cortisol levels are very high, although not quite as great as with paraendocrine tumours. All groups of steroids (Table 2) and many other individual steroids are often also very high. There is no evidence of pituitary dependence. The tumour can usually be localised easily. Secondary deposits may be seen in the lungs, skeleton, liver or elsewhere (Hutter and Kayhoe, 1966).

The only specific forms of treatment available are surgical removal and chemotherapy (Kelly *et al.*, 1979). The primary tumour, or as much of it as possible, should be removed surgically. If the tumour is removed, remission usually follows rapidly and replacement therapy is not needed for long. Recurrence, however, is common. If any primary or secondary tumour is known to have been left behind at operation, or if it recurs after operation, treatment with mitotane should be tried. If the optimal adult dose of 8 g per day is tolerated, the chance of temporary regression of the tumour is good. However, nausea and other side effects are common and prevent effective treatment. Metyrapone may provide symptomatic relief. Long-term survival from operation with or without chemotherapy has been reported occasionally, but few patients survive for more than one or two years (Fig 36.13).

Aldosteronism

Excessive secretion of aldosterone by an adrenal adenoma, causing hypertension, hypokalaemia, intermittent paralysis and polyuria, was first described by Conn in 1955, and this syndrome of primary aldosteronism is now known by his name (Harrison *et al.*, 1975; Montgomery and Welbourn, 1975; Friesen, 1978). The condition is cured by removal of the tumour. About 25% of patients with the same metabolic and clinical features have bilateral adrenocortical hyperplasia or nodular hyperplasia of unknown cause and not a single adenoma, and they form a separate variety of the same syndrome. The adrenals may also secrete large quantities of aldosterone in response to renin and angiotensin, which are formed in excess in some forms of cardiovascular, renal, hepatic and other diseases and during diuretic therapy. This condition is called secondary aldosteronism. The interrelationships between aldosterone, renin and angiotensin are different in the two syndromes (Fig 36.15).

Clinical features

Primary aldosteronism is much more common in women than in men and very rare in children. Hypertension has usually been present for some years before the condition is diagnosed. The clinical features are caused by the metabolic effects of aldosterone. Retention of sodium causes hypertension, which is often mild, but may be severe, is associated with headache

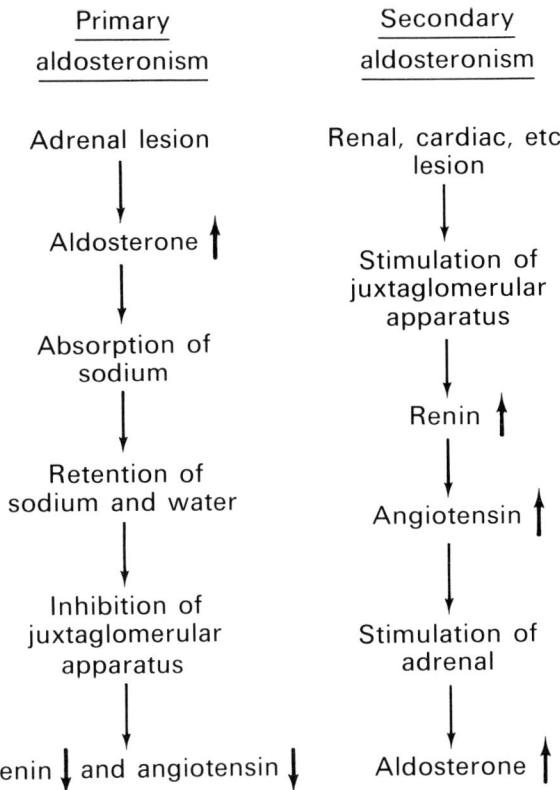

Primary aldosteronism	Secondary aldosteronism
Adrenal lesion	Renal, cardiac, etc. lesion
↓	↓
Aldosterone ↑	Stimulation of juxtaglomerular apparatus
↓	↓
Absorption of sodium	Renin ↑
↓	↓
Retention of sodium and water	Angiotensin ↑
↓	↓
Inhibition of juxtaglomerular apparatus	Stimulation of adrenal
↓	↓
Renin ↓ and angiotensin ↓	Aldosterone ↑

Fig 36.15 Mechanisms of metabolic disturbances in primary and secondary aldosteronism. ↓ = sequence of events; ↑ = high and ↓ = low blood concentration.

and may be complicated by retinopathy and cardio-vascular lesions. Excessive urinary excretion of potassium causes hypokalaemia, muscular weakness, which may be episodic and severe, and alkalosis, which reduces the ionised calcium in the blood, sometimes causing paraesthesia and tetany. Hypokalaemia also damages the proximal renal tubules, causing polyuria, nocturia and polydipsia. The plasma potassium is usually low (<3.8 mmol/l) and sometimes very low indeed. Alkalosis and retention of urea and NPN (non-protein nitrogen) are usual and the plasma sodium is often raised slightly. The urine is alkaline, of low osmolality, and contains an excess of potassium and often some protein.

Investigation

Four questions must be answered in the presence of these clinical and laboratory findings:

1 Does the patient suffer from aldosteronism?
2 If so, is it primary or secondary?
3 If primary, is it due to an adenoma or to bilateral adrenal hyperplasia?
4 If a tumour, which side is it?

1 Other conditions which cause similar features must be excluded. They include the consumption of liquorice and carbenoxolone, Cushing's syndrome and other forms of hypertension. Hypokalaemia from other causes has similar effects, but is usually associated with a normal or low blood pressure (Hunt *et al.*, 1975). Thiazide diuretics, used in the treatment of hypertension increase potassium loss and cause hypokalaemia; they should, therefore, be withheld for 3 weeks before potassium is measured in the blood and urine. It must be established that the hypokalaemia is the result of loss of potassium in the urine. This may be assumed if the daily loss is more than 25 mmol when the plasma potassium is 3.5 mmol/l or less. The diagnosis of aldosteronism is made on the finding of an excess of aldosterone in the blood and/or a 24-h sample of urine. Sodium restriction increases its production in normal people so that an intake of at least 120 mmol/l per day should be ensured for 1 week before the collections.

2 The distinction between the two types of aldosteronism depends first on the exclusion of lesions which may cause the secondary variety. This may be complicated by the fact that the hypertension and hypokalaemia of the primary disease may cause cardiac and renal lesions. Next, while both types cause increased levels of aldosterone in the blood and urine, primary aldosteronism *lowers* the plasma renin and/or angiotensin levels, while the secondary variety *raises* them (Fig 36.15).

3 Adenoma can be distinguished from hyperplasia with reasonable confidence by several methods.

a Posture influences the blood aldosterone concentration independent of the sodium intake. Standing for 4 h causes a mean *fall* of about 33% in those with adenoma and a mean *rise* of about 80% in those with hyperplasia. Blood samples are taken at 08.00 h before the patient rises, and again at 12.00 h after he has been on his feet.

b The biochemical disturbances tend to be greater with adenomas than with hyperplasia and a computer-aided analysis, which takes account of the plasma concentrations of aldosterone, renin, sodium, potassium and PCO_2, has been found to separate the two groups effectively.

c Selective venous sampling of the two adrenal veins, with measurements of aldosterone, shows a much higher concentration on the side of a tumour than on the other, but approximately similar concentrations in veins draining hyperplastic glands.

4   The side of a tumour may have been indicated by the selective venous sampling. Since the tumours are usually small, radioisotope scanning is the best of the other methods (Liebermann *et al.*, 1971).

Treatment

In both varieties of primary aldosteronism, hypokalaemia must be corrected with spironolactone (50–100 mg, 6-hourly *after* meals) and potassium supplements by mouth (Slow-K, Ciba, 2 to 4 g 6-hourly). In an emergency, potassium may be required intravenously.

An adenoma should be removed surgically, together with the whole adrenal, leaving the other gland intact (Ferris *et al.*, 1975). The total body deficit of potassium may be great and it is advisable to prepare the patient for at least 1 week before operation and monitor the electrolyte state postoperatively. Operative mortality is extremely low and removal of adenomas nearly always corrects the metabolic disturbances. The response of the blood pressure to spironolactone gives a fair prediction of the effects of operation (Herf *et al.*, 1979). On average the systolic pressure falls by about 50 mm Hg and the diastolic by about 25; the latter remains below 100 mmHg for years in 90% of patients. The blood pressure may be controlled with drugs in those who remain hypertensive (Clarke *et al.*, 1979).

Bilateral hyperplasia is best treated with spironolactone alone, once the hypokalaemia has been corrected. Total adrenalectomy (with permanent replacement therapy) should be considered if spironolactone causes complications. Prolonged therapy may result in enlargement of the breasts and impotence in men, dysmenorrhoea in women and dyspepsia, constipation and sweating in both. In these circumstances hypotensive drugs and potassium, together with restriction of sodium, may be effective.

Other adrenocortical syndromes

Virilisation

Virilisation is caused by either hyperplasia or a tumour of the adrenal cortex. Hyperplasia, of which there are several varieties, results from enzyme defects which reduce the synthesis of cortisol. This in turn increases the secretion of ACTH, which stimulates adrenal hyperplasia and the excessive production of androgens. Consequently, the patients are both virilised and suffer adrenocortical deficiency. Tumours, which are very rare, may be benign or malignant. The effects of androgens on the tissues vary with the age and sex of the patient, so that different varieties of the syndrome are encountered (Table 5). The term *adrenogenital syndrome* was originally applied to the condition in adult females but is now used for infants of either sex.

Virilising hyperplasia involves the surgeon in the differential diagnosis of virilising states, in the correction of anomalous external genitalia by plastic procedures, and in the complication of acute adrenal crisis if operation is performed without steroid cover. Virilising tumours require surgical removal.

Virilisation of adrenal origin developing in a previously healthy child is almost always caused by a tumour. In the adult female it may be due to hyperplasia or a tumour, while in the adult male there is no clearly defined virilising syndrome. In precocious isosexual pseudopuberty in the male, secondary sex characteristics develop early and growth is excessive. The penis enlarges, but the testes remain small. In precocious heterosexual pseudopuberty in the female, masculine secondary sex characters develop. These include hirsutism, muscular and skeletal growth, deepening of the voice and enlargement of the clitoris. The adult female suffers regression of feminine secondary sex features, namely amenorrhoea and atrophy of the breasts, and also develops masculine secondary sex characters.

Hyperplasia and tumour can be distinguished from each other, from idiopathic hirsutism and from virilising tumours of the testis and ovary on clinical and biochemical grounds and by demonstration of a tumour. Virilising adrenal adenomas are exceptionally rare, but are readily excised. The results are excellent. Adults and children regain their normal appearance, although hypertrophy of the clitoris and some hirsutism remain. Carcinomas, which are commoner, usually cause the mixed Cushing's virilising syndrome, which has been described already.

Table 5
VIRILISING LESIONS AND SYNDROMES OCCURRING IN THE TWO SEXES AT DIFFERENT PERIODS

	Fetus	*Child*	*Adult*
Lesion	Hyperplasia	Tumour	Hyperplasia or tumour
Male syndrome	Precocious isosexual pseudopuberty (macro genitosomia praecox, 'Infant Hercules')		(No clearly defined syndrome)
Female syndrome	Female pseudo-hermaphro-ditism	Virilism	

Feminisation

Adrenal tumours secreting oestrogens predominantly, and causing feminisation in the male, are exceptionally rare and nearly all are malignant. The main clinical features are enlargement of the breasts, testicular atrophy, loss of libido and impotence. Removal of a benign adenoma cures the condition. Carcinomas are managed in the same way as those causing Cushing's virilisation syndrome, except that metyrapone is not helpful. The prognosis is bad.

Silent tumours

Very rarely small functionless benign cortical adenomas are discovered incidentally in life on CAT scanning or perhaps at laparotomy. They are probably harmless and may be left alone, but should be kept under observation and removed if they enlarge or start to secrete.

Sometimes, cortical carcinomas cause general features, such as pyrexia, pain, fatigue and loss of weight, and their secondary deposits may give rise to symptoms, without any specific metabolic or clinical disorder being apparent. They may secrete biologically inactive steroids, which appear in the urine in the 17-OGS and 17-OXOS. Some cause hypoglycaemia, but the mechanism is not understood. They are treated in the same way as the carcinomas already described and have a bad prognosis.

Adrenocortical deficiency in surgery

Surgeons may encounter primary or secondary adrenal insufficiency unexpectedly in patients suffering from other conditions. Chronic failure should be suspected in patients with pigmentation, hypotension, hyponatraemia and hyperkalaemia. An injury or a surgical operation may precipitate an acute adrenal crisis, with severe hypotension, which may prove fatal unless treated immediately with hydrocortisone (100 mg) or its equivalent intravenously. This situation should be avoided, if possible, by assessment of adrenal function with tetracosactrin (a synthetic analogue of ACTH). The plasma 11-OHCS are measured before and 30 min or 6 h after injection. If the response is inadequate, or if there is no time to perform the test, steroids should be used prophylactically over the period of an operation. The prevention of adrenal insufficiency after adrenalectomy is described under Adrenalectomy.

Phaeochromocytoma

Clinical features

Phaeochromocytomas (Harrison *et al.*, 1975; Montgomery and Welbourn, 1975; Manger and Gifford, 1977; Friesen, 1978; Modlin *et al.*, 1979) may develop at any time from infancy to old age, but are commonest between the ages of 20 and 60 years. Their incidence is similar in men and women. About one-third of patients have symptoms for up to 1 year before diagnosis, another third for up to 3 years and the remainder for longer. At least one-third of patients with phaeochromocytomas die from their effects, mainly cardiovascular, and are diagnosed at autopsy.

The main clinical and metabolic features, due to the excessive circulating adrenaline and noradrenaline, are hypertension, paroxysms and diabetes, which is usually mild and rarely requires treatment. Other features, whose causes are not always apparent, are hypercalcaemia and renal artery stenosis. Hypertension is almost invariable and sometimes complicated by retinopathy or strokes. A specific form of cardiomyopathy, induced by catecholamines, may cause tachycardia and cardiac irregularities. It has been estimated that between 0.1% and 1% of the hypertensive population have phaeochromocytomas. Hypertension is paroxysmal only in about 50% of patients, sustained only in about 20%, and sustained with superadded paroxysms in about 30%. The mean blood pressure at rest, when patients are not having paroxysms, is about 200/120 mmHg and is significantly greater in women than in men. It rises much higher during paroxysms.

The main features of paroxysms are, in order of frequency, hypertension, palpitations, sweating, headache, anxiety, and pain in the chest or abdomen. During a paroxysm the blood pressure may swing up and down from very high to very low levels and the patient may die from a stroke or cardiac arrest. Paroxysms are sometimes induced by pressure on a tumour, by the patient or a doctor, and occasionally by minor trauma or a surgical operation for an unrelated lesion. All these procedures are dangerous and should be avoided if possible.

Associated major lesions are neurofibromatosis (von Recklinghausen's disease), in which phaeochromocytomas are particularly common, medullary carcinoma of the thyroid (multiple endocrine neoplasia type II–MEN II), which is familial, and cerebellar haemangioblastoma (the von-Hippel-Lindau syndrome). Phaeochromocytomas in the bladder usually cause haematuria and paroxysms or syncopal attacks on micturition. When phaeochromocytomas are associated with pregnancy, and remain undiagnosed, the maternal and fetal mortality rates are high and many of the fetuses áre deformed. Very rarely malignant phaeochromocytomas metastasise widely to the lungs, skeleton and elsewhere, causing local effects. A very few phaeochromocytomas are paraendocrine tumours, that is they secrete polypeptides characteristic of other endocrine glands, usually of the APUD series. The best known, though very rare, is ACTH, causing Cushing's syndrome.

Investigation

The urinary VMA is raised, at least on occasions, in about 95% of patients, and the urinary metadrenalines in rather more (Fig 36.4). Both these measurements are useful screening tests. The catecholamines, adrenaline and/or noradrenaline in the urine and/or the blood are nearly always raised and should be measured if a phaeochromocytoma is suspected and the screening tests are repeatedly negative. Older methods of investigation allowed nearly 90% of tumours to be localised correctly before operation (Fig 36.16). The proportion is higher now that CAT scanning and ultrasonography are available.

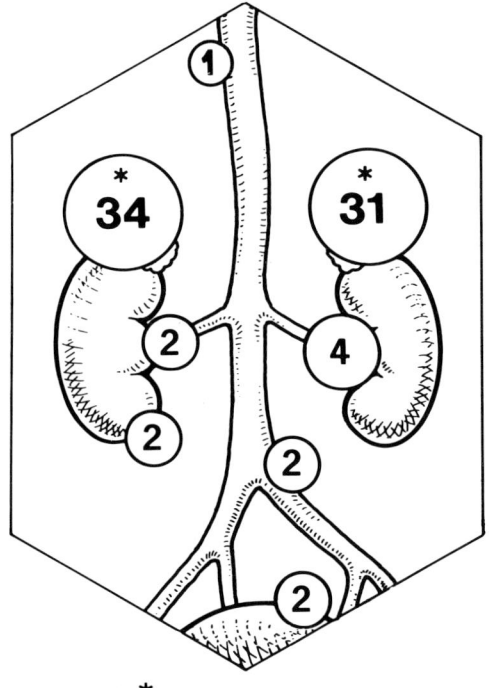

*Bilateral in six

Fig 36.16 Sites of 78 phaeochromocytomas in 72 patients (Modlin *et al.*, 1979).

Management

The best form of treatment for nearly all patients is surgical removal of the tumour. Most patients are hypovolaemic, since noradrenaline in excess constricts not only the arterioles, causing arterial hypertension, but also the great veins, reducing the total capacity of the vascular bed. Before this was appreciated, not only did handling of the tumour at operation cause severe hypertension, but its removal caused profound hypotension, owing to sudden dilatation of the vascular bed. These problems can be overcome by:

1 Preparing the patient for operation with a long-acting adrenergic α blocking agent, such as phenoxybenzamine, which partially restores the blood volume. A suitable dose of phenoxybenzamine is 10 mg 8-hourly, increasing by 10 mg per dose until the diastolic blood pressure is below 100 mmHg. If the patient develops tachycardia or cardiac irregularities before or during operation, a β blocker, such as propranolol, is given also;

2 Injecting a rapidly-acting blocker, such as phentolamine, or a vasodilator, such as sodium nitroprusside, when the pressure rises too high during operation;

3 Infusing rapidly a blood volume expander, such as plasma, to maintain the arterial blood pressure at a normal level as soon as the tumour has been removed. One or two litres may be needed in addition to replacement of the measured blood loss with whole blood (Fig 36.17).

The few malignant tumours require sharp dissection and are more difficult to remove. Any adjacent tissue which is attached should be removed with the tumour and any enlarged lymph nodes in the vicinity excised. It is probably wise to irradiate the area postoperatively. After the tumour has been removed the whole abdomen is searched again. Any remaining adrenal tissue on either side and any lumps are squeezed and the blood pressure is recorded. Sometimes previously unsuspected tumours (rarely more than one) are found in this way.   In patients with MEN II, even if only one tumour is found, both adrenals should be removed completely. Eventually all their adrenal medullary tissue develops phaeochromocytomas, which may be malignant, and it is better to accept the need for replacement therapy than run the risk of malignant recurrence.

If phaeochromocytoma is diagnosed in pregnancy, localisation may be attempted by ultrasound, but not by techniques involving irradiation. In the first 6 months immediate operation is advisable. In the third trimester it is probably best to control hypertension

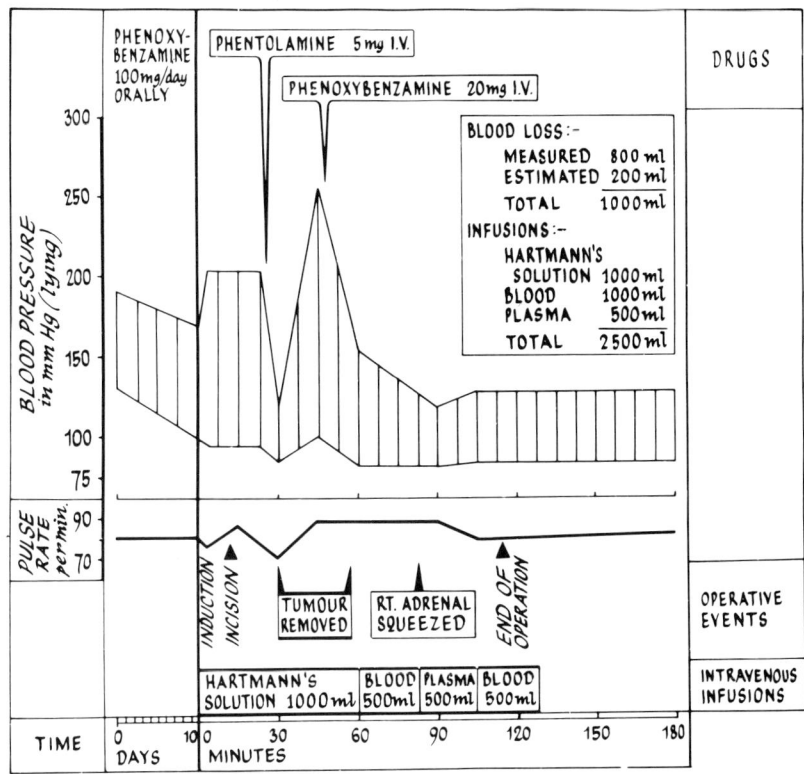

Fig 36.17 Record of blood pressure and management before, during and after surgical removal of phaeochromocytoma (Montgomery and Welbourn, 1975).

with an α blocker and to wait until the fetus is judged mature enough for delivery. Then Caesarian section and removal of the tumour can be undertaken at the same time. If the tumour has not been located, and cannot be found at operation, α blockade must be continued, further localisation studies undertaken and the tumour removed later.

Prognosis

The operative mortality is about 1 or 2% in special centres, but probably still much higher elsewhere. The VMA or other measurements should be repeated 2 or 3 weeks after operation to ensure that they have returned to normal. Measurements made earlier than this may be high as a result of the operative stress and are therefore useless. Persistent high readings indicate the need for further careful investigation for another tumour.

Symptoms are relieved rapidly, paroxysms cease and the blood pressure returns almost to normal in 75% of patients. The remaining 25% are well controlled by anti-hypertensive drugs. Diabetes is cured and hyper-

calcaemia is usually corrected. Those with malignant lesions fare surprisingly well and many survive in health for years. A very few, however, develop widespread metastases and must be treated symptomatically. Irradiation of troublesome deposits may be helpful. When phaeochromocytomas are diagnosed in pregnancy, the outlook for the mother is now excellent, but that for the fetus is still poor.

About 60 to 70% of all patients undergoing operation for phaeochromocytoma survive in good health for 10 years and many live much longer.

Other adrenal medullary tumours

Ganglioneuroma

The patient is usually an adult or an older child. The presenting feature is usually a mass, which grows very slowly, in the abdomen or very rarely in the neck. Occasionally a shadow may be seen in the abdomen or chest on x-ray. The tumour may spread through inter-vertebral foramina, forming dumb-bell masses, and compress nerve roots or even the spinal cord.

Most tumours secrete catecholamines and some resemble phaeochromocytomas clinically. Most, however, are incapable of converting noradrenaline to adrenaline. A very few also secrete excessive amounts of vasoactive intestinal polypeptide (VIP) like vipomas and cause watery diarrhoea, hypokalaemia, which may be profound, and achlorhydria or hypochlorhydria; the WDHA syndrome.

Biochemical investigation shows high excretion of VMA, DOPA, dopamine and HVA (Fig 36.4) in 75% of patients. The plasma VIP level is high in those with the WDHA syndrome, but the level of pancreatic polypeptide is normal (*see* chapter 37). X-rays, as described already, usually reveal the tumour and may show congenital defects of the spine and ribs.

The tumours can usually be excised without dif-ficulty. If catecholamine excretion is increased, they should be managed in the same way as phaeochromo-cytomas. Hypokalaemia may require correction. The prognosis is excellent.

Neuroblastoma

Neuroblastoma (Cohen, 1978; Grosfield *et al.*, 1978) mainly affects infants and young children. The clinical features may be non-specific at first, and include anorexia, vomiting, loss of weight, anaemia, pyrexia and failure to thrive. The primary tumour may be felt as a mass in the abdomen or, in the neck, it can produce Horner's syndrome, tracheal deviation or venous obstruction of the arm. In the chest it may cause respiratory symptoms and, in the pelvis, interference with the urinary tract or bowel. Pain is usual. It may form a dumb-bell tumour like a ganglioneuroma which compresses nerves. Sometimes the primary tumour remains small, while large secondary deposits, espe-cially in the skull or liver, cause symptoms. The secre-tion and excretion of catecholamines is similar to that of ganglioneuromas, and a few neuroblastomas may also secrete VIP.

X-rays show calcification in about 20% of tumours and may reveal depression of a kidney and secondary deposits in the skeleton and elsewhere. Scintigraphy often shows deposits in the liver or skeleton, which are not apparent on x-rays. Myelography may reveal intra-spinal spread. Biopsies of accessible lesions, including those in the bone marrow, provide a histological diagnosis.

The treatment and prognosis depend on the stage of the disease and the age of the child. The tumours may be staged as follows:

I   Confined to organ or structure of origin
II   Unilateral spread to adjacent tissue or lymph nodes
III Spread across the mid-line
IV Remote metastases

A subgroup (IV S), with a surprisingly good prog-nosis, is defined as stage I or II except that the patient has remote disease in the liver, skin and/or bone mar-row, but not in the bony skeleton. ('S' refers to 'soft tis-sues'.)

Treatment involves removal of the primary tumour, if possible, with suitable precautions if it secretes catecholamines. However, attempted removal of an extensive tumour may be hazardous and undue risks should not be taken. When it appears that all the tumour has been removed, the patient should be fol-lowed up carefully. Further treatment in the form of radiotherapy and chemotherapy need only be given if the tumour remains or recurs at the primary or at secondary sites. Chemotherapy with various regimens is under trial and, if continued for at least 2 years, prob-ably prolongs life in those with advanced disease. The prognosis is best in infants less than 1 year old, about 70% of whom survive 2 years. In stages I, II and IV S over 90% survive for that period and 80% for 5 years. In stages III and IV over 70% *die* within 2 years. After the first year, although the stage of the disease still affects the outcome, only about 15% survive 2 years. Some 5% of neuroblastomas, especially in infants, regress completely, perhaps as a result of an immune response. Some others, which mature slowly to ganglio-neuromas, follow a benign course and can be excised.

Adrenalectomy

Removal of one gland is required for a unilateral tumour. Complete removal of both glands may be undertaken for Cushing's syndrome due to hyperplasia or for bilateral phaeochromocytomas (Edis *et al.*, 1975; Welbourn, 1977). Adrenalectomy is rarely used now for patients with advanced carcinoma of the breast (*see* chapters 38, 39).

Three approaches – posterior, anterior and lateral – are available, and each is ideal in certain circumstances. The posterior route is usually best for removal of hyperplastic glands or small tumours (up to 2 or 3 cm in diameter). The anterior is suitable for most patients with phaeochromocytomas, and the lateral for all those with large tumours.

The special preoperative measures required in differ-ent diseases have been described already. In addition, a reliable intravenous drip should be set up, sufficient blood must be available and, if the posterior or lateral approach is to be used, x-rays showing the lower ribs should be in the theatre.

Replacement of steroids

Adequate replacement of steroids is essential to life. They are required for all patients undergoing bilateral adrenalectomy and for those with Cushing's syndrome who are losing one gland. Unilateral adrenalectomy for other conditions rarely requires steroid cover. The following schedule (Table 6) is recommended for adults, except in those with Cushing's syndrome:

Postoperatively all patients undergoing adrenalectomy, and especially those with Cushing's syndrome and phaeochromocytoma, should have the blood pressure and pulse measured continuously, or at least every 15 min, until these have been stable for 2 days. The plasma electrolytes should be estimated daily during this time.

If the systolic blood pressure falls below 100 mmHg during the first 48 h, and if bleeding or other causes can be excluded, the rate of infusion of hydrocortisone should be increased. If the pressure falls suddenly, an extra 100 mg should be injected intravenously at once. The changeover from the intravenous to the oral route depends on the patient's ability to eat food. If he develops anorexia, nausea, abdominal discomfort, tachycardia or slight pyrexia, adrenal insufficiency should be suspected and the dose increased. An additional sign of insufficiency in Cushing's syndrome is severe desquamation of the face, which may spread to the whole body.

The eventual replacement dose for all patients, after bilateral adrenalectomy, which must be discovered by trial and error, is usually about 30 mg of hydrocortisone per day, but in those with Cushing's syndrome it may require several weeks for this dose to be achieved. Withdrawal of steroids in patients with Cushing's syndrome due to benign or malignant tumours has been discussed already.

Not all patients require fludrocortisone, which is a mineralo-corticoid similar in action to aldosterone, for long-term replacement therapy, but some do and it rarely does harm. For this reason it is best to give it routinely. If, however, hypertension persists in patients who had Cushing's syndrome or bilateral phaeochromocytomas, or if there is evidence of sodium retention, it should be withdrawn or given in a smaller dose.

Every patient requiring steroid replacement therapy should carry a card with him at all times, giving the essential information. In the event of stress, such as that caused by an acute illness, accident or operation, the doses should be doubled for the duration of the acute stress and then reduced by stages to the maintenance levels. If for any reason the patient cannot take steroids by mouth – e.g. vomiting or unconsciousness – he must receive them by injection.

Posterior approach

The patient is placed face down, the 12th rib is resected on one or both sides (Fig 36.18), the pleura is displaced upwards and one or both adrenals are removed. The right adrenal vein or veins, which are short and drain into the posterolateral part of the vena cava, are identified with ease, ligated and divided. If the site of a small tumour has not been identified for certain, both glands may be explored before either is removed. The postoperative course is usually remarkably smooth. If the wounds become infected, as they may in Cushing's syndrome, they drain downhill and heal rapidly.

Anterior approach

An anterior abdominal incision allows both adrenals to be examined and removed and the whole abdomen to be explored. This is important with phaeochromocytomas, which may be bilateral, or in extra-adrenal sites, when a mid-line incision is convenient. It is also helpful in Cushing's syndrome due to a paraendocrine

Table 6

Day	Steroid	Dose
Night before operation	Hydrocortisone sodium succinate	100 mg once by i.m. injection
Day of operation	Hydrocortisone sodium succinate	100 mg in 24 h by i.v. infusion
Day 1 after operation	Hydrocortisone sodium succinate	100 mg in 24 h by i.v. infusion
Day 2 after operation	Hydrocortisone sodium succinate	80 mg in 24 h by i.v. infusion
	OR hydrocortisone	20 mg 6-hrly p.o.
Days 3–5 after operation	OR hydrocortisone	20 mg 8-hrly p.o.
Days 6–9 after operation	OR hydrocortisone	15 mg 8-hrly p.o.
Days 10 + after operation	Hydrocortisone	10 mg 8 hrly p.o.
	+ Fludrocortisone	0.1 mg once daily p.o.

For patients with Cushing's syndrome the doses should be about three times greater. In particular, 300 mg of hydrocortisone sodium succinate are needed on the day of operation.

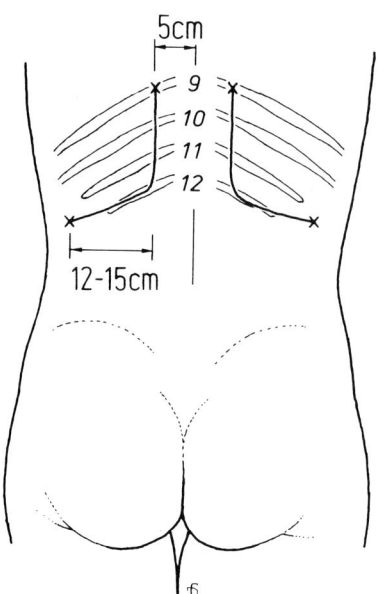

Fig 36.18 Incision for posterior operative approach to adrenals. (Welbourn, 1977.)

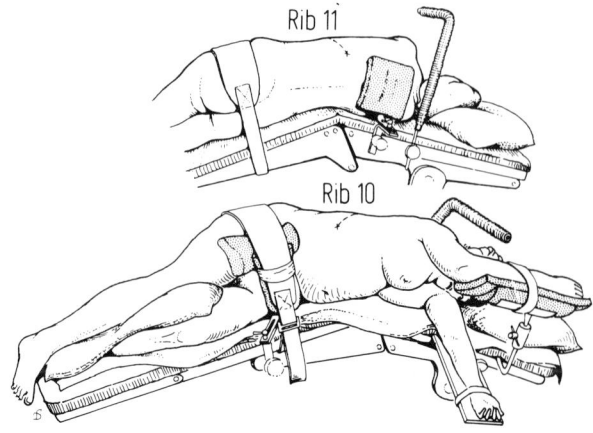

Fig 36.19 Position on table and incisions for lateral operative approach to adrenals. (Welbourn, 1977.)

tumour, when it may be possible to find a primary lesion (e.g. an abdominal carcinoid tumour) or to biopsy secondary deposits in the liver. A bilateral subcostal or roof-top incision gives good access to both glands. However, removing the right adrenal may prove difficult or impossible. The right adrenal is approached directly, above the kidney, and the vein or veins identified and ligated with care. The left gland is exposed best by mobilisation of the spleen and tail of the pancreas. In Cushing's syndrome wound infection may lead to a subphrenic abscess, which is a serious disadvantage.

Lateral approach

The lateral approach provides the best access to large tumours, to adrenals which have been operated on previously and in any circumstances when difficulty is anticipated. On the left side an extrapleural incision through the bed of the 11th rib provides the best access and, on the right, a transthoracic exploration through the bed of the 10th rib is most satisfactory (Fig 36.19).

Adrenalectomy in children

The indications for operations for adrenal disease in children are the same as those in adults, although

malignant tumours are relatively more common. Smaller doses of steroids are required. In operations for Cushing's syndrome, children up to about 5 years of age require 100 mg on the day of operation, those up to about 15 need 200 mg and older children should receive adult doses. Doses on the succeeding days should be calculated accordingly.

A tumour is best approached by a lateral incision and that through the bed of the 11th rib gives good access on each side. For bilateral adrenalectomy the posterior and anterior approaches may provide inadequate access, even in teenagers, and the bilateral 11th rib approach is advised. Children, unlike adults with Cushing's syndrome, withstand being turned from one side to the other during operation. The maintenance dose of hydrocortisone in those requiring permanent replacement must be adjusted regularly with great care, because any excess stops growth.

References

Burke C.W., Doyle F.H., Joplin G.F., Arnot R.N., Macerlean D.P., Fraser T.R. (1973). Cushing's disease: treatment by pituitary implantation of radioactive gold or yttrium seeds. *Quart. J. Med*; **42**:693–714.

Clarke D., Wilkinson R., Johnston I.D.A., Haggith J.W. (1979). Severe hypertension in primary aldosteronism and good response to surgery. *Lancet*; **1**:482.

Cohen S.J. (1978). Operations for neuroblastoma. In *Operative Surgery – Paediatric Surgery* (Rob C., Smith R., Dudley H.A.F., Nixon H.H., eds.). London: Butterworth.

Edis A.J., Ayala L.A., Egdahl R.H. (1975). *Manual of Endocrine Surgery*. Berlin: Springer-Verlag.

Ferriss J.B. *et al.* (1975). Results of adrenal surgery in patients with hypertension, aldosterone excess, and low plasma renin concentration. *Brit. Med. J*; **1**:135.

Friesen S.R. (1978). *Surgical Endocrinology: Clinical Syndromes*. Philadelphia: Lippincott.

Grosfield J.L., Schatzlein M., Ballantine T.V.N., Weetman R.M., Baehner R.L. (1978). Metastatic neuroblastoma: factors influencing survival. *J. Pediatr. Surg*; **13**:59–65.

Harrison T.S., Gann D.S., Edis A.J., Egdahl R.H. (1975). *Surgical Disorders of the Adrenal Gland: Physiologic Background and Treatment.* New York: Grune and Stratton.

Herf S.M., Teates D.C., Tegtmeyer C.J., Vaughan E.D., Ayers C.R., Carey R.M. (1979). Identification and differentiation of surgically correctable hypertension due to primary aldosteronism. *Amer. J. Med*; **67**:397.

Hunt T.R., Schambelan M., Biglieri E.G. (1975). Selection of patients and operative approach in primary aldosteronism. *Ann. Surg*; **182**:353.

Hutter A.M., Kayhoe D.E. (1966) Adrenal cortical carcinoma. *Amer. J. Med*; **41**:572–81.

Jeffcoate W.J., Rees L.H., Tomlin S., Jones A.E., Edwards C.R.W., Besser G.M. (1977). Metyrapone in long-term management of Cushing's disease. *Brit. Med. J*; **2**:215.

Kelley W.F., Barnes A.J., Welbourn R.B. *et al.* (1979). Cushing's syndrome due to adrenocortical carcinoma – a comprehensive and biochemical study of patients treated by surgery and chemotherapy. *Acta Endocrinol*; **91**:303.

Lieberman L.M., Beierwaltes W.H., Conn J.W. (1971). Diagnosis of adrenal disease by visualization of human adrenal glands with ^{131}I-19-iodocholesterol. *New Engl. J. Med*; **285**:1387.

Manger W.M., Gifford R.W. (1977). *Pheochromocytoma.* New York: Springer-Verlag.

Modlin I.M., Farndon J.R., Welbourn R.B. *et al.* (1979). Phaeochromocytomas in 72 patients: clinical and diagnostic features, treatment and long-term results. *Brit. J. Surg*; **66**:456–65.

Montgomery D.A.D., Welbourn R.B. (1975). *Medical and Surgical Endocrinology.* London: Arnold.

Montgomery D.A.D., Welbourn R.B. (1978). Cushing's syndrome: 20 years after adrenalectomy. *Brit. J. Surg*; **65**:221.

Moore T.J., Dluhy R.G., Williams G.H., Cain J.P. (1976). Nelson's syndrome: frequency, prognosis and effect of prior pituitary irradiation. *Ann. Intern. Med*; **85**:731.

Salassa R.M., Laws E.R., Carpenter P.C., Northcutt R.C. (1978). Transsphenoidal removal of pituitary microadenoma in Cushing's disease. *Mayo Clin. Proc*; **53**:24–8.

Sutton D. (1975). The radiological diagnosis of adrenal tumours. *Brit. J. Radiol*; **48**:237.

Thrall J.H., Freitas J.E., Beierwaltes W.H. (1978). Adrenal scintigraphy. *Sem. Nucl. Med*; **8**:23.

Welbourn R.B. (1977). Operations on the adrenal glands. In *Operative Surgery: Fundamental International Techniques,* 3rd edn. (Rob C., Smith R., eds.) pp. 403–19. 'Abdomen'. London: Butterworth.

Welbourn R.B. (1980). Some aspects of adrenal surgery. *Brit. J. Surg*; **67**:723–7.

Welbourn R.B., Montgomery D.A.D., Kennedy T.L. (1971). The natural history of treated Cushing's syndrome. *Brit. J. Surg*; **58**:1.

Wilson C.B., Tyrell J.B., Fitzgerald P. (1979). Cushing's disease revisited. *Amer. J. Surg*; **138**; 77–9.

Further reading

Davies C.J., Joplin G.F., Welbourn R.B. (1982). Surgical management of the ectopic ACTH syndrome. *Ann. Syrg*; **196**:246–58.

Johnston I.D.A., Thompson N.W., eds (1983). *Endocrine Surgery.* pp. 53–75; 182–8; 189–202. London: Butterworth.

Sisson J.C., Frager M.S., Valk T.W., *et al.* (1981). Scintigraphic localization of pheochromocytoma. *N. Engl. J. Med*; **305**:12–7.

Wilson C.B., Tyrrell J.B., Fitzgerald P.A., Forsham P.H. (1982). Cushing's disease: surgical management. In *Hormone-secreting Pituitary tumours* (Givens J.R., ed.) pp. 199–208. Chicago: Year Book.

Endocrine tumours of gut

R.B. WELBOURN and R.B. GALLAND

Anatomy and physiology

The alimentary tract contains more endocrine cells and a greater variety of them than any other organ in the body (Montgomery and Welbourn, 1975; Welbourn, 1977; Bloom, 1978; Friesen, 1978). Those in the stomach and intestines are scattered among the mucosal cells on the luminal surface and in the crypts, while most of those in the pancreas are grouped in clumps in the Islets of Langerhans. At least 18 cell types and 16 products have been identified and more remain to be discovered. The cells belong to the APUD series (with a high **A**mine content and the capacity for amine **P**recursor **U**ptake and **D**ecarboxylation), whose products are peptides and amines (Table 1). Most cells probably secrete one substance only, but some produce both an amine and a peptide and others possibly two peptides. They do not take up conventional histological stains, but some, the enterochromaffin cells, are argentaffin and most of the remainder are argyrophil. Electron-microscopy (Fig 37.1) helps to distinguish the different types of cell, shows them to contain dense secretory granules and reveals microvilli (which are probably sensory) on the luminal surfaces of most of those in the stomach and intestines. The peptide products, which are antigenic, can be seen under ultraviolet light, when subjected to appropriate specific antibodies labelled with fluorescein, and can thus be identified microscopically (Fig 37.2). They can also be extracted from the tissues and measured by radioimmunoassay (RIA).

Table 1

SOURCES AND PHYSIOLOGICAL ROLES OF PEPTIDES AND AMINES ARISING FROM THE GUT WHICH ARE SECRETED BY ALIMENTARY ENDOCRINE TUMOURS

Substance	Cells and organs of origin	Physiological role
Insulin	B cells in islets	Controls storage of energy (anabolism) and lowers blood glucose
Glucagon	A cells in islets	Controls production of energy (catabolism) and raises blood glucose
Somatostatin	D cells in islets, stomach, small intestine and from other parts of body	Widespread (probably paracrine) inhibition of endocrine and other bodily functions
Vasoactive intestinal polypeptide (VIP)	Neural tissue in whole gut and other parts of nervous system, and endocrine cells in colon, etc.	Unknown ? Neurocrine and paracrine
Pancreatic polypeptide (PP)	PP cells in islets	Unknown
Gastrin	G cells in gastric antrum and upper small intestine	Stimulates secretion of gastric acid
5-Hydroxytryptamine (5-HT)	EC, EC1 and EC2 cells in stomach and intestines	?Paracrine stimulation of smooth muscle
Substance P	EC1 cells in stomach and upper small intestine	? Paracrine stimulation of smooth muscle and vasodilatation
Motilin	EC2 cells in upper small intestine	? Endocrine inhibition of gastric emptying, etc.

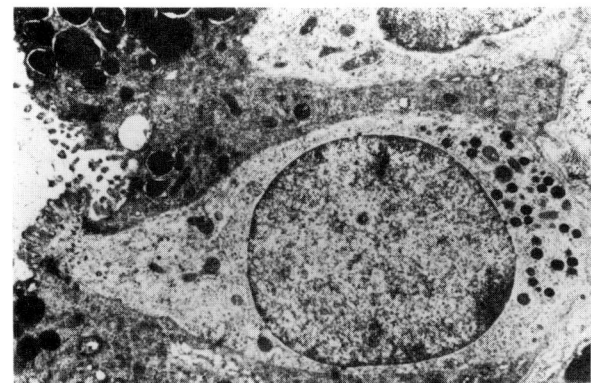

Fig 37.1 Normal endocrine cell of the gut mucosa showing the presence of a tuft of microvilli at the luminal (left) end and numerous electron dense secretory granules in the basal part of the cell. × 4700 (By courtesy of Dr J.M. Polak.)

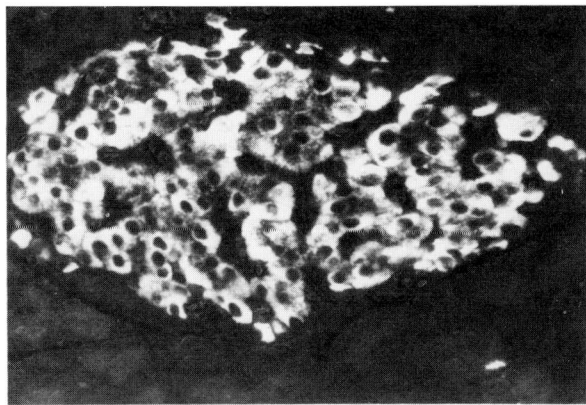

Fig 37.2 Human pancreas immunostained with specific antibodies to insulin. Pancreatic islet. × 170 (By courtesy of Dr J.M. Polak.)

Some of the products are hormones (e.g. insulin, glucagon and gastrin), entering the circulation and exerting remote *endocrine* control of bodily functions. Their concentrations in the blood, which vary in response to physiological requirements, can be measured by RIA. Other products (e.g. 5-hydroxytryptamine and somatostatin), which are present in low concentrations in the blood under normal conditions, are probably local hormones entering the interstitial fluid and exerting *paracrine* control of adjacent cells which may be endocrine, exocrine or muscular. A third group of products e.g. vasoactive intestinal polypeptide (VIP) and substance P is found not only in endocrine type cells, but also in nervous tissue. They may be *neurocrine* in nature, acting as neurotransmitters at synapses.

At least eight peptides secreted by endocrine cells in the gut are present in central and peripheral neural tissue also.

Pathology

The peptides and amines of the gut may disturb alimentary functions, such as secretion and motility in common diseases not usually regarded as endocrine in nature, for example peptic ulceration, Crohn's disease, cholera and paralytic ileus, but little is known of their roles in such conditions.

From the surgical point of view the important lesions are those which secrete peptides and amines in excess, causing characteristic metabolic and clinical disturbances (Bonfils, 1974; Modlin, 1979). These lesions, arising from APUD cells, are known as apudomas and are classified as follows:

Hyperplasia
Neoplasia   – adenoma
                adenomatous hyperplasia
                carcinoid
                carcinoma

In the gut hyperplasia is much less common than neoplasia. Histologically, the tumours usually appear endocrine in nature, but do not always resemble their cells of origin. For instance, the secretory granules may be normal (Fig 37.3), abnormal or of mixed types. Sometimes they are almost absent, indicating that the products are secreted with minimal preliminary storage. On the other hand, the tumour cells usually display APUD characteristics with even greater clarity than their cells of origin.

The secretory capacity (Fig 37.4) of these lesions is great and versatile and single tumours often produce

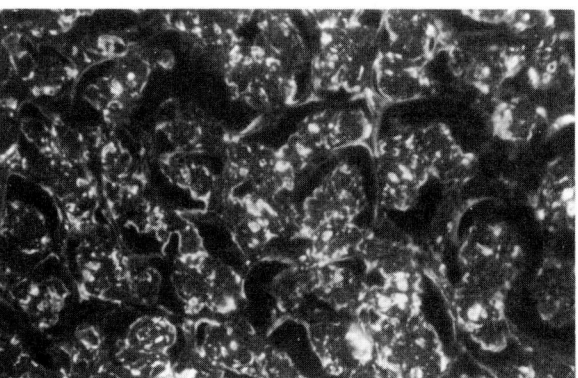

Fig 37.3 Pancreatic insulinoma immunostained with specific antibodies to insulin. × 100 (By courtesy of Dr J.M. Polak.)

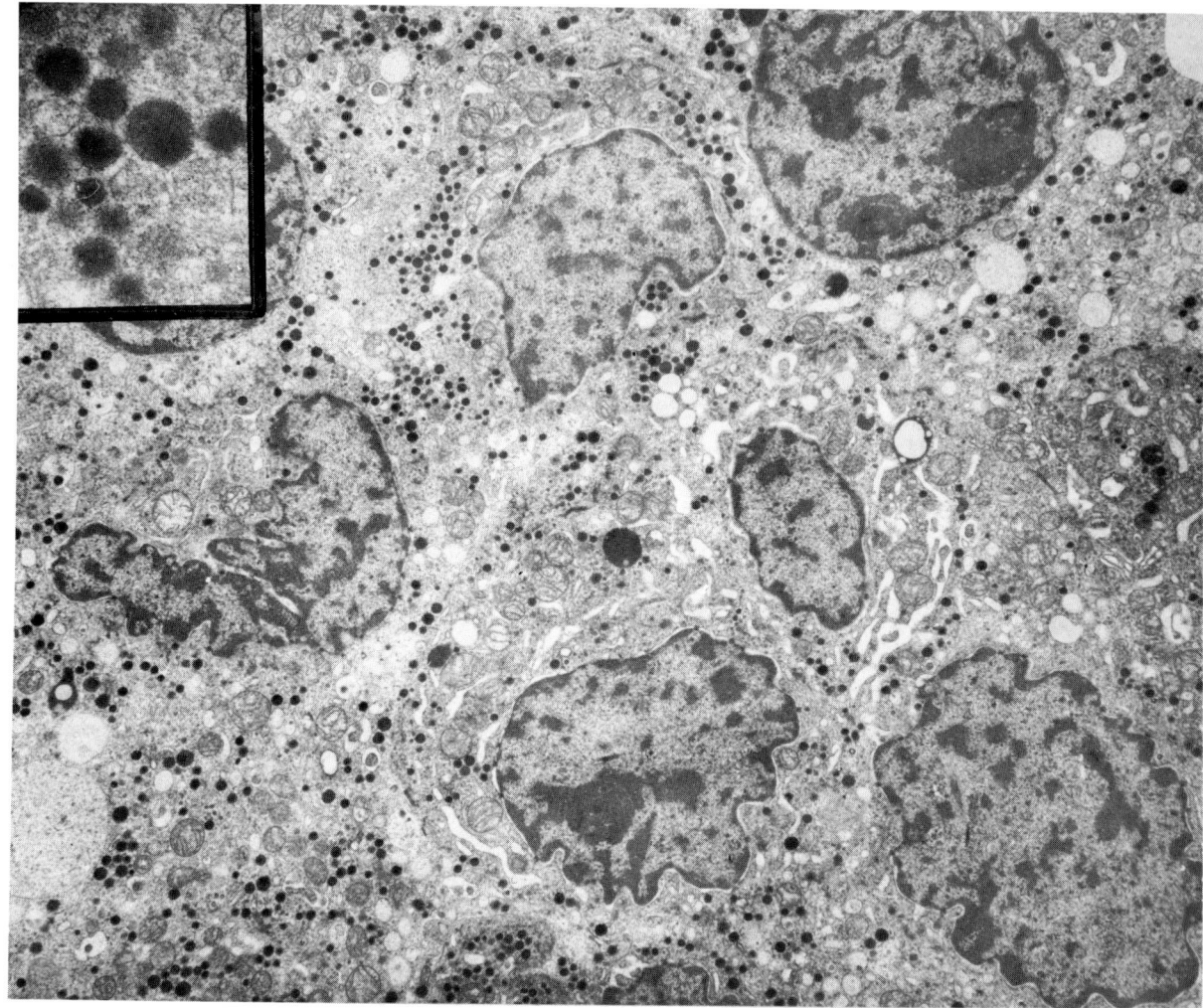

Fig 37.4 Ultrastructural appearance of the same insulinoma showing the presence of numerous electron dense secretory granules. × 7300. *Insert:* Details of the secretory granules. × 33 400 (By courtesy of Dr J.M. Polak.)

more than one, and sometimes many humoral agents, usually from different cells. Often one only causes recognisable effects, the others being apparently inactive. Sometimes the peptides are secreted in abnormal forms. The clinical and metabolic features depend more on the products of the lesions than on their pathological nature. Malignant tumours, however, metastasise to local lymph nodes and the liver, invade surrounding structures and may eventually spread throughout the peritoneal cavity and the rest of the body. When advanced, they display clinical features related to their spread, but they tend to grow very slowly and patients may survive for many years. Metas-

tases usually show the same histological and secretory features as the primary lesions.

Some of the secretions, e.g. insulin, which normally circulate in the blood in physiologically appropriate quantities, appear in much larger amounts under these pathological conditions and exert uncontrolled effects. Others, e.g. VIP, whose normal functions are probably local and which are barely detectable in the blood, are secreted into the circulation in large quantities and exert widespread metabolic effects.

The endocrine lesions may be (1) orthoendocrine, secreting the normal products of their cells of origin; (2) paraendocrine, secreting peptides or amines which are normally produced by other glands or tissues; or (3) they may form part of the syndrome of multiple endocrine neoplasia (adenopathy) type I (MEN I)*, in which these lesions are associated with similar ones in other endocrine glands, in particular the parathyroids and the anterior pituitary.

Diagnosis

All these lesions are rare, but many are missed because they are not suspected. Diagnosis of the syndromes depends on:

1 A high clinical suspicion, based on a knowledge of the syndromes (Table 2)
2 Full clinical examination
3 Non-specific investigations, such as gastric acid secretion, blood glucose and serum potassium
4 Specific investigations, which are chemical or immunological (RIA).

Once the presence of a syndrome has been established, attempts must be made to localise the lesion and to discover its nature. Many methods are available, including barium meal and follow-through, arteriography, selective venous sampling, CAT scanning, ultrasonography, endoscopy, laparotomy and biopsy.

Carcinoid tumours

Carcinoid tumours or agentaffinomas arise from the enterochromaffin (EC or Kulschitsky) cells in the gut and its derivatives. About one-third are in the appendix, where they are benign, one-third in jejunum and ileum, where they usually display low grade malignancy, and the remainder in other parts of the gut (including the pancreas) and in the bronchus, where they may be benign or malignant (Friesen, 1978). Rarely they develop in teratomas of the ovary and have been reported in the testis. They are sometimes multiple and accompanied by a separate carcinoma, especially in the alimentary tract. Occasionally they form a part of MEN I.

Clinical features

The clinical features vary with the site of the tumour, whether or not it has metastasised and what products it secretes. Appendiceal carcinoids are usually diagnosed at operations for suspected appendicitis. Jejunal and ileal tumours often cause intestinal obstruction and are diagnosed at operation. Those elsewhere are found either incidentally or as a result of their secretions.

Carcinoid tumours especially malignant ones arising in the midgut, secrete 5-hydroxytryptamine (5-HT) (Table 3) and kallikrein, an enzyme which causes the synthesis of bradykinin from a plasma globulin. These are mainly responsible for the malignant carcinoid syndrome. Other products are prostaglandin E, substance P and motilin, all of which may contribute to the syndrome, and pancreatic polypeptide, which is a useful

Table 2
CLUES TO THE DIAGNOSIS OF APUDOMAS ARISING FROM THE GUT OR ASSOCIATED WITH MULTIPLE ENDOCRINE NEOPLASIA, TYPE I

Clinical state	Possible apudoma
Peptic ulcer disease	Parathyroid adenoma or hyperplasia* Gastrinoma
Diarrhoea	Carcinoid tumour Vipoma Gastrinoma Glucagonoma
Constipation	Parathyroid adenoma or hyperplasia**
Hypoglycaemia	Insulinoma
Hyperglycaemia	Glucagonoma Gastrinoma Somatotrophinoma Corticotrophinoma (ortho- or paraendocrine) Somatostatinoma
Hypokalaemia Acidosis Alkalosis	 Vipoma Corticotrophinoma (paraendocrine)
Migratory erythema	Glucagonoma
Flushing	Carcinoid tumour Vipoma

*Adapted from Welbourn, 1977
**Parathyroid lesions are not apudomas, although related to them.

Table 3
SYNTHESIS AND METABOLISM OF 5-HYDROXYTRYPTAMINE

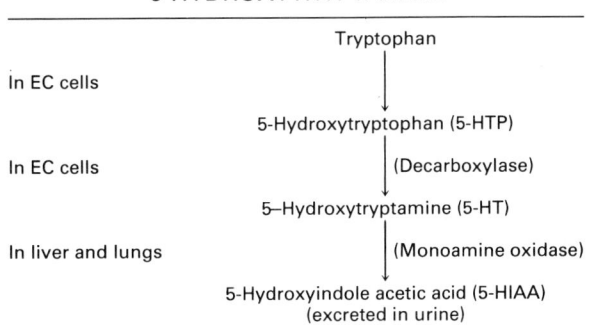

marker for carcinoid tumours and islet cell tumours of the pancreas.

5-HT and possibly the other secretions, which enter the portal vein, are normally metabolised and removed from the circulation by the liver, and 5-HT is also metabolised by the lungs. When tumours have metastasised to the liver, their products enter the general circulation directly via the hepatic veins. They may do so also if the secretion is great enough to overload the liver's capacity or if, as in the case of the gonads, the primary tumour is not in the portal circulation.

The malignant carcinoid syndrome usually develops in patients who have had abdominal operations, which have left visible scars, and palpable deposits in the liver. The syndrome includes acute symptoms, which occur in episodes and worsen with the passage of time, and chronic features, which are steadily progressive. The episodic attacks may be provoked by food (especially cheese) or alcohol, are infrequent at first, lasting a few minutes only, and later become more frequent, lasting for long periods. The acute features are facial and bodily flushing and watery diarrhoea, in nearly all patients, and bronchospasm in a few. The chronic features are right-sided cardiac valvular stenoses (the most lethal lesions), telangiectases and oedema, all of which are common, and pellagra, arthralgia and scleroderma, which are rare. A very severe variety, the 'atypical syndrome', is associated particularly with carcinoids of the foregut, especially the stomach. There is less diarrhoea, but the flush is more intense, may last for days and is accompanied by lachrymation, facial oedema, salivation and sometimes mental, nervous and circulatory disturbances. The mechanism is uncertain, but such tumours have been found to secrete histamine, 5-hdroxytryptophan (5-HTP) and other humoral agents.

Paraendocrine syndromes associated with carcinoid tumours are very rare, but include Cushing's syndrome, due to secretion of ACTH (especially by bronchial carcinoids), the Schwartz-Bartter syndrome (due to ADH) and several others.

Investigation of malignant carcinoid syndrome

The urinary 5-hydroxyindoleacetic acid (5-HIAA) is raised (normal 2–15 mg per 24 h) and is sometimes very high indeed. Urinary 5-HTP may be raised in patients with foregut carcinoids. Attacks may be provoked by ingestion of alcohol, injection of adrenaline or the infusion of calcium salts. Pancreatic polypeptide levels in the blood are raised in about half the patients with secreting carcinoids at all sites. The plasma calcitonin level is frequently raised also, but the cause is uncertain. The localisation of tumours follows general lines.

Treatment

Primary tumours should be removed surgically. Simple appendicectomy cures nearly all appendiceal carcinoids, but if there is any suggestion of malignancy (e.g. local spread or involvement of the caecum), a right hemicolectomy should be undertaken. Tumours in the small intestine should be excised widely, together with adjacent lymph nodes. The five-year survival rate is about 70% for patients with resectable lesions, 40% for those with unresectable tumours, and 20% for those with liver metastases (Welch and Malt, 1977).

Treatment of patients with the malignant carcinoid syndrome involves avoidance of aggravating factors, symptomatic relief with drugs, destruction or removal of metastases, and cytotoxic drugs. None of the methods is curative, but patients may maintain reasonable health for months or years. Several drugs are available. The best are methysergide for diarrhoea and bronchospasm, p-chlorphenylalanine for diarrhoea, α-methyldopa and prednisone for flushing (the most difficult feature to control), and isoprenaline for bronchospasm.

The main bulk of the tumour is in the liver and the metastases (like those of other endocrine tumours) obtain their blood supply principally from the hepatic artery. They may be destroyed by embolisation with various substances, under radiographic control, by the percutaneous route (Allison, 1978). The procedure may be repeated, if required, and the preliminary results are so encouraging that embolisation is probably the procedure of choice. Ligation of the hepatic artery at operation is a bigger undertaking and does not devascularise the liver so effectively. It cannot be repeated when revascularisation occurs and it precludes the possibility of effective embolisation. Surgical removal of large masses of tumour in lymph nodes, the liver or elsewhere may provide symptomatic relief. Cytotoxic drugs may be given systemically or by infusion into the hepatic artery after operation or percutaneously under radiographic control. A few patients have responded well to cyclophosphamide and/or methotrexate, to 5-fluorouracil and/or streptozotocin, and to 5-fluorotryptophan.

Tumours of the pancreas

Orthoendocrine tumours secrete the five known peptide products of the normal pancreas, four of which cause characteristic syndromes (Creutzfeldt, 1977). The tumours presumably arise from the normal cells of origin of these peptides and are equally common in all parts of the gland. Paraendocrine tumours, whose cells of origin are not known, secrete gastrin (causing the Zollinger-Ellison syndrome), corticotrophin (Cushing's syndrome), antidiuretic hormone (Schwartz-Bartter syndrome), and so on. Different types of tumour (Table 4) show different tendencies to malignancy, to multiplicity and to inclusion in the MEN I syndrome. A very small proportion of most types display generalised hyperplasia or adenomatous hyperplasia instead of discrete tumour formation. Benign tumours vary in size from about 5 mm to 5 cm in diameter, but malignant ones may be much larger. Multiple discrete tumours are rarely more than two or three in number.

Most of the lesions arise at all ages from infancy to old age, but usually develop in young and middle-aged adults. Those associated with MEN I tend to develop earlier.

Insulinoma

Clinical features

This tumour, arising from the B or β cells of the pancreas, was described by Mayo and Wilder in 1927 and was the first islet cell tumour to be recognised.

The clinical features are the result of hypoglycaemia, caused by hyperinsulinism. They are usually mild and episodic at first and commonest when fasting, particularly before breakfast or after a meal has been missed. They may become severe and frequent later. The disease usually runs a course of several years, but occasionally is fulminating in onset and rapidly fatal (Le Quesne *et al.*, 1979; Van Heerden *et al.*, 1979).

Symptoms and signs are very variable. Hunger and epigastric discomfort are common and patients may discover that sugar brings relief so that they eat excessively. For these reasons obesity is common.

Mental features range from mild neurotic symptoms, such as tiredness, anxiety, restlessness, confusion and emotional instability, to those of frank psychosis, and some patients behave in a most bizarre manner. Reflex *sympathetic stimulation* often causes sweating, pallor, tremor and palpitation. Signs of *organic nervous disease* include disturbances of speech and vision, vertigo, convulsations, hemiparesis, loss of consciousness and coma. The nervous system sometimes suffers permanent damage and death may ensue.

Many patients are misdiagnosed at first and are thought to be suffering from mental or nervous disease, especially epilepsy. Admission to a mental hospital may occur. Most patients, however, display Whipple's triad, namely (1) attacks of nervous or gastrointestinal disturbances coming on in the fasting state, associated with (2) hypoglycaemia with blood glucose levels below 2.22 mmol/l, (3) which is relieved quickly by the ingestion or injection of glucose. This provides grounds for suspicion, which should lead to full investigation.

Hyperinsulinism in infants may be caused by single insulinomas, but is more commonly due to a form of generalised adenomatous hyperplasia, called nesidioblastosis. If not treated early and effectively, this causes permanent mental damage.

Investigation

The syndrome is diagnosed by a long fast, during which only calorie-free drinks are allowed, and blood for the measurement of glucose and insulin is withdrawn every 3 h. This causes hypoglycaemia together with an inappropriately high level of insulin. A fast of 24 h is usually sufficient, but the syndrome cannot be excluded for certain in less than 72 h. The patient is encouraged to walk about and is observed closely. If hypoglycaemia becomes obvious clinically, a final blood sample is taken and the patient is given 50 g of glucose by mouth or intravenously.

The tolbutamide test may be dangerous in patients with hyperinsulinism, but it may be used cautiously in selected cases to *exclude* the diagnosis. Pancreatic polypeptide is raised in about 20% of patients.

Glucagonoma

Clinical features

This tumour, arising from the A cells, was first described fully by McGavran and colleagues in 1966. It was not recognised often until a RIA for glucagon was developed a few years ago, but nearly 50 patients had been reported by 1979. The tumour secretes excessive

Table 4
PRINCIPAL ENDOCRINE TUMOURS OF PANCREAS (ALL PERCENTAGES ARE APPROXIMATE)

	Insulinoma	Glucagonoma	Vipoma	Gastrinoma
Cell of origin	B	A	?	?
Benign (%)	95	25	50	30
Single (%)	90	70	90	30
Hyperplasia (%)	?1	?	20	5
High blood PP level (%)	20	50	75	25
MEN I found in association (%)*	5	<5	<5	25
Proportion found in MEN I %*	30	————50————		
Cured by single operation (%)	90	25	33	?20

* i.e. About 5% of patients with insulinomas have MEN I, while about 30% of patients with MEN I have insulinomas. About 50% have one of the other named tumours.

quantities of glucagon which causes severe migratory, necrolytic erythema (Fig 37.5) associated with painful glossitis and angular stomatitis. Protein catabolism causes severe loss of weight and deficiency of amino-acids in the blood. Diabetes mellitus, anaemia and mental depression are usual. A few patients suffer diarrhoea. Deep venous thrombosis, sometimes with fatal pulmonary embolism, is common and prophylactic low dosage heparin is advisable until effective therapy has been provided. The ESR may be very high (Higgins *et al.*, 1979).

Investigation

The diagnosis should be suspected in all patients with the characteristic dermatitis, who are usually sent to dermatologists initially, and is confirmed by a high fast-ing level of glucagon in the blood. Pancreatic polypeptide is raised in half the patients.

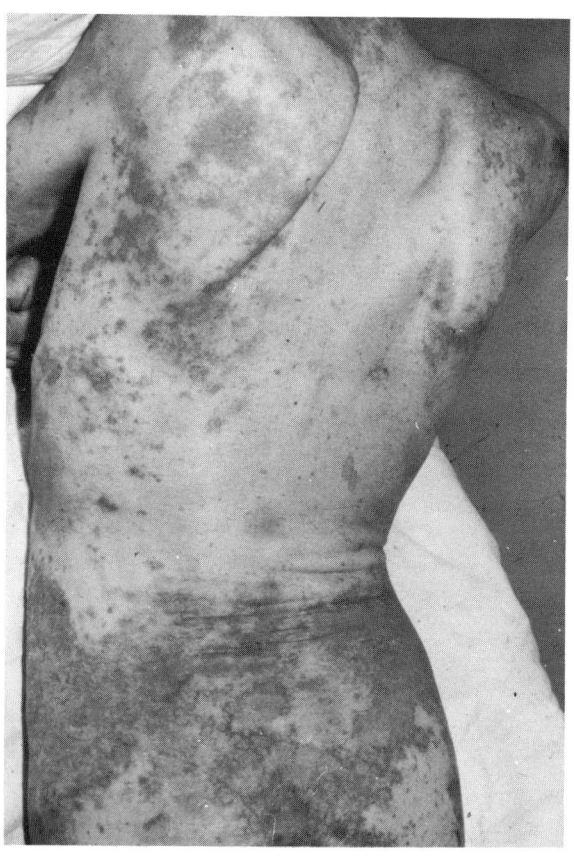

Fig 37.5 Necrolytic migratory erythema in patient with glucagonoma. (By courtesy of Prof S.R. Bloom.)

Vipoma

Clinical features

In 1958 Verner and Morrison described a syndrome of **W**atery **D**iarrhoea, **H**ypokalaemia and **A**chlorhydria, associated with non-βislet cell tumour of the pancreas, and named the condition the WDHA syndrome. More than 50 patients had been reported by 1974, and it is now clear that *hypo*chlorhydria is commoner than achlorhydria and that hypotension is also common (Verner and Morrison, 1974). The syndrome is also called the 'Verner-Morrison syndrome' and 'pancreatic cholera'. Most of the tumours secrete VIP in large amounts, but their cell of origin is not yet known. Simi-larly, most of the patients have very high levels of VIP in the blood and this is almost certainly responsible for the metabolic and clinical features. However, a few patients do not have high VIP levels and some show no correlation between VIP and the clinical course of the disease. Possibly prostaglandins or other substances are sometimes responsible. There are other patients who show the same clinical features without high VIP levels or evidence of pancreatic tumour, a condition known as the 'pseudo-Verner-Morrison syndrome'.

Investigation

The syndrome is diagnosed in the great majority of patients by a very high level of VIP in the blood. About 80% of them also have raised pancreatic polypeptide levels. It should be remembered that some adrenal medullary tumours also secrete VIP and cause the same clinical syndrome (pp. 549, 550). They can be distin-guished by appropriate x-rays and other tests.

Somatostatinoma

A few tumours have been described apparently aris-ing from the D cells and secreting somatostatin alone. All the patients were diabetic and some had steator-rhoea. Somatostatin has such widespread effects, mainly inhibitory, that other features may be recog-nised as a new syndrome when more patients have been described. High blood levels of somatostatin are found (Bloom, 1978; Modlin, 1979).

PPoma (pancreatic polypeptide tumour)

A very few tumours, apparently arising from the PP cells and secreting PP only, have been described, but they had no characteristic metabolic or clinical features (Bloom, 1978; Modlin, 1979).

PP is, however, secreted by separate cells in about half of pancreatic endocrine tumours of other types (especially glucagonomas and vipomas) and is found in high concentrations in the blood (Table 4). It is also found in the blood in a similar proportion of patients with carcinoid tumours at all sites, although its cell of origin in these cases is not known. It is, therefore, a useful tumour marker.

Gastrinoma

Clinical features

In 1955 Zollinger and Ellison described two patients who exhibited the triad of (1) fulminant peptic ulceration, which recurred despite gastric operations, (2) gross basal gastric hypersecretion and (3) a non-β islet cell tumour of the pancreas. This condition is named the 'Zollinger-Ellison syndrome' (ZES) and the tumours are now known to secrete gastrin in various forms (Deveney *et al.*, 1978; McCarthy, 1978). The pancreas is the commonest site of gastrinomas, where they are paraendocrine, but the cell of origin is not known. At least two-thirds are malignant and are a similar proportion multiple. Orthoendocrine tumours are occasionally found in the stomach as G cell hyperplasia or very rarely as carcinoma, or in the duodenum as G cell adenoma or carcinoma. About 25% of gastrinomas are associated with MEN I.

For some years many patients were diagnosed at a late stage with primary and often multiple ulceration low in the duodenum or in the jejunum, or with rapid recurrence, accompanied by serious and often fatal complications, after normally adequate ulcer operations. Diarrhoea and steatorrhoea, due to the gross gastric hypersecretion, often associated with hypertrophic gastric mucosa, and serious loss of weight were other frequent features. Since clinicians became aware of the condition and a RIA for gastrin became widely available a few years ago, patients are being diagnosed earlier and younger, frequently with ulceration in the first part of the duodenum, and more are receiving effective treatment.

Investigation

The possibility of gastrinoma should be *considered* in every patient with duodenal ulceration. Specific investigations should be undertaken in any with ulceration in the 2nd part of the duodenum or lower, with diarrhoea in association with peptic ulceration, in those found to have unusually high gastric acid secretion (e.g. basal acid output >10 mmol/l), especially when accompanied by mucosal hypertrophy, in patients with hyperparathyroidism, in all members of families with MEN I, especially if they have dyspepsia, and in all patients developing recurrence after an operation for duodenal ulcer.

The investigations include:

1 Measurement of gastric acid secretion, at least the basal acid output, since achlorhydria (as in pernicious anaemia) causes hypergastrinaemia.
2 Measurement of the fasting plasma gastrin, which is usually at least twice the upper limit of normal (which varies in different laboratories). If the patient secretes gastric acid and has hypergastrinaemia, there are several possible causes, namely gastrinoma, G-cell hyperplasia, hyperparathyroidism especially in MEN I, a retained excluded gastric antrum after gastrectomy, and chronic renal failure. They may be distinguished by the following tests.
3 An intravenous injection of 1 to 2 iu/kg of secretin (GIH or synthetic) usually increases the plasma gastrin by 50% or more in 5 min in patients with tumorous gastrinomas, especially those in whom the basal level is only slightly raised, but not in other patients with hypergastrinaemia.
4 Endoscopy and biopsy of the pyloric antrum, with special reference to the G cell population, should confirm or exclude the presence of G cell hyperplasia. Endoscopy, biopsy and a barium meal should also reveal the presence of an antral or duodenal tumour.
5 Measurement of the serum calcium and phosphate should exclude or raise the suspicion of hyperparathyroidism.
6 X-ray of the pituitary fossa and other hormonal assays should reveal or exclude a pituitary tumour.
7 If the presence of a retained, excluded gastric antrum has not been recorded in notes of previous operations, it may be revealed sometimes by careful radiological and endoscopic methods.
8 Renal function tests will reveal or exclude chronic renal failure.

Localisation of pancreatic endocrine tumours

A barium meal may reveal large tumours. Ultrasonography, selenium scintigraphy and CAT scanning have not so far proved helpful for detecting small ones. However, selective arteriography, combined with magnification and subtraction, is very valuable and, in skilled hands, about 90% of insulinomas, even less than 1 cm in diameter, can be identified (Fig 37.6). Excellent localisation of other tumours may be achieved also, but for some reason many gastrinomas are difficult to detect (Fulton *et al.*, 1975; Passaro, 1979). Percutaneous

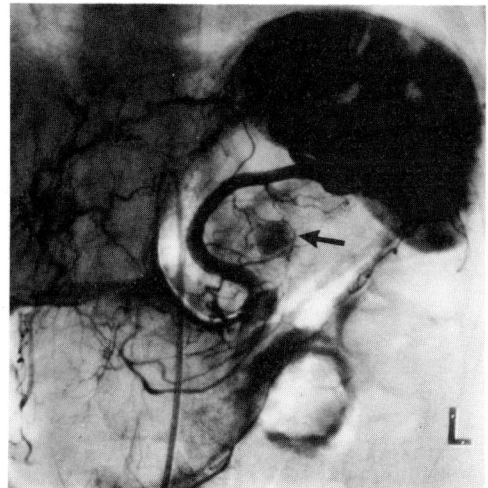

(a)

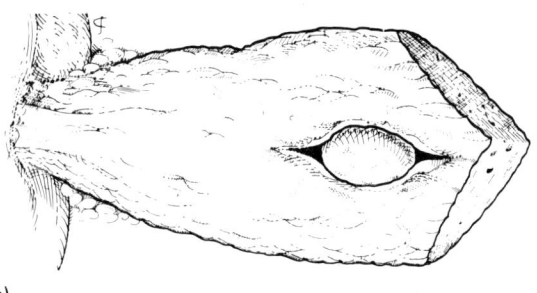

(b)

(c)

transhepatic selective venous sampling is a new technique whose place is not yet decided. When successful, arterio-venous differences in concentrations between the arterial and particular venous samples show the sites of production of specific peptides (including pancreatic polypeptide) by the tumours. Higher concentrations in the hepatic veins than in the portal vein suggest the presence of large metastases in the liver. The method has been very helpful in some patients, but unhelpful in others, and has not been without danger. Perforation of the gallbladder or colon and hepatic bleeding are possible complications. The spread of tumour to the liver and other sites can be determined as in patients with other tumours.

Treatment

The following methods are available:

1 Surgical excision of the primary lesion
2 Cytotoxic drugs for control of malignant tumours
3 Other procedures, which include operations or drugs for individual lesions and measures for the treatment of hepatic metastases

Surgical excision

This is the procedure of choice whenever it is practicable. It is possible to remove and cure in one operation the following approximate proportions of pancreatic tumours:

Insulinomas	90%
Vipomas	33%
Glucagonomas	25%
Gastrinomas	?20%

Perhaps earlier diagnosis and better supportive measures will improve these figures (Edis *et al.*, 1975; Le Quesne and Thompson, 1977).

The following general principles apply to all types of tumour. A transverse incision from one rib margin to the other, curved upwards, halfway between the xiphisternum and the umbilicus, allows access to the whole pancreas (Fig 37.7). The whole abdomen is explored

Fig 37.6 (a) Selective pancreatic angiogram (with subtraction) in patient with insulinoma (→). (By courtesy of Prof D.J. Allison.) (b) Selective venous sampling in same patient. Insulin concentrations in pmol/l. Veins are: A = hepatic; B = portal; C = superior mesenteric; D = splenic; E = inferior mesenteric. The 'hot spot' for insulin corresponds with the tumour circulation seen in the x-ray. (By courtesy of Prof D.J. Allison and Prof S.R. Bloom.) (c) Drawing of resected tissue showing tumour. (By courtesy of Mr D. Simmonds.)

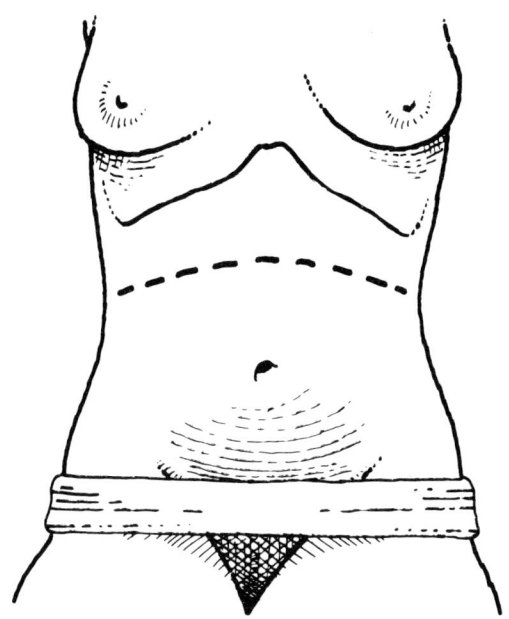

Fig 37.7 Incision for operations on islet cell tumours. (By courtesy of Mr D. Simmonds.)

and a careful search is made for secondary deposits in the liver or regional lymph nodes. The whole pancreas is exposed, inspected in front and behind and palpated between fingers and thumb. The head of the pancreas is exposed by Kocher's manoeuvre. The body and tail are examined by division of the gastrocolic omentum, mobilisation of the spleen and division of the posterior peritoneum along the lower border of the pancreas. Blunt dissection then allows the spleen and the tail and body of the pancreas to be mobilised and drawn over to the right. Systematic inspection and palpation of the organ must include the junction between the head and the body posteriorly and the uncinate process. Many tumours are found readily. However, if none is found and the preoperative x-rays and selective venous sampling suggested a small one at a particular site, an incision should be made into the pancreas, in line with the pancreatic duct.

Apparently benign tumours in the head of the pancreas should be dissected out delicately with minimal damage to the normal tissue. It is easy to tear the pancreatic duct or one of its tributaries and it is helpful to inject secretin (1–2 i.v./kg i.v.), which causes a brisk flow of pancreatic juice within 10 min and reveals any leakage. A tributary of the duct can be ligated or clipped but, if the main duct is injured, it is wise to divide and ligate or clip it and to resect the distal part of the gland. The raw surface is then oversewn. Up to 90% of the pancreas can be removed without serious interference with function.

Benign tumours in the body or tail are best treated by distal pancreatectomy. If it is difficult to see the duct, an injection of secretin shows it up easily if it is open or confirms that it has been closed.

Radical removal of malignant tumours by pancreaticoduodenectomy has little place. It should be attempted only if it is reasonably certain that the whole tumour can be excised, because the operative mortality and morbidity are high and recurrence is likely. However, biopsies of the primary and of secondary deposits should be taken for detailed study of the tumour. Cannulation of the hepatic artery or portal vein is not advisable. The bed of the pancreas should always be drained.

Cytotoxic drugs

Patients with incurable malignant tumours, whose symptoms cannot be controlled by other means, may be treated with cytotoxic drugs (Friesen, 1978). The best for pancreatic tumours is streptozotocin and objective regression is obtained in the following approximate proportions:

Vipomas	90%
Insulinomas	50%
Glucagonomas	25%
Gastrinomas	25%

The drug can be administered in various ways, but intravenous infusion of 2 to 4 g four times on alternate days every month is satisfactory. If the response is good, the intervals between courses may be increased. Acute complications include diarrhoea, nausea and fever, and can be prevented with aspirin and phenothiazines. Haematological and renal damage occur and patients must be observed carefully for these complications. If they develop, treatment must be stopped.

If streptozotocin is ineffective, cyclophosphamide and 5-fluorouracil may be tried and are sometimes effective. Cytotoxic drugs have also been administered effectively by infusion into the hepatic artery, either percutaneously under radiographic control or after cannulation at operation.

Other procedures

Other operations and drugs for individual lesions are discussed separately below. Procedures on the liver, especially hepatic artery embolisation, as described for metastatic carcinoid tumours, may be used with similar effects for islet cell tumours.

Special measures for individual tumours

Insulinomas

It is helpful to know before operation if the hypoglycaemia can be controlled by diazoxide without toxic effects.

Before and during operation glucose should be infused intravenously at a rate which maintains the fasting blood glucose at a constant level (say 5 mmol/l). It has been suggested that frequent measurements will show a rapid rise in the blood glucose when all the tumour tissue has been removed. However, the level may not rise for some hours. Hyperglycaemia for a few days after operation is a good sign and rarely requires treatment with insulin.

It may be possible to localise a tumour *at operation* by selective venous sampling along the splenic and other veins draining the pancreas, together with a rapid RIA for insulin. Opinions differ about the best procedure to follow on the rare occasions when a tumour cannot be found, but it is influenced by the patient's previous response to diazoxide. If control was satisfactory, it is probably best to biopsy the tail of the pancreas, to confirm or exclude generalised hyperplasia, close the abdomen and continue diazoxide therapy. The patient might then be reinvestigated by any available methods of localisation which had not been used before and then, if these showed a small tumour, be re-explored. If control with diazoxide was unsatisfactory, distal pancreatectomy with division of the gland at the neck, may reveal a small tumour or hyperplasia on immediate histopathological examination. If it does not, subtotal pancreatectomy, with removal of all but about 15% of the gland, adjacent to the duodenum, may then be undertaken.

Generalised hyperplasia, adenomatous hyperplasia or nesidioblastosis may be treated by diazoxide or by subtotal pancreatectomy. If this does not control the disease, it may be necessary to remove the whole gland by pancreatico-duodenectomy, but this operation has higher morbidity and mortality rates. Very rarely hypoglycaemia cannot be controlled by any of these methods and a long-acting somatostatin analogue may prove effective (Long *et al.*, 1979). The alternatives are frequent glucose feeds, which cause obesity, and corticosteroids, which cause Cushing's syndrome.

Glucagonomas

Measures to prevent deep vein thrombosis, such as low dosage heparin, should always be used. Incision should be avoided through an area of dermatitis. If the abdomen is involved, an effort should be made to heal the lesion by the administration of zinc. Intravenous hyperalimentation is advisable from the time of operation.

Vipomas

Dehydration and hypokalaemia must be corrected before operation. Diarrhoea should be stopped for several days, if possible, using codeine and prednisone (up to 80 mg per day). Indomethacin is sometimes effective. Malignant lesions nearly always respond well to streptozotocin, as described, and patients may remain well for years.

Gastrinomas

Few gastrinomas are curable by surgical excision and, until recently, the treatment of choice for most patients was total gastrectomy. This is best done with a Roux-en-Y oesophagojejunal anastomosis and a loop at least 40 cm long to prevent oesophageal reflux. Now the situation is changing because drugs, the first of which is cimetidine (up to 3.6 g/d), an H_2 inhibitor, reduce gastric secretion and heal the ulceration rapidly and apparently permanently in nearly all patients. Cimetidine allows treatment to be undertaken electively instead of in the face of an emergency. It seems reasonable to use it to heal the ulceration and then to explore the possibility of removing the pancreatic tumour(s), which may be achieved in, perhaps, 20% of patients. If the plasma gastrin falls, the cimetidine is withdrawn and the patient observed carefully for recurrence. A few who had benign tumours have remained well for many years. If the tumour(s) cannot be removed, the cimetidine is continued indefinitely. Total gastrectomy may still be used if it fails. Occasionally, the presenting feature is an acute complication of ulceration requiring operation. This should be as small a procedure as is needed and treatment with cimetidine started at once.

Patients with MEN I usually have hypergastrinaemia and a tendency to peptic ulceration, whether or not they have gastrinomas. In those (the majority) with hyperparathyroidism, the gastrin level depends directly on the calcium level and the effect of parathyroidectomy should always be tried. This frequently reduces both and may heal the ulceration, sometimes for years. It should not, however, preclude an attempt to remove a gastrinoma.

Patients with proved G cell hyperplasia of the pyloric antrum should be treated by distal gastrectomy (total antrectomy) perhaps with vagotomy. Half of all duodenal gastrinomas are benign and curable by local removal.

Miscellaneous

Other pancreatic tumours must be treated on their merits. For instance bilateral adrenalectomy may be appropriate in a patient with Cushing's syndrome when the tumour cannot be removed.

Multiple endocrine neoplasia type I

Underdahl and his colleagues, in 1953, and Wermer, in 1954, described this familial syndrome, in which two or more endocrine glands undergo hyperplasia or tumour formation in the same person at the same time or consecutively. Hypersecretion is usual and causes various clinical syndromes (Ballard *et al.*, 1964; Harrison and Thompson, 1975). The parathyroids are involved most frequently (about 90% of patients). Pancreatic islet cell tumours develop in about 80% and take the form of gastrinoma, insulinoma, vipoma or other types of tumour in that order of frequency. Conversely, about 20 to 30% of patients with gastrinomas have other endocrine lesions, about 5% of those with insulinomas and still smaller proportions of those with other types of pancreatic tumour. About 65% of patients with MEN I have pituitary tumours and a small proportion have carcinoids in the gut or bronchi. Duodenal ulceration is very common.

It is important to screen every patient with an alimentary apudoma for evidence of MEN and, if other lesions are found, they should be treated on their merits and all blood relations should be screened also. The relationship between hyperparathyroidism and gastrinoma has been discussed already.

References

Allison D.J. (1978). Therapeutic embolization. *Brit. J. Hosp. Med*; **20**:707–15.

Ballard H.S., Frame B., Hartsock R.J. (1964). Familial multiple endocrine adenoma-peptic ulcer complex. *Medicine*; **43**:481–516.

Bloom S.R. (1978). *Gut Hormones*. Edinburgh: Churchill Livingstone.

Bonfils S. (1974). Endocrine-secreting tumours of the GI tract. In *Clinics in Gastroenterology*. London: Saunders.

Creutzfeldt W. (1977). Endocrine tumours of the pancreas. In *The Diabetic Pancreas* (Volk B.W., Wellman K.F., eds.) pp. 551–90. New York: Plenum.

Deveney C.W., Deveney K.S., Way L.W. (1978). The Zollinger-Ellison syndrome – 23 years later. *Ann. Surg*; **188**:384–93.

Edis A.J., Ayala L.A., Egdahl R.H. (1975). *Manual of Endocrine Surgery*. Berlin: Springer-Verlag.

Friesen S.R. (1978). *Surgical Endocrinology: Clinical Syndromes*. Philadelphia: Lippincott.

Fulton R.E., Sheedy P.F., McIlrath D.C., Ferris D.O. (1975). Pre-operative angiographic localisation of insulin producing tumours of the pancreas. *Amer. J. Roentgenol*; **123**:367–77.

Harrison T.S., Thompson N.W. (1975). Multiple endocrine adenomatosis – I and II. In *Current Problems in Surgery*. Chicago: Year Book Medical.

Higgins G.A., Recant L., Fischman A.E. (1979). The glucagonoma syndrome: surgically curable diabetes. *Amer. J. Surg*; **137**:142–8.

Le Quesne L.P., Nabarro J.D.N., Kurtz A., Zweig S. (1979). The management of insulin tumours of the pancreas. *Brit. J. Surg*; **66**:373–8.

Le Quesne L.P., Thompson J.P.S. (1977). Operations on the pancreas for insulinoma. In *Operative Surgery*, 3rd edn. (Rob C., Smith R., Dudley H.A.F., eds.) pp. 301–7. London: Butterworth.

Long R.G., Barnes A.J., Adrian T.E. *et al.* (1979). Suppression of pancreatic endocrine tumour secretion by long-acting somatostatin analogue. *Lancet*; **ii**:765–7.

McCarthy D.N. (1978). Report on the United States experience with cimetidine in Zollinger-Ellison syndrome and other hypersecretory states. *Gastroenterology*; **74**:453–8.

Modlin I.M. (1979). Endocrine tumours of the pancreas. *Surg. Gynaecol. Obstet*; **149**:751–69.

Montgomery D.A.D., Welbourn R.B. (1975). *Medical and Surgical Endocrinology*. London: Arnold.

Passaro E. (1979). Localisation of pancreatic endocrine tumours by selective portal vein catheterisation and radioimmunoassay. *Gastroenterology*; **77**:806–7.

Van Heerden J.A., Edis A.J., Service F.J. (1979). The surgical aspects of insulinoma. *Ann. Surg*; **189**:677–82.

Verner J.V., Morrison A.B. (1974). Endocrine pancreatic islet disease with diarrhoea. *Arch. Intern. Med*; **133**:492–500.

Welbourn R.B. (1977). Apudomas of the gut. *Amer. J. Surg*; **133**:13–22.

Welch J.P., Malt R.A. (1977). Management of carcinoid tumour of the gastrointestinal tract. *Surg. Gynaecol. Obstet*; **145**:223–7.

Further reading

Johnston I.D.A., Thompson N.W., eds (1983). *Endocrine Surgery*. pp. 76–103; 104–24; 144–63; 164–81. London: Butterworth.

Wood S.M., Polak J.M., Bloom S.R. (1983). Gut hormone secreting tumours. In *Proceedings of the Fourth Symposium in a Series on Basic Science in Gastroenterology* (Polak J.M., Bloom S.R., Wright N.A., Butler A.G., eds.). *Scand. J. Gastroenterol*; **18**(suppl.82):165–79.

Tumours of the breast, head and neck

Introduction

Anthropological investigations indicate that human cancer existed long before written history, and bones, estimated to be about 5000 years old and almost certainly affected by metastatic cancer, have been found in Egypt. Neoplastic disease occurs in all animal species and approximately one person in four is affected by cancer at some stage of life. While individual tumours have wide variation in incidence throughout the world, cancer in one form or another is common almost everywhere. Epidemiological research has not only allowed the variable global distribution of cancer to be mapped out, but more importantly the risk factors predisposing to the development of specific cancers have been made clear.

The carcinogenic effects of certain chemicals and the control of potential cancer producing substances has had major social and economic consequences. Viruses have been implicated as carcinogens in man and over 150 different viruses have been demonstrated to produce tumours in animals and plants. The viral causation of certain human tumours has gone in and out of fashion and the evidence, although circumstantial, has at times drawn tantalisingly close to what might be accepted as scientific fact. It seems certain that multiple factors will be found to be involved in the production of tumours.

Late in the 19th century, it became possible to transplant tumours from diseased animals and plants to healthy recipients. This finding led to the concept of autonomy of tumours and opened the way to detailed investigation of their biology. Fundamental data about the behaviour of cancer derives from investigations of tumours in culture and understanding of the genetic code has allowed precise study of biological activities of normal and malignant cells.

One of the main difficulties in observing human tumours is that such growths only become large enough to be observable at a relatively late stage of their life. Technological development has certainly allowed the identification of pre- or subclinical cancer in some tumours and there is now considerable evidence to suggest that treatment of tumours at this earlier stage enhances the prospect of cure. This screening of people who are symptom free has important therapeutic implications. The question of staging the extent of cancer once diagnosed is, likewise, relevant in planning treatment. Developments and refinements in diagnostic imaging have permitted detection of hitherto occult metastatic deposits and has led to newer approaches to treatment. The once dominant role of radical surgery for all but the most advanced cancers has yielded to more discriminating use of such extirpation and to the concept of combined treatment using chemotherapy and radiation, in addition to the operation.

Adjuvant chemotherapy after operation is employed in an attempt to kill cancer cells assumed to have disseminated, even though these microscopic foci of disease are undetectable by present methods. This form of cytotoxic chemotherapy is gaining ground as appropriate treatment in many apparently early cancers. The vulnerability of the cancer cell to radiotherapy and anticancer drugs varies with the phase of the cell cycle. A search continues for components which can sychronise cancer cells into the same drug-sensitive phase of the cycle. The chapter on brain tumours emphasises their biological aspects and the different disciplines which contribute to the management of the patient with cancer is well exemplified by the chapters on the mouth, jaws, neck and larynx. This multispecialty approach has led to the development of better techniques and methods.

Advances in immunobiology of malignant disease have made the diagnosis of primary and secondary tumours by immunological methods possible and the presence and type of certain tumours may be realised with the aid of monoclonal antibodies. Immunotherapy, whether specific or non-specific, has not been associated with great success in cancer therapy, but the prospect remains that such treatment will be applicable to at least some types of malignant disease. While existing biochemical indices may be misleading in the diagnosis of primary cancers, they are of clinical value in following the progress of a disease; for example, rising values of carcino-embryonic antigen (CEA) following resection of a colorectal tumour may be sufficient to justify a second-look laparotomy.

Recent years have seen greater public education about cancer, earlier diagnosis of malignant disease, rationalisation of radical surgery and refinements in radiotherapeutic and chemotherapeutic techniques. The application of technological developments has allowed major surgical excision to be followed by prosthetic replacement in many parts of the body particularly in the extremities.

Major advances in knowledge and management of human cancer have depended upon close working relationships between scientists and clinicians of all disciplins. It is important to maintain and extend these links if the complexities of malignant disease are to be understood.

N. O'H

Tumours of the breast, head and neck

Oncology

NIALL O'HIGGINS

Cancer accounts for about 25% of deaths in people under the age of 75 years and in Western countries is second only to cardiovascular disease as the commonest cause of death. Great variation exists in the incidence of cancer in different parts of the world, but the total incidence of malignant disease is similar in the developing and in the developed countries.

Environmental factors influence cancer risk more commonly than genetic factors. Many instances exist where migrant groups lose their predisposition to certain types of cancer found in their native population and acquire the risk of cancers associated with their new environment. In Japan, there is a high incidence of gastric cancer and a relatively low incidence of colorectal cancer. Conversely, in the United States of America, the incidence of gastric cancer is relatively low and is declining while colorectal cancer is a common disorder. Japanese migrants to the USA tend to have a lower incidence of gastric cancer and a higher incidence of colorectal cancer than their compatriots in Japan. Cancer of the large bowel is commoner in Africans who migrate from rural to urban areas and European migrants to parts of Australia develop a high incidence of cancer of the skin.

Geographical distribution of cancer

Dietary and nutritional factors are of importance in the risk of gastrointestinal neoplasia. Cancers of the buccal cavity, pharynx and oesophagus occur frequently in areas of undernutrition. Gastric cancer is prominent amongst populations whose dietary carbohydrate intake is high and colorectal tumours are linked with communities with high animal fat and protein intake. Bronchogenic cancer is more widely distributed among both rich and poor countries and is closely linked in all populations with cigarette smoking. Specific causal relations have been identified only in a few tumours. As well as cigarette smoking and lung cancer, sunlight is a definite carcinogenic factor in skin cancers in white populations, betel nut chewing predisposes to oropharyngeal cancer and aflotoxin is important in producing primary hepatic tumours.

Oesophageal cancer

No tumour has a more variable incidence than oesophageal cancer which varies about 200-fold in incidence throughout the world. It is particularly common in the Transkei province of South Africa, where it is the commonest cancer. It occurs frequently in China, Scandinavia, Ireland, Scotland and in parts of the USSR and Iran. Conditions known to be associated with oesophageal cancer, such as lye strictures, Paterson-Brown Kelly (Plummer-Vinson) syndrome and achalasia cannot be important factors in epidemiological terms.

Gastric cancer

A striking epidemiological fact in gastric cancer is the progressive and continuous reduction in incidence in the United States of America during the past 50 years. The falling incidence has been attributed to a reduction in intake of dietary carbohydrate and an increased consumption of animal fats and protein. The tumour is common in Iceland, Finland, Poland, USSR, Chile and Japan. The incidence is higher in low socio-economic groups. Chemicals of the alkylnitrosurea group produce gastric carcinoma in experimental animals. Ingested nitrites and nitrates can be converted into potentially carcinogenic nitrosamines in the low pH which exists in the stomach. The dietary intake of nitrates as food preservatives has been reduced in the United States of America while the nitrate level in agricultural produce or in water has been found to be high in some countries where there is a high incidence of cancer of the stomach.

Colonic cancer

Dietary factors appear to be of dominant importance in the aetiology of colonic malignancy. A high dietary intake of fat and protein, beef and a low dietary fibre have been suggested as provocative agents. Fat intake influences cholesterol and bile salt metabolism and affects colonic bacteria which act on these sterols. Colonic bacteria can convert sterols into agents known to be carcinogenic in experimental animals. A delayed intestinal transit time, associated with a low dietary fibre, may enhance the possible carcinogenic actions of these substances. Colonic cancer occurs most commonly in Western Europe and the United States of America and rarely in rural communities in Africa and Asia. The distribution of the tumour is closely connected with economic development.

Breast cancer

The distribution of breast cancer throughout the world reveals a close relationship between incidence and economic development. High rates occur in North America and Western Europe, particularly the Netherlands. The disease now occurs more frequently in Japanese women, who, until recent years, were relatively protected from it. This rising incidence seems to be confined to premenopausal women as there is a sharp decline in the occurrence of disease after the age of 45 years in Japanese women. Although obesity has not been demonstrated to be related to cancer of the breast, dietary fat may be a factor. Within the economically developed countries, the incidence of breast cancer is higher in the colder climates of the Northern Hemisphere.

Bronchus

The predominant factor in the aetiology of bronchogenic carcinoma is cigarette smoking, the incidence of the tumour being 8–15 times higher in smokers compared with non-smokers. It occurs six times as commonly in men as in women. The disease is also associated with exposure to nickel, chromate, uranium and asbestos and painters and woodworkers are at special risk.

Skin

Cancers of the skin are related closely to exposure to ultraviolet light. These tumours occur predominantly on the exposed parts of the body and pigmentation of the skin confers protection. The duration and intensity of exposure to sunlight is a factor and fair-skinned people are at special risk. Malignant melanoma occurs frequently in the State of Queensland in Australia and in the southern states of North America. Light sensitive diseases, such as albinism and xeroderma pigmentosum are especially likely to be associated with malignant skin tumours.

Uterine cervix

The mortality from cancer of the uterine cervix increases with age, but the incidence of the disease is declining in England and Wales and in the United States of America. The incidence is greatly reduced in nuns and in multiparous and Jewish women. The disease is common in Chinese women and in Hindu women in India as well as in American negroes.

Oncogenic viruses

That viruses are responsible for the majority of malignant tumours in animals is supported by considerable experimental evidence (Gross, 1978). Many species of animal are hosts to a great number of transmissable viruses, but there is yet no proof that human cancer can be induced by them. In animals the oncogenic viruses are either based on deoxyribonucleic acid (DNA) or ribonucleic acid (RNA).

DNA viruses

DNA viruses known to be carcinogenic are the *papova* groups and the adeno-viruses, herpes viruses and pox viruses. Papova is an acronym for a group of viruses, which include the papilloma, polyoma, simian vacuolating and simian virus 40 (SV40) viruses. Polyoma virus is apparently harmless in adult mice, but both it and SV 40 produce tumours in new-born rodents. Allen and Cole (1972) suggest that transcription of part of the invading viral DNA occurs in the host cell nucleus to form a viral messenger RNA (mRNA) and that self-assembly of the virus then takes place in the cell nucleus. Adenoviruses produce conjunctival and respiratory symptoms in man, but have not been identified in any human tumours.

Herpes viruses cause renal carcinoma in frogs and lymphomas in chickens (Marek's disease). The Epstein-Barr virus (EBV), another herpes virus, is associated with infectious mononucleosis and also with Burkitt's lymphoma. It can be identified in cell cultures of Burkitt's lymphoma and antibodies to the virus are found much more frequently in patients with the disease than in non-affected persons. Burkitt's lymphoma occurs in areas of endemic malaria, which may render the reticulo-endothelial system susceptible to the effects of the EBV. In the nasopharyneal carcinomas, particularly common in the Cantonese Chinese, antibodies to EBV are identified in almost all of the patients. EBV is commonly found in cervical lymphoid tissue, so its aetiological relationship with nasopharyngeal carcinoma is doubtful. EBV may also be related causally to Hodgkin's disease and has been identified in a cell line cultured from Hodgkin's disease tissue (Stewart *et al.*, 1969). Herpes virus hominis (HVH) causes oral (type 1 virus) or genital herpes (type 2 virus). HVH-2 has been implicated in the aetiology of cancer of the cervix uteri.

RNA viruses

Oncogenic RNA viruses, or *oncorna* viruses, include the chicken sarcoma virus identified by Rous and the mammary-tumour virus of Bittner. It is likely that RNA viruses, if involved in human cancer production, have a supportive or promotional role rather than an initiating one. Viral particles resembling RNA viruses have been identified in the milk of women with breast cancer and in the relatives of patients with mammary cancer more commonly than in controls or in women without a family history of the disease. Most patients with fibrosarcomas and osteosarcomas have antibodies against RNA viruses, a finding which occurs in a much smaller proportion of controls, but viruses have not been identified consistently in these tumours. Viral antibodies are identified in leukaemic patients and viral particles have been identified in leukaemic cells. Such particles are found, however, in the plasma of normal controls as well as in patients with leukaemia.

Two main hypotheses concerning the oncogenesis of viruses have been proposed. Huebner and Todaro (1969) suggested that genetic material for producing an oncogenic RNA virus is present in the gene pool of all vertebrates and is transmitted from generation to generation. This 'oncogene' is normally suppressed, but may be stimulated to produce neoplastic change by other factors such as chemical carcinogens or radiation. Temin's hypothesis (1971) is that a 'protovirus' may be produced from cellular RNA by interaction with reverse transcriptase. The usual mode of transfer of genetic material from DNA to RNA to protein could be altered to DNA to RNA to DNA. In support of this view is the finding that oncogenic RNA viruses are capable of reverse transcriptase activity.

Chemical carcinogenesis

Chemical substances in the environment may play an important part in the genesis of human cancer, but documentation and precise information on the importance of this role is difficult to define at present. The most accurate information derives from studies on occupational hazards associated with exposure to specific chemicals (Symington and Carter, 1976).

Polycyclic hydrocarbons

That polycyclic aromatic hydrocarbons may induce cancer has been recognised for 200 years since the description by Pott of the scrotal cancer which developed in boys exposed to chimney soot. Shale oil workers and cotton spinners developed scrotal and skin cancers when exposed to mineral oils. A high incidence of premalignant dermatosis was found in jute workers habitually exposed to mineral oils. Mists of mineral oils have been associated not only with scrotal and other skin cancers, but with respiratory and gastrointestinal malignancy. Similarly, long contact with tar and pitch has been linked with skin tumours and in recent years, tar fumes have been implicated in skin, scrotal, bronchogenic and bladder tumours in Europe, Japan and North America.

Vinyl chloride

Angiosarcoma of the liver has been reported from many European countries and from the United States of America among workers exposed over periods of 12–30 years to vinyl chloride. The incidence of this rare tumour was highest in workers involved with autoclaves in which polymerisation of vinyl chloride to polyvinyl chloride takes place. In experimental animals, tumours of the lung and kidney as well as liver can be induced by exposure to vinyl chloride in the atmosphere.

Aromatic amines

Carcinoma of the bladder was diagnosed with exceptional frequency in industrial dye workers exposed to the aromatic ámines, α and β-naphthylamine and benzidine. It appears that while all these substances are carcinogenic, β-naphthylamine is the most potent substance inducing tumours and the risk of cancer is higher with exposure to this substance than with the others. Substances used as antioxidants, such as 4-aminobiphenyl in the rubber industry were also found to induce cancer of the bladder. Other groups of workers at increased risk of bladder cancer because of environmental pollution with aromatic amines include those involved in the manufacture of paints and textiles. Gas workers and laboratory workers are also at risk.

Alkylating agents

Employees in the manufacture of mustard gas were seen to develop cancer of the oro- and nasopharynx and bronchus more commonly than would be expected and the chloro-ethers, bis-(chloromethyl)-ether (BCME) and chloromethyl-methyl-ether (CMME) causes bronchogenic and respiratory tract cancer in man and cutaneous and subcutaneous tumours in experimental animals. Their carcinogenicity is presumably due to a mutagenic effect at subcellular level since structural alterations of DNA occurs with exposure to alkylating agents. Other related compounds, dimethylcarbamoyl chloride (DMCC) and diethylcarbamoyl chloride (DECC) have also been implicated as possible carcinogens as they are mutagenic in bacterial strains of *E. coli* and salmonella.

Asbestos

Workers in the mining, industrial processing and manufacture of asbestos products have been found to be at high risk of developing cancer of the respiratory tract. Bronchogenic carcinoma, mesothelioma and possibly gastrointestinal neoplasia, are linked with exposure to asbestos. The risk of developing cancer of the lung appears to be related to the concentration and duration of exposure to asbestos. There are several forms of asbestos – crocidolite, chrysotile, amosite and anthophyllite – in industrial use, and crocidolite seems to be the most potent carcinogen. The carcinogenicity of asbestos and cigarette smoking are synergistic in producing bronchogenic carcinoma, but not mesothelioma. Mesothelioma of the pleura or peritoneum seems to be related more to the crocidolite form of asbestos than to the other forms.

Metals

Arsenic. A list of metals which are known or suspected carcinogens in man is shown in Table 1. Although it has not been possible to induce tumours in experimental animals by the arsenical compounds, its

Table 1
CARCINOGENICITY OF METALS

Metal	Tumours in man	Tumours in animals
Arsenic	Skin Lung Lymphoma Angiosarcoma of liver	None
Beryllium	? Lung	Osteosarcoma Lung
Cadmium	?Prostate ?Kidney ?Lung	Sarcoma Testicular tumours
Chromium	Lung Nasal cavity	Lung
Iron	? Lung	Sarcoma
Nickel	Lung Nasal sinuses ? Larynx ? Gastric ? Soft tissue sarcoma	Sarcoma Lung

role in inducing cutaneous and pulmonary cancer in man is established. Arsenic smelters and others occupationally exposed to arsenic have a 5-fold increased risk of developing bronchogenic carcinoma.

Beryllium. Osteosarcomas can be induced in mice by intravenous injection of beryllium compounds and lung cancers have been identified in rats after inhalation of beryllium aerosols. The evidence implicating beryllium in human lung cancer is conflicting. It may act as a cocarcinogen with other agents.

Cadmium. Cadmium derivatives can produce sarcomas and testicular tumours in experimental animals. It is not clear whether cadmium causes human cancer. Increased incidences of prostatic, renal and bronchogenic carcinoma have been reported among workers involved in the manufacture of alkaline batteries where exposure to cadmium oxide occurs. Synergism in carcinogenicity may take place with exposure to cadmium and cigarette smoking.

Chromium. Increased death rates from cancer of the nasal cavities and bronchus have been reported repeatedly in workers exposed to chromium. A wide variety of different tumours have been produced in animals by this metal.

Iron. Local sarcomas at the site of injection have been produced in rodents by iron-polysaccharide complexes. An increased incidence of lung cancer was reported among workers in iron ore miners in Sweden and England, but because it has been impossible to exclude other carcinogens as contributory causes, the role of iron as a carcinogen in man is uncertain.

Nickel. Nickel produces local sarcomas in rodents after injection and lung tumours after inhalation. A high excess of squamous cell carcinoma of the paranasal, particularly ethmoid, sinuses and of lung cancer was seen among workers in nickel refineries. The latent period of exposure is between 10 and 30 years.

Drugs

Immunosuppressants. Patients who have had renal transplants are treated with immunosuppressant agents and have a high risk, said to be 150 times greater than expected, of developing reticulum cell sarcoma. Lymphomas tend to occur soon after transplantation and affect the brain predominantly. The relative risk appears to be greater for children than adults. Cancers, other than lymphoma, are identified with twice the expected frequency in renal transplanted patients. The precise role of immunosuppressive drugs in inducing tumours is unknown but a number of hypothetical possibilities occur. Infection by oncogenic virus is facilitated by the use of immunosuppressive drugs.

Diethylstilboestrol and oestrogens. In 1971, Herbst and colleagues demonstrated the increased risk of vaginal adeno-carcinoma in adolescent girls whose mothers had been taking relatively large doses of diethylstilboestrol during pregnancy. A suggestion that conjugated oestrogen therapy, prescribed for menopausal symptoms, could induce endometrial carcinoma has been proposed (Smith *et al.*, 1975).

Reserpine. The rauwolfia derivative, reserpine, used as treatment for hypertension, has been implicated in the pathogenesis of cancer of the breast (Armstrong *et al.*, 1974), but this association has not been confirmed consistently.

Radiation carcinogenesis

The association between ionising radiation and cancer has been recognised since 1910 when the experimental production of cancer in rats by means of x-rays was described by Clunet. In the following year Jagie described leukaemia in radiologists. The peak incidence of leukaemia among the atomic bomb survivors in Nagasaki and Hiroshima occurred 6–7 years after the bombing. An increased incidence of leukaemia has been noted in patients with ankylosing spondylitis who were treated by local irradiation and in patients who had pelvic irradiation for menorrhagia.

Controversy exists as to the leukaemic potential for internal radioactive isotopes, such as ^{131}I used to treat hyperthyroidism and ^{32}P in polycythaemia rubra vera. Exposure to ionising radiation in childhood is associated with a higher risk of developing leukaemia than is exposure in adult life. The contrast medium, Thorotrast (thorium dioxide) is also associated with leukaemia.

Ionising radiation causes structural alteration in chromosomal pattern and shape. It may be that the haemopoietic cell chromosomes are especially at risk, as leukaemia seems to be the commonest type of malignancy to develop after exposure.

Survivors of the Japanese atomic bombings were seen to develop cancers other than leukaemia. The appearance of these tumours occurred some 15 years after exposure to the irradiation. A variety of different tumours were attributed to irradiation, including differentiated thyroid tumours, lymphomas, bronchogenic carcinomas, colorectal, breast and salivary gland tumours. The increased risk of differentiated thyroid cancer many years after irradiation to the neck for thymic enlargement, tuberculosis and acne has been clearly demonstrated. Radiotherapy to the breast for benign conditions was noted to be related to an increased risk of cancer of the breast.

Radium dial painters were found to develop osteosarcoma of the jaw and carcinoma of the paranasal sinuses. In addition to leukaemia, people given Thorotrast (thorium dioxide) also developed cholangiocarcinoma and hepatoma 15 to 30 years after exposure. Radon in the atmosphere has been implicated in the genesis of lung cancer.

Bone-seeking radionuclides have a neoplastic potential in certain tissues related to the skeleton. The tissues at risk are osteogenic cells, haemopoietic stem cells in the bone marrow, epithelial cells of the air sinuses of the skull and possibly neuroglial cells. In animals the most frequent types of tumour induced by radioactive isotopes are osteosarcoma, chondrosarcoma, fibrosarcoma, tumours of haemopoietic mesenchymal origin and of the air sinuses of the skull. These tumours appear after administration of isotopes of strontium, calcium, yttrium and radon. Viral and hormonal cofactors may play a part in these types of radiation-induced cancers.

An increased risk of childhood leukaemia and other cancers has been reported in children who have been subjected to prenatal radiation for purposes of diagnostic radiology (Stewart and Knealem, 1970). This finding has not been fully confirmed.

Non-ionising radiation, in the form of ultraviolet radiation is known to predispose to skin cancers, particularly squamous cell carcinomas, to a lesser extent basal-cell carcinomas and to a lesser extent, malignant melanoma.

Hereditary factors in cancer development

Hereditary factors are of undoubted importance in many types of malignant disease (Lynch, 1976). Chromosomal abnormalities have been identified in some forms of cancer. Hereditary conditions predisposing to cancer are numerous and some common types of malignancy have a hereditary element. It may be impossible to distinguish whether a condition, which is apparently familial, has been induced by genetic or environmental factors. For instance, cancer of the breast has a familial component, yet so many aetiological elements are involved that clearcut distinction between inherited and environmental causes is not possible.

Certain conditions associated with chromosomal disorders carry with them an increased risk of cancer. Down's syndrome patients are prone to develop acute leukaemia, those with Klinefelter's syndrome are associated with breast cancer and female patients with gonadal dysgenesis are susceptible to dysgerminoma.

Inherited disorders of the immune system, resulting in immunodeficient states, predispose to malignant disease. Congenital agammaglobulinaemia and IgM deficiency are associated with lymphomas and leukaemia. Cancers of the breast, gut, skin as well as lymphomas occur in IgA deficiency. Cancers of the lymphoreticular system are commonest with inherited immunodeficiency. Other inherited disorders render patients particularly susceptible to certain types of tumour. Polyposis coli and Gardner's syndrome (gastrointestinal polyps, sebaceous cysts, bony and soft tissue tumours) lead to colorectal cancer, xeroderma pigmentosum and albinism predispose to skin cancers and von Hippel-Lindau syndrome (retinal and cerebellar angiomata, hypertension, polycythaemia) is associated with phaeochromocytoma and renal carcinoma. Certain types of endocrine tumour, such as phaeochromocytoma, medullary thyroid cancer and multiple endocrine neoplasia syndromes may occur in the familial form. Retinoblastoma, particularly if bilateral, is often hereditary.

Tumour immunology

Tumour antigens

All cells of the body have antigenic properties which are responsible for the rejection which occurs when an organ is transplanted from one animal to another. The finding that tumours may contain specific antigens on the surface of the neoplastic cell led to the hope that suitable antibodies might be raised and used as cancer therapy. Such tumour antigens were developed in inbred strains of mice with chemically-induced sarcomas (Freedman, 1976). Tumour-specific antigens have been identified in a number of tumours, those spontaneously developing and those induced by viruses or chemical means. Experimentally, the behaviour of tumour-specific transplantation antigens (TSTA) can be studied by eliminating the effects of the histocompatability antigens on the surface of normal cells. This was achieved by the use of strains of mice and other rodents so inbred that they became genetically identical. Chemically-induced tumour tissue, transplanted from one rodent to another, was followed by a specific immunity in the recipient and further tumour transplants were rejected. Antigens from tumours induced by chemical means are highly specific. The recipient animal develops immunity to the transplanted tumour from one animal but acquires no immunity from tumour cells of another, even if the tumours are induced by the same agent and the donors are similarly inbred. Tumours produced by viruses, in contrast, share a common antigen for all tumours produced by that virus.

Immune response

Two types of immune response are evoked in the host by tumour-specific antigens, (a) cell-mediated immunity induced by the T lymphocyte produced by the reticulo-endothelial system and (b) the production of antibodies by stimulation of the B lymphocyte system. Contact of the immune lymphocyte with the tumour cell antigen in some way brings about fracture of the cell membrane and lysis of the tumour cell. Circulating antibodies to tumours are immune globulins synthesised by plasma cells and have variable cytotoxic activity. Rejection of transplanted tumour is mainly related to the cell-mediated response. The immunological responses to these experimentally induced tumours are comparatively weak and can be overcome by transplantation of a large number (10^6) of tumour cells.

Escape mechanisms

Loss of antigenicity. In some experimental tumours, loss of tumour specific antigen results from the repeated passage of tumour cells through strains of inbred mice. It has been postulated that this loss of antigenicity is brought about by a process of immunosolution by which the cells with stronger antigens are destroyed by the antibodies which they evoke, while the less antigenic cells develop into surviving clones.

Specific immunological inhibition. When a tumour is transmitted before the development of the normal immunological mechanisms, it may grow in the host without being rejected in spite of its antigenicity. An example of this is the mammary carcinoma in mice transmitted through RNA virus in the milk. The tumour develops unimpeded in the offspring by the 'immune tolerance' of the undeveloped immune system in the host.

Immune enhancement. It has been demonstrated that where a long time elapses between exposure of animals to tumour-specific antigens and subsequent challenge with the tumour, the growth of the second tumour transplant may, paradoxically, be facilitated rather than inhibited. This enhancement of transplanted tumour cell growth is due to the activity of humoral antibodies which cover the antigenic sites and prevent the formation of cell-mediated immunity by small lymphocytes.

'Sneak-through' phenomenon. Even without tolerance, enhancement or depression of the immune response, tumour growth may continue in transplanted tumours and this is known as the 'sneak-through' phenomenon. It is seen when small numbers of tumour cells are implanted and the suggestion is that the antigenic stimulus is not present until the tumour reaches a certain size. When 'sneak-through' is observed after large numbers of tumour cells are transplanted, it is thought that an excessive amount of tumour antigen overwhelms the immune resistance of the host, allowing uninhibited growth of the tumour.

Allogeneic inhibition

When small numbers of tumour cells are transplanted into syngeneic (genetically identical) recipients, tumour growth occurs more readily than when similar numbers of tumour cells are inoculated into allogeneic (genetically dissimilar) recipients. This syngeneic preference and allogeneic inhibition involves the small lymphocyte, but does not require the activation of the immune response since no prior exposure is required.

Tests of cell-mediated immunity to TSTA

Cell-mediated immunity can be tested *in vitro* by mixing tumour cells with test lymphocytes and by observing the reduction in tumour colonies or the cytotoxicity of the lymphocyte on the tumour cell. Cytotoxicity can be determined by detection of release of radioactive labelled compounds such as chromium-51, ^{3}H-thymidine or ^{125}iododeoxyuridine from the dead cell. If lymphocytes have previously been sensitised by exposure to tumour-specific antigens they undergo 'blast transformation' when exposed again to the

tumour antigen. This lymphocyte transformation is associated with increased DNA and RNA activity which can be demonstrated by tracing the uptake of radioactive substances into cellular components. After contact between tumour specific antigen and sensitised lymphocytes a factor is released which prevents the *in vitro* migration of macrophages or other white blood cells. This observation forms the basis of migration inhibition tests for cell-mediated immunity.

Tests of antibodies to TSTA

Immunofluorescence, immunodiffusion, complement fixation tests and cytotoxicity tests are used for the detection of humoral antibodies to TSTA.

Blocking factors can be identified in the serum of patients with tumours and may explain why tumours grow and spread even when cell-mediated immunity is developed. These blocking factors are identifiable *in vitro*. Sensitised lymphocytes are added to tumour cells and inhibit tumour growth. This inhibition is 'blocked' by the addition of serum from the patient with a developing tumour. Blocking factors act both on tumour cells and on the lymphocytes and are thought to be circulating antigen-antibody complexes.

Carcino-embryonic antigen (CEA)

Antigens produced in the fetus, but not identifiable in serum after the first year of extrauterine life, are found again in the serum of patients with some types of malignant disease. These tumour-associated glycoproteins may be found by radioimmunoassay in the tumour tissue or in the blood. They have been identified in the faeces of patients with colonic carcinoma and in the urine of patients with urothelial tumours. A variety of carcinomas, sarcomas and lymphomas are capable of producing CEA and it has been found in patients with inflammatory bowel disease, cirrhosis of the liver, in cigarette smokers and in other non-malignant conditions. It has not been found consistently with all tumours. While not being specific for cancer, nor present invariably in the presence of tumour, it is a useful test for following the progress or response to treatment in patients who are known to have a raised CEA.

Alpha-feto-protein is another fetal antigen. It is a globulin and appears to be of more discriminating diagnostic value than CEA. It is present in up to 80% of patients with hepatomas, and it has also been found in patients with gastrointestinal and urological malignancies.

Tests of immune competence in cancer patients

The two most commonly employed investigations of non-specific immune competence are skin testing with common antigens and dinitrochlorobenzene (DNCB) sensitisation. A battery of skin tests with antigens to which the patient is likely to have had previous exposure generally includes candida, mumps, purified protein derivative (PPD) of tuberculin and streptokinase-streptodornase. The antigens are injected intradermally and a test considered positive, if 48 hours later, there occurs at the injection site an area of induration measuring at least 1 cm in diameter. The DNCB test involves the application of a sensitising dose of 2000 μg DNCB. Two weeks later, further applications of varying concentrations of DNCB are carried out and the hypersensitivity reaction is seen and recorded. A negative reaction usually accompanies progressive malignant disease. The DNCB test may be used sequentially and the development of anergy in patients with previously positive tests indicates progression or recurrence of tumour and correlates well with clinical deterioration.

Acquired immune deficiency syndrome

More than 2000 cases of acquired immune deficiency syndrome (AIDS) have been reported since the syndrome was first recognised as a clinical entity in 1979. This condition is characterised by abnormalities in T cell function. Lymphopenia, anergy to intradermal antigens, reduced natural killer cell activity and an abnormal lymphocyte response to antigenic stimulation are features of the condition. Opportunistic infections are a common cause of morbidity and mortality in this condition and a striking feature of the syndrome is a marked predisposition to develop unusual malignant neoplasms, such as Kaposi's sarcoma and lymphomas. Approximately 75% of patients with AIDS are homosexuals, 15% are drug abusers and some 5% are haemophiliacs or natives of Haiti and parts of Central Africa. The Kaposi sarcoma in AIDS grows rapidly, invades lymphatics and disseminates extensively. It is usually fatal. The development of a rapidly fatal malignant neoplasm with a possible contagious cause has provoked intensive research.

Immunotherapy in cancer

Immunotherapy in human cancers is still of unproven benefit. Although it has been tried in a variety of human tumours, no clearcut advantage has yet emerged. In principle immunotherapy may be *active*, by attempting to stimulate the patient's own immune system or *passive* or adoptive, by administration of antisera, immunised lymphocytes or subcellular fractions previously immunised. Immunotherapy may be *specific*, by stimulating reaction to TSTA or *nonspecific*, where attempts are made to enhance the immune system of the host (Morton, 1974).

Non-specific active immunotherapy

Non-specific immunity to viruses, bacteria, fungi and tumour antigens can be stimulated in the host by a variety of bacterial toxins, bacillus Calmette Guerin (BCG), Corynebacterium parvum and fractions of the tubercle bacillus. This type of immunotherapy has been widely used in patients with acute leukaemia, malignant melanoma and metastatic mammary cancer.

BCG has been found to be helpful in arresting malignant melanoma when cutaneous, subcutaneous or regional nodal involvement is present, but has little effect when the disease involves multiple viscera. The implication is that such therapy is valuable with limited tumour bulk, but extensive major visceral involvement apparently overwhelms the immune system and limits the effect of BCG. This concept has led to the advocacy of 'debulking' surgical procedures, aimed at resecting major tumour-bearing areas in order to allow the immune system to become efficient and active. It has also led to the idea of adjuvant immunotherapy after primary resection of malignant melanoma in the belief that optimum opportunity for immunotherapy exists when the load of tumour is small. This approach has led to lower rates of recurrence in stage II malignant melanoma. When BCG is injected into a tumour, fever, abscesses, regional lymphadenopathy, hepatitis and even anaphylactoid reactions may occur. Toxicity is much reduced if BCG is administered intradermally.

DNCB. Local immunotherapy with DNCB has been used with success in basal and squamous cell carcinoma of the skin and in local and regional recurrences in carcinoma of the breast.

C. parvum. Heat-killed suspensions of the Gram positive bacterium, *C. parvum*, when injected into patients with tumours have the capacity to stimulate the reticulo-endothelial system. Its place has been well established in experimental animals (Scott, 1974). As it is a killed vaccine, there is no risk of infection and because it may cross-react with different antigens than BCG, it may be active in cases where BCG is not, or it may be used in conjunction with BCG. It may cause fever and gastrointestinal disturbances and this toxicity is probably dose related. It appears to have effects in stimulating macrophage activity when injected intravenously, while the intratumour injection is followed by local effects which are dependent on T lymphocyte activity. Its action is, therefore, almost certainly bimodal.

Levamisole. Levamisole is an antihelminthic drug. It is an imidazole compound and stimulates or potentiates delayed hypersensitivity reactions. Patients with negative responses to DNCB skin test may convert to positive responders after an oral administration of levamisole. It has been used not only in malignant disease, but in patients with chronic inflammatory diseases, such as rheumatoid arthritis. The dose appears to be critical, the usual dose being 150 mg daily for 2–3 weeks and repeated every 2–3 weeks.

Passive or adoptive immunotherapy

Immunity can be transferred from one syngeneic animal to another by transfusion of immune lymphocytes. Potential human donors cannot be injected with cancer cells in order to harvest immune lymphocytes and transfused lymphocytes are rejected. Passive immunity may be transferred by injection of lymphocyte fractions of which transfer factor and immune RNA are the most promising.

Transfer factor. The immunity of the donor can be transferred to a recipient by the injection of transfer factor, a subcellular fraction of lymphocytes. Its action appears to be the facilitation of cell-mediated immunity and it has both antigen-specific and non-specific action in immunopotentiation. Its effect has been demonstrated in immunodeficiency states and it has been reported to be of benefit in some patients with lymphoma and carcinoma, but its place in the treatment of human cancer has yet to be fully established.

Immune RNA. The inoculation of human tumour cells into sheep allows sensitised lymphocytes to be harvested from the sheep's lymph nodes and spleen. The immunised lymphocytic RNA is extracted and injected into the patient. As the immune RNA can be extracted from the tissues of an xenogenic host and causes little toxicity, it has obvious advantages. Evidence of its value in human value is sparse at present.

Thymosin. Thymosin is an extract of calf thymus and, in experimental animals, restores cell-mediated immunity. In immunodeficient mice it restores T lymphocyte function. In patients with cancer, particularly the elderly, there may be a depression of T lymphocyte activity which can be corrected by administration of thymosin. It may, therefore, be shown to be an effective immunotherapeutic agent, either alone or in combination with other specific or non-specific agents.

Plasmapheresis. Plasmapheresis involves the removal of blood, separation of plasma from cells and retransfusion of the packed cells. It removes from the blood substances on the patients tumour cell or in the plasma which might interfere with the immune response. The precise mechanisms governing the undoubted favourable responses to this form of treatment for cancer remain unclear.

Interferon. Interferon inhibits cellular invasion by viruses. It is a protein derivative of lymphocytes. It has an effect in stimulating the immune system in animals and also has a direct anti-tumour action. It is made from tissue culture, but is expensive to produce. Intensive studies of its anti-tumour activity in man are being carried out. Many substances, known to induce production of interferon have been studied and appear to have an effect on immunostimulation.

Cell cycle

If the timing and scheduling of cytotoxic chemotherapeutic agents is to be arranged in the most effective way, knowledge and understanding of the biological cell cycle and the precise mode of action of drugs on the cycle are most important. Chemotherapeutic agents affect normal as well as cancer cells and the life cycle of normal and cancer cells are similar. However, the duration of the cycle in cancer cells and the susceptibility of such cells to anti-tumour agents differ from the normal cell.

After undergoing mitosis, the cytoplasm of the daughter cells enlarges and an initial resting phase occurs. This is known as the 'G1 phase' or 'first-gap phase'. After this, the cell passes into the 'S phase', a period during which active DNA synthesis occurs, associated with chromosomal replication. Most cytotoxic drugs act in the S phase. Before further mitosis (M phase), the cell passes into the 'G2 phase', a second resting phase, otherwise known as the 'second-gap phase'. During this phase, organisation of DNA protein and cell membrane development occur. After mitosis, some tumour cells go into a dormant 'G0 phase', where little biochemical metabolic activity occurs. G0 phase tumour cells may be stimulated at any time to enter the G1 phase in preparation for further tumour cell mitosis (Fig 38.1).

These stages of cell cycle activity have been developed as a result of investigations involving the use of labelled thymidine. Such experiments allowed the incorporation of thymidine into DNA synthesis to be studied and led to the concept of resting phases before and after active chromosomal replication.

Both *in vitro* and *in vivo* studies have yielded similar results in the assessment of the duration of each phase in the cell cycle. Approximate times for each phase are as follows:

M phase	=	1 hour
G 1 phase	=	0 to 30 hours
S phase	=	10 to 20 hours
G 2 phase	=	2 to 10 hours

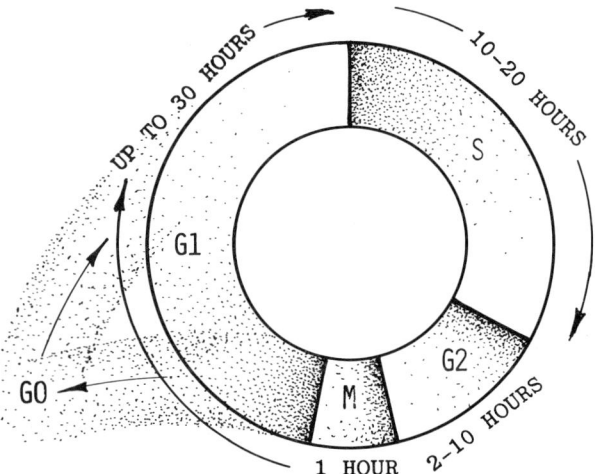

Fig 38.1 Diagrammatic representation of the cell cycle.

The duration of the G 1 phase, being the most variable in terms of time, determines the difference between rapidly and slowly dividing cell populations. The cell cycle time of a tumour cell is not shorter than that of a normal cell and is, in general, considerably longer than that of normal leucocytes or enterocytes. The cell cycle time of a tumour cell tends to be more rapid, and perhaps less predictable in the early stages of tumour growth but once a tumour contains 10^9 cells or is about 1 cm in diameter, the cell cycle time is fairly constant. Tumours increase in size, not because the growth rate of cells is more rapid than normal, but because death of cells does not occur at the same rate as proliferation. The normal controlling mechanisms by which genesis of cells is matched by cell death is lost in cancerous growth.

Rate of tumour growth

In normal tissues, cell replacement is equal to cell loss and the ratio of cells lost to cells produced, the cell loss factor, is 100%. In tumorous growths, this factor is about 95%, so giving rise to a net gain in tumour size. Tumour cells may be: (a) actively involved in the cell cycle (proliferating clonogenic cells); (b) in the G 0 resting phase, capable of joining the active cycle under suitable stimulus (non-proliferating clonogenic cells); (c) dying and being shed from the tumour (non-clonogenic cells). The growth fraction of a tumour is the ratio of the number of actively cycling cells to the total number of cells in the tumour. The growth of a tumour depends on the cell cycle time, the cell loss factor and the growth fraction.

The tumour doubling time refers to the time taken for a tumour to double its volume. Tumour doubling times vary widely and as a tumour enlarges in size its doubling time becomes longer. Most chemotherapeutic agents are directed against actively proliferating cells and are therefore, more likely to be effective against tumours with a high growth fraction. However, as the tumour increases in size, more cells enter the G 0 phase and less go into the G 1 phase directly after mitosis. Treatment of such large tumours involves the use of agents which are not particularly dependent for their cytotoxicity on proliferating cells.

Detection of cancer

As a tumour develops, it may become detectable in several ways:

1 Cancer screening programmes which involve the investigation of people who believe themselves to be free from signs and symptoms of cancer. The value of screening is based on the assumption that earlier diagnosis improves the curability of tumours.
2 An expanding lesion may become apparent by the development of a swelling or by clinical features of obstruction, compression or destruction of organs.
3 Ulceration or haemorrhage occurring in enlarging tumours may lead to the detection of a neoplasm.
4 In about 15% of cases, tumours may be found by the discovery of a metastatic deposit, the primary lesion being clinically 'silent'.
5 Cancer may become apparent because of some systemic manifestation of malignancy.

Hormonal and metabolic factors

Endocrine tumours present with the clinical features of excessive production of the hormone secreted by the tumour of origin e.g. Cushing's syndrome from adrenal carcinoma and Zollinger-Ellison syndrome from non-beta islet cell tumours of the pancreas. Endocrine manifestations may also develop as a result of tumours which secrete hormonal substances not normally synthesised by the organ of origin. ACTH, producing features of Cushing's syndrome, may be synthesised and secreted by tumours of the lung, thymus, pancreas or thyroid and TSH, producing hyperthyroidism, may be secreted by testicular tumours or choriocarcinoma.

Retroperitoneal, mediastinal and hepatic tumours may produce substances which have hypoglycaemic effect while hypercalcaemia due to production of parathyroid-hormone-like substances occurs with carcinoma of the breast, uterus and lung. Hypercalcaemia also develops in myeloma. Hyperuricaemia occurs in leukaemias and lymphomas and other cancers which are associated with a rapid turnover of nucleic acid. It often follows cytotoxic chemotherapy, and urate crystals may be precipitated in the renal tubules causing renal failure. Some pulmonary and prostatic cancers secrete anti-diuretic hormone (ADH). Gonadotrophin secretion by hepatic and pulmonary tumours may give rise to gynaecomastia. Cancer of the kidney may also produce a rise in liver enzymes even when no liver metastases are present.

Neuromusculo-skeletal disorders

Malignant tumours of the lung, breast or ovary may produce a variety of neuromuscular disorders in the absence of discernible evidence of metastatic spread. In particular a progressive polyneuropathy or polymyopathy is found with bronchial and mammary tumours and subacute cerebellar degeneration occasionally accompanies these tumours. Improvement in the syndrome follows removal of the primary tumour in about 50% of patients. Painful hypertrophic osteoarthropathy of bones and joints of the hands and feet is associated with bronchogenic carcinoma and is relieved by resection of the primary tumour.

Blood disorders

Haematological disorders are associated with non-haematological malignancy even when bone marrow infiltration by metastatic disease is not identified. Carcinoma of the kidney, uterus and adrenal medulla producing erythropoietin may cause increase in the red cell mass. Many tumours produce leukaemoid reactions and tumours of stomach, lung and pancreas produce a hypercoagulable state, sometimes with thrombophlebitis migrans, in which thrombocytosis may be found. Some forms of cancer, particularly of the gastrointestinal tract and the breast may be associated with an unexplained disseminated intravascular coagulopathy (DIC).

Cutaneous manifestations

Dermatomyositis may be the presenting clinical feature in patients with carcinoma of the bronchus, breast or stomach and some forms of malignancy, particularly lymphomas, may give rise to a variety of cutaneous conditions such as erythema multiforme and pemphigoid reactions. The condition of acanthosis nigricans is associated with cancer of stomach, breast and bronchus.

Generalised manifestations

Fever, anorexia, and loss of weight leading to malignant cachexia are common features of advanced cancer. This generalised protein and glycogen catabolism may be temporarily reversed by intravenous nutritional support. Such improvement may make cytotoxic chemotherapy possible and may be justifiable in patients who can be expected to obtain remissions from the disease by such chemotherapy.

Pathways of spread of malignant tumours

Local invasion

Tumours have a tendency to spread along fascial sheaths before infiltrating or penetrating them (del Regato, 1977). It is not known what forces determine the invasion of adjacent structures by malignant tumours, but several factors have been identified in experimental studies (Sugarbaker and Ketcham, 1977):

Increased pressure occurs when the growth of tumour cells results in a mass pressure effect on adjacent tissue.

Amoeboid movements. Some tumour cells have the ability to send out pseudopodia between interstices of cells and this may be a mechanism by which cells gain access to the lymphatic and blood vascular compartments.

Loss of normal contact inhibition. This can result in movement around and overlapping of adjacent normal cells.

Severance of intercellular connections.

Proteolytic enzymes produced by cancer cells may favour local tumour spread.

Why an expanding cancer develops finger-like microscopical projections is unknown. Wide excision of a tumour may demonstrate a clear segment of normal tissue around the tumour, apart from areas where the tentacle of the tumour have extended to the margin of the resection. The peripheral parts of growing tumours are more richly vascularised, have a greater oxygen saturation concentration and a more rapid rate of DNA synthesis than has the centre of a tumour.

Distant spread

Tumour cells gain access to the lymphatic and venous systems and rarely enter the arterial system. Once in the circulation, they are carried to distant sites, where metastatic deposits become established.

Lymphatic spread

Malignant cells in a lymphatic channel, may spread to the regional lymph nodes by direct propagation of tumour cell upon tumour cell along the lymphatics or by tumour emboli within the lymphatic channel. These afferent lymphatics convey tumour to the subcapsular sinusoids of the regional lymph node. If not destroyed within the node, tumour cells may pass by efferent channels into the main lymphatic trunks and thence to the venous circulation.

Spread of tumour cells to lymph nodes tends to follow an anatomically logical step-wise sequence. Nodes in the proximity of the tumour are usually affected before more distant nodes, but tumour cells may 'by pass' the proximal nodes and affect more distal nodes in the same group. Intralymphatic tumour cells may gain access to the venous circulation by way of lymphatico-venous anastomoses proximal to the lymph nodes.

Evidence concerning the fate of tumour cells in lymph nodes is variable. Several possibilities exist and have been observed in experimental tumours:

1 The tumour cells reaching the subcapsular sinus may be killed.
2 Cells may be 'trapped' temporarily in lymph nodes and later pass out to efferent lymphatics.
3 Metastatic tumour growth may occur within the lymph node.
4 Cells may pass directly through the nodes into the systemic circulation.

Most tumour cells are killed in the lymphatic circulation and local and general immunological mechanisms may determine the number and pathogenicity of the cells escaping into the venous circulation.

Haematogenous spread

Tumour cells may infiltrate blood vessels by amoeboid infiltration or come to lie with blood vessels during the development of neovascularisation. The periphery of a tumour tends to be its most vascular area. As new capillaries develop in a tumour, they can be seen to be lined by tumour cells which make up the endothelial vessel lining. Such cells can be swept away with the blood stream to other parts of the body. Showers of tumour cells can be identified in the venous system draining tumours when these are incised or manipulated. This phenomenon is seen in many experimental tumours and also in human cancer. In spite of release of large numbers of circulating tumour cells, the number of metastases which develop is small. Tumour cells may survive in organs remote from the primary tumour and yet may not develop into obvious

destructive deposits. In experimental animals, it is estimated that less than 0.1% of tumour cells injected intravenously form metastatic deposits. The overwhelming majority of tumour cells entering the venous circulation are destroyed within it. For tumour cells to become implanted at a distant site and to proliferate as a metastasis probably requires that the cells adhere to the capillary endothelium at the selected site.

The site of metastatic deposits is influenced by the venous anatomy of the tumour-bearing area. Tumours of the gastrointestinal tract with portal venous drainage to the systemic system are more commonly associated with pulmonary deposits. Many experimental tumour models have confirmed specific organ preference for some metastases, but the mechanism for such affinity is unknown. It may be related to local chemical factors at the site of potential bonding of endothelial cell and tumour cell. Immunological factors may also be of importance in determining the location of metastatic deposits since immunosuppression may facilitate the development of metastases and immune stimulation may alter their distribution.

The metastatic potential of metastases from human tumours is controversial because it is extremely difficult to prove such spread. In animal models, it has been demonstrated that metastases can produce metastases (Hoover and Ketcham, 1975) and there is strong circumstantial evidence that such spread also takes place in man (Roth *et al.*, 1976). Arterial invasion by cancer cells is rare, but if a tumour invades a large artery, metastases may result in the area supplied by the artery.

Transcoelomic spread

The incessant movement occurring in the intrathoracic and intra-abdominal compartments, together with the constant flux of fluid in the pleural and peritoneal cavities, favours transcoelomic spread of malignant cells seen commonly with gastric, ovarian and pulmonary tumours.

Cerebrospinal spread

Medulloblastomas and ependymomas spread by way of the cerebrospinal fluid. Fragments of tumour break off and may become adherent to the lining of the sub-arachnoid space. Secondary tumours are found in the ventricles of the brain or in the spinal cord.

Biopsy

Tissue diagnosis is mandatory before staging procedures can be undertaken or treatment planned. Tissue may be obtained by some form of biopsy or cells may be available for cytological examination.

Needle biopsy

Fine needle biopsy

Needle biopsy may be carried out with a fine 18- or 21-gauge needle and syringe. Cellular contents are aspirated from the lesion, a smear made and is examined immediately. This aspiration-biopsy-cytology (ABC) technique has been found to be useful in cystic and solid lesions, particularly of the breast, lymph nodes, thyroid and salivary glands. An unequivocal diagnosis of malignancy can be obtained and allows treatment to be planned, but an aspirate which contains no malignant cells does not exclude the diagnosis of cancer. For example, in mammary lesions, a 'negative' aspirate from a solid lesion does not confirm that the lesion is benign, because sampling errors occur. One cannot be certain of having obtained a representative biopsy and a formal excision biopsy must then be advised.

The fine needle technique has been used extensively for deeper lesions such as liver, lung, pancreas, ovary, bone and even brain and spleen. With guidance by radiological image intensification or by ultrasound examination, the fine needle can be inserted into the desired area. There is little risk of haemorrhage or visceral damage with this technique. For example, when percutaneous biopsy of the pancreas is being carried out by this technique, the stomach is often punctured without adverse clinical consequences.

Large-bore needles

Several types of large-calibre biopsy needles are available and provide tissue for full histological examination. A core of tissue is obtained and its architecture is undamaged. This type of needle, such as the Tru-Cut, is widely used for biopsy of superficial lesions and also for the liver. Special needles for bone marrow aspirate for cytological study, or bone and marrow biopsy, are widely used for investigation of haematological disorders. The same caution regarding unrepresentative samples must be exercised with large-bore needles as with fine needles. Although rare, serious bleeding may result from percutaneous liver biopsy and pancreatic haemorrhage and fistula have been reported. The high-speed air-powered drill biopsy, which drives a trephine of 1.5 mm internal diameter into the lesion, is also used for diagnostic purposes. As the trephine has a cutting edge and rotates at high speed, the procedure is less uncomfortable for the patient than are the manually-controlled large-calibre needles and produces a better specimen.

Excision biopsy

Excision biopsy involves complete removal of the tumour and can be used for most lesions.

Wide excision may also be the definite treatment in some forms of malignant disease, such as squamous or basal cell skin tumours. More usually, excisional biopsy for cancer is carried out for diagnosis alone and more radical operative treatment carried out if malignancy is confirmed. In some conditions, such as lymph node biopsy, the pathologist is aided if the specimen is sent to him in its entirety, undistorted and undisturbed. With other lesions, for example, large soft tissue sarcomas, excision biopsy may be harmful, because of possible contamination of a large operative area by tumour cells.

Incision biopsy

Incision for biopsy has the same disadvantage as using a needle in that sampling errors can occur and the tumour may be overlooked by an unrepresentative sample. Because incision of a tumour implies local spillage of cells into the operative field, the subsequent operation should not be delayed longer than necessary and the biopsy operative field should be removed completely. A frequent type of incision biopsy is endoscopic biopsy of gastrointestinal, genitourinary and respiratory tract lesions, where the specimen is partially removed by a forceps under direct inspection. If adequate tissue for histological examination cannot be obtained in this way, cell brushings for cytology are usually available to the endoscopist. Oesophageal, bronchial, bladder, gastroduodenal and colonic brushings often provide the diagnosis of malignancy when a histological diagnosis has not been obtained. Cytological smears have been used in the detection of gynaecological carcinoma for over 50 years.

Another form of incision biopsy is curettage which is carried out for diagnosis of endometrial lesions and for soft masses of tumour such as sarcomas of soft tissue or bone or in some cerebral tumours.

Staging of cancer

The definition of 'the staging of malignant disease' is 'the assessment of the extent of the disease before primary treatment'. If all stages of a malignant condition were treated in the same fashion, the value of staging would be in allowing some assessment of prognosis. Because different stages of a cancerous process may require different types of treatment, staging in some cancers has become of therapeutic as well as of prognostic importance. For many tumours the prognosis depends on the stage and also on the treatment, while the treatment also depends on the stage. Planned staging before treatment is recognised as being essential for accurate treatment of many forms of malignant disease.

The staging of a particular cancer is ascertained by:

1　clinical examination
2　histological examination
3　special investigations

Several different types of clinical staging or classification or different types of tumours have been described, but the TNM system of staging devised by the Union Internationale Contre le Cancer (UICC) has the merit of having international agreement. Such agreement is indispensible for exchange of information between different centres.

The system is based on an assessment of:

1　extent of the primary tumour　　　T
2　condition of the regional lymph nodes　　N
3　absence or presence of distant metastases　　M

A TNM classification has been devised for many tumours at different sites (Table 2).

T1, T2, T3 and T4 refer to increasing degrees of size and local extent of the primary tumour. T0 means that there is no evidence of primary tumour, as in patients in whom metastatic disease has been identified while the primary tumour is occult. TX signifies that it is not possible to assess fully the extent of the primary tumour when surgical operation is not done. TIS refers to carcinoma *insitu* (preinvasive carcinoma) and must be distinguished from T0.

N1, N2, N3 signifies the condition of the regional lymph nodes as ascertained by clinical examination e.g. lymphangiography. If the nodal status is impossible to assess, NX is used and N0 means that the regional nodes are impalpable clinically or that they appear normal on lymphangiography.

M0 means that no metastases can be detected clinically and MI refers to the presence of metastases.

On histological grounds, additional information may be obtained and histopathological staging (P) based on the extent of infiltration by the tumour and pathological grading (G) based on the histological appearance, have been laid down by UICC. For example in gastric cancer, P1 indicates tumour confined to mucosa, P2 involves gastric wall but not including serosa, P3 indicates extension through the serosa with or without invasion of adjacent structures and P4 refers to diffuse involvement of the entire gastric wall without obvious boundaries.

G1 refers to low-grade malignancy, G2 to medium-grade malignancy and G3 to high-grade malignancy.

Further definitions are used for certain tumours. L refers to lymphatic invasion, L0 being no invasion of lymphatics while L1 and L2 refer to invasion of the superficial and deep lymphatics respectively.

Venous invasion is defined by V, e.g., for renal tumours V0 signifies that the veins do not contain tumour, V1 that the renal vein contains tumour and V2 that the vena cava contains tumour.

Like all staging systems, the TNM system of clinical staging poses some difficulties in interpretation. For example, the size of a tumour in the breast is often difficult to define on clinical examination if it is deeply placed and assessment of axillary lymph node status on clinical grounds may be misleading. However, the system is universally understood and accepted and this allows uniformity of recording and accurate comparisons of the results of treatment from different centres.

Staging by special investigation

It is well recognised that tumours may spread to distant sites without any clinical sign of metastatic disease and that clinically occult metastases can be demonstrated by specialised investigations. Conventional radiography is relatively crude in detecting osseous metastases and nuclear imaging techniques are more sensitive. Nuclear scintigraphy has been widely used for bone, liver and brain as preliminary investigations to search for secondary deposits. Sonography in the chest or abdomen is helpful in the detection of hepatic metastases and for mass lesions, such as enlarged retroperi-

Table 2
TNM CLASSIFICATION

Head and neck	Lips
	Buccal cavity
	Oropharynx
	Nasopharynx
	Hypopharynx
	Larynx
	Thyroid
Alimentary canal	Oesophagus
	Stomach
Breast	
Gynaecological sites	Cervix uteri
	Corpus uteri
	Ovary
	Urethra
	Vagina
	Vulva
Urological sites	Kidney
	Bladder
	Prostate
	Testis
	Penis
Lung	
Skin (excluding melanoma)	

toneal lymph nodes. Computerised tomographic scanning is now being used in selected centres to screen the patient for evidence of metastatic disease.

Laparoscopy and laparotomy have been used occasionally in the staging of carcinoma of the breast and have become routine in many centres for the staging of Hodgkin's disease. Extensive investigations in search for metastases is expensive and takes time, but it may alter treatment. In Hodgkin's disease the staging, and therefore the treatment, is altered by staging laparotomy in about 20% of patients. It may alter the stage by identification of unsuspected intra-abdominal disease or by excluding the presence of nodes in areas thought to be involved. Lymphangiography of the iliac and para-aortic nodes is a valuable complementary investigation to laparotomy since it helps identify possible sites of nodal disease, which the surgeon can confirm or disprove at operation. It is important to ensure that the radiologically suspect nodes have been removed by taking specimen radiography of the removed tissue and comparing the film with the pre-operative lymphangiogram.

Staging laparotomy for Hodgkin's disease

The spectacular improvement in treatment of patients with Hodgkin's disease has been due to improved diagnosis of the extent of the disease and improvements in radiotherapy and chemotherapy. The prognosis in Hodgkin's disease is related to the histological type of the tumour and to the stage of the disease, the Rye histopathological classification has widest acceptance and is now in general use (Lukes and Butler, 1966).

Lymphocyte predominance type has the best prognosis. Typical Reed-Sternberg cells are few and there is dense infiltration by normal lymphocytes.

Nodular sclerosing. Hodgkin's disease is made up of nodules of lymphoid tissue, separated by collagen strands. The size of the nodules is quite variable.

Mixed cellularity type of Hodgkin's disease is associated with a mixture of Reed-Sternberg cells, eosinophils, plasma cells, fibroblasts and lymphocytes within a variegated stroma.

Lymphocyte depleted type has the worst prognosis. Reed-Sternberg cells are plentiful, lymphocytes are few and fibrosis is irregular and diffuse.

Ann Arbor classification

The clinical staging of the disease most widely used is the Ann Arbor classification (Carbone *et al.*, 1971):

Stage I   refers to involvement of one anatomical lymph node site or, rarely, to a single extralymphatic primary site.

Stage II   indicates involvement of two or more lymph node regions on the same side of the diaphragm, either above or below with or without localised extralymphatic disease. Where localised extralymphatic disease is present, the stage is called II_E.

Stage III indicates involvement of lymph nodes on both sides of the diaphragm with or without involvement of the spleen (III_S) or localised extralymphatic disease (III_E) or both (III_{SE}).

Stage IV   signifies diffuse extra-nodal disease, liver involvement being indicated IV_H and bone marrow disease IV_M.

Any stage may be described A or B depending on the absence (A) or presence (B) of any of the following symptoms:

1 Night sweats
2 Unexplained loss of more than 10% of body weight in the previous 6 months
3 Unexplained rise in temperature above 38°C

Any one of these symptoms places the patient into category B.

The extent of the disease cannot be assessed by clinical examination alone since nodal or visceral disease may not be clinically detectable. Routine chest radiography is carried out to check for hilar lymph node involvement or pulmonary infiltration. Whole lung tomography is done if there is doubt and mediastinoscopy and biopsy may be needed in some to confirm or exclude mediastinal Hodgkin's disease. Skeletal scintigraphy may indicate bone disease, but marrow and bone biopsy of the iliac crest is also important. Needle marrow aspirates are of little value in this regard, open biopsy of bone with a cutting trephine being required. Nuclear imaging of liver and spleen and gallium scanning are of limited value. Liver scanning may reveal falsely positive and falsely negative information. An enlarged spleen may not be involved by Hodgkin's disease while a normal sized spleen may be heavily infiltrated. Scanning of the spleen is unreliable because it may indicate disease where none exists and fail to demonstrate tumour where it is present. Gallium scanning is difficult to interpret below the diaphragm because uptake of the isotope in the liver and the bowel may obscure identification of intra-abdominal disease.

Lymphangiography is of considerable help in staging. Bi-pedal intralymphatic infusions are carried out and the size, shape, distribution and architecture of the inguinal, iliac and para-aortic nodes evaluated. The accuracy of interpretation varies. If the lymphangiogram indicates retroperitoneal nodal involvement, this is confirmed at laparotomy in about 80% of cases. When lymphangiography is normal, the surgeon identifies involved nodes in some 10% of patients. Lymphangiography and operative biopsy at laparotomy should be considered complementary rather than competitive investigations. Preliminary lymphangiography allows the surgeon to excise radiologically suspicious nodes and specimen radiography of the removed nodes provides important proof that the nodes under question have been excised.

The purpose of the operation is to search for and localise areas of disease below the diaphragm. It is normally carried out through a mid-line or paramedian incision although occasionally a left subcostal incision may be preferred. The peritoneal cavity is examined for signs of disease, the spleen is removed, wedge biopsies are taken from each lobe of the liver and needle biopsies are taken from the depths of each lobe. The retroperitoneum is explored, lymph nodes are removed from the para-aortic and para-iliac regions and the area is marked with metal clips. Nodes are also removed from the small bowel mesentery, from the porta hepatis and the coeliac axis if they are enlarged and accessible. The ovaries may be displaced medially to the fundus of the uterus or to the lateral pelvic wall so as to reduce the risks of ovarian irradiation should radiotherapy to the para-aortic, iliac and inguinal nodes be needed later.

Advantages

1　Removal of the spleen allows full histological examination to be carried out and allows far more accurate assessment of splenic involvement than can be obtained by other less invasive means. Histological examination of the spleen should be 100% accurate in determining intrasplenic Hodgkin's disease, but multiple sections through the spleen 3 mm apart are needed ('Bread-loaf slices') to demonstrate small foci of disease.

2　Splenectomy eliminates the need for irradiation of the spleen with its hazards of damage to the base of the left lung and kidney.

3　Splenectomy may help counteract the haemopoietic suppression induced by cytotoxic therapy and may increase the haemopoietic tolerance of chemotherapy.

4　Splenectomy may have some therapeutic advantage if hypersplenism exists.

5　Several liver biopsies and gross examinations of the liver are more accurate than current nuclear imaging techniques. However, some centres have discontinued the use of deep needle biopsy because the yield of positive Hodgkin's disease is so low with these samples. The presence of disease in the spleen appears to be a more reliable indicator of hepatic disease than liver biopsy. Liver involvement never occurs without splenic involvement.

6　Retroperitoneal node biopsy can be confirmatory in the diagnosis of radiologically suspicious nodes and sometimes identifies retroperitoneal nodal disease which is unsuspected radiologically.

7　Laparotomy allows assessment of nodes in the porta hepatis, small bowel mesentery and splenic hilum. Preoperative lymphangiography of these nodes is not feasible.

8　Laparotomy permits displacement of the ovaries.

Disadvantages

1　Laparotomy involves a major surgical operation with its attendant morbidity and discomfort. The perioperative mortality associated with the procedure is about 1% and the incidence of major complications is about 3%.

2　Venous thrombosis may occur in the lower limbs or in the splenic and portal veins. A high platelet count and increased platelet adhesiveness are known to occur after splenectomy, but there seems to be no correlation between the incidence of venous thrombosis and the level of the platelet count.

3　Transient, unexplained tachycardia may occur after operation, particularly in patients who have mediastinal nodal disease.

4　Pulmonary complications, especially atelectasis of the base of the left lung is common and there is an increased risk of pulmonary embolism consequent on venous thrombosis. Prophylactic subcutaneous heparin is generally advised for patients undergoing staging laparotomy.

5　Infection in the wound or under the left lobe of the diaphragm can occur, particularly if the stomach or the pancreas have been damaged. Such damage predisposes to pancreatitis or to leakage of gastric or pancreatic juice.

6　The possibility of overlooking sites of disease by sampling errors, particularly in the para-aortic nodal area, is always present but should be reduced to a minimum with the aid of preoperative lymphangiography.

7　The delay in treatment of 2 or 3 weeks, necessitated by the operation, may be important and, in some patients with rapidly advancing disease, may not be justifiable.

8　There is strong evidence linking splenectomy with severe subsequent pneumococcal infection in children with and without underlying disease. Overwhelming infections, particularly with *Haemophilus influenzae*, *pneumococcus* and *meningococcus* have been reported in adults with Hodgkin's disease after splenectomy and removal of the spleen may predispose to herpes zoster in these patients. Because there are many reasons why patients with Hodgkin's disease are prone to infections, it is not yet possible to attribute such predisposition to the splenectomy. Evidence that healthy adults who undergo splenectomy for traumatic rupture are at special risk of overwhelming infections is uncertain. The question, at present, remains open.

Because about 30% of patients with clinical Stage I and II supradiaphragmatic disease have subdiaphragmatic involvement discovered at operation, staging laparotomy is probably advisable for these patients, especially if they have 'B' symptoms. Operation appears to be of marginal value in patients with IA or IIA nodular sclerosing type Hodgkin's disease (Stein, 1978). Patients with widespread, clinical stage IV disease do not require staging laparotomy since Stage IV has already been ascertained. Controversy exists about Stage III patients; those with B disease are usually treated by chemotherapy, but there is a difficulty in deciding treatment in patients with Stage IIIA disease. Radiotherapy is used for this group of patients in many centres, but chemotherapy is required if the liver is involved. The question of liver involvement is best solved by staging laparotomy and many centres, therefore, advise this procedure for clinical Stage IIIA disease as well as for patients with clinical Stage I and Stage II disease.

Use of computerised tomography has undoubtedly led to identification of intra-abdominal disease and it remains to be seen if this form of investigation will be sufficiently reliable to render staging laparotomy obsolete in Hodgkin's disease.

Treatment of cancer

The aim of cancer therapy varies with the stage of the disease. In 'early' cancer the aim of treatment is to 'cure' the patient and in order to accomplish this the therapist treats the patient as aggressively as he considers necessary. For many forms of primary cancer radical resection of the tumour with all the lymphatics and all the regional lymph nodes en bloc was considered to be standard therapy. Such procedures were considered justifiable and the undesirable cosmetic and functional sequelae were deemed unavoidable. This approach to cancer therapy has gradually changed in recent years as a result of clinical trials and a fuller understanding of tumour biology. Clinical trials in cancer of the breast, for example, have failed to demonstrate superiority of radical mastectomy procedures over more conservative mastectomy in terms of recurrent disease or survival. Improved modalities of investigation have demonstrated metastatic disease in many ostensibly 'early' tumours and there is now substantial evidence that many forms of malignant disease are systemic diseases at the time of diagnosis. Although the technology of clinical investigation has not yet developed to the stage of allowing identification of small foci of tumour at distant sites, the concept of 'micrometastases' has been accepted universally for many forms of cancer. While radical local surgery still has a place as the sole form of therapy, combinations of surgery and radiotherapy or surgery or chemotherapy for primary tumours are coming into more general use.

In advanced cancer, whether locally advanced or metastatic, the aim of treatment is control of the disease, palliation of symptoms and prevention of distressing complications. There are notable exceptions to this approach, as in metastatic choriocarcinoma, which may still be deemed 'curable'. In general, however, aggressive and radical procedures for the primary tumour may be quite inappropriate, even if they are technically feasible. Recognition of the different approaches to the treatment of potentially curable cancer and to that of incurable disease is of fundamental importance and emphasises the need for accurate staging of disease before any treatment is undertaken.

Surgical treatment

For most types of early cancer, surgical treatment offers the best prospect of cure and is the most effective form of therapy in eradicating local disease and preventing local recurrence. Operations for potentially curable disease are determined by the biological behaviour of the tumour and the condition of the patient. They may be conveniently divided into four groups:

1 Wide local excision
2 Extensive local resection
3 Extensive local resection with regional lymphadenectomy
4 Extensive regional resection.

With whatever type of procedure is adopted, care is taken to avoid the risks of tumour dissemination and local tumour cell implantation. The risk of dispersal of tumour cells into the lymphatic or venous system is reduced by:

1 ligating the draining veins at an early stage of the operation
2 avoiding manipulation of the tumour until the vascular pedicle has been ligated
3 reducing the vascularity of the tumour where possible before operating, for example by exsanguinating a limb by tourniquet pressure.

Local implantation of tumour cell is reduced to a minimum by:

1 avoiding unnecessary handling of the tumour
2 incising healthy tissue around the tumour rather than incising the tumour itself
3 discarding scalpels, other instruments and gloves which are likely to have come into contact with the tumour.

Wide local excision

Basal-cell carcinomas of the skin are treated satisfactorily in this fashion. Wide resection involves excision of healthy tissue in all planes, length, breadth, and depth around the tumour. For many lesions, particularly for surface tumours, it is possible to carry out this type of treatment without touching the tumour. Many expanding tumours have a pseudocapsule of compressed cells, both neoplastic and normal; 'enucleation' of such tumours from within the capsule leaves cancer cells *in situ*. With some tumours, it is not possible to determine the extent of a tumour on macroscopic grounds and the use of frozen-section histology is then useful. This applies particularly to soft tissue sarcomas. Spreading as they do along tissue planes of fascia, nerve and vascular sheaths, intermuscular septa and organ capsules, these tumours may ramify widely into and around adjacent structures. Frozen section histology then provides an assurance as to the extent of resection required.

En-bloc resection

The aim of this type of operation is to remove the primary tumour, all the lymphatic channels draining the tumour and the regional lymph nodes. Dissections of this kind involve removal of all the tissue intervening between the tumour and the regional nodes. In removing the nodes, the most distant glands from the tumour are dissected first and the operation carried down to more proximal nodes in the belief that this order of dissection reduces the risk of distant dissemination of tumour cells. Likewise dissection, both sharp and blunt, should proceed towards and not away from, the tumour.

The original application of this kind of operation was the Halsted-Meyer radical mastectomy for carcinoma of the breast. The technical success of the operation led to its wide adoption in the belief that by removal of affected lymph nodes en bloc with primary lymphatics and tumour, all the cancer cells could be extirpated. That this operation is now carried out less frequently is due, not to rejection of the principle but to:

1 knowledge that dissemination of cancer beyond the regional nodes has often occurred when the nodes are infiltrated by tumour
2 demonstration by prospective trials that involved nodes are treated equally well by radiation as by surgical removal
3 doubts about the possible harmful effects of removing uninvolved or sparsely involved lymph nodes, which might have an immunological role in containing the disease
4 recognition that morbidity and cosmetic disfigurement associated with the procedure could be reduced by less extensive operations without increasing the risks of clinical recurrence.

En bloc excision for other tumours is established practice, as in cervical lymphadenectomy for tumours of the oral cavity metastatic to local nodes, or abdomino-perineal resection of the rectum, where the rectum, a wide margin of adjacent tissue, the mesorectum and the regional lymph nodes are removed together.

More extensive resections

Improvements in monitoring, anaesthesia and pre- and postoperative care have allowed very extensive resections to be carried out. These are occasionally justifiable for removal of massive, locally-growing tumours, particularly of the extremities. Fore-quarter or hind-quarter amputations have a definite place in extensive local malignancy such as low-grade bony or soft-tissue sarcomas while pelvic exenteration procedures are occasionally required for locally-infiltrating adenocarcinoma of the uterus or rectum.

Palliative surgery

Local resection of a primary tumour often provides the patient with advanced disease with good palliation. In obstructing or bleeding gastric tumours, for example, local excision of the tumour provides better palliation than does gastrojejunostomy. Biliary or gastro-intestinal by-pass procedures are commonly carried out for obstructing and unresectable tumours. 'Debulking' procedures are being advised for some unresectable primary tumours or for extensive lymphatic nodal disease. Effectiveness of radiotherapy and chemotherapy are enhanced by reducing the tumour mass to a minimum. When this kind of operation is being carried out, incisions are inevitably made through tumour. The macroscopic extent of the tumour is defined by radio-opaque markers so that radiotherapy can be accurately directed.

Isolated metastases, particularly in the lung, are sometimes removed especially if there is no other evidence of metastatic disease. In some instances, notably with testicular tumours, the 5-year survival after such operations exceeds that of resection for primary bronchogenic carcinomas. Calculation of tumour doubling times allows a realistic evaluation of the likelihood of success. Serial chest films are taken and the diameter of the pulmonary lesion is plotted against time on a semi-logarithmic scale. If the tumour doubling time exceeds 40 days, the 5-year survival after resection of the lesion is about 65% which compares favourably with the 5% 5-year survival with unresected lesions. There is no advantage in resection if the tumour doubling time is less than 20 days. Isolated or apparently solitary hepatic metastases are removed sometimes in patients with secondary deposits especially from colonic tumours. Where feasible, this operation gives results which are better than hepatic artery ligation or infusion of 5-fluorouracil.

'Second-look' laparotomy procedures or reoperation is sometimes advised for intra-abdominal malignancy. The problem usually occurs when a rising value of CEA or other tumour marker suggest the presence of recurrence. Reoperation is sometimes advised when chemotherapy has induced clinical remission. For example, in ovarian malignancy the oncologist may need to know whether any residual disease is detectable before advising further treatment.

Operations on endocrine glands provide worthwhile palliation in patients whose tumours are influenced by hormonal factors. Oophorectomy, adrenalectomy and pituitary ablation are carried out for advanced mammary cancer if clinical and biochemical factors indicate a likelihood of improvement.

Radiotherapy

Ionising radiation provides an important form of treatment for many forms of malignant disease, either alone or combined with surgical treatment or chemotherapy. Radiotherapy is employed as primary curative management in some forms of cancer and is also widely used in the palliation of advanced malignancy. Shrinkage of large unresectable tumours, control of haemorrhage, relief of pain and obstruction are frequent results of radiation therapy and over half of all cancer patients require this mode of treatment at some stage. The effect of radiation on cancer cells is brought about either by destroying the tumour cell or by interfering with its potential for replication.

Electromagnetic radiation

In the electromagnetic spectrum, radiation is produced in different wavelengths of the spectrum, but only the x-ray and gamma-ray wavelength is capable of producing radiation which is ionising.

Particle radiation

Alpha rays, beta rays, electrons, neutrons, protons and pi (π) mesons are ionising particles.

Alpha particles consist of two protons and two neutrons and are identical with the helium nucleus. These particles are intensely ionising and cause considerable tissue damage. They have little penetration and consequently are not used in radiotherapy.

Beta particles are electrons of variable penetrating potential. Their penetration depends upon the isotope emitting them. Isotopes which emit β-rays are used in cancer as surface therapy, interstitial therapy or as systemic or intracavitary treatment.

Electron therapy applies to electrons which are produced by electron generators rather than by decay of radioisotopes. They are otherwise identical with β particles.

Neutron beams have become available as a form of treatment in recent years. Neutrons release densely ionising particles and their effect is much less dependent on oxygen than is the case with x-rays. Fast neutrons have an energy above 10 keV by definition. In cancer therapy neutrons of high energy (over 1 MeV) are used. A major advantage of fast neutron therapy is that it is more effective than x-rays on hypoxic cells. Slow neutrons have little radiotherapeutic applicability.

High energy proton particles can be delivered in narrow beams. At the end of their path the radiation released increases greatly and then decreases rapidly. Intense radiation to a small area is possible by this type of radiation which has been used in radiotherapy to the pituitary gland. Negative pi (π) mesons (pions) are charged subatomic particles. Like protons, they exhibit the Bragg peak effect with intense and rapid radiation emission near the end of their path followed by an abrupt fall in radiation. This type of therapy is suitable for deep tissues with a low entrance dose and a negligible exit dose.

External beam therapy

Superficial therapy units. The Grenz Ray unit refers to x-rays of low voltage, between 10 and 60 keV. The Grenz (or 'border') unit is so-called because the rays are at the border between x-rays and ultra-violet light on the electromagnetic spectrum. These rays cause no damage to subcutaneous structures and are used for skin lesions and for accessible mucosal lesions. In the 60 to 160 keV range, superficial x-ray machines are used for malignant lesions of the skin.

Deep x-ray therapy machines (orthovoltage) x-rays of 200 to 300 keV are produced by these machines which, although largely superseded by megavoltage radiation, are still used for relatively superficial lesions.

Megavoltage (or supervoltage) units (greater than 1 million volts) have advantages over orthovoltage therapy. The high energy beam of short wavelength x-rays allows correspondingly higher penetration, more circumscribed and defined edges of beam permits more precise distribution of dosage, bone absorption is reduced and the maximum absorbed dose is deep to the skin, thus reducing undesirable radiation effects on the skin itself.

Linear accelerators produce x-rays between 4 and 20 MeV, the usual therapeutic operating range being between 4 and 8 MeV. A filament gun fires bursts of electrons along a tube. The electrons are accelerated by electromagnetic radar waves and photons produced by a target. Resulting interaction with the target of high atomic number such as gold allows x-rays to be produced. An electron beam can be produced by removing the target.

Betatrons are machines producing electrons of up to 40 MeV. Electrons are accelerated in a circular orbit. With electron beam therapy, there is an abrupt fall-off in the absorbed dose, making this form of treatment suitable for lesions in or close to the surface of the body.

Gamma ray beam units are also used for megavoltage therapy, the two radio-isotopes in most frequent use being cobalt 60 and caesium 137. The gamma ray produced by the cobalt 60 unit is equivalent to 2 MeV and those produced by caesium 137 equivalent to about 1 MeV.

Units of radiation*

The Roentgen (R) is the unit of radiation in a beam of x-rays or gamma rays emerging from the generating source. The radiation exposure refers to the radiation dose to which a patient is exposed over a period of time and is measured in roentgens. The roentgen refers to radiation in air and is the amount of x-radiation or gamma radiation producing one electrostatic unit of charge in 1 ml of air at standard temperature and pressure.

Of more importance in radiotherapy is the amount of radiation absorbed by tissues. Radiation is absorbed by air in its path from source to tissue. The rad is the unit of dose absorbed by the tissue. It is applied to all types of ionising radiations. Absorption of 10 μJ per gram (units of energy) is equal to one rad. In some tissues, for example, muscle, the absorption of radiation is similar to that of air, but the absorption in other tissues, such as bone, may be much greater. Thus the relationship of rads to roentgens depends on the energy of the radiation and on the nature of the irradiated tissue.

* In SI unit system 1 Gray (Gy) = 100 rad and 1 rad = 1 cGy.

Effects of radiation on tissues

Ionising radiation may exert its effect either directly or indirectly. Rapidly dividing cells may undergo necrosis, but the more usual direct effect is interference with cell division by fragmentation of chromosomes or by inhibition of mitosis. Indirect effects on cells may be brought about by interference with the blood supply of the irradiated tissue and by the phagocytic action of the reticulo-endothelial system. The nucleus appears to be the most vulnerable part of the cell to the effects of radiation. Damage to tissues is related to the quantity of energy delivered to the tissues and the intensity of energy transfer is referred to as the linear energy transfer (LET). The LET varies with different types of ionising radiation.

The effect of oxygen

The dose of radiation required to produce death of hypoxic cells is two to three times that required to kill well oxygenated cells. The presence of hypoxic cells in many tumours is well-known and may account for their relative radio resistance. The proportion of hypoxic cells in tumours varies and is usually in the region of 20 to 40%. Reoxygenation of hypoxic cells occurs in some animal tumours and possibly in human tumours also. It may be that fractionated radiotherapy regimens can be arranged to best effect by pulsing therapy during reoxygenation. Fast neutron irradiation is much more effective in killing hypoxic cells than are x-rays. Neutrons displace protons and other heavy particles which are more densely ionising than electrons and the cellular damage caused by these interactions is affected only slightly by the presence of oxygen. The difference in cell kill between hypoxic and oxygenated tissues is known as the oxygen enhancement ratio (OER). The presence of oxygen modifies the effect of x-rays by a factor of about 3 while modifying that of fast neutrons by a factor of about 1.6.

Patients have been exposed to hyperbaric oxygen at three atmospheres of oxygen in an attempt to reduce the proportion of hypoxic cells in tumours. It appears that local tumour control is more effective with hyperbaric oxygen when given in large fractions.

High LET radiation occurs with neutrons, heavy particles and pi mesons, which cause dense ionising radiation in tissues and the effect of this type of radiation on tissues appears to be relatively independent of oxygen.

Chemical sensitisation

Many agents have been used in an attmept to sensitise cells to the effects of radiation. Some of these, such as metronidazole, p-aminoacetophemone (PNAP) and derivatives of nitrofuran, sensitise hypoxic cells to radiation in a selective way while others, such as actinomycin-D, bleomycin and doxorubicin, enhance the effects of radiation on normal as well as tumour tissue. Enhancement of the radiation effect of these substances depends on their delivery to the target tumour cells by an adequate blood supply. The poor vascularity in the case of many tumours may reduce their value.

Fractionation

Radiotherapy is conventionally given in fractions, the total dose being given over several days with the low dose rates of interstitial therapy or in several fractions over several weeks with external beam therapy. Fractionation results in better tolerance of normal tissue and in progressive damage to the cancer cells which are more sensitive to the effects of radiation. The timing and organisation of the fractionation varies widely, schedules often being arranged to suit the condition and the convenience of the patient rather than based on proven radiobiological factors since the optimal methods of fractionation are unknown.

Radiosensitivity of tumours

Tumours are described as being radiosensitive or radioresistant, but this is a matter of degree. A radiosensitive tumour is destroyed by a relatively small dose of radiotherapy while a radioresistant tumour is unresponsive to doses which cause death of normal cells. Apart from the oxygen effect, the degree of differentiation of a tumour is of importance in radiosensitivity, an anaplastic tumour being in general more vulnerable than a well-differentiated tumour. The tolerance of the normal tissue in the region of a tumour is often the factor which limits treatment.

Chemotherapy

The demonstration of the significant antitumour effect of nitrogen mustard in 1946 led to intensive research in cytotoxic chemotherapy for cancer. Discovery of new and effective drugs has been accompanied by an increased knowledge of the biology of the normal cell and the cancer cell. Developments in cell kinetics have allowed the mode of action of anticancer agents to be studied and have led to rationalisation in the use and timing of drugs (Dorr and Fritz, 1980).

Gompertzian growth

When tumours are small, the cells divide more rapidly than when they are large. Tumour doubling time is short with small tumours and the growth frac-

tion is large because of the large number of proliferating cells in small tumours. When tumours become large, the tumour doubling time lengthens, the growth fraction decreases and the number of cells in the G0 resting phase increases. This biological pattern of alteration in cell numbers with time is known as Gompertzian growth. With small tumours, anticancer agents which are effective against proliferating cells are appropriate, while with large tumours the use of agents active against both proliferating and resting cells seems to be more rational. Drugs which are active against cells in the G0 phase are 'cycle non-specific' and drugs active in the stage where DNA synthesis occurs are 'S-phase specific'. Other drugs are active at the stage when mitosis occurs. Thus the action of drugs on a specific tumour depends on the proportion of proliferating and resting cells in the tumour.

In 1964, Skipper and his colleagues, on the basis of observations on L 1210 leukaemia cells in mice, demonstrated that a single malignant cell could proliferate and cause death. They also laid down a principle that the percentage of leukaemia cell populations of varying size killed by a cytotoxic agent was fairly constant. Thus cytotoxic agents kill not a certain fixed number of cancer cells, but a certain proportion of the total tumour cell mass irrespective of tumour size. Moreover, the proportion of tumour cells killed is closely related to the dose of the cytotoxic drug and the larger the number of tumour cells injected, the shorter the survival.

The cytotoxic effect of drugs is not specific to cancer cells, but as tumour cells have diminished ability for repair after damage compared with normal cells, while both normal and tumour cells are damaged by cytotoxic drugs, normal cells recover relatively quickly once the drug is discontinued. This advantage is used by administering antitumour chemotherapy in 'pulsed' or intermittent, rather than in continuous fashion.

After treatment, utilising the slower recovery of tumour cell populations, a second course of treatment should be given when the normal cell population has returned to its pretreatment value. In theory, it should be possible to eradicate all tumour cells in this way. If the interval between courses of treatment is too long, the tumour cell population has time to overcome its disadvantage of slower recovery and treatment becomes ineffective. When drugs are given too frequently, toxicity to normal cells occurs and there is insufficient time for restoration of the normal cell population to pretreatment values. Most modern cytotoxic programmes are based on this high-dose intermittent treatment.

Some concern exists about the possible carcinogenetic effect of anticancer drugs as many of them are carcinogenic in experimental animals (Harris, 1976), and the development of new cancers in patients treated with anticancer drugs is well-known (Davis *et al.*, 1975).

Patients with renal transplants who have been treated with immunosuppressive drugs have an increased risk of developing epithelial and connective tissue tumours, while epithelial changes, possibly premalignant, have been identified repeatedly in patients undergoing treatment with anticancer drugs (Schramm, 1970).

Low dose single agent chemotherapy was the earliest and most widely practised form of treatment. Although it has been of proven benefit in some forms of chronic leukaemia and ovarian tumours, it is intrinsically unsatisfactory because (a) it fails to utilise the kinetic differences in recovery between normal cells and tumour cells, (b) may lead to tumour cell resistance and (c) kills a smaller proportion of tumour cells than would a larger dose.

Combination chemotherapy

Because different drugs have different modes of action on the normal and tumour cells and because toxicity of drugs differs with different types of drugs, it should be possible to devise a combination of drugs which are synergistic in their antitumour effect without increasing toxicity. Combinations of two, three, four and even seven or eight drugs have been used in various cytotoxic regimens. While the use of a combination of drugs implies uncertainty about the sensitivity of a tumour to all the drugs, combination chemotherapy has been demonstrated to be far more effective than single agent therapy in many malignant diseases. In general, combined regimens are made up of drugs which are known to be effective against the tumour when used alone, which do not share undesirable side-effects and which have different modes of action against the cancer cell.

Adjuvant chemotherapy

In clinical practice cytotoxic chemotherapy was used at first for advanced malignant disease and only in recent years has it been used as an adjuvant to surgery or radiotherapy for potentially curable cancer. Even after apparently adequate treatment of the primary tumour, metastatic disease often occurs later and causes death. The idea that micrometastases were present, although undetectable, at the time of primary treatment, seems inescapable. Both the oxygenation and the growth fraction of cells are greater with smaller tumours; hence chemotherapy, in theory, would be expected to be more effective when dealing with a small tumour load than a large tumour mass. This type of therapy has been widely used in recent years and results of careful trials attesting its objective value are becoming available. There is no doubt, however, that many patients with malignant disease enjoy a long and recurrence-free survival after primary treatment.

Clinicians have been cautious in using adjuvant therapy on a wide scale, not because of doubts about its theoretical value, but because of (a) difficulty in selecting patients for such treatment (b) reluctance to treat unrecognised disease with powerful agents which have unpleasant and distressing side-effects and (c) the unknown, possibly harmful sequelae of long-term use of antitumour agents.

Agents used in cytotoxic chemotherapy

In 1966, antitumour agents were classified on the basis of their different effects on the kinetics of normal and neoplastic cells. Class I agents are non-specific in action affecting cells at all stages of the cell cycle as well as in the resting phase and having equal destructive effect on normal and cancer cells. Class 2 drugs are cell-cycle stage specific (CCSS) or phase-specific and affect the cell during the 5 phases of DNA synthesis. Resting cells, whether normal or tumorous, are not influenced by such drugs. These drugs are given in repeated doses so that all tumour cells become targets when they enter into the sensitive stage of the cell cycle. They are not given continuously because prolonged therapy places the normal cells at risk of destruction (as well as the tumour cells) when they enter the vulnerable S-phase of the cycle. Class 3 agents are cycle specific or cell cycle stage non-specific (CCSNS) and have a more destructive effect on proliferating than on non-proliferating cells. Cycle-specific drugs are given at high-dose and are administered relatively infrequently. If proliferating tumour cells are destroyed by Class 3 agents, resting $G0$ cells may be 'recruited into the cell cycle where phase-specific drugs would be effective.

Thus the combined approach of CCSNS and CCSS drugs may produce maximal cell kill. Valeriote and Edelstein (1977) apply generalisations for single-agent regimens:

1　CCSS drugs should be given in fractionated schedules or infusions.
2　CCSNS agents should be given in large single doses and scheduled intermittently.
3　Many courses should be scheduled if tumour cell populations of more than 10^4 cells are present. (A tumour mass of 1 cm diameter contains about 10^9 cells while a tumour containing 10^{12} cells weighs about one kilogram.)
4　Courses of treatment should be separated by intervals of at least 2 weeks to allow recovery of normal cells.

Although it might be more appropriate in the clinical context to divide the cytotoxic agents into phase specific and cycle specific drugs, it has become standard to group them into biochemical groups:

1 Alkylating agents
2 Antimetabolites
3 Antitumour antibiotics
4 Vinca alkaloids
5 Miscellaneous drugs

Alkylating agents

The cardinal features of an alkylating agent is the presence of an alkyl grouping (CH_2) capable of combining by covalent binding with other constituents of cells. Of the thousand or so alkylating agents which have been synthesised, perhaps a dozen are used in clinical practice as anticancer agents.

Nitrogen mustard. Nitrogen mustard was first used in clinical medicine in 1947. As with all alkylating agents, nitrogen mustard alkylates DNA at the guanine position and inhibits cell growth at the G2 phase. It acts rapidly and has a particular effect on lymphoid tissue. The toxic effects are considerable. Depression of the haemopoietic system, nausea, vomiting, diarrhoea and alopecia are commonplace. If injected outside the vein, it produces an intense local cellulitis and sloughing of the overlying skin may occur. Nitrogen mustard is widely used in lymphomas, chronic leukaemias and in bronchogenic, mammary and ovarian tumours.

Phenylalanine mustard (L-PAM, Melphelan) may be administered orally, intravenously or occasionally by intra-arterial injection for perfusing isolated organs or limbs. It has been widely used in multiple myeloma and in carcinoma of the testis and ovary, as well as in adjuvant therapy in mammary cancer. As with nitrogen mustard, depression of the bone marrow is its most marked toxic effect and it also produces hair loss and gastrointestinal disturbance.

Cyclophosphamide is converted into a biologically active metabolite in the liver by the action of hepatic enzymes. It is more selective in its actions than nitrogen mustard, probably because normal cells can detoxify the active metabolite more efficiently than can tumour cells. Although marrow suppression and gastrointestinal symptoms occur, they are less marked than with nitrogen mustard and thrombocytopenia is rarely a problem. Metabolites of cyclophosphamide produce inflammation of the bladder and haemorrhagic cystitis occurs. An interstitial type of cystitis can result, leading to fibrosis of the bladder wall and a contracted bladder. These complications can probably be avoided by ensuring adequate diuresis during therapy. Cyclophosphamide may also cause testicular atrophy and ovarian fibrosis. It is effective against lymphomas, leukaemias, and carcinoma of breast, ovary and bronchus.

Chlorambucil (Leukeran) is also active against lymphomas and leukaemias and also ovarian carcinoma, seminoma of the testis and Waldenstrom's macroglobulinaemia. Marrow toxicity is the major drawback to long-term therapy.

Thiotepa, derived from triethylene melamine, is used intraperitoneally to control ascites, and intrapleurally for malignant effusions. Like other alkylating agents it may cause marrow toxicity. As an intracavitary agent it is occasionally used in bladder tumours.

Busulphan (Myeleran) is an alkylating agent containing two sulphur atoms. Its principal use is in chronic myeloid leukaemia as its main effect is on granulocytes. Increased pigmentation of the skin occurs with the drug, but the main unwanted effect with long-term usage is interstitial pneumonitis leading to pulmonary fibrosis. Patients on this medication should have serial pulmonary function tests and chest radiographs. The drug is discontinued and steroid therapy commenced at the first evidence of deteriorating lung function.

Nitrosureas. Nitrosureas are sometimes effective against tumours which have failed to respond to alkylating agents or antimetabolites. Their mode of action is by inhibiting the synthesis of purine and its incorporation into DNA. They also appear to function as alkylating agents and are sometimes linked with them. BCNU (1,3-bis (2-chloroethyl-1-nitrosurea), CCNU (1-(2-chloroethyl)-3-cyclohexyl-1-nitrosurea and methyl CCNU (1-(chloroethyl)-3-(4-methyl cyclohexyl)-1-nitrosurea) are the three most widely used nitrosureas. Fat-soluble, they penetrate the blood-brain barrier, and their effect on marrow suppression is delayed when compared to the alkylating agents. They function by inhibiting the synthesis of nucleic acids and DNA. BCNU is given intravenously, but CCNU and methyl-CCNU may be given by mouth. They are used in the treatment of lymphomas and in malignancy of the gastrointestinal and respiratory systems. They may also be effective in primary and secondary brain tumours (*see* Chapter 40).

All the nitrosureas may cause hepatic and renal damage and lead to alopecia and gastrointestinal tract upset.

Antimetabolites

These drugs interfere with nucleic acid synthesis and are cell cycle specific having greatest effect against proliferating cells.

Methotrexate. After folic acid has been converted to folinic acid, dihydrofolate is converted to tetrahydrofolate by the action of dehydrofolate reductase.

Methotrexate is a competitive inhibitor of this enzyme and its action results in defective nucleic acid synthesis. The toxic effects of methotrexate on the marrow, skin, gastrointestinal tract and liver may be offset by administration of folinic acid (Citrovorum factor). The drug is absorbed by the gastrointestinal tract and in part bound to plasma proteins. It is excreted unchanged in the urine. It may also be given by intramuscular or intravenous injection and is sometimes administered intrathecally, since it crosses the blood-brain barrier in unpredictable fashion. The drug is used widely in many conditions; it is particularly valuable in the treatment of choriocarcinoma where cure can be brought about. It is used in leukaemias and in tumours of the breast, bronchus, testis and bone. It is also used in severe psoriasis. Resistance to its effects can occur either by interference with the transport of the drug or an accumulation of dihydrofolate reductase activity.

5-fluorouracil. The active compound into which 5-fluorouracil is converted after metabolism is 2- deoxy -5-fluorouridine. The drug prevents DNA synthesis by interfering with the enzyme thymidylate synthetase which catalyses the production of thymidylic acid. Thymidylic acid is an essential step in the synthesis of pyrimidine. The drug is given in intravenous doses of 10–15 mg/kg for about 5 days. It is poorly absorbed by the gut; it may be administered topically or by intra-arterial perfusion. It is metabolised in the liver. Its greatest effect is in gastrointestinal and gynaecological malignancies as well as in bladder tumours. Mild to severe gastrointestinal tract disturbances are frequent and the drug may also cause hair loss, dermatitis increased pigmentation of the skin and myelosuppression.

Cytosine arabinoside by inhibiting the enzyme DNA polymerase interferes with pyrimidine synthesis. It is used in the treatment of leukaemia and its toxic effects on the bone marrow and gastrointestinal tract limit its use.

6-mercaptopurine inhibits purine synthesis, is also used in leukaemia and choriocarcinoma and is toxic to the marrow and gut. It is often used with allopurinol which lowers serum uric acid because the rapid rate of cellular destruction by 6-mercaptopurine may result in serious hyperuricaemia.

Antitumour antibiotics

Actinomycin-D, like many of the antimitotic antibiotics, is derived from strains of Streptomyces. By binding irreversibly with DNA strands it inhibits RNA synthesis. It is administered intravenously and its main use has been in the treatment of Wilm's tumour, soft tissue sarcomas, choriocarcinoma and testicular tumours. It is often combined with radiation therapy particularly in patients with Wilm's tumour. It is toxic to the skin, marrow and gut.

Mithramycin is a potent cytotoxic agent used particularly in patients with testicular tumours and in the management of hypercalcaemia which has been unresponsive to other forms of treatment. It can cause severe thrombocytopenia and a haemorrhagic tendency. The toxic effects are more likely to occur in patients who are in poor general condition.

Bleomycin, given intramuscularly or intravenously is used in testicular and squamous cell tumours, particularly of the head and neck, and for some lymphomas. It is toxic to skin and gastrointestinal tract, but relatively little marrow suppression occurs. A transient hypersensitivity pneumonitis, responsive to steroid therapy, is associated with it and interstitial pneumonitis leading to fibrosis also occurs with prolonged use.

Daunorubicin is used in leukaemia, is toxic to skin, hair, marrow and gastrointestinal tract. In addition it is cardiotoxic, especially in elderly patients or those with pre-existing cardiac disease. It causes cardiomyopathy.

Doxorobicin has similar toxic effects to daunorubicin and is probably even more cardiotoxic. Its effect on the heart is probably dose related and reversible at lower doses. It is used in a wide variety of solid tumours such as lymphomas, soft tissue sarcomas and carcinomas, especially breast cancer.

Streptozotocin, also derived from species of streptomyces, is a nitrosurea and has proven to be effective in malignant endocrine tumours. Given intravenously or by regional arterial perfusion, it is effective against insulinoma and carcinoid tumours. It has little effect on the marrow, but is toxic to the gut and kidney.

Vinca alkaloids

The vinca alkaloids are derived from the periwinkle (*Vinca rosea*). They act as cytotoxic agents by binding with cytoplasmic precursors of the protein spindle in the S phase of the cell cycle.

Vincristine is used in the treatment of leukaemias and lymphomas. It has neurotoxic effects causing paraesthesiae and peripheral neuropathy and paralysis. Administration should be discontinued once neurological symptoms or signs appear. Alopecia and constipation, probably due to a neurotoxic effect on bowel motility are common. Vincristine is given intravenously and is usually combined with other cytotoxic drugs.

Vinblastine is used in Hodgkin's disease and in other solid tumours. It is much less neurotoxic than vincristine, but its suppressive action on the bone marrow is more prominent.

Miscellaneous drugs

Procarbazine is a monoamine oxidase inhibitor. Its mode of action is unclear, but it is useful in Hodgkin's disease, almost always in combination with other drugs. It is also used in melanoma. It causes myelosuppression and gastrointestinal upset and may lead to mental confusion.

Cis-platinum diaminedichloride was introduced into clinical practice after its inhibitory effect on bacteria and transplantable tumours had been verified in the laboratory. It is toxic to the marrow, gastrointestinal tract and nervous system. It is ototoxic and may cause renal tubular damage, an effect which may be reduced by infusing crystalloid solutions with the drug. It is of greatest value in ovarian and testicular tumours.

Razoxane (ICRF-159) is related to ethylenediamine tetra-acetic acid (EDTA). It probably acts in the G2 phase of the cell cycle and is used in leukaemias, non-Hodgkin's lymphomas and advanced colorectal carcinoma. Its main toxic actions are on the bone marrow and to a lesser degree on the gut.

Imidazole carboxamide (DTIC) probably affects the cell in the G2 phase. *In vitro* it inhibits DNA synthesis in bacteria. In man its mode of action may involve dimethylation in the liver leading to release of a carbonium ion. It is given intravenously and is of value in melanoma, soft tissue sarcoma and Hodgkin's disease, where it is usually given in combination with other drugs. Vomiting, diarrhoea and myelosuppression occur with this drug which also produces a fever and eosinophilia in some patients.

L-asparaginase activates the conversion of the essential amino-acid asparagine to aspartic acid and ammonia. The normal cell has the ability to synthesise asparagine, but malignant cells need exogenous asparagine for their growth. In practice, 1-asparaginase is of limited value because of hypersensitivity reactions associated with it and because resistance to the drug develops. Its main use has been in acute lymphoblastic leukaemia.

The use of specific chemotherapeutic agents in the management of brain tumours is discussed in Chapter 40.

Regional chemotherapy

High concentration of cytotoxic chemotherapeutic agents can be delivered to the tumour-bearing area by means of intra-arterial perfusion. Systemic toxicity should be reduced by this approach if the drug is rapidly metabolised or taken up by the tumour. Several systems for intermittent and continuous arterial perfusion have been devised. Extracorporeal equipment can be used to perfuse the isolated limb with drugs. The main artery and vein to the area are isolated and perfusion is maintained by a pump oxygenator and blood warmer. In general, regional perfusion techniques have proven to be disappointing in the treatment of malignant disease and their use is confined currently to melanoma of the limbs, primary or secondary liver tumours and carcinoma of the head and neck. In these cases, intra-arterial infusion can be strikingly, but inconsistently, effective. Hepatic arterial ligation and infusion chemotherapy is followed by regression of hepatic tumours in about 50% of patients with metastatic liver disease. Intra-arterial infusion pumps have been refined. Portable pumps can be carried in a shoulder holster with little inconvenience to the patient and special pumps for subcutaneous implantation are now available.

Selected chemotherapeutic regimens in the management of certain tumours

HODGKIN'S DISEASE

MOPP regimen				
Nitrogen Mustard	6	mg/m²	i.v.	Days 1 to 8
Vincristine (Oncovin)	1.4	mg/m²	i.v.	Days 1 and 8
Prednisone	40	mg/m²	oral	Days 1 to 14 (incl.)
Procarbazine	100	mg/m²	oral	Days 1 to 14 (incl.)

Vinblastine 6 mg/m² i.v. may be used instead of vincristine unless there is severe marrow depression
6 to 12 courses at monthly intervals are usually given.

RESISTANT HODGKIN'S DISEASE

ABVD programme				
Adriamycin	25	mg/m²	i.v.	Days 1 and 14
Bleomycin	10	mg/m²	i.v.	Days 1 and 14
Vinblastine	6	mg/m²	i.v.	Days 1 and 14
DTIC*	375	mg/m²	i.v.	Days 1 and 14

* Imidazole carboxamide.

NON-HODGKIN'S LYMPHOMA

1. COP

Cyclophos- phamide	650–1000	mg/m^2	i.v.	Day 1
Vincristine (Oncovin)	1.4	mg/m^2	i.v.	Day 1
Prednisone	40	mg/m^2	oral	Days 1 to 5 (incl.)

Repeat course every 3 weeks for 12 courses.

2. BACOP

Bleomycin	5	mg/m^2	i.v.	Days 15 to 22
Adriamycin (Doxo rubicin)	25	mg/m^2	i.v.	Days 1 and 8
Cyclophos- phamide	650	mg/m^2	i.v.	Days 1 and 8
Vincristine (Oncovin)	1.4	mg/m^2	i.v.	Days 1 and 8
Prednisone	60	mg/m^2	oral	Days 15 to 28 (incl.)

Repeat course every 4 weeks for 12 courses.

ADVANCED MAMMARY CARCINOMA

1. CMF

Cyclophos- phamide	100	mg/m^2	oral	Days 1 to 14 (incl.)
Methotrexate	40	mg/m^2	i.v.	Days 1 and 8
5-Fluorouracil	600	mg/m^2	i.v.	Days 1 and 8

Repeat monthly for 1 year.

2. CMFVP

Cyclophos- phamide	60	mg/m^2	oral	Daily for 1 year
Methotrexate	15	mg/m^2	i.v.	Weekly for 1 year
5-Fluorouracil	300	mg/m^2	i.v.	Weekly for 1 year
Vincristine	0.625	mg/m^2	i.v.	Weekly for 10 weeks
Prednisone	30	mg/m^2	oral	Daily for 14 days
→	20	mg/m^2	oral	Days 15 to 28 (incl.)
→	10	mg/m^2	oral	Days 29 to 42 (incl.)

3. LMF

Chlorambucil (Leukeran)	10	mg	oral	Days 1 to 10 (incl.)
Methotrexate	100–200	mg	i.v.	over 2 hours followed by
5-Fluorouracil	750	mg	i.v.	over 2 hours
Leucovorin	15–30	mg		orally6 and 12 hours after infusion.

TESTICULAR TUMOURS

1.

Cis-platinum	20	mg/m^2	i.v.	Daily for 5 days Repeat course at 3 weeks and 6 weeks
Vinblastine	0.2	mg/kg	i.v.	Daily for 2 days
Then	0.3	mg/kg	i.v.	every 3 weeks for 2 years
Bleomycin	30	units	i.v.	weekly for 12 weeks

2.

Vinblastine	4	mg/m^2	i.v.	Day 1
Bleomycin	20	mg/m^2	i.v.	Daily for 7 days
Cyclophos- phamide	600	mg/m^2	i.v.	Day 1
Actinomycin-D	1	mg/m^2	i.v.	Day 1
Cis-platinum	120	mg/m^2	i.v.	Day 8

Maintenance dose of Vinblastine 4 mg/m^2 and Actinomycin-D 1 mg/m^2 every 3 weeks and Chlorambucil 4 mg/m^2 orally daily for 2 of every 3 weeks.

ASSESSMENT OF SUBJECTIVE RESPONSE TO CYTOTOXIC CHEMOTHERAPY

The Karnofsky scale

Normal	100%
Minor signs and symptoms	90%
Normal activity with effort	80%
Unable to carry out normal activity, but can care for self	70%
Occasional help required for personal needs	60%
Disabled	50%
Requires considerable aid and medical care	40%
Severely disabled and hospitalised	30%
Very sick; active support therapy needed	20%
Moribund	10%
Death	0%

RADIATION UNITS AND MEASUREMENTS

	Old unit	SI unit	Special name (symbol)	Relationship
Exposure	röntgen (R)	C kg^{-1}	——	1 R = 258 × 10^{-6} C kg^{-1} 1 C kg^{-1} = 3.876 × 10^{3}R (approx.)
Absorbed dose Kerma*	rad (rad)	J kg^{-1}	gray (Gy)	1 rad = 0.01 Gy 1 Gy = 100 rad 1 rad = 1 cGy
Dose equivalent	rem (rem)	J kg^{-1}	sievert (Sv)	1 rem = 0.01 Sv 1 Sv = 100 rem
Activity	curie (Ci)	s^{-1}	becquerel (Bq)	1 Ci = 37 × 10^9 Bq 1 Bq = 27.03 × 10^{-12}Ci (approx.)

* Acronym for 'Kinetic Energy Released per unit MAss'.

References

Allen D.W., Cole P. (1972). Viruses and human cancer. *New Engl. J. Med*; **286**:70.

Armstrong B., Stevens N., Doll R. (1974). Retrospective study of the association between use of Raufolfia derivatives and breast cancer in English women. *Lancet*; **ii**:672.

Carbone P.P., Kaplan H.S., Musshoff, K., Smithers D.W., Tubiana M. (1971). Report of the committee of Hodgkin's disease staging classification. *Cancer Res*; **31**:1860.

del Regato J.A. (1977). Pathways of metastatic spread of malignant tumours. *Semin. Oncol*; **4**:33.

Dorr R.T., Fritz W.L. (1980). *Cancer Chemotherapy Handbook*. London: Henry Kimpton Publishers.

Freedman, S.O. (1976). Antigens in tumours. In *Scientific Foundations of Oncology* (Symington T., Carter R.L., eds.) pp. 505. London: Heinemann Medical.

Gross L. (1978). Viral etiology of cancer and leukaemia: a look into the past, present and future. *Cancer Res*; **38**:845.

Harris C.C. (1976). The carcinogenicity of anticancer drugs: a hazard in man. *Cancer*; **37**:1014.

Herbst A.L., Ulfelder H., Poskanzer D.C. (1971). Adenocarcinoma of the vagina: association of maternal stillboestrol therapy with tumour appearance in young women. *New Engl. J. Med*; **284**:878.

Hoover H.C.Jr., Ketcham A.S. (1975). Metastasis of metastases. *Amer. J. Surg*; **130**:405.

Huebner R.J., Todaro G.J. (1969). Oncogenes of RNA tumour viruses as determinants of cancer. *Proc. Nat. Acad. Sci. U.S.A*; **64**:1087.

Lukes R.J., Butler J.J. (1966). The pathology and nomenclature of Hodgkin's disease. *Cancer Res*; **26**:1063.

Lynch H.T. (1976). *Cancer Genetics*. Illinois, Springfield: Charles C. Thomas.

Morton D.L. (1974). Cancer immunotherapy: an overview. *Semin. Oncol*; **1**:297.

Roth J.A., Silverstein M.J, Morton D.L. (1976). Metastatic potential of metastases. *Surgery*; **79**:669.

Schramm G. (1970). Development of severe cervical dysplasia under treatment with azathioprine (Imuran). *Acta Cytol*; **14**:507.

Scott M.T. (1974). Corynebacterium parvum as an immunotherapeutic anticancer agent. *Semin. Oncol*; **1**:367.

Skipper H.E., Schabel F.M.Jr., Wilcox W.S. (1964). Experimental evaluation of potential anticancer agents. XII. On the cirteria and kinetics associated with curability of experimental leukaemia. *Cancer Chemother. Rep*; **35**:1.

Smith D.C., Prentice R., Thompson D.J., Herrmann W.L. (1975). Association of exogenous estrogen and endometrial carcinoma. *N. Engl. J. Med*; **293**:1164.

Stein R.S. (1978). Staging laparotomy in Hodgkin's disease: a critical appraisal of its value. *South Med. J*; **71**:1553.

Stewart S.E., Mitchell E.Z., Whang J.J. *et al.* (1969). Viruses in human tumours. J. Hodgkin's Disease. *J. Natl. Cancer Inst*; **43**:1.

Stewart A., Knealem G.W. (1970). Radiation dose effects in relation to obstetric x-rays in childhood cancers. *Lancet*; **i**:1185.

Sugarbaker E.V., Ketcham A.S. (1977). Mechanisms and prevention of cancer dissemination: an overview. *Semin. Oncol*; **4**:19.

Symington T., Carter R.L., eds (1976). *Scientific Foundations of Oncology*. London: Heinemann Medical.

Temin H.M. (1971). The protovirus hypothesis: speculations on the significance of RNA – directed DNA synthesis for normal development and for carcinogenesis. *J. Nat. Cancer Inst*; **46**:3.

Valeriote F.A., Edelstein M.B. (1977). The role of cell Kinetics in cancer chemotherapy. *Semin. Oncol*; **4**:217.

Further reading

Copeland E.M. (1983). *Surgical Oncology*. New York: John Wiley.

Holland J.F., Frei E. (1982). *Cancer Medicine*. Philadelphia: Lea and Febinger.

De Vita V.T., Hellman S., Rosenberg S. (1982). *Cancer. Principles and Practice of Oncology*. Philadelphia, Toronto: J.B. Lippincott.

del Regato J.A., Spjut H.J. (1977). *Ackerman and del Regato's Cancer Diagnosis: Treatment and Prognosis*. St. Louis: C.V. Mosby Co.

Breast

NIALL O'HIGGINS

Development

In the 6th week of embryonic life a thickened ridge of ectoderm appears and extends from the axillae to the groins. At stages along this milk line areas of increased thickening appear. In man the lower ridge and thickening disappear and the pectoral ridge becomes more substantial to form the rudimentary pectoral breast. At about the 20th week the breast develops solid cords which become canalised and supported by a connective tissue stroma. These cords become confluent at the areola and when channels are developed, they open at tiny orifices at the nipple. At birth some 20 channels open at the rudimentary nipple, which becomes slightly everted. The areola develops some modified subaceous glands of Montgomery. In the first week of extrauterine life, about 70% of infants develop swelling in the breast and secrete a small amount of cloudy fluid. There is an associated increase in vascularity of the breast. These changes are probably due to increased secretion of prolactin, stimulated by the reduction in the infant's blood stream of circulating maternal oestrogens. In the second and third week of life the swelling subsides and the secretion ceases. Thereafter the breast remains quiescent until adolescence. At adolescence, there is often an enlargement of one or both breasts in the male which persists for months or years before the breast returns to its prepubertal stage. Throughout the remainder of life, under normal circumstances, the male breast undergoes little or no further change apart from the deposition of fatty tissue which increases with age. The female breast, however, undergoes great change at puberty and in adult life related to the menstrual cycle, pregnancy, lactation and the menopause.

Physiological changes in the female breast

Adolescence

In the prepubertal stage, the nipple and areola become slightly raised and everted from the surrounding skin to form a 'bud'. These changes are associated with dilatation and elongation of the duct system, each duct drawing with it an outer sleeve of connective tissue as it stretches. The fatty tissue in the stroma of the breast becomes displaced backwards to lie against the pectoral fascia. Breast lobes, separated from each other by fascial sheaths, develop in relation to each main duct. At ovulation, with the development of a branching system of ducts, several lobules are formed in each lobe and early acinar formation occurs. Lobular and acinar formation remains underdeveloped in multiparous women. These changes occur under the influence of ovarian oestrogens and progestogens and of trophic hormones from the pituitary gland. A slight increase in pigmentation occurs in the areola and smooth muscle becomes apparent in the nipple and under the areola.

Adult resting gland

Tiny ducts surrounded by alveoli remain rudimentary before pregnancy. The ducts become interconnected with each lobe to form larger ducts. The confluence of the 20 or so ducts, each emanating from a lobe of the breast, occurs at the milk sinus, immediately beneath the areola. From the milk sinus several short excretory ducts open on to the surface of the nipple. The excretory ducts and milk sinus are lined by squamous epithelium and the collecting ducts by cuboidal or columnar epithelium.

Under the influence of many hormones which affect the organ, the breast undergoes changes during the menstrual cycle. Direct stimulation from the pituitary and hypothalamus occurs due to growth hormone, oxytocin and prolactin, while indirect stimulation from the anterior pituitary takes place under the influence of TSH, releasing thyroxine from the thyroid gland, FSH, releasing ovarian oestrogens and progesterone and ACTH causing secretion of adrenal oestrogen. After the first week of the menstrual cycle the female breast increases in size progressively until menstruation occurs. Most of the increase is due to fluid retention and increased vascularity but there is also a transient proliferation of lobules and parenchyma. In the premenstrual period the breasts often become painful, tender and nodular to palpation. With the onset of menstruation the swelling begins to subside and a week later the breasts become softer and smoother to palpation and the tenderness usually disappears.

Pregnancy and lactation

From the start of pregnancy, the breast increases in size, the nipple becomes more prominent and more deeply pigmented. The vascularity of the organ increases, veins become prominent, the overlying skin becomes stretched so that striae appear, Montgomery's follicles in the areola become prominent and raised from the surface as tubercles and the breasts become tender, engorged and nodular to palpation. The ducts in the lobules and alveoli develop, acini are formed at ends of ducts and secrete a small amount of clear or opalescent fluid known as colostrum. This secretion increases progressively throughout pregnancy. After delivery, the acinar cells increase in size and the acini fill with milk. Under the stimulus of suckling the myoepithelial subareolar cells allow the milk flow from the nipple. After lactation the lobular tissue involutes to an extent and the areola subsides.

Menopause

At and after the menopause the entire breast undergoes involution in a gradual fashion. The lobules shrink and become fibrosed so that distinction between parenchyma and stroma is lost, although a few isolated lobules remain scattered throughout the breast. Fat becomes deposited as the glandular element involutes and the breasts become more pendulous as the supportive stroma of connective tissue and interlobular fascia becomes lost. The breast becomes soft, smooth and homogenous and the tenderness associated with hormonal effects disappears.

Anatomy

The breast, being a modified intradermal gland, lies predominantly on the pectoral fascia overlying the muscles of the upper chest wall. It extends from the second to the sixth ribs; its medial boundary is at the lateral margin of the sternum and it extends at its upward and outward extremity into the axilla across the anterior axillary lines as the axillary tail of Spence. The axillary tail extends around the lateral border of the pectoralis major muscle where it dips under the deep fascia. The cyclical premenstrual mastodynia associated with overall enlargement is most noticeable in this part of the breast, confined as it is by its fascial envelope.

Arterial supply

Three groups of arteries supply the breast. The perforating branches of the internal mammary artery sends branches through the first four intercostal spaces lateral to the sternum. These vessels pierce the medial fibres of the pectoralis major muscle, supply the medial part of the breast and form an anastomotic network with the other arteries. The lateral thoracic artery, a branch of the axillary artery, runs along the lateral border of the pectoralis minor muscle and sends branches to enter the breast on its lateral side. The thoraco-acromial, another branch of the axillary artery, pierces the clavipectoral fascia. Its mammary branches enter the breast from above and anastomose with the other arteries. Smaller contributions to the arterial supply of the breast come from the intercostal and subscapular arteries and from the superior branch of the axillary artery.

Venous drainage

The superficial veins of the breast drain mainly into the internal mammary veins by perforating branches through the upper intercostal spaces. In the upper part of the breast, superficial veins drain into the superficial veins of the lower cervical area. The deep veins drain to three main areas, firstly to the internal mammary veins, secondly to the axillary vein by several small tributaries and thirdly to the posterior intercostal veins which anastomose freely with each other.

Lymphatic drainage

A rich lymphatic meshwork exists in the breast. Lymphatics in the skin overlying the breast communicate freely with each other, having no valves, and open out into the subareolar plexus. From this plexus, lymphatic channels course in the periductal planes along with draining veins of the breast towards the lymph nodes. The major drainage is towards the axillary nodes of which there are between 50 and 60 (Fig 39.1). Many lymph nodes lie within the breast substance in the upper outer quadrant of the breast. Lymphatics from the lower outer quadrant of the breast drain into the lateral lower axillary nodes while the areola, the upper outer quadrant and the axillary tail of the breast drain into the superior and medial axillary nodes. The inferior and lateral nodes drain into the superior and medial nodes by way of second lymphatic channels.

The apical nodes extend to the infraclavicular nodes. Lymphatics from the posterior part of the breast drain into the interpectoral (Rotter's) nodes between the pectoralis major and pectoralis minor muscle and thence to the apical axillary, supraclavicular or the uppermost internal mammary nodes. The medial half of the breast is drained by lymphatics which pass through the upper intercostal spaces to internal mammary nodes, four or five in number, which lie along the internal mammary artery. Part of the areola also drains to these nodes. From the apical and internal mammary nodes, lymph is carried to the node at the junction of the internal jugular and subclavian veins and thence into the venous system. Retrograde tumour extension in lymphatics is often associated with visible or palpable enlargement of the supraclavicular nodes. The internal mammary nodes also connect with the anterior mediastinal nodes and lymphatics from the lower inner quadrant of the breast may drain into the system on the anterior rectus sheath.

Breast examination

Self-examination

Routine self-examination of the breasts has been widely advocated through channels of public communication and education. Advice and guidance of this kind are based on the belief that malignant disease can be detected sooner by routine self-examination than by the accidental finding of an abnormality in the breast. In 9 patients out of 10 with cancer of the breast, the patient herself finds the lesion. By careful routine self-examination, small lumps and minor degrees of asymmetry can be detected. As the prognosis for carcinoma of the breast is directly related to the size of the tumour, efforts have been directed at detecting lesions when they are small. It has not been demonstrated clearly yet whether such public education has had a major beneficial effect in improving the survival statistics. Such instruction by way of radio, television and printed matter must be carried out with extreme care lest harmful and unnecessary anxiety be engendered in those women who are overly anxious. To be helpful, self-examination should be carried out during the 2nd week of the menstrual cycle and the breasts should be examined in a systematic fashion.

Examination

Inspection

Inspection of the breasts is a most important part of the physical examination, as lesions which may be over-

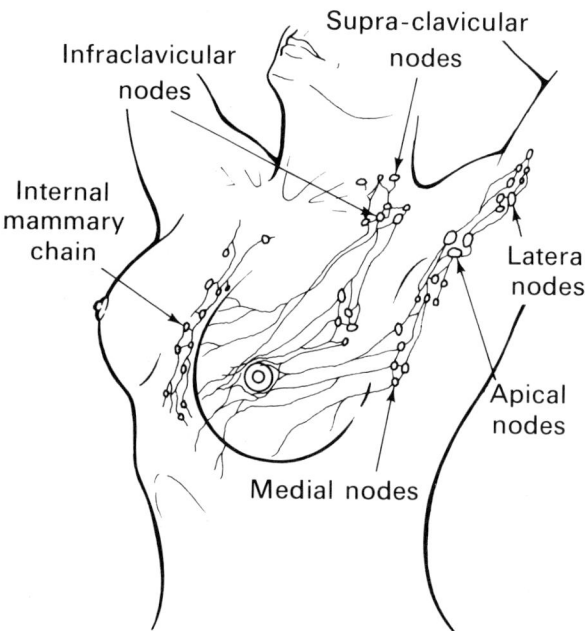

Fig 39.1 Lymphatic drainage of the breast.

looked on palpation, can be detected easily by inspection. The breasts should be looked at directly from in front at eye-level, rather than from the side of an examination couch. The patient should be examined with her arms by her side and inspection is continued while she is asked to raise her arms fully above the head. During this movement, minor degrees of asymmetry, dimpling or tethering of the skin can be detected and movement of the breast on the pectoral muscle and chest wall can be identified. Abnormalities of the nipple, such as retraction, discharge, ulceration or encrustation are noted. The skin over the breast is examined for signs of thickening, oedema, erythema, ulceration or prominent veins.

Palpation

Because some lumps in the breast are more easily detectable when the patient is sitting forward, palpation should be carried out with the patient in the upright as well as in the supine position. Gentle palpation of the breast involves systematic examination of each quadrant and the central part using the volar aspect of the fingers. When the patient is reclining, the breast can be examined more readily if she is asked to turn slightly away from the examiner with the arm held above the head on the examination couch. This position allows the axillary tail of the breast to be examined easily. If a lump is detected in the breast, the overlying skin is pinched gently to ascertain whether it is tethered or not to the lump. The mobility of the lesion on the pectoralis major muscle from side-to-side and from above downwards is then assessed. The muscle is put on tension by asking the patient to abduct the arm and to press the hand into the flank. The mobility of the lump should be checked when the muscle is both contracted and relaxed. Should the mobility of a lump be restricted when the pectoralis major muscle is contracted, tethering or fixity of the mass to the muscle is implied. If a mass in the breast is adherent to the chest wall, its mobility is restricted even when the pectoralis major muscle is relaxed.

Physical examination of the regional lymph nodes is routine during the time of examination of the breast. The medial, anterior, posterior and lateral walls of the axilla are first examined followed by examination of the apical area. During axillary examination, the patient's forearm rests on the examiner's forearm, so that the muscles about the shoulder joint are relaxed. The presence or absence of palpable axillary nodes is noted. If nodes are palpable, an assessment must be made as to whether they are fixed to each other or to adjacent structures. The infraclavicular and supraclavicular nodes are then examined, usually and most conveniently while standing behind the patient. When examining the right axilla, the medial and anterior walls

are palpated with the left hand, using the volar aspect of the extended fingers. The lateral and posterior walls are examined with the right hand. The apical nodes are evaluated last of all as this is the most uncomfortable part of the examination for the patient and the most difficult area to assess for the examiner. If left until the end of assessment, the patient tends to be more relaxed and cooperative.

Mammography

A mammogram, or soft tissue radiograph of the breast, has become a valuable adjunct to physical examination in evaluating the presence or absence of malignant disease in the breast. In recent years, mammographic techniques have become refined so that definition of clinically undetectable lesions is possible. Improved techniques have resulted in a reduced radiation dose being required and mammography is becoming less expensive. Mammography can be carried out in the conventional way with ordinary film or by xeroradiography, which involves exposure to x-rays using an aluminium plate with charged metal particles of selenium. The resultant image can be transferred to photographic paper or to conventional radiographic film. The radiation dose of xeroradiography is lower than with conventional mammography, but in recent years, low dose film mammography has become available so that the radiation doses with both methods have become comparable. The advantages of xeroradiography are said to be that the edge of a lesion is better defined (edge enhancement), the retromammary space is well visualised and the axilla and its contents are often more clearly seen (Fig 39.2).

Mammography is especially useful in older women with large breasts which contain a higher content of fatty tissue than in the young. Radiological identification of lesions is easier in fatty breasts while in young women with dense breasts, mammograms are more difficult to interpret and are, therefore, of more limited use. The interpretation of mammograms requires special experience but a correct evaluation can be made in about 90% of cases. False positive and false negative results occur occasionally. Characteristics of benign mammary lesions on mammography are that the abnormalities are circumscribed, homogeneous and surrounded by a layer of fat. If calcification is present, it is coarse or ring-shaped, indicating ductal or vascular calcification. In cancer of the breast, mammography reveals a lesion which is poorly defined. The edges are irregular and spiculated. Calcification, when present, is fine, stippled and arranged in small clusters. The overlying skin is often thickened and pulled inwards and there may be associated retraction of the nipple. Dilated veins may be seen in the vicinity of the lesion. When carcinoma of the breast is found

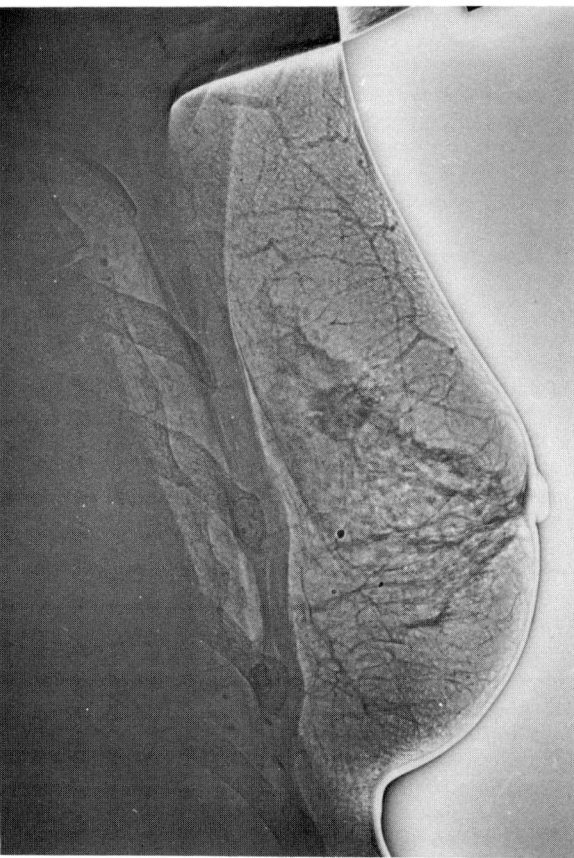

(a)

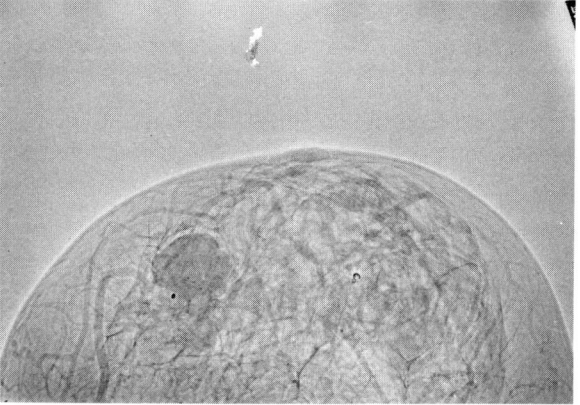

(b)

Fig 39.2 Xeromammograms of breast. (a) Showing malignant tumour mass (lateral view). (b) Showing a tumour with speckled calcification and dilated veins consistent with carcinoma and coarse benign calcification around the tumour (cranio-caudal view).

on mammography alone, in the absence of any clinical evidence of disease, axillary lymph node involvement by tumour is rare. In addition to its use in screening for cancer of the breast, discussed later, mammography is also of value in the following groups of patients:

1   Those with proven mammary carcinoma, to check if (a) there is a second tumour in the same breast or (b) another primary neoplasm in the opposite breast.
2   Patients with marked fibroadenosis, where nodularity in the breasts makes evaluation of abnormalities difficult and in whom there is a slightly increased risk of cancer compared to those without fibroadenosis.
3   Those over the age of 35 with large breasts in whom small lesions are often impalpable.
4   Patients who have had previous mastectomy, who form a group at the highest risk of developing a new cancer.
5   Other patients at special risk, discussed later.
6   In patients with excessive anxiety, the added reassurance of a mammogram may be of value.
7   In patients with metastatic carcinoma to axillary or cervical lymph nodes or to distant organs, where the site of the primary lesion is unknown.
8   Patients with abnormalities of or discharge from the nipple or with changes in the skin or doubtful areas in the breast on palpation.
9   In some patients with mastodynia.

Apart from its limitations in the younger woman, the use of mammography is restricted by its possible hazards. Repeated mammograms carry the theoretical risk of delivering a dangerous level of ionising radiation to the breast and of inducing neoplasia. The possible carcinogenic effects of repeated mammography have resulted in continuing changes and refinements in technique so that the radiation dose delivered to the breast per mammogram is being reduced constantly.

Thermography

Malignant tumours of the breast are generally associated with an increased temperature in the overlying skin. The radiation of heat from the skin can be detected by an infrared camera which can be used to scan the skin of the breast and record temperature changes on the surface. The technique requires a special temperature-controlled room so that fluctuations in the ambient temperature can be eliminated. While thermography is non-invasive and safe, it is unreliable as a method of screening because of the high incidence of false positives and false negatives. Benign conditions of the breast, such as inflammatory disease are also associated with an increased temperature in the overlying skin and malignant conditions may not reveal any demonstrable alteration in temperature in the skin of the breast. Thus, thermography may indicate malignant disease where it does not exist and fail to reveal tumours where they are present. It is, therefore, insufficiently reliable to justify widespread use.

Sonography

The use of specialised sonographic equipment has allowed improved diagnostic accuracy for lesions in the breast by the use of ultrasound. The diagnostic accuracy exceeds 90% in skilled hands and the method is free of hazard and can be carried out repeatedly.

Various *screening* programmes have been carried out in different countries and the frequency with which cancer is detected at screening depends upon the methods used and the selection of women screened. The average detection rate by screening is about 6 per thousand at the initial examination. Screening of large populations for mammary cancer is feasible, but requires special clinics. The examinations can be carried out by trained non-medical personnel.

Routine screening of female population over the age of 40 on a regular basis for signs of carcinoma of the breast is an expensive undertaking and there is still some disquiet about the possible hazards of repeated radiation to the breast. The theoretical risk of radiation-induced cancer of the breast exists and there is yet no agreement as to whether or not a safe dosage of radiation can be accepted. The risk of inducing cancer by radiation is likely to be greater in younger women. The National Cancer Institute *ad hoc* working groups on mammography in screening for breast cancer calculated that in a woman age 35 with one rad radiation exposure, there is an increased lifetime risk of breast cancer of less than 1%. For older patients the risk is much less. On this assumption it has been calculated that the screening of women under the age of 50 would result in 18–30 breast cancers per 100 000 women screened. There is a calculated increased incidence of 0–12 cancers per 100 000 women screened over the age of 50 with an estimated 10–14 lives saved per 100 000 women screened. With improving techniques the dose to the breast can be reduced to below 0.8 rads per examination for conventional mammography and to 0.5 rads for xeroradiography. With these lower doses, the carcinogenic risks in women over 50 years of age are probably negligible.

Benign breast disease

Congenital abnormalities

Congenital absence of the breast (amazia) is rare and may be unilateral or bilateral. Accessory breast tissue commonly occurs and may be found anywhere along the milk line from the axilla to the groin. Such accessory tissue is most often in the axilla. Accessory nipples are common and, if there is underlying breast tissue, mammary ducts may open on to the surface of the nipples and lactation may occur after pregnancy.

Disparity in the size of the developed breast is quite common and may be quite marked. The nipples may be bifid and this may interfere with breast feeding. Massive hypertrophy of the breasts occasionally occurs at puberty and may require surgical treatment by mammary reduction.

Fat necrosis

This condition presents in the breast as a hard lump which does not change in size. In about 50% of patients there is a history of injury with associated bruising of the overlying skin. The condition is commonest in middle-aged or elderly women and may be impossible to distinguish from cancer on clinical grounds. The overlying skin may be oedematous and tethered. The centre of the mass may undergo liquefaction and there is often surrounding infiltration with lymphocytes and plasma cells. Excision of the lump is required to confirm the diagnosis.

Acute bacterial mastitis

This condition usually occurs in the puerperium and is due to staphylococcal or streptococcal infection. The organisms penetrate through a mucosal or dermal abrasion in the nipple area or may supervene on rupture of a milk duct. Cellulitis often occurs and with suitable antibiotic treatment, the condition often resolves. When a localised mass occurs, there are systemic signs of abscess formation and surgical drainage is advised. At operation, multiple abscess cavities are often encountered, separated from each other by the fibrous septa of the breast. Adequate drainage is required and involves the breaking down of all loculations. Abscesses can be associated with extensive destruction to the breast tissue. Deep abscesses in the breast are very uncommon in women who are not lactating. Should they occur, an underlying tumour should be suspected. In some localised cases it may be possible to excise the abscess. Subareolar abscesses can occur at any age and are not necessarily associated with lactation. They are often related to minor degrees of anatomical abnormality in the nipple and occur frequently in women with retractile nipples. They tend to recur after incision and result in a mammillary fistula. Excision of the duct or ducts from which the track arises is important to prevent recurrence.

Chronic abscesses are rare in the breast and may be tuberculous. Areas of induration and chronic sinus formation opening to the surface are usually found in this condition, which is secondary to tuberculosis of the lung or chest wall.

Fibroadenoma

Fibroadenomas are benign tumours of the breast and present most commonly in young women after puberty. In 15% of patients, they are multiple. While they may be multilobular on palpation, they are usually smooth, hard and rounded. They are not adherent to the skin or underlying structures and are freely mobile within the breast and usually not tender. They are well encapsulated and homogeneous. Pericanalicular and intracanalicular types have been described. The pericanalicular type is dense and fibrous while the intracanalicular type is larger and less homogeneous. Fibroadenomas can be induced by the administration of oestrogen and occur in postmenopausal women after oestrogen therapy.

Fibroadenosis

This term refers to a spectrum of conditions, characterised clinically by discomfort, generalised or localised nodularity in the breasts often more noticeable in the premenstrual period and by discrete single or multiple cystic masses. The microscopic features of the condition are also varied, but there are signs of epithelial hyperplasia of the ducts, sometimes with papillary or cystic formation. There is also hyperplasia of the periductal connective tissue and of the fibrous stroma of the breast. If these changes are exaggerated there may be loss of orientation of the epithelial cells and the condition is known as sclerosing adenosis. It may be difficult to distinguish this from carcinoma and the condition may in itself be premalignant.

Fibroadenosis is also known as fibrocystic disease of the breast or cystic hyperplasia. The changes seem to be an extreme form of the normal changes which occur during the menstrual cycle related to the influences of many hormones on the breast. Patients complain of mastodynia or of a lump in the breast. The pain is often unilateral, on examination there is frequently widespread nodularity in both breasts. It is particularly com-

mon for the nodularity to be most marked in the upper outer quadrants of the breasts, which are deep to the deep fascia. The nodularity, usually most marked just before the menstrual period, may subside in mid-cycle. Localised, discrete, hard, mobile lumps in the breasts usually represent cysts. These cysts may be small or large and single or multiple. They are usually so tense that fluctuation is rarely possible on clinical examination. Transillumination cannot be demonstrated unless the cyst is large. Because both fibroadenosis and carcinoma are common and may coexist, it is impossible to be certain about the diagnosis of fibroadenosis when the patient presents with a single lump, until biopsy has been carried out.

Cysts of the breast

Cysts associated with fibroadenosis may be large or small. Cysts may be treated by needle aspiration provided that certain guidelines are followed:

1 The cystic aspirate is not blood-stained.
2 The cyst does not refill.
3 There is no residual lump.
4 There are no suspicious cells on cytological examination.

If the fluid is blood-stained or if there is a residual lump, open biopsy should be carried out. Recurrent cysts should also be treated by excision. Cytological examination of breast cyst fluid is rarely positive for cancer cells, but the occasional abnormal result justifies this practice. Needle aspiration is carried out through a 21-gauge needle using a 20 ml syringe. The patient is re-examined two weeks later to check that the cyst has not refilled and is examined periodically afterwards. The condition of fibroadenosis nearly always improves after the menopause.

Breast pain

The management of patients with breast pain associated with mammary dysplasia is often difficult. Physical examination and mammography should be carried out to exclude serious disease. The reassurance that no serious disease is present often helps the patient to cope with the pain. Simple analgesia may be tried and, if the pain is predominantly premenstrual, a diuretic, such as frusemide may be given daily for a week or 10 days before the period is due. Should this be ineffective, progestational agents may be tried for a week before the period and repeated monthly for 3 months. Inhibitors of follicle-stimulating hormone (FSH) have also been used for mastodynia and are effective in about 50% of patients. Bromocriptine therapy (2.5 mg twice daily) has been used recently for pain in the breast and has also been found to be effective in about 50% of patients, even if the serum prolactin value is not elevated. The agent, Danazol, which selectively inhibits gonadotrophin release, is useful in patients with mastalgia, abolishing pain in about 90% of patients if it is taken for six months or more. It diminishes nodularity and may reduce the rate of large cyst formation. It produces amenorrhoea in some 20% of women. It causes weight gain and nausea in some patients and is at present a very expensive agent. If intractable, oophorectomy is effective in abolishing pain in the breasts in patients with benign disease, but should be reserved for those who are within a few years of the menopause. Subcutaneous mastectomy with internal prostheses is carried out in some hospitals for this complaint. Care must be taken to ensure the emotional stability of the patient before this procedure is undertaken as those with neuropsychiatric disorders may continue to complain of similar symptoms afterwards.

Galactocele

This condition follows lactation and is due to occlusion of a milk duct beneath the areola. Inspissated milk and desquamated epithelium causes the obstruction. A spherical mass, less than 1 cm in diameter is found immediately deep to and at the periphery of the areola. The lump is often tender. At first, it contains milk and later the contents become viscid and consist of a greenish-yellow sterile material.

Mammary ductal ectasia

Mammary duct ectasia is a common condition characterised by unilateral or bilateral discharge from the nipple. It usually occurs after the age of 40 years. The discharge may be serous or thick and may be colourless, yellow or green and usually emanates from several ducts. There is often some erythema of the surrounding nipple, which may become retracted as a result of the condition. There is often some induration of the tissue beneath the nipple. The milk ducts in the subareolar area are dilated and full of liquid or semisolid material. The degree of dilatation varies and as the condition progresses, the dilatation extends deeper into the breast tissue. The periductal tissues are involved by subacute inflammation and the consistent appearance of plasma cells in the periductal fat led to the alternative name of plasma-cell mastitis. Whether the condition is primarily an inflammatory one with secondary dilatation of the ducts or whether ductal obstruction leads to an inflammatory process is unclear. It may be impossible to distinguish the condition from carcinoma

on clinical grounds, particularly if the condition is unilateral and if it is associated with retraction of the nipple or oedema of the skin. A subareolar exploration of the breast with removal of a segment of tissue is commonly required.

Lipoma

As elsewhere, lipomas can occur in the breast, although they are comparatively rare. They are difficult to diagnose on clinical grounds, but may be suspected when there is a single, discrete, smooth, rounded, mobile and softish mass with an otherwise normal breast. Excision is required to confirm the diagnosis and to exclude malignant disease. Pseudo-lipoma refers to a condition due to cancer of the breast. A scirrhous tumour may cause retraction of the fatty tissue in the breast, which may then appear as a mass or localised swelling. It is important to bear this possibility in mind when a lipoma of the breast is encountered.

Galactorrhoea

Excessive secretion of prolactin, usually due to a microadenoma, gives rise to a bilateral milky discharge from multiple ducts in both breasts. The condition may be suspected when a milky discharge continues after breast feeding has stopped or when the discharge appears outside of the puerperium. Galactorrhoea occurs in less than 50% of women with hyperprolactinaemia. Raised levels of prolactin occur not only with prolactin-secreting tumours of the pituitary, but also in hypothalamic disorders which result in a decrease in prolactin-inhibiting factor (PIF), renal disease, hypothyroidism, malignant neoplasms which occasionally produce prolactin, and with a number of drugs, including phenothiazines, metoclopramide, reserpine, methyldopa, oestrogens, monoamine oxidase inhibitors and cimetidine. The treatment of galactorrhoea depends on the cause. If there is a large pituitary tumour, treatment may involve radiation or operation on the pituitary. In a small tumour, bromocriptine in a dose of 2.5 mg t.d.s. will contain the symptoms.

Intraduct papilloma

Unilateral blood-stained or serous discharge from a single duct in the breast is usually due to an intraduct papilloma. The condition is due to hyperplasia of ductal epithelium. It is unifocal within a duct, in contrast to the diffuse papillomatosis which occurs in fibroadenosis. The papillomas are often palpable as rounded nodules adjacent to the nipple. Pressure on the nodule is often followed by a discharge of blood or serous material from the related duct. Treatment is by micro-dochectomy. A fine probe is passed from the discharging orifice, an incision is carried down on to the probe, the papilloma is identified and the entire duct removed. In some centres ductograms are used to locate the lesion accurately, especially where no lump is palpable.

Cystosarcoma phylloides

This condition is a variant of a fibroadenoma, occurring typically in middle-aged women. It may become very large and is often referred to as a giant fibroadenoma. It may recur after local excision and may become so large that the overlying skin becomes thick, stretched and red. Venous distension in the skin occurs with the mass which may grow rapidly. The central area of these lesions is often cystic or necrotic. Wide, local excision is required for treatment. About 20% of these tumours are malignant. Re-excision of local recurrence is advised as radiotherapy is not generally effective. Blood borne metastases, usually to the lung, may occur in about one-third of patients with malignant cystosarcoma.

Incisions for the breast

For removal of lesions in the vicinity of the nipple a periareolar incision is best as it heals well leaving a scar which becomes scarcely noticeable (Fig 39.3). In microdochectomy operations, a radial incision is made in the nipple and areola along the line of a duct which has previously been defined by insertion of a probe along its length. For excision biopsy of lumps, curved incisions in the breast along the lines of Langer heal well, but may interfere with the planning of subsequent mastectomy incisions if the lump is malignant. If mastectomy is likely to follow an excision biopsy, a radial incision is preferable. When excising the lump considered to be malignant for biopsy, an ellipse of skin should be removed if the lesion lies adjacent to the skin.

The classical Halsted-Meyer radical mastectomy involves an oblique elliptical incision from the xiphisternum to the anterior aspect of the shoulder 2 cm above the axillary border of the pectoralis major muscle. The incision involves a wide ellipse around the tumour and the areola. Modifications include a less extensive upper component, the incision being taken to the level of the coracoid process, and a shorter lower end of the incision describing a curved course rather than tapering to a point. With modified radical mastectomy, the elliptical skin incision is placed more trans-

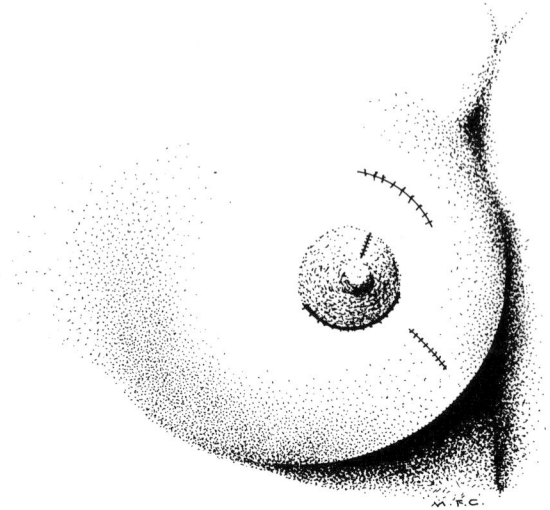

Fig 39.3 Incisions for the breast.

versely and good exposure to axillary contents is achieved if the arm is elevated and held across the trunk. A simple mastectomy, transversely placed ellipse results in a scar which is horizontal. Subcutaneous mastectomy, for extensive benign disease, leaves the nipple and areola and is carried out through a curved, peripheral submammary incision in the inferior part of the breast.

Breast cancer

Carcinoma of the breast is the commonest malignant condition occurring in women in the United Kingdom and is the commonest cause of death from cancer in women. Of all female patients with cancer, 25% have primary breast cancer. If the current incidence of mammary carcinoma continues, one of thirteen women in the United Kingdom will develop cancer of the breast at some stage during her lifetime. About 13000 women in England and Wales die of cancer of the breast annually. The standardised mortality rates for cancer of the breast have increased over the past 50 years, the rate now exceeding 25 per 100000 of the female population. In women between 40 and 50 years of age, it is the commonest cause of death and it is only in women under 35 and over 75 that its role as the major fatal cancer in women is exceeded by leukaemia and colorectal cancer respectively (Fig 39.4).

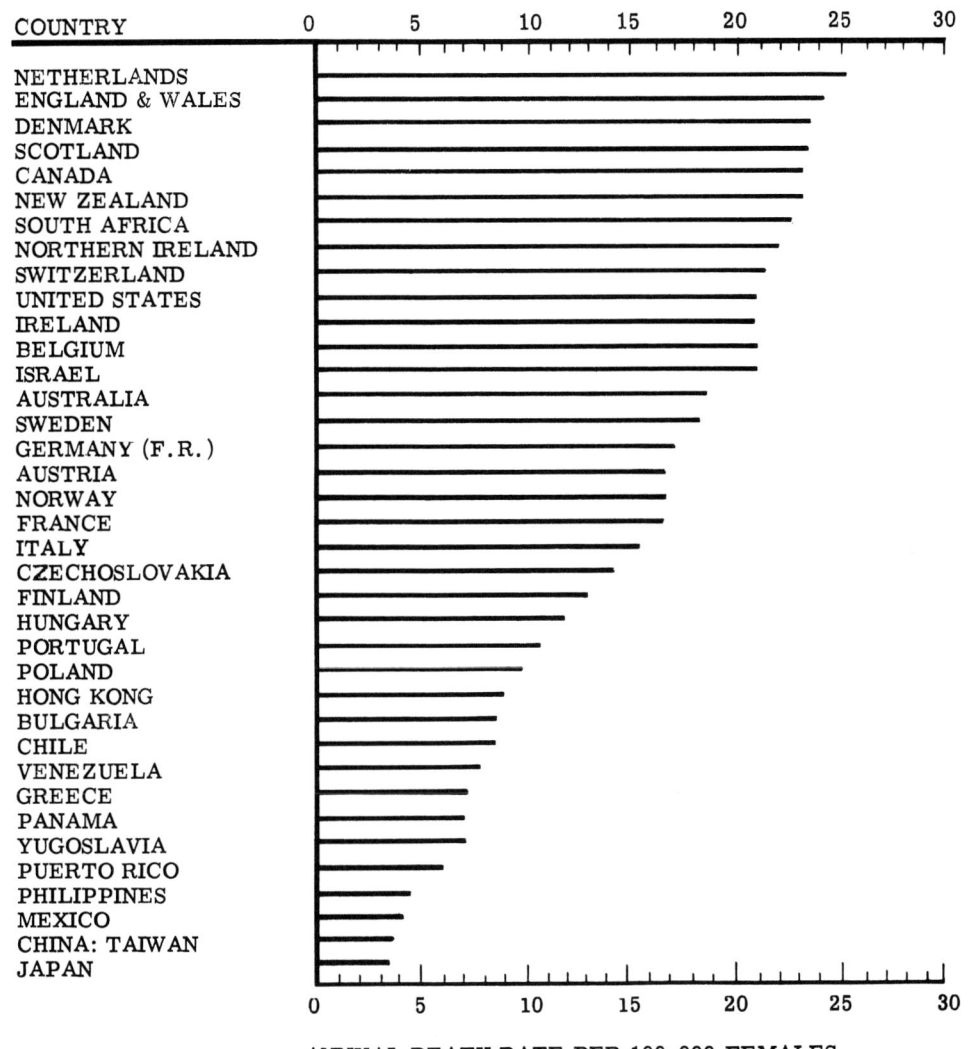

Fig 39.4   Cancer of the breast. Annual death rate per 100 000 females.

Aetiological and risk factors

Sex

Cancer of the breast is overwhelmingly commoner in women than in men; slightly less than 1% of cancers of the breast occur in men.

Age

The disease is rare under the age of 20. Between the ages of 20 and 45 there is a steady rise in incidence to about 125 new cancers diagnosed annually for every 100 000 women aged 20–45. Between the ages of 45 and 55, the incidence reaches a plateau. This plateau is maintained for about 10 years, when the incidence rises again to the age of 80. The break in the rising slope (Clemmensen's hook) suggests that hormonal factors occurring at the menopause contribute to the development of this tumour.

Race

Racial differences in the incidence of cancer of the breast are well known, the standardised annual death rate from breast cancer per 100 000 women being less in Japan compared with the 25 in England and Wales. This striking disparity is probably determined by environmental factors, because the mortality rate for cancer of the breast in Japanese women who live in the United States of America is higher than in those living in their homeland. Moreover, the mortality rates for Japanese women born in the United States is higher than for those born in Japan.

Geographical location

The highest death rate for carcinoma of the breast has been reported from the Netherlands and the disease is much commoner in Europe, North America and Australia than it is in Africa and Asian countries.

Family history

There is little doubt that the daughter of a woman with mammary cancer runs a two- to three-fold risk of developing mammary carcinoma. When the daughters of patients with cancer of the breast develop such tumours themselves, they do so on an average 12 years earlier than their mothers. No constant pattern of inheritance has been identified and the risk among relatives is variable. The risk appears to be increased in relatives whose cancers are diagnosed in premenopausal, but not postmenopausal, life. When cancer of the breast is bilateral the risk of the disease to relatives is higher and may be increased to nine-fold. The risk of relatives of patients with breast cancer developing the tumour is highest for daughters, lower for sisters and least for mothers.

Genetic factors

Klinefelter's syndrome. This condition, associated with an extra X chromosome is characterised by gynaecomastia, small testes, azoospermia and high urinary excretion of gonadotrophins in men. Cancer of the breast in these patients is said to be 66 times commoner than in normal men.

Wet cerumen. Since both the breast and the wax glands in the ear are modified sebaceous glands, the cerumen in the ear has been investigated in patients with cancer of the breast. Whether one has wet or dry wax in the ear is genetically determined and the wet type of wax is associated with increased risk of cancer of the breast. The predominant type of wax is wet in women in the Western hemisphere and dry in Japanese women where cancer of the breast occurs much less commonly.

Multiple hamartoma syndrome (Cowden's disease). Cowden's disease is characterised by soft tissue hamartomas and is associated with an increased risk of cancer of the breast. It is a genetically transmitted condition and follows an autosomal dominant inheritance.

Diet

Mammary tumours in the rat, induced by dimethylbenzanthracene (DMBA) are promoted when the animals are fed with a high fat diet and there is a direct relation between the consumption of fat and the mortality from cancer of the breast in women. In a study carried out by Carroll (1975), involving 39 countries this relationship was demonstrated clearly. Moreover, there is some evidence that overweight postmenopausal women are more prone to develop breast cancer than those of normal weight.

Pregnancy and lactation

Pregnancy at an early age confers some protective effect against the development of cancer of the breast, but when the first pregnancy occurs after the age of 35, this protection is lost. Elderly primipara run a higher risk of developing cancer of the breast than do nulliparous women. Breast feeding and lactation seem to have no protective influence.

Menstrual history

Prolonged ovarian activity may be a risk factor for cancer of the breast. The risk of the disease is higher in women who have had an early menarche and a late menopause, compared with women who have a late menarche and early menopause. Moreover, oophorectomy at a young age markedly reduces the risk, but ovarian ablation after the age of 40 years confers no protection.

Thyroid function

There appears to be a relationship between thyroid status and cancer of the breast, although the basis for this connection is unclear. There seems to be a higher incidence than expected of thyroid disease in patients with cancer of the breast and there appears also to be a higher frequency of mammary cancer in patients on thyroid medication. Allied to this is the finding that patients with cancer of the breast as a group may be subclinically hypothyroid.

Previous history

The patient most at risk of developing carcinoma of the breast is the patient who has had a previous mastectomy. While there may be difficulty in deciding whether the second cancer is a new primary or a metastasis, the risk of developing a new primary in the opposite breast is about 1% per year of survival. Therefore, a new primary is more likely to develop in patients whose mastectomy had been carried out for tumours of good prognosis, as these patients may live long enough to develop a second neoplasm on the opposite side. The incidence of such new tumours depends on the diligence with which they are sought, the detection rate being consistently higher in centres where serial radiology is carried out in addition to clinical examination at follow-up.

Patients with cancer of the breast have a two-fold risk of developing endometrial carcinoma and patients with cancer of the uterine corpus have a two-fold risk of developing cancer of the breast. There is an association between cancer of the breast and cancer of the ovary. Tumours of other sites, such as thyroid, larynx and bone have been found more frequently than would be expected in breast cancer patients, although firm evidence for these associations is difficult to demonstrate.

Benign breast disease

Because both cancer of the breast and fibroadenosis or fibrocystic disease are common, the two conditions often co-exist in the same patient. In appears that the risk of a patient with fibroadenosis developing cancer of the breast is about two to three times that of the general female population. It is not known what particular element in fibroadenosis accounts for the risk, but it is likely that the proliferative elements constitute the risk factor. Epithelial hyperplasia or epitheliosis, particularly if associated with papillomatosis, may lead to cancer. A spectrum of proliferative development from flat ductal epithelium through hyperplasia, epitheliosis, papillomatosis, carcinoma *in situ* to invasive cancer can be demonstrated. Whether this progression occurs in the development of all infiltrating cancers of the breast or not is speculative.

Hormonal metabolism

The oestrogens, oestrone and oestradiol, are known to be carcinogenic for mammary cancer in rats while another oestrogen, oestriol, is not. There have been suggestions that patients with carcinoma of the breast excrete a lower fraction of oestriol compared to oestradiol and oestrone. Androgen metabolism may play a part, the relatively low urinary excretion of the androgen metabolite, aetiocholanolone, compared to the total 17-hydroxycorticosteroid (17-OHCS) excretion providing the basis of the discriminant function devised by Bulbrook and his colleagues (1960). Using the formula 80–80 (mg 17-OHCS/24 h + μg aetiochol-

anolone/24 h), a positive or negative result was obtained. Patients without breast cancer almost always showed a positive result while over half the patients with carcinoma of the breast had negative discriminants. If such low urinary excretion of aetiocholanolone precedes development of carcinoma of the breast, it might be used as a test to detect groups of people at risk of the disease. Such an investigation is being carried out in the island of Guernsey.

Whether or not prolactin is involved in the induction of cancer of the breast, is unknown. Serum levels of the hormone have not been shown to differ in patients with cancer of the breast and control populations, but it does stimulate the growth of experimentally induced cancer in rats.

Viruses

Bittner observed that spontaneous cancers of the breast in mice could be transmitted to their offspring. This transmission occurred through the milk. The milk factor responsible for the tumour was shown to be a virus and became known as the mouse mammary tumour virus (MMTV). Transmissible mammary cancers have also been observed in the milk of monkeys and rat, and virus particles have been found in human milk. Whether this virus is oncogenic is unknown. No correlation exists between breast feeding and an increased risk of developing cancer of the breast. Moreover, the incidence of mammary cancer has remained the same or increased in those countries where the incidence of breast feeding has declined.

Radiation

There is general agreement that ionising radiation can induce cancers of the skin, thyroid and bone. There is probably a two-fold risk of cancer of the breast in women who have previously undergone radiation to the breast for benign disease. The question of the risk of radiation to the breast has become highly important since the advent of breast cancer screening clinics using mammography. The maximum safe dose of radiation has not been determined, but the carcinogenic affects of radiation are likely to be greater in younger women. The National Academy of Sciences has reported that when carrying out mammography, a skin dose of less than one rad in a woman over 50 is unlikely to represent a significant risk.

Pathology

The histological classification of carcinoma of the breast is divided conveniently into invasive and non-invasive tumours of the mammary ducts and lobules,

Paget's disease of the nipple, sarcoma and other rare types of malignancy, including cancer metastatic to the breast.

Invasive ductal carcinoma

Infiltrating carcinoma of the mammary ducts is by far the commonest form of cancer of the breast, occurring in 80% of patients. These tumours are poorly defined, and firm to very hard on clinical examination. At time of presentation they may be large or small and adherent to the skin or pectoralis major muscle. They may be well- or poorly-differentiated on histological grounds and the degree of surrounding fibrosis is extremely variable. When cut, these tumours feel hard and gritty, have a greyish appearance and are called scirrhous.

Papillary carcinoma

Papillary carcinomas account for about 1% of mammary malignancies. They are often multilobular and soft. They sometimes contain a central cystic cavity. A papillary network of cells, usually well-differentiated, is arranged in a pattern so that differentiation from benign papillomatosis may be difficult. The prognosis for patients with this type of cancer is somewhat better than for invasive ductal carcinoma. The tumours are well defined and may become quite large before axillary lymph node metastases occur.

Colloid carcinoma

This condition is also associated with a better prognosis than is usually the case in cancer of the breast. It is an uncommon type of carcinoma, making up some 2% of all mammary malignancies. It occurs typically in older women and may grow to a very large size before detection. It is gelatinous on cutting, due to extensive mucin production.

Medullary carcinoma

Some 5% of mammary carcinomas are of the medullary type. The tumour is rounded and soft to palpation. When cut, it bulges like a fibroadenoma. The lesion is well defined and is made up of large cells arranged in sheets or cords. There is a rich surrounding infiltrate of lymphocytes and plasma cells. When the lymphocytic infiltrate is predominant, lymph node metastases to the axilla occurs less commonly than in other types of cancer and the prognosis is better. Not all types of medullary carcinoma have a better prognosis and local immune factors may play a part in containing the spread of this tumour.

Non-invasive ductal cancer

Carcinomas of the mammary duct may be non-infiltrative when diagnosed. This type of tumour accounts for about 1% and is curable. The diagnosis is often difficult to distinguish from benign ductal hyperplasia, the histological difference being the degree of nuclear pleomorphism and the numbers of mitotic figures seen with a rather disorderly pattern to the cells. A form of this type of tumour is the comedocarcinoma, where the duct is totally occluded by neoplastic cells. Areas of non-infiltrating intraductal carcinoma may be found in scattered foci throughout the breasts and may be associated with an area of infiltrating carcinoma in the vicinity. Intraductal carcinomas often contain areas of microcalcification, visible on mammography as tiny specks of calcification arranged in groups or clusters.

Lobular carcinoma

Invasive. About 6% of invasive cancers of the breast are lobular tumours. They contain small cells distributed in a linear or concentric fashion. Areas of non-invasive lobular carcinoma *in situ* often appears in the area and the two types of tumour are related. The prognosis for invasive lobular carcinoma is similar to that of invasive ductal cancer.

Lobular carcinoma *in situ*. This is a microscopic lesion, often visible on mammography by fine speckled calcification. The lobules are enlarged and the ducts dilated. There are few mitoses and the condition affects the opposite breast in more than half of the patients. Another feature of the condition is that it is multifocal within the breast in about 75% of those in whom it occurs.

Paget's disease of the nipple

Paget's disease accounts for about 1% of all carcinomas of the breast. Patients present with a unilateral eczema-like scaling lesion of the nipple, at times moist and at times dry and encrusted. The condition usually occurs in postmenopausal women. The condition is due to a primary carcinoma of the terminal mammary ducts in the nipple with associated Paget's cells in the adjacent skin. These cells are large with clear cytoplasm and are considered to be intradermal metastatic cells from the underlying tumour, which is usually of the intraduct type. Even where the underlying tumour is invasive, the prognosis is better than average.

Sarcoma

Sarcomas rarely occur in the breast and must be distinguished from cystosarcoma phylloides which, although locally infiltrating, rarely metastasise and are otherwise known as giant fibroadenomas. About 20% of these are truly malignant producing metastatic deposits in the lungs and bone as well as extending locally. The malignant form of the tumour does not usually metastasise to the axillary lymph nodes and is generally unresponsive to radiotherapy.

Inflammatory carcinoma

This condition has the clinical features of inflammation with redness, swelling and tenderness in the overlying skin. The swelling is due to occlusion by tumour cells of the dermal lymphatics. The tumours are often poorly differentiated and the prognosis is worse than for most other types of mammary cancer.

Metastatic deposits

Metastatic deposits in the breast occur rarely from tumours such as melanoma. Lymphomas are sometimes deposited in the breast tissue and metastatic cancer, often bilateral is occasionally seen in patients with cancer of the prostate, especially those treated with oestrogens.

Screening

In an attempt to improve the results of treatment for primary cancer of the breast, attention has been directed to methods of earlier diagnosis. Cancer in a breast is clearly present for some time before it becomes discernible clinically. In an attempt to detect cancer in the 'silent period', mass screening programmes have been set up in selected areas. By screening for mammary cancer is meant the investigation of women who believe themselves to be free from symptoms and signs of mammary disease. The screening methods that have been most widely used have been the combination of physical examination and mammography. It should be stressed that screening by clinical examination alone or by mammography alone is dangerously misleading as tumours may be overlooked by either method. When physical examination is combined with mammography, the risk of overlooking tumours is less than 1%.

A prospective study was started in 1963 to find out whether earlier detection of breast cancer was possible by screening methods and, if so, whether such earlier diagnosis was followed by improved survival. Investigation was carried out by the Health Insurance Plan of New York (HIP) under contract with the National Cancer Institute. 62 000 women, aged between 40–64 were studied in paired groups of 31 000 each. Half of the patients served as a control group and were followed through the HIP records while the other 31 000 women,

the study group, had physical examination and mammography carried out at the outset of the study and annually for 3 years. After 7 years of follow-up, 70 patients in the study group had died of cancer of the breast, while 108 women in the control group had died of this disease. After 9 years of follow-up this one-third reduction in mortality had been maintained. Twenty per cent of all cancers were not detected by clinical means but seen on mammography only and 22% were identified on clinical examination only. This stresses the need for combining the two modalities of investigation. Over 70% of the cancers detected by screening were associated with uninvolved axillary lymph nodes at the time of operation, while only 46% of the control patients had axillary nodes which were free of tumours. While it is likely that the improved results in patients whose tumours were detected by screening can be attributed to earlier diagnosis, it is possible that the earlier diagnosis in the screened group did not alter the natural outcome of the disease, but merely allowed doctor and patient to be aware of the disease at an earlier stage. In this study, the apparent benefits of screening were confined to women over the age of 50 (Strax, 1978).

Clinical features

Lump in the breast

In over three-quarters of the patients with cancer of the breast, the first clinical feature is a lump. This is usually found accidentally during bathing or dressing, but may be found during routine self-examination or routine clinical examination by a medical practitioner. In nine cases out of ten, the lump is first detected by the patient. While in most instances the mass is painless, the presence of pain or tenderness by no means excludes cancer, as some 15% are tender. The predominant site for a tumour is in the upper outer quadrant of the breast. The fact that about 45% of cancers occur in this region is probably due to the fact that there is more breast tissue in this quadrant than the others. About a quarter of the tumours occur in the central area of the breast, while malignant tumours are infrequent (about 5%) in the lower inner quadrant.

Skin abnormalities

Retraction of the skin overlying a lump strongly suggests that the lesion is malignant. The skin may demonstrate major degrees of puckering which is seen more clearly when the patient elevates her arms. Minor degrees of skin dimpling or tethering may easily be overlooked unless sought carefully. Close inspection of the breasts at eye-level may reveal slight degrees of asymmetry which may call attention to an underlying tumour. While this type of skin tethering is typical of carcinoma, it is not pathognomonic as it occurs also with fat necrosis, Mondor's disease and tuberculosis. The nipple may be retracted by a tumour and it is important to distinguish between a retracted and retractile nipple. Unilateral nipple retraction of recent origin is usually due to cancer, but may also be due to duct ectasia.

Inflammatory carcinomas may produce reddening and thickening of the overlying skin with small pits visible in the oedematous skin (*peau d'orange*). The same appearance occurs in the absence of inflammation and is due to obstructive lymphopathy of the dermal lymphatics. This results in swelling of the skin except in the areas where the breast tissue is fixed to the skin by Cooper's ligaments. These are tiny fibrous strands which connect the breast lobules to the skin. Because of their insertion in the skin, no swelling occurs at the site of attachment while the skin around the ligaments is swollen. This is another explanation for *peau d'orange*.

Large tumours may be associated with distended or prominent veins coursing in the skin of the breast and advanced lesions may ulcerate. Paget's disease presents with a unilateral nipple discharge and encrustation.

Discharge from the nipple

A unilateral blood-stained discharge from the nipple, if not due to trauma during breast feeding, is most often related to intraduct papilloma or carcinoma. It is important to ascertain whether the discharge is coming from one or many ducts. Exploration and excision of a single duct (microdochectomy) is an excellent operation for diagnosing and treating an intraduct papilloma. When a bloody discharge occurs in the middle-aged or elderly woman, cancer of the breast is more likely than when it occurs in the younger age group. A small intraduct carcinoma (2 to 3 mm) or papilloma may be detectable in the subareolar area.

Deep fixation

Some advanced tumours may present at a stage when the tumour is fixed or tethered to the underlying pectoralis major muscle or to the chest wall. Fixation to the pectoralis major muscle can be confirmed when mobility of the tumour is restricted, when the muscle is contracted, but unrestricted when the muscle is relaxed. When a tumour is adherent to the chest wall, its mobility is limited whether the pectoralis muscle is relaxed or not.

Regional lymphadenopathy

As cancer commonly spreads to the axillary lymph nodes, enlargement of these nodes is a common finding. Systematic examination of the medial, lateral, anterior and posterior walls of the axilla should be carried out together with examination of the apex of the axilla. In addition, the infraclavicular and supraclavicular lymph nodes should be examined. The regional lymph nodes may be mobile or fixed to each other or to adjacent structures. With advanced tumours, the entire upper limb may be swollen, in which case the axillary lymph nodes, though heavily infiltrated by tumour, may be impalpable.

Distant metastases

Sometimes carcinoma of the breast is first identified when patients present with signs of metastatic deposits in the lung, bones, liver, peritoneal cavity, pleura, skin or brain.

Confirming the diagnosis

While the diagnosis of primary cancer of the breast may be made with a certain degree of confidence on clinical grounds, histological or at least cytological proof is required before treatment is planned. Such a tissue diagnosis can be made by needle cytology (ABC) or needle histology, using a Tru-Cut or an air powered drill. Tissue biopsy, as carried out in the Tru-Cut or drill methods, allows the histologist to describe the type of tumour. Another type of biopsy is the excision biopsy with or without immediate frozen section analysis. An immediate frozen section diagnosis following excision of the mass allows the surgeon to proceed with mastectomy while the patient is anaesthetised for the excision biopsy. Such a system allows rapid treatment of the patient, but has the drawback of preoperative uncertainty, which is often a considerable additional strain on the patient and her family. In addition, unless all patients with suspicious lumps in the breast have routine comprehensive investigation for asymptomatic metastases, the 'frozen section ? proceed to mastectomy' policy does not allow thorough preoperative routine clinical investigation.

Fine needle biopsy (ABC)

Needle biopsy using no. 18 gauge needle and a 20 ml syringe allows aspiration of cells for cytological examination. A skilled cytologist can give a definite diagnosis of malignant disease and this investigation, widely used for the aspiration of cysts of the breast, can be carried out readily in the outpatient department. Even in the best hands, false negative and false positive results occur. False negative results occur when the fine needle misses the tumour and an unrepresentative specimen is obtained. No difficulty occurs as a result of a false negative cytological report, provided that the clinician realises that excision biopsy of the lump must be carried out. A greater problem arises with the occasional false positive diagnosis, when mastectomy may be carried out on cytological appearance of cancer cells in a needle aspirate and where no tumour is found in the mastectomy specimen.

Large bore needle biopsy and histology

The use of the large bore needle biopsy, such as the Tru-cut needle or the air-powered drill has the advantage over the fine needle aspiration in that the histological structure of the tumour can be discerned and reported before treatment. Both these techniques can be done in the outpatient department and require an intradermal injection of local analgesic. A small incision is made in the skin to allow the needle to be manipulated to the level of the tumour. In many cases, the large calibre needle is found to be distinctly uncomfortable by the patient because pressure may be required to penetrate the tumour. The air-powered drill, using a trephine of 1.5 mm internal diameter and a cutting edge, is less uncomfortable as the rapid rotation of the needle (5000 rpm) allows the trephine to slice through the tumour without pressure. The drill is controlled by manipulation of a trigger with the finger. A core of tissue can be obtained by applying a 20 ml syringe to the trephine and by aspirating as the trephine is withdrawn.

Either of these methods allows the pathologist to make a statement of the type and differentiation of a tumour and is not associated with any false positive result. It should be emphasised that a negative or benign result from a needle biopsy does not relieve the surgeon of the responsibility of removing a distinct lump within the breast. The advantage of preliminary needle biopsy diagnosis is mainly a logistic one, as it allows the surgeon to explain and discuss the diagnosis and treatment with the patient and her family. It eliminates the additional worry for the patient engendered by doubt as to whether she will recover from the anaesthetic with or without her breast, permits as extensive a search for metastatic deposits by preoperative investigations as is thought justifiable and allows operating lists to be planned without the uncertainty that surrounds frozen section analysis.

The question of dissemination of tumour as a result of invasive needle biopsy arises. A theoretical risk of dissemination exists with all types of biopsy, whether excisional or incisional and yet proof of malignancy is probably mandatory before mastectomy is carried out for mammary cancer. In experimentally-induced tumours, no deleterious effect was observed by the use of the biopsy drill.

Staging

Many different forms of staging of cancer of the breast have been used throughout the world; because of this, difficulties have arisen in comparing results. As clinical staging may differ from the postoperative classification, clinical and pathological staging systems have been devised. In an attempt to gain universal acceptance of a single system, the International Union against Cancer, known as UICC (Union International Contre le Cancer), devised the TNM staging system. T refers to the tumour, N for the regional lymph nodes and M for metastases. The American Joint Committee for Cancer Staging and End Results reporting (AJC) agreed on a common TNM clinical staging system (c TNM). The AJC had also devised a pathological staging system (p TNM). The UICC clinical TNM classification is shown in Table 1, the Columbia classification in Table 2 and the Manchester system of staging in Table 3.

Table 1
CLINICAL TNM CLASSIFICATION OF CANCER OF THE BREAST

T	— Primary tumour	
TIS	— Preinvasive carcinoma (carcinoma *in situ*) non-infiltrating intraductal carcinoma or Paget's disease of the nipple with no demonstrable tumour	
T0	— No demonstrable tumour in the breast	
T1	— Tumour of 2 cm or less in its greatest dimension	
	T1a	With no fixation to underlying pectoral fascia and/or muscle
	T1b	With fixation to underlying pectoral fascia and/or muscle
T2	— Tumour more than 2 cm but not more than 5 cm in its greatest dimension	
	T2a	With no fixation to underlying pectoral fascia and/or muscle
	T2b	With fixation to underlying pectoral fascia and/or muscle
T3	— Tumour more than 5 cm in its greatest dimension	
	T3a	With no fixation to underlying pectoral fascia and/or muscle
	T3b	With fixation to underlying pectoral fascia and/or muscle
T4	— Tumour of any size with direct extension to chest wall or skin	
	T4a	With fixation to chest wall
	T4b	With oedema, infiltration or ulceration of skin of breast (including *peau d'orange*) or satellite skin nodules confined to the same breast
	T4c	Both of above

Table 2
COLUMBIA CLASSIFICATION OF CANCER OF THE BREAST

Stage A — No skin oedema, ulceration or solid fixation of tumour to chest wall; axillary nodes not clinically involved

Stage B — No skin oedema, ulceration or solid fixation of tumour to chest wall; clinically involved axillary nodes, but less than 2.5 cm in transverse diameter and not fixed to overlying skin or deeper structure of axilla

Stage C — Any one of five grave signs of comparatively advanced carcinoma:
1 Oedema of skin of limited extent (less than one-third of the skin over the breast)
2 Skin ulceration
3 Solid fixation of tumour to chest wall
4 Massive involvement of axillary lymph nodes (2.5 cm or more in transverse diameter)
5 Fixation of the axillary nodes to overlying skin or deeper structures of the axilla

Stage D — All other patients with more advanced breast carcinoma, including:
1 A combination of any two or more of the five grave signs listed in stage C
2 Extensive oedema of skin (involving more than one-third of the skin over the breast)
3 Satellite skin nodules
4 The inflammatory type of carcinoma
5 Supraclavicular metastases, clinically
6 Parasternal metastases, clinically
7 Oedema of the ipsilateral arm
8 Distant metastases

Table 3
MANCHESTER STAGING OF CANCER OF THE BREAST

Stage 1 — A tumour confined to the breast. The skin directly over the tumour may be involved, but is small in relation to the size of the breast

Stage 2 — Growth as in Stage 1, but axillary nodes are palpable and mobile

Stage 3 — The skin is invaded, fixed or ulcerated over a large area in relation to the size of the breast, or the tumour is fixed to the underlying muscle or pectoral fascia. If axillary nodes are palpable they must be mobile

Stage 4 — The tumour has extended beyond the breast:
1 Fixation of axillary nodes
2 Fixation of tumour to chest wall
3 Metastatic deposits in the supraclavicular lymph nodes
4 Metastases in the opposite breast
5 Metastases in the skin wide of the tumour
6 Distant metastases

The importance of clinical staging of cancer of the breast lies in its prognostic value. There is a direct relationship between the size of the primary tumour and the prognosis, small tumours in general having a much better outlook than large. The presence of tumour in the axillary lymph nodes is also directly related to the size of the tumour, larger tumours being more often associated with involved nodes than small tumours. The number and degree of involvement of the axillary lymph nodes is directly related to survival in patients with cancer of the breast. A preoperative staging of all patients with malignant disease of the breast is desirable because it allows the clinician to decide whether his mode of therapy should be potentially curative or palliative.

Treatment

For the purposes of treatment, the clinician must decide whether the patient has *early* or *advanced* carcinoma of the breast. While advanced disease may be clinically apparent or detected on investigation before any treatment has been carried out, it is not possible to be certain about whether a tumour in any individual can be deemed 'early'. Even after apparently adequate local therapy for primary carcinoma of the breast, recurrent disease becomes evident and the patients die of disseminated metastatic deposits at a later time. The inescapable conclusion is that micrometastases are present at the time of primary treatment, but are not clinically discernible and not detectable by current investigative methods. For this reason, there is now widespread use of cytotoxic chemotherapeutic agents or other forms of systemic therapy immediately after potentially curative surgery for carcinoma of the breast. The intention is to strike at and eliminate micrometastases, presumed, although not proven, to be present at the time of primary therapy.

In the clinical context, most surgeons would recommend curative surgery in patients with T0, T1 and T2 tumours and in patients with N0 or N1 disease, provided that no metastases were apparent (M0). Curative treatment is not advised for patients with T4 lesions or for N2 or N3 disease, nor in patients with proven metastases (M1). Difficulty sometimes arises with T3 tumours and a clinical decision must be made whether to recommend curative surgery or not. T3 lesions in a large breast may be considered *curable*, whereas a T3 tumour in a small breast, particularly if on the medial aspect, may be considered *advanced* and deemed to be unsuitable for curative treatment (Fig 39.5).

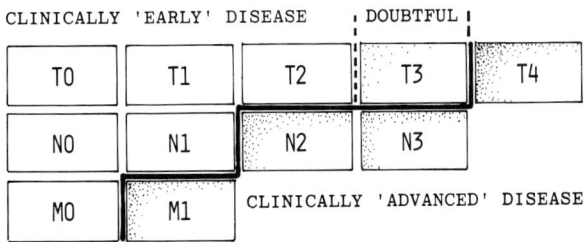

Fig 39.5 Patients with primary lesion T0–T2, with N0 or N1 nodes and M0 disease are deemed 'early', while T4 lesions and those with N2 or N3 nodes or M1 disease are considered 'advanced'. T3 lesions are designated 'early' or 'advanced' depending on their position and the size of the breast.

The value of bone scanning early breast cancer

Disseminated disease is often present at the time of primary diagnosis of carcinoma of the breast, but metastatic deposits may be clinically silent. As investigative techniques become more refined, occult metastatic deposits are being found with increasing frequency in patients with ostensibly early disease. As the skeleton is the commonest site, much attention has been devoted to skeletal scintigraphy as a method for detecting silent secondary deposits. Radiological skeletal survey is relatively crude, as over 50% of bone must be destroyed before a lesion is apparent by conventional x-ray. Bone scanning with bone-seeking radioactive isotopes has been demonstrated to be considerably more sensitive than radiology in the detection of such occult lesions. Strontium-85, Fluorine-18, Technetium-99 have all been used and have variously been reported as finding metastatic disease in between 5 and 24% of patients. Agreement exists that a positive bone scan, unexplained by other conditions such as arthritis and Paget's disease of bone, indicates an extremely poor prognosis. Routine preoperative bone scanning has not yet gained universal acceptance, mainly because of lack of uniformity in interpretation and the relatively small yield of truly positive scans.

Urinary hydroxyproline

Urinary hydroxyproline reflects collagen turnover and the predominant site of collagen is in bone. Increased urinary hydroxyproline excretion may thus indicate metastatic destructive bone disease and has been shown to correlate well with positive bone scans. The hydroxyproline/creatinine ratio, may, therefore, indicate bone disease from cancer of the breast before

it is apparent clinically and may be useful in the staging of mammary cancer. A raised urinary hydroxyproline excretion indicates a poor prognosis and has been shown to correlate well with lymph node involvement. Urinary hydroxyproline excretion is affected by pregnancy, diet, hormones, vitamins and many drugs such as anti-inflammatory and cytotoxic agents.

Other investigations

Scintigraphy and sonography of the liver have also been carried out in an attempt to detect clinically occult deposits, but have not become routine because they may fail to reveal deposits when they are present. These investigations demonstrate unsuspected hepatic metastases in about 7% of patients. When deposits cause structural damage to an organ, the biochemical abnormalities indicating such destruction can be measured and form the basis of a number of investigations currently carried out in patients with apparently early carcinoma of the breast. Abnormal biochemical liver function tests, raised serum calcium related to bone disease and other biochemical tests, if carried out routinely, may indicate metastatic disease. More invasive investigation, such as laparoscopy or even laparotomy, have been carried out in some centres in an attempt to stage the disease before treatment.

Treatment of early carcinoma

Many operations and treatments have been devised for patients with early carcinoma of the breast in an attempt to cure the disease. These forms of treatment include (1) radical mastectomy, (2) extended radical mastectomy, (3) modified radical mastectomy, (4) simple mastectomy, (5) simple mastectomy plus axillary nodal biopsy or superficial axillary clearance, (6) wide local excision of the tumour. In addition, radiotherapy has been used either before or after any of the above-mentioned operations and even as primary treatment after biopsy or local excision of the tumour.

Radical mastectomy

At the end of the 19th century, both Halsted and Meyer independently devised and described the operation of radical mastectomy. The principle of this operation was based on the knowledge that carcinoma of the breast spreads by lymphatic channels to regional lymph nodes before spreading to distant sites. When the tumour is deemed early, removal of the tumour, the regional lymph nodes and all the intervening tissue en bloc is advised. Radical mastectomy, therefore, involves removal of the entire breast, pectoralis major and pectoralis minor muscles and all the axillary lymph nodes together with a wide margin of surrounding tissue.

Extended radical mastectomy

Because tumours of the breast, particularly those situated in the medial half, may spread to the internal mammary nodes, the operation of extended radical mastectomy was devised. This involves, in addition to the classical radical mastectomy, removal of the internal mammary nodes by dividing the costal cartilages in the region of the internal mammary lymph glands. This extended mastectomy often involved removal of the supraclavicular lymph nodes in addition, as these nodes drain the upper part of the breast. Logically, full monobloc excision of regional nodes in the treatment of cancer of the breast involves removal of axillary, supraclavicular and internal mammary nodes in addition to all the breast tissue and pectoralis major and pectoralis minor muscles. The morbidity associated with extended radical mastectomy was considerable and the results found not to be superior to less radical methods.

Modified radical mastectomy

This operation involves monobloc removal of the breast, pectoral fascia, pectoralis minor muscle and the axillary contents while preserving the pectoralis major muscle with its blood and nerve supply. Its advantages over the classical radical mastectomy lie in the cosmetic and functional results. It avoids the unsightly hollow under the clavicle which is associated with removal of the pectoralis major muscle and is followed by less shoulder stiffness and arm swelling.

Simple mastectomy

Simple, or local, mastectomy implies removal of the breast without interference with the axillary lymph nodes. Swelling of the arm and shoulder stiffness should not occur with this procedure, which is cosmetically more acceptable than more extensive operation. Although there are lymph nodes within the breast tissue, the state of the axillary lymph nodes cannot be determined histologically. Because axillary lymph node status is important both from the point of view of treatment and of prognosis, simple mastectomy is usually combined with axillary node sampling to a greater or lesser degree.

Simple mastectomy with superficial axillary clearance

In this operation, the breast is removed, the axilla is explored and the lymph nodes removed up to the axillary vein. As a result of this procedure, not only is axillary nodal involvement by tumour ascertained, but the degree of infiltration can be evaluated.

Wide excision of the tumour

Wide excision of the tumour, including removal of a wide area of apparently normal tissue around the lesion, is sometimes known as extended tylectomy. The purpose of this procedure is to clear all local disease with minimal cosmetic damage. Such an operation, however, is not always acceptable cosmetically, because of the distortion and disparity in size of the breasts after the operation. In addition, the risk of local recurrence after such a procedure is higher than with other methods of primary treatment, even if radiotherapy is carried out after operation. The place of this treatment in potentially curable breast cancer will remain uncertain until the results of prospective controlled studies are known.

Radiotherapy

In potentially curable cancer of the breast, radiotherapy is usually carried out as an adjunct to surgical treatment, either before or after operation. Supervoltage therapy is used, the purpose of which is to prevent local recurrence before or after operation and to kill any metastatic tumour in the regional lymph nodes. Postoperative irradiation is, therefore, often given to chest wall and the axillary, supraclavicular and internal mammary nodes. If the tumour is confined to the breast and has not spread to the nodal areas, radiation is unnecessary. When there is doubt that the tumour has been completely excised surgically or when regional lymph nodes are likely to be, or proven to be, involved by tumour, postoperative radiotherapy is advised. If the axilla has been cleared surgically, however, subsequent radiation to the axilla is unnecessary even if nodal metastases are present. Delay in wound healing and pneumonitis or pulmonary fibrosis are not likely to occur if the radiotherapy is fractionated and spread over several weeks in a dose of 5000 to 5500 rads.

Radiotherapy without mastectomy

Radiotherapy following extended tylectomy has been compared to radical mastectomy and radiotherapy in a randomised trial (Atkins *et al.*, 1972). While there was no difference in survival between the two groups after 10 years follow-up in patients without axillary nodal involvement, the local recurrence rate was much higher in patients who had extended tylectomy and radiation. In patients with involved nodes, radical mastectomy and radiation was the superior treatment in terms of survival at 10 years. Radiation therapy has also been carried out as definitive local treatment, especially in patients who have refused surgical treatment. Improved techniques have allowed delivery of 6000 to 7000 rads without excessive damage to normal tissue.

In patients with stage 1 or stage 2 tumours, the local recurrence rate at 5 years has been reduced to less than 10% and the occurrence of transient pneumonitis reduced to below 10%.

Reconstruction of the breast after mastectomy

If subcutaneous mastectomy, with preservation of nipple and areola, were carried out and an internal prosthesis implanted at the same operation, the grave, and sometimes disabling, psychological effects of mastectomy could be avoided. Because all of the breast tissue cannot be removed by this technique and because of the risk of locally recurrent disease, this type of operation has not gained acceptance. Immediate or delayed reconstruction of the breast after total, radical or modified radical mastectomy is under evaluation in selected groups of patients. As the likelihood of local recurrence is greatest within 2 years of mastectomy, most surgeons advise postponement of reconstructive surgery until at least 2 years have elapsed after mastectomy. By this time many women will have become accustomed to an external prosthesis and may not wish further operation. However, if reconstruction is postponed in this fashion, body image may be so altered that the delayed placement of an internal prosthesis may not be psychologically acceptable or beneficial to the patient. Immediate prosthetic reconstruction poses greater risk of haematoma, seroma, skin necrosis and sepsis and an internal prosthesis may interfere with and delay recognition of locally recurrent cancer. The primary aim of surgery in early breast cancer is to eradicate local disease, cosmetic considerations, although of great importance, being secondary. The dilemma cannot be solved without a prospective controlled trial.

Results of treatment of early carcinoma

A great number of randomised trials have been carried out in primary carcinoma of the breast and the results of many of these are now available (Table 4). Difficulties are always encountered when assessing the results of clinical trials and many of the studies mentioned below are subject to the criticism that the patients were not fully investigated for occult metastatic disease before treatment. Another problem is that many of these trials involved many centres and it is impossible to guarantee the uniformity of treatment in multicentric trials.

In the radical mastectomy and 'watching policy' trial, radical mastectomy was carried out on all the patients, half of whom had additional postoperative radiotherapy while the other half had radiotherapy if and when they developed signs of locally recurrent disease. There was no significant difference in survival between the two groups, although it appeared that immediate postoperative radiotherapy reduced the incidence of local recurrence. There was, however, no difference in the incidence of local disease at the time of death, because delayed radiation was effective in many patients (Easson, 1968). When extended radical mastectomy was compared with simple mastectomy plus 4500 rads the recurrence rates and survival at 15 years was almost identical (Kaae and Johansen, 1968). A comparison of radical mastectomy plus 3250 rads was compared with simple mastectomy with excision of accessible axillary nodes and 3250 rads. There was no difference in survival or recurrence rates at 10 years. The Guy's Hospital study compared classical radical mastectomy for patients with stage 1 and 2 cancer of the breast with extended tylectomy, both groups of patients having radiotherapy. The incidence of local recurrence was much higher in the group who underwent wide excision, a finding that may be related to the relatively low dose of postoperative radiotherapy. This difference was noted at 5 and 10 years in both stage 1 and stage 2 patients. In relation to distant metastases or in survival, there was no significant difference between the two groups in patients with stage 1 disease. However, in patients with stage 2 disease the incidence of distant metastases was higher in the patients treated by extended tylectomy, but the difference in survival rates after the two operations was not found to be statistically significant (Atkins *et al.*, 1972).

A Cancer Research Campaign study (1976) where the patients were randomised into two groups having simple mastectomy plus radiotherapy or simple mastectomy followed by a watching policy demonstrated that radiotherapy reduced the incidence of local recurrence, but did not increase survival. In relation to local recurrence, postoperative irradiation reduced the incidence only in those patients with positive lymph nodes in the tail of the breast or pectoral region, but not those with negative nodes. There was also a suggestion that radiation increased the mortality during the first year of treatment.

The conclusions to be drawn from all these trials demonstrate no advantage for the more radical procedures over the more conservative operations. They show that radiotherapy after operation can reduce the incidence of locally recurrent disease in patients with involved lymph nodes, but has not been shown to prolong life. Indeed, a number of these trials suggest that postoperative irradiation may encourage distant metastases. Moreover, involved axillary nodes can be treated equally well by radiation or by surgery. The standard against which all operations for primary cancer of the breast are measured has been the classical radical mastectomy, the results of which have not been bettered in terms of recurrence or survival. In terms of morbidity and cosmetic result, however, there is a distinct

Table 4

Treatment	Follow-up time in years	Percentage survival	Reference
Radical mastectomy + watching policy *versus* Radical mastectomy + DXT	10	44	Easson, 1968
Radical mastectomy + DXT *versus* Wide excision + DXT	10	Stage 1 58 Stage 2 43 Stage 1 52 Stage 2 30	Atkins *et al.*, 1972
Extended radical mastectomy *versus* Simple mastectomy + DXT	15	37 36	Kaae and Johansen, 1977
Radical mastectomy + DXT ± oophorectomy *versus* Simple mastectomy + DXT ± oophorectomy	8	54 47	Burn, 1974
Radical mastectomy + DXT *versus* Simple mastectomy + DXT	3–5	55 61	Forest *et al.*, 1977
Radical mastectomy *versus* Radical mastectomy + DXT	5	62 56	Fisher *et al.*, 1977
Modified radical mastectomy *versus* Modified radical mastectomy + DXT	5	73 77	Wallgren, 1977
Simple mastectomy + DXT *versus* Simple mastectomy	5	Stage 1 80 Stage 2 78	Cancer Research Campaign, 1976
Simple mastectomy + DXT *versus* Simple mastectomy		Stage 2 77 Stage 2 72	Cancer Research Campaign, 1976
Radical mastectomy *versus* Simple mastectomy + DXT	Clinical N1 B	62 62	Fisher, 1977
Radical mastectomy *versus* Simple mastectomy *versus* Simple mastectomy + DXT	Clinical N0	79 76 81	Fisher, 1977

advantage in the lesser procedures. Adjuvant ovarian ablation is probably not beneficial and adjuvant chemotherapy has been demonstrated to be effective in reducing the incidence of recurrent disease 5 years after radical mastectomy, particularly in premenopausal women, and probably also in postmenopausal patients.

Postoperative complications

When handling the skin flaps, great care must be taken to reduce trauma to a minimum, control all bleeding points and avoid tension. Excessive handling or other injury to the flaps may predispose to infection and tension may give rise to ischaemic necrosis. Antibiotic therapy is advised after radical mastectomy if there is any sign of inflammation. In the younger patient, the arm is kept in a sling for 4 or 5 days until the suction drains have been removed. In the older patient, however, where arm stiffness may occur rapidly, gentle physiotherapy to the shoulder joint is started shortly after operation.

Some degree of swelling of the arm occurs in up to 80% of patients after radical mastectomy as measured by water immersion techniques, but disability occurs in less than 10% of patients. Such arm swelling does not occur after lymphadenectomy alone. It appears that there must also be some interference to venous drainage and therefore great care must be taken to avoid damage to the axillary vein. Patients who have undergone radical mastectomy are at risk of spreading sepsis should they develop an infection of the homolateral limb. They should be advised to protect the hands when they are exposed to sources of infection, such as housework or gardening. Swelling of the arm may occur not only after operation, but also after radiotherapy due to perilymphatic or perivenular fibrosis. Recurrent tumour may also be associated with swelling of the arm. Long-standing arm swelling may result in lymphangiosarcoma, an unusual neoplasm visible as one or multiple raised purple patches in the skin. The endothelial lining of the dilated vascular channels becomes invasive and metastatic deposits in the lung occur frequently in this condition.

Adjuvant chemotherapy

Even after adequate local surgery, patients die from metastatic cancer of the breast. In those with involved axillary lymph nodes, the 10-year survival is in the region of 25%. Adjuvant chemotherapy is designed to destroy micrometastases presumed to be present at the time of primary operation. During the past 10 years a number of trials of adjuvant therapy have been instituted. The cytotoxic treatment used has been either a single agent or combination therapy. Comparing the effect of adjuvant 1-phenylalanine mustard (L-PAM) with that of placebo following conventional or modified radical mastectomy, Fisher and his colleagues gave patients 0.15 mg per kg per day of L-PAM for 5 consecutive days ever 6 weeks for 2 years after surgical treatment. There seemed little doubt that the disease-free interval was prolonged in premenopausal women taking L-PAM when compared to those taking placebo. In postmenopausal women, the difference was not significant. Bonadonna and his colleagues used cyclophosphamide, methotrexate and 5-fluorouracil in combination for 2 years after radical mastectomy and confirmed that the disease-free interval and the survival was significantly greater in premenopausal women treated by chemotherapy when compared with controls. The value of the drug treatment was not significant in postmenopausal women. Offset against the advantages of therapy in relation to clinical recurrence of tumour has been the toxic effects of therapy, including alopecia, leucopenia, thrombocytopenia and gastrointestinal tract disturbances (Bonadonna *et al.*, 1976). Moreover, nearly full doses may be required if benefit is to be achieved (Bonadonna and Valagussa, 1981). At present, there is little evidence to support adjuvant chemotherapy in node negative patients.

The antioestrogen compound tamoxifen is now being used as an adjuvant to mastectomy in primary carcinoma of the breast, and early results of this form of treatment suggest that it may be of value.

Adjuvant ovarian ablation

Adjuvant systemic therapy, other than by cytotoxic drugs, has been used in the past and ovarian ablation by irradiation following radical mastectomy has been the subject of a controlled, randomised trial (Cole, 1970). The dose of irradiation to the pelvis (450 rads) may have been too low to effect total ovarian ablation, but the results demonstrated a prolonged disease-free interval between mastectomy and recurrence, but no significant effect on survival. No benefit from adjuvant ovarian ablation has been recorded in later randomised studies (Ravdin *et al.*, 1970).

The prognosis of early carcinoma

Axillary nodal status

The presence or absence of involved lymph nodes in the axilla is of great prognostic importance (Table 5) and the degree of nodal involvement is also relevant to survival. The 5-year survival of patients with uninvolved nodes is in the region of 75%. When involved

Table 5
AXILLARY NODES NEGATIVE AND POSITIVE

Percentage 5-year survival	Percentage 10-year survival	Reference
	NEGATIVE	
87.1	64.9	American Joint Committee, 1978
–	60	Handley, 1976
80	–	Robinson *et al.*, 1976
74.2	50.2	Brinkley and Haybittle, 1977
–	69	Haagensen and Cooley, 1969
–	56	Butcher, 1969
70	52	Donegan, 1979
	POSITIVE	
46.5	24.9	American Joint Committee, 1978
–	42	Handley, 1976
48	–	Robinson *et al.*, 1976
74.2	50.2	Brinkley and Haybittle, 1977
–	37	Haagensen and Cooley, 1969
–	30	Butcher, 1969
41	22	Donegan, 1979

nodes are found only in the lower part of the axilla below the lower border of the pectoralis minor muscle, the 5-year survival is 65%. Involved nodes behind the pectoralis muscle are associated with a 5-year survival of 45% and if the patient has apical nodal involvement, the 5-year survival is less than 30%.

The absolute number of involved lymph nodes is highly significant, the survival in patients with more than three involved nodes being much poorer than in patients with three or less involved axillary nodes. (Table 6).

Table 6

	5-year survival	10-year survival
Negative axillary nodes	78.1%	64.9%
1–3 positive axillary nodes	62.2%	37.5%
4 or more positive axillary nodes	32.0%	13.4%

Histology

The histological type of tumour has some bearing on the outcome, mucoid and infiltrating papillary carcinomas having a more favourable prognosis than infiltrating ductal carcinomas. Dense lymphocytic infiltration around the tumour and reactive sinus histiocytosis in the axillary lymph nodes also confer a somewhat better prognosis than when these features are absent.

Oestrogen and progesterone receptors

It has now become part of established clinical practice to examine the oestrogen-binding properties of breast cancer specimens; 50–60% of patients whose tumours contain oestrogen receptors are likely to respond favourably to endocrine therapy should this be needed for metastatic disease. Conversely, less than 10% of receptor-negative patients improve on hormonal treatment. The cytosol fraction of homogenised tumour is made 0.5 nmol in tritiated oestradiol. The homogenate is then ultracentrifuged in a sucrose gradient. The oestrogen receptor appears as the 8S and 4S sedimentation peaks. The 8S peak correlates best with clinical response. The precise distinction between receptor-positive and receptor-negative tumours is not clear. It is generally accepted that a value less than 10 femtomoles of bound oestradiol per milligram of total protein indicates a receptor-negative tumour, but the 'cut-off' point varies widely among laboratories.

Progesterone receptors can be identified in breast tumours, usually in those with high levels of oestrogen receptors. In patients who have both oestrogen and progesterone receptors, the response rate to hormonal therapy is 75%. It is usual, but not invariable, for metastases from receptor-positive tumours to be receptor-positive and deposits from receptor-negative tumours are usually receptor-negative. It is not known whether endocrine therapy alters the oestrogen receptor status. As well as being helpful in predicting the response to hormonal treatment, oestrogen receptor status has prognostic significance, receptor-negative patients having a shorter recurrence-free interval and shorter survival than patients with receptor-positive tumours (Fletcher *et al.*, 1978; Blamey *et al.*, 1980).

Carcino-embryonic antigen (CEA)

CEA, a tumour-associated glycoprotein, has been identified in blood and tumours in many malignant and non-malignant conditions. It is neither specific for cancer nor is it found in all patients with tumours. Elevated plasma values of CEA are commonly identified in patients with advanced carcinoma of the breast and may be a guide to prognosis of the disease. Remissions after therapy are often followed by a fall in the CEA value and recurrence or advancing disease is frequently heralded by a rising value. This rise may precede clinical deterioration. CEA is of no value in diagnostic screening for breast cancer, but elevated levels after mastectomy are associated with a poor prognosis.

Other biological tumour markers

A variety of non-specific tumour-associated substances have been identified in patients with carcinoma of the breast. Among these are human chorionic gonadotrophin (HCG), alpha-fetoprotein, raised serum fucose : protein ratio, polyamines, high serum ferritin, cadaverine, putrescene and transfer RNA nucleosides. No single one of these factors is consistently reliable, but when taken together, may be of some help in identifying patients with a poor prognosis. The search continues for a biochemical marker which is tumour-specific, which is readily detectable at an early stage of the disease and which acts as a reliable index to the progression or regression of the disease.

Advanced carcinoma

When mammary cancer is advanced, either locally or systemically, the patient must be deemed to have incurable disease. By locally advanced disease is meant a tumour which is extensive by virtue of its size or fixation to the chest wall or skin or by heavy fixed infiltration of the axillary, infraclavicular or supraclavicular lymph nodes. Demonstrable metastases also indicate advanced disease. Once the patient has been identified as suffering from advanced carcinoma of the breast, major mutilating local surgery may be quite unsuitable. Many forms of systemic therapy are available for patients with such advanced disease and they may be strikingly successful, albeit purely palliative and temporary. The types of systemic therapy available are either endocrine or cytotoxic while radiotherapy may provide excellent palliation for local disease. Endocrine therapy, in turn, may be subdivided into simple endocrine treatment, either ablative or additive, or major endocrine ablation. Cytotoxic chemotherapy may be grouped into single agent and combination chemotherapeutic regimens.

No unanimous agreement exists as to what is meant by a favourable response to treatment in advanced carcinoma of the breast. Subjective and objective criteria have been used and it is difficult to evaluate and compare the results of various forms of therapy when different criteria are used in different centres for the reporting of results. For comparison of results, objective criteria should be used. Stringent guides for favourable response are:

1 measurable regression of all known lesions,
2 the development of no new lesion, and
3 the maintenance of such improvement for at least 3 (or 6) months.

There exists a need for universal agreement on a definition of a 'favourable response' in advanced carcinoma of the breast in order that the relative place of each form of therapy can be assessed fairly and clearly.

Endocrine therapy in advanced carcinoma

Ovarian ablation. In premenopausal women with advanced carcinoma of the breast, ovarian ablation either by oophorectomy or irradiation, may induce remission of the disease in about one-third of patients. Oophorectomy provides a more immediate ablation than radiotherapy, but involves a surgical operation. Irradiation is probably equally effective as operation in reducing urinary levels of oestrogen, although it may take a longer time to do so. Some months after ovarian ablation, the urinary oestrogen levels rise again and fall to zero only after bilateral adrenalectomy. The mechanism of action of ovarian ablation is unknown but after effective therapy, a smaller fraction of cells synthesise DNA when compared with patients who fail to respond. In responsive patients, tumours regress, lytic skeletal lesions become sclerotic and positive bone scans may become negative. The age of the patient and her menopausal status is of importance. Patients under the age of 35 years and perimenopausal patients respond less favourably than do other premenopausal women. An unexplained observation is that women whose ovaries contain metastatic cancer have a better chance of responding well to ovarian ablation than women whose ovaries are free of tumour. About 25% of premenopausal patients with metastatic mammary cancer have ovarian metastases. Operative oophorectomy has the additional advantage that intraperitoneal metastases can be identified at laparotomy.

Oestrogens. Oestrogen therapy, either in the form of diethylstilboestrol, 5 mg t.d.s., or ethinyloestradiol 0.1 mg t.d.s., is used in patients who are well beyond the menopause. The best response rates are obtained in women who are more than 5 years postmenopausal. While some patients on high doses of diethylstilboestrol (150 mg per day) may respond better than patients on smaller doses, oestrogen therapy has its own difficulties. Sodium and fluid retention commonly occur and may give rise to hypertension, cardiac dysrrhythmias, congestive cardiac failure or cerebrovascular accidents. These risks are particularly apt to occur in the elderly patient, who is most likely to respond to this kind of treatment. A noteworthy feature of oestrogen treatment is the 'withdrawal response'. A patient whose disease regresses on oestrogen therapy and who then relapses, may undergo a second remission on withdrawal of the treatment by some unexplained mechanism. Oestrogens also cause increased pigmentation, especially in the areolas and sudden withdrawal of treatment may result in vaginal bleeding.

Androgens. Perimenopausal patients, who are not as a group very likely to respond to endocrine therapy, may be given androgen treatment. This may also be prescribed for premenopausal patients who fail to respond to ovarian ablation or postmenopausal patients, unresponsive to oestrogens. Testosterone and fluoxymesterone are the androgens most commonly used. Fluoxymesterone may be preferable as it is less virilising than testosterone, but androgenic effects, sometimes quite depressing, also occur with this drug. Calusterone may be less upsetting in this regard.

Progestogens. Progestational agents, sometimes combined with oestrogens have been associated with a response rate equal to that of androgen treatment. Medroxyprogesterone acetate 100 to 300 mg orally per day or 300 mg i.m. three times a week or norethisterone acetate 5 to 10 mg t.d.s. by mouth are among the commoner agents used in the control of advanced carcinoma of the breast. Although fluid retention and venous thrombosis do occur, these conditions are less common than with oestrogens. While receptors, specific to progesterone have been identified in human breast cancer tissue, there is as yet no direct relationship between the presence of such receptors and the response of patients with advanced cancer of the breast to progestational therapy. When oestrogen and progestogen therapy is combined, the patient often responds favourably, even when she has not responded to oestrogen therapy alone. Such responses have occurred even in patients who have relapsed after adrenalectomy.

Antioestrogens. Two synthetic antioestrogenic compounds have been widely used in recent years for the treatment of advanced carcinoma of the breast: they are nafoxidine 60 mg t.d.s. and tamoxifen 10 or 20 mg b.d. The mode of action of these agents is by inhibiting the synthesis of oestrogen receptors in the cytoplasm of tumour cells where such receptors are present and also by competing with oestradiol for the receptors. Depending on the criteria for defining response, objective remissions have occurred in between 25 and 40% of patients on this treatment. As nafoxidine may cause marked skin thickening and photosensitivity, tamoxifen is being used more widely. It, in turn, can cause a transient thrombocytopenia, but the unwanted effects of these drugs are uncommon, mild and transitory.

Aminoglutethimide. By inhibiting conversion of cholesterol to pregnenolone, aminoglutethimide inhibits synthesis of cortisol and adrenal androgen and oestrogen. The resultant fall in cortisol is followed by an increased secretion of adrenocorticotrophic hormone (ACTH). This effect can, in turn, be suppressed with dexamethasone or hydrocortisone. By inhibiting the steroid hormone production of the adrenal cortex in such a way, it was hoped that 'pharmacological adrenalectomy' would be comparable to surgical adre-

nalectomy in patients with advanced carcinoma of the breast. Early results of this kind of therapy indicate that it is as effective as adrenalectomy.

Adrenalectomy. Total bilateral adrenalectomy was carried out in 1945 by Huggins and Scott as treatment for patients with advanced carcinoma of the prostate gland. Since then there have been numerous reports of good response to this form of treatment when carried out for advanced carcinoma of the breast. The operation has been shown to bring about excellent and even dramatic response in premenopausal and postmenopausal women, although only one woman in three has a worthwhile regression of the tumour after this procedure. The preoperative mortality from the operation has fallen steadily and is now about 3–5%. The operation can be carried out by separate incisions in the flank, but the transabdominal approach is the more usual one at present. This route allows assessment of the presence and degree of intraperitoneal disease and may be carried out by a mid-line or transverse incision. Bilateral subcostal incision, resulting in an inverted V, gives good exposure provided that the liver is not enlarged. Careful supervision of steroid replacement is required after operation. Selection of patients for adrenalectomy is based on clinical and biochemical criteria. By such selection of patients improved remission rates can be obtained. The likelihood of objective remission after endocrine therapy is discussed below. There is no advantage in carrying out adrenalectomy at the first sign of recurrent carcinoma of the breast. Simpler methods of endocrine therapy and chemotherapy may be tried first and adrenalectomy is usually reserved for patients who have failed to respond to other forms of treatment or who relapse after having obtained a remission.

Pituitary ablation. The pituitary may be destroyed surgically, by irradiation, cryosurgery or ultrasound. Transfrontal hypophysectomy involves a craniotomy and carries the risks associated with a major neurosurgical operation. The olfactory nerve and visual pathways may be damaged and it may be difficult to remove the normal pituitary gland completely. The mortality is less than 5%. Trans-sphenoidal hypophysectomy is being carried out more commonly now and is associated with a lower mortality. The operation is easier on the patient and is carried out through the ethmoid sinuses. It appears to be equally effective as the transcranial operation in terms of completeness of the ablation. Because the pituitary gland is rather radioresistant, external irradiation to the normal pituitary cannot be carried out because of risk of injury to the surrounding brain tissue. External proton beam therapy overcomes these risks largely, but is available in only a few centres. Internal irradiation by implantation of radioactive gold or yttrium rods has also been widely used. By carrying out the procedure under radiological control the radioactive rods can be passed through the sphenoid bone into the pituitary fossa. For total ablation at a consistent rate, a dose of about 300 000 rads is required. Cryotherapy, using a 3 mm probe of liquid nitrogen at a temperature of minus 100 to minus 180°C may be utilised to destroy the normal pituitary. It is carried out either through a transsphenoidal or transfrontal approach under radiographic control. Nerve injuries and leakage of cerebrospinal fluid have been reported after the procedure. Pituitary ablation by ultrasound, involving the application of a probe, delivering an ultrasonic beam at high frequency to the pituitary capsule has been used, but is not widely employed.

Whether to choose pituitary ablation or adrenalectomy for patients with advanced cancer of the breast depends largely on the availability of facilities and specialists. Available evidence suggests that transfrontal hypophysectomy is slightly preferable to adrenalectomy as the proportion of patients undergoing remission has been found to be slightly greater. Adrenalectomy, however, seems superior to ablation of the pituitary by irradiation.

Corticosteroids. Corticosteroid therapy is often administered for patients with advanced carcinoma of the breast. Symptomatic improvement often occurs and the mode of action is usually non-specific. Objective response does, however, occur in about 20% of patients, that is considerably less than after adrenalectomy. The duration of remission is also less than after surgical adrenalectomy. Steroid therapy is indicated for hypercalcaemia, often a preterminal event in patients with skeletal metastases. Steroid therapy as dexamethasone in doses up to 40 mg a day may relieve symptoms of raised intracranial pressure.

Predicting response to endocrine therapy. A number of clinical and biochemical variables are helpful in predicting a favourable response to endocrine therapy.

Clinical. Patients who are many years before or after the menopause are more likely to respond to hormonal therapy, either additive or ablative, than are perimenopausal women. A patient with a long 'free interval' between mastectomy and recurrence tends to respond more often than a patient with a short free interval. Women who have responded previously to endocrine treatment are likely to respond again to different hormonal therapy. Finally, patients with local or regional recurrences, locally advanced disease or skeletal metastases tend to respond more often than patients with visceral metastases.

Biochemical. The most important biochemical factors favouring response to endocrine therapy are positive oestrogen and progesterone binding activity of the tumour. *In vitro* hormonal sensitivity to various hormones has been found by some workers to be of help as have the Bulbrook discriminant function, the pattern of tryptophan metabolism and pregnenolone metabolism. The ability of tumours to conjugate steroids is also thought to be of value in predicting hormonal responsiveness (Dao and Libby, 1969).

Chemotherapy

Cytotoxic chemotherapy is widely used in the treatment of cancer of the breast either as an adjuvant to primary treatment or for established metastatic or advanced local disease. Many drugs have been used, either singly or in combination. With the use of single agents, objective remissions are obtained in 20–35% of patients, while 50–75% of patients respond when drugs are used in combination, but it is not possible to state at present that combination chemotherapy is more successful than single agent therapy. It is usual to treat metastatic disease with chemotherapy when simpler less toxic endocrine measures have failed or in patients who are most unlikely to respond to hormonal therapy, e.g. perimenopausal women or those with receptor-negative tumours. If effective drugs, such as cyclophosphamide or doxorubicin are given in high, frequent dosage, they produce toxicity but result in remissions similar to those achieved by multiple agents. The combination of cyclophosphamide, methotrexate and 5-fluorouracil with or without prednisone is the most widely used and effective combination regimen. Toxic effects of these drugs, such as marrow suppression, alopecia, nausea, vomiting, diarrhoea and malaise are reversible once the drugs are discontinued. The neurotoxicity associated with vincristine is also temporary, but may take several months to clear and cardiomyopathy produced by doxorubicin may not be reversible.

While series reporting remission with combination chemotherapy show complete remission in up to 50% of patients (Table 7), partial responses are seen in up to 80% of patients on this treatment. These improvements are offset to a considerable extent by the serious physical and psychological sequelae, as well as the inconvenience to the patient, of this type of treatment. For these reasons, with the exceptions mentioned above, endocrine therapy is usually the first line of treatment for metastatic breast cancer in the United Kingdom and Ireland.

Radiotherapy

Apart from its role in the management of primary cancer of the breast, radiotherapy has an important

Table 7

Authors	Drugs	Number of patients	Number responding completely	Number responding partially
Decker et al., 1979	Cyclophosphamide Flucytosine Prednisone	146	14 (9.6%)	
Decker et al., 1979	Doxorubicin	20	4 (20%)	
Legha et al., 1979	Doxorubicin Cyclophosphamide	619	116 (19%)	
Muss et al., 1977	Cyclophosphamide Methotrexate 5-fluorouracil Cyclophosphamide Methotrexate 5-Fluorouracil – Vincristine Prednisone	38 34	13 (24%) 17 (50%)	
Jones et al., 1975	Doxorubicin Cyclophosphamide	50	6 (12%)	40 (80%)
Bull et al., 1978	Cyclophosphamide Methotrexate 5-Fluorouracil Cyclophosphamide Doxorubicin 5-Fluorouracil	40 38	3 (7.5%) 7 (18%)	22 (55%) 24 (63%)
Rainey et al., 1979	Doxorubicin Vincristine Cyclophosphamide	32	9 (28%)	14 (44%)

place in advanced disease. Control of advanced local lesions by radiotherapy alone can be achieved by giving up to 6000 rads over a period of several weeks by external radiation. For loco-regional recurrences radiotherapy is also effective. Survival studies indicate that loco-regional recurrence is but a manifestation of advanced systemic disease and that some form of systemic treatment, in addition to local irradiation, is justified in these patients (Karabali-Dalamaga, *et al.*, 1978). For painful skeletal deposits, radiotherapy provides excellent relief of pain and fractionated doses of up to 3000 rads are given. A striking feature of this treatment is the early relief of pain. Pathological fractures are treated by internal fixation followed by radiotherapy. Both modalities of treatment are complementary, allowing bone healing to occur. Intradermal and subcutaneous nodules as well as lymph node and other soft tissue masses are amenable to radiotherapy, which affords excellent palliation of symptoms and reduction in the lesions. Its effect in relieving pain make it useful in patients who are undergoing endocrine treatment or chemotherapy in whom rapid improvement of symptoms may be needed. Intracranial metastases are also treated by radiotherapy in a dose of 2000–3000 rads over a period of 2 weeks, usually combined with dexamethasone 2–4 mg 6 hourly.

Immunotherapy

Cell-mediated immunotherapy has been shown to exist in patients with cancer of the breast and non-specific stimulation of cell-mediated immunity to BCG (Bacillus Calmette Guérin) has been tried. This type of immunity has been assessed by evaluating the response to recall antigens, such as tuberculin and streptokinase-streptodornase, or to new antigens, such as dinitrochlorobenzene (DNCB). Levamisole is a synthetic substance known to restore cell-mediated immunity and has been used in anergic patients with mammary cancer. Rojas and his colleagues (1976) found that this substance, when given after a course of radiation for locally advanced cancer, prolonged the clinical disease-free interval. Regimens of immunotherapy combined with chemotherapy are on trial at present. Preliminary information suggests that while the remission rates are similar in patients treated by chemotherapy alone and those treated by immunotherapy-chemotherapy in combination, the duration of remission and survival after treatment may be longer in those treated by both.

Carcinoma of the second breast

The patient most likely to develop cancer of the breast is the woman who has had a previous mastectomy. It is sometimes difficult to decide whether a tumour in the remaining breast is a new primary or a metastatic deposit from the opposite side. The histological appearances may be similar in metastases and new primary tumours, but metastases are often multiple, tend to appear in the periphery of the breast and lack the adjacent carcinoma *in situ* change, so commonly seen in new primary tumours. Bilateral primary breast cancers are sometimes diagnosed and treated at the same time (synchronous), but it is more usual for the second tumour to be identified later (metachronous). On clinical grounds, about 1% of second cancers are synchronous and about 5% metachronous. Women most at risk of developing a second breast cancer are premenopausal patients with a family history of mammary cancer who have lobular carcinoma *in situ*. Lobular carcinoma *in situ* is non-invasive and is responsible for only about 10% of all cancers of the breast, but is very likely to be bilateral. Whether these tumours have the malignant potential for invasion and metastasis is controversial. Some surgeons adopt a watching policy once the diagnosis of lobular carcinoma *in situ* is made, but McDivitt *et al.* (1967) reported that 35% of such women develop invasive cancer if followed for 20 years. The question of prophylactic mastectomy to prevent invasive cancer developing in the opposite breast arises, but has not been found to be superior to a watching policy in this condition.

The prognosis in synchronously occurring bilateral cancers is similar to that of unilateral cancer (Donegan and Spratt, 1979). Urban and his colleagues (1977) have carried out random biopsies on the contralateral breast in patients with mammary cancer at the time of primary treatment and found carcinoma in the opposite breast in 12.5% of patients. While such contralateral tumours may be detected by mammography, there is often no clinical or radiological sign of malignancy. Most of these occult tumours are small, deemed to be minimal, and are associated with a 96% 10-year survival (Wanebre *et al.*, 1974). It has been estimated that the risk of developing a new primary cancer in the opposite breast in women who have had mastectomy is about 1% per annum (Robbins and Berg, 1964).

Breast cancer and pregnancy

The prognosis for breast cancer occurring during pregnancy has generally been considered to be particularly poor. There is no doubt that the diagnosis of cancer is often delayed in pregnancy and the decision to remove breast lumps in pregnant women is often deferred. Perhaps related to this is the finding that the incidence of axillary node metastases is higher in pregnant women than in non-pregnant women. However, when the survival of pregnant women with breast cancer is compared with that of age and stage-matched non-pregnant women with the disease, no gross differences have been found. Breast cancer, when diagnosed and treated in the first half of pregnancy, has a prognosis similar to that occurring in non-pregnant women. Accordingly the mangement of carcinoma of the breast in the first half of pregnancy is the same as would be advised for any patient, except that investigation by radiology and bone scanning is deferred until after pregnancy.

Controversy exists about the treatment of women in the third trimester. Peters (1968) recommends that these patients be allowed to proceed to delivery before the cancer is treated, if the delay is not too long and the tumour not rapidly progressive. A more general view is that mastectomy be carried out whatever the stage of the pregnancy. Peters found that the patients who became pregnant after mastectomy had longer disease-free intervals and longer survival than those who did not become pregnant again after mastectomy. As the risk of recurrence after treatment for carcinoma of the breast is highest during the 2 years after mastectomy, it is generally considered that pregnancy should be avoided during this time, but the other prognostic factors as well as the patient's wishes and other circumstances must be considered when giving advice in this highly individualised situation.

Sarcoma

About 20% of cystosarcoma phylloides are malignant and other forms of sarcoma occurring in the breast are the lymphosarcomas, fibrosarcomas and rhabdomyosarcomas.

Malignant cystosarcomas

These often grow to very large size and cause visible venous distention in the overlying skin. As they enlarge in size, they cause ulceration of the skin due to pressure necrosis from their bulk. The tumours are vascular and metastasise frequently to the lung, while axillary nodal metastases are uncommon. Local recurrence after excision is influenced by the type of local surgery, being less common after radical than after simple mastectomy. Perhaps a more important determinant of local recurrence, however, is the histological grading of the tumour. Adequate local surgery offers the only prospect of cure, since the tumours are relatively radioresistant and are unresponsive to endocrine therapy and, with very few exceptions, to chemotherapy. Apart from the lung, malignant cystosarcomas metastasise to bone, mediastinum and to the heart.

Primary lymphosarcoma

Primary lymphosarcoma of the breast occurs in elderly women and has a worse prognosis than primary carcinoma, even when axillary nodes are not involved by tumour. The prognosis does not seem to be affected by local therapy, whether radical mastectomy or excision followed by radiotherapy.

Fibrosarcoma

This has a better prognosis than lymphosarcoma with a 5-year survival rate of about 60%. A wide margin of healthy tissue around the lesion must be excised if local recurrence is to be avoided and simple or radical mastectomy are preferred to local excision.

Liposarcomas

These are divided into well-differentiated and poorly-differentiated groups. Local recurrence, sometimes many years after primary treatment, tends to appear with the well-differentiated tumours, while distant metastases to lung and liver are seen with the poorly-differentiated tumours.

Rhabdomyosarcomas

Because rhabdomyosarcomas may spread to axillary nodes, regional nodal irradiation after simple mastectomy or else radical mastectomy is advised with these lesions. Radiotherapy induces regression of recurrent tumour and chemotherapy is more effective with disseminated disease than it is in malignant cystosarcomas.

Lymphangiosarcoma

Lymphangiosarcoma occurring in a swollen arm after radical mastectomy was described by Stewart and Treves in 1948. The condition is seen in women who develop significant arm swelling soon after mastectomy. Many years later the tumour appears as multiple, raised, red or purple patches on the skin of the arm or forearm. This lesion has a propensity to ulcerate, heal and ulcerate again and is often associated with considerable pain. Radiotherapy and chemotherapy have unpredictable results in this condition and forequarter amputation may be indicated in patients with a painful, useless and ulcerated limb. Patients rarely survive more than 2 years after the development of this tumour.

Mammary cancer in men

The aetiological factors in cancer of the breast in men have not been evaluated fully. It is an uncommon tumour. It accounts for less than 1% of cancers found in men and less than 1% of all breast cancers occur in men. A family history of breast cancer in female relatives is probably of aetiological significance, as is previous exposure to ionising radiation. Patients with Klinefelter's syndrome are much more likely to develop cancer of the breast than normal men and a history of testicular atrophy or orchitis may have some aetiological role. Abnormalities in oestrogen metabolism have been found in men with cancer of the breast, but exogenous oestrogen has not been demonstrated to be a factor. Patients with prostatic cancer, treated by oestrogens, may develop mammary tumours, often bilaterally, but almost all of these are metastatic deposits from the prostate and not primary breast cancers. Whether gynaecomastia is premalignant or not is uncertain.

Breast cancer in men is usually diagnosed by the presence of a mass in the breast, associated with skin puckering or ulceration, bleeding from the nipple, an axillary nodal mass or signs of disseminated metastases. While it has been diagnosed in a child of 5 years, it is generally a disease of elderly men with a peak incidence at the end of the sixth decade of life. The delay between first symptom and diagnosis is usually longer than in women. About 25% to 30% of men are found to have advanced local disease at the time of presentation. The best form of primary treatment for this condition is unknown, the usual treatment being either simple mastectomy and radiotherapy or radical mastectomy. As with women, axillary nodal metastases worsen the prognosis and over 50% of patients have such involvement at the time of diagnosis. While 5-year survival is about 80% of those with negative nodes, it is less than 30% in node-positive patients.

For advanced disease, response to additive hormonal therapy is disappointing, but response to orchiectomy is much more frequent and more prolonged than oophorectomy in women. Between 50% and 75% of patients respond favourably to this treatment and response is not confined to any age group.

Gynaecomastia

Gynaecomastia signifies enlargement of the male breast with histological features resembling that of female mammary tissue. Ducts and periductal tissue proliferate, but it is rare for alveoli and acini to become developed. It should be distinguished clinically from fatty deposition around the normal male breast tissue, a common finding in elderly men. The changes may be induced by exogenous or endogenous oestrogen or androgen excess.

Gynaecomastia commonly occurs as a transient phenomenon in neonates, presumably due to stimulation by maternal oestrogens. It is a frequent, and often embarrassing, accompaniment of puberty and is thought to be due to secretion of growth hormone and gonadotrophins. The only therapy required is reassurance and specific operative treatment or biopsy is neither necessary nor desirable. In older patients, gynaecomastia must be distinguished from a lump in the breast. Lumps in the breast require excision, but gynaecomastia after puberty should be investigated for a cause.

Hypogonadism

Hypogonadism is associated with raised gonadotrophin levels which cause gynaecomastia. It, therefore, occurs in Klinefelter's (XXY genotype, high gonadotrophin secretion, small testes, azoospermia) and Reifenstein's (hypospadias, testicular atrophy, azoospermia) syndromes. Gynaecomastia also occurs in hypogonadism when treated with androgens.

Other hormonal factors

Treatment with progestational agents, gonadotrophins, oestrogens or androgens all give rise to gynaecomastia and the condition is also seen in patients with acromegaly and hyperthyroidism. Testicular and adreno-cortical tumours, as a source of excessive circulating endogenous oestrogen, produce the condition while defective metabolism of normal amounts of oestrogen by a cirrhotic liver frequently gives rise to gynaecomastia.

Drugs

Enlargement and proliferation of male mammary ducts and stroma follows administration of many drugs, the commonest being digoxin, spironolactone, phenothiazines, amphetamines, reserpine and, more recently, cimetidine. It is noteworthy that long-term medication with reserpine has been implicated as a factor in inducing mammary cancer in women.

Tumours

Gonadotrophin – secreting tumours, particularly choriocarcinoma of the testis and some forms of bronchial carcinoma, cause gynaecomastia, which may be the first symptom of such neoplastic disorders.

Miscellaneous conditions

Friedrich's ataxia, syringomyelia and dystrophia myotonica are associated with gynaecomastia and the condition is also seen in patients on chronic dialysis for renal failure and in the refeeding phase after starvation. Many patients with gynaecomastia have no cause discovered for their condition, but benefit from bilateral subareolar mastectomy for social reasons.

References

American Joint Committee for Cancer Staging and End-Results Reporting. (1978). *Staging of Cancer of the Breast; Manual for Staging of Cancer*, pp. 101. Chicago: Whiting Press.

Atkins H., Hayward J.L., Klugman D.J., Wayte A.B. (1972). Treatment of early breast cancer: a report after 10 years of clinical trial. *Brit. Med. J*; **1**:423.

Blamey R.W., Bishop H.M., Blake J.R.S. *et al.* (1980). Relationship between primary breast tumour receptor status and patient survival. *Cancer Suppl*; **46**:2765.

Bonadonna G., Brusamolino E., Valagussa P. *et al.* (1976). Combination chemotherapy as an adjuvant treatment in operable breast cancer. *N. Engl. J. Med*; **294**:405.

Bonadonna G., Valagussa P. (1981). Dose-response effect of adjuvant chemotherapy in breast cancer. *N. Engl. J. Med*; **304**:10.

Brinkley D., Haybittle J.L. (1977). The curability of breast cancer. *World J. Surg*; **1**:287.

Bulbrook R.D., Greenwood F.G., Hayward J.L. (1960). Selection of breast cancer patients for adrenalectomy by determination of 17-OHCS and aetiocholandone. *Lancet*; **i**:1154.

Bull J.M., Tormey D.C., Li Shou-Hua *et al.* (1978). A randomized comparative trial of adriamycin versus methotrexate in combination drug therapy. *Cancer*; **41**:1649.

Burn J.I. (1974). 'Early' breast cancer: the Hammersmith Trial: an interim report. *Brit. J. Surg*; **61**:762.

Butcher H.R.Jr. (1969). Radical mastectomy for mammary cancer. *Ann. Surg*; **170**:883.

Cancer Research Campaign (1976). Management of early cancer of the breast. Report on international multicentre trial supported by the Cancer Research Campaign. *Brit. Med. J*; **1**:1035.

Carroll K.K. (1975). Experimental evidence of dietary factors and hormone-dependent cancers. *Cancer Research*; **35**:3374.

Cole M.P. (1970). Prophylactic compared with therapeutic x-ray artificial menopause. In *Clinical Management of Advanced Breast Cancer*. (Joslin C.A.F., Gleave E.N., eds.). 2nd Tenovas Workshop. Cardiff: Alpha Omega Alpha.

Crichlow R.W. (1972). Carcinoma of the male breast. *Surg. Gynae. Obstet*; **134**:1011.

Dao T.L., Libby P.R. (1969). Conjugation of steroid hormones by breast cancer tissue and selection of patients for adrenalectomy. *Surgery*; **66**:162.

Decker D.A., Ahmann D.L., Bisel H.F., Edmonson J.H., Hann R.G., O'Fallon Judith. (1979). Complete responders to chemotherapy in metastatic breast cancer. Characterization and analysis. *J. Amer. Med. Ass*; **242 (19)**:2075.

Donegan W.L. (1979). Staging methods, primary treatment option and end results. In *Cancer of the Breast*, 2nd edn. (Donegan W.L., Spratt J.S., eds.) pp. 242. Philadelphia, London, Toronto: Saunders.

Donegan W.L., Spratt J.S. (1979). Cancer of the second breast. In *Cancer of the Breast*, (Donegan W.L., Spratt J.S., eds), 2nd edn. Philadelphia, Toronto, London: Saunders.

Easson E.C. (1968). Post-operative radiotherapy in breast cancer. In *Prognostic Factors in Breast Cancer* (Forrest A.P.M., Kunkler P.B., eds.). Edinburgh: E. & S. Livingstone.

Fisher B. (1977). United States trials of conservative surgery. *World J. Surg*; **1**:327.

Fisher B., Slack N.H., Cavanagh P.J., Gardner B., Ravdin R.G. (1977). Comparison of radical mastectomy with alternative treatments for primary breast cancer: a first report of results from a prospective randomised clinical trial. *Cancer*; **38**:2827.

Fletcher W.S., Leung B.S., Davenport C.E. (1978). The prognostic significance of oestrogen receptors in human breast cancer. *Amer. J. Surg*; **135**:372.

Forrest A.P.M. (1982). Beatson: hormones and the management of breast cancer. *J. Roy. Coll. Surg. Edin*; **27**:253–62.

Forrest A.P.M., Roberts M.M., Cant E.L.M. *et al* (1977). Simple mastectomy and pectoral node biopsy: the Cardiff-St Mary's trial. *World J. Surg*; **1**:320.

Haagensen C.D., Cooley E. (1969). Radical mastectomy for mammary carcinoma. *Ann. Surg*; **170**:884.

Handley R.S. (1976). The conservative radical mastectomy of Patey: 10 year results in 425 patients. *Breast*; **2, No.3**: 16.

Henderson C., Canellos G.P. (1980). Cancer of the breast. The past decade. *N. Engl. J. Med*; **302**, 17, 78.

Jones S.E., Durie B.G.M., Salmon S.E. (1975). Combination chemotherapy with adriamycin and cyclosphosphamide for advanced breast cancer. *Cancer*; **36**:90.

Kaae S., Johansen H. (1968). Simple versus radical mastectomy in primary breast cancer. In *Prognostic Factors in Breast Cancer* (Forrest A.P.M., Kunkler P.B., eds.) pp. 93. Edinburgh: E. & S. Livingstone.

Kaae S., Johansen H. (1977). Does simple mastectomy followed by irradiation offer survival comparable to radical procedures? *Int. J. Radiat. Oncol. Biol. Phys*; **2**:1163.

Karabali-Dalamaga S., Souhami R.L., O'Higgins N.J., Soumalis A., Clark C.G. (1978). Natural history and prognosis of recurrent breast cancer. *Brit. Med. J*; **2**:730.

Legha S.S., Buzdar A.V., Smith T.L. *et al.* (1979). Complete remissions in metastatic breast cancer treated with combination drug therapy. *Ann. Int. Med*; **91**:847.

McDivitt R.W., Hutter R.V.P., Foote F.W.Jr., Stewart F.W. (1967). *In-situ* lobular carcinoma. *J. Amer. Med. Ass*; **201 (2)**:96.

Muss H.B., White D.R., Cooper M.R., Richards F., Spurr C.L. (1977). Combination chemotherapy in advanced breast cancer. A randomised trial comparing a three – vs a five – drug program. *Arch. Intern. Med*; **137**:1711.

Peters M.V. (1968). The effect of pregnancy in breast cancer. In *Prognostic Factors in Breast Cancer* (Forrest A.P.M., Kunkler P.B., eds.) pp. 65. Edinburgh: E. & S. Livingstone.

Rainey J.M., Jones S.E., Salmon S. (1979). Combination chemotherapy for advanced breast cancer utilizing vincristine, adriamycin and cyclosphosphamide (VAC). *Cancer*; **43**:66.

Ravdin R.G., Lenison E.F., Slack N.H., Gardner B., State D., Fisher B. (1970). Results of a clinical trial concerning the worth of a prophylactic oophorectomy for breast carcinoma. *Surg. Gynae. Obstet*; **131**:1055.

Robbins G.F., Berg S.W. (1964). Bilateral primary breast cancers. A prospective study – clinical pathological. *Cancer*; **17**:1501.

Robinson G.N., Van Heedren J.A., Spencer Payne W., Taylor W.F., Gaffney T.A. (1976). The primary surgical treatment of carcinoma of the breast. A changing trend towards modified radical mastectomy. *Mayo Clin. Proc*; **51**:433.

Rojas A.F., Feirstein J.M., Glait H.M., Olivari A.J. (1976). Levamisole action in breast cancer stage III. In *Immunotherapy of Cancer: Present Status of Trials in Man*, pp. 35. Bethesda: Md Clinical Centre National Institutes of Health (Abstract).

Stewart F.W., Treves N. (1948). Lymphangiosarcoma in post-mastectomy lymphedema. A report of six cases in elephantiasis chirugica. *Cancer*: **1**:64.

Strax P. (1978). Evaluation of screening progams for the early diagnosis of breast cancer. *Surg. Clin. N. Amer*; **58:**667.

Urban J.A., Papachristou D., Taylor J. (1977). Bilateral breast cancer. Biopsy of the opposite breast. *Cancer*; **40(4):** 1968.

Wallgren A.A. (1977). A controlled study: pre-operative versus post-operative irradiation. *Int. J. Radiat. Oncol. Biol. Phys*; **2:**1167.

Wanebre H.J., Huvos A.G., Urban J.A. (1974). Treatment of minimal breast cancer. *Cancer*; **33:**349.

40

Brain tumours

DAVID G.T. THOMAS

Brain tumours comprise a diverse group of neoplasms which occur at almost any intracranial site and which arise from brain and its surrounding structures in patients of all ages. Brain tumours differ in important respects from tumours in other organs of the body.

The pathological classification of brain tumours by cell of origin is complex. The wide variety of cells within the brain and its coverings, as well as in embryological rests, gives rise to a miscellany of histological tumour types, and this has caused consequent difficulty in uniform classification and pathological diagnosis. The grading of malignancy in such tumours by histological examination and the staging of these malignant tumours has required modification of the concepts developed and generally applied in the study of other solid tumours. This is largely because primary malignant brain tumours do not metastasise, with only rare exception, and TNM staging has to be replaced by other approaches which rely more on the locally malignant behaviour of these tumours.

In the normal brain there is localisation of function in specific areas and only a limited reserve exists for recovery after brain damage due to any cause. This has two important consequences in the management of brain tumours. Firstly, the clinically observed manifestations of brain tumours, whatever their histological nature, are due both to local brain dysfunction, at the site of the lesion, and also to raised intracranial pressure within the closed volume of the skull. Secondly, damage caused by growth of the tumour itself, or by

operative surgical treatment to remove it, may be irrecoverable. The neurosurgeon's inclination to attempt radical surgery has, therefore, to be tempered by consideration of the likely quality, as well as length, of survival in the patient after operative insults to the brain. However, the prognosis in malignant brain tumours has been so poor that all modes of adjuvant treatment with radiotherapy, chemotherapy or immunotherapy have been explored. Radiotherapy and chemotherapy have become established as effective modes of therapy for certain types of brain tumour, and immunotherapy has shown some promise.

Types of brain tumours

Classification

'Brain tumours' comprise not only those which arise from brain cells, but also those arising from the meningeal coverings of the brain, the nerve sheaths of the cranial nerves, the pituitary gland, developmental rests and malformations, as well as local extensions of tumours at the base of the skull and metastases from tumours of other organs.

Earliest attempts at classification of these tumours and grading of their malignancy recognised a 'bewildering' variety of histological types. For over 60 years there has been active discussion and controversy on how best to classify brain tumours. A recent classification which incorporates all these types and which is likely to gain wide acceptance has been proposed by the World Health Organisation (1976). A simplified form of this classification is shown in Table 1.

Table 1
CLASSIFICATION OF BRAIN TUMOURS

I Tumours of neuroepithelial tissue
  Gliomas
    astrocytoma, oligodendroglioma, ependymoma, glioblastoma, medullo-blastoma, choroid plexus papilloma, pineal cell tumours, neuronal tumours

II Tumours of nerve sheaths
  Neurilemmoma (schwannoma), neurofibroma

III Tumours of meninges
  Meningiomas, meningeal sarcomas, primary melanotic tumours

IV Primary cerebral lymphomas

V Tumours of blood vessel origin
  Haemangioblastoma

VI Germ cell tumours
  Germinoma, teratoma

VII Other malformative tumours
  Craniopharyngioma, epidermoid, dermoid, colloid cyst

VIII Vascular malformation
  Arteriovenous malformation, cavernous angioma

IX Tumours of anterior pituitary
  Pituitary adenoma, pituitary adenocarcinoma

X Local extensions from regional tumours
  Chordoma, glomus jugulare tumour

XI Metastatic tumours

(Modified after World Health Organisation, 1976.)

Gliomas

The majority of brain tumours arise from cells of neuroepithelial embryonic origin, which include the different glial cells, that is astrocytes, oligodendrocytes and ependymal cells as well as neurones. The tumours which arise from glial cells are termed collectively gliomas. Together gliomas amount to about 40% of all brain tumours (Table 2) and they are all, to a greater or lesser extent, malignant tumours.

Grading of malignancy in gliomas

Criteria for diagnosing the degree of clinical malignancy in gliomas and other brain tumours are different from those applicable to other neoplasms, that is if one interprets *malignancy* as the ability of a tumour to

Table 2
COMPARATIVE INCIDENCE OF DIFFERENT TYPES OF BRAIN TUMOUR*

Glioma	38%
Meningioma	16%
Pituitary adenoma	8%
Neurilemmoma	6%
Craniopharyngioma	3%
Haemangioblastoma	2%
Metastases	12%
Other	15%

* 14 958 cumulated cases.
(From Zimmerman H.M., 1969, Brain tumors: their incidence and classification in man and their experimental production. *Ann. N.Y. Acad. Sci;* **259**:337–59.)

cause the patient's death directly by growth or indirectly by other mechanisms.

The skull forms a closed compartment so that even the most slowly enlarging brain tumour, irrespective of its cytology, ultimately causes an elevation of intracranial pressure with characteristic related symptoms and, if not successfully relieved, eventual fatal outcome. Secondary hydrocephalus may supervene and rapidly enhance the mass effect exerted by small tumours at critical points in the CSF pathways. The local effects of tumour on vital functions may result in similar clinical malignancy, whatever the histological type of tumour. The intact brain depends on regional differentiation to carry out specialised activities, coupled with integration of the whole to achieve normal function. Tumours affecting some specific vital sites in the brain, e.g. mid-brain or brain stem can, therefore, give rise quickly to serious, progressive, permanent neurological deterioration, with early death of the patient. This contrasts with many tumours in certain less critically important sites in the brain and with most other body organs, where normal organ function may continue for longer in the natural history of tumour growth. Even the capacity of an individual glioma for infiltrative growth, and its ability to seed within or outwith the brain, have to be interpreted critically when estimating its degree of clinical malignancy.

The degree of malignancy of a brain tumour is often, but not always, best judged by its propensity for local recurrence and progressive infiltration of nearby vital normal structures. However, in contrast to tumours of many other organs, lack of a circumscribed capsule and presence of diffuse infiltration into surrounding normal brain are features not necessarily accompanied by cellular anaplasia, nor associated with poor clinical prognosis. This kind of infiltrative behaviour is exemplified by many well differentiated astrocytomas which may carry a relatively good prognosis. Primary brain tumours do not tend to metastasise to other parts of the body. They spread by local infiltration, or by seeding in the subarachnoid space. Usually distant meningeal or ventricular metastases are encountered with highly malignant anaplastic tumours e.g. medulloblastoma, but they may also sometimes be seen in oligodendroglioma, a tumour which may have a relatively good clinical prognosis.

In spite of these special considerations, which apply to the behaviour of individual brain tumours, it is necessary also to adopt a form of grading of gliomas based on conventional cytological and histological features. The earliest attempts at histological classification and grading recognised an ascending grade of malignancy up to sarcoma, within the varieties of glioma. Necrosis and vascular hyperplasia in this series of tumours from the National Hospital for Nervous Diseases, Queen Square, between 1902 and 1911 were found to carry unfavourable prognosis. Most subsequent modern classifications of brain tumours are based on the histogenetic method of classifying tumours by their resemblance to different types of normal embryological cells, introduced by Bailey and Cushing (1926). They proposed a scheme consisting of 14 main groups, from medullo-epithelioma, the most primitive, to mature astrocytic glioma, the most differentiated.

A simpler system of classifying gliomas was introduced by Kernohan and Sayre (1952). This was based on the premises that glial tumours developed by dedifferentiation of mature glial cells and that microscopic histological appearances of gliomas could be graded and correlated with prognosis. Their system classified astrocytomas, oligodendrogliomas and ependymomas into four grades, I, II, III, IV, indicating increasing degrees of malignancy. The histological criteria of malignancy which were used are similar to those applied to other neoplasms. They include increase in cellularity, the presence of increased number of mitotic figures, the presence of atypical mitotic figures, pleomorphism of both cells and of tissue architecture with necrosis, abnormally prominent, disordered, stromal reaction and overgrowth and formation of hyperplastic pathological blood vessels in the tumour.

Additional difficulties arise in brain tumours because a small biopsy may be unrepresentative of the whole tumour, and purely cytological considerations are often less important than site of origin and extent of growth of tumour, which cannot be determined from a small sample. Some gliomas contain mixed cell types making it difficult to fit neatly into one grade. In some, the appearance of tumour vessels or the reaction of covering leptomeninges may raise the histological diagnosis of sarcoma.

In spite of these difficulties useful clinico-pathological correlations have been made by relating retrospective assessments of the postoperative progress and survival with histological grade. Typically relatively benign, relatively malignant or highly malignant clinical behaviour is found in, respectively, Grade I (well differentiated), Grades II–III (intermediate) and Grade IV (anaplastic) gliomas (Kernohan and Sayre, 1952).

Glioblastoma

Glioblastoma multiforme (Table 1) is a term sometimes used synonymously with Grade IV glioma, to include those astrocytomas, oligodendrogliomas or, rarely, ependymomas which have areas of malignant change with total anaplasia, although other areas of the tumour permit diagnosis of the original glial cell type. More often it is a term reserved for cerebral tumours with no evidence whatever of a more differentiated tumour.

Medulloblastoma

Medulloblastoma (Table 1.I) is a form of glioma occurring characteristically in the cerebellar vermis or roof of the 4th ventricle, most commonly in children. It contains poorly differentiated cells, corresponding to Grade IV histologically. Choroid plexus papilloma and tumours of the pineal cells or of neurones are very rare tumours of neuroepithelial tissue (Table 1.I).

Other brain tumours

Neurilemmoma

The most common tumour occurring in the nerve sheath is the neurilemmoma or schwannoma (Table 1.II), and it gives rise to about 6% of brain tumours (Table 2). It most frequently arises on the 8th cranial nerve, i.e. acoustic neurilemmoma, although it can affect less commonly 5th, 6th or 9th cranial nerves. It is a well encapsulated, sometimes cystic, benign tumour of Schwann cells.

Meningiomas

Meningiomas, after the gliomas, are the next most common primary brain tumours (Table 2). These arise from the meningeal covering of the brain, including the arachnoid, pia or dura mater and their associated blood vessels (Table 1.III). Most are attached to the dura, particularly close to venous sinuses, possibly arising from arachnoid villi which are numerous in this area. Others arise in the cerebral substance, probably from perivascular cells, or within the ventricles from the tela choroidea of the choroid plexus. Meningiomas may invade bone, producing osteolytic or osteoblastic reactions. Usually they are well encapsulated, but sometimes they grow in a diffuse sheet over the brain (en-plaque). They are typically slow growing, benign tumours, although malignant change, usually sarcomatous, may occur with local invasion or, rarely, metastasis.

Primary cerebral lymphomas

Primary cerebral lymphomas are rare malignant brain tumours (Table 1.IV). The cell of origin of the tumour is subject to controversy. The group includes microglioma and reticulum cell sarcoma. The development of such malignant lymphomas has been observed in patients on long-term immunosuppression, particularly the recipients of organ transplants. Histologically they are in Grades III and IV.

Haemangioblastoma

Haemangioblastoma (Table 1.V) is composed of blood vessels and intervening fat staining stromal cells. The tumour may occur as a well encapsulated tumour, most commonly in the cerebellum and occurs alone or in association with congenital anomalies of Hippel-Lindau disease. Histologically, the tumour is Grade I.

Germ cell tumours

Germ cell tumours (Table 1.VI) occur most often in the pineal region. The germinoma is the most common tumour in this region. It is a malignant embryonic tumour, Grade II–III, identical in histological appearance to seminoma of the testis, and comprises about 60% of tumours at this site. The teratoma, containing tissue derived from more than one embryonic cell layer, is the next most common tumour, after the germinoma, in the pineal region. Histologically it is generally Grade I.

Other embryonic malformations

Other embryonic malformations can result in brain tumours (Table 1.VII). The craniopharyngioma arises from the remnants of the craniopharyngeal duct (Rathke's pouch), in the suprasellar region or within the pituitary fossa. It consists of cyst wall, often associated with some calcified contents as well as cyst fluid, which resembles engine oil in colour and consistence. Epidermoid cysts contain white, pearly fluid, while dermoid cysts contain soft cheesy material as well as hair, or rarely, teeth. The colloid cyst occurs within the 3rd ventricle, close to the foramen of Monro which it may obstruct, causing acute hydrocephalus. These tumours are slowly growing and histologically benign. Vascular malformations (Table 1.VIII) are congenital abnorma-lities in the vascular tree and include the arteriovenous malformation and cavernous angioma. These lesions may behave as expanding brain tumours, as well as causing vascular syndromes due to haemorrhage.

The pituitary adenomas

The pituitary adenomas arise from the cells of the anterior part of the gland (Table 1.IX). They may be classified by conventional histology as acidophil or basophil, according to the standing of their contained hormones, or as chromophobe. Immunohistochemical techniques have made it possible to investigate the endocrine hormones produced by cells in these tumours and to correlate this with pituitary function in the patient.

Local extensions from the skull base which behave as brain tumours include chordoma and glomus jugulare tumours (Table 1.X).

Metastatic brain tumours (Table 1.XI), due to intracranial secondary deposits from distant visceral tumours in the body, are increasingly commonly diagnosed and not infrequently are the presenting lesion in patients with cancer in other organs.

Incidence and epidemiology

Brain tumours are not uncommon and about 2% of deaths in Western Europe and the USA are due to brain tumours. Extracts made from published national statistics from 27 countries using the World Health Organisation Classification of Diseases show an incidence of brain tumours at approximately 5 per 100 000, with a range of 1 per 100 000 in Mexico to 7 per 100 000 in Israel. More rigorous studies in defined populations have tended to show rather higher rates, for example Brewis *et al.* (1966) reported an incidence 11.7 per 100 000 for all intracranial tumours and 6 per 100 000 for primary cerebral tumours in Carlisle, a city with a population of 71 101.

A recent study (Percy *et al.*, 1972) achieved both complete ascertainment of all cases in a defined population and accurate diagnosis in individual cases. In Rochester, Minnesota between the years 1935 to 1968 they found 15.8 per 100 000 primary tumours of the central nervous system, 36% of all cases being first diagnosed at postmortem. In this undiagnosed group, 38% had neurological syndromes which were misinterpreted and the remaining 62% were asymptomatic prior to death. This study showed that the age specific incidence of brain tumour increases with age and revealed no overall sex preponderance, taking 'brain tumours' as a whole. However, there is probably a slightly increased frequency in males over females of medulloblastoma, most astrocytomas, oligodendrogliomas, ependymomas, haemangiomas, craniopharyngiomas, epidermoids, dermoids and vascular malformations. Metastatic carcinoma, particularly from bronchus, is found more frequently in men. Germinoma and teratoma in the pineal show an overwhelming majority in men. There is a slightly greater incidence of intracranial meningiomas in women. The frequency of occurrence of brain tumours at postmortem examination in one series of 64 142 was found to be 1.4%. In another series of postmortem examinations in 1594 patients with systemic cancer, 18% were found to have intracranial metastases. The incidence of cerebral metastasis varied with type of primary tumour. In patients with malignant melanoma 63% of patients had intracranial metastases. In carcinoma of the breast the rate was 28% and in lung 23%, whereas in cancer of the ovary the rate was only 3%.

As yet, there are few clues from epidemiology to the aetiology of brain tumours. Toxoplasma infection, radiotherapy, head injury and chemicals used in rubber industry have all been suggested as possible aetiological factors in brain tumours of varying types, but no causal link has yet been demonstrated.

Brain tumours at different ages

The incidence of different types of brain tumours varies with age. In childhood and adolescence the great majority of brain tumours are primary neuroepithelial tumours of structures in the posterior fossa. The most frequent are medulloblastoma of the cerebellar vermis or 4th ventricle and cystic astrocytoma of the cerebellar hemisphere. Rather less frequent are ependymomas in the region of 4th ventricle and choroid plexus papillomas. Pilocytic astrocytomas are also characteristic of childhood, arising in the optic nerve or chiasm, in 3rd ventricle and hypothalmus, or in the pons and midbrain. The brain stem gliomas are particularly prone to malignant change and rapid progression.

Other tumours which often present in adolescence are the germinoma and teratoma of the pineal region and craniopharyngioma, which is the most common tumour affecting the pituitary fossa at this age. Supratentorial gliomas are rare in children and adolescents. Meningioma, neurilemmoma and pituitary adenoma are virtually unknown.

This pattern changes after adolescence. In adults, the majority of brain tumours occur in the supratentorial compartment. In the middle decades of life (3rd and 4th) astrocytoma and oligodendroglioma in the cerebral hemispheres are the most common brain tumours. Medulloblastoma and ependymoma are rare, and the most frequent cerebellar tumour encountered in this age group is the haemangioblastoma.

In the older age groups, in the 5th to 7th decades, less differentiated gliomas of the cerebral hemispheres (anaplastic astrocytoma, glioblastoma) and cerebral metastases become more common. Meningiomas, neurilemmomas of the acoustic nerve and pituitary adenomas are also most frequently encountered in patients of this age group.

Clinical management

The neurologist or neurosurgeon first makes an anatomical diagnosis of the site of a tumour by the presenting clinical symptoms and signs, which are confirmed by radiological evidence. An informed estimate can then be made of the differential diagnosis, based on knowledge of characteristic natural history, age of onset and favoured site of development of the various pathologically distinct tumours. Operative surgical treatment is then carried out. This may range from biopsy alone to confirm the pathological diagnosis to radical removal of tumour. Subsequent management depends on neuropathological diagnosis, and frequently entails radiotherapy and chemotherapy.

Presentation

Patients with brain tumours present with symptoms due to generally raised intracranial pressure (ICP), to focal change in brain function, or, most frequently, to a combination of both factors (McKeran and Thomas, 1980).

Symptoms of raised intracranial pressure

Raised ICP, due to brain tumour, causes the symptom triad of headache, vomiting and visual failure due to papilloedema. The intracranial volume is approximately 1500 ml in an adult, and only 10% of this is easily displaceable CSF or blood. Brain is incompressible and as a brain tumour expands, normal brain is displaced and distorted. A supratentorial tumour can force the uncus of the temporal lobe to herniate through the unyielding dura of the tentorial hiatus, so causing compression of the midbrain and occlusion of the posterior cerebral arteries, leading to a fatal outcome. In the infratentorial compartment, a brain tumour of the posterior fossa can cause the herniation of the cerebellar tonsils through the foramen magnum, causing fatal compression of the medulla. Short of such dramatic terminal effects, the raised pressure and shift cause headache. This is due to vascular distension and distortion as well as the local effect on pain-sensitive intracranial structures including the dura which is innervated by the 5th cranial nerve. Often the headache is on the same side as the tumour. The headache is commonly intermittent and worse in the early morning, probably due to redistribution of body water while the patient is recumbent during sleep. Commonly, the headache is frontal and occipital. As time progresses it becomes more severe and lasts longer. At times, particularly with tumours causing intermittent hydrocephalus, the pain may be so severe as to cause attacks of screaming. If the patient is examined during such hydrocephalic attacks there is very marked neck stiffness. Generally, however, it is not so severe, although it may reach a stage where the patient lies still to avoid any movement which may increase the pain. This stage often coincides with increasing apathy and drowsiness. Terminally, the depression of conscious level increases until the patient is in coma, terminated by respiratory arrest. In young children the headache may manifest as head holding or restlessness.

Vomiting associated with raised ICP often occurs in the morning and may not be preceded by any feeling of nausea. The mechanism is probably central within the medulla and brain stem. Vomiting is often more marked with posterior fossa tumours, which are most common in children.

Visual failure, particularly if it comes on gradually, may be accepted uncomplainingly by the patient. In some cases papilloedema or consecutive optic atrophy due to long-standing raised ICP is detected when the patient notes a change in vision and consults an optician to obtain a changed prescription for spectacles. Transient visual obscurations are of serious significance and may sometimes not be reversible. They indicate the need for urgent investigation. Specific visual defects may be caused by tumours at specific sites. Pituitary tumours cause chiasmal compression, with generally gradual reduction bilaterally of the temporal visual field. This may come to notice only after an accident at a road junction, or failure at a ball game, due to loss of peripheral vision.

Diplopia, a symptom which generally brings the patient early to medical attention, is also of grave significance. It indicates that the 6th cranial nerve has been distorted by herniation at the tentorial notch and that the imbalance of pressures within the intracranial compartments is close to causing uncal herniation, with possible fatal outcome. When 'coning', that is a tentorial or foramen magnum herniation does occur, the patient lapses into coma and becomes apnoeic, often not reaching hospital alive. Sometimes there can be spontaneous reversal of this pressure cone and the patient may improve to become conscious once more. Such an attack is an indication for urgent investigation.

Symptoms of focal brain dysfunction

The second category of presenting symptoms is due to brain dysfunction brought about by the presence of the tumour. This may be either a breakdown in specific local function or in the general integrated function of the brain. In adults with glioma almost 40% of patients present with epilepsy as the first symptom, and by the time of diagnosis over 50% have experienced an attack (McKeran and Thomas, 1980). The epileptic attacks may have the form of either a generalised convulsion, or of a focal fit affecting the face or limbs. Temporal lobe tumours can cause temporal lobe attacks with short absences, déjà vu or olfactory and gustatory hallucinations.

Focal symptoms other than epilepsy and appropriate to the anatomical site of the tumour also occur. Loss of smell with olfactory groove meningiomas, dysphasia and right sided hemiparesis with gliomas of the posterior frontal region in the dominant left hemisphere, gaze palsies with pineal region tumours, unilateral deafness and ataxia with acoustic schwannoma and multiple lower cranial nerve palsies in brain stem glioma are examples of focal changes in brain function which cause characteristic clinical syndromes.

Special investigations

Patients with symptoms suggestive of brain tumour and with objective neurological signs like papilloedema or hemiparesis are first investigated by non-invasive, screening investigations to determine whether a lesion is present or whether it can be excluded with a reasonable degree of certainty. Further, more hazardous, investigations may be required for technical reasons when planning surgery, or when clinical suspicion is strong and screening tests prove equivocal or negative. A general scheme for the way in which intracranial investigations are planned is shown in Table 3. Usually tests are commenced on an out-patient basis, and may later proceed to in-patient admission. The investigations include specialised clinical investigations, blood tests and, most importantly, neuroradiology.

Clinical examination

Neuro-otology; neuro-ophthalmology; electro-encephalography. The neuro-otologist and neuro-ophthalmologist contribute special skills in the examination of patients thought to be harbouring certain kinds of brain tumour.

Audiometric and calorimetric examination of the acoustic and vestibular function of the 8th cranial nerve may suggest a neuronal lesion, frequently an acoustic neurilemmoma, or alternatively suggest that the

Table 3
APPLICATION OF SPECIAL INVESTIGATIONS TO DIAGNOSIS OF BRAIN TUMOUR

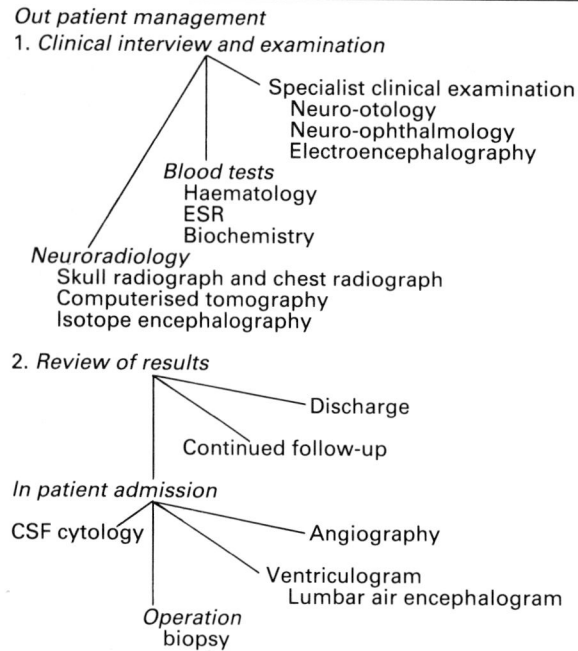

Out patient management
1. *Clinical interview and examination*

                Specialist clinical examination
                Neuro-otology
                Neuro-ophthalmology
                Electroencephalography
         Blood tests
         Haematology
         ESR
         Biochemistry
Neuroradiology
    Skull radiograph and chest radiograph
    Computerised tomography
    Isotope encephalography

2. *Review of results*

                Discharge
      Continued follow-up

In patient admission

CSF cytology   Angiography
          Ventriculogram
          Lumbar air encephalogram
   Operation
    biopsy
    craniotomy

patient's symptoms are due either to primary ear disease or to a brain stem lesion caused by demyelination or vascular accident (Doig, 1972).

Neuro-ophthalmological examination of the ocular fundus can document the presence or absence of papilloedema, and detailed analysis of the defect in acuity and fields of vision of the two eyes may strongly suggest the most probable site, and hence pathology, of a lesion in the visual pathway. This is particularly important in patients with gliomas or meningiomas situated in the optic nerve or chiasm, and with tumours arising from the pituitary fossa, that is pituitary adenomas and craniopharyngiomas.

The electroencephalogram is a further special examination often undertaken at this stage to screen for focal brain abnormality, particularly in patients presenting with epilepsy.

Blood tests

Routine haematological and biochemical analysis of patients' blood samples seldom contribute to the diagnosis of primary brain tumours. However, the finding of a high erythrocyte sedimentation rate, leucocytosis or anaemia may be helpful in the differen-

tial diagnosis of cerebral metastasis or cerebral abscess. Specific tests, for example acid phosphatase in carcinoma of the prostate, may be indicative of a metastatic rather than primary tumour. Endocrinological assessment is important in the preoperative diagnosis of functional pituitary adenomas, as well as in the pre- and postoperative management of patients with chromophobe adenomas or craniopharyngiomas who present with visual symptoms and who may have no symptoms due to endocrine imbalance.

Neuroradiological tests

Plain skull radiograph. Plain skull radiography is the initial, classical and still very important step in the investigation of a patient with a brain tumour. Non specific changes may reveal erosion of the dorsum sellae indicative of raised ICP, or shift of the normal calcified pineal gland due to supratentorial tumour. Certain changes may be found pathognomonic of particular brain tumours. These include erosion of the pituitary fossa due to pituitary adenoma (Fig 40.1), erosion of the internal auditory meatus (Fig 40.14a,b, p. 644), due to neurilemmoma of the 8th nerve, enlargement of the optic foramen due to optic nerve glioma or meningioma, sclerosis of the sphenoid ridge or skull vault associated with meningioma (Fig 40.2), suprasellar calcification in a craniopharyngioma, and lytic or sclerotic lesion of the cranial vault due commonly to metastases.

Chest radiograph. Chest radiography may demonstrate primary or metastatic lung tumours, or lung abscess, which can on occasion simplify intracranial diagnosis. Skeletal survey may also assist in the differential diagnosis of brain metastases by revealing bone secondaries. Frequently specialised radiology of the gastrointestinal or renal tracts may be required in an attempt to identify a latent primary tumour in a patient with suspected brain metastases.

Scans: computerised tomography, isotope encephalography. Computerised axial tomography (CAT) has revolutionised the investigation of brain tumour since its introduction only a few years ago (Huckman, 1975). It is non-invasive in cooperative patients, although restless patients may require sedation or general anaesthesia. In order to obtain maximum information about some brain tumours, or to exclude confidently certain other lesions, enhancement of the scan by intravenous injection into the patient of iodine containing contrast materials may be required (Fig 40.3). This introduces a small risk of hypersensitivity reactions. However, the method is highly reliable as a 'screening' technique, and can also be used as frequently as necessary during follow-up in known brain tumours to detect recurrence (Fig 40.4).

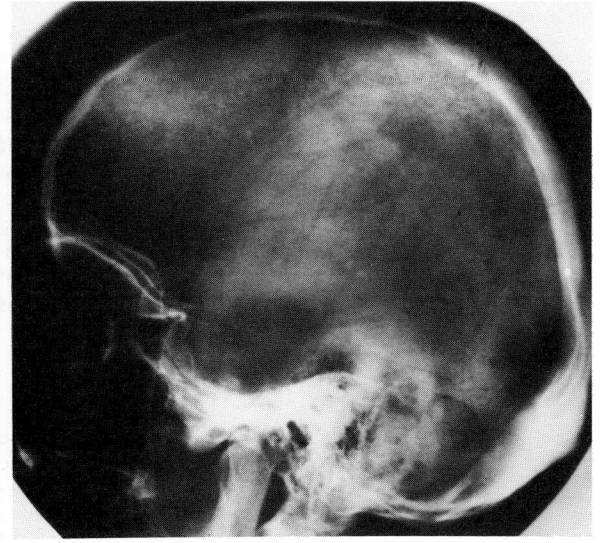

Fig 40.1 Pituitary adenoma. Plain lateral skull radiograph. Gross erosion of pituitary fossa.

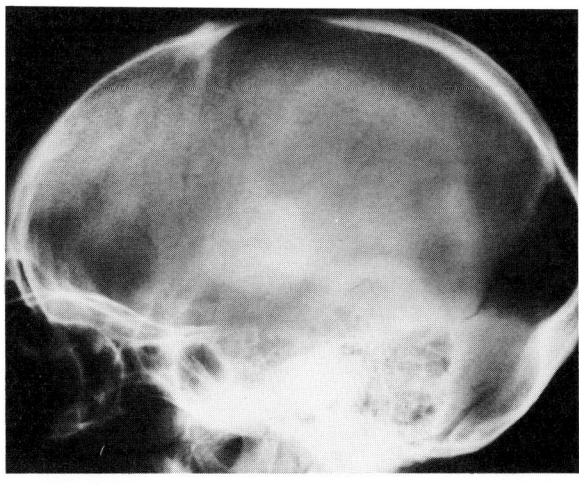

Fig 40.2 Meningioma of cranial vault. Plain lateral skull radiograph. Calcification in rounded tumour in posterior frontal region (same case as Fig 40.9a).

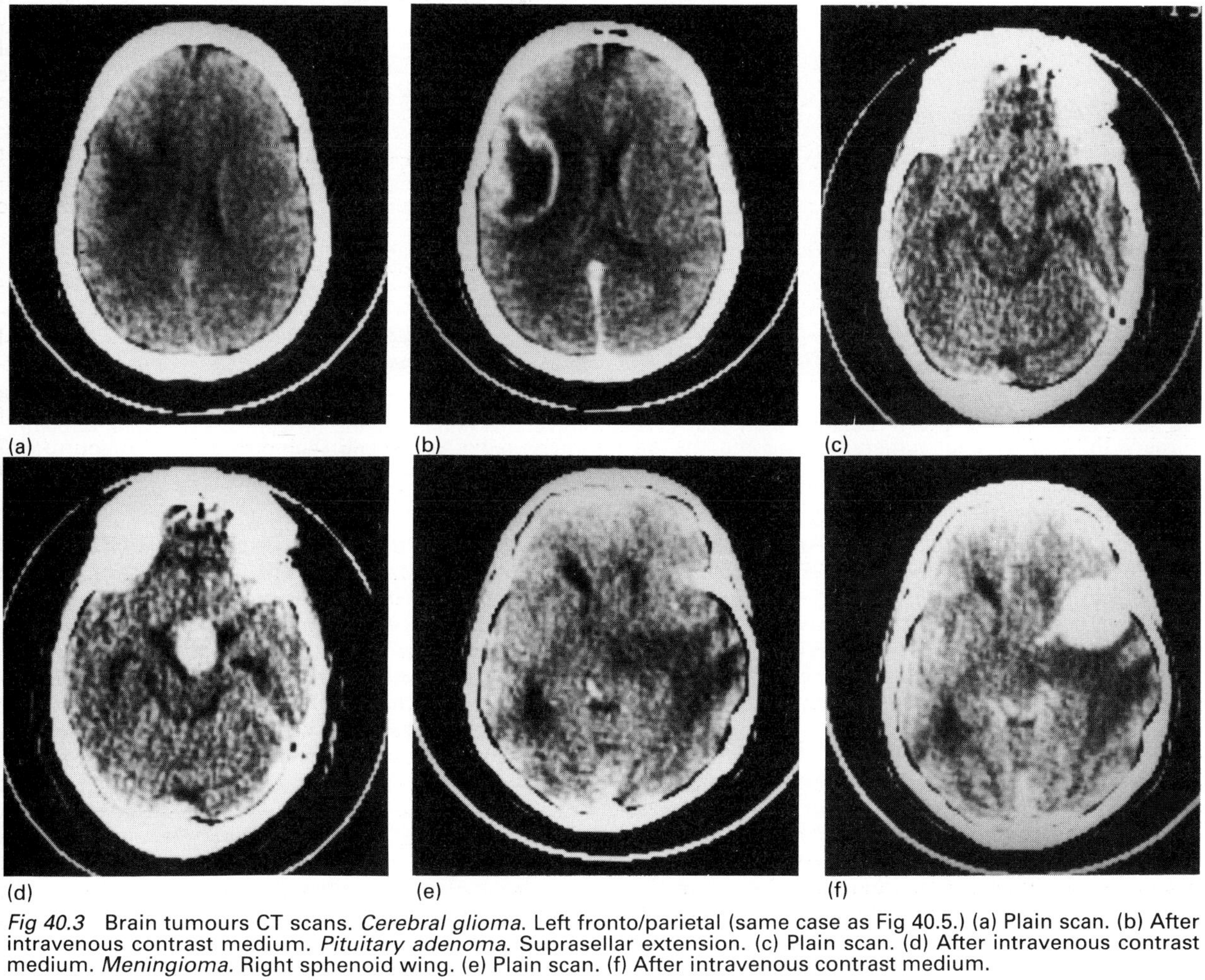

(a) (b) (c)

(d) (e) (f)

Fig 40.3 Brain tumours CT scans. *Cerebral glioma*. Left fronto/parietal (same case as Fig 40.5.) (a) Plain scan. (b) After intravenous contrast medium. *Pituitary adenoma*. Suprasellar extension. (c) Plain scan. (d) After intravenous contrast medium. *Meningioma*. Right sphenoid wing. (e) Plain scan. (f) After intravenous contrast medium.

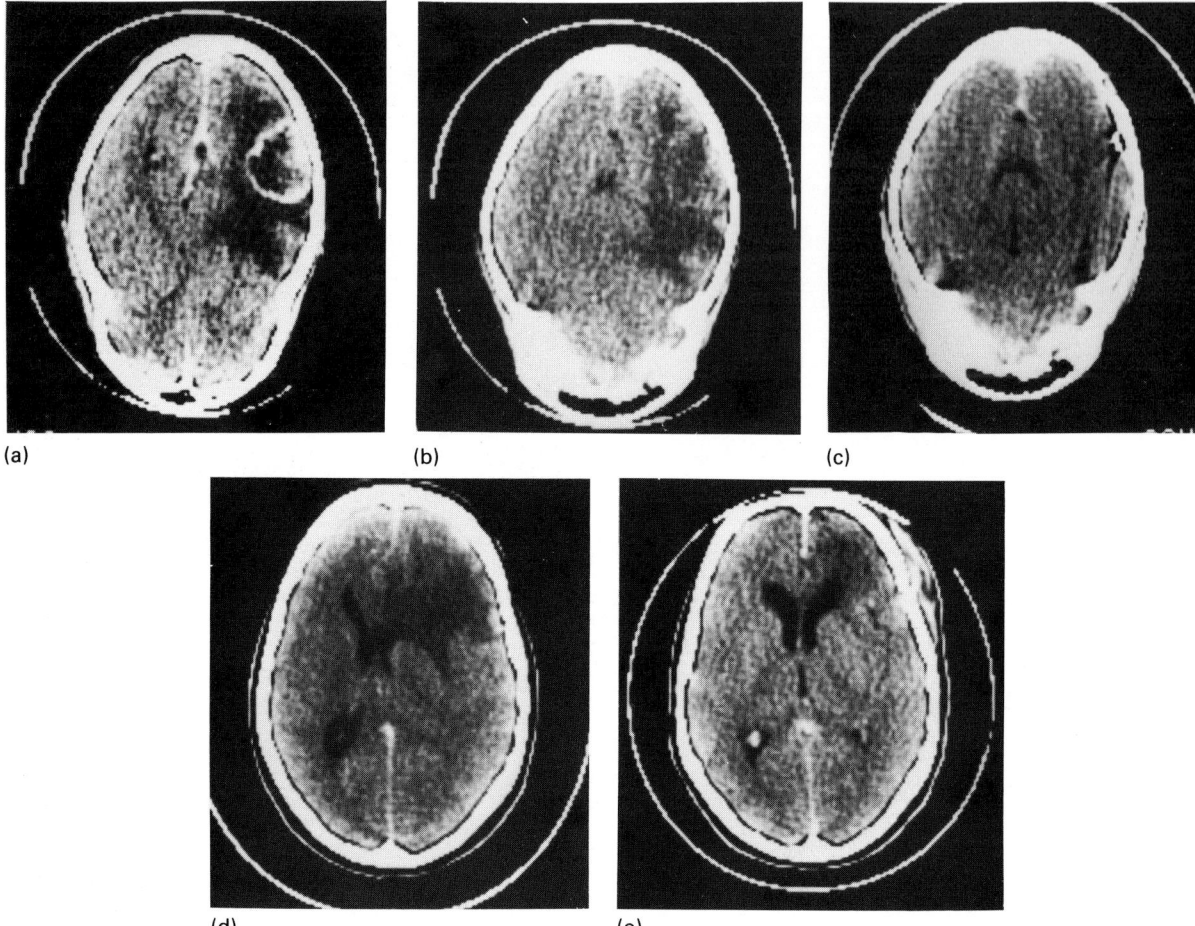

(a)   (b)   (c)

(d)   (e)

Fig 40.4 Cerebral glioma with treatment. CT scans, with intravenous enhancement. (a) Left occipital glioma before surgery. (b) 2 weeks after surgery. (c) At 6 months, after surgery, radiotherapy and chemotherapy. (d) Right frontal glioma before surgery. (e) 2 weeks after surgery.

Isotope encephalography depends on the entry into brain tumours, by selectively increased permeability, of a radioactive label administered by injection. It has been largely superseded by computerised tomography, although it may be useful for technical purposes in planning operative surgery in some cases (Fig 40.5).

Angiography

Injection of contrast into the vessels of the neck by direct puncture or by catheterisation of femoral vessels, demonstrates the vascular anatomy of the carotid and vertebral arterial trees. This method can in some cases reveal vascular tumours in great detail, occasionally allowing a virtually certain pathological diagnosis to be made preoperatively (Fig 40.6). In the majority of cases, however, it does not reveal a diagnostic pathological tumour circulation. The method carries a small, but definite, morbidity consisting of temporary neurological deficits in 2–3% and permanent deficits in 0.1–0.5%, as well as a very small mortality. It is, therefore, generally reserved for patients in whom the previous screening tests indicate the presence of a tumour and where the surgeon is concerned with the specific details of vascular anatomy in planning the operative treatment.

Ventriculography: lumbar air encephalography

These methods are invasive and involve use of contrast material, either air or positive contrast material like myodil, in the CSF pathways. This may be injected

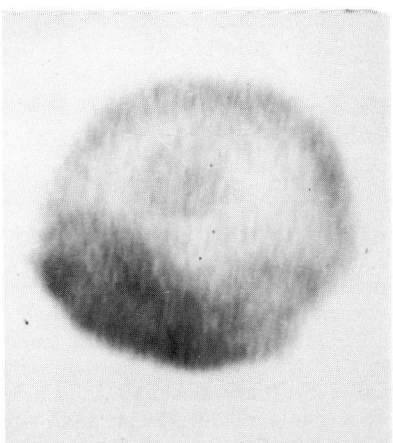

Fig 40.5 Cerebral glioma. Isotope scan. Increased uptake in tumour in left posterior frontal/parietal region (same case as Fig 40.3a,b.)

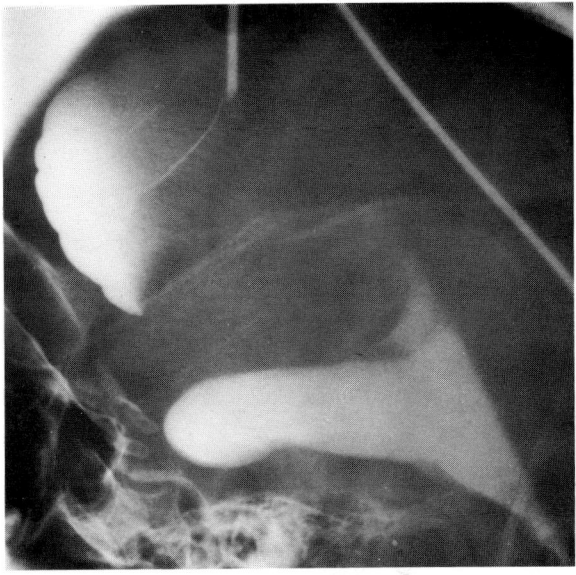

Fig 40.7 Cerebral glioma. Ventriculogram. Large intraventricular extension of glioma in 3rd ventricle region.

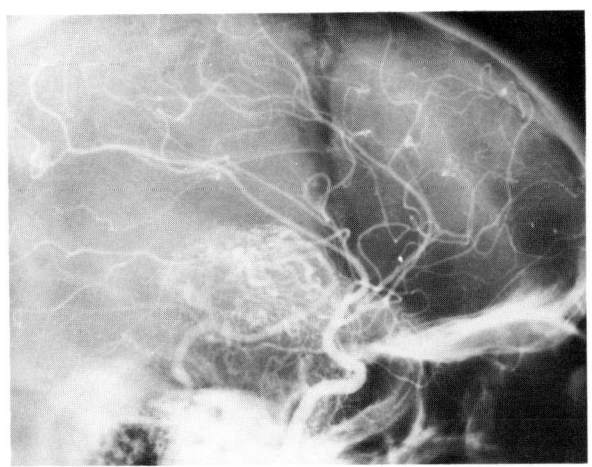

Fig 40.6 Cerebral glioma. Carotid angiogram. Extensive pathological circulation shown in right temporo-parietal region.

through a burrhole in the skull into the lateral ventricle of the brain or, by lumbar puncture, into the spinal theca. Both methods involve appreciable morbidity and mortality and their use has declined very markedly since the introduction of computerised tomography. However, in some cases, particularly in tumours of the 3rd ventricle or pineal regions (Fig 40.7) and also in tumours of the suprasellar and cerebello-pontine angle regions (Fig 40.8), they still have a place.

Cytology of cerebrospinal fluid

Lumbar puncture is unsafe in the presence of brain tumour, but may on occasion be reasonably undertaken, although only in a neurological unit when preparations have been made to proceed urgently to surgery if the patient develops a pressure cone due to brain herniation. Ventricular puncture, through a burrhole is an alternative, often safer, route for obtaining CSF. Cytological examination of the CSF may be diagnostic, particularly in cases of secondary carcinomatous infiltration of the meninges, but also in some cases of glioma or medulloblastoma and, frequently, in germinoma of the pineal region.

Surgical management of specific brain tumours

When the special investigations have been completed, and taking clinical features like the age of the patient and site of the lesion into account, the surgeon can in the vast majority of cases make a differential diagnosis of the pathological type of the brain tumour. However, even when the diagnosis of a highly malignant tumour seems virtually certain, most neurosurgeons feel it vital to obtain histological confirmation. This is important to avoid leaving untreated patients with curable benign tumours. It is also important in

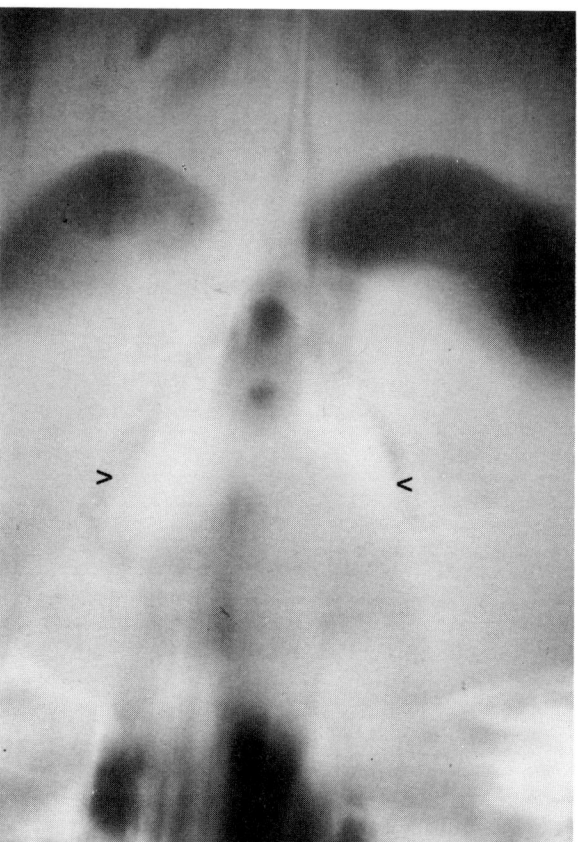

Fig 40.8 Brain stem glioma. Lumbar air encephalogram. Tomographic cut in coronal plane through brain stem; >< indicates lateral margins of brain stem. Asymmetrical enlargement by intrinsic lesion of brain stem, more extensive on left side.

order to provide the optimal currently available palliative treatment to those with incurable malignant tumours.

In general the surgical approach to brain tumours depends on accurate preoperative anatomical localisation of the tumour, because once the bony skull is opened further change in direction of access is very difficult. The basic surgical principles of aseptic technique, gentle handling of tissue and meticulous haemostasis are particularly important in the neurosurgery of brain tumours. This is because meningitis, cerebral abscess, cerebral contusion or intracerebral haematoma due to forcible retraction and postoperative subdural or extradural haematoma all carry serious and sometimes fatal consequences to the patient. The operative techniques for approach to brain tumours comprise craniotomy and burrhole exploration in the supratentorial cranial compartment, occipital craniectomy in posterior fossa exploration and transphenoidal or transcranial approach to the pituitary fossa. The uses of these methods are exemplified in the surgical treatment of specific types of brain tumour.

Craniotomy and burrhole exploration

A burrhole can be cut under local or general anaesthesia. Through a 3 cm scalp incision a hand operated bit and brace is used to perforate and burr the bony skull. Such a burrhole is a very limited opening in the skull, exposing less than one square centimetre of brain surface. This allows needle biopsy and aspiration of cyst fluid, as well as passage of shunt tubing for prolonged drainage of a ventricle or a cyst cavity.

A standard osteoplastic craniotomy can expose a much greater area of brain, in the region of 10 to 100 square centimetres. It is generally performed under general anaesthesia. The neuroanaesthetist makes an invaluable contribution to modern surgery of brain tumours by the use of smooth induction techniques, by the avoidance of factors which raise intracranial pressure, e.g. hypoxia, raised $Pa\text{co}_2$, certain inhalational anaesthetic agents, and by the control of blood pressure and respiration. The hair is shaved from the scalp and the position of the proposed scalp flap is marked out accurately to overlap the region of the tumour demonstrated in lateral angiographic radiographs or on isotope or CT scans. The scalp is incised and reflected, with the widest possible vascular pedicle at its base. Multiple burrholes are cut and joined up, using a hand operated flexible rope saw or power driven craniotome. The bone flap can then be elevated off the underlying dura. It may be left hinged to the remaining skull by pericranium or removed as a free flap. If the dura is tense and bulging, mannitol may be administered peroperatively to reduce cerebral swelling, or a brain needle used to aspirate tumour cyst fluid or CSF from the ventricle, so reducing intradural pressure, before dural opening. During closure of the craniotomy the dura is tightly closed and 'hitched' up to the pericranium by interrupted sutures. This latter manoeuvre tamponades the meningeal vessels against the internal surface of the skull and prevents postoperative extradural haematoma. The bone flap is fixed back in position and the scalp closed in layers. It is also possible to remove the bone flap and to leave the dura open before closing the scalp. This allows space for tumour growth in the case of malignant tumour, or accommodates temporary brain swelling in the case of benign tumours. However, these manoeuvres are not generally required and most surgeons prefer to restore the normal contour of the head by replacing the bone flap.

Cerebral glioma

The extent of tumour resection is often a matter of judgement and is dependent on the site of the tumour in relation to vital structures. A glioma in the cerebral hemisphere generally consists of a tumour 3 to 5 cm in diameter at the time of surgery (Figs 40.3; 4). There is an outer rim of actively proliferating tumour cells, intermingled with oedematous normal brain which may still be functionally recoverable. Inside this, there is a further actively growing shell of tumour and, inside this, an area of poorly vascularised, frankly necrotic and degenerating tumour. In some cases radical surgery is possible and macroscopically total removal of the tumour can be performed without unacceptable neurological damage to the patient (Ransohoff and Lieberman, 1978). Even in these cases there remains tumour which has infiltrated microscopically into the normal brain at the edges of the resection. This continues to grow by further diffuse infiltration of normal brain and causes disability and eventually death.

A tumour arising in the dominant hemisphere, beneath the speech area (Figs 40.3a,b) is often subject to biopsy or very limited removal, while those in the non-dominant frontal lobe may be extensively resected (Fig 40.4d,e). Tumours in the frontal, temporal or occipital lobes are amenable to lobectomy. In the frontal lobe, this entails resection of the cerebral hemisphere from frontal pole to the sphenoid ridge. The method is to coagulate vessels in the pia at the proposed line of section and then to deepen the cut into brain using suction to divide white matter. The resection in the frontal lobe is tapered off medially to spare the anterior cerebral vessels at the midline. Haemostasis is achieved by diathermy or application of metal clips to the normal and tumour vessels. Often the line of resection is seen to pass through the tumour and in every case some residual tumour remains. In the dominant, left temporal lobe, brain can be resected with reasonable safety back to 5 cm from the tip of the lobe provided the superior temporal gyrus is spared. In the right, non-dominant, temporal lobe, the lobectomy can be carried back 6 cm from the temporal pole, and include the superior temporal gyrus. Occipital lobectomy is taken 6–7 cm from the occipital pole and always results in hemianopia in the contralateral visual field. The purpose of partial removal, with or without expendable normal brain in the case of lobectomy, is to lower intracranial pressure and to facilitate postoperative adjuvant radiotherapy and chemotherapy and so by combination therapy to yield improved survival. With surgery alone, the median survival is under 6 months, with fewer than 10% of patients alive at 2 years.

A vigorous surgical resection, within the bounds of good judgement, will usually result in relief of the patient's symptoms, achieve histological diagnosis, and allow radiotherapy to commence within 2–3 weeks, which may or may not be followed by chemotherapy. Gliomas which arise in the thalamus, or in the 3rd ventricle, as well as those in the brain stem (Figs 40.7;8) and pineal region tumours, are generally not amenable to resection or biopsy. Where diagnosis can be made with reasonable confidence on the basis of radiological studies, it is often best to forgo histological confirmation. In such cases a shunt may be required to relieve hydrocephalus, prior to radiotherapy. This consists of a hollow tube, fitted with a pressure regulating valve, led from the ventricular system through the jugular vein to the atrium of the heart or subcutaneously to the peritoneal cavity.

Meningioma

This tumour occurs over the convexity of the brain, in the skull vault (Figs 40.2;9a), along the sphenoid ridge (Figs 40.3e,f) and olfactory groove at the base of the skull, in the dural septa of the falx or tentorium (Figs 40.9b; 10) or inside the ventricle. The degree of difficulty in surgical access by craniotomy, and consequently the hazards of surgery and the feasibility of complete removal of this benign tumour vary with site and with the degree of local invasion by the tumour.

Meningiomas arising in the dura of the cranial vault are the most common and the most accessible (Fig 40.2; 9a). At craniotomy the dura is incised at a distance of about 2 cm from the tumour. This leaves a wide cuff of normal dura around the attachment of the meningioma to be removed with the tumour in order to minimise the possibilities of recurrence. The centre of the tumour is 'gutted' with rongeurs, cutting diathermy and suction, so that only a thin pliable capsule of tissue is left adherent to brain. This can then be removed with the minimum of traction and retraction on the underlying, compromised cerebral tissue. Large vault meningiomas are associated with severe oedema of the underlying cerebral hemisphere and it is frequently advisable to leave out the bone flap at the initial operation and replace it some weeks later at a second operation when swelling has settled. With a small tumour and little cerebral oedema, immediate replacement of bone flap is possible with uneventful recovery.

Similar principles are applied to meningiomas at other sites, in order to minimise both brain damage during surgery and recurrence due to incomplete removal. Where the meningioma involves the major venous sinuses, or if it has invaded bone at the skull base, total removal may be impossible. Meningiomas are not radiosensitive but, in some of these cases, radiotherapy is used, with occasional success, in subsequent management.

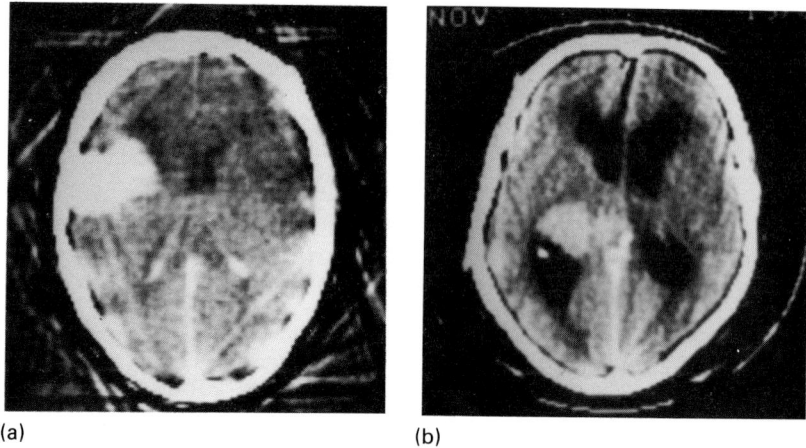

(a)   (b)

Fig 40.9   Meningioma. CT scans after intravenous contrast medium. (a) Left vault meningioma (same case as Fig 40.2). (b) Left tentorial meningioma (same case as Fig 40.10).

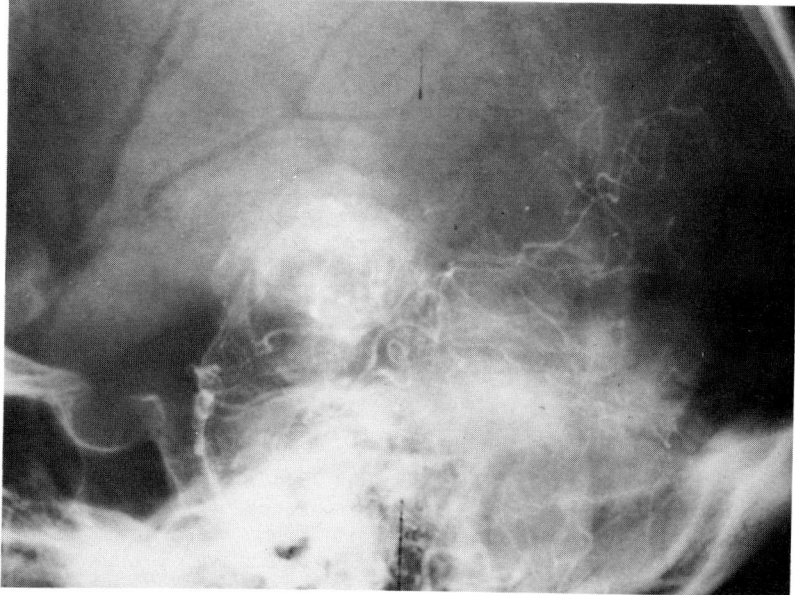

Fig 40.10   Meningioma. Vertebral angiogram. Left tentorial meningioma (same case as Fig 40.9b). Shows blush in tumour circulation.

Cerebral metastasis

In cases of solitary cerebral metastasis, with latent primary tumour, the preoperative differential diagnosis may include glioma, meningioma, metastasis and abscess, so that burrhole exploration or craniotomy is essential to achieve histological diagnosis. Solitary metastases can be approached by craniotomy with an apparent subtotal removal achieved in some cases. Often there is a pseudocapsule which gives a plane of cleavage between the tumour and compressed normal brain. In other cases either partial removal by resection

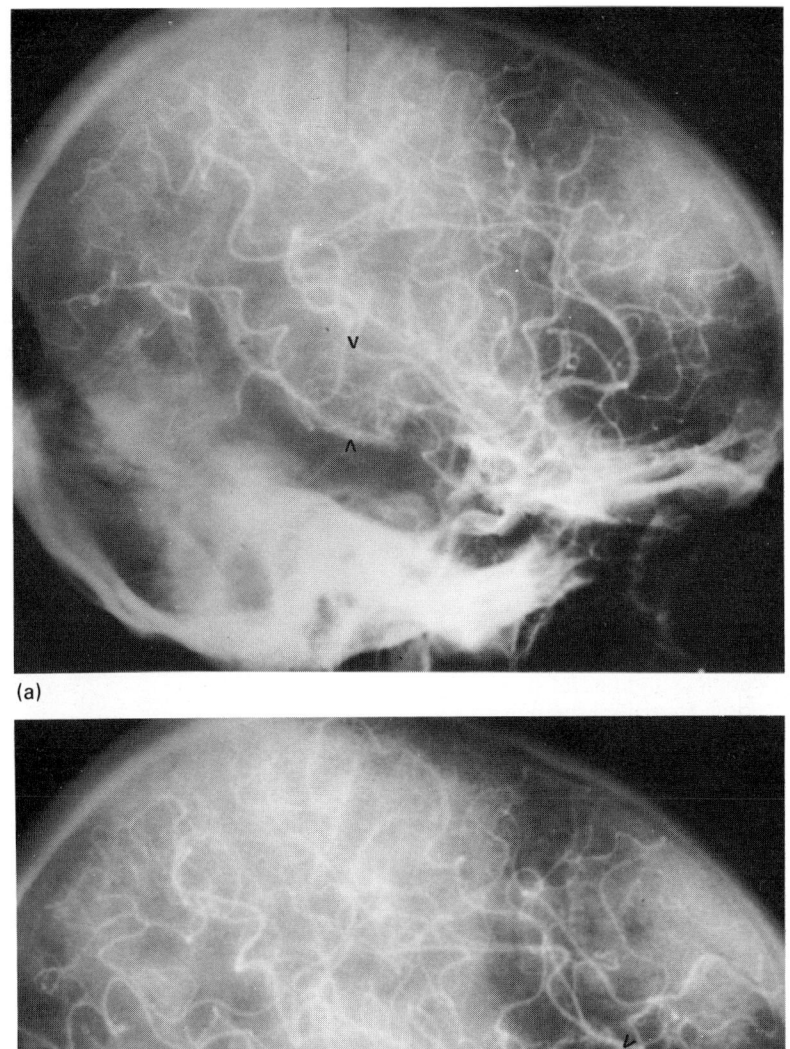

(a)

(b)

Fig 40.11 Cerebral metastases. Carotid angiograms. (a) Right carotid circulation; pathological circulation shown ( ) in temporoparietal region. (b)
Left carotid circulation; pathological circulation shown ( ) in frontal region.

of the necrotic, often cystic, centre of the tumour or lobectomy may be appropriate. Such surgery usually relieves neurological symptoms and increases worthwhile survival (Goran and Murthy, 1977). Further palliation is yielded by postoperative radiotherapy.

In patients with multiple metastases (Fig 40.11a, b) often with known primary carcinoma, it is usually best to relieve raised intracranial pressure by administration of synthetic steroids (*see below*), coupled with palliative radiotherapy.

Occipital craniectomy in posterior fossa exploration

Surgical access in the posterior fossa is more awkward than in the supratentorial compartment. The space is restricted and many vital structures are packed into a small volume. Posterior fossa exploration is usually carried out under general anaesthesia with the patient in one of three positions. With the patient prone, and the neck flexed, the midline structures are accessible. With the patient in a lateral recumbent 'park bench' position the more laterally placed structures can be explored. The sitting position provides excellent access both to midline and lateral structures, but carries the risk of fatal air embolism due to air entering venous channels in bone or venous sinuses, during the extradural approach. This risk can be reduced by using a 'G' suit to elevate venous pressure. In any of these positions a scalp incision, carried down through the cervical and occipital muscles, is required to expose the occipital bone. Usually the occipital bone is opened with one or more burrholes and is then removed piecemeal by rongeurs. In addition to occipital craniectomy, the posterior arch of the atlas is generally removed to increase the ease of access to the lower part of the fossa and to reduce the possibility of impaction of the cerebellar tonsils at the foramen magnum in the postoperative period. Many patients with posterior fossa tumours have hydrocephalus, and a supratentorial burrhole in the occipital or frontal regions, with cannulation of the ventricle and drainage of CSF is required preoperatively. Scrupulous closure of the wound is required to prevent CSF fistula. Often lumbar puncture is carried out daily for some days in order to drain bloodstained CSF and to encourage drainage through the outlets of the 4th ventricle to prevent development of hydrocephalus.

Medulloblastoma and ependymoma

These midline tumours lie within the 4th ventricle or in the cerebellar vermis (Fig 40.12). They are accessible through a midline exposure. Often the tumour involves important structures in the floor of the 4th ventricle and

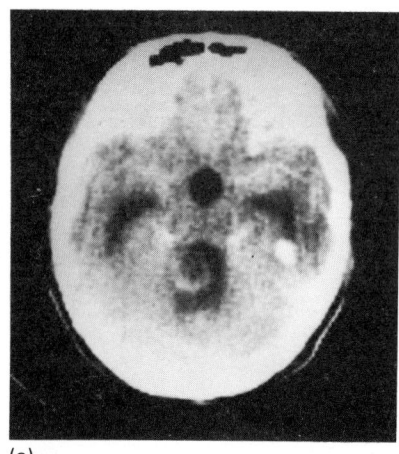

(a)

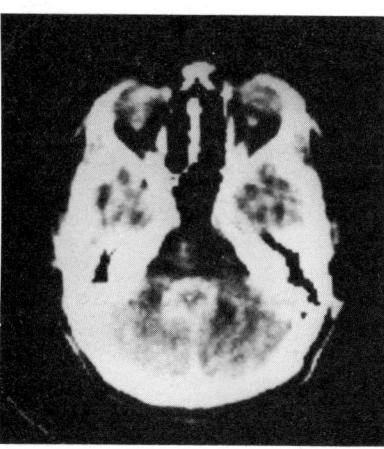

(b)

Fig 40.12 Cerebellar ependymoma. CT scan. (a) Plain scan. (b) After intravenous contrast medium. Tumour shown in 4th ventricle.

the safest surgical procedure is a limited partial removal by rongeurs and by suction. This is sufficient to remove local pressure and to unblock the outlets from the 4th ventricle allowing CSF to drain. Residual tumour which is attached to the vital centres in the floor of the 4th ventricle which control respiratory and cardiac reflexes is left *in situ*. Meticulous haemostasis is essential, as postoperative haematoma is generally fatal. If the CSF pathways remain blocked, external CSF drainage through a catheter in the lateral ventricle is continued postoperatively and subsequently an internal shunt is inserted. Postoperative radiotherapy is generally given, both to the local area and to the whole neuraxis. The latter is necessary in order to prevent seeding of tumour in the CSF pathways, which is otherwise common with these tumours. Chemotherapy is also of use in the primary management, and is also sometimes beneficial later, when tumour recurrence occurs.

Cerebellar astrocytoma, haemangioblastoma, cerebellar metastasis

These tumours lie in the hemisphere of the cerebellum, lateral to the midline (Fig 40.13). When the cerebellum is exposed at posterior fossa exploration these tumours can be located by needling the cerebellar hemisphere with a brain cannula. Frequently, a cyst is encountered and can be aspirated. The associated solid

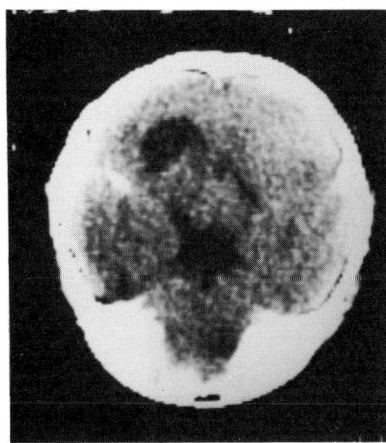

(a)

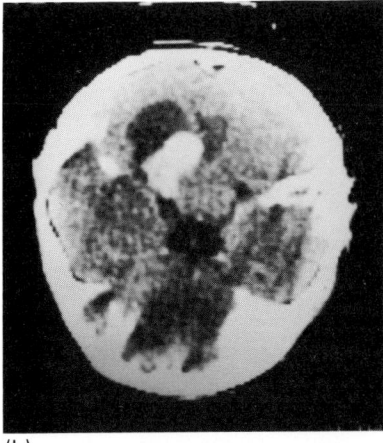

(b)

Fig 40.13 Cerebellar astrocytoma. CT scan. (a) Plain scan. (b) After intravenous contrast medium. Cystic tumour, with mural nodule (enhancing) shown in right cerebellar hemisphere.

tumour can be visualised by widening the cannula track.

It is possible to achieve a total, curative resection in most cases of cerebellar astrocytoma and haemangioblastoma. In some cases of astrocytoma and in cerebellar metastasis a partial removal only is achieved, and subsequent radiotherapy is performed.

Acoustic neurilemmoma

These tumours arise from the acoustic nerve, and growth of the intracanalicular portion of the tumour enlarges the internal auditory meatus (Fig 40.14). If the patient presents early, with only unilateral deafness, and at a stage when the tumour is very small, it is sometimes possible to perform a total removal through the labyrinth of the ear. In the vast majority of cases, however, the tumour has enlarged to fill the cerebellopontine angle giving rise to ataxia and hydrocephalus before diagnosis is made. Investigations show a mass, often cystic, anterior and lateral within the posterior fossa (Fig 40.15), which necessitates a relatively lateral surgical approach. Operation is commonly performed in the lateral recumbent position, through a laterally-placed oblique incision, midway between the mastoid process and external occipital protuberance. Retraction of the cerebellum exposes the lower cranial nerves. After drainage of any associated cyst, piecemeal removal of the interior of the tumour is carried out. The capsule can then be dissected off the side of the brain stem and freed from the adjacent 7th cranial nerve, which enters the internal auditory meatus with the 8th nerve. Postoperatively a lateral tarsorraphy is required to protect the cornea during the period of facial palsy pending recovery of the 7th nerve. Not infrequently the facial palsy is permanent and facio-hypoglossal nerve anastomosis may then be performed in order to improve the appearance by restoring some function in the facial muscles.

Pituitary fossa

Functioning pituitary tumours can present while still small microadenomas (diameter less than 10 mm) with endocrine syndromes, rather than symptoms due to mass effect. Those producing growth hormone present with acromegaly, while those producing prolactin may present with amenorrhoea, galactorrhoea or with infertility in women. Non-functioning pituitary adenomas, as well as some of the functioning tumours, generally present with symptoms due to the space occupying effect of the tumour, although they can present with features of hypopituitarism. Suprasellar extensions of the adenoma impinge on the optic chiasm, and characteristically affect first those fibres from the nasal part of

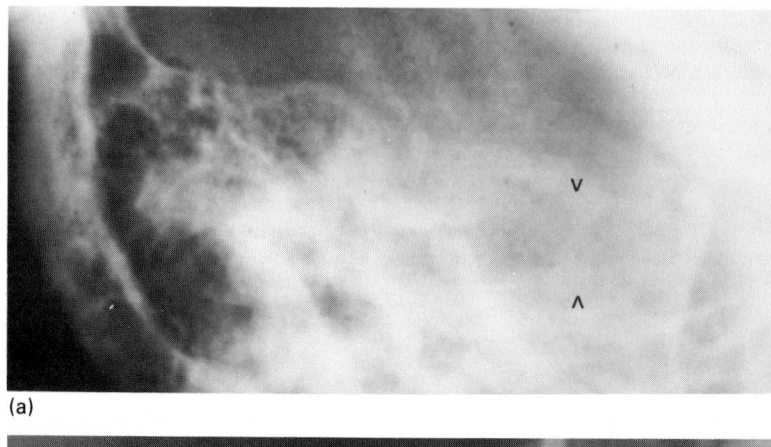

(a)

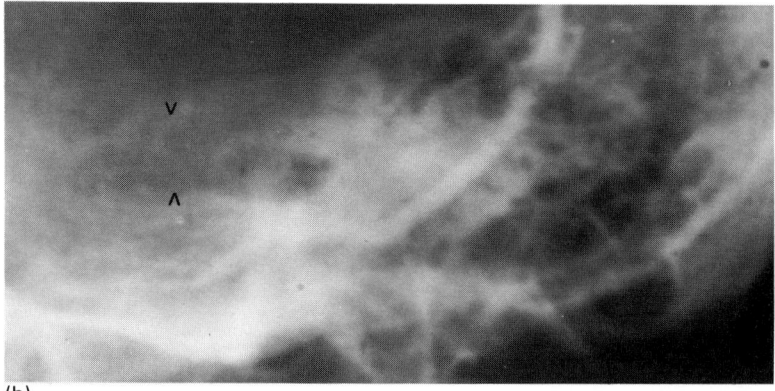

(b)

Fig 40.14 Acoustic neurilemmoma. Skull radiograph of internal auditory meatus ( ). (a) Right. (b) Left. Erosion of right internal meatus by tumour (same case as Fig 40.15).

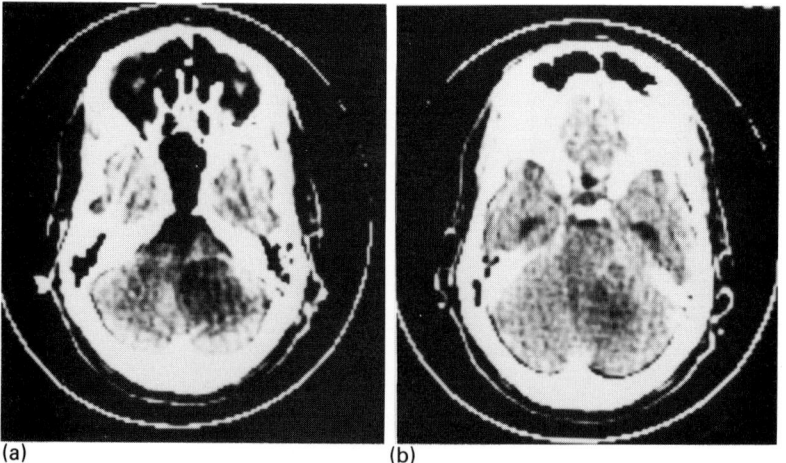

(a)   (b)

Fig 40.15 Acoustic neurilemmoma. CT scan. (a) Plain scan. (b) After intravenous contrast medium. Large tumour shown with a cystic component impinging into cerebellar hemisphere and an area of enhancing solid tumour at right cerebello-pontine angle (same case as Fig 40.14).

the retina which decussate at the chiasm (Figs 40.3c,d). The functional effect of this is a bitemporal hemianopia, often associated with headache and optic atrophy. The pituitary gland can be approached transsphenoidally or transcranially (Guiot and Derome, 1976). Generally the functioning tumours, which are often microadenomas located in the anterior inferior part of the anterior pituitary, are best approached from below by the trans-sphenoidal route. The larger tumours, particularly if there is an irregular, or a lateral and an anterior suprasellar extension, are usually approached from above (Figs 40.1; 3c,d). However, particularly in the elderly patient, it may be advisable to decompress even larger pituitary tumours by partial removal from below (Fig 40.16), rather than accept the greater morbidity involved with transcranial operation.

Trans-sphenoidal approach

Trans-sphenoidal approach to the pituitary is carried out through an intraoral incision of the gingival mucosa just above the maxilla, followed by submucous resection of the cartilaginous nasal septum. With the aid of the operating microscope, the anterior wall of the sphenoid bone is visualised through a nasal speculum. Using bone chisels and punches an opening is made into the sphenoid sinus and the mucosa removed. A window is

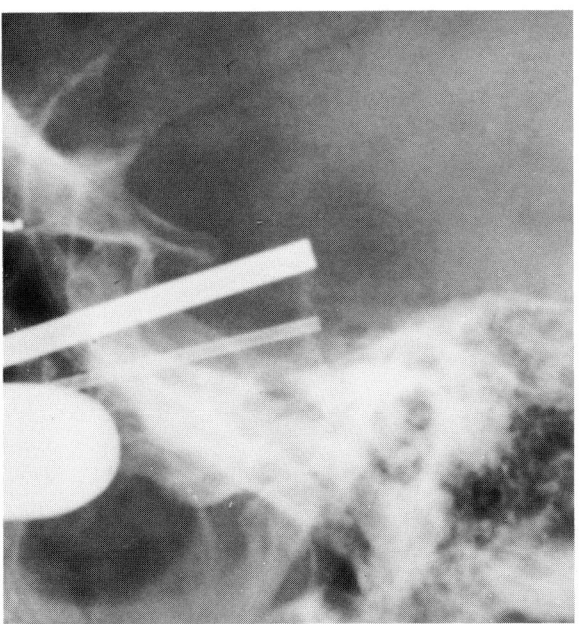

Fig 40.16 Pituitary adenoma. Plain lateral skull radiograph (peroperative). Trans-sphenoidal approach to large pituitary adenoma with suprasellar extension.

cut through the anterior wall of the pituitary fossa and the dura over the gland then opened (Fig 40.16).

A frequent site for a microadenoma is in the anterior inferior part of the anterior pituitary and it may be seen as soon as the dura is open. In many cases the microadenoma can be removed completely, leaving behind normal, but compressed, pituitary tissue. In larger tumours a progressive partial tumour removal can be carried out as the tumour descends gradually from the suprasellar region during the course of surgery. Closure is with a muscle graft taken from the thigh and held in place by struts of nasal cartilage. An alternative approach from below to the pituitary is the trans-ethmoidal route, carried out through a skin incision at the lateral margin of the nose. Both the transoral, transnasal trans-sphenoidal and the transethmoidal routes avoid the risk of intracranial haematoma and of postoperative epilepsy, but there is, instead, a small risk of postoperative CSF fistula and meningitis. The other main advantage is that under optimal conditions it often proves possible to remove totally a functioning microadenoma and still retain satisfactory pituitary function postoperatively, with return of fertility.

Transcranial approach

The transcranial route to a pituitary adenoma is generally through a right frontal craniotomy, although a left-sided approach may be used if there is a lateral extension of the tumour on that side or in the presence of a blind left eye. Under direct vision, anterior to the chiasm and subtemporally, posterior to the carotid artery, the tumour is partially removed using rongeurs and suction. Although the chromophobe adenoma of the pituitary is benign, it is not generally possible to remove it completely and in most clinics it is routine to carry out postoperative radiotherapy. The combined modes of therapy, surgery with radiation, give effective cure with a low rate of recurrence.

Visual failure is generally arrested, and in some cases there is gratifying improvement both in fields and visual acuity. There is an appreciable risk of postoperative clot in the tumour cavity, with grave risk to vision, and of intracerebral haematoma in the frontal lobe following retraction. There is also a risk of postoperative epilepsy, which although present after any craniotomy, seems to be rather more common in this tumour than many others.

Pre- and postoperative care

Steroids

Synthetic glucocorticoids, particularly dexamethasone, are used widely in neurological practice to control cerebral oedema associated with brain tumours. In patients with symptoms of raised ICP or severe local deficits, dexamethasone, typically in a dose 4 mg six hourly in adults either by oral or by intramuscular routes, is administered during preoperative investigations. It is continued for some days postoperatively, and as cerebral oedema settles after tumour removal, gradually tapered off. Replacement therapy with steroid is required acutely after pituitary surgery, and in some patients has to be continued indefinitely.

Anticonvulsants

Those patients with brain tumours who present with epilepsy are started on anticonvulsant therapy, generally with phenytoin as drug of first choice, when first seen. Postoperatively this is usually continued indefinitely as, following even total removal of a benign tumour, a craniotomy results in residual scarring and gliosis which remain to irritate the brain. In those patients who have not been subject to epilepsy before surgery, the policy of individual surgeons concerning prophylactic anticonvulsants varies. Any supratentorial craniotomy for tumour may be complicated by epilepsy and some surgeons prescribe prophylactic anticonvulsants for one or two years postoperatively. Others do not employ the drugs routinely and only commence treatment if a seizure develops at some stage later in management.

Intensive care

Following craniotomy for brain tumour all patients are carefully observed for at least 24 h. During this period life threatening complications can occur. Postoperatively bleeding either in the tumour bed, or from pial vessels in the subdural space, or from meningeal vessels in the extradural space, can cause haematomas which require reoperation. The first sign of this may be increasing restlessness with subsequent onset of focal deficits e.g., hemiparesis or dilation of a pupil. There may be bradycardia associated with rise in blood pressure. The cardinal sign, however, is deterioration in level of consciousness, as defined in terms of verbal response, eye opening and limb response to command or stimulation. Early postoperative epilepsy can cause sudden alterations in consciousness. When there is doubt about the presence of a postoperative clot, reinvestigation with computerised tomography, or reexploration is necessary.

Adjuvant therapy

Radiotherapy

Radiotherapy is of value following surgery in the treatment of malignant brain tumours, and has a place also in the postoperative treatment of pituitary adeno-

mas and craniopharyngiomas which have been partially removed. It has little or no place in the treatment of meningioma or acoustic neurilemmoma, although it may sometimes be given for these tumours when surgery has failed or cannot safely be undertaken.

Results of radiotherapy for malignant brain tumours

Cerebral glioma; lymphoma; metastasis; medulloblastoma. Patients with glioma in the cerebral hemispheres who have undergone partial tumour removal at craniotomy or burrhole biopsy and who remain without severe neurological disabilities are usually treated with radiotherapy. There is evidence that such treatment improves slightly, but significantly, the results at 1–5 years. In one report patients with grade III astrocytoma were found to have a 5-year survival of 2% in those without irradiation compared with 16% in those having radiotherapy. In patients with grade IV astrocytoma the 1-year survival figures were 8% without and 24% with irradiation, and at 3 years 6% of those receiving radiotherapy were alive. However, there were no 5-year survivors in either the non-irradiated or irradiated groups with this grade of tumour (Sheline, 1976).

The range of results in glioma for radiotherapy combined with surgery is for astrocytoma Grade I–II, 58–86% 1-year survival, 31–64% at 3 years and 20–50% at 5 years and for Grade III–IV tumour, 20–44% at 1 year, 0–16% at 3 years, and 0–9% at 5 years (Salazar *et al.*, 1976).

The principal factor which limits the amount of radiotherapy which can reasonably be given to brain tumours is the relative radiosensitivity of tumour and normal brain. Areas of necrosis, haemorrhage, demyelination and gliosis, causing progressive neurological deficit, but without raised ICP, can occur due to radiation damage at anytime from 3 months to 5 years after radiotherapy. The brain stem and the hypothalamus are particularly sensitive. When radiation therapy is planned, the chief aim is to deliver the maximum dose to the tumour that is compatible with acceptable risk of radiation injury to the surrounding brain. Doses above 5000 rads to the whole brain in five daily fractions for 5 weeks are likely to be associated with late changes of radiation necrosis, (or 5500 rads in five daily fractions for 6 weeks).

Most commonly the treatment is delivered from a megavoltage radiation source using multiple fields crossing the target area from different positions around the patient's head. In general, although there are variations in individual radiotherapist's techniques, the policy is one of irradiation to the whole brain with a higher dose in the tumour area (Capra, 1980).

Anaplastic astrocytomas in the cerebral hemispheres, which spread widely and diffusely, are treated by the use of high doses, 6000–8000 rads. This does not appear to prevent later recurrence in the Grade IV tumours, although there is an increase in survival time by combining radiotherapy with surgery.

One possible reason for failure is that hypoxic cells are relatively radio-resistant, and the necrotic areas of gliomas may contain viable but hypoxic cells. Even if the tumour shrinks in response to radiation, these protected cells can repopulate the tumour and cause recurrent growth. One avenue which is being explored to circumvent this form of radio-resistance is the use of neutron radiation (Jones, 1978), as hypoxia seems to be less of a barrier with this form of irradiation. The use of hyperbaric oxygen has been tried and found impractical and ineffective. A more promising approach to treating gliomas, which contain hypoxic areas, is the use of chemical radiosensitising agents. One such radiosensitiser, metronidazole, has been used in the treatment of Grade IV astrocytomas and found to delay the time of tumour recurrence, although not to increase overall survival (Urtasun *et al.*, 1977). The dose of radiation used in this trial was low, 3000 rads in nine fractions in 18 days. A new radiosensitiser, misonidazole has also been used and shown promise in the treatment of malignant astrocytoma (Wiltshire *et al.*, 1978).

Radiotherapy for malignant posterior fossa tumours, like medulloblastoma, ependymoma or brain stem glioma, and for pineal region tumours is performed in a way similar to that for cerebral hemisphere gliomas, that is with consideration given to total volume of brain to be irradiated and total dose applying equally. However, with medulloblastoma, ependymoma and germinoma of the pineal region there is an appreciable risk of seeding along the CSF pathways with seedlings particularly likely to spread to the spinal canal or subfrontal regions. In these cases, prophylactic total neuraxis radiation may be performed simultaneously with radiation of the primary site within the brain, or sequentially thereafter. The best results in medulloblastoma for surgery with adjuvant radiotherapy are in the range 25–40% 5-year survival, and 10–25% at 10 years.

Solitary cerebral metastasis after surgery, or multiple metastases, may be treated with palliative radiation to the whole brain. Where indicated radiation is also given to the primary tumour.

Radiotherapy for benign brain tumours

Pituitary adenoma and craniopharyngioma. Radiotherapy following partial surgical removal of pituitary adenoma may be delivered by external radiation, or, less commonly, by implanted radioactive seeds. The avoidance of radiation necrosis of brain, by restricting the total volume of brain irradiated and by limiting the total dose, are particularly important considerations in these benign tumours. In non-functioning chromophobe adenomas postoperative irradiation has a major place in treatment and significantly reduces the risk of recurrence, which may otherwise occur many years later. Radiotherapy may also be effective in controlling hormone levels in some cases of functioning pituitary adenomas where surgery alone has not achieved this result.

Craniopharyngioma is not as radio-sensitive as pituitary adenoma, but it does respond to radiation. The recurrence rate of this tumour can be diminished by the therapy and frequently the best management is by partial surgical excision of the tumour followed by radiotherapy, rather than by attempted radical surgery.

Chemotherapy

Chemotherapy for malignant brain tumours has been investigated in many clinical trials during the past two decades in attempts to improve on the results provided by surgery alone or in combination with radiotherapy.

Clinical chemotherapy trials have been conducted mainly in primary malignant glioma of the cerebral hemispheres in adults. Posterior fossa tumours of childhood, especially medulloblastoma, but also including ependymoma and brain stem glioma, have also been treated in chemotherapy trials, as have metastatic cerebral tumours. No one drug has yet been discovered which is highly effective against these tumours. However, in carefully designed clinical trials, the best agents so far obtained, the nitrosoureas and procarbazine, have exerted a beneficial response, either by delaying recurrence when given as a primary treatment or by inducing remission at the time of recurrence. They may increase survival to a modest, but significant, extent. The special factors which arise in the chemotherapy of brain tumours have become better understood as a result of such clinical trials, and from basic studies in pharmacology and cell biology of these neoplasms.

Pharmacology

Blood brain barrier. In the normal brain there is a barrier to the entry of large molecules, posed by the intact membrane junctions of the endothelial cells of brain capillaries. This blood brain barrier excludes water soluble drugs of molecular weight in excess of 180, as well as fat soluble agents of molecular weight above 450. If a drug is carried in the blood bound to a protein, it takes on the transport properties of the carrier protein which may be excluded by the blood brain barrier. In brain tumour tissue, there is alteration of the capillary cell junctions causing breakdown of the normal blood brain barrier, although at the point where the growing, infiltrating edge of the tumour meets normal brain, the barrier may be maintained. These factors

have important implications for delivery of chemotherapeutic drugs into brain tumours, particularly their
infiltrative peripheral regions.

Any drug which does not cross the normal blood
brain barrier, but only the abnormal tumour capillary,
enters the tumour's extracellular space and rapidly
passes to the cerebrospinal fluid along a steep concentration gradient. The CSF acts as a 'sink' and returns
the drug into the venous circulation. However, a drug
which can cross the normal brain capillary as well as the
abnormal tumour vessel enters the important
peripheral region of the tumour directly and does not
tend to diffuse so rapidly out of the tumour to the CSF,
because there is no such steep concentration gradient,
although there is some return of the drug to the venous
capillary circulation and passage into CSF. In the nec-
trotic centre of a glioma, even such drugs may not
achieve delivery, due to poor perfusion and the
relatively large distances of tumour cells from capillaries.

Routes of administration

The most commonly used routes for chemotherapy
for malignant brain tumours have been by mouth or by
intravenous or intramuscular injection. Intra-arterial
infusion into the carotid or vertebral arteries offers the
theoretical advantage of high initial drug concentration
in the brain tumour, as well as potentially less exposure
of the rest of the body to the toxic effects of the drugs.
The advantage is not sustained after the first passage
through the circulation, and cannot be considered for
those drugs which require enzymatic activation in the
liver. In spite of the technical success of ingenious
methods which have delivered drugs by intra-arterial
infusion, this method, with agents available at present,
offers no advantage over the less invasive ones. The
intrathecal route has a place in drug delivery in treatment of leukaemic or carcinomatous infiltration of the
meninges, but has not proved superior to systemic
administration for solid tumours. Direct infusion of
drug into the tumour bed has been tried, with few complications, but no improvement in clinical results. At
present, the more invasive methods seem to offer no
advantage over systemic administration.

Cell biology of malignant brain tumours

In malignant gliomas, as in other solid tumours,
there exist populations of cells which are either proliferating or resting. The number of cells within a
tumour, and therefore its size, increases, primarily due
to an increase in the proportion of cells in the proliferating pool, rather than by more rapid cell division.
There is also increase in tumour bulk due to cell loss
exceeding the capacity of the brain to remove dead

cells. The cell kinetics of glioma cells have been investigated by a variety of methods (Hoshino, 1979). The
growth fraction, that is the ratio of proliferating cells in
cell cycle to non-proliferating ($G0$) cells, is 15–40%,
(average 30%) at the proliferating tumour edge of
human malignant gliomas. In the central necrotic
tumour area, the growth fraction approaches zero, and
a value of 10–15% is probably representative of the
neoplasm as a whole. The cell cycle time, T_c, of glioma
cells is remarkably consistent in the region of 2–3 days.
These kinetic characteristics have implications for
chemotherapy of human glioma. Certain drugs, the cell
cycle specific agents, can act only on the proliferating
cell population. Therefore, such a drug, maintained at
effective levels throughout one cell cycle, that is about
2–3 days, could at best kill only 10–15% of the malignant tumour cells. This would reduce tumour diameter
by less than 10%, and it is therefore unlikely, on cell
kinetic grounds, that such cell cycle specific agents
would achieve a significant reduction in the size of a
glioma.

Cell cycle non-specific drugs can kill both proliferating and resting cells and are, therefore, more likely to
exert a cell kill in the region of 90% or more, following
one course of treatment. However, assuming the cell
kinetic properties of the glioma are not changed, such a
tumour could repopulate in 53 to 78 days. It is possible
that the growth fraction may increase in response to
effective treatment with associated cell killing, and
replacement of dead cells may take place even more
quickly, even in 20–30 days. Unfortunately, the
cumulative toxic effects of most chemotherapy agents,
particularly on bone marrow, generally preclude their
being given in repeated doses at the short intervals
which would be necessary to achieve progressive step-
wise reduction in tumour size by overcoming rapid
regrowth of this sort. However, intermittent, high dose
chemotherapy with cell cycle non-specific drugs at
maximum tolerated dose, repeated as soon as the toxic
effects have worn off, combines the optimum antitumour effect with least toxicity.

Specific drugs

Chemotherapy drugs are not selective in killing
tumour cells and tissue in the same way as are surgery
or radiotherapy. In their effective doses all known
oncolytic agents have toxic side effects on normal body
cells or organs, most commonly seen in their effects on
bone marrow and gut. They may be classified by their
mode of action when it is known, by their source of production, and by whether they are cell cycle specific or
cycle-non-specific in their activity.

Nitrosoureas. BCNU   (1,3-bis-(2-chloroethyl-1-
nitrosourea), CCNU, (1(2-chloroethyl)-3-cyclohexyl-1-

nitrosourea) and methyl-CCNU (MeCCNU) are drugs which are cell cycle non-specific. They act both as alkylating agents, damaging desoxyribonucleic acid strands in the nucleus of the cell, as well as carbamoylating agents causing inhibition synthesis of proteins and purine bases. They are highly fat soluble, and penetrate cell membranes and the blood brain barrier easily. They are at present the most effective agents for chemotherapy of glioma.

BCNU is administered by intravenous injection, while CCNU and MeCCNU can be given orally. The dose (mg/m²) is calculated according to the body surface area of the patient, read off a histogram relating body weight, height and area. There is often transient nausea and vomiting on the day of treatment, which is controlled by antiemetics where necessary. The principal toxic effect is relatively late bone marrow depression, with a nadir in the white blood cell and platelet count at 4–5 weeks, recovering at 6–8 weeks. Treatment can then be repeated, usually to a total of 12 courses when possible.

Vinca alkaloids. Vincristine and vinblastine are derived from the plant, vinca rosea. They are cell cycle specific drugs which act at the mitotic spindle and arrest cell division. Vincristine has been used effectively in treatment of medulloblastoma, and in combination chemotherapy of gliomas.

Vincristine is administered by intravenous injection, and does not have depression of the bone marrow as a toxic effect. However, in some patients it can cause peripheral neuropathy.

Methotrexate. This is a cell cycle specific antimetabolite which blocks the normal pathways of folic acid conversion to tetrahydrofolic acid, thus interfering particularly with purine synthesis necessary for nucleic acid production. It is water soluble and delivery to brain is difficult. It can be administered by intrathecal injection for effective treatment of carcinomatous or leukaemic infiltration of the meninges. Other, more lipid soluble antifolate drugs have been developed but, as yet, have not proved effective against brain tumours.

5-fluorouracil. 5-fluorouracil (5-FU) is an analogue of the pyrimidine bases of nucleic acids, and interferes in normal nucleic acid metabolism. Although it is hydrophilic, it enters the brain following systemic administration, and has been used in treatment of brain tumours, with little effect.

Procarbazine. Procarbazine (N-isopropyl-(2-methyl-hydrazino)-P-toluamide monohydrochloride) is a derivative of the monoamine oxidase inhibitors. It is a cell cycle non-specific drug which has a complex action on synthesis of both nucleic acids and proteins, as well

as damaging desoxyribonucleic acid strands in the nucleus. It is lipophilic and has proved clinically effective against brain tumours.

The drug is administered orally, in a course of divided daily doses for 10 days. Bone marrow depression, and sometimes nausea, are side effects.

Corticosteroids. It is possible that the synthetic glucocorticosteroids, which are widely used to reduce the cerebral oedema associated with brain tumours, may have an oncolytic effect in their own right (Gutin, 1975). They are used in chemotherapy of some other forms of cancer but it is not yet established whether or not they inhibit or even enhance either effect on growth of brain tumours.

Clinical chemotherapy trials

Most active chemotherapeutic agents which have been developed so far have been prepared by chemical extraction from biological sources or by chemical synthesis, and then their antitumour effects have been detected by screening programmes carried out in the treatment of a panel of various animal tumours. Promising drugs, after vigorous toxicological investigation in animals, have then to pass through distinct stages in human investigations.

Alternative methods of determining drug effects by assay tissue culture of chemosensitivity are being developed and applied to brain tumours (Thomas et al., 1979). These may make screening for active agents easier, and possibly allow identification of particularly sensitive individual patient's tumours.

Phase I is the initial trial of a drug in man, aimed at demonstrating some anti-tumour effect, and establishing the maximum tolerated dose and the side effects in humans. The patients who are investigated in such a study have failed to respond to all conventional treatment, although they are not necessarily in a terminal state. Usually a small number of patients, approximately 20, with a variety of different cancers will be studied in great detail. Often brain tumours are not included in this human 'screen'. Phase II consists of testing a drug which has shown acceptable, low toxicity in Phase I, as well as some promise of tumour effect against a particular type of human tumour. Generally, patients in such a trial have recurrent tumours, and conventional treatment has been exhausted. The drug is given to them looking for any response to therapy. In Phase II trials several drugs have been tested against malignant brain tumours, and in some cases as many as 50% of the patients have shown a favourable response with a remission sustained for 6 months or more. If a drug appears to be useful in Phase II studies, further prospective, randomised, controlled trials are undertaken. In this kind of Phase III study, careful statistical design is employed to compare the effect of the new drug treatment with the results of the best conventional methods in a prospective, randomised trial. The purpose is to show definitely whether chemotherapy with a particular drug is beneficial, and to estimate whether the benefit is large or small.

Phase II and Phase III chemotherapy trials in patients with brain tumours present special difficulties. As the tumours are relatively uncommon and as the natural history of the various types of tumour varies widely, it is necessary to stratify the patients entering the study carefully by all known prognostic factors, for example histological grade and site, before randomising them between treatment groups. It is also necessary to establish defined criteria for assessing results following chemotherapy. Survival time from surgery to death can be measured comparatively easily, and in patients with malignant glioma treated with surgery and radiotherapy it is commonly short, in the region of 6 months. However, simple measurement does not indicate the quality of survival in patients with brain tumour, and can be easily affected if one treatment group is usually treated terminally at home, while another, receiving chemotherapy, is nursed for a longer time in hospital. The Karnofsky scale (Karnofsky et al., 1951; see Ch. 38, p. 594), which estimates functional ability of the patients on a numerical scale, allows changes during follow-up to be measured and the quality of survival to be assessed objectively. The non-invasive neuroradiological tests, CT scan and isotope scan, may also be repeated at regular intervals during therapy to measure the response of the tumour itself to chemotherapy. Differences in approach to measurement of results are probably the main cause of conflicting reports which have come from different groups using chemotherapy for brain tumours. Other factors include different criteria for acceptance of patients for chemotherapy as well as variation in dosage and timing of drugs used in different trials. These difficulties are particularly pronounced in the chemotherapy of brain tumours since the drugs which are available so far have shown, even in carefully conducted clinical trials, only modest activity against these tumours.

Results of chemotherapy

Malignant glioma. Phase II trials using BCNU, CCNU and MeCCNU used alone as single agents showed objective remissions in 50% or more of patients with recurrent cerebral glioma, lasting up to 6 to 9 months (Fewer et al., 1972; Young et al., 1973). Phase II trials of Procarbazine also show rates of remission in the region of 50% in patients with recurrent glioma (Kumar et al., 1974). A Phase III study (Walker et al., 1978) has shown that BCNU prolongs median survival time in patients with cerebral glioma when given as adjuvant therapy combined with radiotherapy, but not when used alone. 303 patients with anaplastic glioma were randomised into four groups in this study. Of these, 222 met the criteria of confirmed neuropathological grading as well as receiving therapy strictly according to the treatment protocol, and they formed the Valid Study Group (VSG). Patients received either BCNU alone (80 mg/m^2/day on 3 successive days every 6–8 weeks), radiotherapy alone (5000 to 6000 rads to the whole brain), BCNU and radiotherapy in combination, or best conventional care, but neither chemotherapy nor radiotherapy.

Some patients in the VSG died before treatment proceeded far and a further subgroup, the Adequately Treated Group (ATG), was defined as those who had received at least two or more courses of BCNU, 5000 rads of radiation, or to have survived 8 weeks or longer without chemotherapy or radiation. The median survival of patients in the VSG was, best conventional care 14 weeks (ATG:17 weeks); BCNU alone 18.5 weeks (ATG:25.0 weeks); radiotherapy alone: 35 weeks (ATG:37.5 weeks); BCNU with radiotherapy 34.5 weeks (ATG:40.5 weeks). All treatment groups showed a statistical benefit compared with best conventional care. BCNU alone was less effective than radiotherapy alone. Although addition of BCNU to radiotherapy only marginally increased median survival in the ATG, it had a significant effect in increasing the fraction of patients (18%) surviving at the end of 18 months (p = 0.01), where nearly all those who had received either chemotherapy or radiotherapy alone had died. MeCCNU proved less effective than BCNU in the hands of the same group of workers in a similar study (Walker and Strike, 1976).

A Phase III study of CCNU found an increase in median survival time, but not an increase in the disease-free interval before tumour recurrence occurred, in patients with cerebral glioma (EORTC Brain Tumor Group, 1976). However, another group found an increase in mean time to tumour recurrence (Band et al., 1974), while a third group using different treatment regimes as well as different patient selection was unable to show an increase in survival with CCNU (Brisman et al., 1976).

Combination chemotherapy

The rationale for combining different chemotherapy drugs is that by choosing agents with different mechanisms of antitumour effect and differing types of toxic effects, it should be possible to maximise the former and minimise the latter. One such triple agent combination is Procarbazine, CCNU and Vincristine. This appears a promising regime which has attained a projected median survival of over 50 weeks in one trial (Shapiro and Young, 1976).

Medulloblastoma. The principal treatment of medulloblastoma is surgery with adjuvant radiotherapy and this management can result in some long-term survivors in children who develop this tumour. The total neuraxis radiation required to prevent spread of this tumour in the subarachnoid space causes bone marrow depression and for this reason it may be difficult to give the patient chemotherapy in addition to radiotherapy. It is not desirable to reduce the craniospinal irradiation to ineffective levels simply to allow chemotherapy to be administered. In spite of these difficulties some trials of chemotherapy for medulloblastoma have been reported (Levin and Edwards, 1980). It seems probable that the drug combination Procarbazine, CCNU and Vincristine, used at the time of primary treatment does not show an improvement over radiotherapy alone, although it may induce remissions at the time of tumour recurrence.

Drug resistance

It is evident that several drugs can induce remissions lasting 6–9 months in approximately half of patients with cerebral glioma when given at the time of tumour recurrence. However, these same drugs appear only to increase median survival and disease-free interval by a matter of weeks when given as adjuvants at the time of primary treatment with surgery and radiotherapy. The reason for this discrepancy is not known, but it may be that those tumour cells which respond to radiation are the same 'sensitive' cells which respond also to drugs, and that the remaining viable fraction is 'resistant' to both modes of treatment, used alone or combined. This could explain why the majority of tumours recur at about the same time whether given radiotherapy alone or with chemotherapy, while a minority some, perhaps 18–20%, with a fraction particularly sensitive to chemotherapy, show prolonged survival.

Immunotherapy of malignant brain tumours

Histological examinations of operative biopsies or of autopsy material from patients with anaplastic cerebral gliomas have revealed lymphocyte infiltration in between one and two-thirds of cases. The perivascular infiltration is most marked at the periphery of the tumour, and is less pronounced in Grade IV than in Grade III astrocytoma. These findings suggest that some form of spontaneous immune response is taking place in patients with gliomas, although they do not provide evidence of specific antiglioma tumour immunity. Some tests of delayed type cutaneous hypersensitivity in patients with glioma, as well as *in vitro* tests of blood lymphocyte response or of serum factors have

suggested that in some cases there may be immunisation to glioma related antigens. Although these observations have to be interpreted with caution, because histocompatibility reactions may interfere in the tests, they suggest that immunotherapy of glioma may be feasible.

A number of clinical trials of immunotherapy for cerebral glioma have been undertaken. It has proved possible to cause an immune reaction in human glioma by immunotherapy, either by injection into tumour of lymphocytes or by active immunisation of the patient with tumour cells emulsified with Freund's adjuvant.

Passive immunotherapy by transfer of lymphocytes to the tumour bearing patients has shown some encouraging results. Using as donors healthy, non-tumour bearing volunteers, it was possible in one trial to treat patients with glioma either by bone marrow transplants administered intravenously or by white blood cells given directly into the tumour bed after surgical resection (Takakura *et al.*, 1972). In this series of 18 patients with malignant glioma, who had previously undergone surgery and radiotherapy, a 1-year survival of 85% and 2-year survival of 60% was obtained. It is possible to prepare by leucophoresis from a glioma patient's own peripheral blood a white cell fraction containing mixed autologous lymphocytes and leucocytes, which can be injected back into the patient either directly into the tumour bed or intrathecally into the subarachnoid space. In a series of 17 patients treated by intratumoural instillation of these cells, 8 showed clinical improvement (Young *et al.*, 1977). Following immunotherapy by intrathecal injection of such cells into the subarachnoid space, lymphocytic infiltration of the tumour has been demonstrated, but it is not yet established whether survival has been increased.

Active immunotherapy, by immunisation of the patient with the putative tumour antigens contained in intact tumour cells or in tumour homogenates has also been attempted. Some workers have been able to induce positive skin tests to an extract from glioma, and have achieved a small, but significant, increase in survival in patients with malignant glioma by such methods. Others have failed to demonstrate changes either in cutaneous reactivity to tumour extract or survival in patients receiving this form of immunotherapy. The results achieved may be due to variations in technique, particularly in methods of antigen preparation, choice of adjuvants used and immunisation regime employed.

Although it has proved possible to induce in some patients by immunotherapy an immune reaction to glioma using such methods, it must be recognised that the effects of immunotherapy are weak. However, if other modes of treatment, surgery, radiotherapy and chemotherapy can reduce the tumour mass to a low level, it may in future prove that immunotherapy will be useful clinically.

Further advances

In operative neurosurgery technique has advanced greatly during the past 20 years, due largely to the widespread introduction of the operating microscope and to concurrent advances in neuroanaesthetic techniques. The latter have improved with increased understanding of the physiology of raised intracranial pressure and cerebral blood flow so that operating conditions can be ideal for the surgeon at time of craniotomy. Powerful synthetic glucocortico steroids have been developed which can control cerebral oedema pre- and postoperatively. In this way the results of surgery for many benign tumours, particularly acoustic neurilemmoma, meningioma at the skull base and pituitary microadenoma, have improved dramatically in terms of morbidity and mortality. Newer technical methods are being developed which may be of use with malignant brain tumours. These include the use either of an ultrasonic probe disintegrator combined with an irrigating sucker or of a laser beam capable of both tissue vaporisation and haemostasis, in order to facilitate removal of cerebral glioma accurately and with minimum damage to surrounding brain. A further surgical innovation which is currently the subject of clinical trial in malignant glioma is the use of chemotherapy 4–6 weeks prior to craniotomy. The rationale for this, in cases where the diagnosis is established with reasonable certainty by radiological evidence or by burrhole biopsy, is to allow the surgeon to remove not only the portion of the tumour normally removed, but also those cells killed by the first course of drug treatment. It is also hoped that chemotherapy and surgery performed in this sequence may favourably alter the cell kinetics of the residual tumour by increasing its growth fraction and improving response to postoperative radiotherapy and further chemotherapy.

In radiotherapy new forms of radiation, neutrons and protons, have been explored. These can be delivered within a confined volume at a depth within the skull and may be of use in management of certain benign brain tumours, like pituitary adenoma and craniopharyngioma, and even some cases of neurilemmoma. A special class of radio-sensitising drugs, including metronidazole and misonidazole, has been developed. This can increase the radiation sensitivity of the normally radioresistant hypoxic cells in a brain tumour without increasing damage to the normal brain. It is possible that other classes of radiosensitising drugs may be developed in the future, for example agents which delay repair of what is otherwise sublethal radiation damage to tumour cells. The optimum way of frac-

tionating total radiation dose may also be changed. In the treatment of malignant brain tumour there is a trend towards whole brain irradiation using doses above brain tolerance with, in some cases, total neuraxis treatment. Interstitial radiation directly by stereotactically placed radioactive seeds is also under investigation.

In the field of chemotherapy new effective agents are being sought, both by rational synthesis on the basis of predicted biochemical target points in the tumour cell as well as by screening natural biological products of all kinds. Further variations in molecular structure of the nitrosourea group of drugs may improve their usefulness in the treatment of glioma. Experimental work with animal brain tumour models and with tissue cultured tumour cells may aid in development of new drugs and in selection of a particular agent for an individual patient according to the sensitivity of his tumour. Variations on the regimens and routes of delivery of chemotherapy drugs for brain tumours are also being investigated. Preliminary clinical studies suggest that massive doses of chemotherapeutic drugs, in otherwise fatal doses, coupled with autotransfusion of the patient's own marrow cells, which have been removed and stored before treatment, may be particularly effective against glioma.

Methods of immunodiagnosis and immunotherapy of brain tumour are being explored. Antigens specific to normal brain have been isolated and these can be assayed in blood, CSF and tissue. It is hoped that brain tumour specific antigens, if they exist, can be isolated and these may prove to be sensitive markers for diagnosis and follow-up during treatment. Immunotherapy with HLA mismatched, but live, glioma cells is being employed. If this method can be demonstrated to induce specific antitumour immunological responses, it may eventually supplement other modes of therapy.

References

Band P.R., Weir B.K.A., Urtasun R.C. *et al.* (1974). Radiotherapy and CCNU in Grade III and IV astrocytoma. ASCO Abstracts; **25:**161.

Bailey P., Cushing H. (1926). *A Classification of Tumors of the Glioma Group*. Philadelphia: Lippincott.

Brewis M., Poskanzer D.C., Rolland C., Miller H. (1966). Neurological disease in an English City. *Acta. Neurol. Scand.* Suppl; **42, 24:**1–89.

Brisman R., Houseplan E.M., Chang C., Duffy P., Balis E. (1976). Adjuvant nitrosourea therapy for glioblastoma. *Arch. Neurol*; **33:**745–50.

Capra L.G. (1980). Radiotherapy of cerebral gliomas. In *Brain Tumours: Scientific Basis, Clinical Investigation and Current Therapy* (Thomas D.G.T., Graham D.I., eds.). London: Butterworth.

Doig J.A. (1972). Auditory and vestibular function and dysfunction. In *Scientific Foundations of Neurology* (Critchley M., O'Leary J.L., Jennet W.B., eds.) pp. 138–47. London: Heinemann Medical.

EORTC Brain Tumor Group. (1976). Effect of CCNU on survival rate of objective remission and duration of free interval in patients with malignant brain glioma – first evaluation. *Europ. J. Cancer*; **12**:41–5.

Fewer D., Wilson C.B., Boldrey E.B., Enot K.J. (1972). A phase II study of 1-(2-chloroethyl)-3-cyclohexyl-1-nitrosourea (CCNU). *Cancer Cemother. Rep*; **56**:421–7.

Goran A., Murthy K.K. (1977). Solitary cerebral metastasis. Long-term survival following surgery. *N.Y. State J. Med*; **77**:1780.

Guiot G., Derome P. (1976). *Surgical Problems of Pituitary Adenomas. Advances and Technical Standards in Neurosurgery.* New York: Springer-Verlag; **3**:1–33.

Gutin P.H. (1975). Cortico-steroid therapy in patients with cerebral tumors: benefits, mechanisms, problems, practicalities. *Sem. Oncol*; **2**:49–56.

Hoshino T. (1979). Therapeutic implications of brain tumor cell kinetics. In *Modern Concepts in Brain Tumor Therapy, Laboratory and Clinical Investigations* (Evans A.E., ed.) pp. 27–33. London: Castle House.

Huckman M.S. (1975). Computerised tomography in relation to diagnosis of gliomas. In *Recent Results in Cancer Research: Gliomas* (Hekmatpanah J., ed.) p. 79. New York: Springer-Verlag.

Jones A. (1978). Cerebral astrocytoma – trends in radiotherapy and chemotherapy: a review. *J. Roy. Soc. Med*; **71**:669–74.

Karnofsky D.A., Burchenal J.H., Armistead G.C. *et al.* (1951). Triethylene melamine in the treatment of neoplastic disease. *Arch. Int. Med*; **87**:477–516.

Kernohan J.W., Sayre G.P. (1952). Tumours of the central nervous system. *Atlas of Tumour Pathology*, Fasicle 35. Washington D.C: Armed Forces, Institute of Pathology.

Kumar A.R.V., Renaudin J., Wilson C.B., Boldrey E.B., Enot K.J., Levin V.A. (1974). Procarbazine hydrochloride in the treatment of brain tumours. Phase 2 study. *J. Neurosurg*; **40**:365–71.

Levin V.A., Edwards M.S. (1980). Chemotherapy of primary malignant gliomas. In *Brain Tumours: Scientific Basis, Clinical Investigation and Current Therapy* (Thomas D.G.T., Graham D.I., eds.). London: Butterworth.

McKeran R.O., Thomas D.G.T. (1980). The clinical study of gliomas. In *Brain Tumours: Scientific Basis, Clinical Investigation and Current Therapy* (Thomas D.G.T., Graham D.I., eds.). London: Butterworth.

Percy A.K., Elveback L.R., Okazaki H., Kurland L.T. (1972). Neoplasms of the central nervous system: epidemiologic considerations. *Neurology* (Minneap) **22**:40–8.

Ransohoff J., Lieberman A. (1978). Surgical therapy of primary malignant brain tumours. *Clin. Neurosurg*; **26**:403–11.

Salazar O.M., Rubin P., McDonald J.V., Feldstein M.L. (1976). Patterns of failure in intracranial astrocytomas after irradiation: analysis of dose and field factors. *Amer. J. Roentgenol: Radium Ther. Nucl. Med*; **126**: 279–92.

Shapiro W.R., Young D.F. (1976). CCNU alone and combined with vincristine sulfate (VCR) and procarbazine (PCZ) as chemotherapy for malignant glioma. *Proc. Amer. Soc. Clin. Oncol*; **17**:258.

Sheline G.E. (1976). The importance of distinguishing tumor grade in malignant gliomas: treatment and prognosis. *Int. J. Radiat. Oncol. Biol. Phys*; **1**:781–6.

Takakura K., Miki Y., Kubo O., Owaga N., Matsutani M., Sano K. (1972). Adjuvant immunotherapy for malignant brain tumours. *Jpn. J. Clin. Oncol*; **12**:109.

Thomas D.G.T., Darling J.L., Freshney R.I., Morgan D. (1979). *In vitro* chemosensitivity assay of human glioma by scintillation autoflurorography. In *Proceedings of the International Symposium on Multidisciplinary Aspects of Brain Tumour Therapy*. Brescia, Italy (Paoletti P., ed.). Amsterdam: Elsevier/North Holland Biomedical Press.

Urtasun R., Band P.R., Chapman J.D., Feldstein M.L. (1977). Radiation plus metronidazole for glioblastoma. *N. Engl. J. Med*; **296**:757.

Walker M.D., Alexander E., Hunt W.E. *et al.* (1978). Evaluation of BCNU and/or radiotherapy in the treatment of anaplastic gliomas. A co-operative trial. *J. Neurosurg*; **49**:333–43.

Walker M.D., Strike T.A. (1976). An evaluation of methl-CCNU, BCNU and radiotherapy in the treatment of malignant glioma. *Proc. Amer. Ass. Cancer Res*; **17**:652.

WHO (1979). *Histological Typing of Tumours of the Central Nervous System.* (Zulch K.J., ed.) Geneva: World Health Organisation.

Wiltshirc C.R., Workman P., Watson J.V., Bleehan N.M. (1978). Clinical studies with misonidazole. *Brit. J. Cancer*; **37** Suppl III: 286–9.

Young H., Kaplan A., Regelson W. (1977). Immunotherapy with autologous white cell infusions ('lymphocytes') in the treatment of recurrent glioblastoma multiforme. *Cancer*; **40**:1037–44.

Young R.C., Walker M.D., Canellos G.P., Schein P.S., Chabner B.A., DeVita V.T. (1973). Initial clinical trials with methl-CCNU 1-(2-chloroethyl)-3-(4-methylcyclohexyl)-1-nitrosourea (MeCCNU). *Cancer*; **31**:1164–9.

41

Neck, pharynx, larynx, oral cavity

J. HIBBERT, A.G.D. MARAN and P.M. STELL

The neck

In the surgery of the neck one of the most important considerations is the correct management of the patient who presents with a lump in the neck. Most of these lumps can be correctly diagnosed by history and clinical examination. Radiological and serological examination may on certain occasions be valuable, but the concept of excisional biopsy is not to be recommended except to confirm the diagnosis of a lymphoma. The dangers of excisional biopsy without careful investigation beforehand are two-fold. Firstly metastatic squamous carcinoma from the upper respiratory tract is always a possibility in any patient with a lump in the lateral neck and excision biopsy of a lymph node containing metastatic squamous carcinoma seriously jeopardises the chance of curing the patient. In general a squamous carcinoma of the upper respiratory passages which has metastasised to cervical lymph nodes is most successfully treated by an incontinuity resection of the primary tumour and the neck glands and the integrity of this resection may be breached by a previous excision biopsy. Thus where the characteristics of a lump in the neck even remotely raise the possibility of a metastatic carcinoma a full examination of the upper respiratory tract should be performed under anaesthesia. The second situation in which excision biopsy of a lump in the neck may lead to problems is when the lesion is a carotid body tumour. Thus when a lump in the neck is closely related to the carotid artery, such a diagnosis should be borne in mind and either excluded or confirmed by a carotid angiogram. In this way the potentially dangerous situation of biopsy of a carotid body tumour will be avoided.

The diagnostic possibilities in a patient who presents with a lump in the neck are shown in Table 1.

Table 1
CLASSIFICATION OF NECK SWELLINGS

1. Congenital	lymphangiomas
	dermoid cysts
	thyroglossal duct cysts
	branchial cysts
2. Infective	tuberculosis
	sarcoidosis
	suppurative neck space infectious
	infectious mononucleosis
	toxoplasmosis
	brucellosis
3. Tumours of nervous tissue	peripheral nerve tumours
	carotid body tumours
	glomus vagal tumours
4. Developmental neck masses	laryngocoeles
	pharyngeal pouches
5. Thyroid and parathyroid swellings (*see* chapters 34, 35)	
6. Salivary gland swellings (*see* chapter 42).	
7. Lymphomas (*see* chapter 38)	
8. Metastatic lymph nodes	

The lesions of surgical interest will be described below. Thyroid, parathyroid and salivary gland swellings are discussed in chapters 34 and 35.

Congenital neck swellings

Lesions included under this heading are thought to arise because of abnormalities of development of the cervical region and are usually, though not always, present in childhood.

Lymphangiomas

These usually occur alone, but occasionally may be associated with haemangiomas. Three pathological types are recognised. The lymphangioma simplex consists of capillary-sized lymphatic vessels and is most commonly found in the oral cavity, particularly the lips, tongue and cheek. Cavernous lymphangiomas are composed of dilated lymphatic vessels with a fibrous adventitia. They are the most frequent of the lymphangiomas and occur mainly in the tongue either on its lateral border or at the base where they may be confused with a lingual thyroid. Cystic hygromas consist of multilocular cystic masses, each loculus being lined by a single layer of flattened endothelium and containing cholesterol crystals. The individual cysts may be isolated or may communicate with each other. Cystic hygromas usually occur in the neck, but often extend into the mouth and occasionally into the axilla or mediastinum.

Clinical features. Most lymphangiomas are obvious at or soon after birth, although those restricted to the mouth may not be diagnosed until adult life. The presenting symptom and sign is usually that of a mass, possibly associated with pressure symptoms due to displacement or compression of the trachea. Occasionally these lesions may give rise to sudden onset of stridor due to haemorrhage into the cysts. Surgical excision is the treatment of choice, but they may be much more extensive than at first appears. In lesions of the neck a chest radiograph is necessary to identify a mediastinal component. Once the diagnosis has been established, surgery should be performed because delay will nearly always result in increase in size and increased mortality or morbidity. This is especially true in lesions of the neck. The operation is difficult because of the extent of these swellings, but the aim should be complete excision with preservation of normal structures. The lesion will often be closely related to the internal jugular vein within the carotid sheath and the structures within the sheath should be dissected free from the cystic mass. Extension into the parotid region may occur and excision should only follow after superficial parotidectomy and identification of the facial nerve. Lymphangiomas in the oral cavity are often very extensive and usually require an external approach through the submandibular triangle. Lymphangiomas of the base of the tongue may be controlled by coagulation diathermy, cryosurgery or laser surgery. Macrocheilia due to a lymphangioma of the lip is treated by a lip shave, i.e. elevation of the vermilion and excision of sufficient cyst and vermilion to reduce the lip to a normal size.

Recurrence of a lymphangioma may occur within months of surgery or may be delayed until adult life, following excision of a lesion in infancy. Incision and drainage of lymphangiomas, or injection of sclerosing agents is not advisable as it does not cure the lesion and only makes subsequent surgery more difficult. Irradiation has been suggested as one form of treatment but, because of growth retardation and the risks of inducing malignancy in adjacent organs in adult life, it is not to be recommended.

Dermoid cysts

Three varieties of cyst can be included under this heading:

1 Epidermoid cysts are lined by squamous epithelium and contain cheesy keratinous material. No adnexal structures occur in these cysts and that is their distinguishing feature.
2 True dermoid cysts are lined by squamous epithelium associated with skin appendages such as hair, sebaceous glands and sweat glands. The congenital type of dermoid cyst occurs along lines of fusion of ectoderm; the traumatic type occurs at the site of a puncture wound which has implanted epidermis into the underlying tissues.
3 Teratoid cysts are lined either by squamous epithelium or respiratory epithelium and contain tissues derived from all three embryonic germ layers. Thus nails, teeth, glandular structures and even nervous tissue may be present.

Clinical features. Teratoid cysts nearly always present in the first year of life, whereas dermoid cysts, though probably present from birth, usually present in the second or third decades. Dermoid cysts give rise to painless swellings which, when large, can cause obstructive symptoms. The most common site is in the midline of the neck from suprasternal notch to the submental region. Treatment is by surgical excision and usually there is an easy plane of dissection between the cyst wall and surrounding tissues.

Thyroglossal duct cyst

This is the most common variety of midline neck cyst and arises from a remnant of the thyroglossal duct. The thyroid gland precursor arises from the floor of the pharynx between the first and second pharyngeal pouches and this site of origin is represented by the foramen caecum of the tongue. The thyroglossal duct atrophies at the 6th week of intrauterine life, but on occasions persists, opening at the foramen caecum. Since the tongue and hyoid bone develop later than the thyroid gland the persistent duct is buried deep in the muscle of the tongue and has a variable relationship with the hyoid bone, lying behind or in front or occasionally passing through the body of the bone. Thyroglossal duct cysts occur anywhere from the foramen caecum to the suprasternal notch and are attached to the base of the tongue by the duct.

Clinical features. The age of presentation is anything from infancy to old age, but most cysts present in childhood at about the age of 5 years. Most are in the midline, but 10% occur to one side of the midline as far lateral as the anterior border of the sternomastoid. For no apparent reason laterally situated cysts are much more common on the left than the right. The level of the cyst in the neck is variable though most occur in the region of the hyoid bone (75%). The lesion usually presents as a painless cystic swelling which rises on swallowing and on protrusion of the tongue. If the cyst is low in the neck, the persistent duct may be visible as a subcutaneous tract. An external fistula occurs only as a result of infection or more commonly following previous surgery. Treatment of these cysts is surgical and the cyst and duct should be removed in their entirety to avoid recurrence. This invariably means removing the central part of the body of the hyoid bone.

A thyroglossal duct cyst can occasionally be the site of a papillary thyroid carcinoma which is usually diagnosed on histological examination of the excised cyst.

Branchial cysts

The origin of branchial cysts is a subject of debate and a number of theories have been put forward (Maran and Buchanan 1978). One theory is that these cysts arise from developmental anomalies occurring in the branchial apparatus as remnants of pharyngeal pouches or branchial clefts. Thus in a 2-week-old embryo there are six branchial arches and between them five branchial clefts and five pharyngeal pouches. The first pouch forms the middle ear, the second the palatine tonsil, the third and fourth contribute to the parathyroid glands and thymus. A downgrowth from the second pouch meets the fifth arch and lies lateral to the second, third and fourth clefts, forming the cervical sinus of His. It is possible that a branchial cyst is a remnant of part of this developmental system. It is also conceivable that a cyst could arise from the first pharyngeal

pouch as cysts do occur related to the parotid gland with an internal opening into the external auditory meatus. Origin from the second pouch or from the cervical sinus of His would explain those cysts which have an internal opening in the region of the tonsil. Origin of cysts from the third pouch is unlikely as the internal opening would have to be in the pyriform fossa and this has not been described. Similarly, fourth pouch remnants would have to lie inferior to the branchiocephalic artery on the right and aortic arch on the left. Origin of a cyst from the thymopharyngeal duct has been suggested, but in this case one would expect to find cysts deep to the thyroid or related to the thymus and these have never been described.

The main objection to the origin of cysts from the primitive branchial apparatus is that only the occasional lesion has any connection with the pharynx, the vast majority being totally isolated. It is probable that those cysts with an internal opening or a fibrous tract connected to the external auditory meatus or pharynx do arise from the first or second pharyngeal pouches, but most cysts probably have a different origin. The alternative explanation is the inclusion theory in which it is postulated that the squamous epithelium of branchial cysts is derived either from the epithelium of lymph nodes, or from epithelial inclusion at the time of formation of the lymph nodes. This would explain why branchial cysts have lymphoid tissue in their walls. This theory also agrees better with the peak age of incidence of branchial cysts which is later than would be expected for a congenital condition (cf. thyroglossal duct cyst).

Clinical features. Branchial cysts most commonly present in the 3rd decade as a lump in the lateral neck. They are more common (66%) in the left neck than the right and the majority are situated along the anterior border of the sternomastoid muscle in the upper third of the neck. They can occur in the parotid region, in the lower neck and, occasionally, in the parapharyngeal space adjacent to the oropharynx. Most cysts present as a painless lump in the neck, some give rise to intermittent swelling and others are painful or tender with obvious signs of infection. On palpation, 70% of cysts are fluctuant but 30% feel solid. On occasions, transmitted pulsation can be felt and in this case carotid angiography is necessary to exclude a chemodectoma. Branchial cysts are usually lined by stratified squamous epithelium, but some have non-ciliated columnar epithelium. Most cysts have lymphoid tissue in their walls and contain straw-coloured fluid in which cholesterol crystals can be found.

The treatment of branchial cysts is by excision (Deane and Telander, 1978). Those cysts presenting with obvious infection should be treated with antibiotics rather than by incision and drainage which complicates subsequent removal. When the cyst is in the parotid region, facial nerve identification and superficial parotidectomy are necessary to avoid damaging the nerve. If a tract is found arising from a cyst it should be traced inwards though, as previously stated, this is a rare event.

Infective neck swellings

The infective swellings of surgical interest are tuberculous cervical adenitis and suppurative neck space infections.

Tuberculous cervical adenitis

This condition is still common in Asia and Africa but uncommon in the UK. The organism involved is usually the human tubercle bacillus and since less than 5% of patients have evidence of coexistent pulmonary tuberculosis the probability is that the bacillus reaches the lymph node via the lymphatic tissue of the upper respiratory tract. In the UK the peak age incidence is 5–9 years but a significant proportion of patients are adults (about 30%).

Clinical features. Most patients have a fairly long history of a lump in the neck which may have become painful. Usually the condition is unilateral and as a rule only one group of lymph nodes is involved, the commonest being the deep jugular, followed by the submandibular and the nodes of the posterior triangle respectively. The differential diagnosis is between a lymphoma and metastatic cancer, thus a search should be made for a possible primary carcinoma in the upper respiratory tract. The diagnosis of tuberculosis is made by histology or bacteriology and a positive tuberculin skin test is suggestive. Treatment is excision followed by chemotherapy. When the glands are large and fixed, local removal is hazardous and the safest approach is to perform a functional neck dissection with preservation of the sternomastoid muscle, accessory nerve and internal jugular vein. Chemotherapy should immediately follow excision, otherwise a sinus will develop with a poor cosmetic result.

Neck space infections

The division of the neck into numerous spaces bounded by fascia is of little more than anatomical interest now that antibiotics effectively control the spread of infection. From a surgical point of view three neck spaces are important as sites of abscesses. The retropharyngeal space lies between the pharynx and the prevertebral fascia. The lateral pharyngeal space or parapharyngeal space lies lateral to the pharynx and communicates posteriorly with the retropharyngeal space. It is limited laterally by the lateral pterygoid muscle, the carotid sheath and the stylohyoid and digastric muscles. The submandibular space lies between the mucous membrane of the tongue and floor of mouth and the fascia between the hyoid bone and mandible. It is divided by the mylohyoid muscle into the sublingual space and the submaxillary space containing the glands of the same name.

Clinical features. *Retropharyngeal abscess.* This can occur in children or adults. In children the abscess is due to infection of one of the retropharyngeal lymph nodes which usually lie to one side of the midline. The infection is bacterial and usually secondary to an upper respiratory tract infection. The abscess arises at first to one side of the midline and the posterior pharyngeal wall swelling may be sufficient to cause laryngeal obstruction. The diagnosis is confirmed by a lateral radiograph of the neck and treatment is by incision and drainage through the pharyngeal mucosa. In the adult a retropharyngeal abscess is usually behind the prevertebral fascia due to spread of tuberculous disease of the cervical vertebrae. The diagnosis is confirmed by a lateral radiograph and treatment is by incision and drainage via the neck followed by antituberculous chemotherapy.

Parapharyngeal abscess. An abscess in this space is a complication of tonsillitis or tonsillectomy in 60% of patients and the result of infection of the lower third molar tooth in 30%. Ingested foreign bodies, infection of the petrous apex or mastoid tip complicating otitis media account for the remainder. Clinically the patient is ill with fever and trismus. The tonsil is pushed medially by the swelling and there is swelling of the neck at the posterior part of the middle third of the sternomastoid muscle. Treatment is by intramuscular penicillin with incision and drainage from a cervical approach in those patients where a discrete abscess has formed.

Ludwig's angina. This is the name given to a rapidly spreading cellulitis of the floor of the mouth and submandibular space. The usual cause is dental infection and in these patients the lower molars are placed eccentrically so that their roots lie close to the lingual surface of the mandible. When the roots of the teeth are inferior to the mylohyoid line, the infection occurs initially in the submaxillary space later spreading to the sublingual space. The floor of the mouth becomes grossly oedematous and brawny with the tongue pushed upwards and backwards so that respiratory obstruction is a danger. Treatment is with antibiotics with extraction of the tooth responsible. Incision and drainage of the submandibular space is rarely necessary as pus is not usually formed.

Tumours of nervous tissue

These tumours arise from tissues derived from the neural crest and the different types are summarised in Fig 41.1.

Neurofibromas, schwannomas and ganglioneuromas give rise to peripheral nerve tumours and are considered together. Paragangliomas will be considered separately.

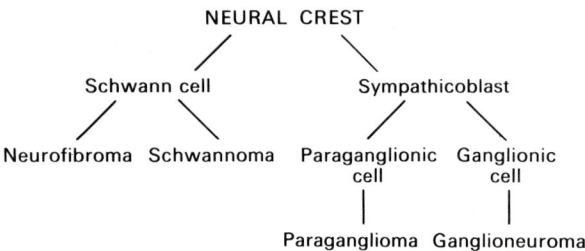

Fig 41.1   Tumours of nervous tissue.

Peripheral nerve tumours

Peripheral nerve tumours occur more commonly in the head and neck than in any other region and can arise from the cervical and brachial plexus, IX to XII cranial nerves and in the case of ganglioneuromas from a sympathetic ganglion. Schwannomas and neurofibromas arise from the inner and outer sheaths of nerves respectively and differ histologically and clinically. Schwannomas consist of Schwann cells and connective tissue fibres which may be regularly arranged with palisading of nuclei (Antoni type A) or loosely arranged (Antoni type B). Schwannomas tend to be single, painful, well encapsulated and very rarely subject to malignant change. Neurofibromas consist of a dense arrangement of spindle shaped cells arranged in streams or whorls. They are often multiple, forming part of von-Recklinghausen's syndrome, and are seldom painful unless malignant change has occurred and this is liable to happen in 10–15%.

Clinical features. These tumours present as a slow growing, usually painless, mass in the neck. Pressure on the sympathetic chain may give rise to a Horner's syndrome, but the other nerves involved are usually only paralysed when malignant change has occurred. Diagnosis of a solitary nerve tumour is confirmed by excision biopsy, but this is only undertaken after endoscopy of the upper respiratory tract to exclude a silent primary carcinoma with a secondary metastatic deposit, though a patient with the latter usually has a much shorter history. At excision, the nerve of origin of the

tumour should be preserved if possible. A malignant peripheral neuroma presents as a painful, rapidly growing swelling in a previous painless swelling and may be associated with a palsy of the brachial plexus or cranial nerves IX to XII. Treatment is by wide excision if possible.

Paragangliomas (chemodectomas)

These arise from non-chromaffin paraganglionic cells which occur in the neck at the carotid bifurcation, the ganglion nodosum of the vagus nerve, or the jugular bulb. Lesions at the first two sites present as a mass in the neck, lesions at the jugular bulb present with tinnitus and cranial nerve palsies. There is an increased incidence of paragangliomas in populations living at high altitude and there is a familial tendency. Multiple or bilateral tumours are found in 25% of patients and a phaeochromocytoma may occur in the same patient. Malignant paragangliomas have been described though less than 10% of patients have obviously malignant lesions (Conley, 1965).

Clinical features. All patients present with a painless lump in the neck which has usually been present for a number of years. The carotid body tumour presents as a swelling in the mid-neck at the level of the carotid bifurcation. Vagal body tumours are a little higher at the angle of the jaw and can be confused with a parotid swelling. About 30% of patients, as well as having a swelling in the neck, have an obvious swelling in the oropharynx displacing the tonsil medially and this must be distinguished from other causes of a parapharyngeal mass including a deep lobe parotid swelling. On occasions the tumour may not be palpable in the neck and only visible in the oropharynx. The mass, when palpable in the neck, is usually pulsatile and in large tumours may be associated with IX to XII cranial nerve palsies or a Horner's syndrome. Any patient with a swelling in the lateral neck adjacent to the carotid artery should be suspected of having a carotid body tumour, and an angiogram should be ordered. This usually shows a highly vascular tumour with separation of the internal and external carotid arteries. In addition to demonstrating the tumour, angiography is important to demonstrate cerebral cross-circulation (Palacios, 1970) so that if the carotid artery needs to be ligated or grafted the risks of a neurological deficit can be assessed. A useful investigation to identify possible complications of surgery is cerebral blood flow measurement after carotid compression.

The treatment of these lesions is surgical, but because of the mortality and morbidity of carotid artery ligation this is not recommended in all patients. In general, patients in the following three groups should be advised to have surgical treatment (Conley, 1963):

1   Tumours which are growing rapidly and appear to be clinically malignant.
2   Patients under the age of 50 years in good health.
3   Patients with a tumour which because of pharyngeal extension is interfering with swallowing, speech or breathing.

Patients who refuse operation or those who are elderly and have symptoms related to the tumour should be treated with radiotherapy as some of these lesions are radiosensitive.

The technique of operating on carotid body tumours is initial control of the carotid arteries above and below the lesion followed by dissection of the tumour from adjacent structures. The attachment of the tumour at the carotid bulb is the final part of the dissection since this is the most likely point at which the carotid system will be damaged. In 80% of patients the carotid artery will not be damaged by the procedure (Farr, 1967). In the others, some form of arterial surgery is necessary, either primary closure of a defect in the artery or replacement of a segment of artery by a vein graft (Ward *et al.*, 1978).

Developmental neck masses

Included in this group are laryngoceles and pharyngeal pouches which 'develop' by dilatation of existing structures.

Laryngocele

A laryngocele is an air-containing sac which arises by dilatation of the laryngeal saccule, a structure which opens into the laryngeal ventricle between the true and false cords and lies on the medial surface of the thyroid cartilage. Laryngoceles are more common in men than women (5:1) and the peak age incidence is 50–60 years. They have been said to be more common in trumpet-players or glass blowers, but this is not confirmed. A small proportion of laryngoceles is secondary to a laryngeal carcinoma which has obstructed the laryngeal saccule. The laryngocele may expand laterally and present in the neck by passing through the thyrohyoid membrane at the point of entry of the internal laryngeal vessels and nerve. Alternatively the laryngocele expands internally displacing the ventricle, aryepiglottic fold and pyriform fossa. Approximately 50% of laryngoceles have both an internal and external element, 30% are purely external and 20% internal.

Clinical features. The most common presenting symptoms are hoarseness and swelling in the neck, which may be bilateral. Some patients present with stridor and the danger of laryngoceles is that they can seriously impair the laryngeal airway. Laryngoceles feel cystic and can be filled by the patient performing a Valsalva manoeuvre and emptied by compression. On occasions, a laryngocele may become infected which results in rapid increase in size, pain, dysphagia and respiratory distress. If the diagnosis is suspected, it can be confirmed by an antero-posterior radiograph of the neck which shows an air-filled sac, often with a fluid level.

Laryngoceles should be treated by excision after the larynx has been examined by direct laryngoscopy. A temporary tracheostomy may be necessary. At operation the thyroid cartilage on the side of the lesion is exposed and its external perichondrium is incised along the upper border and turned inferiorly as a flap. In this way the upper half of the thyroid cartilage can be removed and the neck of the laryngocele identified and transected (Stell and Maran, 1975).

Pharyngeal diverticulum

Although this very rarely gives rise to a palpable mass in the neck it is discussed here for the sake of completeness (*also see* chapter 4.)

Pathology. The most common pharyngeal diverticulum is a pulsion diverticulum of the mucosa of the posterior pharyngeal wall between the cricopharyngeal and thyropharyngeal components of the inferior constrictor muscle. It occurs most frequently in the elderly. Manometric and cineradiographic studies show a region of increased pressure at the cricopharyngeus with a failure of relaxation at the time of swallowing. Sometimes a second swallow against a closed cricopharyngeus can be demonstrated. It is, therefore, considered that the diverticulum develops as a result of increased pressure in the hypopharynx as a result of uncoordinated swallowing.

Clinical features. Most patients complain of dysphagia, regurgitation of undigested food and a gurgling sensation on swallowing. In some patients weight loss, cough and pneumonia will be the result of dysphagia and overspill. Only rarely will a mass be palpable in the neck though a gurgling sensation may be felt if the patient is asked to swallow fluid. A barium swallow will demonstrate the pouch and this can be confirmed by oesophagoscopy which is often difficult because the oesophagoscope tends to pass into the pouch and the anterior lying oesophageal opening may be difficult to identify. Occasionally, a carcinoma develops in a pharyngeal pouch and this can be biopsied at oesophagoscopy.

Treatment. On occasions the pouch will be very small and not giving sufficient symptoms to warrant treatment, particularly in the elderly. However, most pouches ought to be treated and this can either be by endoscopic diathermy or by surgical excision. The rationale for endoscopic diathermy is that it saves the patient a neck exploration and is, therefore, said to be safer in the elderly. At endoscopy the partition between the pouch and oesophageal wall is destroyed by diathermy. Although this procedure gives good results in experienced hands (Dohlmann and Mattson, 1960), the danger is that too enthusiastic diathermy will perforate the pouch and oesophagus with the risk of mediastinitis which carries a high mortality. The alternative procedure is to explore the neck, excise the pouch, perform a cricopharyngeal myotomy and close the defect in the pharynx. This is probably the safer procedure even in the elderly.

Lymphomas

The cervical lymph nodes are the most frequent site for lymphoma in the head and neck. Other sites are in the nasopharynx, the oropharynx and the paranasal sinuses.

Clinical features. The patient will present either with a lump in the neck or with symptoms related to a mass in the nasopharynx, oropharynx or paranasal sinuses. In those patients who present with a lump in the neck, the main differential diagnosis is of a primary carcinoma of the upper respiratory tract with a metastatic lymph node. This should be excluded by endoscopy. The diagnosis of lymphoma is made by biopsy of the mass in the nasopharynx, oropharynx or paranasal sinuses or by excision biopsy of a lymph node when this is the only site. A chest radiograph, pedal lymphangiography and liver and spleen scan are important in the staging of the disease. In general, lymphoma which is restricted to the head and neck is treated by radiotherapy and disseminated disease by local radiotherapy and systemic chemotherapy (*see* chapter 38.)

Metastatic cervical lymph nodes

A common clinical situation is the one in which a patient presents with a single swelling in the neck and the possibility arises as to whether this is a secondary malignant node. The importance of the correct handling of this clinical situation is that biopsy of a secondary deposit from a primary carcinoma in the head and neck seriously jeopardises future curative treatment and should be avoided. The commonest primary sites in the head and neck which present with metastases in cervical glands are nasopharynx, oropharynx and pyriform fossa: 60%, 20% and 10% of patients respectively with a lesion in these sites have a lump in the neck as a pre-

senting symptom. Occasionally, a tumour from below the clavicle may present as a swelling in the neck; bronchus, stomach and breast being the commonest primary sites.

The investigation of a patient with a lump in the neck which is suspected of being a lymph node mestastasis should be by history, clinical examination, radiology and endoscopy, all performed before contemplating excisional biopsy. In the clinical examination, particular attention should be paid to mirror examination of the nasopharynx, hypopharynx and larynx and careful examination of the oral cavity, (particularly the retromolar trigone) and oropharynx. Radiological examination should include a chest radiograph and a barium swallow. The final stage in diagnosis is endoscopy under anaesthesia of the nasopharynx, oropharynx, hypopharynx and larynx with examination under magnification and palpation of these sites. If inspection is negative some authorities would advocate biopsy of the nasopharynx, base of tongue and excision of the tonsil on the side of the lesion. If all these investigations are negative the likelihood is that the lump will be a lymphoma and the patient should be prepared for excision biopsy. As an alternative to excision biopsy, drill biopsy is performed in some centres with positive results in 70–90% of patients. Where skilled histology is available, fine needle aspiration biopsy cytology (ABC) can provide immediate diagnosis. Incisional biopsy with subsequent local spread of tumour should not be performed. At excision biopsy a frozen section should be performed and if the gland contains metastatic squamous carcinoma a radical neck dissection should be done. Careful follow-up of these patients with repeated endoscopy will reveal a primary tumour in about 40%, and a further 40% will die of distant metastases with no evidence of a primary lesion. In those patients in whom a primary lesion is subsequently discovered the site of the primary will be in the head and neck in 60% (Table 2).

At one time there was a vogue for the diagnosis of branchiogenic carcinoma assuming that squamous carcinoma in the lateral neck had arisen from a branchial remnant. Many of the patients diagnosed as having a

Table 2
RELATIVE FREQUENCY OF TUMOUR SITES IN PATIENTS WITH A METASTATIC GLAND AND AN OCCULT PRIMARY

Oropharynx	15%
Nasopharynx	15%
Thyroid	20%
Hypopharynx	10%
Lung	20%
Gastrointestinal tract	10%
Miscellaneous distant sites	10%

branchiogenic carcinoma had inadequate search for a primary tumour, and it is likely that most of the patients had secondary carcinomas from an occult primary in the head and neck.

Classification of metastatic cervical lymph nodes

Many carcinomas of the head and neck metastasise to the cervical nodes, but spread beyond these nodes may be delayed for long periods or may never occur. Head and neck cancers are staged by a system depending upon the extent of the primary tumour, the presence and extent of the involved cervical lymph nodes and the presence or absence of distant metastases. The present classification (UICC, 1978) of malignant lymph nodes is shown in Table 3.

Table 3
CLASSIFICATION OF METASTATIC CERVICAL LYMPH NODES

N_0	Regional lymph nodes not palpable
N_1	Mobile homolateral lymph nodes
N_2	Mobile contralateral or bilateral lymph nodes
N_3	Fixed nodes

N_1 and N_2 categories can be divided into *a* or *b* as to whether they are considered not to contain a growth or to contain growth respectively. These divisions are of little value in practice as this is a clinical not histological classification. The progression from N_0 to N_3 implies a worsening prognosis, whereas this is not true, in that the prognosis for bilateral nodes is nearly always worse than that for fixed nodes.

Management of cervical lymph nodes in patients with head and neck cancers

Patients with no palpable nodes (N_0). It has been suggested many times that in order to improve the survival rates of patients with head and neck cancer, treatment should be directed to both the primary lesion and cervical nodes even when no nodes are palpable. This is based upon the concept that a proportion of patients will have tumour in the cervical lymph nodes when these are not palpable. The incidence of occult nodes with primary tumours at various head and neck sites is shown in Table 4.

Table 4
INCIDENCE OF OCCULT NODES

Pyriform fossa	40%
Base of tongue	20%
Supraglottic larynx	15%
Transglottic larynx	10%
Glottic with fixed vocal cord	5%

Though theoretically an advantage to the patient with a high risk of occult nodes, prophylactic neck dissection has never been shown to give superior survival rates over patients treated by neck dissection when nodes become palpable. This assumes a careful follow-up of patients and it may be that prophylactic neck dissection is of value for those patients with a high risk of occult nodes who are unlikely to return for follow-up. The alternative approach is the use of prophylactic neck irradiation in patients with a high risk of metastases but no palpable nodes, and it may be that prophylactic neck irradiation may reduce the number of patients needing neck dissection for nodes which become palpable after successful treatment of the primary lesion (Johnson *et al.*, 1980).

Unilateral cervical metastases (N_1). It is generally, though by no means universally, accepted that once a head and neck tumour has metastasised to the cervical lymph nodes the best chance of cure is surgery. This means an *en bloc* resection of the primary tumour and cervical lymph nodes. It also means surgical treatment of lymph nodes which appear after the successful treatment of a primary lesion. The standard operation of radical neck dissection was first described by Crile in 1906 and the basic surgical procedure remains unchanged since that time. Certain modifications of the operation have been suggested, namely preoperative radiotherapy in an attempt to improve the cure rate and certain technical modifications to reduce the complications of operation.

Preoperative radiotherapy. Most patients who die of head and neck cancer do so because of recurrence of tumour either at the primary site or in the neck. After surgery, recurrence of tumour may occur either because tumour was left behind at the margins of the excision, or because tumour cells were implanted into the raw surfaces exposed by surgery. A small dose of radiotherapy (1000–2000 rads) is known to destroy 98% of cells in sensitive tumours and this given preoperatively would theoretically reduce the recurrence rate without increasing complications. This theoretical advantage remains to be substantiated by controlled trials.

Prevention of complications. Major complications after radical neck dissection are of the order of 20% and these result in a significant mortality as well as morbidity. The main lethal complication is skin necrosis with exposure and then rupture of the carotid artery. The frequency of this complication is increased by radiotherapy, and it is more frequent in those patients who develop a salivary fistula after resection of a lesion in the oral cavity, pharynx or larynx. In order to avoid this complication particular attention should be paid to the skin incision. In patients particularly at risk the carotid artery should be protected.

The skin incision. Crile in his original description advocated a Y-shaped incision and since that time many different incisions have been described. A modification of Crile's original Y-shaped incision is still in widespread use today (Fig 41.2). This modification incorporates a wavy vertical limb to reduce the likelihood of scar contracture. The disadvantage of this incision is that if wound breakdown occurs, this is most likely at the three point junction and along the vertical limb which often overlies the carotid artery. The McFee incision avoids a vertical component by using two horizontal incisions, one at the level of the hyoid bone and the other just above the clavicle (Fig 41.3). Recent experimental work (Rogers and Freeland, 1976) suggests that the skin of the neck derives its blood supply from above and below from vessels running vertically. The watershed between these two vascular supplies is an approximately horizontal line running from the middle of the anterior border of the trapezius towards the medial end of the clavicle. An incision which avoids interrupting the blood supply to the neck skin should run along this watershed. A ⊣ shaped incision with the vertical limb at the anterior border of the trapezius and the horizontal limb running forwards from the middle of the trapezius and then turning superiorly to the point of the chin would seem to be the most suitable (Fig 41.4). The other advantage of this incision is that if wound breakdown does occur at the three point junction this is well behind the carotid artery.

Carotid artery protection. In a patient who has been irradiated and particularly when the operation is combined with a major oral, pharyngeal or laryngeal resection when fistula formation is likely, the carotid artery should be protected. This can be done either by a muscle flap or by a free dermal graft. The former method is probably the more satisfactory. The levator scapulae is incised posteriorly and inferiorly to develop a triangular flap hinged anteriorly and turned forward to protect the artery (Figs 41.5; 41.6).

Functional neck dissection. In order to reduce the morbidity after radical neck dissection, modified techniques preserving the sternomastoid muscle, accessory nerve and internal jugular vein have been described (Bocca *et al.*, 1980). How much these techniques compromise the chance of cure is unkown and probably depends on the size and number of the metastatic nodes. Certainly this type of modified neck dissection is the one of choice for papillary carcinoma of the thyroid gland, a tumour which although it metastasises to local lymph nodes does not transgress the capsule of the node, unlike metastases from squamous carcinomas of the head and neck.

Bilateral neck glands (N₂). Bilateral cervical metastases are not common; perhaps 5% of all patients have bilateral nodes at presentation. This is fortunate because a tumour which has metastasised bilaterally is rarely curable. Tumours of the base of the tongue, the supraglottic larynx and the hypopharynx are the primary tumours which most commonly give rise to bilateral metastases. Of these tumours with bilateral metastases, supraglottic laryngeal lesions carry the best prognosis,

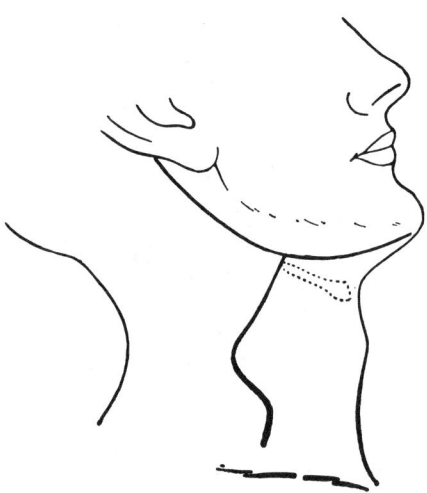

Fig 41.2 Y-type incision.

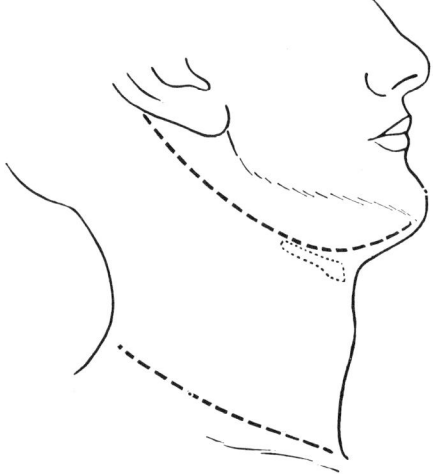

Fig 41.3 Double horizontal incision (McFee).

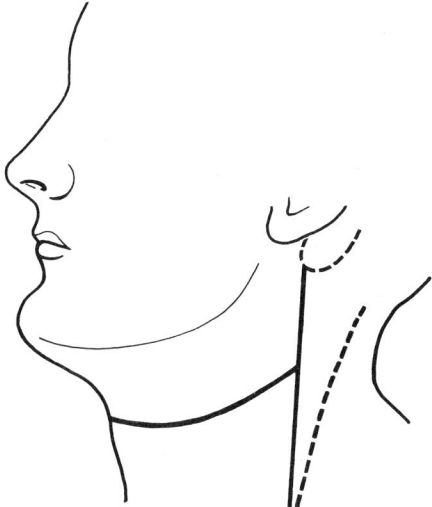

Fig 41.4   Recommended incision for radical neck dissection.

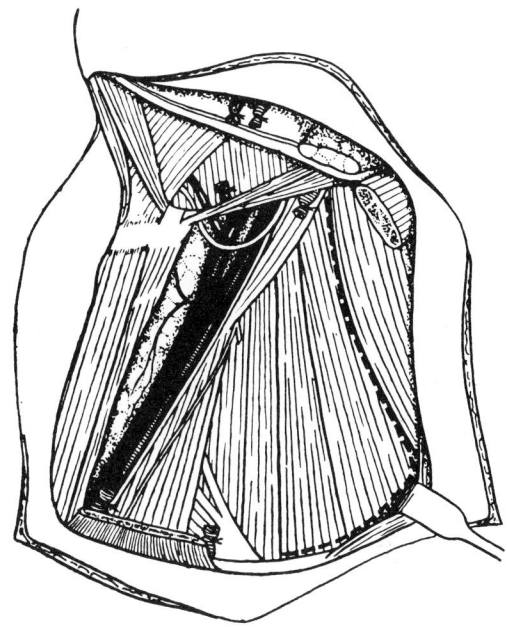

Fig 41.5   Levator scapulae flap marked out.

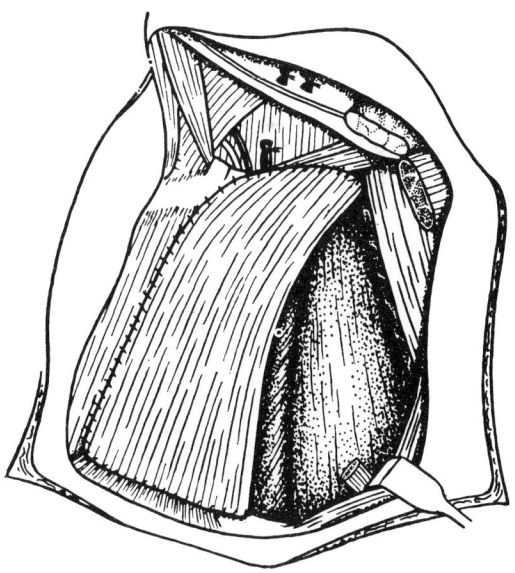

Fig 41.6   Levator scapulae flap stitched into place.

and it may be that patients with tumours at other sites with bilateral neck metastases are best left untreated and certainly not treated surgically. This is not true of patients who develop a node in the contralateral side of the neck following treatment of a primary tumour and ipsilateral neck metastasis. These patients do very well with a second neck dissection. The complication rate with bilateral simultaneous neck dissection is very high with an increased incidence of skin necrosis, fistulas and facial oedema. Perhaps the most lethal complication after bilateral simultaneous neck dissection is cerebral oedema. The intracranial pressure rises threefold after ligation of one internal jugular vein whereas if both are ligated the pressure rises fivefold. The value of hypertonic mannitol, steroids and diuretics are unknown, but certainly patients who have had bilateral neck dissection should be nursed sitting up and there should be no dressings on the neck. A second neck dissection performed some time after the first side, although associated with temporary facial oedema, is not associated with these complications. A temporary tracheostomy, however, should be performed because of laryngeal and pharyngeal oedema.

Fixed neck gland (N$_3$). Fixation of metastatic neck glands is very difficult to assess and is subject to wide observer variation. A gland is most unlikely to be fixed unless it is large (i.e. 6 cm or more in diameter) and even then it can usually be dissected free. Fixation to the base of the skull or brachial plexus almost certainly means that the patient cannot be cured. Fixation to the skin is not common, but if it occurs without fixation to

other structures, resection can be performed with replacement of the skin with a delto-pectoral flap. A gland fixed to the mandible can be removed either by subperiosteal dissection or perhaps more safely by a marginal resection of the involved bone. A tumour fixed to the common carotid artery is an unusual situation which can be overcome by resection of the common carotid artery and vein grafting, but the operative morbidity and mortality is high and the chance of cure very low, although an occasional survivor has been described.

The pharynx

The pharynx consists of three parts the nasopharynx, the oropharynx and the hypopharynx (laryngopharynx) which lie behind the nasal cavities, the oral cavity and the larynx respectively. These divisions are shown in Fig 41.7. The only lesions of the pharynx which are of general surgical interest are neoplasms and the vast majority of these are malignant.

Nasopharynx

This, the most superior division of the pharynx, lies behind the posterior choanae of the nose and above the soft palate.

Malignant tumours

Pathology. Most of the malignant tumours are squamous carcinomas, with 10% of non-Hodgkin's lymphomas and small numbers of adenocarcinomas, rhabdomyosarcomas, fibrosarcomas and plasmacytomas. Nasopharyngeal cancer is particularly common in China where it forms 80% of head and neck cancers, compared with 6% of head and neck cancers in Europe. The EB virus has been implicated in nasopharyngeal cancer, raised antibody being demonstrable in 40% of patients with early disease and 100% with advanced disease. The disease is about twice as common in men as women and the maximum age incidence is 30–60 years.

Clinical features. One of the most important features of nasopharyngeal carcinoma is that lymph node metastasis is frequent (N_1 30%, N_2 15%) and nasopharyngeal carcinoma is a strong possibility in a patient presenting with an enlarged cervical lymph node and no obvious primary tumour. As well as presenting with a lump in the neck, patients with nasopharyngeal cancer present with local symptoms (nasal obstruction, epistaxis), aural symptoms (deafness due to middle ear effusions) and cranial nerve symptoms (pain and anaesthesia in the distribution of the maxillary nerve, ocular palsies and IX, X, XI and XII nerve palsies). The tumour may be visible on postnasal mirror examination, and a skull radiograph may show bone destruction in relation to the foramen caecum, carotid canal, greater wing of the sphenoid and the petrous apex. The diagnosis is made by examination of the nasopharynx under general anaesthesia, when a biopsy is taken.

Treatment. Treatment is by radiation for both squamous carcinomas and lymphomas, and the field should include the upper neck whether palpable metastases are present or not. A small proportion of patients may be helped by radical neck dissection, when either the primary has been controlled by radiotherapy and the cervical metastasis persists, or when a cervical metastasis appears after control of the primary tumour. The overall 5-year survival is of the order of 35%.

Benign tumours

The most important benign tumour is the juvenile angiofibroma which occurs in adolescents and virtually never occurs in girls. Histologically the tumour consists of vascular spaces with no contractile elements in their walls and surrounded by fibrous tissue. The tumour expands locally into the orbit, the nasal cavity, the antrum, the pterygopalatine and infratemporal fossae and into the cheek. The tumour may be visible in the postnasal space as a fleshy vascular mass. Biopsy of the tumour is dangerous and may result in severe haemorrhage. It is, therefore, avoided and the diagnosis made by a carotid angiogram which shows a highly vascular tumour. The treatment is surgical. Tumours confined to the nasopharynx can be removed by a transpalatal approach. Larger tumours are exposed by both transpalatal and lateral rhinotomy approaches, and very

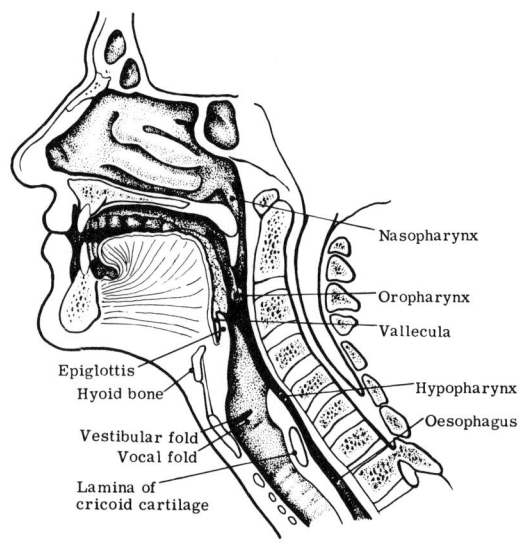

Fig 41.7 Sagittal section to show the divisions of the pharynx.

Nasopharynx

Oropharynx

Vallecula

Epiglottis
Hyoid bone

Hypopharynx

Oesophagus

Vestibular fold
Vocal fold

Lamina of
cricoid cartilage

large tumours may require a Weber Fergusson incision elevating the whole of one side of the face and cheek.

Oropharynx

The oropharynx extends from the hard palate above to the level of the hyoid bone below and is limited anteriorly by the anterior faucial pillars which separate it from the oral cavity. The oropharynx therefore comprises the posterior one-third of the tongue, the vallecula and anterior surface of the epiglottis, the faucial pillars and tonsils, the posterior pharyngeal wall and the antero-inferior surface of the soft palate. Tumours of the anterior surface of the epiglottis and vallecula behave like supraglottic laryngeal lesions and are considered later.

Pathology

Although papillomas and occasionally other benign tumours occur in the oropharynx the vast majority of tumours in this region are malignant. Most of the tumours are squamous carcinomas (75%), 15% are non-Hodgkin's lymphomas, 5% lymphoepitheliomas (an undifferentiated squamous carcinoma in close relation to lymphoid tissue) and 5% miscellaneous including salivary tumours. The maximum age incidence of squamous carcinoma of the oropharynx is 70 years and the sex ratio is 10:1 men to women. 65% of oropharyngeal cancers have a palpable cervical metastasis at presentation and this is true for both squamous carcinomas and lymphomas.

Clinical features

These lesions present with one or more of the following symptoms: sore throat, pain on swallowing, earache and a lump in the neck. Oropharyngeal cancer is one of the tumours in the head and neck which can present with a cervical metastasis, the primary tumour being symptomless.

Treatment

Non-Hodgkin's lymphoma. This tumour is treated by local radiotherapy to the oropharynx and cervical lymph nodes, with chemotherapy being reserved for systemic disease.

Squamous carcinoma. Primary tumours which have not metastasised to cervical lymph nodes are treated by radiotherapy. Patients who on presentation have a palpable cervical gland are treated by primary surgery – the composite resection. This involves a radical neck dissection in continuity with primary resection of the

body and ramus of the mandible, part of the tongue, tonsil, lateral oropharyngeal wall and soft palate. The defect can be closed primarily, or by a pedicled distant flap depending on the extent of the resection (Stell, 1976). If a significant amount of soft palate has been resected, a flap is usually necessary to prevent unintelligible speech due to nasal escape. The flaps available are similar to those for reconstruction of the oral cavity and are discussed in that section.

The hypopharynx

This is the lowest division of the pharynx and extends from the oropharynx above at the level of the hyoid bone to the oesophagus below at the level of the cricoid cartilage. The hypopharynx is divided into three sites: the pyriform fossae (a pair of wedge-shaped spaces on each side of the larynx between the thyroid cartilage laterally and the aryepiglottic folds medially), the postcricoid region (on the posterior surface of the cricoid cartilage) and the posterior pharyngeal wall (Fig 41.8).

Pathology

Virtually all tumours of the hypopharynx are squamous carcinomas. The site incidence of these lesions varies from series to series mainly because of geographical variation in the incidence of these tumours. In the UK the pyriform fossa is the most common site (50–60% of the total), the postcricoid region

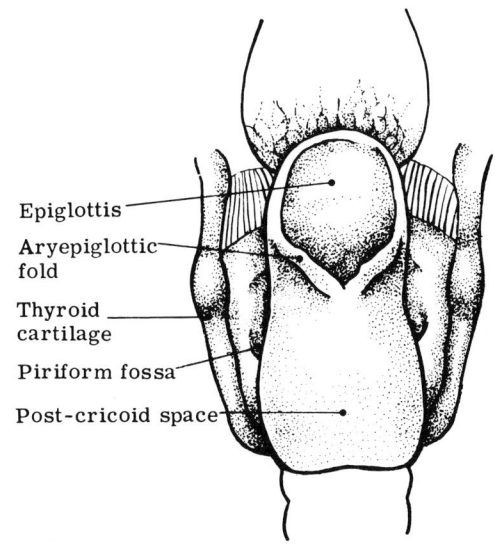

Epiglottis

Aryepiglottic fold

Thyroid cartilage

Piriform fossa

Post-cricoid space

Fig 41.8 Divisions of the hypopharynx as viewed from behind.

the next most common (30–40%) and the posterior pharyngeal wall the least common site (about 10%). Most of the tumours of this region are extensive when first seen. Pyriform fossa lesions extend medially to involve the larynx and fix the glottis. They also extend laterally through the thyrohyoid membrane, producing a palpable mass in the neck. About 75% of patients with pyriform fossa cancer have a palpable lymph node in the neck on presentation.

Carcinomas of the postcricoid region extend inferiorly to involve the cervical oesophagus, anteriorly to involve the party wall between the trachea and oesophagus and laterally to involve the recurrent laryngeal nerves and thyroid gland. At presentation about 20% of patients with postcricoid carcinoma have a palpable lymph node in the neck; 5% of patients have bilateral lymph nodes. Carcinomas of the posterior pharyngeal wall are usually exophytic as opposed to infiltrative and about 50% of patients have a palpable lymph node on presentation.

Clinical features

Tumours of this region are often diagnosed very late, and this is one of the reasons why cure rates are so poor. Vague symptoms such as the feeling of a crumb in the throat or persistent sore throat may be the first sign, but are often neglected or are diagnosed as being due to globus hystericus. Such a diagnosis cannot safely be made without a normal barium swallow and a normal pharyngoscopy and oesophagoscopy. Dysphagia, first for solids and then for liquids, hoarseness due to direct laryngeal infiltration or recurrent nerve involvement, or a lump in the neck are symptoms which indicate advanced disease. Mirror examination of the pharynx may show pooling of saliva, oedema, or obvious tumour of the arytenoids, or immobility of one or both vocal cords. The diagnosis is confirmed and the extent of the tumour defined by barium swallow and endoscopy.

Treatment

A good deal of controversy exists regarding the treatment of patients with this disease. A certain proportion, perhaps 25%, are probably not curable, and extensive surgery or radiotherapy may simply increase their misery (Clinical Otolaryngology, 1979). On the other hand a patient with severe dysphagia may be relieved of this symptom by surgery or radiotherapy even if he is not cured of the disease and this may provide useful palliation. The most important reasons for not treating a patient are: advanced age, poor general condition, an inoperable local tumour or fixed or bilateral neck nodes. Local causes of inoperability are invasion of the base of the tongue, extension into the

tracheo-oesophageal groove, or involvement of the recurrent laryngeal nerves.

Although different treatment plans are advocated by different centres the following is a reasonable plan of action: small tumours (say less than 3 cm in diameter) may be amenable to radiotherapy. Patients with large tumours or those who have a palpable lymph node in the neck on presentation should be treated by primary surgery the extent of which depends upon the size and site of the lesion. When cervical metastases are present the operation should include a radical neck dissection in continuity with the primary resection.

The surgery of pyriform fossa lesions is a total laryngectomy and partial pharyngectomy, reconstituting the pharynx with the pharyngeal mucosa remaining after the resection. Approximately 30% of patients with a pyriform fossa cancer have involvement of the upper end of the oesophagus, and when this occurs a total pharyngolaryngectomy is necessary. Reconstitution of the pharynx after this operation is discussed below.

Tumours of the posterior pharyngeal wall which have recurred or are not suitable for radiotherapy may be resected through a lateral pharyngotomy, preserving the larynx. The defect is closed either primarily or by a pedicled skin flap. If the larynx or pyriform fossa is involved by the tumour, then the larynx cannot be preserved and a total pharyngolaryngectomy is necessary.

Postcricoid tumours which have recurred or which are not suitable for radiotherapy are treated by a total pharyngolaryngectomy; the problem is then pharyngeal replacement. Although a variety of methods has been used in the past, three operations are currently in vogue: replacement with a deltopectoral flap, replacement with stomach, or with colon.

Replacement with a deltopectoral flap. This method, originally described by Bakamjian (1965) involves replacement of the hypopharynx with a tube of skin created from a deltopectoral flap. After the pharyngolaryngectomy, a tubed deltopectoral flap is anastomosed to the oropharynx superiorly and to the oesophageal remnant inferiorly (Fig 41.9). The lower anastomosis is done end-to-side incorporating the oesophageal remnant into the longitudinal suture line by which the skin flap is tubed (Fig 41.10). After 3 weeks the pedicle of the flap is divided and the temporary fistula closed (Figs 41.11; 41.12). The advantage of this operation is that it is a less formidable undertaking for the patient than visceral replacement (Stell *et al.*, 1978). The disadvantages are that it is a two-stage procedure and that local complications, e.g.fistula and stenosis are frequent, though usually only temporary.

Gastric transposition. The pharynx may be replaced by mobilising the stomach, preserving the right gastric

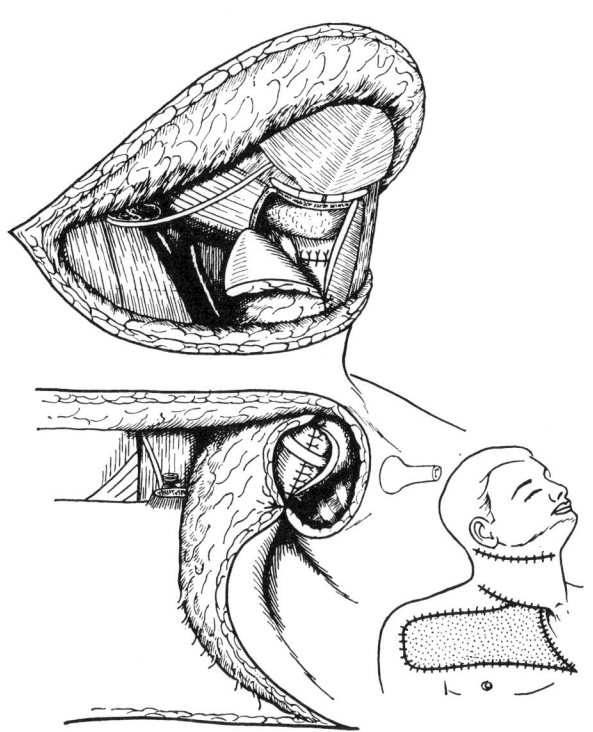

Fig 41.9 Anastomosis of skin tube to orostome and oesophagostome.

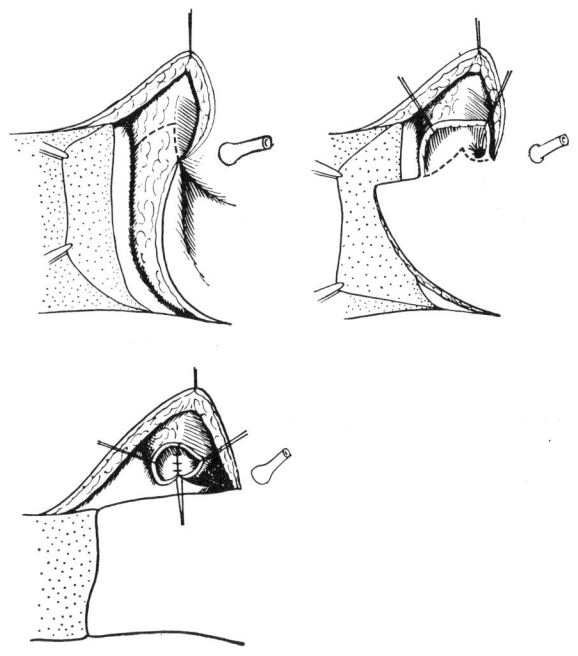

Fig 41.11   Division of lower end of skin tube and return of pedicle.

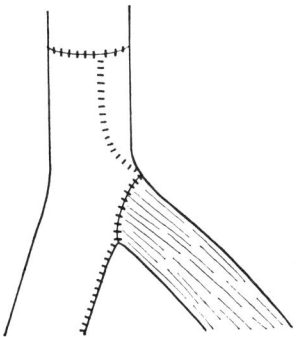

Fig 41.10 End-to-side anastomosis of skin tube to oesophagus.

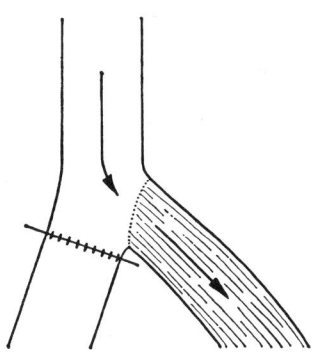

Fig 41.12   Diagram of division of skin tube.

and right gastro-epiploic vessels (Fig 41.13). The stomach is passed into the neck through the posterior mediastinum and the fundus anastomosed to the oropharynx. In this way a total laryngopharyngo-oesophagectomy is performed (Ong and Lee 1960; LeQuesne and Ranger, 1966). The disadvantage of this procedure is that it is a massive surgical undertaking with a high mortality.

Colon transplantation. In this operation a portion of the colon is mobilised, usually based on the left colic vessels (Fig 41.14). The segment of colon is anastomosed to the oropharynx above and after passing through a subcutaneous, retrosternal or posterior mediastinal tunnel, it is anastomosed to the stomach below (Brain and Reading 1966; Fairman and John, 1966). Like gastric transposition this is a major surgical

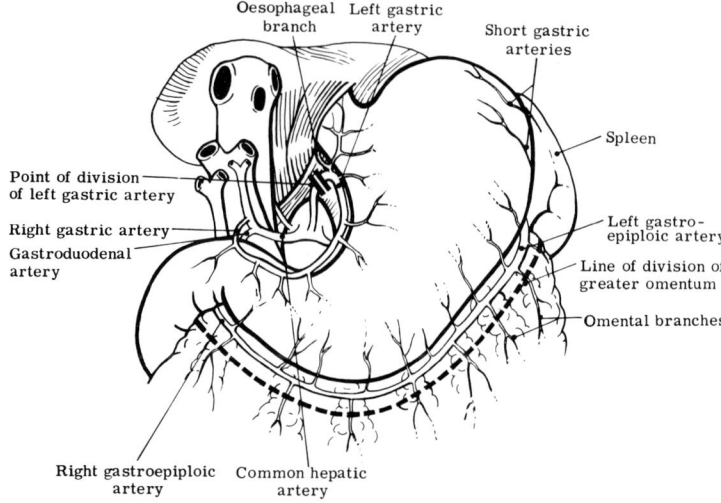

Fig 41.13 Stomach mobilisation.

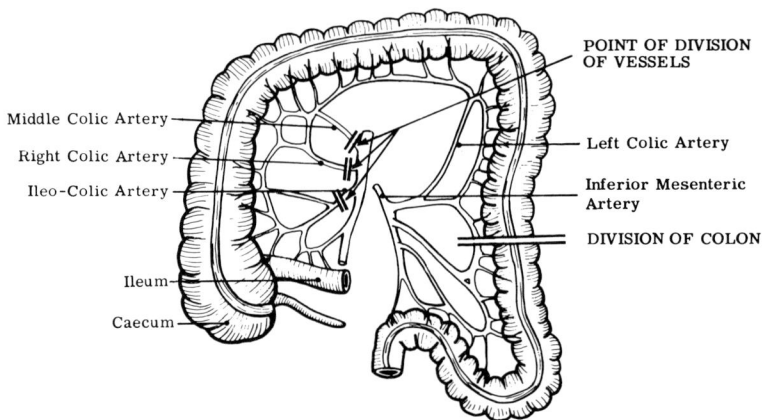

Fig 41.14 Mobilisation of the colon.

undertaking, though if the patient survives, good swallowing usually results with freedom from local complications.

Diseases of the larynx

The larynx is an important organ whose functions include phonation, the protection of the lower respiratory tract from the inhalation of food, and the initiation of the cough reflex. For descriptive purposes it is often divided into three areas: the supraglottis, the glottis and the subglottis. The disorders of the larynx of interest to the general surgeon are trauma, paralysis and tumour.

Acute laryngeal trauma

The importance of laryngeal trauma is that in the acute phase it is life threatening and in the long-term it causes functional impairment of respiration and speech. Direct trauma is most commonly due to road traffic accidents; if other injuries are present the laryngeal trauma may be unrecognised, at least initially.

The type of injury depends upon the type and severity of the trauma and also upon the extent of calcification of the laryngeal cartilages. If the thyroid cartilage is minimally calcified, and therefore flexible, it is compressed against the cervical spine and this results in a linear fracture between the thyroid laminae (Fig 41.15).

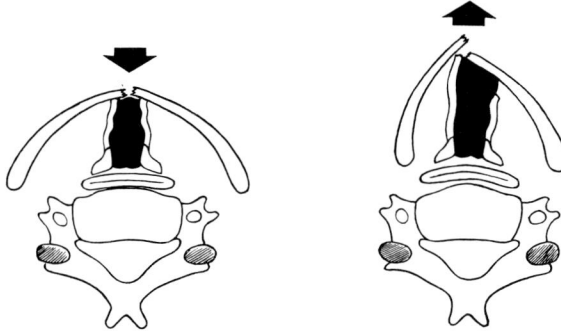

Fig 41.15 Compression of an uncalcified cartilage leads to a linear thyroid fracture and possible detachment of vocal cord and/or epiglottis.

In addition to the fracture of the thyroid cartilage, the epiglottis may be partially detached to fall back into the airway, the vocal cords may be detached anteriorly or the arytenoids may be dislocated. If the blow is directed from an inferior direction, the cricoid cartilage may be fractured, usually anteriorly, or the crico-tracheal membrane may be torn, detaching the larynx from the trachea. If the thyroid cartilage is well calcified, and as a result less flexible, it is shattered by the injury (Fig 41.16) and this may also result in injuries to the epiglottis, vocal cords and arytenoids.

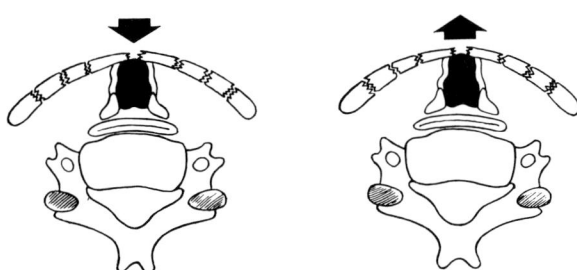

Fig 41.16 Compression of a calcified cartilage causes flattening of the neck due to shattering of the cartilage.

Clinical features

If the trauma is severe and the laryngeal injury extensive, there will be immediate, often fatal, airway obstruction (*see* chapter 44). Usually, however, the patient may be symptom free initially, but as a haematoma develops, hoarseness and stridor appear. (Other symptoms and signs of laryngeal injury are pain on swallowing, haemoptysis, surgical emphysema and loss of the laryngeal prominence.) If the patient has other injuries, little attention will be focussed on the larynx and a significant injury may be overlooked. This may

subsequently give rise to airway embarrassment or much later to laryngeal scarring and stenosis. If a laryngeal injury is suspected, mirror examination may be helpful in assessing the injury and the airway. In an unconscious or uncooperative patient, direct laryngoscopy under anaesthesia may be necessary, but the possibilities of a cervical spine injury must be considered and great care must be exercised in positioning the patient. A patient with multiple and serious injuries should always be examined for:

1 Stridor
2 Surgical emphysema of the neck
3 Loss of the laryngeal prominence

Any of these indicates a severe laryngeal injury which should be treated in the *acute* phase. The importance of this is that the surgery of acute injuries is nearly always successful in the restoration of good function. If the larynx is allowed to heal with gross disorganisation of the normal anatomy, the scarring which occurs is much more difficult to treat and the results of surgery of chronic laryngeal stenosis are much less satisfactory.

Treatment

If the injury is not severe, observation is all that is necessary, bearing in mind that haematoma formation and laryngeal oedema may be progressive. In more extensive injuries a tracheostomy will be necessary and the larynx will need to be explored through a collar incision and its lumen inspected by separating the thyroid laminae in the midline (laryngofissure). An attempt is made to restore the anatomy to normal and to remove obviously devitalised tissue. Fractures are reduced and stabilised by internal fixation using a solid laryngeal stent which is left in place for at least 6 weeks. In less severe injuries with mucosal lacerations a sheet of tantalum (McNaught keel, Fig 41.17) or of silastic is fixed between the vocal cords to prevent the formation of adhesions.

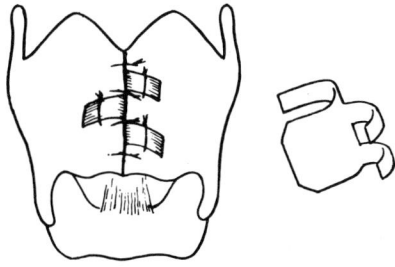

Fig 41.17 Right, a McNaught keel: *left*, the keel in position between the vocal cords with the flanges sutured to the thyroid cartilage.

Chronic laryngotracheal stenosis

Pathology and aetiology

Chronic stenosis of the larynx may follow acute laryngeal trauma, and this is the reason that laryngeal injuries should be treated in the acute phase. Even after careful repair, a proportion of patients will develop stenosis, the site depending upon the region of maximal damage, though this will usually be subglottic or glottic and rarely supraglottic. Another cause of chronic laryngeal stenosis is prolonged endotracheal intubation: here the stenosis is usually at the subglottic level or less commonly at the site of the inflatable cuff. Tracheostomy can also be the cause of stenosis, particularly when the incision in the trachea is high and the cricoid cartilage is damaged.

Clinical features

In patients with mild stenosis the only symptom may be difficulty in clearing bronchial secretions, but in those patients with severe stenosis there will be stridor which may be progressive. Alternatively, it may be found that the patient who needed a tracheostomy at the time of the original injury cannot breathe adequately when the lumen of the tracheostomy tube is occluded. The extent of the stenosis is assessed by indirect and direct laryngoscopy, and by laryngography, a radiographic technique in which a contrast medium, e.g. Dionosil, is introduced into the larynx.

Treatment

The correction of an established laryngeal stenosis is difficult. If the patient has a satisfactory airway and his only symptom is hoarseness, there may be little that can be done. If the airway is impaired, so that a tracheostomy is necessary, one solution is a valved tracheostomy tube enabling the patient to phonate. If the idea of long-term tracheostomy is unacceptable to the patient, surgical treatment of the stenosis will be successful in a proportion of patients.

Stenoses at the glottic level are explored through a laryngofissure, the adhesions divided and the raw areas kept apart by the insertion of a keel. If the stenosis is due to fixation of the arytenoid cartilage in a medial position, this can be excised and the vocal cord sutured laterally to establish an airway. Stenosis at the subglottic level is more difficult to treat and the results are less satisfactory (Bryce, 1975). Simple excision of the scar tissue with application of a stent is usually unsatisfactory and the two most popular methods of dealing with this situation are to excise the stenosed segment completely and perform an end-to-end anastomosis, or to split the cricoid cartilage in the midline, separate the

segments and splint them apart, thus opening the airway. The disadvantages of excision are that the recurrent laryngeal nerves may be damaged as they pass behind the crico-thyroid articulations and also that restenosis is very liable to occur. Splitting the cricoid in the midline in a stepways fashion and splinting the fragments has been described (Evans and Todd, 1974). Alternatively, a pedicled graft of cartilage from the thyroid cartilage or bone from the hyoid is inserted between the two segments (Fearon and Cotton, 1972). Tracheal stenosis is dealt with by excision and end-to-end anastomosis; again the recurrent laryngeal nerves are vulnerable. Up to 4 cm of trachea can be excised and the defect closed by mobilisation of the remaining trachea. Various procedures have been described to 'drop the larynx' to assist primary closure (Dedo and Fishman, 1969), but these may well disturb laryngeal function and increase the patient's problems. Replacement of segments of trachea with prosthetic materials, e.g. dacron or marlex are usually unsuccessful because of crust formation on their inner surface.

Laryngeal paralysis

Pathology

The intrinsic laryngeal muscles are innervated from the nucleus ambiguus of the vagus. The crico-thyroid muscle receives its supply from the superior laryngeal nerve, the remaining muscles being innervated via the recurrent laryngeal nerve. The crico-thyroid muscle is a tensor and adductor of the vocal cord but it is difficult to assess the disability associated with isolated paralysis; it is probably minimal or non-existent in a majority of patients. Paralysis of the recurrent laryngeal nerve causes an immobile vocal cord. The position which a paralysed vocal cord takes up is dependent on a number of factors and varies from patient to patient. If the abductor muscles only are paralysed, the cord can still be adducted and occupies a position close to the midline (paramedian). This may be the case when the recurrent nerve is paralysed and the superior laryngeal nerve is functioning. When both abductor and adductor muscles are paralysed the cord takes up a more lateral position (the cadaveric position). The superior laryngeal and recurrent laryngeal nerves are also sensory nerves to the supraglottis, glottis and pharynx and paralysis also results in swallowing difficulties, particularly of fluids, with inhalation. Laryngeal palsies may be unilateral or bilateral; the various causes and their incidence are as follows:

1 *Malignant disease – 25%.* Most of these paralyses are due to bronchial carcinoma affecting the left recurrent laryngeal nerve in the chest, but some

are due to oesophageal, thyroid or naso-pharyngeal carcinoma affecting the vagus or recurrent laryngeal nerves in the neck.

2 *Surgical trauma – 20%*. The vagus or, more usually, the recurrent laryngeal nerves may be damaged during oesophageal, pulmonary, vascular or thyroid surgery, and also in partial laryngectomy, radical neck dissection and excision of a pharyngeal pouch.

3 *Idiopathic causes – 15%*. A number of patients develop a vocal cord palsy for which no cause is found. A viral neuropathy has been postulated as the cause.

4 *Inflammatory causes – 15%*. Pulmonary tuberculosis with mediastinal lymphadenopathy is the commonest cause in this group.

5 *Non-surgical trauma – 10%*. Laryngeal injury in road traffic accidents, stretching of the nerve by an aortic aneurysm or an enlarged left atrium may occasionally cause a recurrent laryngeal nerve paralysis.

6 *Miscellaneous causes – 10%*. Haemolytic anaemia, subclavian vein thrombosis, rheumatoid arthritis, syphilis and collagen diseases may occasionally be responsible.

7 *Neurological causes – 5%*. Central causes such as brain stem ischaemia, multiple sclerosis, syringobulbia and amyotrophic lateral sclerosis may result in a palsy of the vagus nerve. Alcoholism, diabetes and the Guillain-Barré syndrome may cause a peripheral neuropathy affecting the vagus or recurrent laryngeal nerves.

Clinical features

A unilateral vocal cord palsy may cause few symptoms if the cord is paralysed in the paramedian position, but results in a hoarse, breathy voice with difficulty in swallowing and aspiration of fluids (because of the loss of laryngeal sensation) if the cord is in the abducted position. Bilateral vocal cord paralysis results in stridor and dyspnoea. Examination and investigation are aimed at identifying the aetiology. A full head and neck examination, chest radiograph and endoscopy are usually essential.

Treatment

Unilateral vocal cord palsy. If the cord is in the midline or close to it, the hoarseness is minimal and no treatment is necessary. When the cord is in a more lateral position the patient will have a weak voice, an inefficient cough and will complain of aspiration of food. Speech therapy may help, but an injection of Teflon paste or implantation of cartilage to move the paralysed cord medially is usually needed to improve the voice and restore laryngeal competence.

Bilateral vocal cord palsy. Usually a tracheostomy is necessary to provide an adequate airway. If a valved tube is used, the patient will also have a good voice. If long-term tracheostomy is unacceptable to the patient, a variety of surgical procedures have been devised in order to improve the airway. These operations, with one exception, inevitably impair the voice by virtue of the fact that one of the vocal cords is moved to a more lateral position. This can be done by excising the arytenoid cartilage and suturing the vocal cord laterally and a number of surgical approaches have been described.

The arytenoid can be identified by dissection along the posterior border of the thyroid cartilage identifying the arytenoid cartilage at its articulation with the cricoid cartilage. The arytenoid cartilage is dissected free and removed and the vocal cord sutured laterally with a stitch through the thyroid cartilage, assessing the position of the cord laryngoscopically (Woodman, 1953). Alternatively, the thyroid cartilage can be split in the midline by laryngofissure and the arytenoid dissected out by an internal approach. Dissection of the arytenoid endoscopically using a microscope and a laryngoscope has also been described. As an alternative to arytenoidectomy, a reinnervation of the posterior arytenoid muscle has been described using a portion of the omohyoid muscle in a neurovascular pedicle (Tucker, 1978). This operation, theoretically, would seem to be the most satisfactory approach as the voice would not suffer as a result of the operation.

Laryngeal tumours

The majority of laryngeal tumours are malignant, though benign tumours are occasionally encountered.

Benign

The benign tumours and their relative incidence are shown in Table 5. The papillomas which occur are of two distinct types: juvenile papillomas are multiple and recurrent, but adult papillomas are single and do not usually recur. The juvenile papillomas occur in childhood and commonly regress before or at puberty. They present with hoarseness and/or stridor and spread throughout the upper respiratory tract, even down into the bronchi. Recurrence following removal may be very rapid and tracheostomy may be required to maintain an airway.

Table 5

Papilloma	85%
Adenoma	5%
Chondroma	5%
Miscellaneous	5%
(granular cell myoblastoma, lipoma, haemangioma, neurofibroma)	

Granular cell myoblastoma is an uncommon lesion of the larynx, the important features being that the overlying epithelium may show pseudoepitheliomatous hyperplasia which may be mistaken for a squamous carcinoma so that radical treatment may be incorrectly advised. Local removal is sufficient for this lesion.

Malignant

Approximately 90% of laryngeal carcinomas occur in men with a peak age incidence between 55 and 65 years. Most of the lesions (85%) are squamous carcinomas, usually moderately to well differentiated. Occasionally verrucous and undifferentiated carcinomas, adenocarcinomas and sarcomas occur in the larynx, but these are rare. Laryngeal carcinoma may arise from the supraglottic, glottic and subglottic regions of the larynx. The relative incidence of supraglottic, glottic and subglottic carcinoma in the UK is 40%, 55% and 5% respectively.

Supraglottic carcinoma. The commonest site of a carcinoma in this region is the infrahyoid epiglottis, but tumours may also arise from the vestibular folds and the aryepiglottic folds. The rate of lymph node metastasis is high and varies from site to site (Table 6).

Table 6
LYMPH NODE METASTASIS IN SUPRAGLOTTIC CARCINOMA

N_0	65%
N_1	20%
N_2	7.5%
N_3	7.5%

Glottic carcinoma. The glottis is the most common site for laryngeal carcinoma. Glottic carcinoma may be divided into those small tumours occurring on one vocal cord and remaining localised to this site for a long period and those tumours (named 'transglottic') which involve a wide area on one side of the larynx crossing the vocal cord and extending into the subglottis and supraglottis. These two tumours are almost certainly not different stages of the same disease, but transglottic carcinoma probably represents a wide field malignant degeneration. Small glottic carcinomas spread along the vocal cord across the anterior commissure onto the other cord, but only spread very late superiorly and inferiorly to the supraglottis and subglottis and laterally to the intrinsic musculature of the larynx. Transglottic carcinoma spreads widely invading the cartilagenous framework of the larynx. Lymph node metastases are rare in true glottic carcinomas but occur in about 30% of transglottic carcinomas.

Subglottic carcinoma. These are uncommon lesions which invade the thyroid and cricoid cartilages and give rise to cervical lymphadenopathy in about 20% of patients.

Clinical features

The two prime symptoms of laryngeal disease are hoarseness and stridor. Small glottic lesions cause hoarseness very early, whereas supraglottic and subglottic do not affect the voice until they are fairly well advanced. Stridor due to compromise of the airway is a late sign of disease, but in some patients (characteristically those with subglottic lesions) it is the presenting symptom. Pain is also a relatively late symptom in laryngeal carcinoma, and the pain may be confined to or radiate to the ear. The diagnosis of laryngeal carcinoma is made by mirror examination (indirect laryngoscopy) and confirmed by endoscopy (direct laryngoscopy) and biopsy.

Treatment

Laryngeal cancer is eminently suitable for curative treatment: 95% of patients can be treated, many with a hope of cure. The prognosis depends to a large extent on the stage of the disease when the diagnosis is made. A small glottic carcinoma limited to one vocal cord is cured by radiotherapy in about 90% of patients, whereas an advanced carcinoma involving all regions of the larynx, with bilateral or fixed nodes has a cure rate of less than 5%, even when surgery is advised.

In general, the treatment policy in the UK is to irradiate the vast majority of tumours and to carry out a total laryngectomy for those patients with recurrent or residual disease. To be successful, this policy depends upon meticulous follow-up; if this is not possible for patients with advanced laryngeal tumours at presentation, primary total laryngectomy can be a safer policy. Two situations arise where a policy of irradiation and follow-up are contraindicated. The first is in those patients who at presentation have a cervical metastasis and these are best treated by primary surgery. The second situation in which primary radiotherapy is inadvisable is when a patient with a laryngeal tumour presents with stridor. A tracheostomy to provide an airway carries a high risk of recurrent cancer at the site of the tracheostomy, so that the best policy for this patient is an emergency total laryngectomy.

Supraglottic tumours. Primary supraglottic tumours with no palpable cervical metastases should be treated by radiotherapy. When palpable nodes are present, the patient should be treated by primary surgery. When the vocal cords are involved by the tumour, total laryngectomy and neck dissection should be advised. When the vocal cords are fully mobile and are not involved by the supraglottic tumour, partial surgery in the form of a supraglottic laryngectomy may be applicable. This partial surgery is not advisable when there is any cartilage destruction, and is also contra-indicated in elderly patients or those with severe bronchitis, as swallowing after the operation is difficult and inhalation occurs in most patients. In a supraglottic laryngectomy, the tissue between the base of the tongue and the vocal cords is excised, (including the pre-epiglottic space), and the base of the tongue is anastomosed to the remaining part of the larynx. The advantages of the operation are that the patient avoids a permanent tracheostomy, and retains his voice.

Glottic tumours. Most glottic tumours are cured by radiotherapy. In the unlikely event of a small glottic tumour recurring after radiotherapy and remaining localised to one vocal cord, a vertical partial hemilaryngectomy may be applicable. In this operation the thyroid ala and the true vocal cord are excised. Here again, the patient retains his voice. Vertical partial hemilaryngectomy should not be done when there is supra or subglottic extension of the tumour, when there is limitation of vocal cord mobility or when there is a palpable node in the neck, in which instances a total laryngectomy is necessary. In transglottic tumours, cartilage destruction and cervical metastases usually mean that radiotherapy is contra-indicated and total laryngectomy is necessary.

Subglottic tumours. In those patients with subglottic cancer who have an adequate airway and no cervical metastases, radiotherapy with close follow-up is suitable treatment. When the airway is significantly impaired, cervical lymphadenopathy is present or the tumour has recurred after radiotherapy, total laryngectomy with or without neck dissection is advised.

Oral cavity

Lesions of the upper and lower jaw have been dealt with earlier, so discussion in this section will be limited to the tongue, floor of mouth and buccal mucosa. There are many lesions of the epithelium lining the oral cavity and classification is difficult, but most conditions can be considered under the following headings:

1   Benign ulcers of the oral mucosa
2   Specific benign lesions of the tongue
3   Benign tumours of the oral mucosa
4   Leukoplakia and erythroplakia
5   Malignant tumours

Benign oral ulceration

Traumatic ulcers

Ulceration can be caused by ill fitting dentures or the sharp edge of a broken tooth. When the underlying cause has been eliminated, a traumatic ulcer should heal in a week; if not, a biopsy must be taken.

Recurrent oral ulceration

Recurrent oral ulcers for which no cause is found are very common. Usually these are small single or multiple ulcers which heal within a week or two. Occasionally a major ulcer may persist for many weeks and here it is most important to exclude malignancy by biopsy. The aetiology of recurrent aphthous ulcers is unknown, although it has been suggested that this may be an autoimmune phenomenon as in 75% of patients it is possible to demonstrate antibodies against oral mucosa. Vascular, joint, neurological and gastrointestinal lesions may also occur. Topical steroids are useful in recurrent aphthous ulceration in both increasing the rapidity of healing and possibly also reducing the number of new ulcers forming. When ulceration occurs in association with genital ulceration and iridocyclitis the condition is known as Behcet's syndrome.

Other causes of oral ulceration

Oral ulceration occurs as a result of herpes simplex, various vitamin deficiencies (B_{12}, folic acid and iron deficiency) and on occasions may be drug induced (e.g. propanalol). Severe oral ulceration is seen in agranulocytosis and acute lymphocytic leukaemia.

Specific benign lesions of the tongue

A number of unrelated conditions are included under this heading.

Median rhomboid glossitis

This is a smooth red area on the dorsum of the tongue in front of the foramen caecum. It is said to be a remnant of the tuberculum impar, but also seems to arise in adult patients where it may represent a candidal infection.

Geographic tongue

In this condition areas of the tongue take on a red, smooth appearance due to atrophy of the filiform papillae. The cause is unknown, but areas may return to normal with regeneration of the papillae.

Black hairy tongue

This condition is of unknown aetiology, although it may in some patients be related to smoking. The discoloration and hairiness of the dorsum of the tongue can be removed by rubbing with fresh pineapple or probably just as efficiently with a tooth brush.

Benign tumours of the oral mucosa

Squamous papilloma

These lesions are moderately common particularly on the soft palate or uvula. Occasionally they may be multiple, but never become malignant.

Salivary tumours

Most tumours which arise from salivary tissue in the mouth are malignant. Pleomorphic adenomas do occur and are most common on the hard palate, occasionally occurring on the buccal mucosa or floor of the mouth (*see* Chapter 42).

Haemangiomas and lymphangiomas

These lesions may be well localised or very extensive and occur particularly on the lateral border of the tongue and in the cheek.

Ranula

The simple ranula is not a tumour, but a retention cyst of a minor salivary gland and usually occurs in the floor of the mouth. On occasions the so-called plunging ranula extends deeply into the musculature of the floor of the mouth and even into the neck. This extension may be due to extravasation of mucus. Treatment is best effected by marsupialisation of the cyst.

Granular cell myoblastoma

This may be a true tumour or may represent a degenerative lesion of striated muscle. The most important feature is that the overlying epithelium shows changes known as pseudo-epitheliomatous hyperplasia which can be mistaken for a squamous carcinoma. The lesion occurs most often on the tongue or in the larynx and should be treated by local excision.

Leukoplakia and erythroplakia

Leukoplakia simply means a white patch, but has been accepted as meaning an epithelial abnormality of

unknown aetiology. It shows a variety of histological appearances;

1 Simple keratosis
2 Hyperkeratosis perhaps with parakeratosis or acanthosis
3 Hyperkeratosis with dyskeratosis

It is the third category which is particularly liable to malignant change (perhaps in about 10% of patients), but the clinical appearance is not a reliable guide to the histological features. Thus all these lesions should be biopsied and those showing dyskeratosis should be excised and replaced with a split skin graft. Cryosurgery or laser excision are possible alternatives. It is reasonable simply to observe those which do not show dyskeratosis, but repeat biopsy is necessary if the lesion changes in character, becomes ulcerated, bleeds, or is painful.

Erythroplakia is an epithelial abnormality similar to leukoplakia, being red as opposed to white. Dyskeratosis is much more common in erythroplakia and these lesions should be excised.

Malignant tumours

The incidence of oral cancer in men in England and Wales has fallen considerably in the last 20 years (a fall of 3% per annum) and now constitutes only about 1% of cancer deaths. This falling incidence is difficult to reconcile with the increase in smoking and consumption of alcohol, factors thought to be related to oral cancer. The disease now affects men and women with almost equal frequency and the peak age incidence is in the sixth decade.

About 95% of malignant tumours of the oral cavity are squamous carcinomas, the remainder being salivary tumours (mostly adenoidcystic carcinoma) with small numbers of malignant melanomas and soft tissue sarcomas. One rather rare but important variant of the squamous carcinoma is the verrucous carcinoma which forms about 5% of oral cancers. Its importance lies in its different clinical behaviour in that it is radioresistant and radiotherapy is liable to induce an anaplastic change. Clinically, the appearances are of a florid, warty area resembling leukoplakia and histologically the lesion is a well-differentiated squamous carcinoma arranged in compressed invaginated folds.

The site incidence of squamous carcinoma of the oral cavity is shown in Table 7.

The majority of lesions of the tongue occur on the lateral borders. Lymph node metastases are common in oral cancer, about 40% of patients having an enlarged node at first presentation. The commonest nodes to be involved are the submandibular and jugulo-digastric. The jugulo-omohyoid node may be the only palpable

Table 7
SITE INCIDENCE OF ORAL CAVITY CARCINOMA

Tongue	50%
Buccal mucosa	15%
Floor of the mouth	15%
Lower alveolus	15%
Upper alveolus	5%

metastasis in lesions of the tip of the tongue and anterior floor of the mouth. Lymph node metastases seriously affect the prognosis of the disease. About 60% of patients with oral cancer and no metastases will be cured, but this falls to 30% when unilateral nodes are involved and close to zero with bilateral node involvement.

Clinical features

Most mouth cancers present with a painful ulcer, but a proportion present with unilateral earache or a lump in the neck with no symptoms referable to the mouth. Palpation is an essential part of the investigation, the true extent of the tumour often being considerably larger than the visible ulcer. Palpation of the primary tumour after treatment is also essential in that residual tumour is much more easy to feel than to see. The neck must also be palpated to determine the state of the cervical lymph nodes as this affects the treatment plan.

The treatment of oral cancer depends upon the site and involvement of adjacent structures. Floor of mouth and tongue lesions can be considered together, buccal cancer is managed slightly differently as is upper and lower jaw cancer which was considered earlier.

Cancer of the tongue and floor of the mouth

This is a very extensive and controversial subject and only a broad outline can be presented here. In general small lesions, that is up to 3 cm in largest diameter with no palpable metastatic nodes can be treated by radiotherapy or surgery. The best form of radiotherapy is the implantation of iridium wires locally into the tumour designed to deliver 7000–8000 rads. External beam irradiation is unsatisfactory in lesions of the tongue and if facilities for implantation are not available surgery is preferable. The lesion is excised with a 2 cm margin of clearance and the resulting defect can be closed primarily or can be covered with a split skin graft using the technique of quilting (McGregor and McGrouther, 1978). These considerations also apply to floor of mouth lesions, but when the lesion reaches the mandible, radiotherapy is not applicable and surgery should be advised.

In larger lesions of the tongue and floor of the mouth

(i.e. 3 cm and greater) and in those with a metastatic lymph node, radiotherapy is almost certain to fail and the best treatment is primary surgery. Failed radiotherapy increases the complication rate after salvage surgery to an alarming degree with a high rate of wound breakdown and orocutaneous fistula formation. This is the main reason for the policy of primary surgery for patients with large tumours or with metastatic nodes.

Patients with a unilateral metastatic node at the time of presentation are best treated by a radical neck dissection in continuity with resection of the primary tumour. Patients with bilateral nodes at the time of presentation are so unlikely to be cured that it is very doubtful whether it is justifiable to inflict upon them the miseries of a massive surgical procedure.

The problems of surgery of the oral cavity are firstly adequate surgical access and secondly the repair of the defect resulting from the excision (McGregor, 1977). Access to the primary tumour depends upon the site and size of the lesion. Small anterior lesions can be excised entirely through the mouth. Larger lesions can be approached by a combination of a peroral excision and a submandibular approach and the access can be improved by a temporary mandibulotomy. This approach is made easier when the tumour is involving the mandible and a hemimandibulectomy is also being performed. The best exposure of oral tumours involves a midline split of the lip with a mandibulotomy, but the disadvantage of this is that the resulting scar is often very noticeable. Repair of the defect resulting from the surgery of oral cancer is a challenging problem and the important considerations are healing without fistula formation and the functional and cosmetic result. The two main alternatives in repair are primary closure i.e. suturing of tongue remnant to cheek, or the interposition of a flap. The difficulties of primary closure are that if this is done under tension, wound breakdown is likely and also the tethering of the tongue which results is liable to affect speech and deglutition. The alternative approach is to fill the defect with a flap and although this adds its own problems, it has the advantage of probably a more mobile tongue remnant and a better functional result. The flaps used may be either local or distant. The two main local flaps are the lingual flap (Chambers *et al.*, 1969) and the nasolabial flap (Cohen and Theogaras, 1975). The lingual flap is developed from the tongue (Fig 41.18) and is only applicable for floor of mouth and alveolar lesions when the tongue is not involved in the resection. Nasolabial flaps (Fig 41.19) provide a limited amount of tissue and are most useful in anterior floor of mouth defects which are difficult to close in any other way. Distant flaps include the forehead (McGregor, 1963) (Fig 41.20), the deltopectoral (Bakamjian *et al.*, 1971) (Fig 41.21) and the more recently described myocutaneous flaps (Ariyan and Clono, 1980).

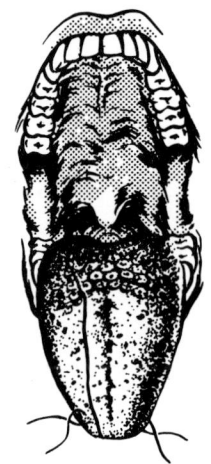

Fig 41.18 Lingual flap cut.

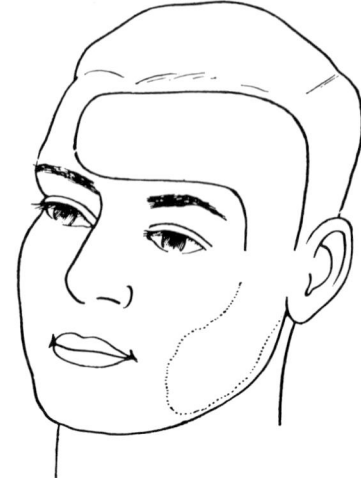

Fig 41.20 Forehead flap marked and based on the superficial temporal artery.

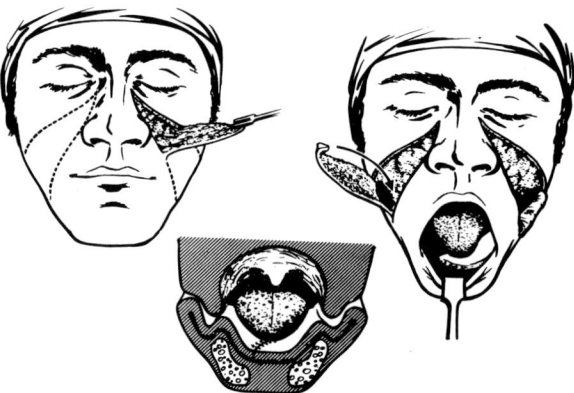

Fig 41.19 Technique of elevation and transposition of naso-labial flap.

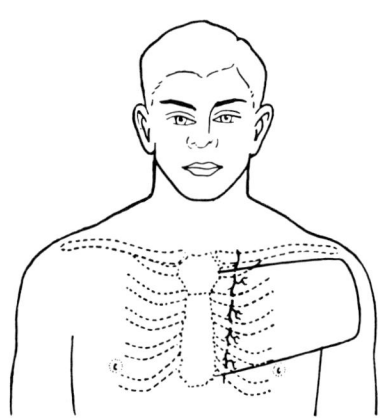

Fig 41.21 Delto-pectoral chest flap.

Buccal carcinoma

Small tumours (i.e. 2 cm diameter) of the buccal mucosa are best treated by local excision either with primary closure or a split skin graft. Because of the difficulties of repair, larger lesions are probably best treated by radiotherapy reserving surgery for recurrences. Surgery of larger lesions involves a through-and-through excision of cheek and facial skin and subsequent repair usually needs either a lined forehead flap or a combination of distant flaps.

References

Ariyan S., Clono C.B. (1980). Myocutaneous flaps for head and neck reconstruction. *Head Neck Surg*; **2**:321–45.

Bakamjian V.Y. (1965). A two stage method for pharyngo-oesophageal reconstruction with a primary pectoral skin flap. *Plast. Reconstr. Surg*; **36**:173–84.

Bakamjian V.Y., Long M., Rigg B. (1971). Experience with the medially based deltopectoral flap in reconstructive surgery of the head and neck. *Brit. J. Plast. Surg*; **24**:174–83.

Bocca E., Pignataro O., Sasaki C.T. (1980). Functional neck dissection. *Arch Otolaryngol*; **106**:524–7.

Brain R.H.F., Reading P.V.F. (1966). Colon transplantation into the pharynx and cervical oesophagus. *Brit. J. Surg*; **53**:933–42.

Bryce D.P. (1975). The laryngeal subglottis. *J. Laryngol. Otol*; **89**:667–85.

Chambers R.G., Jacques D.A., Mahoney W.D. (1969). Tongue flaps for intra-oral reconstruction. *Amer. J. Surg*; **118**:783–6.

Clinical Otolaryngology (1979). Treatment of postcricoid carcinoma (editorial). *Clin. Otolaryngol*; **4**:85–6.

Cohen I.K., Theogaras D. (1975). Nasolabial flap reconstruction of the floor of the mouth after extirpation of oral cancer. *Amer. J. Surg*; **130**:479–80.

Conley J. (1963). The management of carotid body tumours. *Surg. Gynaecol. Obstet*; **117**:722–32.

Conley J. (1965). The carotid body. *Arch. Otolaryngol*; **81**:187–93.

Crile G. (1906). Excision of cancer of the head and neck. *J. Amer. Med. Ass*; **47**:1780–6.

Deane S.A., Telander R.L. (1978). Surgery of thyroglossal duct and branchial cleft anomalies. *Amer. J. Surg*; **136**:348–53.

Dedo H.H., Fishman N.H. (1969). Laryngeal release and sleeve resection for tracheal stenosis. *Ann. Otol. Rhinol. Laryngol*; **78**:285–96.

Dohlmann G., Mattsson O. (1960). The endoscopic operation for hypopharyngeal diverticula. *Arch. Otolaryngol*; **71**:744–52.

Evans J.N.G., Todd G.B. (1974). Laryngo-tracheoplasty. *J. Laryngol. Otol*; **88**:589–97.

Fairman H.D., John H.J. (1966). Treatment of cancer of the pharynx and cervical oesophagus. *J. Laryngol. Otol*; **80**:1091–101.

Farr H.W. (1967). Carotid body tumours. *Amer. J. Surg*; **114**:614–9.

Fearon B., Cotton R. (1972). Surgical correction of subglottic stenosis of the larynx. *Ann. Otol. Rhinol. Laryngol*; **81**:508–13.

Johnson J.T., Leipzig B., Cummings C.W. (1980). Management of T_1 carcinoma of the anterior aspect of the tongue. *Arch. Otolaryngol*; **106**:249–51.

Le Quesne L.P., Ranger D. (1966). Pharyngo-laryngectomy with immediate pharyngogastric anastomosis. *Brit. J. Surg*; **53**:105–9.

Maran A.G.D., Buchanan D.R. (1978). Branchial cysts, sinuses and fistulae. *Clin. Otolaryngol*; **3**:77–92.

McGregor I.A. (1963). The temporal flap in intra-oral cancer; its use in repairing the post-excisional defect. *Brit. J. Plast. Surg*; **16**:318–35.

McGregor I.A. (1977). Problems of reconstructive surgery of the oral cavity. *J. Laryngol. Otol*; **91**:445–65.

McGregor I.A., McGrouther D.A. (1978). Skin graft reconstruction in carcinoma of the tongue. *Head Neck Surg*; **1**:47–51.

Ong G.B., Lee T.C. (1960). Pharyngogastric anastomosis after oesophago-pharyngectomy for carcinoma of the hypopharynx and cervical oesophagus. *Brit. J. Surg*; **48**:193–200.

Palacios E. (1970). Chemodectomas of the head and neck. *Amer. J. Roentgenol*; **110**:129–39.

Rogers J.H., Freeland A.P. (1976). Arterial vasculature of cervical skin flaps. *Clin. Otolaryngol*; **41**:325–32.

Stell P.M. (1976). Tumours of the oropharynx. *Clin. Otolaryngol*; **1**:71–90.

Stell P.M., Carden E.A., Hibbert J., Dalby J.E. (1978). Postcricoid carcinoma. *Clin. Oncol*; **4**:215–26.

Stell P.M., Maran A.G.D. (1975). Laryngocoele. *J. Laryngol. Otol*; **89**:915–24.

Tucker H. (1978). Human laryngeal re-innervation. *Laryngoscope*; **88**:598–604.

Ward P.H., Jenkins H.A., Hanaffe W.L. (1978). Diagnosis and treatment of carotid body tumours. *Ann. Otol. Rhinol. Laryngol*; **87**:614–21.

Woodman De G., (1953). Bilateral abductor paralysis. *Arch. Otolaryngol*; **58**:150–3.

UICC (1978) *TNM Classification of Malignant Tumours.* Geneva: UICC.

42

Salivary glands

JOHN MAYNARD

The oral cavity is bathed with saliva from the secretions of three main paired salivary gland masses – the parotid, submandibular and sublingual, as well as numerous minor salivary glands scattered throughout the cavity. The parotid is the largest of the salivary glands and is distinguished by the presence of the peripheral branches of the facial nerve which pass through its mass and complicate surgical procedures. The submandibular gland has a superficial and deep portion. From the latter arises the main duct which has an intimate relation to the lingual nerve.

The sublingual gland is the most variable of the major glands. It drains by a varying number of separate ducts into the floor of the mouth and in 50% of cases by a major duct into the main submandibular duct.

The minor salivary glands are found in labial and buccal mucosa, in the tongue and hard and soft palates.

The total salivary secretion is between 1000 and 1500 ml daily and is almost all the result of stimulation. The bulk of the secretion, 90%, is shared by the parotid and submandibular glands. The sublingual gland contributes 5% of the total as do the minor salivary glands.

The parotid gland clinically is predominantly affected by tumour formation, 20% of which are malignant and rarely by acute infection, obstruction or calculous disease. The submandibular gland is most commonly affected by calculous obstruction and only 5% of all salivary tumours are found here, but nearly 50% are malignant. The sublingual gland rarely produces clinical problems and then almost entirely tumours, 75% of which are malignant. However, they account for less than 1% of all salivary tumours. The minor salivary glands are occasionally involved by neoplasms, about 10% of the total, and 50% are malignant.

To put the clinical problem finally in perspective, salivary tumours form less than 3% of all neoplasms and the incidence is low – between 1 and 3 per 100 000 in all regions of the world with a slightly higher incidence of malignant neoplasms in Eskimos (Thackray, 1969).

Investigations

Radiology

Plain x-rays of the parotid gland may rarely show a simple calculus or multiple tiny peripheral calculi in obstructive disease. Plain x-rays of the submandibular gland and its duct may demonstrate one or more calculi and occlusal films are much more satisfactory for this purpose. Twenty percent of salivary calculi are non-opaque to x-rays.

Injection into the parotid or submandibular duct orifice of oily radio opaque fluid produces a sialogram depicting the main duct and branch duct. Following injection, further x-rays after stimulation by lemon juice or citric acid may show failure of complete emptying of the duct system which is significant in certain diseases of both major glands. Aqueous solutions are absorbed more rapidly and do not demonstrate delayed emptying so satisfactorily. Because of their low viscosity the acini are filled and such parenchymal images are more useful for demonstrating tumours as filling defects. Water soluble substances are generally more useful. Malignant tumours infiltrate the duct system and sialography may then show gross distortion, localised obstruction and destruction of ducts with pooling of the radio opaque medium. Tomography may help to diminish the surrounding and overlying bony structures and produce more detailed films.

Radiology is helpful in the diagnosis of:

Calculi
Degree of glandular damage in obstruction
Tumours, particularly deep parotid tumours not easily detectable clinically
Differentiation between benign and malignant tumours
Duct strictures
Duct fistulas and sialocoeles

Radioisotopes

Technetium 99m is taken up sufficiently by salivary tissue for scanning and evaluation of the glandular parenchyma. At present it is impossible to differentiate tumours below 1 to 2 cm in diameter. Warthin's tumours may take up more of the isotope and appear as 'hot' lesions. Carcinomas take up very little and appear cold. Patients with Sjögren's disease have a very low uptake of the isotope.

Ultrasound

Distinguishes solid tumours from the rare cysts and sialocoeles.

CAT scanning

Computerised axial tomography has a definite place in the assessment of the extent of deep parotid tumours.

Constituents of saliva

The measurement of salivary constituents may be of diagnostic help. In inflammatory disease the sodium level may be as much as 10 times higher while the phosphate level is depressed up to 50%. In Sjögren's disease the sodium is often much higher and the phosphate more depressed than in obstructive parotitis and therefore may help in distinguishing the two. These changes are always bilateral in Sjögren's disease, but unilateral in those cases with intermittent obstruction in one parotid. The albumen content of saliva is usually very low,

but albumen and the immunoglobulins IgA and IgM are three to ten times the normal level in Sjögren's disease. In 75% of patients with Sjögren's disease antibodies to salivary duct epithelium can be demonstrated.

Parotid

A painless swelling in the parotid must be assumed to be neoplastic until proved otherwise. A painful swelling in the parotid must arouse the suspicion of a malignant neoplasm. Unless there are obvious physical signs of malignancy it is not possible to distinguish various neoplasms clinically, a fact which considerably influences management. Swellings such as sialosis, oncocytosis and benign lymphoepithelial lesions are discussed later. Neoplasms may be classified as follows (Table 1):

Table 1

Benign	Intermediate
Adenolymphoma (Warthin)	Pleomorphic adenoma (mixed parotid tumour)
Other monomorphic tumours	Low grade mucoepidermoid tumour
Sebaceous adenomas	Acinic cell tumour
Sebaceous lymphadenoma	Adenoid cystic tumour
Oncocytoma	
Basal cell tumour	
Clear cell adenoma	
Haemangioma	
Lymphangioma	
Lipoma	
Neural tumour of VII nerve	

Malignant
Carcinoma in a pleomorphic adenoma
High grade mucoepidermoid carcinoma
Adenocarcinoma
Squamous cell carcinoma
Undifferentiated carcinoma
Metastatic carcinoma
Lymphoma

Benign tumours

Pleomorphic adenomas, the so-called mixed parotid tumours are often classified under this heading, but for clinical reasons, apparent below, they should be included in the intermediate group.

Warthin's tumour

This accounts for 5% of all salivary neoplasms. It is more commonly found in the 6th decade, the male to female ratio is 5 to 1, 10% are bilateral and they appear to be multifocal. They are always benign and almost confined to the parotid. Isolated examples have been reported in the submandibular glands and in minor glands in the lips, larynx and pharyngeal wall. The histological appearance is characteristic and easily recognised. Delicate papillary fronds of a well-differentiated double- or treble-layered finely granular epithelium are separated from each other by lymphoid tissue containing germinal centres. The current theory of aetiology is that the tumour develops from ductal inclusions in adjacent lymph nodes. Such ectopic salivary ducts are normally found in lymph nodes following the course of development of the parotid gland. This then explains the virtual confinement of adenolymphomas to the parotid. An alternative theory supposes that the lymphatic and lymphoid stroma is an inflammatory or even auto-immune response to leakage from blocked ducts resulting from proliferation of the adenoma. Both theories are not necessarily mutually exclusive and would explain the occasional adenolymphomas in sites other than the parotid.

Macroscopically the tumours are well encapsulated, partly cystic and often exude a clear or opaque brownish or yellowish fluid, not unlike pus, if damaged during mobilisation. This feature is almost diagnostic.

Oncocytomas

These are rare, constituting less than 1% of salivary tumours and are most often found in the parotid and usually in patients over the age of 50. The large eosinophilic granular cells are found in other tumours and may represent hyperplasia rather than neoplasia; the existence of a malignant oncocytoma is doubtful.

Other monomorphic tumours are also rare, accounting perhaps for 2% of all salivary tumours and found in patients in the 6th and 7th decade. Sebaceous cells are found in normal glands and sebaceous adenomas and lymphadenomas may be metaplastic rather than neoplastic. Basal cell adenomas are occasionally found in the parotid and in minor glands in the upper lip and behave as benign tumours. Clear cell adenomas are rare.

Intermediate tumours

Certain salivary tumours, particularly the low grade mucoepidermoid and acinic cell types, metastasise late and if adequately removed have an excellent prognosis. Patey refused to distinguish them by the name carcinoma, but preferred to classify them as acinic cell and low grade mucoepidermoid tumours (Patey *et al.*, 1965). Adenoid cystic tumours, although more aggressive initially, often run a benign course and metastatic deposits may remain unaltered for years. Pleomorphic adenomas might be included in this group. Although benign they easily recur and a small

proportion after many years become aggressive malignant carcinomas.

Pleomorphic adenomas

These form no less than 70% of 'benign' salivary tumours, 84% in the parotid, 8% in the submandibular gland (Rauch, 1959), 0.5% in the sublingual and 5% in minor salivary glands of which 4% are found in the hard and soft palate.

They are firm, mobile smooth tumours which characteristically grow very slowly and most commonly are found in the lower pole of the parotid. This is probably the result of their slow growth and the confined space in which the deeper part of the gland is enclosed. They are not multifocal as has been so frequently reported. This apparent feature is the result of inadequate initial surgery and the resulting multi-focal recurrences are due to spillage. Macroscopically they appear to be encapsulated and multilobulated, grey, white and yellow in colour with patches of translucency corresponding to the cartilage-like material. If the capsule is inadvertently ruptured, the tumour tissue exudes as a grey/white rather granular toothpaste-like substance. Microscopically two types of cells predominate, an inner layer of epithelial cells and an outer of myoepithelial cells. The general appearance is pleomorphic with a variable pattern of papillary, trabecular or cystic arrangement of epithelial cells and varying amounts of mucoid and cartilaginous-like stroma. The cartilaginous appearance is the result of mucinous degeneration of myoepithelial cells (Mylius, 1960) and is not true cartilage. Willis (1960) was moved to say 'anyone who doubts the epithelial origin of pleomorphic adenomas is pathologically incorrigible'. Close examination of the capsule shows that it is defective in places and buds or satellites of adenoma may be seen apparently infiltrating the surrounding normal tissue, but most authorities agree that such outgrowths are merely part of a benign tumour. However, enucleation is bound to leave small areas of adenoma behind which accounts for the multifocal recurrences after inadequate surgery. Malignant change in an epithelial component of the pleomorphic adenoma is well documented. The incidence varies in different series up to 5%. Such malignant transformation may not occur for many years and the average length in Patey's series was 19 years (Patey *et al.*, 1965). This feature of pleomorphic adenomas is another excellent reason for adequate initial excision.

Mucoepidermoid tumours

These account for 33% of all malignant salivary tumours and are the commonest malignant tumours of the parotid and also the commonest malignant salivary tumour in children. Forming 9% of all salivary tumours, 6% of them are found in the parotid. The degree of malignancy varies considerably and attempts have been made, by correlating histological appearances and clinical behaviour, to classify them in three or more categories. It is simpler to differentiate between low grade tumours with 90% survival if adequately treated and the less common high grade tumours with only a 20% survival.

Macroscopically these tumours are firm, greyish red in colour and often contain small cysts. They are poorly encapsulated and may be seen to be infiltrating locally. Microscopically, they arise from duct epithelium and contain varying proportions of squamous cells and glandular mucus-secreting cells. Circumscribed tumours which are well-differentiated and easily identified behave as low grade tumours. Diffuse infiltration of the whole tumour by mucin indicates the probability of recurrence and, therefore, a high grade tumour.

Acinic cell tumours

These were originally thought to be benign adenomas. They are, however, unpredictable in their behaviour. They grow slowly, metastasise late and have an overall good prognosis when adequately treated; 20% metastasise and a 10% 5-year mortality has been reported by Eneroth *et al.*, 1966. They account for 1% of salivary tumours and are nearly all found in the parotid gland.

Macroscopically these tumours are firm multinodular greyish white, solid and partially encapsulated. Histologically the cells are predominantly granular and resemble serous acini.

Adenoid cystic tumours

These are included in this section as they are slow growing tumours with a long period of survival after treatment even with metastases. Foote and Frazell (1954) prefer to call them adenoid-cystic carcinomas. They form 5% of all salivary tumours and nearly 25% of tumours of minor glands in which they are more common, particularly the hard palate. The instance of metastases varies up to 50% and increases with time after treatment up to 10 years or more. In one series (Conley and Dingman, 1974) the mortality was 62% after 15 years. Undoubtedly the prognosis is worse when minor glands are involved, perhaps due to inadequate excision or relative inaccessability. Adequate wide surgical excision initially is probably the most important factor involving prognosis.

They are firm pinkish grey tumours, incompletely encapsulated and often attached to surrounding structures with evidence of local infiltration. The cut surface is wet and shiny like a pleomorphic adenoma. Micro-

scopically, the predominant cells are small with little cytoplasm and darkly staining nuclei; in the past they were often called cylindromas. A tendency to invade perineural spaces can lead to x-ray appearances of enlargement of foramina at the base of the skull. It is possible to correlate histological features with estimates of prognosis. Clinically detectable metastases may remain unchanged for years and if solitary may be excised with benefit.

Malignant tumours

Carcinoma in pleomorphic adenomas represents a malignant change, the incidence of which is 5% in one series (Patey *et al.*, 1965). Seventy-three percent occur in the parotid and 23% in the submandibular. Such malignant changes in a pleomorphic adenoma may take many years to occur, an average of 19 years in one series (Patey *et al.*, 1965) and 47 years in one of my own cases. Adequate initial management of the frequently occurring pleomorphic adenoma will prevent the occurrence of this disease with its poor prognosis.

Metastases occur in as many as 70% of patients and a 5-year mortality is greater than 50% overall. Other primary carcinomas, including high grade mucoepidermoid tumours have a rapid clinical course with frequent recurrence and a high mortality. Squamous cell carcinomas which presumably result from malignant change in metaplastic duct epithelium occur more frequently in men in the 6th and 7th decade. The five-year survival is less than 20%. Metastatic squamous cell carcinoma from other sites must be considered in the differential diagnosis. Adenocarcinomas run an inexorable clinical course with 50% dead in 5 years. Metastatic carcinoma in the 20 or 30 lymph follicles in the parotid come predominantly from melanomas and squamous cell carcinomas. Finally, a lymphoma may present in the parotid. In Patey's series (1965) there was a 1% incidence of such tumours.

Clinical features of tumours

Benign and intermediate tumours that have not metastasised cannot be distinguished clinically. Those occurring in the superficial part of the parotid present as firm, smooth or lobulated mobile masses. They are all slow growing and the size of the tumour mass is related to the length of history, which in the past was often many years. Those arising in the deep lobe are often diagnosed much later unless they obviously bulge into the palate or tonsillar region. They may produce diffuse enlargement of the parotid and the gradual enlargement of the gland is often unobserved by the patient.

The clinical features of malignant tumours are very different. Rapid growth, hardness, skin attachment and even ulceration, together with deep fixity and lymph node enlargement, produce an obvious picture. Facial nerve involvement leads to rapid diagnosis. However, in the early stages of development these tumours infiltrate sensory nerves and produce vague pain in the distribution of the great auricular and auriculo-temporal. The combination of pain and enlargement of the parotid must be regarded as sinister. If there is no evidence of obstructive parotid disease or inflammation, biopsy or parotidectomy is essential.

Investigations

Tumours in the superficial lobe of the parotid require no special investigations unless there are features suggesting malignancy. Diffuse enlargement of the gland or clinically detectable enlargement into the oropharynx requires further investigation to establish the correct diagnosis.

Sialography may show a deep space occupying lesion displacing the duct system and may suggest a malignant tumour. Tomography and CAT scanning may help in defining the extent of the tumour and in planning treatment. Plain x-rays of the base of the skull may show widening of cranial nerve foramina in cases of adenoid-cystic carcinoma.

Management

Tumours arising in the superficial part of the parotid, unless there are obvious signs and symptoms of malignancy, are treated by superficial parotidectomy as discussed below. This procedure need not necessarily mean a formal removal of the whole of the superficial lobe; the aim is wide excision of tumour tissue with a generous cuff of surrounding normal gland. Ideally, the specimen should be sent immediately for frozen section. Tumours in the deep part of the parotid require mobilisation of the facial nerve before excision unless the nerve is apparently involved in tumour tissue when frozen section biopsy should be performed. In all low grade tumours the facial nerve should only be sacrificed if involved by tumour. Radical neck dissection and postoperative radiotherapy is not necessary.

Poorly differentiated mucoepidermoid, malignant pleomorphic tumours, squamous cell and undifferentiated carcinomas require more radical treatment. Obviously, infiltrating tumours with facial nerve involvement should be biopsied for frozen section before conservative excision. High grade tumours must be treated by a radical parotidectomy combined with block dissection of the homolateral lymph nodes and postoperative radiotherapy. There seems little doubt that the best chance of cure is the first radical operation. Surgery for recurrences has a poor prognosis (Fig 42.1).

Operation

The incision is made in front of the ear and curves below the angle of the mandible and then anteriorly into a skin crease in the neck (Fig 42.2). The Y incision formerly practised is unnecessary. The anterior skin flap is dissected forward nearly to the anterior border of the parotid, but not beyond because the finer branches of the facial nerve leave the gland superficially and may be damaged.

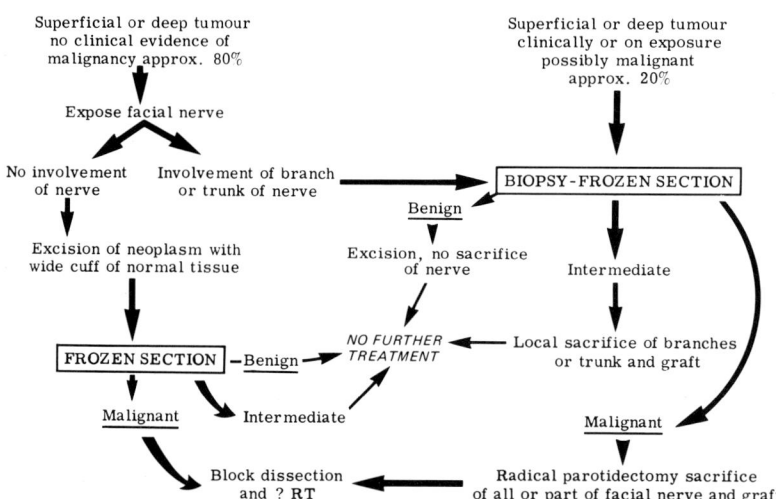

Fig 42.1 Flow diagram: surgical management of neoplasms.

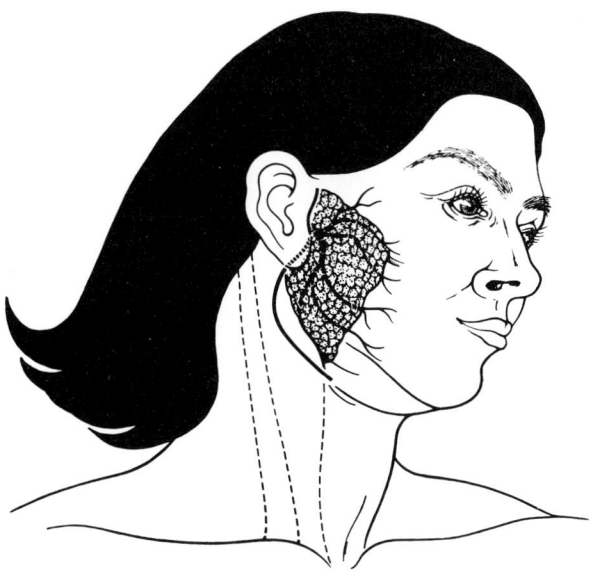

Fig 42.2   Parotidectomy – incision.

The facial nerve should be identified by dissection just anterior to the posterior border of the gland opposite the apex of a 'V' sulcus made by the lower border of the external auditory meatus above and the anterior surface of the mastoid below (Fig 42.3). The sulcus is easily palpable rather than visible (Maynard, 1978). Once the main trunk and branching of the facial nerve is identified (Fig 42.4) the superficial lobe or part of it containing the tumour is dissected from the nerve and its branches (Fig 42.5). Tumours arising in the deep lobe will require anterior mobilisation of the superficial lobe. The branches of the facial nerve may then be lifted from the deep lobe to allow excision of the latter. Low grade tumours including pleomorphic adenomas, but not benign tumours, which are ruptured during dissection or when there is doubt concerning adequate excision, should be treated with postoperative irradiation.

Radical parotidectomy for high grade tumours entails sacrifice of the facial nerve. The trunk should be identified well behind the tumour, if necessary removing part of the mastoid process. The tumour is excised widely with surrounding normal tissue if possible and the branches of the facial nerve identified well anterior to the tumour limits, and marked. A radical block dissection of the homolateral posterior triangle is then carried out and the cervical plexus, removed with the block, is preserved. Thus more than sufficient amount of nerve tissue is available to fashion a new facial nerve which is then sutured to the main trunk and peripheral branches using 8/0 virgin silk or 10/0 nylon (Maynard, 1978).

In as many as 50% of patients following parotidectomy Frey's syndrome of gustatory sweating may develop. Flushing and sweating in the distribution of the auriculotemporal nerve occurs following gustatory stimulation. Division of the tympanic branch of the glossopharyngeal in the middle ear may relieve the symptoms in those few patients whose symptoms are excessive (Frey, 1923; Harrison and Donaldson, 1979).

Inflammatory and obstructive diseases of the parotid

Acute parotitis

Viral parotitis or mumps causes few problems in diagnosis. Acute bacterial parotitis is now rarely seen, but at the turn of the century it was one of the commonest complications of abdominal surgery. The combination of dehydration and poor oral hygiene in a debilitated patient allowed retrograde spread of infection from the mouth to the gland. Such acute parotitis today almost always responds dramatically to antibiotics and drainage is only occasionally necessary. A small incision in the line of a routine parotidectomy incision in front of the ear will expose the gland. A transverse incision through the capsule over a fluctuant area allows drainage without risk of damage to the facial nerve.

Recurrent swellings of the parotid gland

Calculus

Recurring swellings of the gland with subsequent decompression sometimes related to eating and chewing and sometimes spontaneous, suggests the calculous obstruction familiar in the submandibular gland. However, the parotid gland is serous secreting and calculi are rare and usually secondary to obstruction.

Autoimmune

Mikulicz (1892) first described unexplained swellings of salivary and lacrimal glands in one patient as did Sjögren (1933), an ophthalmologist. There now seems little doubt that the so-called Mikulicz disease in the past was a collection of misdiagnosed cases of sarcoidosis, lymphoma, tuberculosis and an autoimmune disease affecting salivary and lacrimal tissue. The latter is still called Sjögren's disease. We now recognise a spectrum of diseases with or without obvious swelling of the parotid, often with xerostoma, decreased lacrimal secretion and associated arthritis and 75% of such patients have antibodies to salivary duct epithelium

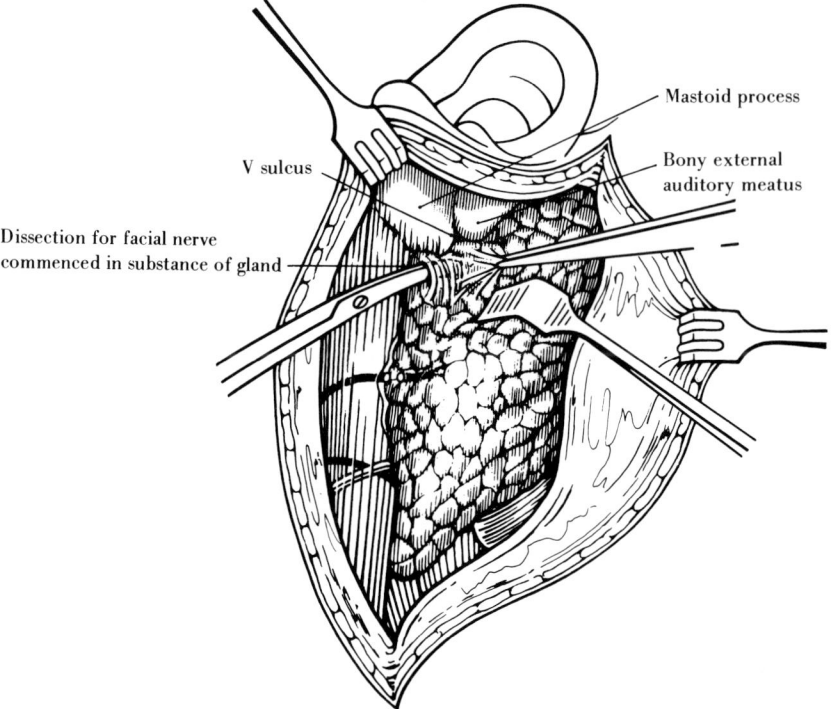

Fig 42.3 Parotidectomy – exposure of facial nerve and beginning of dissection.

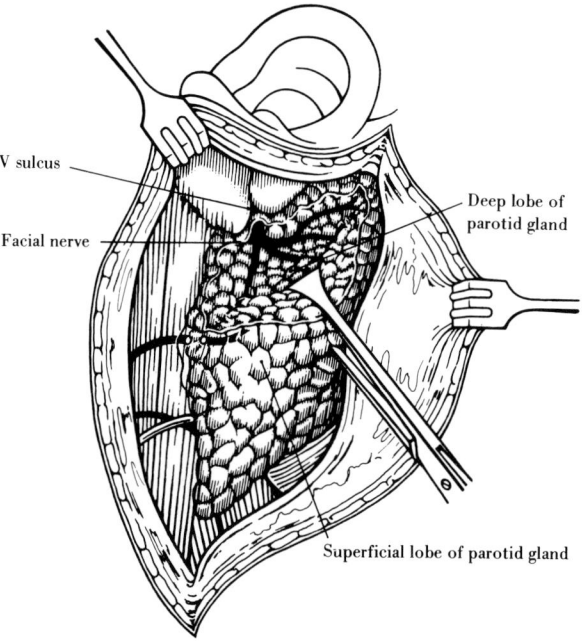

Fig 42.4 Parotidectomy – dissection for facial nerve.

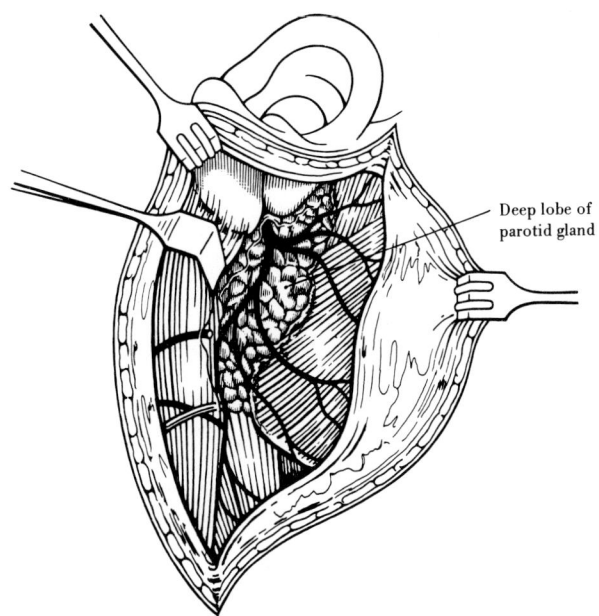

Deep lobe of parotid gland

Fig 42.5 Parotidectomy – completion of dissection.

detectable in their serum. Antinuclear factors are present in 70%. Histologically the salivary glands show acinar destruction and infiltration with lymphocytes and plasma cells. The benign lymphoepithelial disease of Godwin (1952) is histologically identical and part of the same disease process (Morgan and Castleman, 1953). Among this group there are a number of patients with recurrent parotid swellings and no other stigmata of an autoimmune process. They apparently do not ultimately develop Sjögren's disease and the swellings either spontaneously remit or may be successfully treated (Maynard, 1965, 1979).

Diagnosis. Clinically this rests on a combination of dry eyes, a dry mouth, associated arthritis with or without recurrent swellings or permanent enlargement of one or both parotid glands.

Investigations. A positive Schirmer test (measurement of lachrymal secretion) and a low stimulated parotid secretion rate, less than 0.5 ml/min., suggests the diagnosis. Analysis of salivary content from both parotids shows a bilateral raised sodium and depressed phosphate; the albumin is also raised. Serum protein studies show a marked elevation of gammaglobulin. The rheumatoid factor is consistently found and antinuclear factors in 68% of patients (Bloch *et al.*, 1960).

Biopsy of a labial salivary gland shows the characteristic histology. Sialography merely illustrates the degree of duct damage and is discussed below.

Decreased uptake of technetium may in future help in diagnosis.

Management. So far there appears to be no adequate treatment other than symptomatic. The eyes must be lubricated with methylcellulose drops and the mouth with glycerine and mouthwashes. Frequent dental treatment and attention to oral hygiene is important.

Painful swollen parotid glands may be treated by superficial parotidectomy. Such apparently aggressive treatment may become justified as increasing reports appear of the development of malignant lymphoma and carcinoma in cases of long standing Sjögren's disease (Azzopardi and Evans, 1971; Hornbaker *et al.*, 1966). Irradiation should not be used as it may act as a trigger in the development of such tumours.

Recurrent parotid swellings (non autoimmune)

Patients with recurrent swellings of one or both parotids with no evidence of autoimmune disease appear to be a distinct group. Nearly 300 such patients have been treated over the last 15 years and none has so far developed the stigmata of Sjögren's disease (Maynard, 1979). Shearn (1971) suggests that such patients represent an incomplete form of Sjögren's. The natural history and suggested aetiology is illustrated in Fig 42.6. Investigations reveal none of the changes associated

ADULTS

Autoimmune disease
(Sjögren's)

Abnormally low
secretion rate
(unknown aetiology)

Decreasing
parotid function

Retrograde infection

Mucus metaplasia, excess mucus
and periodic obstructive symptoms

Spontaneous
recovery 20%

Main duct changes, stricture calculi
and symptoms

Irreversible structural damage
and symptoms

Xerostomia

CHILDREN

Abnormally low
secretion rate

Retrograde infection

Mucus metaplasia, excess mucus
and periodic obstruction

Duct growth

Main duct change

Spontaneous
recovery

Irreversible damage and symptoms

Fig 42.6 Aetiology of Sjögren's disease and recurrent parotid swelling.

with Sjögren's. Sialograms show merely progressive stages of damage to the duct system (Figs 42.7–42.10). Main duct dilatation is associated with a significantly low secretion rate and probable irreversible changes.

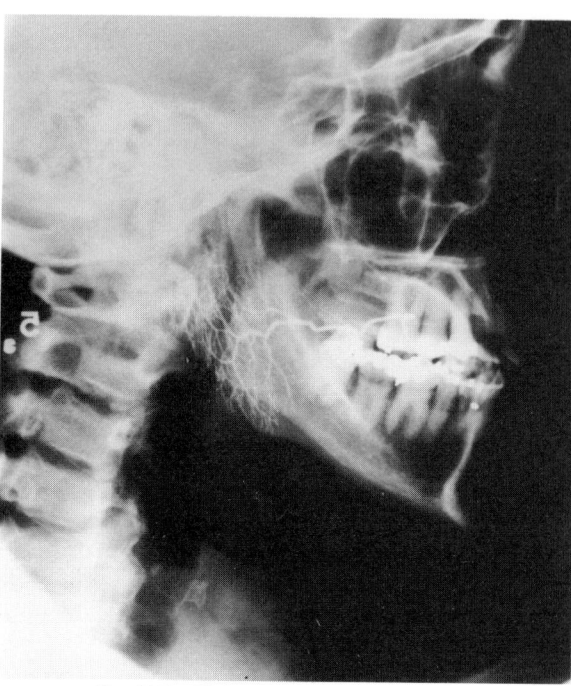

Fig 42.7 Sialogram or normal parotid.

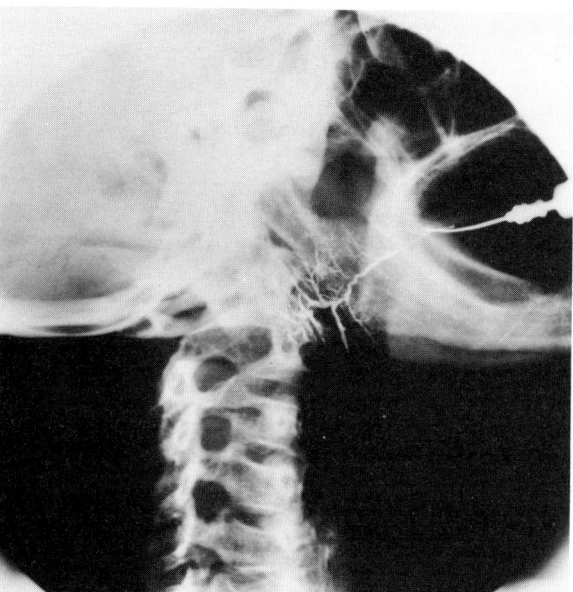

Fig 42.8 Branch duct dilatation.

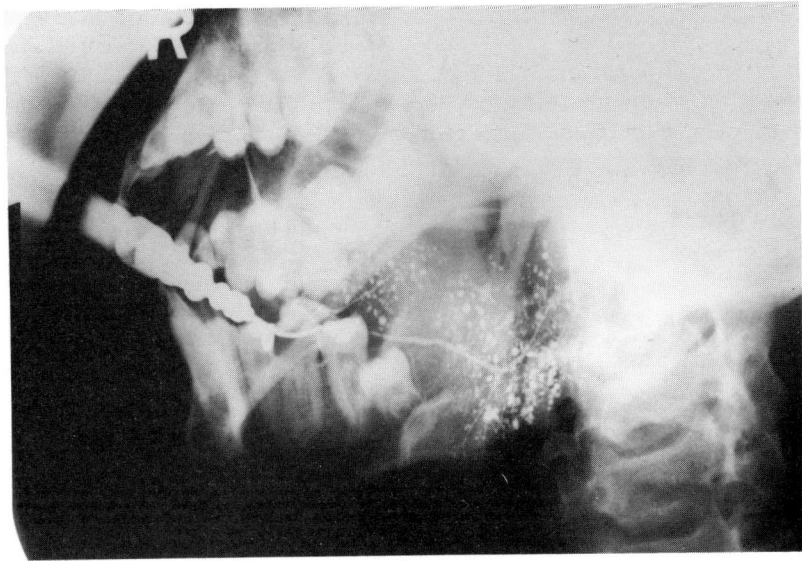

Fig 42.9   Sialectasis.

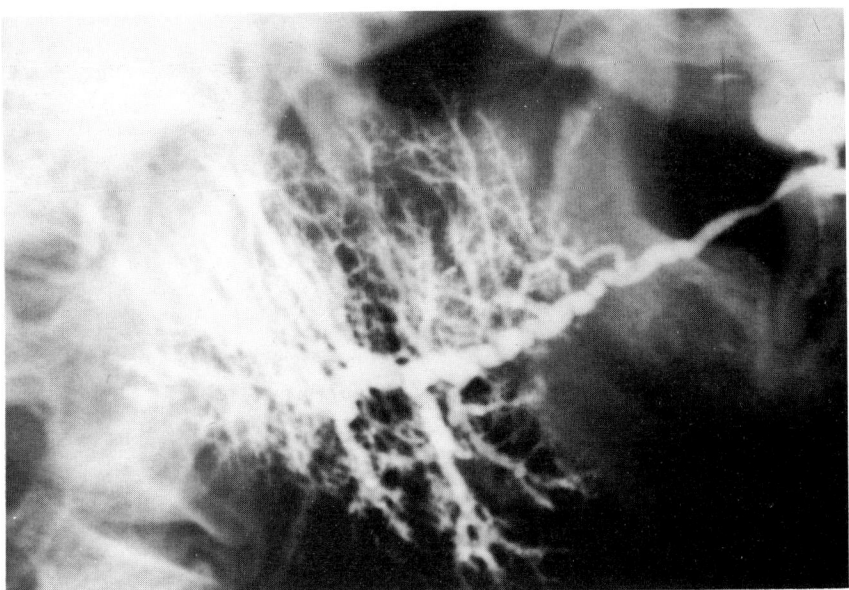

Fig 42.10   Main duct dilatation and strictures.

Management. Conservative treatment consists of stimulation of the parotid secretion by intermittent chewing of apples or carrots and was successful or partly successful in 77 out of 90 patients in one series (Maynard, 1979). Destructive surgery may, however, be necessary. Parotidectomy is curative, but carries the risk of damage to the facial nerve. The much lesser procedure of intraoral duct ligation may lead to parotid atrophy and cessation of symptoms but is successful in only a third of patients. The situation can then be retrieved by parotidectomy. A plan of management is illustrated in Fig 42.11.

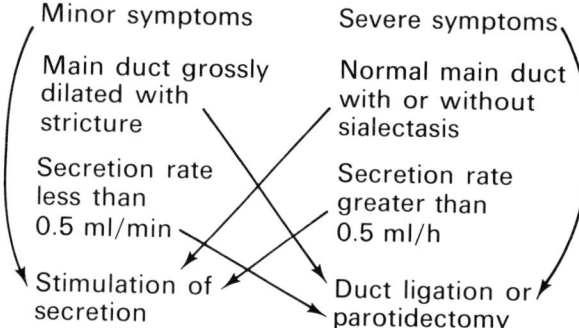

Fig 42.11 Plan of management of patients with recurrent parotid swelling.

Salivary fistulas and sialoceles

Fistula

The parotid duct is much more frequently injured as a result of facial trauma than the submandibular gland and the resulting fistula is usually external. Injury to the submandibular duct produces an intraoral fistula which is of no consequence.

Parenchymal fistula

A parotid parenchymal leakage of saliva is inevitable after partial parotid resection. A sialocele results which becomes an external fistula if, as usual, the operation site is drained. Provided there is no main duct blockage such fistulas and sialoceles invariably heal within a few days. Repeated aspiration of the sialocele through the healing wound hastens this resolution.

Traumatic parotid, parenchymal or fine duct fistulas as a result of facial injury usually heal in a few days. If there is associated main duct disease, as in recurrent obstructive parotitis and Sjögren's disease, the fistula may persist. A persistent external fistula leads to local inflammation and this, in turn, may aggravate the obstruction. The only treatment is parotidectomy.

Main duct fistula

Injury to the main duct in facial trauma should lead to reconstruction of the duct as soon as possible following the injury. The distal end of the duct is cannulated with a fine silastic tube and the latter advanced until it appears in the wound. The proximal end of the severed duct is often difficult to find. Magnification with a loupe or dissecting microscope is an advantage. Pressure over the gland may identify the proximal end by the flow of saliva or an injection of B methyl choline (Diamant *et al.*, 1957) intravenously may stimulate secretion. The cannula may then be advanced into the proximal end and the duct reconstructed over the cannula using fine interrupted submucosal Dexon sutures. The cannula should be stitched to the buccal mucosa as it leaves the duct orifice and retained as a splint for 7 days.

In certain circumstances the distal part of the duct is destroyed in the injury. A distal reconstruction is possible by marking out a strip of buccal mucosa and suturing it over a cannula or splint to make a tube. The adjacent mucosa is then undermined and sutured over the mucosal tube to bury it. After a week the mucosal tube is retrieved by incision through the overlying buccal mucosa and partly mobilised to allow its proximal end to be passed through the buccinator and sutured to the proximal end of the duct over a cannula. Such procedures may be difficult or fail. The situation can always be retrieved by parotidectomy. Proximal duct ligation may lead to gland atrophy in a proportion of cases (Maynard, 1979) if parotidectomy is contraindicated.

Trauma to the parotid or submandibular ducts may lead eventually to pooling of saliva in the interstitial tissues of the cheek or neck without an external fistula. Reconstruction is difficult and such sialoceles are best controlled by opening them into the mouth by incising the buccal mucosa and draining the cavity with a silastic tube which should be retained for at least a week. The resulting intraoral fistula resolves the problem. Failure is managed by excision of the gland.

Submandibular gland

Calculus

Submandibular calculi are primary and responsible for the subsequent inflammatory changes in the gland and duct. Parotid calculi, which are much less common, are the result of inflammatory and obstructive changes in the gland.

Aetiology and pathology

Stagnation, a matrix for calculous formation and changes in saliva influencing the precipitation of calcium and phosphates are the probable factors involved. The long uphill course of the submandibular duct and much narrower duct orifice compared to the parotid may produce stagnation. Mucus as a result of stagnation and perhaps subclinical retrograde infection from the mouth, alters and coalesces to form a gel which acts as a matrix. The calcium and phosphate hydroxyl apatites and phosphatases, which are in higher concentration than in parotid saliva, favour the precipitation of salts, aided perhaps again by low grade infection. Calculi are commonly found where the first part of the duct curves around the posterior border of the mylohyoid. They are often multiple and bilateral.

Clinical findings

Commonly, patients complain of intermittent swelling and pain when chewing or eating especially tart or spicy food. The swelling subsides after eating, only to recur on repeated stimulation. Less commonly, an acute inflammatory episode occurs with constitutional symptoms, pain and swelling in the floor of the mouth and also a painful swollen submandibular gland. One or more calculi may be symptomless, never give rise to obstructional swelling of the gland and are only found on incidental examination or radiography. Inspection of the floor of the mouth may show signs of inflammation in the region of the duct. This may not have given rise to symptoms necessarily. Stretching the mucosa with the finger sometimes allows the yellowish calculus to be seen more easily. The diagnosis is dependent mainly on digital examination bimanually with one finger in the floor of the mouth. Calculi are easily palpable in the anterior part of the duct, and the gland itself often feels firmer and larger in comparison with the other side.

Investigations

Extra-oral radiographs are unsatisfactory because of the surrounding bony structures and the faint calcification in many calculi. Twenty per cent of submandibular calculi are non-opaque. Occlusal films are more satisfactory but radiographs of the posterior part of the duct with occlusal films may be too uncomfortable for the patient. Sialography may demonstrate a filling defect with non-opaque impalpable calculi and also distinguish calcification not related to the gland and its duct.

Management

Acute obstruction with painful inflammation should be treated initially with antibiotics, but may resolve spontaneously with ulceration and extrusion of the calculus. If not, a calculus in the anterior part of the duct should be removed by simple incision over the duct under local anaesthetic. Recurrent obstructions due to calculus are treated in the following way:

Calculi in the anterior part of the duct. Under local anaesthetic or general anaesthetic a stitch is placed around the duct proximally and distally to fix the floor of the mouth and prevent the calculus moving back into the posterior part of the duct. (Fig 42.12) The area in the region of the calculus is then infiltrated with 1/300 000 adrenalin. A small incision is made through the

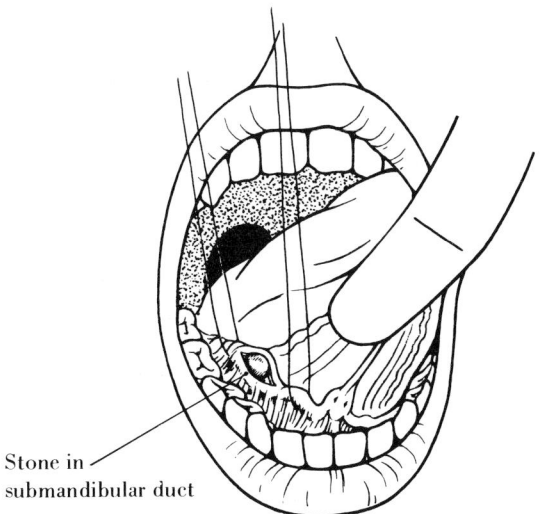

Stone in
submandibular duct

Fig 42.12   Excision of calculus from anterior part of submandicular duct.

mucosa and a longitudinal incision in the duct over the calculus allows removal. It is unnecessary to repair the duct but the patient should be warned that there is approximately a 20% recurrence rate.

Calculi in the posterior part of the duct or gland. It is difficult to remove a calculus from the posterior part of the duct where it curves around the posterior edge of the mylohyoid. The lingual nerve is a close relation here and is liable to damage. A stricture of the duct at this site following operation increases the chances of recurrent calculi. Operations on the gland itself to remove calculi leave a damaged duct system favouring stagnation and further calculus formation. Therefore, posterior duct and glandular stones should be treated by excision of the gland.

A 5 cm incision is made directly over the gland 2 cm below the lower border of the mandible (Fig 42.13). The dissection should keep within the fascia enclosing the gland. The mandibular branch of the 7th nerve must be protected in the upper leaf of the wound. The facial artery is often buried in the posterior part of the gland and supplies it. The lingual nerve is a close relation to the deeper part of the gland and the duct. The duct should be traced forward as far as possible and excised, as a calculus may otherwise be left behind in the anterior part of the duct (Fig 42.14) (Maynard, 1978).

Neoplasms

Only 5% to 10% of salivary tumours are found in the submandibular gland (Eneroth, 1971). Unfortunately

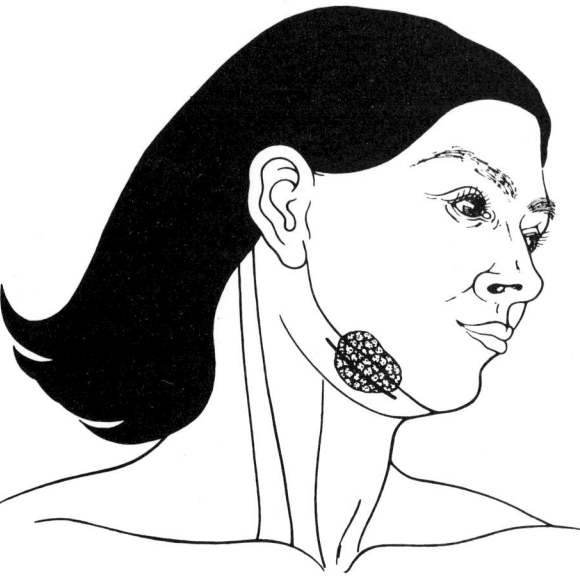

Fig 42.13   Excision of submandibular gland. Incision.

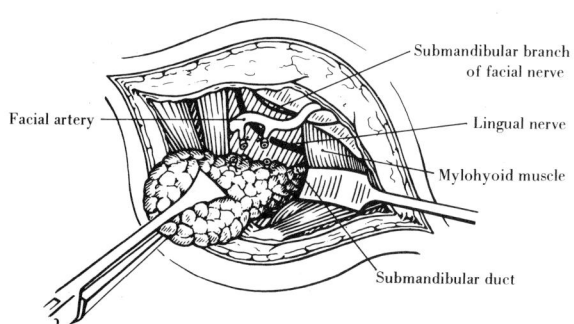

Submandibular branch
of facial nerve

Facial artery

Lingual nerve

Mylohyoid muscle

Submandibular duct

Fig 42.14   Excision of submandibular gland. Completion
of dissection.

nearly 50% of them are malignant. The duration of
symptoms and incidence of metastases (75%) are
greater at this site, probably because of the much
higher incidence of calculous disease leading to delay in
diagnosis. They are classified in descending order of
frequency of occurrence:

Adenoidcystic
Mucoepidermoid
Malignant change in pleomorphic adenoma (23%
submandibular, 73% parotid)
Pleomorphic adenoma (8% submandibular, 84%
parotid)
Undifferentiated carcinoma

Acinic cell tumours are rarely found in the submandibular gland and adenolymphomas are exceptionally
rare.

Pain and swelling in one submandibular gland naturally suggests calculous obstruction but bimanual
examination may reveal enlargement of the whole
gland or part of it and it feels hard and may be fixed.
However, all these physical signs may also be present in
inflammatory disease. Suspicion must be aroused if
there is no satisfactory history of recurrent swelling or
fluctuation in size on eating or chewing. The presence
of enlarged lymph nodes in the cervical region and the
absence of calculi on radiology of the region should
increase suspicion.

Treatment

Once suspicion has been aroused, the only satisfactory treatment is complete excision and the best chance
of surgical cure is the first operation. The prognosis
after operation for recurrence is unsatisfactory.

The gland is explored in the way described above.
Suspicion is increased or first awakened if the gland is
hard, infiltrating surrounding structures, or has a gross
appearance of neoplastic tissue. Management now
depends on the type of neoplasm and frozen section is
essential. It is helpful to divide the neoplasms found
here into high and low grade tumours (Table 2).

Table 2

Low grade	High grade
Well differentiated mucoepidermoid	Poorly differentiated mucoepidermoid tumours
Adenoidcystic	Malignant mixed tumours
(Acinic cell tumours)	Squamous cell and un-differentiated carcinomas

If frozen section indicates a low grade tumour then
complete excision of the gland and surrounding infiltrated tissue must be performed. The lingual and
hypoglossal nerves may be preserved unless, in the case
of adenoid cystic tumours, there appears to be any suggestion of infiltration of the nerves. It is unnecessary to
combine excision with a block dissection of the cervical
nodes and postoperative radiotherapy is also unnecessary, certainly with well-differentiated mucoepidermoid or the rare acinic cell tumours. The commonest
benign tumours are pleomorphic adenomas which
should be excised intact with the whole gland.

In the case of high grade tumours the only hope of
cure is radical excision with sacrifice of nerves. As over
40% of these tumours have already metastasised to
regional nodes, a block dissection of the cervical nodes
on that side should be carried out at the same time.
Postoperative radiotherapy is probably wise.

Sublingual gland

This least of the major glands is rarely involved in disease. Tumours occasionally develop here, nearly 80% were malignant in most series. The most frequently occurring are adenoidcystic and mucoepidermoid. Treatment is complete excision after frozen section. There is no place for biopsy or partial excision. Patients with low grade tumours are then potentially cured, but those with high grade tumours also require block dissection and radiotherapy.

Minor salivary glands

Ranula

A soft bluish painless cyst in the floor of the mouth may be the result of partial duct blockage, perhaps originally the result of local inflammation. They are more commonly seen in neonates and children and may, if large enough, be a cause of respiratory embarrassment. They are best treated by total excision of the sublingual gland. Certain ranulas extend from the floor of the mouth to the neck and are generally considered to be branchogenic in origin (*see* chap. 41).

Mucous cysts

These are commonly found arising in a minor mucus secreting gland in the lower lip. They sometimes spontaneously disappear, but should otherwise be excised and if found to be solid, widely excised since adenoidcystic tumours sometimes present in this way (*see below*).

Tumours

There is a high incidence of malignancy in tumours of minor salivary glands, 50% or greater. They appear as masses beneath the mucosa and are occasionally mistaken for cysts. In order of frequency of recurrence they are found in the hard and soft palates, the lips, buccal mucosa and tongue. Adenoidcystic and mucoepidermoid tumours are most frequently found and they must be initially treated by wide excision. Spread is unpredictable and excision of lymph nodes not justified. The prognosis is not good because of late diagnosis and sometimes the difficulty of wide excision.

Salivary diseases in childhood

Mumps

Viral sialadenitis is a common disease of young children. Both parotid glands become painful and swollen in 90%; the submandibular glands only occasionally. The pain, swelling and accompanying general malaise is diagnostic and subsides in a few days. Lifelong immunity results from the infection which helps distinguish mumps from recurrent bouts of obstruction.

Recurrent swellings of the parotid

Recurrent bouts of obstruction of one or both parotids occasionally occurs in children. Symptomatic treatment and reassurance of the parents is all that is necessary. There is no place for surgical tampering. The majority of these attacks spontaneously remit by puberty although a small proportion persist with symptoms into adult life (Fig 42.6).

Tumours

The commonest tumour of the parotid in infants is a haemangioma. The rapid growth spurt in the first two or three years of life is characteristic of all haemangiomas. The tumour is soft, compressible and often bluish sometimes accompanied by an overlying cutaneous haemangioma. These tumours nearly always undergo natural resolution and should not be interfered with. If, by school age, no further resolution has occurred, or there is a persisting lymphangiomatous element, operation may be resorted to.

Lymphangiomas

Lymphangiomas are less common than haemangiomas and do not regress. They have a tendency to enlarge and are prone to infection. When the parotid is involved, the lymphangioma is not usually confined to the gland, but extends into the deeper tissues in the neck. Complete resection may not be technically possible, partial resection with preservation of the nerve is satisfactory. The technique of parotidectomy in children is similar to adults except that the mastoid is not completely developed and the facial nerve trunk is consequently much more superficial.

Neoplasms

Pleomorphic adenomas are the commonest benign neoplasm and mucoepidermoid carcinoma the commonest malignant tumour. Fortunately they only occur rarely. The acinic celled tumour is the second commonest potentially malignant tumour. Rhabdomyosarcoma, fibrosarcoma and aggressive undifferentiated carcinomas have been reported. Management, including radiotherapy if necessary, is the same as for adult neoplasms.

References

Azzopardi R., Evans W. (1971). Malignant lymphoma of parotid in association with Mikulicz's disease. *J. Clin. Path*; **24:**744.

Bloch K., Bunim J., Wohl M. *et al.* (1960). Unusual occurrence of multiple tissue component antibodies in Sjögren's syndrome. *Trans. Ass. Amer. Physician*; **73:**166.

Conley J., Dingman D.L. (1974). Adenoidcystic carcinoma in the head and neck (cylindroma). *Arch. Otolaryngol*; **100:**81–90.

Diamant B., Diamant H., Holmstedt B. (1957). The salivary secretion in man under the influence of intravenously infused acetyl B methyl choline iodide. *Arch. Int. Pharmacodyn*; **111:**86–97.

Eneroth C.M. (1971). Salivary gland tumours in the parotid gland, submandibular gland and the palate region. *Cancer*; **27:**1415.

Eneroth C.M., Hamberger C.A., Jakobsson P.A. (1966). Malignancy of acinic cell carcinoma. *Ann. Orol. Rhinol. Laryngol*; **75:**780–92.

Foote F.W., Frazell B.L. (1954). *Atlas of Tumour Pathology*, Fascicle 11. Washington D.C.: Armed Forces Institute of Pathology.

Frey L. (1923). Le syndrome du nerf auriculotemporal. *Rev. Neurol*; **30:**97–104.

Godwin J.T. (1952). Benign lymphoepithelial lesion of the parotid gland (adenolymphoma, chronic inflammation, lymphoepithelioma, lymphocytic tumour, Mikulicz disease). Report of 11 cases. *Cancer*, **5:**1089–1103.

Harrison K., Donaldson I. (1979). Frey's syndrome. *J. Roy. Soc. Med.* **72:**503–8.

Hornbaker J., Foster E., Williams G. *et al.* (1966). Sjögren's syndrome and reticulum cell sarcoma. *Arch. Int. Med*; **118:**449.

Maynard J.D. (1965). Recurrent parotid enlargement. *Brit. J. Surg*; **52:**784.

Maynard J.D. (1978). Contemporary surgery: submandibular and parotid gland resection. *Hosp. Med*; **20:**70-9.

Maynard J.D. (1979). Recurrent swellings of the parotid gland, sialectasis and Mikulicz's syndrome. *J. Roy. Soc. Med*; **72:**591.

Mikulicz J. (1892). Uber Eine Eigenartige Symmetrische Erkrankung der Thranenund Mundspeicheldriesen. *Beitr A. Chir. (Festschr. f. Theodor Billroth)* Stuttgart 610.

Morgan W.S., Castleman B. (1953). A clinico pathologic study of 'Mikulicz's disease'. *Amer. J. Path*; **29:**471.

Mylius E.A. (1960). The identification and the role of the myo-epithelial cell in salivary gland tumours. *Atlas Pathol. Microbiol. Scand.* **50** Suppl. 139:1.

Patey D.H., Thackray A.C., Keeling D.H. (1965). Malignant disease of the parotid. *Brit. J. Cancer*; **19:**712–37.

Rauch S. (1959). *Die Speicheldrusen des Menschen.* Stuttgart: Thieme.

Shearn M. (1971). *Sjögren's Syndrome.* Philadelphia: WB Saunders.

Sjögren H. (1933). Zur Kenntnis der Keratoconjunctivitis Sicca. *Acta Ophthal*; Suppl.2.1.

Thackray A.C. (1969). Salivary gland tumours. *Proc. Roy. Soc. Med.* **61:**1089–92.

Willis R.A. (1960). *Pathology of Tumours*, 3rd edn. pp. 327. London: Butterworth.

Upper and lower jaws

D.F.N. HARRISON and A.D. CHEESMAN

Surgery of the upper jaw

D.F.N. HARRISON

The bony skeleton of the face is suspended from the skull and consists of fixed and moveable portions – the upper and lower jaws. In its widest topographical sense the upper jaw consists of a facial component, the maxilla being the largest of the 12 paired bones; and a cranial component formed by the frontal, ethmoid and sphenoidal bones where they are related and joined to the facial bones. Contained within these bones or closely related to them are a number of important cavities or regions, such as the maxillary sinus and the pterygo-palatine fossa. Although the term upper jaw is, therefore, a clinical rather than an anatomical concept, surgery of this region is of necessity complex demanding both knowledge of the relevant anatomy and mastery of many varied surgical techniques (Lederman, 1970).

Prior to the availability of antibiotics, acute infection of the upper jaw was frequently accompanied by serious or life threatening complications. Involvement of adjoining structures such as orbit or brain caused blindness or cerebral abscess and cavernous sinus thrombosis was an ever present danger. Such complications are rare today although still seen in undeveloped countries or with unusually virulent organisms.

Emergency surgery to deal with acute infections of the paranasal sinuses or osteomyelitis of the maxilla is now a rarity and will not be considered. Neither will odontogenic infections since this is a problem best left to dental specialists. Chronic infection still poses an occasional problem although this is becoming less common and most major upper jaw surgery is now carried out for removal of benign or malignant neoplasms. Maxillofacial trauma is a specialised subject and will be covered elsewhere (see chap. 44).

Clinical evaluation of much upper jaw pathology is restricted by the relative inaccessibility of many of the cavities contained within the bony framework. Presenting symptoms of both benign and malignant tumours are largely dependent upon the site and extension of the lesion. Pain, facial swelling or nasal obstruction with purulent or sanguineous discharge occur in most cases. None of these symptoms is specific for neoplasia and the early case of malignancy is usually detected accidentally during nasal or antral exploration for some other purpose or where the tumour arises in a readily accessible or detectable site such as nasal passages or alveolar buccal sulcus. Unilateral epistaxis, epiphora or variations in sensation over the cheek must, therefore, be viewed as highly significant symptoms (Harrison, 1973).

Most upper jaw surgery is designed to provide access for diagnosis or removal of benign tumours, or for the wide removal of malignant tumours, although the latter is limited by the anatomical complexities of the region.

Unfortunately, these varied procedures have been bedevilled by loose terminology and inadequate appreciation of the technical problems to be faced. A fundamental surgical principle is that 'the operation should fit the patient', and not *vice versa*. This does not mean that every minor modification in technique requires or deserves an eponymous title, e.g. Dargent *et al.* (1948) recorded fourteen variations of partial maxillectomy and seven variations of total maxillectomy!

Radiological assessment

Pathological conditions affecting the upper jaw will produce bone destruction or alterations in translucency of the paranasal sinuses or nasal passages. Obstruction to normal sinus drainage channels occurs in both inflammatory, benign and malignant disease. Therefore, loss of translucency on conventional radiological positions may be inadequate for diagnosis and may conceal underlying bone destruction. Standard positions used to demonstrate paranasal sinuses by plain x-ray are occipito-mental and frontal, submento-vertical and lateral positions. Any suspicion of malignancy will certainly require tomography utilising coronal, lateral and axial planes. Specialised tomographic units capable of pluridirectional or circular movements such as the Philips Massiot Polytome have greatly enhanced the value of these techniques. Axial tomography (Lloyd, 1971) is the optimum method of demonstrating the ethmoid cells radiologically providing a plan view of the whole of the ethmoidal labyrinth on a single film. The value of this in determining the operability of malignant disease in this region and the degree of orbital involvement cannot be overestimated (Fig 43.1).

Introduction of radio-opaque media into the nose or paranasal sinuses is seldom used although the former is useful in infants with choanal atresia.

Ultrasound and thermography are occasionally useful for specific problems whilst selective angiography supplemented with magnification and subtraction can provide useful, and at times, essential information. It is doubtful if embolisation of the internal maxillary artery is of proven value in any upper jaw tumour except perhaps for angiofibromata in the pterygopalatine fossa.

The increasing availability of computerised tomography has provided a means of determining intracranial extensions of upper jaw tumours as well as showing soft tissue abnormalities in the nose and paranasal sinuses (Fig 43.2). Such delineation (without contrast enhancement) depends upon the demonstration of bony destruction; this is no better than with conventional polytomography. Orbital and retro-orbital areas are ideal for delineation of soft tissue masses since no large contrasts in density exist, but in the maxillary sinus, CT scanning is less effective. Artifacts produced by teeth fillings may cause confusion.

My personal experience of a wide variety of both benign and malignant tumours in which these various radiological techniques have been evaluated by a specialised radiologist, indicates that they can provide some indication of the minimal extent of tumours affecting the upper jaw. Evaluation of 260 patients with various malignant bony and mucosal tumours,

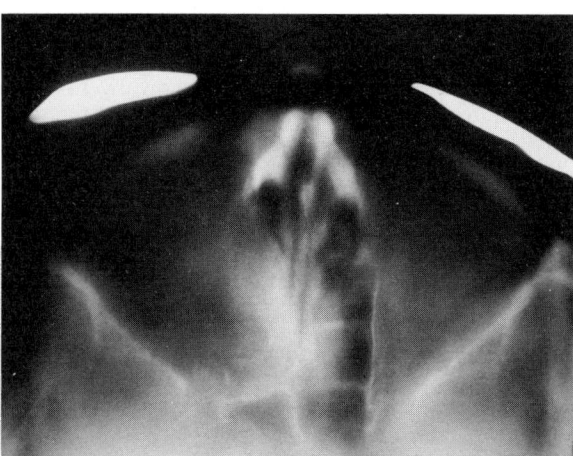

Fig 43.1 Axial submentovertical tomography showing destructive lesion in right ethmoidal labyrinth and maxillary antrum.

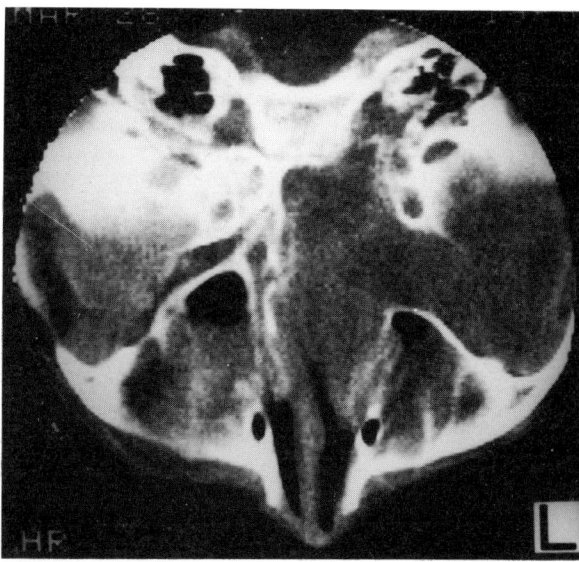

Fig 43.2 CAT scan to show neoplastic mass in left nasal passage extending into maxillary antrum and pterygopalatine fossa.

however, showed that in over 60% of patients surgical excision demonstrated that tumour extent was greater than suspected. However, radiological assessment is essential in planning surgical management.

Histological assessment

The problems inherent in classification of upper jaw tumours will be discussed later, but planning of any surgical procedure must take account of the natural history of the pathological condition under treatment. A wide variety of both benign and malignant conditions arise within the confines of the upper jaw. Adequate and representative biopsy is essential, though not always easy, and the subsequent surgical operation must take account of histopathological findings together with existing knowledge of pathways of spread. Fortunately, regional metastases are uncommon for most upper jaw neoplasms and long-term cure is largely related to the efficacy of local control.

Surgery of the nasal passages

Apart from polypi, which are not tumours but the product of dependent oedematous mucosa, most intranasal tumours are difficult to evaluate. Even when benign, they can produce local destruction and site of origin may be impossible to determine without exploration. Surgery of nasal polypi is dependent upon intimate knowledge of the ethmoidal labyrinth and details are best found in more specialised textbooks.

Successful management of the less common, but much more serious, true tumours of the nasal cavities depends upon direct visualisation and adequate exposure of the operative field. When confined to the nasal septum, complete removal is possible by a sublabial incision which, if extended bilaterally, allows 'degloving' of the nose (Conley and Price, 1979). Complete removal of the septum can be carried out and skin can be lifted from underlying bone as far as the root of the nose and infraorbital foramina. Bleeding is brisk but a wide variety of benign and low grade malignant tumours can be effectively removed without the need for skin incisions. I have used this for such lesions as chondrosarcoma, pleomorphic adenoma and carcinoma of the septum as well as primary melanomas of the nasal passages.

Lateral rhinotomy

In the early years of this century tumours arising within the nasal passages were invariably treated by intranasal removal and electrocauterisation. Cure rates were low and complications frequent. In 1902, E.J. Moure of Bordeaux published his external approach to the ethmoid labyrinth thus introducing a new concept to nasal surgery. His operation has undergone minor modifications and is now an essential technique in the management of nasal tumours (Harrison, 1977).

The skin incision extends from the medial palpebral ligament along the nasomaxillary groove around the ala of the nostril to enter the nose. If necessary, extension superiorly to the eyebrow or inferiorly to divide the upper lip allows even greater exposure. The nasal skin and cartilages are displaced laterally allowing excision of the lateral nasal wall from the front of the turbinals to the eustachian tube and from the cribriform plate to the nasal floor.

In the past there has been some reluctance to remove the entire lateral nasal wall for fear of causing drastic disturbances of nasal physiology. Despite removal of most of the medial orbital wall and transection of the naso-lachrymal duct there is rarely postoperative epiphora and after a period of crusting the whole cavity re-epithelialises. Occasionally, this procedure is referred to as 'en bloc ethmoidectomy and medial maxillectomy'. This is both confusing and inaccurate! Without removal of the cribriform plate and the most posterior of the ethmoidal cells (which may be intimately related to the optic canal) total ethmoidectomy is not feasible. 'Medial maxillectomy' is so imprecise as to be valueless. The surgical approach of choice is by a lateral rhinotomy, accompanied by a detailed account of the tissues removed. This will depend upon the nature and extent of the neoplasm under treatment.

Benign lesions such as neurofibromas can be resected with minimal loss of tissue. Primary malignant melanomas are best approached by removal of all nasal mucosa where possible. Invasive tumours may require more extensive resection. External deformity is minimal if the incision is sited correctly and is not affected by preoperative radiotherapy.

Craniofacial resection

Some mention must be made of the combined craniofacial approach for tumours involving ethmoidal sinuses and cribriform plate area. The inaccessibility of this region has prevented en bloc resection in the past and tumours have of necessity been treated primarily with radiotherapy. Cure rates have been low, although the natural history of neoplasms such as adenocarcinoma or olfactory neuroblastoma suggested that adequate local resection would be rewarding. Ketcham *et al.* in 1963 described a combined intracranial facial approach for such tumours and this operation has now been refined and accepted as a standard technique for localised invasion of the anterior cranial fossa. Use of operating microscope and modern bone cutting drills allows the experienced head and neck surgeon to carry out the intracranial approach without need for neuro-surgical help. Dural involvement can be assessed, excised and repaired. Reinforcement with skin graft or fascia lata prevents herniation of brain and morbidity is low. Acceptance of this procedure as both safe and effective has encouraged early primary resection of many ethmoidal cancers previously treated primarily with radiotherapy followed by limited resection by lateral rhinotomy. Evaluation of the feasibility of intracranial resection can be assisted by CT scanning, but exploratory craniotomy is essential. Limits of resection are clearly defined (Clifford, 1977) and long-term cure is primarily influenced by the size of the tumour.

Surgery of the maxilla

Not only is the maxilla an essential part of the facial contour, but it contains the largest of the paranasal sinuses, and the one most commonly involved in neoplasia. On reviewing the surgical operations performed on this bone, one is impressed by the wide variety of techniques used as well as the differing nomenclatures. However, these reflect personal rivalries as well as intellectual confusion for, in essence, maxillary surgery is either exploratory, for the purpose of diagnosis, or excisional. The latter is either partial, total or if accompanied by removal of eye etc. – 'extended'.

The most commonly used procedure for the treatment of benign disease of the maxillary sinus or for diagnostic purposes is the Caldwell-Luc operation. First described by George Caldwell of New York in 1893, and later in 1897 by Henri Luc of Paris, this allows inspection of the maxillary antrum via a window cut in the anterior wall of the maxilla. Care must be taken in positioning this opening to avoid damage to the roots of permanent teeth or the anterior superior alveolar nerve. A drainage window is fashioned in the medial wall of the antrum beneath the inferior turbinal. In cases of chronic infection the antral lining is completely removed; in suspected neoplasms, tissue can be removed for histological examination and the bony walls examined for erosion. The incision in the gingivo-buccal sulcus is closed loosely with a single suture allowing drainage of blood.

This approach allows removal of part of the ethmoidal labyrinth (Janson Horgan or transantral ethmoidectomy) or after removal of the posterior bony wall – exploration of the pterygopalatine fossa for ligation of the internal maxillary artery or vidian neurectomy.

Partial maxillectomy

It is the surgeon's responsibility to clear as widely as possible by the most appropriate means the whole tumour-bearing area, although this may be difficult to determine following radiotherapy. With adequate knowledge of plastic surgical procedures and the availability of skilled prosthetic help it is nonsensical to talk of upper jaw surgery as being 'mutilating'.

Before the era of external radiation, partial removal of the maxilla, frequently – but erroneously – referred to as a palatal fenestration, was used to provide access to the maxillary sinus for usage of local radium applicators. Unfortunately, most malignant tumours involving the maxillary sinus present at an advanced stage, being difficult to contain by even the most radical of surgical procedures. To jeopardise survival by inadequate surgery is inexcusable and partial maxillectomy is only indicated in small localised neoplasms of the maxillary infrastructure extending no further than the tuberosity posteriorly, certain nasal fossa malignancies and as part of a routine lateral rhinotomy. Occasionally, the orbital floor is left in a total maxillectomy. This is rarely wise, but would at least justify regrading the operation as a partial procedure. It is, of course, suitable for extensive benign tumours of the maxilla requiring only local removal.

Total maxillectomy

Unfortunately, classical total maxillectomy is rarely indicated being suitable only when disease is confined within the bony walls of the maxillary sinus or to the maxilla itself. More frequently, this operation must be extended to remove orbital contents, ethmoid, cheek or malar bone. It is probably the oldest of all 'monobloc' operations but is not the procedure commonly accredited to Sir William Fergusson. The description published in *The Times* in February 1842 of the removal of a large maxillary tumour in a girl aged 12 years indicates that that operation was a partial maxillectomy. Obviously, a formidable task which required removal of part of the orbital floor as well as the malar bone. Operating time was 16 minutes.

The technique is standardised and uncomplicated, exposure being obtained by the creation of a flap from the middle of the face. Bleeding is rarely severe and easily controlled. Care must be taken when using the Weber-Fergusson incision after radiotherapy to ensure that the upper end of the lateral rhinotomy and the transverse arm is as obtuse as possible. Removal of the underlying bone leaves this thin skin unsupported and necrosis is common. Resection of the bony attachments is best accomplished with an oscillating saw which minimises danger of fragmentation in a maxilla weakened by malignant bone erosion. Reconstruction of the palatal defect is unwise with malignant tumours since the defect is adequately filled with a prosthesis. Removal allows complete inspection of the cavity. It is usual to pack the operation cavity with gauze impregnated with Whitehead's varnish. This valuable preparation, containing iodoform, benzoin and balsam of Tolu (Pig. Iodof. Co. BPC), first appeared in Martindale in 1881 and was used by William Whitehead (1840–1913) to pack the oral cavity after total glossectomy. It has the advantage of remaining uninfected for several weeks when left *in situ*.

Complete removal of the orbital floor should not result in noticeable sinking of the eye unless the attachments of Tenon's capsule are disturbed. Reinforcement of the suspensory sling with temporalis muscle or silastic sheeting is usually effective, but is difficult as a secondary procedure (Som, 1974).

Extended maxillectomy

An important step in the standard total maxillectomy is detachment of the orbital periosteum away from the underlying maxilla to ensure that bony erosion has not occurred. Although involvement of the globe is most unusual, erosion of the thin inferior and medial orbital walls is common. Even though the eye be otherwise normal, radical excision of the tumour is impossible with the eye *in situ*. Indeed, if it is left, extension of tumour soon produces painful proptosis and visual loss.

With postradiotherapy patients, the problem may be complicated by evidence of bony erosion but no determinable neoplasm. In my personal experience of 130 patients with maxillary tumours, such patients invariably have evidence of bony erosion or residual tumour elsewhere.

Removal of the orbital contents should not include loss of the eyelids. Their preservation, with loss of tarsal plate and lash margins, allows primary suture and the socket is now lined with a sheet of well vascularised skin allowing early fitting of a prosthesis (Fig 43.3). Conley and Baker (1979) have suggested a more complex closure of the orbital defect allowing the wearing of a 'free' prosthesis. However, radiotherapy whether pre- or postoperatively is a contraindication and this must surely limit the number of suitable patients. Extension into facial skin is not invariably followed by cervical lymph node metastases and wide resection can be repaired by local flaps after histological control of the residual defect (Fig 43.4). During this time the intra-oral prosthesis can be held in place with suspensory wires to minimise pressure on the transposed skin. Extension posteriorly into the pterygoid region is usually visible on coronal tomography and carries a poor prognosis. If such extension is suspected, radical

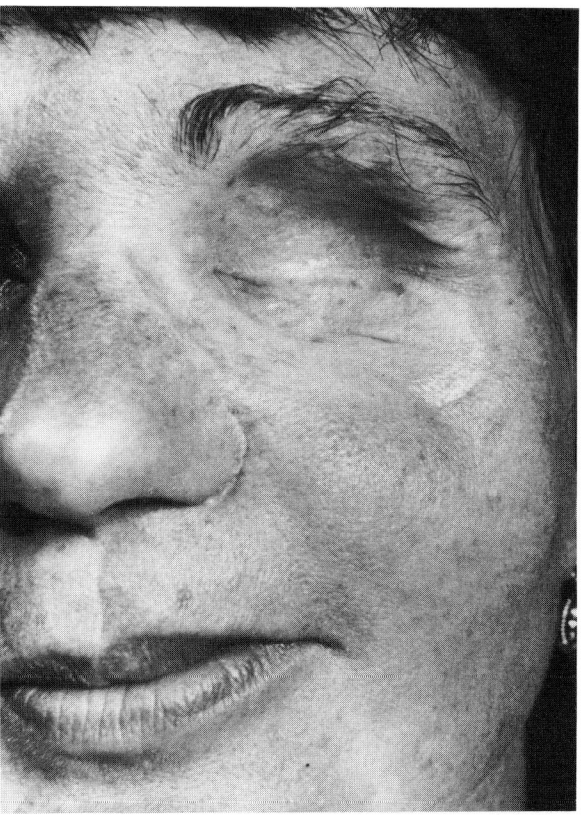

Fig 43.3 Primary reconstruction of the orbit using eyelids following removal of orbital contents.

maxillectomy should be accompanied by exploration of the pterygoid fossa. In the standard operation, separation of the maxilla from the pterygoid plates is often accomplished by a chisel placed in the pterygomaxillary sulcus – a blind and often bloody procedure.

Worthington (1977) has examined the various surgical approaches to the pterygoid region and recommends a modification of that described by Crockett in 1963. This is the approach I have used; extension of the Weber-Fergusson incision over the zygomatic arch gives adequate exposure. After sectioning of bone the temporalis fascia is cut along the upper border allowing the attached masseter to be turned downwards. Division of the coronoid allows the temporalis muscle to be turned upwards allowing access to the pterygoid region from the lateral aspect. Pterygoid plates and muscles can be sectioned under direct vision although it is obviously not possible to carry out a wide resection if gross tumour is present.

The intimate relationship between the ethmoid cells and the maxillary sinus results in many neoplasms

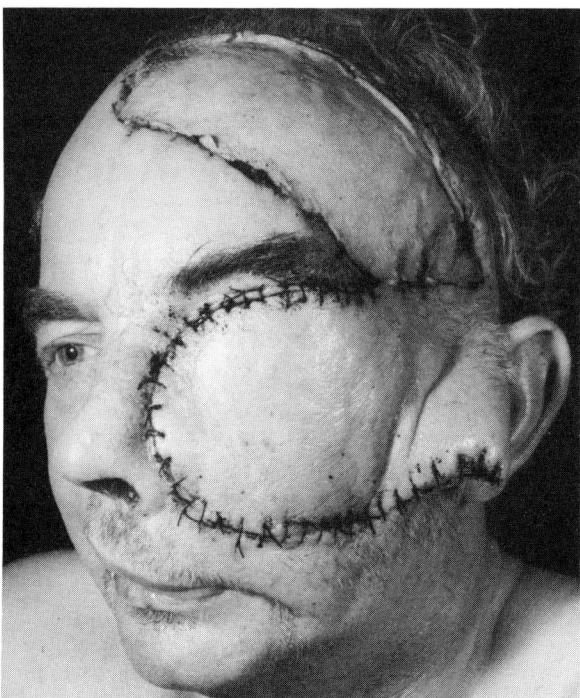

Fig 43.4 Repair of full thickness skin defect in cheek with rotated forehead flap.

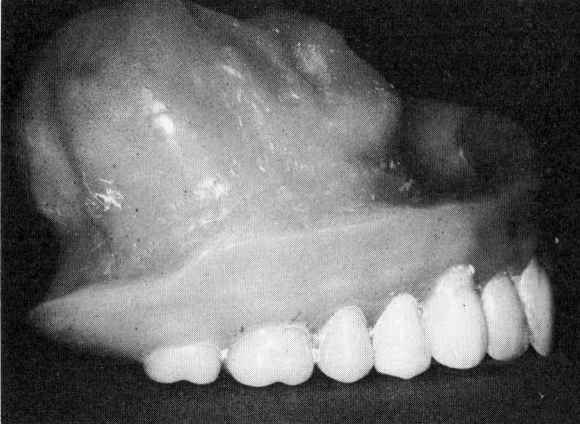

Fig 43.5 Acrylic intra-oral prosthesis following total maxillectomy. This should be light and self retaining.

involving both regions. Craniofacial resection is now an integral part of some extended maxillectomies provided that extension elsewhere is controllable.

Prosthetic care

To be deemed successful, radical surgery of the upper jaw requires complete removal of disease with maximal preservation of appearance and function. This necessitates careful preoperative planning and co-ordination by surgeon and prosthodontist (Harrison, 1979). The immediate surgical obturator is constructed on the basis of a preoperative dental impression and may have to be wired in place to achieve stability, particularly in edentulous patients. Placement of the bony cuts, amount of residual soft palate, presence of a skin graft on the raw surface of the facial flap and absence of teeth on the unoperated side, will all affect lateral retention of the prosthesis.

A comfortable, appropriately sized intra-oral prosthesis enabling the patient to eat, talk and face the world is an essential part of the surgical management of upper jaw tumours (Fig 43.5).

Problems in classification

The practice of dividing cancer cases into groups according to so-called 'stages' arose from the observation that crude survival, or apparent recovery rates were higher for patients in whom the disease was localised than when the tumour had extended beyond the organ of origin. There are inherent weaknesses in this philosophy since prognosis is influenced by rate of growth, histological type, tumour-host relationship and the true site of origin.

Most sites within the head and neck have now been classified, but confusion and disagreement remains regarding the paranasal sinuses. Only Lederman (1970) has actually proposed a system suitable for the whole upper jaw, all others confining themselves to the maxillary sinus, the commonest site for paranasal sinus cancer. A critical analysis of the existing systems was published by Harrison in 1978 who emphasised that if histology was ignored, failure to cure upper jaw malignancy was primarily failure to eradicate extension of tumour outside the bony walls of sinus or nasal passages. Few patients present or develop regional lymph node metastases and even less, systemic spread. Since limitations in clinical assessment are well recognised, there can be little justification for erecting a complex system of classification based upon unstable foundations. Clinical experience emphasises the importance of certain directions of tumour extension in relation to subsequent prognosis and it would seem logical to base future classifications upon such premises. Posterior ethmoids, nasopharynx, orbital apex and pterygopalatine fossa all present formidable or impossible surgical problems. Primary surgery followed by radiotherapy or chemotherapy will be necessary. Extension to the cribriform fossa area is now of less prognostic significance if unaccompanied by less accessible disease and a maxillary sinus full of neoplasm, but without bone erosion, is less serious than a small extension into ethmoidal labyrinth or pterygopalatine fossa. In considering and reporting the end results of the surgical management of upper jaw neoplasia, these matters are of considerable importance and relevance.

Surgery of the lower jaw

A.D. CHEESMAN

The use of prosthetic repair following radical resection of the upper jaw usually results in successful rehabilitation of the patient with little cosmetic or functional defect. Unfortunately this is more difficult to achieve following similar surgery to the lower jaw. The results of simple excision and direct suture were so poor, that many surgeons turned to radiotherapy for the treatment of tumours involving the mandible. However, experience with radiotherapy has failed to show an improvement in cure rates and radical radiotherapy can result in quite severe complications. Furthermore the improvement of anaesthesia, and reconstruction techniques, over the last decade has resulted in successful surgical methods of rehabilitation, and there has been a resurgence of interest in surgery of the lower jaw. These newer techniques use the skills of various specialists and considerable experience of the problems involved is needed, consequently, such patients are best managed in specialised Head and Neck Units.

Surgical anatomy

The anatomical relations of the horizontal ramus and floor of mouth are complex, and must be clearly understood prior to any surgery in the region. Several aspects need special emphasis.

The tongue and floor of mouth are supported by a muscular diaphragm comprising the supra-hyoid muscles and the mylohoid with its lateral insertion into the mylohoid line on the inner table of the mandible. Contraction of this diaphragm is important in the primary phase of swallowing, resulting in obliteration of the oral cavity and elevation of the larynx. Any loss of continuity of the mandibular arch results in loss of function of this diaphragm and crippling of both speech and swallowing. Furthermore, the loss of arch disturbs normal mastication and may alter facial contour. If loss of anterior mandibular arch occurs the problems are particularly severe, the so-called Andy Gump deformity.

Loss of support to the oral sphincter gives continual drooling of saliva, the tongue prolapses back into the pharangeal airway and the cosmetic defect is particularly severe.

The vertical ramus of the mandible is surrounded by the insertions of the powerful masticatory muscles. Should it become free, due to loss of continuity with the horizontal ramus, these muscles tend to move it upwards and medially towards the oral cavity.

The cross-sectional shape of the mandible changes with age, the loss of teeth and absorption of the alveolar bone leaving only the narrow basal portion, this is the typical 'pipe-stem' mandible.

Pathological conditions

The mandible may be involved by a variety of pathological conditions. Some are obviously related to the teeth and are best managed by the dentist or oral surgeon. However, it is important to remember that several of the cysts and tumours of the mandible are of odontogenic origin, such conditions are best managed in conjunction with the oral surgeons, and full details will be found in the specialised texts. Similarly the mandible may be involved as part of a generalised metabolic disorder such as Paget's Disease, or hyperparathyroidism, and diagnosis will be made on the results of the appropriate investigations.

More commonly, the mandible is involved by secondary spread of squamous cell carcinoma from other areas of the oral cavity, and this will be our main concern.

Osteosarcoma

Osteosarcoma is used as a generic term to cover the various types of sarcoma occurring in bone. It is an unusual tumour, usually formed in long bones, but does occur in the jaws especially the mandible.

It presents as a rapidly expanding mass usually accompanied by pain. X-rays show central destruction with the radiating osseous laminae giving the typical 'sun ray' appearance. Both local and distant metastases are common, but inadequate local control is often the cause of failure in treatment. Biopsy is essential to confirm histological diagnosis.

Treatment is by radical resection of the involved mandible and any locally involved tissues, with block dissection in the presence of metastatic lymph nodes. Postoperative radiotherapy and chemotherapy have also been suggested.

Squamous cell carcinoma

Primary carcinoma of the mandible is rare, but squamous cell carcinoma of the alveolar mucosa accounts for 15% of all oral malignancies. The mandible is often involved by secondary spread from the adjacent regions of buccal mucosa and floor of mouth.

It used to be thought that the lymphatics from the tongue and floor of mouth passed through the periosteum of the mandible and 'in-continuity' resection of the mandible was performed with all surgical resections of these regions, the 'commando' operation. However, there is an increasing amount of clinical and histological evidence to dispute this view (Marchetta *et al.*, 1971) and it is now thought that involvement of the mandible results from direct spread. Consequently, careful assessment of any tumour adjacent to the mandible is mandatory.

Pretreatment assessment

Careful radiological examination is performed to detect the presence of bone involvement. The patient is assessed by the dentist and oral hygienist, and appropriate treatment is initiated. We then routinely review all cases under general anaesthesia, allowing assessment of mucosal fixation.

Palpation of oral cavity and neck and routine endoscopy of the rest of the upper air and food passages is performed to exclude a second primary tumour. A margin of 1.5 cm is tatooed with Indian ink around the tumour (Baluyot and Shumrick 1972), and biopsies are taken at different sites. Finally, diseased teeth are extracted, especially those near the tumour. Joint consultation is then held with the radiotherapist to decide the treatment programme.

Treatment philosophy

Tumours of this region can be managed by either surgery or radiotherapy, or a combination of both with possible adjunctive chemotherapy. The traditional role of radiotherapy has undergone critical review over the last few years, hence the vital importance of initial joint consultation by both surgeon and radiotherapist.

Most surgeons agree that radiotherapy in skilled hands is effective in curing the exophytic tumour without bone erosion. The technique of irradiation will depend on the radiotherapist, but use of interstitial irradiation requires considerable expertise and is generally accompanied by less complications. Use of external irradiation by a mega-voltage source tends to have a wider effect and the incidence of radiotherapeutic and subsequent surgical complications is greater, especially radionecrosis of the mandible.

The more invasive type of tumour, particularly with bone involvement, does poorly with radiotherapy, and is probably best managed surgically. However, with an extensive invasive growth the use of a small dose of preoperative irradiation may improve cure rates without causing undue surgical complications.

Our current practice is to use interstitial irradiation where appropriate, but when an external source is used the tumour response must be carefully monitored. If there is little response after 4000 rads, it is unlikely that the tumour is radiosensitive and resection is indicated. Following radiotherapy, a careful monthly follow-up is essential and all suspicious areas must be biopsied. A pessimistic attitude is necessary if surgical salvage is to have any chance of success.

In the absence of adequate radiotherapy, surgical resection, possibly followed by irradiation to the healed area, is probably the treatment of choice, as the complications of poor radiotherapy can render subsequent surgery almost impossible.

Radionecrosis of the mandible

This is the main complication of radiotherapy and results from endarteritis of the already tenuous mandibular blood supply. This is generally associated with decreased salivary secretion, and often increased carbohydrate intake. The mandible is more susceptible to infection and the teeth to caries. If exposure of bone occurs, either from necrosing tumour or dental extraction, osteomyelitis rapidly develops. The best method of treatment is prevention, hence our careful procedure on the mandible following radiotherapy should be done under antibiotic cover including Metronidazole, as there is some evidence implicating co-existent anaerobic infection (*see* chap. 54).

Radionecrosis is recognised by a painful swelling or ulceration of the overlying mucosa. It must be managed surgically, but care must also be taken to ensure sequential necrosis of bone does not occur. The principles are surgical excision of the sequestrated bone under full and prolonged antibiotic cover. The mandible must be carefully isolated from the saliva of the oral cavity by the use of local flaps if necessary. Any drainage and sequestrectomy is best performed via the neck, the necrotic bone being excised back to the healthy bone, but with careful preservation of periosteum. No reconstruction with autogenous bone or prosthesis should be performed primarily. Hyperbaric oxygen and closed wound irrigation have been used with variable success.

Surgical techniques

This will be considered in terms of excision and repair of both soft tissue and bone.

Soft tissue excision

Wide exposure of the area is essential for accurate excision and is best achieved by splitting the lower lip and reflecting a full thickness cheek flap. Careful closure of the lip in three layers gives a minimal cosmetic defect, but a superior result may be obtained by the more experienced surgeon with only partial division of the lip and superior reflection of the cheek flap. However, there are few occasions when a pull through type of procedure is justifiable due to the poor exposure obtained. (Conley, 1967).

The principle of wide local resection in all planes to encompass the original tumour margins prior to irradiation is well accepted and facilitated by pretreatment tattoos. Similarly, in the presence of nodal disease an en-bloc resection of the cervical lymphatics should be performed. In the absence of nodal metastases, most surgeons limit themselves to a suprahyoid block dissection as they have to enter this area for the primary excision.

In those patients where salvage surgery is attempted without assessment, prior to radiotherapy, it is often difficult to distinguish between tumour and radiation fibrosis. In such cases we perform a wide through-and-through excision to leave a large orostome with skin to mucosa closure. The specimen is then studied by serial sections and the histological extent of the tumour ascertained (Gregory and Cheesman, 1976). This can generally be achieved within the period of delay of a nape flap and delayed primary closure is achieved some 3 weeks later with a sure knowledge that the excision is adequate. In such cases, prior gastrostomy assists the nutrition of the patient and defunctions the area.

Bone excision

The importance of maintaining mandibular arch continuity in order to minimise functional and cosmetic defects has forced the surgeon to review the types of surgical resection, and he has become more conservative! The normal shape of the mandible lends itself to partial resections, conversely the elderly 'pipe stem' mandible can rarely be subjected to partial resection. Three basic surgical techniques are available, marginal resection, segmental resection and hemimandibulectomy. Marginal resection is achieved by partial removal of the mandible, either in a horizontal plane

removing the lingual plate, or by some combination of both techniques. Mandibular arch is maintained by the residual bone. This type of resection is easily achieved by use of the dental fissure burr, but following radiotherapy there is a danger that radionecrosis of the remaining bone may occur.

Segmental resection implies total removal of part of the mandibular arch and depending on site may be followed by reconstruction. Hemimandibulectomy entails removal of one complete half of the mandibular arch including the condyle.

The type of mandibular resection used depends on the degree of bone involvement by tumour. Deep invasion requires full hemimandibulectomy, but local involvement may be treated by segmental resection or occasionally marginal resection. Tumours of the anterior arch are best treated by marginal resection or by segmental resection with immediate autogenous bone graft. In both cases prior irradiation will jeopardise the result and many surgeons treat tumours in this site with primary surgery. Segmental resection of the lateral arch, especially if placed posteriorly, does not cause much defect and reconstruction can often be omitted.

Soft tissue repair

Following wide local resection, primary closure by advancement of buccal and lingual mucosa is rarely satisfactory with poor healing and often tongue fixation, particularly following radiotherapy.

Although McGregor (1977) has emphasised the value of Thiersch grafts in the treatment of multifocal disease of the mucosa, they have little part to play in the resurfacing of more major defects.

Local flaps of oral mucosa, especially lingual flaps have their advocates (De Santo, 1974), but, in practice, the amount of cover provided is limited and may give rise to unacceptable tongue fixation. For secondary repair following necrosis of the tip of a regional flap they are of considerable value.

Another type of local flap is the nasolabial skin flap (Cohen and Egerton, 1971), which is raised on the face and then introduced into the oral cavity by a temporary fistula. This provides excellent cover for anterior defects and if a pair of these flaps is used, quite large areas of cover may be obtained in the region of the anterior arch. Subsequent division of the pedicle and closure of the fistula is performed after 3 weeks.

For the repair of large defects, particularly following radiotherapy, regional skin flaps are used. Initially, the use of cervical skin flaps was popular but they have several disadvantages. They are generally hair-bearing skin, and are usually covered by one of the portals of irradiation. Considerable skill is required in their planning. However, more importantly, the use of Thiersch grafts to cover the donor defects in the neck does not give adequate protection to the underlying carotid artery system, and further local flaps are needed to cover it.

Consequently the more popular regional flaps for lining the oral cavity are the forehead and medially based deltopectoral flaps. For cover, the deltopectoral flap is useful, but our current preference is for the myocutaneous nape of neck flap.

The forehead flap has an excellent reputation for effective repair of oral defects. It is raised without delay and if the whole width of the forehead is used the flap will reach any part of the oral cavity. It may be introduced into the mouth by a variety of routes. Initially a tunnel through the cheek was popular, but the more usual route depends on the reconstruction problem. For most mandibular resections where the coronoid process has been removed the preferred route is deep to the zygoma after prior displacement of the temporalis muscle. The pedicle is divided 3 weeks later and partially returned to give a symmetrical defect. Alternatively the carrier portion may be de-epithelialised and left *in situ*. The major disadvantage of this flap is the cosmetic defect of the motionless forehead although this can be concealed by a fringe in women.

The defect can be reduced by attention to detail in planning the flap. The whole of the forehead unit must be removed to give a symmetrical defect, and any excess pedicle must be discarded on return. The decreased thickness of the donor area can be overcome by allowing the bed to granulate over 2 to 3 weeks before grafting. Alternatively, the edges of the defect may be deliberately bevelled to give a smooth contour. Delayed Thiersch grafting with one large piece of skin gives a better cover of the defect and also reduces operating time. However, care must be taken to ensure that the donor bed does not dry with subsequent necrosis of the periosteum, and it should be dressed with lyophilised porcine dressings covered with many layers of tulle gras. An important aspect of the use of the forehead flap is to ensure that an excessive amount of flap is not used within the mouth, and although the whole forehead is raised only a small portion of it, containing the artery, is used for the actual repair (Wilson, 1967).

The medially based deltopectoral flap is an excellent regional flap, although not quite as safe as the forehead flap. In about 10% of cases some minor necrosis of the tip occurs, but this does not generally cause problems. The flap is best used undelayed since delay does not appreciably improve its viability, and adversely affects its extensibility. Generally, this flap is used for the repair of posterior defects and the need for a temporary fistula may be used with advantage in the heavily irradiated patient. In such cases the creation of a deliberate orostome by suturing skin to the mucosa minimises complications and speeds healing.

Secondary closure is usually accomplished after 3 weeks. A less common use of the deltopectoral flap is for the repair of large anterior defects associated with loss of anterior mandibular arch. In these cases the flap is introduced via an orostome in the anterior floor of the mouth. Usually the flap is sutured anteriorly over the mandibular reconstruction, the tongue mucosa being sewn to cervical skin. Secondary closure is achieved by dividing the pedicle and using its skin for lining of the anterior floor of the mouth, cover being provided by the existing cervical skin.

The particular flap used depends on the reconstructive problem, but the forehead flap is the most popular, giving closure in one stage particularly for lateral and anterior defects.

Mandibular reconstruction

The large number of papers concerning techniques of mandibular reconstruction indicates the inadequacies of current methods (Behringer and Schweiger, 1977; Harashina *et al.*, 1978). In all successful series the one common factor is absence of irradiation. Following radiotherapy, it is unlikely that bone grafting will be successful, and some form of prosthetic repair is then necessary.

In the absence of irradiation and with careful technique it is possible to achieve a successful bone graft for a mandibular defect provided the following criteria are observed:

1 Absence of infection
2 A well vascularised bed with little scar tissue
3 Complete soft tissue cover
4 Wide, close contact between graft and mandible
5 Total immobilisation of mandibular fragments

With localised resection of bone alone, primary grafting is generally successful using autogenous bone, either large cancellous chips or block bone from the iliac crest. When wide local soft tissue resection has occurred, secondary grafting is more successful (Snow *et al.*, 1976), but in practice patients learn to accept the deformity and refuse secondary bone grafting unless well motivated.

Following irradiation most surgeons use some form of primary prosthetic repair. Lee and Wilson (1973) have discussed the major techniques in detail; unfortunately, they commonly end up with extrusion or infection of the prosthesis, needing its removal. Fortunately fibrosis in the intervening period often stabilises the mandibular fragments and if soft tissue replacement is adequate, surprisingly little deformity is left.

Our own preference for prosthetic repair is a Teflon rod. It is totally inert and its flexibility removes the stresses from the junction between bone and prosthesis, a common site of prosthetic failure. It is easily cut to the correct length with a scalpel, and then wired into a tunnel in the basal portion of the mandible. Slip-on ends have been constructed for condylar replacement or for wiring to the flat vertical ramus. Provided good soft tissue lining and cover exists, this type of prosthesis gives moderately successful results.

Adjunctive surgery

Some form of disturbance in swallowing generally results from surgery of the mandible and floor of mouth and this may be aggravated by inco-ordination of the cricopharyngeal sphincter. Consequently we routinely perform a cricopharyngeal myotomy at the time of primary excision.

End result evaluation

It is difficult to assess the results of tumour surgery involving the jaws. Success in terms of 5-year cure rates is relatively unimportant as many patients are elderly and there has been no major improvement in cure rates over the last four decades. The great advances have been in terms of rehabilitation, so important where deformity is clearly visible and interferes with speech and swallowing. Disturbance of these facilities leads to as much social isolation as cosmetic defects, for clear speech and trouble-free eating in company are vital for normal social intercourse. The available surgical techniques are adequate for full rehabilitation, and surgical mutilation should be a feature of the past.

The present problem concerns the role of radiotherapy. Successful radiotherapy is excellent, but failed radiotherapy may be a disaster as it can rarely be followed by successful surgical salvage with full rehabilitation. Our approach is a more critical appraisal of tumour response during irradiation, but other centres have concentrated on primary surgery including reconstruction, followed by a full course of irradiation. With this approach McGregor (1977) has obtained improved surgical rehabilitation with intra-oral tumours without adversely affecting prognosis. Primary resection followed by radiotherapy concentrating on residual or high risk areas, is now the treatment of choice for most upper jaw tumours. These philosophies, whilst not necessarily improving long-term cure rates will at the very least, improve the prospect of effective reconstruction with well planned rehabilitation.

References

Baluyot S.L. Jr., Shumrick D.A. (1972). Pre-irradiation tattooing. *Arch. Otolaryngol*; **96**:151–9.

Behringer W.H., Schweiger J.W. (1977). Mandibular replacement after resection for tumour. *Laryngoscope*; **87(II)**:1922–31.

Clifford P. (1977). Transcranial approach for cancer of the antroethmoidal area. *Clin. Otolaryngol*; **2**:115–30.

Cohen I.K., Egerton M.T. (1971). Transbuccal flaps for reconstruction of the floor of the mouth. *Plast. Reconstr. Surg*; **48**:8–10.

Conley J. (1967). *Cancer of the Head and Neck*, pp. 270–7. New York: Appleton-Century-Crofts.

Conley J., Baker D.C. (1979). Management of the eye socket in cancer of the paranasal sinuses. *Arch. Otolaryngol*; **105**:702–5.

Conley J., Price J.C. (1979). Sublabial approach to the nasal and nasopharyngeal cavities. *Amer. J. Surg*; **138**:615–18.

Crockett D.J. (1963). Surgical approach to the back of the maxilla. *Brit. J. Surg*; **50**:819–21.

Dargent M., Gignoux M., Gaillard J. (1948). *Le Traitment des Tumeurs Malignes Primitives due Maxillaire Superieur*. Paris: Masson.

De Santo L.W. (1974). Lingual flap reconstruction after resection for cancer. *Trans. Amer. Acad. Opth. Otolaryngol*; **78**:1135–9.

Gregory M.M., Cheesman A.D. (1976). Clinico-pathological co-operation in the management of primary reconstruction in maxillary carcinoma, p. 45. Proc. 3rd Congress of European Ass. for Max. Fac. Surg.

Harashina T., Nakayima H., Imai T. (1978). Reconstruction of mandibular defects with revascularised free rib grafts. *Plast. Reconstr. Surg*; **62**:514–22.

Harrison D.F.N. (1973). Management of malignant tumours affecting the maxillary and ethmoidal sinus. *J. Laryngol*; **87**:749–72.

Harrison D.F.N. (1977). Lateral rhinotomy: a neglected operation. *Ann. Otol. Rhinol. Laryngol*; **86**:1–4.

Harrison D.F.N. (1978). Critical look at the classification of maxillary sinus carcinomata. *Ann. Otol. Rhinol. Laryngol*; **87**:1–7.

Harrison R.E. (1979). Prosthetic management of the maxillectomy patient. *Head, Neck Surg*; **1**:366–9.

Ketcham A.S., Wilkins R.H., Van Buren J.M. (1963). A combined intracranial facial approach to the paranasal sinuses. *Amer. J. Surg*; **106**:698–703.

Lederman M. (1970). Tumours of the upper jaw: natural history and treatment. *J. Laryngol*; **84**:369–407.

Lee S.E., Wilson J.S.P. (1973). Carcinoma involving the lower alveolus, an appraisal of past results, and an account of current management. *Brit. J. Surg*; **60**:85–107.

Lloyd G. (1971). Axial tomography of the orbits and paranasal sinuses. *Brit. J. Radiology*; **48**:460–70.

Marchetta F.C., Sako K., Murphy J.B. (1971). The periosteum of the mandible and intra-oral carcinoma. *Amer. J. Surg*; **122**:711–3.

McGregor A.J. (1977). Reconstruction following excision of intra-oral and mandibular tumours. In *Reconstructive Plastic Surgery*, vol. 5, 2nd edn., ch. 62. Philadelphia: WB Saunders.

Moure E.J. (1902). Traitment des tumeurs malignes primitives de l'ethmoide. *Rev. Laryngol. Otol. Rhinol.* (Bord); **23**:401-12.

Snow G.B., Kruisbrink J.J., Van Slooten E.A. (1976). Reconstruction after mandibulectomy for cancer. *Arch. Otolaryngol*; **102(4)**:207–10.

Som M.L. (1974). Surgical management of carcinoma of the maxilla. *Arch. Otolaryngol*; **99**:270–3.

Wilson J.S.P. (1967). The application of the two centimetre pedicle flap in plastic surgery. *Brit. J. Plast. Surg*; **20**:278–96.

Worthington P. (1977). Surgical approach to the pterygoid region. *Brit. J. Oral Surg*; **15**:135–46.

Trauma and technique

Introduction

The importance of trauma in surgical practice is unlikely to diminish. Whether due to war, civil violence or road accidents, trauma is the leading cause of death in adolescents and young adults in almost all western communities. Public education programmes about road accident prevention have probably not had much effect in reducing accidents, but there is considerable evidence that compulsory wearing of seat belts for motorists, crash helmets for motor cyclists and the introduction of speed limits on highways have reduced mortality from road accidents. Significant contributions to the prevention of childhood road accidents have been made in Scandinavian countries and in the Netherlands by specific legislation and urban planning designed to protect children, whether they are pedestrians, cyclists or car occupants.

All surgeons are involved in caring for injured patients so that understanding the metabolic consequences of trauma is germane to all surgical practice. Rapid increase in our knowledge of the pathophysiology of trauma has been associated with major developments in applied technology for monitoring and supporting damaged organs. Organisation of Accident and Emergency Departments has resulted in clearer definition of priorities in situations involving multiple casualties. Almost every hospital now has a policy or code of action to be followed in the event of major disaster. In individuals with multiple critical injuries, it is appreciated that immediate effective resuscitation precedes diagnosis of the nature and extent of the injury.

The proliferation of Intensive Care Units has been responsible to a great extent for the improved prognosis for patients who have sustained major trauma. Rapid transfer to hospital, improvements in diagnostic technology, developments in the continuous monitoring of vital function and the training of medical and nursing staff in the care of the injured have all contributed to the improved survival rates. Ventilatory support and intravenous nutrition are now commonplace and while sepsis is still a major cause of death in the injured patient, the recognition and control of infection is being facilitated by newer diagnostic tests and drugs.

It is clear from the chapters which follow that the best results from treating trauma depend on an understanding of the mechanisms by which tissue damage occurs and on the optimum primary treatment. Secondary repairs, no matter how expert, are almost always less satisfactory than skilled and appropriate primary care. The superiority of microsurgical techniques in the repair of nerves and small blood vessels is now widely accepted. Training in the use of the operating microscope may well become an essential part of training for all surgeons in the future.

Because the patient with multiple injuries may require many different specialists, the establishment of responsibility is essential. Speed and accuracy of communication also becomes important and a clear line of authority is required for decision-making and triage. A specific individual, whether physician, surgeon, anaesthetist or intensivist must have ultimate responsibility for the major decisions in management.

N. O'H.

Trauma and technique

Emergencies and catastrophes

D. W. YATES

Immediate care

The basic principles of assessment and initial management of the acutely injured patient are discussed in detail in this chapter. The first part is concerned with the clinical care of individual patients at the scene of the accident and in the Accident and Emergency Department, and the second part with the organisational problems created by catastrophes. Subsequent management of specific injuries is discussed elsewhere.

Expert medical assistance at the scene of an accident is considered by some to be an essential first step in resuscitation. Others feel that it wastes valuable time and that it is safer to transfer the patient to hospital as quickly as possible, applying en route the basic principles of first aid. Such views may be influenced by considerations of difficulty of extraction, journey time, terrain and availability of staff. Nevertheless there are wide differences of opinion on the usefulness of 'immediate care'.

Most casualties in the UK are treated at the scene and transported to hospital by ambulance crews trained in the basic principles of airway control, external cardiac massage and limb splintage. Until quite recently in North America many patients were transferred from accident scene to hospital by the local undertaker. Often no other vehicles would have been available to accomodate stretchers. This difference may explain why there has been so much support for the creation of 'paramedics' in the US and why there has been some reluctance to develop a similar service in the UK.

The weakness of the present British system is the low exposure rate of the ambulance crews to life threatening situations – under 5% of their calls are to emergencies. This could be overcome if the ambulance service was divided into two parts – one concerned with emergency work, the other providing a form of taxi service for out-patients. The provision of medical aid at the accident scene to supplement ambulance crews has been encouraged in recent years by general practitioners (Easton, 1970) and hospital doctors.

The common aims of the various types of immediate care schemes are to stabilise the cardiorespiratory system, to splint fractures and to make a quick assessment of the patient before and during transfer to hospital (Table 1). To achieve this in the field is often very difficult. Doctors will find that it takes time to gain the

Table 1
IMMEDIATE CARE OF INJURED PATIENT

1 Establish and maintain an adequate airway and if necessary provide assisted ventilation
2 Prevent further injury – apply cervical collar and if possible move patient to safety
3 Begin to correct hypovolaemia by intravenous infusion of plasma expander
4 Reduce pain and anxiety by splinting fractures and giving gaseous analgesic (e.g. Entonox)

necessary expertise. Ambulance crews must have comprehensive instruction courses supplemented by occasional refresher sessions (Stewart, 1977). Table 2 lists the techniques and skills commonly taught. (The management of acute myocardial infarcts by these paramedical crews is not considered here.)

Table 2
SKILLS OF THE 'PARAMEDIC'

Care of the airway, administration of oxygen
Artificial respiration, endotracheal intubation
External cardiac massage, ECG recording
Intravenous fluid therapy
Splintage of cervical spine and limb fractures
Administration of inhalational analgesics
Extraction techniques
Good working relationship with base hospital
Radio communications

The indiscriminate use of immediate care schemes can weaken the provision of medical care elsewhere. It is important, therefore, to restrict their activities to those situations where benefit is most likely to be obtained. Unfortunately, there has been very little scientific work carried out in this field. Indeed, there are some indications that greater benefit will be achieved by improving resuscitation inside hospital than en route to the hospital or at the scene (Hoffman, 1976; Yates, 1979).

Skilled on-site resuscitation is probably of maximum benefit to trapped patients and those requiring long ambulance journeys. It is important to link this provision with the reorganisation of the ambulance service mentioned previously. The skills acquired by the ambulance crews would otherwise be used rarely, leading to low morale and poor performance.

Equipment

Location does not influence priorities in resuscitation, but it may influence some of the techniques and equipment used. A detailed consideration of primary resuscitation will be found on p. 711. However, it is more appropriate to discuss at this point recent developments of potential importance to on-site care.

Protection of the airway from blood and vomit remains one of the most difficult tasks for the resuscitation team. Endotracheal intubation can be difficult to perform, even with all the facilities available in the emergency room. At the accident scene it may be impossible. The oesophageal obturator airway was developed by Don Michael *et al.* (1968) to overcome this problem. It can be introduced into the oesophagus blindly, when the neck is flexed, the inflatable cuff pre-

venting regurgitation of stomach contents (Fig 44.1). However, removal of the device may be associated with copious reflux. Recently a modification has been developed to prevent this complication (Fig 44.2). Gastric contents can be aspirated through a nasogastric tube whilst the obturator is in use.

The oesophageal obturator airway is used extensively by paramedics in North America and it is perhaps not surprising that an increasing number of complications associated with its use are now being reported. Nevertheless, this device would seem to have a place in the management of the trauma patient at the accident scene. Perhaps it is because it is so easy to insert that problems are being encountered. Restriction of its use to doctors and ambulance crews who have received advanced training should reduce the number of complications. A modified tube which can be inserted into either oesophagus or trachea has been introduced recently by Eisenberg (1980). Preliminary experience suggests that it overcomes some of the problems associated with the oesophageal obturator airway. In the hospital environment, however, endotracheal intubation will remain the ideal method of airway control.

Other field aids to ventilation include the hand operated self-expanding bag with valve and mask (Fig 44.3) and oxygen powered ventilators. Pressure cycled

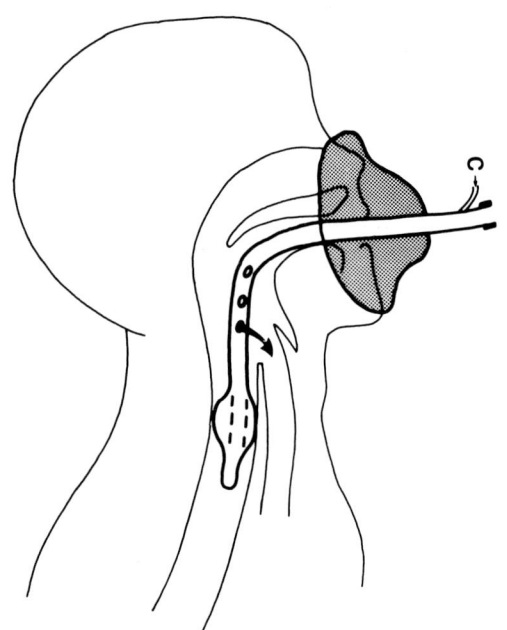

Fig 44.1 The oesophageal obturator airway. C = cuff inflation point.

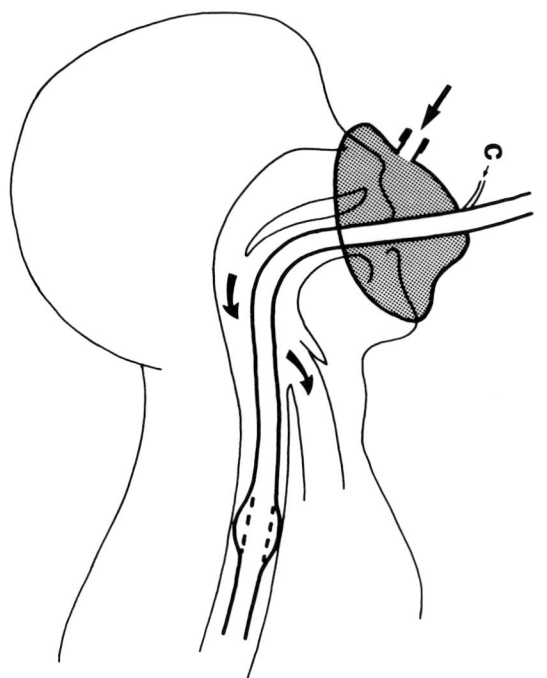

Fig 44.2 Modification of the airway to allow aspiration of gastric contents. C = cuff inflation point.

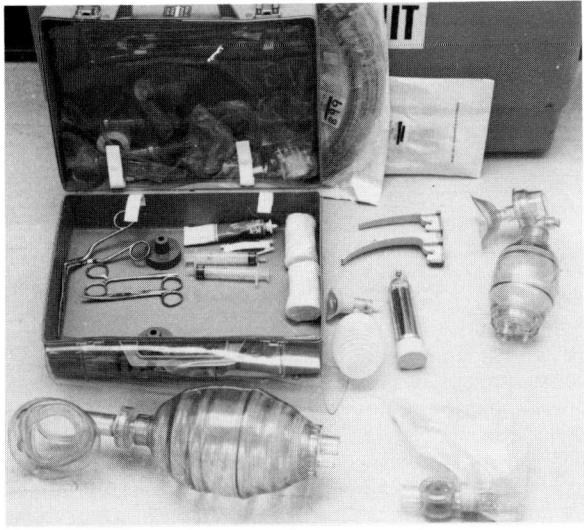

Fig 44.3 Airway equipment for field use.

machines are incompatible with the reversed intrathoracic pressures associated with external cardiac massage and should not be used as aids to resuscitation. The ideal oxygen powered ventilator should be hand-triggered and give a very high flow rate (100 litres of oxygen per minute). The mechanical ventilators avail-able for field use have been evaluated by Harber and Lucas (1980).

Rapid blood loss and the prospect of a long delay before the patient arrives in the emergency room present difficulties for the rescue team. Autotransfusion from the legs and pelvis will provide short-term correction of hypovolaemia. This may be achieved by applying pneumatic tourniquets. (e.g. medical anti shock trousers). These suits have been used with encouraging results in North America, but have not become popular in Great Britain. Pressures above 50 mmHg are unnecessary and can be dangerous. Prolonged use may lead to muscle ischaemia. However, they must only be removed when transfusion facilities are available to treat the consequent local hyperaemia and systemic hypotension.

Primary transport

The casualty should be moved from the scene of the accident to the emergency room in the receiving hospital as soon as possible, but speed must not be pursued to the exclusion of medical care. An uneven ride for the patient with inadequately splinted limb fractures is extremely painful. Anxiety expressed in the actions and attitudes of the ambulance crews is quickly transmitted to the patient. Pain and panic will, in turn, impair the normal homeostatic responses to circulatory fluid loss.

Splintage of fractures need not be complex to be effective and should be achieved before the patient is moved (p. 728). The patient must, in turn, be secured to his stretcher, in a position determined by the injuries sustained. If he is unconscious but breathing spontaneously, he should be held in the recovery or semi-prone position with a Guidel airway *in situ*. Effective suction and a bag respirator must be immediately available. It is wise to apply a cervical collar to all patients with a head injury and to those with suspected cervical trauma.

Within the above constraints, it is helpful to apply pressure to major limb wounds and to elevate them to reduce bleeding. Tourniquets must not be used. The temptation to apply haemostats to bleeding wounds must be resisted. Direct pressure will suffice. The head down position must be avoided as it reduces lung volume by allowing the abdominal contents to press against the diaphragm.

Helicopters are now used with increasing frequency in the primary transport of injured patients (Oxen, 1975). The smooth ride and short journey time must be weighed against the problems of access in urban areas and their great expense.

The resuscitation area

The resuscitation area must be an integral part of a large Accident Unit or Accident and Emergency Department. Doctors and nurses would never become acquainted with an isolated resuscitation unit because of the paucity of major emergencies and the need to employ the team elsewhere during quiet periods. It would be difficult to provide an efficient resuscitation service in these circumstances. Even an integrated unit will not provide sufficient clinical experience and familiarity with equipment unless it is in use several times everyday. This can be achieved in urban areas by limiting the number of such units and improving ambulance services to them. In rural areas the deleterious effects of a long journey and the possible delay in providing resuscitation must be balanced against the advantages of centralisation.

In order to reduce the movement of the casualty once he has arrived at the hospital, the ambulance bay should be adjacent to the resuscitation room, and x-ray facilities close at hand (or even within the department). Similarly, the intensive care unit, operating theatres and surgical wards should be within easy reach in the same building.

The resuscitation room should have an open plan with the capacity to take up to four patients at any one time. However, under normal circumstances only one or two patients should be in the area simultaneously. Such a policy encourages speedy resuscitation and the rapid formulation of priorities for definitive treatment, which will be carried out elsewhere. Some consider that the provision of an additional room, capable of receiving only one patient, is useful for the care of the critically ill. Certainly, this ensures that other patients in the resuscitation area are screened from what can be a very disturbing experience.

Table 3 lists the equipment required in the resuscitation area. This should be arranged in functional units, e.g. airways, endotracheal tubes, suction tubing and tracheotomy sets on one wall unit, and all the equipment necessary to set up intravenous and central venous pressure lines on another wall unit. One section should be devoted to paediatric resuscitation equipment.

Doctors should not be encouraged to write copious notes in the resuscitation area, but a small desk is useful where brief clinical notes can be entered on the Casualty Card and where charts and request forms can be completed. The relevant forms, specimen tubes, telephones and x-ray viewing boxes should be clustered around this desk (Fig 44.4).

In addition to the small stores mentioned above, a basic set of emergency equipment should be provided at the head of each trolley, including airway, bag resus-

Table 3
RESUSCITATION AREA EQUIPMENT

Airway	Suction equipment, mouth gag Guidel airway, oxygen Face mask and self expanding resuscitation bag Laryngoscopes (adult, child and infant) Endotracheal tube, introducer and McGill forceps Needle for crico-thyroid stab Tracheotomy set Bronchoscope
Heart	Electrocardiograph Defibrillator Intracardiac needles Pacing equipment
Circulation	Short wide bore cannulae Central venous pressure lines and manometers Isotonic saline, colloid solution Dried plasma, plasma protein fraction Blood warmer Blood filters Pump
Drugs	Atropine, adrenaline, lignocaine, rhythmadon Calcium gluconate, salbutamol, 50% glucose Diazepam, naloxone, dexamethazone Morphine sulphate, entonox Sodium bicarbonate 8.4%
Miscellaneous	Chest drain and Heimlich valve Urinary catheter Nasogastric tube Peritoneal lavage set Insulating blanket Splints and cervical collars Thermometers oral, rectal and subnormal Suture material with large needles Heparinised syringes Specimen tubes Emergency buzzer Clock with sweep second hand

citator, laryngoscope and endotracheal tube. A large bore cannula is kept on this head board and a 0.9% saline intravenous infusion is set up ready for direct connection to the cannula. To reduce the number of poles and floor mounted equipment the drip can be suspended from an overhead rail. A spotlight can be suspended similarly and one of the rails used to store a cervical collar (Fig 44.5). An emergency call button should be situated in each trolley bay so that extra staff can be summoned at once from other parts of the department.

Each patient trolley must have a radiolucent base to accommodate an x-ray cassette and be adjustable into the 'head down' and 'back up' positions. Oxygen should be available from a wall fixture and from a cylinder under the trolley.

Finally, some thought should be given to moving the patient from the resuscitation room to another part of

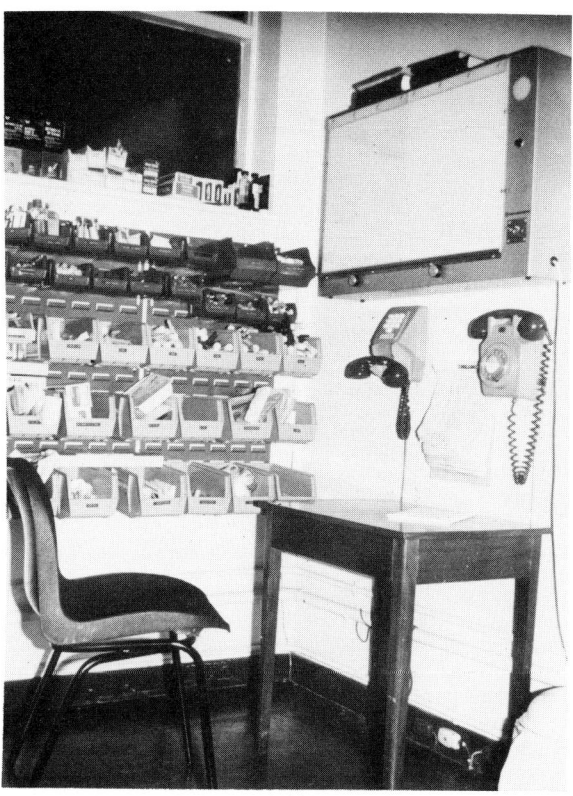

Fig 44.4   Strategically placed desk in resuscitation area.

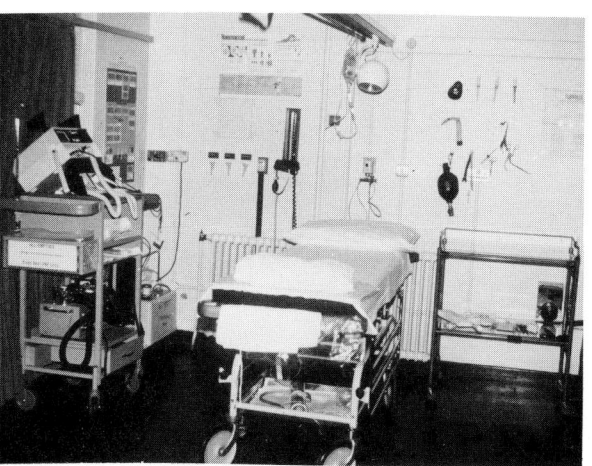

Fig 44.5   Resuscitation trolley.

the hospital. This can be a hazardous affair (Waddell, 1975). The patient may vomit in a lift or become apnoeic whilst being wheeled along a corridor. Equipment must be carried on the trolley which will allow the accompanying nurse to deal with such an emergency. A pressurised canister with venturi device will provide adequate emergency suction. The provision of emergency telephones in corridors and lifts will facilitate the prompt arrival of the resuscitation team at such incidents.

Primary resuscitation

The principle aim of primary resuscitation is rapid stabilisation of the cardiorespiratory system. Some progress may have been made towards achieving this goal at the scene of the accident and on the journey to hospital but, in any event, it must be the first concern of the resuscitation team in the emergency room. Local treatment of limb injuries and even of serious head injuries must not be allowed to delay the first priority which is immediate attention to the airway and the circulation.

Airway

The basic principles of airway management feature prominently in instruction courses for First Aiders. Until recently a similar emphasis was unusual in undergraduate medical curricula. There has been a consequent tendency for newly qualified doctors to begin specific management of individual injuries before ensuring that the upper airway is clear. This omission has been shown to affect significantly the mortality rate associated with major trauma (Yates, 1977). Surprisingly, airway control is sometimes more effective en route to hospital than it is within the hospital.

The effect of poor management of the airway on morbidity is more difficult to establish, but it is, for example, thought to be a significant factor in the pathogenesis of cerebral oedema after head injury (Jennett and Carlin, 1978). Table 4 summarises the management of the upper airway in the unconscious patient who is breathing spontaneously. Artificial ventilation is essential in the apnoeic patient (Table 5).

The oesophageal obturator airway (Figs 44.1 and 44.2) may have some place in prehospital care if the technical skills necessary for endotracheal tube insertion are not available (p. 708). However, it is not the simple answer to airway control that some have suggested. Endotracheal intubation should remain the ideal, and is essential when the gag reflex has been lost and blood may be aspirated. Intubation can be difficult if the patient is not deeply unconscious. The associated complication rate is much higher than that experienced

Table 4
UPPER AIRWAY MANAGEMENT

Unconscious, breathing spontaneously

Clear mouth	Dentures ⎱ manually Debris ⎰
	Vomit ⎱ by suction Blood ⎰
Maintain airway	Draw jaw forward Insert Guidel airway
Give oxygen	If blue, breathless or severely injured
Avoid further obstruction	Put patient in semiprone position

Table 5
UPPER AIRWAY MANAGEMENT

Unconscious apnoeic

Clear mouth	Dentures ⎱ manually Debris ⎰
	Vomit ⎱ by suction Blood ⎰
Maintain airway	Place patient supine Draw jaw forward Extend upper cervical spine (dangerous if neck injury)
Artificial respiration	Mouth to mouth or Guidel airway bag and mask or Oesophageal obturator airway and bag or Endotracheal intubation and bag Connect bag to oxygen line

in the more formal environment of the operating theatre. Particularly troublesome are laryngeal stridor and breath holding, which result in raised intracranial pressure and aggravate the effects of head injury. When laryngeal spasm causes difficulty in a restless patient, a short acting muscle relaxant may be given immediately prior to intubation. This is not without risk and should be performed only by a senior member of staff with anaesthetic experience. Intubation is also difficult if a cervical collar has been applied. However, the challenge must be accepted and the collar left in position.

Injuries to the facial skeleton may dislodge teeth, which may be inhaled. Usually teeth can be detected on subsequent radiographs, but fragments of dental prostheses are not radio-opaque. Their inhalation may go unrecognised until segmental collapse and infection occur. To avoid these problems, very loose teeth should be fixed or removed and an attempt made to account for all missing teeth and dentures.

Many patients who present with difficult airway problems have full stomachs and are likely to vomit shortly after arriving in the resuscitation area. This can be prevented by emptying the stomach with a wide-bore nasogastric tube. The smaller tubes used to drain gastric juices postoperatively are of no value for this purpose. However, the insertion of a large gastric tube is not without risk. There have been case reports of their inadvertent introduction into the cranial cavity via an extensive fracture of the skull base (Fig 44.6) (Wyler and Reynolds, 1977).

Tears of the hypopharyngeal wall are a well recognised complication of endotracheal intubation, especially in patients with prominent osteophytes on the cervical vertebrae. Similar damage can be caused by direct trauma, swallowed dentures and foreign bodies. The tear may go undetected as the patient will have minimal symptoms for the first few hours. However, retropharyngeal air will be seen on a lateral cervical spine radiograph (Fig 44.7). Early recognition is essential if fatal mediastinitis is to be prevented.

Tracheotomy

Emergency tracheotomy is very rarely necessary, but relevant instruments and tubes must be available in the resuscitation area. Indications are listed in Table 6 and an example is shown in Fig 44.8. The procedure is particularly difficult and dangerous in infants and small

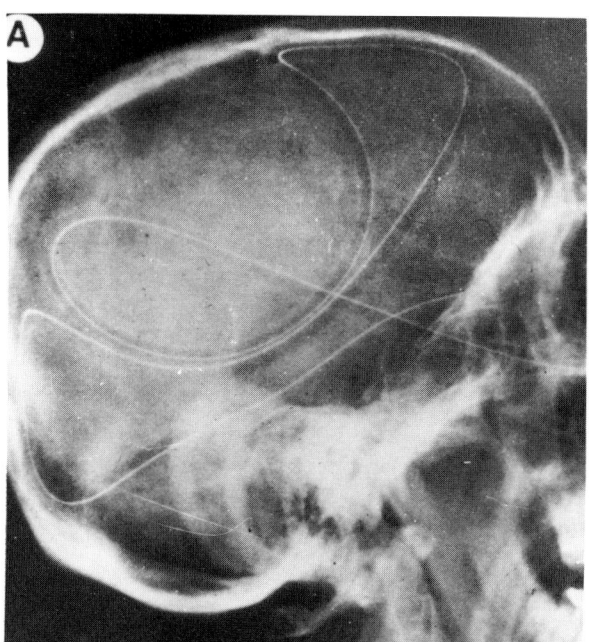

Fig 44.6 Radiograph showing gastric tube in cranial cavity (From Wyler and Reynolds, 1977. *J. Neurosurg*; **47**:297–8 by courtesy of the Editor.)

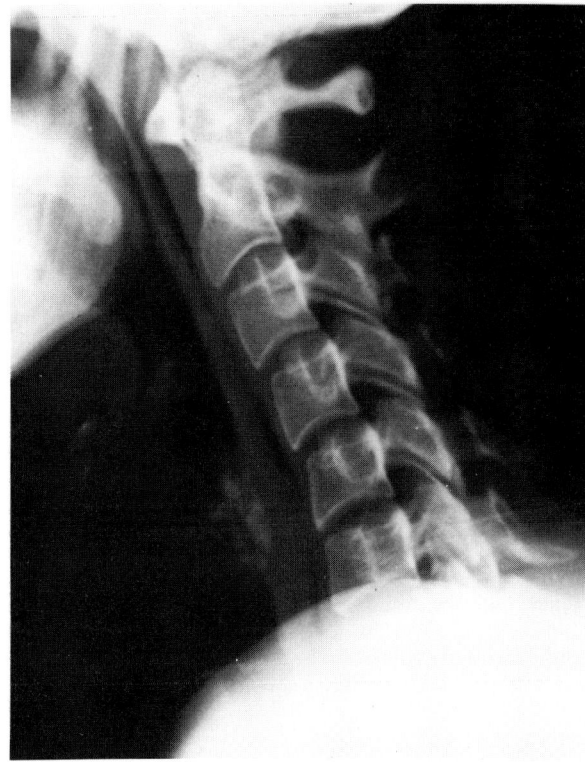

Fig 44.7   Note retropharyngeal air due to tear of pharyngeal wall.

Table 6
SURGICAL INDICATIONS FOR EMERGENCY TRACHEOTOMY

Extensive trauma to the larynx
Open wounds of the upper trachea
Impaction of foreign body across larynx
Very extensive facial injury

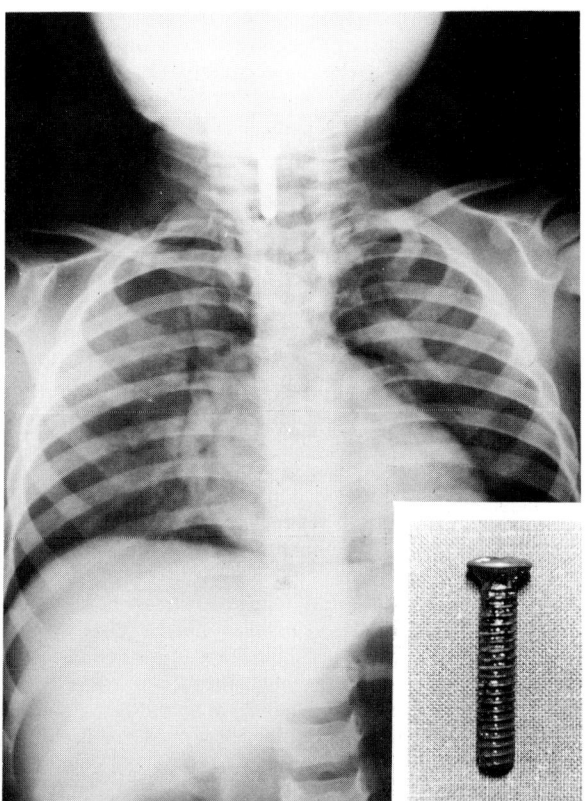

Fig 44.8   Infant requiring emergency tracheotomy. Note screw (*inset*) obstructing trachea.

children because of the short neck and more cranial position of the left brachio-cephalic vein. A good account of the operative technique is given by Griffith (1976).

An alternative to emergency tracheotomy, if the obstruction is above the thyroid cartilage, is the insertion of a wide bore cannula percutaneously at the level of the crico-thyroid membrane. This manoeuvre can be life saving until definitive treatment is undertaken. Larger obturators designed for percutaneous insertion into the upper trachea have not gained wide acceptance.

Bronchoscopy

The rigid and possibly the fibreoptic, bronchoscope should be considered an appropriate instrument for the resuscitation area. It is essential for the removal of inhaled foreign bodies, teeth and fluids from the main bronchi. It can be used also as a diagnostic tool to give information on the source of bronchial bleeding and on the state of the main bronchi in patients who have inhaled fumes, gastric contents or corrosives.

Cardiac arrest

If the patient has had a cardiac arrest, it is common practice to stop external cardiac massage after every 5 compressions, to inflate the lungs. The need for this pause is now being questioned. Rudikoff *et al.* (1977) have shown that improved oxygenation can be achieved if the lungs are inflated during a cardiac compression. Simultaneous cardiac massage and lung inflation has been claimed to improve blood gas tensions (Chandra *et al.*, 1980). Mechanical external cardiac compressors may provide a more consistent and continuous cardiac output but are rarely of value in the management of trauma patients.

Hypovolaemia

Early correction of hypovolaemia is an essential part of primary resuscitation. However, it may not be appreciated on initial clinical examination that the patient *is* hypovolaemic. A previously fit person can maintain a normal blood pressure with only a modest tachycardia in the early stages of active blood loss. For this reason all seriously injured patients must have at least one large bore intravenous line set up irrespective of the apparent state of the circulation.

Isotonic saline is quite suitable for this first line. There is little point in adding to the hyperglycaemic response to injury by giving a sugar solution. The blind initial administration of a colloid is unwise, as it may transpire that the patient is normovolaemic with, for instance, a serious head injury. Saline has the added advantages of being cheap, having a long shelf life and not precipitating out in the giving set or causing phlebitis. A 500 ml bag can be set up over the resuscitation room trolley to await the patient. Unused sets should be replaced every 12 h to avoid the risk of contamination.

The establishment of this first intravenous line should be considered as a first aid measure. Other initial steps include direct pressure to reduce any major external bleeding and elevation of the injured part if practicable. Tilting the patient head down is not recommended as it allows the abdominal viscera and diaphragm to fall towards the chest and reduce total lung volume. However, redistribution of some lower limb blood into the trunk can be achieved by elevating the legs and keeping them in pneumatic trousers (*see* p. 709).

Once these preliminaries have been completed, attention can be turned to estimating the amount of fluid loss, and the type of fluid to be used as replacement.

Amount of fluid loss

Shock can be regarded as a failure of perfusion of the microcirculation in vital tissues. To measure its progress by the time honoured estimation of the arterial blood pressure is to ignore well established principles of cardiovascular physiology. The arterial blood pressure is often irrelevant – even misleading. It is ironic that it is so easy to measure the blood pressure and that many of the more useful parameters either require invasive techniques or defy arithmetic precision.

Early evidence of hypovolaemic shock will be obtained by taking a general clinical view of the patient, as discussed on p. 716). This will include the level of cerebral and renal function and the extent of peripheral circulatory shutdown. The level of consciousness as an index of circulatory competence is rarely of value, as many victims have sustained a direct head injury, and all will be influenced by pain and anxiety. However, urine output will reflect renal and, indirectly, core circulation. Adequate perfusion produces a urine output of at least 1 ml/kg/h. Great toe temperature and the gradient between it and the core temperature relates fairly closely to the degree of hypovolaemia (Henning *et al.*, 1979). The environmental temperature influences this relationship and complicates interpretation of the results. But, in any given patient, the trend can be most valuable and has been shown to be of greater prognostic value than blood pressure.

A rough estimate of potential blood loss can be obtained by considering the sites of injury (Table 7). Although many variables will influence the exact amount of blood loss in any individual patient, certain general observations can be made. Occult bleeding into the thoracic, abdominal and pelvic cavities is often underestimated, as is the loss into contused muscle surrounding a femoral shaft fracture. In contrast, external bleeding is usually overestimated and injuries to the forearm are rarely important in this respect.

The central venous pressure (CVP) responds more quickly to loss of blood volume than arterial blood pressure. A short catheter can be introduced into the subclavian or internal jugular vein or a longer line into the antecubital vein. Whichever route is employed, the patient must be tilted head down to fill the neck veins and prevent air embolus, and an aseptic technique employed. Whilst the success rate with the antecubital approach is not as high as with the more direct route, the complication rate is lower. A chest radiograph must

Table 7
GUIDE TO BLOOD LOSS

Injured site	Blood loss
Head and scalp	Usually overestimated except in infants
Chest and abdominal cavities	Usually underestimated often over 2 l
Chest wall	Isolated fractures ¼–½ l extensive fractures 1–2 l
Lumbar area	½–2 l
Pelvis	½–3 l
Femoral shaft	1–2 l
Tibial shaft	½–1 l
Shoulder	¼–1 l

In theory, a 2 cm overall increase in thigh diameter will accommodate 4 l of blood. Blood loss is significantly greater if limb fractures are compound.

be taken immediately after CVP line placement to exclude a pneumothorax and to determine the site of the catheter tip. Subsequent films may also be necessary as late complications from CVP lines are now recognised. The response pattern of the CVP to a fluid load is of more importance than its absolute value. It will provide information about right heart performance as well as the capacity of the venous system.

A knowledge of the left atrial pressure is particularly important when the response to hypovolaemic shock is compromised by cardiogenic shock. Direct measurement of left atrial pressure is rarely appropriate in the acute resuscitation phase, but indirect measurement is feasible using a balloon-tipped catheter with pressure transducer to obtain the pulmonary artery wedge pressure. Unfortunately the constant relationship between pulmonary artery wedge pressure and left heart performance (Pardy and Dudley, 1977) no longer holds when myocardial function is compromised. Transcutaneous aortovelography, a new non-invasive Doppler ultrasound technique has been shown to give reproducible measurements of aortic flow and should resolve these difficulties (Hanson et al., 1980).

Type of fluid replacement

The injured patient initially loses blood from the plasma space, but soon the continued loss of 'blood' is modified by fluid moving into the vessels from the extracellular space and later from the intracellular space. Replacement fluids must be capable of restoring all these deficits, although replenishment of the plasma space must take priority.

The initial aim of transfusion is to correct hypovolaemia; concern about oxygen-carrying capacity is secondary. Indeed a slight reduction of the packed cell volume to about 35% is beneficial – the less viscous blood reduces heart work. The enzyme 2,3 diphosphoglycerate concerned with oxygen uptake by red cells has a much reduced activity in stored blood. It is reactivated only slowly after transfusion. Hence a blood transfusion will not bring about a dramatic improvement in oxygen carrying capacity – although it is better in this respect than colloid or crystalloid. Oxygen by mask will increase slightly the amount transported in physical solution.

To replenish the plasma space, it is necessary either to transfuse a colloid which is osmotically active and is essentially restricted to this space, or to give a very large amount of crystalloid which will be distributed throughout the plasma space and extracellular space. The administration of large volumes of crystalloid gained popularity during the Vietnam War and was undoubtedly responsible for the successful resuscitation of many critically ill patients (Moss, 1972). However, the associated interstitial oedema, particularly in the lungs, can be difficult to disperse. The development of improved colloid solutions has coincided with a decline in popularity of high volume crystalloid therapy.

In Great Britain, the dextrans have been the most extensively used plasma expanders. High molecular-weight, inert polysaccharides, they are available in solutions of isotonic saline and glucose and with different average molecular weights. The most popular dextran for acute resuscitation has an average molecular weight of 70 000 and will remain osmotically active in the plasma space for at least 6 h, its precise rate of excretion depending on the state of the circulation. Anaphylactic reactions have been reported (Ring and Messmer, 1977), presumably due to the formation of large immune complexes. Pretreatment with hapten to occupy antibody binding sites is a theoretically appealing preventative measure and is now the subject of research. Oozing from small vessels occurs when large volumes of dextrans are transfused. They also cause rouleaux formation *in vitro*, interfering with cross matching of blood. A sample of blood for laboratory use must be taken, therefore, before starting a dextran transfusion. The lower molecular weight dextrans (e.g. 40 000) may cause renal tubular stasis in low flow states and should not be used in hypovolaemic shock.

Gelatin solutions have been used for many years as plasma expanders, but have not been popular in Great Britain until the recent advent of Haemaccel and Gelofusine. These solutions do not impair renal function – indeed they enhance it. There is no interference with blood cross matching. Starch is well established as a good volume expander, and recently a safe derivative, hydroxyethyl starch has been developed (Rudowski, 1980). The trend in emergency room practice over the past few years has been to move away from the dextrans towards the gelatins. A typical fluid replacement regime is given in Fig 44.9.

Blood should be warmed prior to transfusion and passed through a millipore filter. If these precautions are not taken the core temperature will fall significantly and micro aggregates will impair lung and renal function (Buley and Lumley, 1975). Blood is becoming increasingly expensive and we can expect to see greater use of plasma-poor red cells in the future. The problems of long term storage are being resolved by the use of hydroxyethyl starch and deep freezing techniques although the latter are still at an experimental stage.

Equipment for autotransfusion (reinfusion) of shed blood is now available (Sterling *et al.*, 1975). The problems of air emboli, clotting and micro-aggregates have been largely overcome. The use of blood from a soiled peritoneal cavity is said not to be associated with any septic complications. This technique has been used with considerable success in the resuscitation of the severely hypovolaemic patient (O'Riordan, 1977).

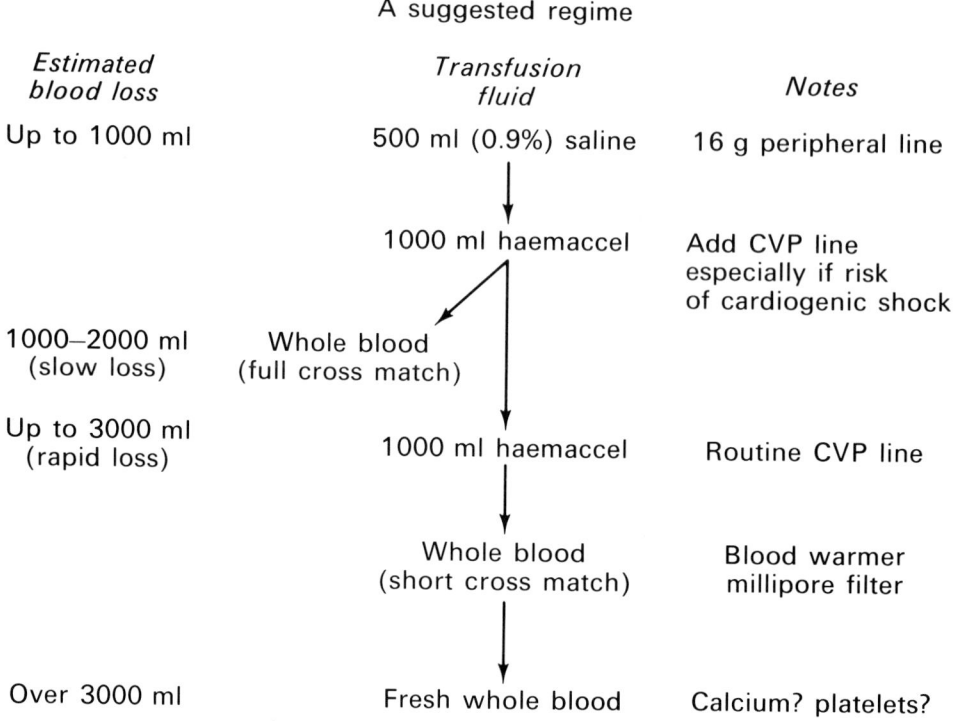

Fig 44.9 Fluid replacement after blood loss.

Time for reflection

As soon as the immediate threat to life has been overcome it is useful for a senior doctor to dissociate himself from active treatment for a few moments to make an overall assessment of the situation. It is essential to identify priorities at this stage. Hasty decisions made in the resuscitation area will commit the patient to a pattern of investigations and treatment which may not be in his best interests. It may be many hours before these decisions are challenged.

An assessment of the injuries sustained is, of course, central to the determination of priorities and this will be discussed in detail in later sections. However, other information will also influence management. The age and previous medical history of the patient may be relevant. Sometimes, aggressive and active intervention may be considered inappropriate in the frail and elderly. The history of the accident is usually helpful. The full extent of the injuries sustained is rarely evident initially and a knowledge of the mechanism of the accident may point to occult injury. Certain evident injuries are known to be associated with lesions elsewhere. Table 8 lists the commonest associations. Management will be influenced also by the number of patients demanding treatment when resources are limited. This problem is discussed in the second part of this chapter.

It is helpful for the senior doctor assessing priorities to summarise the injuries sustained. The development of the Injury Severity Score (ISS) has simplified this process (Table 9; Baker et al., 1974). The ISS has been developed for research use and is not intended as a prognostic indicator, but its use in individual cases has been found to be of value in giving an overall impression of severity. This increases awareness of transfusion requirements which may have been underestimated.

Clinical priorities are determined by the threat to life which is posed by the individual injuries. Hence obstruction of the airway will have the first priority followed closely by the surgical repair or removal of damaged tissues responsible for massive haemorrhage. Tension pneumothorax and flail chest have equally high priority. Once the cardiorespiratory system has been stabilised, attention can be turned to head and limb injuries. Neither of the latter will benefit from hastily-arranged surgery if due attention has not been given to the airway and the circulation.

Even in the best run and most frequently used resuscitation areas, the combination of an infinite variety of

Table 8
ASSOCIATED INJURIES

Evident	Maybe occult
Head injury	Cervical spine injury
Sternal fracture	Crush fracture of upper thoracic vertebrae
	Cardiac contusion
Lower rib fracture	Liver/spleen injury
Pelvic fracture	Urethral injury
Knee injury	Posterior dislocation of hip
Os calcis fracture	Crush fracture lumbar spine
	Fracture base occiput
Wrist fracture	Dislocated shoulder/rotator cuff injury
	Fracture of clavicle

Table 9
THE INJURY SEVERITY SCORE

1 Determine the scores of individual injuries using the *Abbreviated Injury Scale*.
2 Identify the highest score in each of the following six areas:

Head and neck	Face
Abdomen and pelvic contents	Chest
Bony pelvis and limbs	Body surface

3 Add together the squares of the three highest scores.

Example
A car occupant sustains a minor head injury, fracture of mandibular ramus, extensive facial lacerations, a fracture of one clavicle, 5 fractured ribs with underlying pneumothorax, a ruptured liver, an extraperitoneal rupture of the bladder associated with pubic rami fractures and a compound tibial fracture.

		AIS	Highest AIS	AIS^2
Head and neck:	unconscious <15 min	2	2	
Face:	mandibular ramus fracture	1	1	
Chest:	5 rib fractures	2		
	pneumothorax	3	3	9
Abdomen:	ruptured liver	5	5	25
	ruptured bladder	3		
Bony pelvis and limbs	clavicle fracture	2		
	pelvic fracture	2		
	compound tibial fracture	3	3	9
Body surface:	facial lacerations	2	2	
			ISS =	43

† Over 400 injuries are listed and scored from 1 to 6 in the AIS booklet obtainable from 40 Second Avenue, Arlington Heights, IL 60005, USA.

clinical presentations and the evident need for urgent action can lead to errors of omission and commission. Most of the problems arise because possibilities have not been considered. With this in mind some departments have developed reminder charts or 'check lists' for display in the resuscitation area (Table 10). In addition a small library of reference works in the accident unit is invaluable.

Notes and charts

Advanced resuscitation cannot be carried out by a single person. There is the need, therefore, to record and to communicate to others information about the patients changing clinical state. Unfortunately, documentation of events during an emergency is often poor, sometimes non-existent. The initial assessment of a patient with multiple injuries may contain important clues about the underlying pathology (e.g. clothing imprints, state of the airway, level of consciousness). Such information is lost if this assessment has been carried out by someone who does not have any long-term involvement with the patient and who has left the tedious business of taking notes to someone else. Similarly, recordings on charts may be so intermittent as to be of no value in assessing progress. Inadequate documentation not only hinders patient care, but also makes any form of retrospective research impossible.

There is usually some time during any emergency to write concise problem-oriented notes and collect data. This task should be delegated to one member of the team to avoid omissions and duplications. While it is better to have too much data rather than not enough, all members of the resuscitation team must realise that the collection of data is not an end in itself – an attitude all too easy to adopt with the recent development of patient monitors. Clinical observation remains central to patient care, but for it to be valuable in the long term it must be recorded and timed.

When more than one intravenous line is in use and drugs are being given by various routes and different personnel, it is useful to have a double check on the records. This can be accomplished by putting all the empty ampoules and intravenous packs in a special container and listing the contents before the patient moves out of the resuscitation area (Fig 44.10).

Initial management of chest injuries

Chest injuries may disrupt the mechanism of respiration, produce hypovolaemic and/or cardiogenic shock and may impair gas exchange. These events can pose a threat to life within minutes of the accident, but some of them can be prevented by prompt and often fairly simple treatment. It is essential, therefore, to examine the chest as soon as the upper airway has been cleared and an intravenous infusion started. The management of the profound hypovolaemic shock which may be associated with chest injuries is described on p. 714.

Table 10

MAJOR INJURY CHECK LIST

Airway	Remove false teeth. Sucker Airway – nurse on side Intubate – careful with neck Cricothyroid stab – 12G medicut × 2 Oxygen	**Record**	Details of accident Time of arrival BP, pulse, temp. Abdominal girth Nasogastric tube Glasgow Coma Scale Marks of external violence Drugs given Past history – ? Diabetic Catheterise bladder
Cervical spine	Protect with rigid collar	**Abdomen**	Bowel sounds? Peritoneal lavage (after erect abdo. film)
Circulation	Femoral pulse? – External cardiac massage Large bore drips. N.saline→colloid ECG – continuous and print out for record CVP	**Locomotor**	Back injury? Paraplegia? Pelvis and hips Peripheral pulses Splint fractures – Entonox. Never narcotics initially Estimate total potential blood loss
Chest	Tamponade? Tension pneumothorax? Trial tap→Chest drain Flail chest? IPPR (can cause T. pneumothorax) Erect CXR Indication for bronchoscopy? Danger of delayed pulmonary oedema?	**Head**	Maxillo – facial injury? Basal skull fracture with pharyngeal bleeding? Vault lacerations and depressed fractures – thorough search Re-examine neck carefully
Investigate	Hb. group and cross match blood Urea and electrolytes. Blood gases. Drug levels?		

General   Stabilisation of the cardiorespiratory system, clinical observation and good records are our initial concern. An erect chest film is usually the only helpful x-ray during this first stage of resuscitation. However if there appear to be several injuries there are probably even more. Damage to the abdomen and spine is easily overlooked. Always x-ray cervical and dorsolumbar spine and pelvis later when the patient's general condition permits. Do not ask for stress views. Remember tetanus.

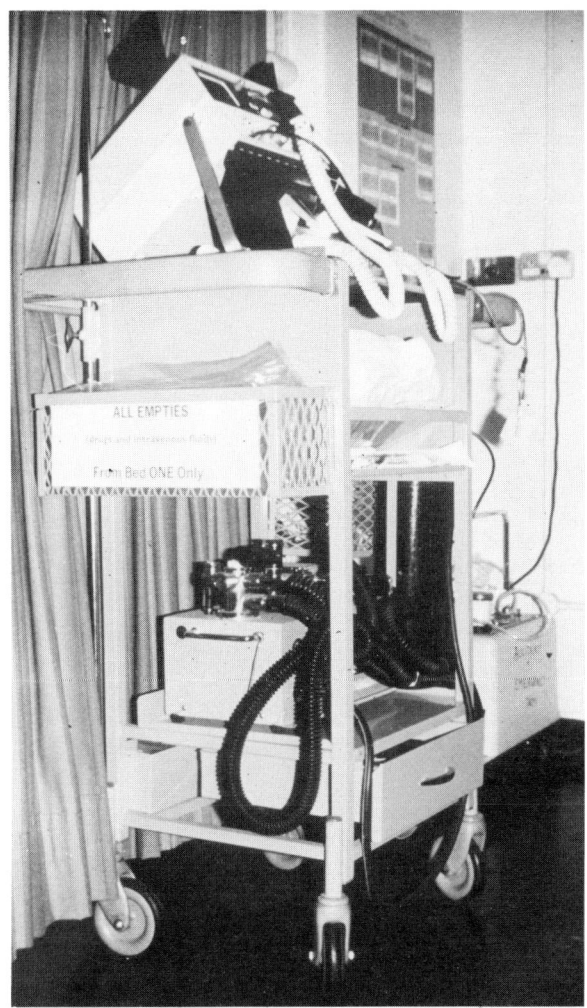

Fig 44.10 Convenient method for checking empties from an individual bed.

Respiratory problems

An external examination of the chest, which must include the back, may reveal bruises, clothing imprints or friction burns. This can help to determine the direction and severity of the injuring agent. Large open sucking wounds must be made airtight by the application of large dressings. Smaller lacerations may also penetrate the parietal pleura, and the site of all such lesions should be noted. The pattern of breathing may be paradoxical in the presence of a flail rib segment, or be decreased unilaterally with a pneumothorax. These signs may not be present initially due to the slow onset of some complications of chest injury. Repeated physical examination is essential.

Arterial blood gas analysis should be performed in all patients with a chest injury. Apparently minor degrees of paradoxical respiration may cause significant hypoxaemia. This can be reversed by endotracheal intubation and intermittent positive pressure ventilation with oxygen enriched air.

Mediastinal shift due to a pneumothorax may be detected clinically by deviation of the trachea in the suprasternal notch and displacement of the apex beat. Careful palpation of the chest wall may identify sites of suspected rib fracture and the presence of surgical emphysema. The latter is a most useful sign as it may precede other evidence of damage to air containing structures (usually the lung or oesophagus). Impaired lung function will be assessed initially on the degree of central cyanosis and the respiratory rate. However, sequential measurements of arterial blood gas concentrations and the tidal and minute volumes will be more valuable in measuring subsequent progress.

In the initial period of resuscitation, the presence of a tension pneumothorax must be considered, if central cyanosis and dyspnoea persist despite adequate oxygenation through a clear airway, and the stabilisation of any flail segments. Venous return is impaired, the central venous pressure is high and cardiac output falls. Usually the abnormal side is evident and a chest drain is inserted as described in Table 11. In an emergency an ordinary needle will quickly reduce the intrapleural pressure. If there is any uncertainty as to the presence or side of a pneumothorax, a trial tap should be performed initially. In the short term, it is acceptable and indeed most convenient to attach the drain to a Heimlich valve (Fig 44.11). These tend to block with blood and it is advisable to change to an underwater seal later.

Intermittent positive pressure ventilation increases the tendency for a small pneumothorax to enlarge and 'tension'. It is sound practice to insert bilateral chest drains in any seriously injured patient who is to be ventilated whenever there is the slightest suggestion of a pneumothorax. (Fig 44.12.)

When the chest is crushed petechial haemorrhages may develop over the upper chest and face. This *traumatic asphyxia syndrome* is caused by retrograde venous flow from the right side of the heart. No treatment is necessary and the prognosis is good if there is no associated structural damage. However, extensive crushing of the chest will cause lung contusion and alveolar collapse, leading to severe respiratory embarassment. Unfortunately, there are few signs initially to suggest lung damage, and it may be a few hours before pulmonary oedema·develops. A similar sequence of events may follow exposure to blast and toxic vapours. A knowledge of the nature of the accident will be useful

Table 11
HOW TO INSERT A CHEST DRAIN

Side	Determined clinically – *see text* In emergency don't wait for chest x-ray If in doubt, especially when positive pressure respiration is to be used, insert bilateral drains
Site	A Mid clavicular line, second intercostal space (especially useful for pneumothorax) B Mid axillary line, sixth intercostal space (especially useful for haemothorax) C Other sites as determined by chest x-ray when pleural, adhesions restrict lung collapse
1*	Using surgical gloves and drapes infiltrate local anaesthetic down to the parietal pleura. Aspiration of air bubbles confirms pleural puncture
2*	Insert loose purse string suture around intended incision
3	2 cm incision down to parietal pleura
4	Insert chest drain with trochar. In adult use at least 20 G. Maximum depth 8 cm initially – use flange or calibrations on drain
5	Remove trochar and attach Heimlich valve quickly.
6	Advance drain up to 20 cm, tie securely with purse string and cover wound with water-proof dressing
7	Check position of drain on x-ray.

* Omit in emergency

in these circumstances. Patients at risk must be admitted and their arterial blood gases monitored. Bronchodilators given by nebuliser with oxygen are very useful in such cases.

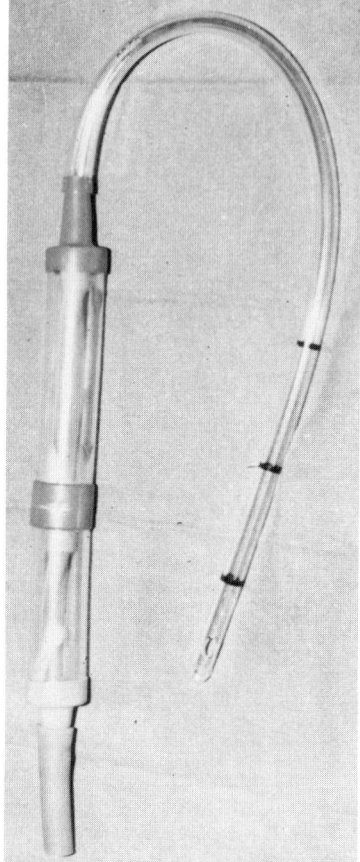

Fig 44.11 Heimlich valve.

Cardiovascular problems

Damage to the heart and great vessels may be inflicted by gunshot or by stabbing or may be produced by sudden changes in velocity, as for example in high speed transport accidents and in falls from buildings. Often the injury will remain undetected. The paucity of specific signs precludes early and precise diagnosis in the majority of patients. These difficulties could be considered to be of little importance if rapid deterioration and death were inevitable with most injuries to heart and great vessels. However, this popular belief is not borne out by fact. Many serious injuries remain latent for hours or even weeks and it is now possible to provide advanced cardiovascular support for such patients until a cardiac team can be assembled. The major stumbling block to establishing a diagnosis still appears to be lack of appreciation that a patient with a pulse can, nevertheless, have an injured heart or a transected aorta.

Cardiac injuries

Ventricular rupture is usually immediately fatal, but survival after rupture of the atrial or septal wall is recorded (Parmley et al., 1958). Valvular lesions produce variable signs of heart failure and can be identified by contrast radiography (Kimbler, 1977). Cardiac contusion and disturbances in conduction are much more common, though largely unrecognised. High frequency analysis of ECGs of such patients has shown abnormalities not recognised on conventional recordings. Cardiac scanning after ^{99m}Tc injection reveals a high incidence of cardiac contusion after chest injury. Although the majority of such patients do not develop important complications, cardiac dysrhythmias and cardiogenic shock may occur. Continuous cardiac monitoring is advisable.

A haemopericardium is frequently associated with these injuries and, depending on the speed of formation, may produce tamponade. The clinical presenta-

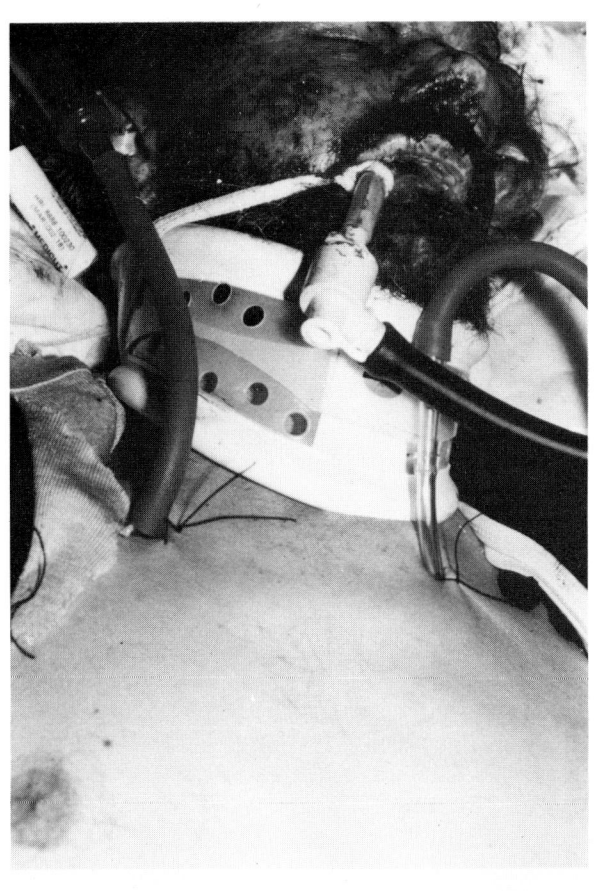

Fig 44.12 Bilateral chest drains for pneumothorax.

stages of resuscitation. The diagnosis is usually made because the clinician suspects it and finds, in the patient, a rapidly rising central venous pressure. Treatment in the resuscitation area includes aspiration of the pericardial sac and circulatory support. Definitive treatment of the underlying condition may be required subsequently as a matter of great urgency. Aspiration is best done with the patient semi-recumbent. A wide bore needle is inserted just to the left of the xiphisternum and aimed at the right shoulder. An ECG lead connected to the needle may help determine the position of the needle tip (Pories and Gaudiani, 1975).

Aortic injuries

Immediate survival after aortic injury is dependent on the formation of an acute false aneurysm. The intima and media rupture, most commonly at the level of the isthmus, but the adventitia and adjacent mediastinal structures may provide a sufficiently strong sheath to contain the arterial pressure for a few hours or indeed many years. These injuries can be occasionally overlooked at thoracotomy because of a normal external appearance of the aorta. In one series, only 50% of patients found to have aortic rupture, at thoracotomy had presented with clinical signs of hypovolaemic shock (Mattox *et al.*, 1978); but, significantly, all had sustained multiple injuries. Precordial pain is not commonly associated with aortic injury. Pain radiating to the back is more significant.

Inequalities in upper limb and neck pulses and blood pressure may be observed if the injury involves the aortic arch. Aortic obstruction causing proximal hypertension and systolic murmur has also been described. A plain chest radiograph will usually show a widened mediastinum (>8 cm on AP film taken at 100 cm), but this may be obscured by coincidental lung injury. The trachea is usually displaced to the right, and the left main bronchus depressed. The aortic knob may be absent and there may be separation of calcium deposits in the aortic wall. Aortography is essential to confirm the site and nature of an aortic rupture preoperatively (Keen, 1972). The retrograde femoral route is quite safe in these patients.

tion may be insidious or dramatic. Many signs have been attributed to a pericardial effusion. Pulsus paradoxus (falling blood pressure and flow during inspiration) is usually present and may be so marked that the pulse disappears on full inspiration. Unfortunately, Beck's Triad – falling arterial pressure, rising venous pressure and a 'small quiet heart' – may be modified by coincidental injuries. ECG and chest radiographs do not show pathognomonic changes in most cases. Echocardiography is the most accurate means of diagnosis (Horowitz *et al.*, 1974), but is rarely used in the early

Chest wall injuries

Hypovolaemia may develop in a patient with chest injury as a result of damage to the intercostal arteries associated with rib fractures. This is the usual cause of the haemothorax which may accompany a traumatic pneumothorax. Conservative treatment with one or two (apical and basal) chest drains is indicated. Whereas bleeding from a minor lung laceration will usually stop if the lung collapses, bleeding from the chest wall may continue.

Management will vary depending on the speed of development of the haemopneumothorax. Chest wall lacerations must be explored under good anaesthesia. Most will be found to penetrate the parietal pleura, but previous pleurisy and adhesions may prevent the appearance of lung collapse. In such instances delayed pneumothorax has been reported so it is important to repeat examination and chest radiographs regularly in the first few days after injury. Thoracotomy is indicated after any stab injury if bleeding continues at a rapid rate, or if a large bronchopleural fistula has developed preventing resolution of a tension pneumothorax.

Initial treatment is based on clinical examination alone. Subsequent radiological examination should be restricted to an erect chest film. An antero-posterior film taken with the patient supine is of very limited value. A haemothorax may be missed because blood collects in the paravertebral gutter without a demonstrable fluid level (Figs 44.13 and 44.14).

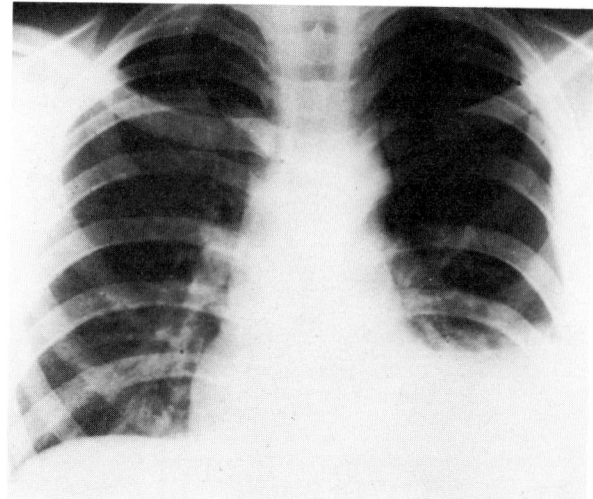

Fig 44.13 Supine chest x-ray. Haemopneumothorax: blood in paravertebral gutter.

Initial management of abdominal injuries

Injuries to the abdomen may be remarkably painless in the initial stages, in contrast to injuries of the chest and limbs, which are usually associated with bone fracture and considerable pain. However, when these latter injuries occur, the abdomen is frequently injured also – particularly after deceleration/acceleration incidents. Consequently, it is possible to overlook an abdominal injury. Those involved in such accidents should be assumed to have sustained occult abdominal injury and the history, examination and monitoring should be directed at its exclusion. At least one large bore intravenous line is established and measures taken to prevent hypovolaemic shock as discussed on p. 714.

Paralytic ileus may occur after extra-abdominal injury and is particularly common in children with head injury. Much of the resulting distention can be avoided by passing a nasogastric tube. If this is of wide bore, it will remove also partially digested food and reduce the risk of its aspiration into the lungs.

Small lacerations on the abdominal wall may represent stab wounds. Although they may appear superficial, they usually penetrate the peritoneum. Injury to the intestine and mesentery may not be accompanied by the rapid clinical deterioration usually associated with stab wounds to the liver, spleen, or major vessels. Indiscriminate laparotomy in all these patients has an associated morbidity which can be reduced by a selective approach. All patients are admitted for observation, although a significant proportion will settle spon-

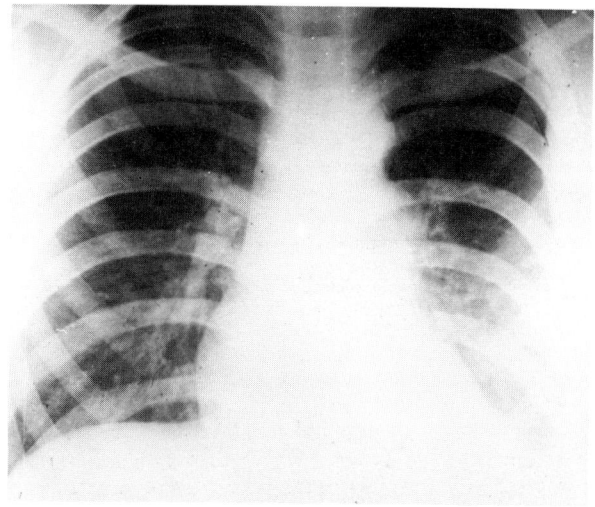

Fig 44.14 Erect chest x-ray. Haemopneumothorax: demonstrable fluid level.

taneously. The delay before laparotomy in other cases has not been shown to influence outcome adversely (London, 1979). Preoperative administration of antibiotics is recommended to reduce the risk of septic shock when bowel perforation is suspected.

The indications for laparotomy after blunt abdominal trauma are less well defined. The details of the accident should be sought. From this, and an examination of the clothing and skin, it may be possible to determine the direction and approximate force of the injuring agent. Clothing imprints on the anterior abdominal wall suggest a blunt impact, which commonly causes damage to relatively immobile structures such as liver, spleen, duodenum and pancreas (Fig 44.15).

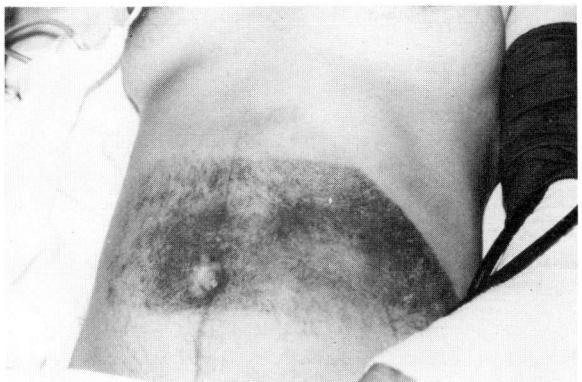

Fig 44.15   Clothing imprint on anterior abdominal wall.

Renal damage can be produced in this way, and from rear impact, with damage to the lumbar transverse processes (Fig 44.16) and paravertebral muscles (Fig 44.17). The latter may lead the patient to flex his hip joints and experience pain on attempted hip extension. Urinalysis to detect haematuria must be carried out routinely in all patients with abdominal injuries. Whenever renal damage is suspected, an intravenous urogram must precede exploration. Indications for laparotomy after blunt trauma are listed in Table 12. The decision to operate may be taken with confidence when there are compelling physical signs. Occasionally, however, the general condition of the patient will be so good that equivocal local signs will not be sufficient to warrant anything other than continued observation.

There are many patients between these extremes in whom it is difficult to determine the correct line of management. Problems arise particularly if there is an associated head injury, or the patient is thought to be intoxicated or abusing drugs. When there are other very major injuries threatening survival and the resuscitation team is undecided as to whether to abandon or redouble their efforts, some information on the state of the abdomen can be most valuable in formulating an overall plan of care. Abdominal paracentesis was advocated to improve diagnostic accuracy in these 'intermediate' and 'extreme' cases, but has fallen into disrepute because of the high frequency of false negative taps. Peritoneal lavage has replaced it in popularity (Gill *et al.*, 1975). The technique is outlined in Table 13. Figure 44.18 shows a patient with lower limb injuries and abdominal grazing – a negative lavage demonstrated that the low CVP was due to skeletal rather than abdominal blood loss. False negatives have been reported, particularly with diaphragmatic and pel-

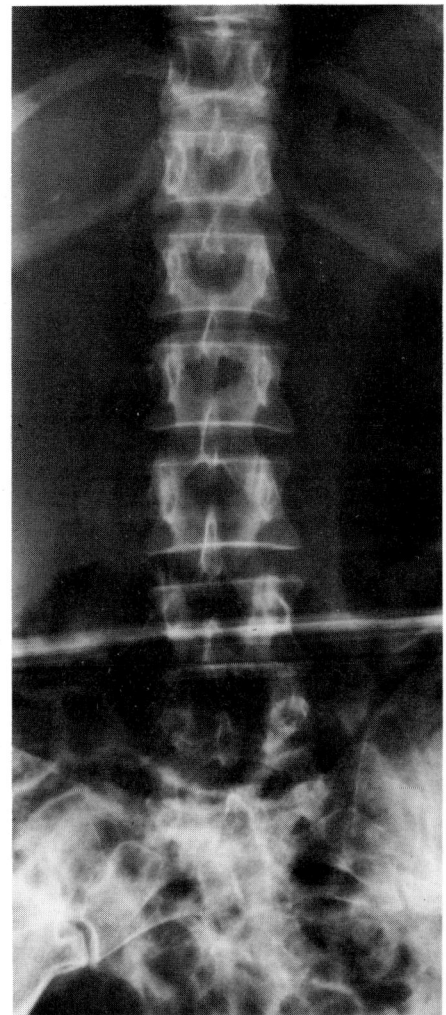

Fig 44.16   Fractured lumbar transverse processes.

vic injuries, but are relatively uncommon. Iatrogenic damage to bowel, and false positives due to blood vessel damage during insertion are also rare but have led some to introduce the catheter under direct vision at a 'mini-laparotomy', but this procedure may occasionally produce local complications. Lazarus and Nelson (1979) have suggested introducing the catheter over a floppy wire previously passed down an 18G needle and claim no complication with this method.

Pregnancy

Abdominal injury in pregnant women is unusual. Maternal behaviour probably reduces exposure to

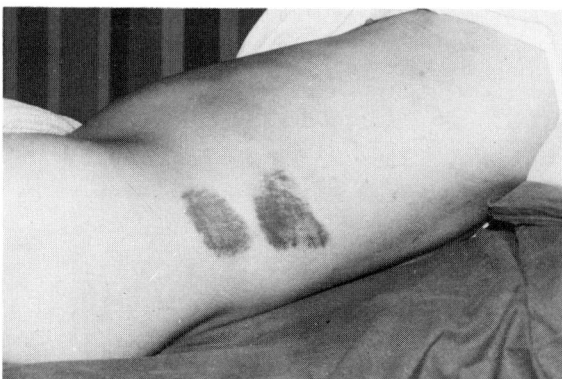

Fig 44.17 Signs of damage to paravertebral muscles.

Table 12
INDICATIONS FOR LAPAROTOMY AFTER
BLUNT ABDOMINAL TRAUMA

1 Shock persisting or recurring, with clinical evidence of abdominal injury
2 Free gas
3 Increasing girth (not due to acute gastric distention)
4 Increasing peritonism
5 Shoulder pain, fractured lower rib and hypochondrial pain

dangerous environments and extra protection is afforded by the gravid uterus. However, when blunt trauma does occur, it presents diagnostic problems. Signs of intraperitoneal bleeding tend to be reduced or modified. The maternal circulation is protected somewhat by the physiological hypervolaemia, but the fetus is very vulnerable to anoxia. Diagnostic peritoneal lavage has been shown to be just as accurate in pregnancy. In late pregnancy it may be necessary to insert the catheter above the umbilicus, but no other modifications or problems have been reported. Buchsaum (1968) has reviewed all aspects of accidental injury in pregnancy.

Initial management of pelvic injuries

The pelvis is fractured frequently in patients with multiple injuries. Gross instability can be detected clinically and is very painful, but minor fractures of the pubis or ischium may be masked by more severe pain from other injuries. Comminuted fractures of the lateral and posterior parts of the pelvic ring and those

Table 13
DIAGNOSTIC PERITONEAL LAVAGE

Procedure
1 Plain abdominal x-ray (to exclude free gas)
2 Catheterise bladder
3 Anaesthetise skin in midline 5 cm below umbilicus
4 Introduce catheter towards pelvis, with trochar, or under direct vision
5 Flush in 500 ml warm isotonic saline
6 Turn patient, allow to mix for 20 min
7 Drain off fluid, avoiding airlocks

Positive result
1 At 4 above; heavily blood stained non-clotting fluid
2 At 7 above – PVC $> 1\%$
$\quad$ – $> 100\,000$ RBC/CC
$\quad$ – > 17.5 μ/ml amylase
3 Lavage fluid exits from other sites (e.g. bladder catheter, chest drain)

associated with central dislocation of the hip joint will result in severe blood loss from the pelvic veins. Damage to the femoral vessels by bone fragments from more anterior fractures is less common and the resulting haemorrhage usually self-limiting. However, anterior fractures may be associated with injury to the urethra and bladder. Damage to the bladder is more common if it is full at the time of the accident.

A plain antero-posterior radiograph of the pelvis is an essential part of the initial assessment of the multiply injured patient. Frequently a totally unsuspected fracture is thereby identified.

The first priority in management is to treat the associated hypovolaemic shock. This is discussed in detail on p. 714. Immobilisation of a very unstable pelvic fracture should be attempted using sandbags and an encircling inelastic bandage.

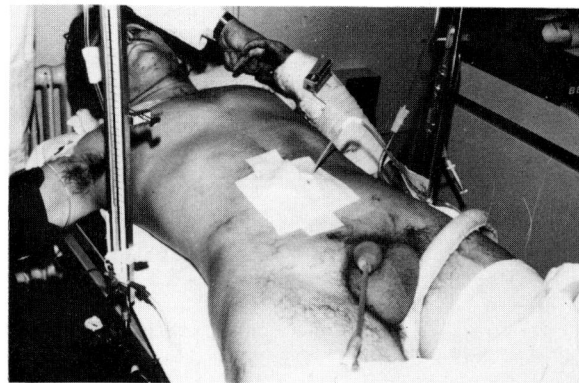

Fig 44.18 Peritoneal lavage of a patient with lower limb injuries, abdominal grazing and minor head injury.

Catheterisation of the bladder has been recommended previously as a routine procedure in the initial period of resuscitation. When injury to the genito-urinary tract is suspected, this manoeuvre must be preceded by careful examination of the external urethral meatus and perineum, and by a rectal examination. Blood at the meatal tip is pathognomonic of urethral injury. In males the 'missing prostate' sign on rectal examination suggests that a complete rupture of the membranous urethra has allowed the bladder to draw the prostate up into the abdomen. More commonly, injuries involve only part of the urethral wall and management must be directed towards preserving the remaining urothelial continuity. A clumsy urethral catheterisation will usually complete a partial urethral rupture and pave the way for long-term stricture formation and its attendant complications. On the other hand the gentle introduction of a small catheter per urethram by a skilled clinician is quite safe in most cases. If any obstruction is encountered the procedure is abandoned. Metal introducers and force must be avoided. Useful information about the position of the catheter during introduction can be obtained by simultaneous rectal or vaginal examination. However, if urethral damage is thought to be extensive or the skills of a suitably experienced clinician are not available, it is essential to insert a suprapubic catheter and leave the urethra alone. Once the bladder has been catheterised contrast radiography is used to determine the extent of any bladder injury (Clarke and Prudencio, 1972).

Perineal injuries may be overlooked either because the area is not examined or because the significance of small lacerations is not appreciated. Apparently trivial lacerations in this area can be very deep and may communicate with the peritoneal cavity. Whenever the full extent of a perineal injury cannot be determined with ease, a full exploration under general anaesthetic is essential. This should not be carried out in the resuscitation area as it may be necessary to proceed to laparotomy and colostomy. To reduce the risk of gas gangrene and septic shock, prophylactic benzyl penicillin, a broad spectrum antibiotic and metronidazole should be started at the earliest opportunity.

Initial management of head and neck injuries

Head injuries

The initial objectives of head injury management are to prevent the development of complications and to determine, if possible, the nature of the underlying lesion. These aspects are discussed at this stage to emphasise their importance within the more general context of primary resuscitation. A full account of head injury management will be found in Chapter 45.

Unconsciousness may not be a direct consequence of injury. Indeed, the onset of coma may have caused the accident. Known diabetics should be given 20 ml 50% glucose into a large vein to exclude hypoglycaemia as the cause of unconsciousness. Blood should be withdrawn for subsequent analysis before infusion of glucose. Knowledge of the presenting blood glucose level aids later management of the unconscious diabetic. Breath alcohol estimations should be obtained if alcohol abuse is suspected. However, it is unwise to attribute neurological signs to alcohol intoxication below 300 mg% breath alcohol.

Prevention of complications

It is useful to distinguish between 'primary brain injuries' which are produced at the time of impact and 'secondary brain injuries' which may develop later (Fig 44.19). Many of the secondary lesions are avoidable (Rose *et al.*, 1977). Vasogenic brain oedema is the most important secondary brain injury to concern the resuscitation team. Its development as a direct consequence of injury can be exacerbated in various ways. Inadequate airway control will produce hypercarbia and acidosis, leading to cerebral vasodilatation and a rise in intracerebral pressure. Epileptic fits cause a rapid rise in central venous pressure and impair gas exchange in the lungs. Laryngeal stridor, often associated with poor airway control and unsuccessful endotracheal intubation has a similar effect. Intracranial venous pressure rises and oedema formation increases. These pressure changes can be monitored by subdural or extradural

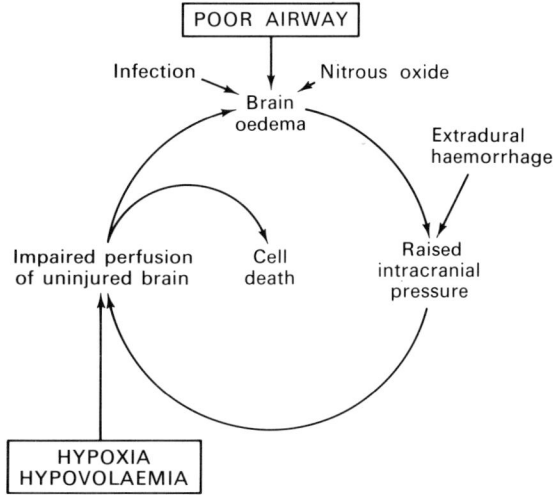

Fig 44.19 Effects of secondary brain injuries.

transducers (McDowall, 1976). While not appropriate to the emergency resuscitation area this should be considered when the patient is transferred to the intensive care unit.

To prevent the tendency to develop high intracranial pressure, it is necessary to have immaculate control of the airway and treat convulsions promptly with intravenous valium. The nitrous oxide/oxygen mixture 'Entonox' has been found to produce a rise in intracranial pressure, thought to be due to a cerebral vasodilatory action. This gas should not be used as an analgesic in head injured patients.

The administration of very high doses of dexamethazone (e.g. 48 mg) is claimed to reduce cerebral oedema after severe head injury. Animal work shows best results with pretreatment, and in clinical practice very early treatment seems to be important. However, the effect is not as dramatic as in patients with tumours and many remain sceptical about the value of steroids in head injured patients.

There is no disagreement, however, about the effect of hyperventilation. The resulting lowered Pco_2 and raised Po_2 are independently beneficial, although excessive lowering of Pco_2 (<20 mmHg) is detrimental, causing cerebral ischaemia.

The use of osmotically active agents such as mannitol should be considered only as a temporary expedient when the above methods of reducing oedema have failed and early neurosurgical intervention is planned. Mannitol does not reduce oedema, it causes a fall in intracranial pressure by dehydrating healthy brain tissue.

'Secondary brain injury' can also be caused by hypovolaemic shock. A low blood pressure should not be attributed to a head injury unless there are massive scalp lacerations or a large haematoma in an infant. Usually the cause of the hypovolaemia can be found elsewhere. Its correction will improve the oxygen supply to the uninjured parts of the brain and move the potential for recovery towards the limits set by the primary brain injury.

The most frequently quoted, though uncommon, secondary brain injury results from compression of uninjured brain by an expanding extradural haematoma. The identification of such a lesion has been made much easier with the development of computerised axial tomography and some authorities recommend installation of this equipment in A & E departments. A full discussion of the diagnosis and management of intracerebral haematoma will be found in Chapter 45.

Intracerebral infection may complicate a compound skull fracture, be it a vault fracture with overlying scalp laceration, or basal fracture extending into an air sinus, the middle ear or nasopharynx. Patients with such injuries should receive intramuscular injections of penicillin and sulphonamide whilst in the A & E department to reduce the chance of this complication.

Assessment

The secondary component having been thus identified and hopefully reduced, attention is focussed on assessment. This has been facilitated by the recent introduction of coma scales, but, inevitably, the more precise and detailed the observations that they require, the more difficult it is to ensure that th information is obtained and recorded. The Glasgow Coma Scale (Teasdale and Jennett, 1974) appears to have overcome this problem and is now used in many centres in Europe and North America. Clinical progress can be observed from the chart at a glance (Fig 44.20). Subjective interobserver error is minimal.

The scalp should be examined for lacerations and haematoma, and the ears and nose for evidence of CSF leak. An auroscope may introduce infection and must not be used. Scalp haematoma can appear very rapidly (e.g. on the forehead of young children) or much more slowly (e.g. in hypothermia) and be hidden by a mass of blood soaked hair. Repeated examination is essential. The external appearance of the scalp can give valuable information about the nature of the injuring force and help to explain the nature of the underlying brain injury.

Information obtained from radiographs of the skull does not influence the primary resuscitation of the patient with head injury. Good quality radiographs are, of course, important because of the association between skull fracture and brain injury. However, the reversible sequelae of brain injuries are not fatal within minutes of the injury. Very rarely will a patient, with a head injury amenable to neurosurgical correction, die from his brain injury within the first hour. Prevention of secondary injury in this hour may well be life saving, but does not require skull radiographs for its accomplishment. Those who die despite such care will usually have primary irreversible brain damage.

Cervical spine injuries

Injury to the cervical spine is sustained frequently when the moving head strikes a stationary object – as in the majority of road traffic accidents and falls. It is less common when the immobile head is struck by a moving object such as a falling roof tile or during an assault.

When injury has occurred, it is unlikely that the force of impact will have rendered the cervical vertebrae grossly unstable yet left the spinal cord intact. However, a difficult endotracheal intubation or excessive flexion and rotation of the neck may further damage partially torn ligaments, producing instability and cord damage where neither existed previously. It is wise, therefore, to stabilise the cervical spine with a semi-rigid collar in all multiply injured and head

COMA SCALE		Date								
		Time								
EYES OPEN Eyes closed by swelling = C	Spontaneously									
	To speech									
	To pain									
	None									
BEST VERBAL RESPONSE Endotracheal tube or tracheostomy = T	Orientated									
	Confused									
	Inappropriate words									
	Incomprehensible sounds									
	None									
BEST MOTOR RESPONSE	Obey commands									
	Localise pain									
	Flexion to pain									
	Extension to pain									
	None									

Fig 44.20 The Glasgow coma scale (*see also* p. 747).

injured patients before they are moved. When this has been done it is unusual for neurological deterioration to occur and when it does, it may well have a vascular rather than a traumatic aetiology. However, some centres consider that urgent decompression and stabilisation of cervical cord injuries is beneficial. The advantages of such treatment are not universally accepted at present. The resuscitation team should be aware of the policy of the regional spinal injuries unit on this matter.

Soft tissue injuries to the neck

Lacerations of the neck are often deeper than a casual examination might suggest. The airway may be compressed by an enlarging haematoma, creating difficulties in endotracheal intubation. Direct damage to the pharynx, larynx or trachea may demand early tracheostomy. Prompt attention to the airway in this manner must be followed by prevention of massive bleeding by direct pressure. The usual practice of 'elevating the bleeding part' must be avoided because of the danger of air embolism. Any attempt to arrest arterial bleeding by the application of haemostats will usually fail in its objective and nearly always cause further damage.

Vascular injuries in the neck may remain clinically occult for many hours or days and cannot be excluded by the palpation of a normal carotid pulse. The exploration of such wounds under local anaesthetic in the resuscitation area may produce catastrophic haemorrhage. The main difficulty is to decide which wounds should be merely closed and observed and which are worthy of full exploration in a well equipped theatre after arteriography and the cross matching of blood. Some advocate routine exploration of all wounds which penetrate the platysma. Others are more conservative, operating only when there is definite evidence of deep structure injury. It is claimed that exploration when there is circumstantial but not necessarily conclusive evidence of injury to major vessels or oesophagus reduces the number of unnecessary operations yet prevents delay in the repair of major injuries.

Initial management of limb injuries

The sight of a compound tibial fracture has a much greater emotional impact on the rescuer than the subtle deterioration of an unconscious patient who is bleeding from a ruptured spleen. The dangers inherent in the disparity between first impressions and actual threat to life must be appreciated by all those concerned with the initial management of patients with multiple injuries. Before examining the injured limb, it is essential to secure the airway and examine the chest, to establish an intravenous line and assess the extent of hypovolaemic shock, and to protect the cervical spine. Thereafter, assessment and initial management of limb injuries is relatively straightforward when contrasted with the problems posed by injuries elsewhere.

Circulation

The most important immediate effects of limb trauma are local and systemic alterations in the cardiovascular system. Local blood loss is particularly important in lower limb injuries (Table 7). Systemic effects are related to the pain produced by fractures. Pain impairs the normal CNS response to circulatory fluid loss and thereby reduces the effectiveness of peripheral vasoconstriction and the maintenance of a core circulation.

The blood supply to the distal part of the injured limb may be jeopardised if there has been damage to the main vessels by spikes of bone, stab wounds or shearing forces. Distal pulses, capillary circulation and venous drainage must be assessed routinely in all limb injuries. This is particularly important in relation to injuries around the elbow and knee.

Not all arterial injuries are produced by direct trauma. High velocity gunshot wounds may cause intimal damage and occlusion at some distance from the bullet track, leaving the adventitia and media intact (*see* chapter 46).

Bleeding into a confined fascial compartment, such as that containing the pretibial muscles, will restrict venous return and, eventually, arterial supply. The swelling of contused muscles within such compartments following crushing injuries will have a similar effect. An early and extensive fasciotomy is essential to reduce extramural pressure and permit flow through undamaged vessels.

All limb injuries producing major vascular occlusion should be explored within 4 hours.

Splintage

Mobile fractures are painful, continue to promote blood loss from damaged muscle and possibly increase the subsequent risk of fat embolism. Early splintage reduces these complications. Strapping the upper limb to the trunk or the lower limb to its fellow is adequate as a first aid measure, but should be replaced with definitive splintage as soon as possible, and certainly on arrival at hospital.

Upper limb fractures can be held between two rigid gutter splints, which are then bound together and held in a sling. Femoral shaft fractures should be immobilised in a Thomas's Splint or one of the more easily

applied derivatives. Skin traction is adequate as a first aid measure. Application of the splint can be carried out with minimal additional discomfort if the patient breathes Entonox and steady manual traction is applied to the limb. Manipulating the leg without traction allows the bone ends to come together and is extremely painful. Tibial fractures should be stabilised on a rigid posterior support extending from mid-thigh to toes.

Inflatable splints and vacuum splints are easy to apply, particularly to lower leg and forearm fractures, and are popular with some rescue services. It is important that the former are not over inflated, thereby impeding the blood supply. This is unlikely to happen if they are blown up by mouth. A foot or hand pump should not be used. Technical problems with both types or splint are common. One or two carefully applied malleable backsplints can give as much support at a fraction of the cost.

Soft tissues

Some closed fractures may distort the soft tissues and press up under the skin. This is particularly common in ankle fractures (Fig 44.21). Immediate reduction of such fractures will prevent skin necrosis and thereby simplify subsequent treatment, which usually involves internal fixation.

Two other aspects of soft tissue injury are of concern to those working in the resuscitation area.

Contused open wounds provide a good culture medium for bacteria. The viability of the area around the wound, and indeed of the whole limb, may be jeopardised if all dead tissue and foreign material is not removed. This will be done in the operating theatre, but early recognition is important so that priorities can be determined and appropriate antibiotics started. Prevention of tetanus is similarly achieved by a combina-

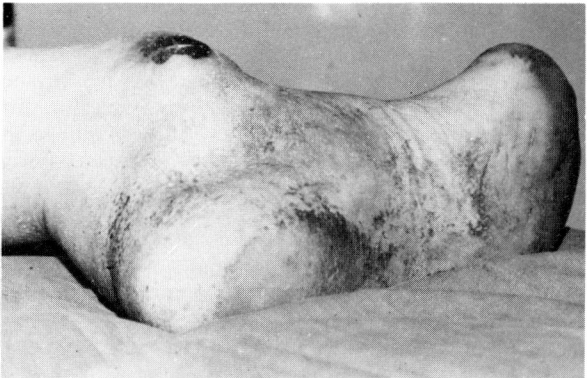

Fig 44.21 Ankle fracture dislocation with distortion of overlying tissues.

tion of excision of all dead tissue and injection of anti-tetanus toxoid or human immunoglobulin as appropriate (Table 14) (Smith *et al.*, 1975). Many contused and contaminated wounds will be left open after initial toilet, to allow tissue oedema to develop and then resolve, without increasing interstitial pressures or impairing the blood supply.

Table 14
PREVENTION OF TETANUS
The most **effective** way to prevent tetanus is to remove all dead tissue and clean the wound thoroughly.

	Additional treatment	
Immune status	*If clean wound* No contusion No penetration < 6 hours old	*All other wounds*
Good	Nil	Nil
Fair	Toxoid booster	Toxoid booster
Poor	Toxoid booster	Toxoid booster plus HTI
Bad or unknown	Toxoid course	Toxoid course plus HTI

NOTES
Good = Complete course of toxoid or booster within previous 5 years.
Fair = Complete course of toxoid booster between 5 and 10 years ago.
Poor = Complete course of toxoid or booster more than 10 years ago.
Bad = Never had toxoid course or booster.
HTI = Human tetanus immunoglobulin.

Finally a careful examination of nerve and tendon function must be conducted and the results recorded prior to anaesthesia.

Pain relief

Pain modifies the normal CNS response to circulatory fluid loss, reducing the peripheral vasoconstriction which is so essential for the maintenance of a core circulation. Unpleasant sights, disturbing noises and emotional distress may have a similar effect. Reduction of the pain and relief of the anxiety associated with trauma has, therefore, a pathophysiological as well as a compassionate base.

The injured patient should be sheltered from the chaos and conflict which can permeate the accident scene. Evacuation to hospital should be quick but controlled. A calm approach to resuscitation will reassure the patient and create an atmosphere which is conducive to good decision making.

Major limb fractures are a potent cause of pain and should be immobilised as soon as possible. When there is suspicion of a spinal injury, extraction of the patient is made much safer and less painful if a spinal board or cervical collar is applied.

Analgesia may be used regionally or generally. Infiltration of local anaesthetic around a limb fracture has been advocated, but is usually only successful in the hand. Regional anaesthesia for limb trauma may not be appropriate to the initial resuscitation phase, requiring a standard of patient cooperation and a period free from interruption rarely available at this stage of treatment. However, low brachial plexus blocks may be useful in upper limb trauma. Intercostal blockade will reduce the pain associated with rib fractures and will improve lung function.

Opiates produce the most effective general analgesia. However, they must not be used in patients with multiple injuries until the clinical state of the patient is established and a series of base line recordings of cardiorespiratory function are obtained. Their respiratory depressant properties, influence on pupil size and effect on the level of consciousness make them unsuitable at any stage in the management of head and chest injuries. In other patients, and in those with only trivial head injuries, opiates should be given by titration, in small intravenous doses. An intramuscular injection is dangerous. It will not be absorbed initially being washed into the systemic circulation later when the muscle capillary beds open up, producing unexpected hypotension and respiratory depression.

If the patient has sustained limb fractures but there is no possibility of injury to the head or trunk, intravenous opiates can be used immediately. However, it is usually impossible to exclude such injuries within the first hour after a transport accident or a fall. The immediate administration of intravenous opiates is best reserved for relatively low velocity injuries where a good consecutive account of the accident is given by the patient – for example a tibial fracture sustained on the football field.

Pentazocine has less respiratory and CNS depressant effects than the opiates, but its analgesic effect is variable and sometimes disappointing. It has not found wide acceptance in the management of pain during the early resuscitation phase after injury.

Entonox – a mixture of equal volumes of nitrous oxide and oxygen – has become popular in recent years as an inhalational analgesic for use at the scene of the accident and during resuscitation in hospital. The administration set popularly used incorporates a demand valve preventing release of the gas until the patient creates a negative pressure at the mouthpiece. It has the advantage of rapid action and rapid excretion, but its analgesic properties are inferior to those of the opiates. There is some evidence that nitrous oxide raises intracranial pressure, presumably by producing cerebral vasodilation. This would appear to preclude its use in head injured patients.

Radiographs

The initial stabilisation of the cardiorespiratory system does not involve radiography. The x-ray department is a dangerous place for the injured patient and he should not be introduced to it until basic resuscitation has been completed (Table 15). Even if x-ray equipment is available in the resuscitation area, emergency

Table 15
RESUSCITATION AND RADIOGRAPHS

Time	X-ray
During stabilisation of cardiorespiratory system	None
After basic resuscitation	Erect chest
	Pelvis
	Cervical spine
Before leaving resuscitation area	Skull
	Lumbar spine
	Long bones
	Abdomen
Later	Distal limbs
	Minor joints

management should be based on clinical judgement and not await the development of radiographs. For example, a deformed and painful thigh is placed in a Thomas's splint with the help of an inhalational analgesic and a drip is set up before radiographs are taken.

Later management may be influenced by radiological findings. An erect chest film may show a haemothorax, pneumothorax or unsuspected rib fractures. The film most probably will have been taken anteroposteriorly and some magnification of mediastinal structures is to be expected, but the possibility of great vessel or cardiac injury should be considered (*see* p. 720). A supine film is of much less value, in particular it will not show a haemothorax (Figs 44.13 and 44.14). Early radiographs will not reveal any evidence of the profound changes in perfusion and ventilation which occur after lung contusion. This again emphasises the secondary role of radiology in resuscitation.

Pelvic and cervical spine films must be obtained in all cases of multiple trauma and can be taken at the same time as the erect chest film. Fractures in these areas may not be suspected clinically, but their discovery will, naturally, have an immediate influence on management. There is no such association between radiological investigation and emergency management of injuries to the skull and limbs. Here clinical observations will dictate initial management. If a skull table is not immediately available, it may be wise to wait until the patient can be moved with safety to a neuroradiology suite. In any event, stress views of the cervical spine and views of the base of the skull must not be taken

without expert advice, as the manipulation required may damage the cervical cord.

Detailed radiography has much to offer the patient with multiple injuries after the initial resuscitation phase. An authoritative review of the available techniques has been compiled by Ayella (1978).

Secondary transport

The concept of regional centres with specialist interests is now firmly established in neurosurgery, spinal injuries, burns, thoracic surgery and microsurgery. Increasingly, patients are moved from the receiving hospital to such centres either by ambulance or helicopter. This 'secondary transport' can be planned more carefully than can the primary movement of the patient from the accident scene. The key to success is thorough preparation before the journey and comprehensive monitoring en route.

Hypothermia and trauma

Temperature and injury are related in various ways. The metabolic and clinical responses to trauma are modified by core temperature (Stoner, 1976). Conversely, these responses tend to alter the temperature gradients between core and periphery. Thirdly, exposure after injury and the intravenous transfusion of cold fluids have a significant effect on core temperature.

When core temperature falls, fluid shifts from the plasma space into the extracellular space and eventually into the intracellular space. If intravenous fluids are used during the rewarming phase there is a danger of fluid overload. Below 32°C cardiac dysrrhythmias are common – particularly ventricular fibrillation. External signs of injury, such as bruises, haematomas and grazes are very slow to develop at low temperature. Depressed cerebral function further confuses the clinical picture. Indeed, even major trauma may go unrecognised initially if there are no witnesses of the accident or its circumstances. A knowledge of the core temperature is essential if these problems are to be appreciated and taken into consideration in the management of the critically injured patient.

The most convenient and accurate method of determining the core temperature uses a thermistor in the external auditory meatus. The pinna is covered with a servo-controlled heating pad incorporated into head phones (Fig 44.22). The pad warms the pinna to within 0.2°C of the thermistor temperature, thereby eliminating any thermal gradient around the thermistor (Yates and Little, 1979).

Prolonged exposure at the scene of the accident, in the resuscitation area and in the operating theatre will

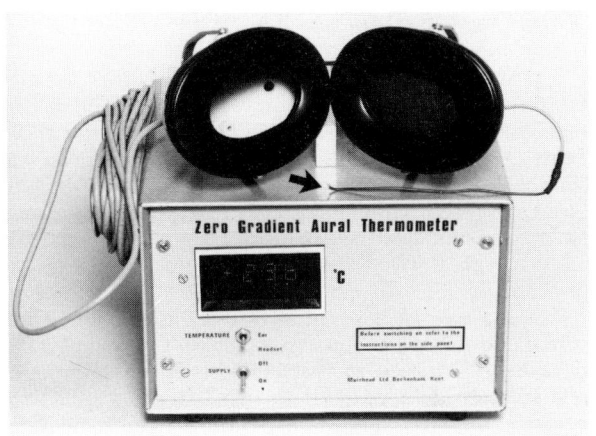

Fig 44.22 Aural thermometer. Thermister (arrowed) is held in external meatus with cotton wool.

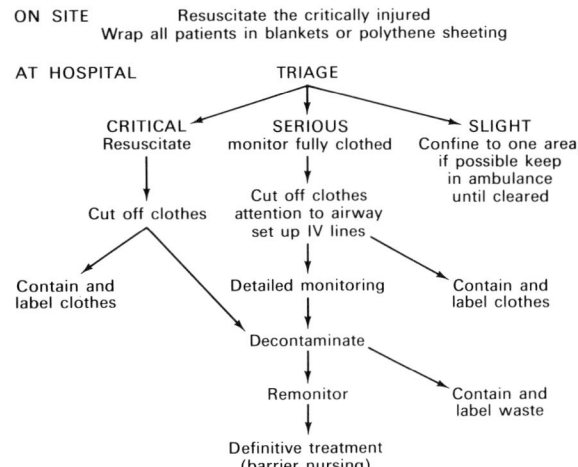

Fig 44.23 Radiation casualties: a system for their reception and initial management.

result in significant heat loss, especially in children. This can be prevented by the use of underblanket heating pads and aluminium foil blankets. A heating element should be incorporated into the giving set if more than one litre of fluid is to be given to an injured patient. Similarly diagnostic peritoneal lavage should be carried out using fluid at body temperature. Rewarming may be achieved passively or by applying heat either to the core (Yates and Little, 1979) or to the surface (Ledingham and Mone, 1972).

Radiation and trauma

Very high doses of radiation produce profound central nervous system disruption and death. Lower doses impair the function of the gastrointestinal tract and the haemopoeitic and immune systems, modifying the normal pathophysiological responses to trauma. While these effects are of importance when planning the treatment of individual patients, of more immediate concern to the rescuers will be the possibility of spread of radioactive surface contaminants.

Overall management will be a compromise, but primary resuscitation of critically ill patients must take absolute priority over all other considerations. A system for the reception and initial management of irradiated casualties is outlined in Fig 44.23.

Surface contamination is best removed by dry or slightly moist swabs. A shower or washing down a wound will produce further problems; contaminated fluids are difficult to contain and hold until monitored. The patient should be kept on a polythene sheet or newspaper. Movement of both patient and staff should be kept to a minimum and logged by an independent member of the team. Staff should wear surgical gloves,

aprons and gowns – masks are probably unnecessary. Spread of contamination is thereby kept to a minimum and the potential routes for such spread are known.

Prognosis is a function of the direct tissue trauma sustained and radiation dose absorbed. An impression of severity of physical trauma can be obtained fairly quickly in the usual way, but the extent of irradiation is much more difficult to assess. The time of onset and extent of CNS, gastrointestinal and haemopoietic abnormalities are useful guides to severity, but of no use to the surgeon assessing patients immediately after the incident. Information about the size of the radiation source and its type is unlikely to be accurate and the dose received by individual patients is influenced as much from their protection by buildings, for example, as by their distance from the source. It is wrong to assume that patients who have not sustained major injuries will not have received high doses of radiation. Some nuclear weapons are capable of producing high radiation levels outside a relatively small blast zone (Eiseman and Bond, 1978).

Fluid balance, red cell function, haemostasis, tissue repair and infection become major problems if the patient survives the first few days. It follows that treatment based on clinical judgement must be accomplished with speed. The irradiated patient will never be more fit to withstand surgical intervention than he is during the first 24 h after injury.

Auditing emergency care

Informal reviews of clinical work have been considered an essential part of medical care for many years (Irving and Temple, 1976). Only recently have they become formal and inevitably attracted a new name – Medical Audit. Irving (1976) described methods of reviewing regularly the performance of surgical departments and suggested that their adoption has led to improved patient care. The unstructured and sometimes unsupervised conditions encountered in the emergency department provide plenty of opportunities for mistakes. The need to reduce their number is perhaps more urgent here than anywhere else in the hospital.

Most emergency departments seek to improve patient care by providing teaching sessions and guidance notes for junior staff. Unless these efforts are supplemented by daily reviews of a department's work, errors in diagnosis and management may continue to go unnoticed. Such reviews are now widely accepted with respect to radiographs. Combined reviews by senior clinician and radiologist are particularly helpful and can be used to teach junior staff and students. The regular review of ECGs is less frequently undertaken and clinical notes are very rarely audited systematically.

A full audit of the department's clinical notes for the previous 24 hours can be completed in less than an hour. This should be an essential part of the day's routine. Mistakes can be picked up at an early stage, interesting clinical material retained for subsequent teaching sessions, and trends in individual performance identified.

CATASTROPHES

Natural disasters and warfare continue to take their toll of human life and civilian disasters appear to be increasing in number. Perhaps the latter are an inevitable consequence of man's tendency to live in conurbations, to travel in large groups at high speed, to work in dangerous environments and to indulge in urban warfare. Prevention should be our first concern in these areas, but it seems unlikely that there will be an early reversal of this upward trend. Rutherford (1973) has estimated that at least two major incidents occur in the UK every year and there are many occasions when somewhat smaller incidents overload, temporarily, the rescue and medical services available.

Compared with the number of patients injured and killed in other accidents, the total involved in these incidents remains very small. However, the organisation of medical services necessary to deal with mass casualties raises difficulties that are not encountered in routine civilian medicine. These include the assessment of priorities for evacuation and treatment, the administrative arrangements required to deal with a sudden influx of patients, their relatives and the media, and communications within and without the hospital (Richardson, 1975).

The disaster plan

Every hospital in the UK which has facilities for the treatment of casualties is required to have a plan for reception and management of patients from major accidents (MOH, 1954). Many plans have been drawn up simply to comply with this requirement only to be filed away and forgotten. Conversely, many major incidents have been managed satisfactorily without referral to any such plan. What, then, is the value of a disaster plan and what are its limitations?

The authors of a hospital disaster manual will be stimulated to look at the experience of colleagues who have been involved in real disasters. They will soon realise that detailed planning is counterproductive because of the enormous variety of incidents. However, they will learn also that there are common sites of confusion where advanced planning could be helpful. For example, the alert procedure is often not understood. Communications to, and within, the designated hospital frequently break down due to pressure on the switchboard. If the flow of patients into the receiving area is not structured, it is impossible to assess and compare priorities for urgent medical care. Patients may be lost between departments because of poor documentation and the inadequate provision of signs.

A disaster plan must be simple if it is to be assimilated quickly by anxious staff working under pressure. It must use existing hospital routines wherever possible for the same reason. It must be flexible to allow for very considerable variations in the type of disaster and should mention staff by position rather than by name. A suggested list of contents is given in Table 16.

A concise and unambiguous style is essential, with lists and diagrams rather than descriptive prose. A loose leaf format encourages frequent revision at low cost. 'Action cards' giving details of the individual responsibilities of members of staff have been advocated. They can be distributed routinely with the plan

Table 16
**HOSPITAL DISASTER MANUAL
LIST OF CONTENTS**

Definition and aims
Alert procedure
Implementation procedure
List of staff duties
(including guide lines on priorities for medical staff)
Role of site medical officer
Role of mobile medical team
Hospital reorganisation in very large incidents
(including use of designated areas and role of
co-ordinating team)
Telephone numbers

or held centrally until action is required. Their use by medical staff is not widely supported, but they are an attractive device for ensuring a consistent response from staff with a high turnover rate who are, nevertheless, essential for the success of the plan – for example, portering staff and telephonists. The information printed on the action cards must also appear in the main disaster plan.

It is useful to rehearse those parts of the plan which deal with communication and the alert procedure. However, the costly and disruptive ritual of moving theoretical casualties about the hospital and vacating wards and out-patient departments has little to commend it. Almost certainly the characteristics of the real disaster will differ markedly from those of the rehearsed version. To encourage adherence to a rigid protocol dampens initiative – an essential attribute for those involved in disaster management.

The alert procedure

Rarely has the theory of the hospital disaster plan been adhered to in recent major disasters in the UK. Some parts of most plans have been useful, but the alert procedure has been the part most commonly mishandled, with consequent confusion and delay in the provision of staff and facilities.

A good alert procedure should be capable of using information from a variety of sources and bringing together a group of 'key personnel' as quickly as possible. They can then plan the medical and administrative response and establish good communications.

Most commonly, the ambulance authority will be the first to contact the hospital, using the nationally agreed phrase 'Major Incident – Alert'. The hospital response should be limited to bringing together the consultant in the accident and emergency department, the divisional nursing officer, the senior administrator and the head porter. No further action is required unless the ambulance authority uses the phrase 'Major Incident – Implement'. Seriously injured patients have arrived at inner-city hospitals in cars, taxis and even on foot before the ambulance authority has been informed of the accident. It may be necessary, therefore, to implement the plan from within the hospital on the instructions of the senior doctor in the A & E department.

The implementation stage is not well thought out in some plans, again resulting in a discrepancy between theory and practice, with inevitable confusion. To progress from the alert to a consideration of redesignation of hospital wards and departments is unrealistic. It is unusual for such major reorganisation to be necessary. More commonly only 10 to 20 patients will require admission and the out-patient load will be no greater than that occasionally dealt with by the A & E depart-

ment at very busy times. In these incidents the problems are medical priorities, documentation and communication. A rigid all-or-none response may be considered so disruptive to normal hospital routine that staff actually delay its implementation. It is necessary, therefore, to phase the extent of the response according to the pressures imposed by the incident. This can be achieved by dividing the plan into three stages as in Fig 44.24. (The terms used in disaster management are now standardised to avoid confusion. They are explained in Table 17.)

Table 17
GLOSSARY OF TERMS USED IN DISASTER MANAGEMENT

At the scene
Police Incident Officer
   Senior policeman in overall charge
Fire and Ambulance Incident Officers
   Responsible for respective emergency serices
Incident Control
   Communications centre and base for incident officers
Site Medical Officer
   Assesses medical involvement and decides priorities for evacuation
   Identifies casualties requiring on-site care
Mobile Medical Team
   Stabilises cardiorespiratory system, relieves pain and prepares patients for transfer to hospital

At the hospital
Police and Ambulance Liason Officers
   Establish communication with respective units at incident site. (Sited in A & E department and/or Recovery Area)
Police Documentation Team
   Establishes list of casualties, with personal details, and notes their movement within the hospital. (Sited in A & E department)
Reception Area
   Entrance to A & E department. Triage Point for assessment of priorities of incoming patients by senior doctor
Major Treatment Area
   Seriously injured patients only. Management restricted to stabilisation of cardiorespiratory system and splintage of fractures – high turnover. X-ray discouraged.
Minor Treatment Area
   Definitive treatment for less severe injuries in patients to be discharged home
Reception Ward
   Previously cleared ward receives all patients from Major Treatment Area
Recovery Area
   All patients pass through this area for final medical and administrative check before discharge
Co-ordinating Team
   Doctor, Nurse and Administrator oversee the hospital response and maintain contact with incident scene. (Site near or in switchroom)

Elsewhere
Police Central Enquiry Bureau
   Deals with all enquiries from the public

First stage

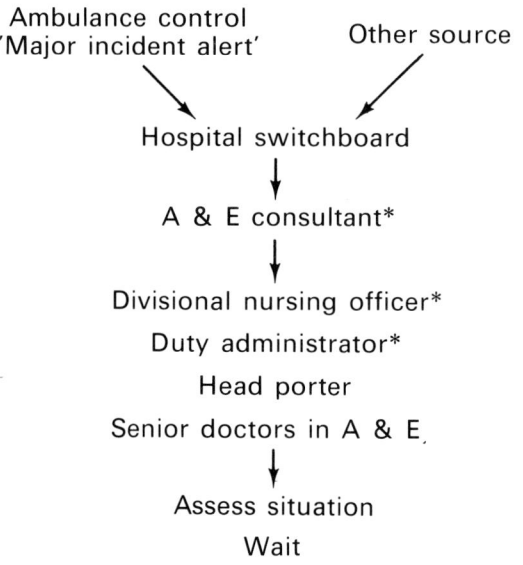

Ambulance control
'Major incident alert'   Other source

Hospital switchboard

A & E consultant*

Divisional nursing officer*
Duty administrator*
Head porter
Senior doctors in A & E

Assess situation

Wait

Second stage

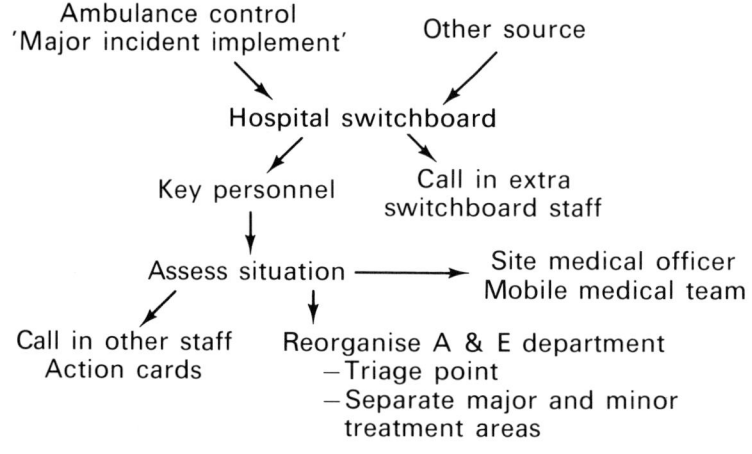

Ambulance control
'Major incident implement'   Other source

Hospital switchboard

Key personnel   Call in extra
switchboard staff

Assess situation ⟶ Site medical officer
Mobile medical team

Call in other staff   Reorganise A & E department
Action cards   —Triage point
—Separate major and minor
treatment areas

Third stage

Implemented only by key personnel
—establish coordinating team
—prepare reception ward
—use A & E department as triage point and major treatment area
—prepare minor treatment area elsewhere
—establish recovery area
—make provision for press, television etc.

(* = Key personnel)

Fig 44.24   Three-stage implementation.

Communications

Poor communications create a lot of confusion in the first few hours after a disaster. Good planning and occasional rehearsals will shorten this period of confusion and lead to a more efficient use of manpower and resources.

Communication at the incident scene is the responsibility of the rescue services. Much has been achieved in recent years to provide good quality radio contact and to integrate radio and telephone to give a comprehensive network. It is now possible for a rescue worker to use a pocket transmitter to talk to a doctor on a hospital telephone extension. Land lines can be established very rapidly and are particularly useful in tunnels and mines where conventional radio contact is difficult. New low frequency equipment is being developed to improve radio communication in tunnels (Bromage, 1976).

Communications between workers at the scene and those in the hospital may be a problem, especially if the latter's switchboard becomes overloaded. The hospital plan must be developed in such a way as to reduce pressure at this point. Extra telephone operators will be amongst the first additional staff to be called in. The switchboard should have a few exdirectory lines which can be reserved for out-going calls. Arrangements can be made to connect permanently one or two important extensions to the external system. Coin operated mobile ward telephones and fixed public call boxes are other useful sources of external lines. The police documentation team will require a base in the A & E department and should be given their own direct outside line. Details of the siting of these special telephones must be given in the disaster plan. A further reduction in the use of the hospital switchboard can be achieved by encouraging staff to use the 'snow ball system' for calling in colleagues – the person contacted at home being asked to alert a specific list of members of staff using his own telephone.

Communication within the hospital may be via a separate internal telephone system or by the use of messengers. Unskilled but enthusiastic help is usually in abundance in disaster situations and the establishment of a messenger service can mop up many volunteers, keeping them away from clinical areas where they are often counter-productive.

When very large numbers of patients are expected it is useful to set up a coordinating team to integrate the hospital response and strengthen links between the hospital and the scene (Fig 44.24, Stage 3). The team should be sited near the hospital switchboard and comprise a senior hospital doctor, nursing officer and administrator.

Documentation

People under stress work most efficiently when they are in familiar surroundings performing familiar tasks. Special stationery and a strange documentation system will confuse even the most experienced receptionist, but it is necessary to have some special forms. The overall system should be as simple as possible and follow closely the normal pattern of the department.

Labelling patients at the scene of the incident is essential, to indicate priorities for evacuation, drugs given and possibly brief details of clinical state. The UK ambulance service uses labels with colour codes as detailed in Table 18.

The dead must be identified and marked to prevent time-consuming re-examination by other doctors (Milner, 1976).

Medical Records staff should be stationed near the hospital triage point (p. 738). Name bands or numbers should be attached to patients' wrists and as many details as possible entered in the standard receptionist's ledger and on the Casualty Card.

A separate list of patients involved in the incident can be used to keep a check on admissions, discharges and movements within the hospital (Savage, 1975). The Police Documentation Team and the Ambulance Liaison Officer will find such a list valuable. The administrator on duty must ensure that extra Medical Records staff are called in as soon as the disaster plan is implemented, so that this list can be kept accurate and up-to-date.

Table 18
AMBULANCE PRIORITY CODES

Red	Major injury. Top priority
Blue	Moderate or minor injury. Low priority
Black	Dead

The medical response

The structured flow of patients which will have been developed by the rescue services at the disaster scene must be maintained within the hospital. Triage sites should be established as indicated in Fig 44.25. It will take some time to develop and man all the areas detailed in the plan, so it is important to direct staff initially to those points where they are most urgently needed. These are numbered in order of priority in Fig 44.25. The first instructions to medical staff, whether contained in the disaster plan or on separate 'actions cards', should be to procede to the A & E department,

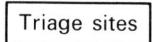

(Numbers refer to manning priorities in hospital)

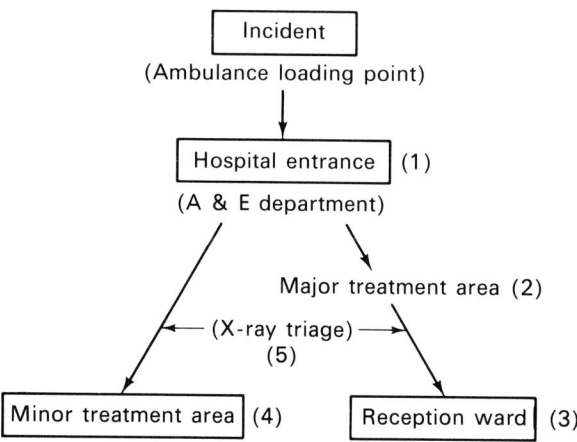

Fig 44.25   Triage sites.

contact the senior doctor there and make sure that the triage point and major treatment areas are manned. The next priorities are the minor treatment area and the reception ward. Once these places are manned, decisions can be taken about interchanging doctors to match more closely their experience with their tasks. It is unwise to be too specific about doctors' functions in the disaster plan without mentioning this first essential of manning the reception and primary treatment areas.

In a large incident it is useful to send out a doctor to assess the extent of the medical involvement. The 'Site Medical Officer' should be a mature person with some administrative experience – he need not be a practicing clinician. His first task of medical assessment is conducted with the Police Incident Officer. Links are established with the receiving hospitals. With the assistance of the Police and the Ambulance Liaison Officers a system is developed for the appropriate distribution of casualties among the designated receiving hospitals. This reduces the impact of the disaster on any one hospital (Jacobs *et al.*, 1979). The next step is to identify those patients who are in greatest need of urgent medical attention and to arrange for their despatch to hospital. When the number of critically ill patients greatly exceeds the resources available – an unusual event – it is vital to distinguish those who may respond to treatment from those who will inevitably die. Precious ambulance facilities must be reserved for the former.

A list of those who have volunteered to act as Site Medical Officer should be held in the hospital switch-room. It is useful to introduce these doctors informally to the senior rescue service personnel when the disaster plan is being drawn up.

If the Site Medical Officer considers that some patients should receive treatment before and during transfer or there are seriously injured trapped patients, the A & E consultant must be asked to send out a Mobile Medical Team. Potential members of this team will have been selected previously, lists being available in the hospital switchroom and the A & E department. They will be transported to the site by police or ambulance vehicles and wear protective clothing and identification tabards. A typical 'disaster kit' is shown in Fig 44.26a,b.

On site resuscitation demands skills which are not easy to acquire within the hospital. Senior doctors and nurses from the A & E department would make an ideal team. However, this would deplete the A & E department of essential staff if the team is requested from the hospital designated to receive the casualties. A new development in conurbations, whereby Mobile Medical Teams are requested from hospitals not so designated, will overcome this objection. If this arrangement is not possible, team members should be selected from the middle grades of surgical, medical and anaesthetic departments.

The mobile Medical Team will work under the direction of the Site Medical Officer, concerning itself with critically injured patients. Its medical role is restricted, therefore, to stabilising the cardiorespiratory system and relieving pain.

Triage sites

In the first few hours after a sudden influx of new casualties the available medical resources may be overwhelmed. In its simplest form the triage procedure aims to ease this pressure by identifying the critically injured, who should have priority over the less seriously wounded and those who are so seriously injured as to be beyond hope of recovery, and by identifying the dead. This is a skilled task and must be carried out by a senior doctor. He is most effective if extending his normal role, and it is appropriate, therefore, that the consultant in accident and emergency medicine should assume responsibility for the initial sorting of patients at the hospital entrance, because he is familiar with this process in his everyday work. Similarly, consultants in general and orthopaedic surgery and in anaesthetics have appropriate experience in triage within the hospital. The task must not be left to junior medical staff or members of the rescue services.

The aim of triage is to preclude unnecessary loss of life. The most important patients to identify are those whose critical condition will benefit most rapidly from

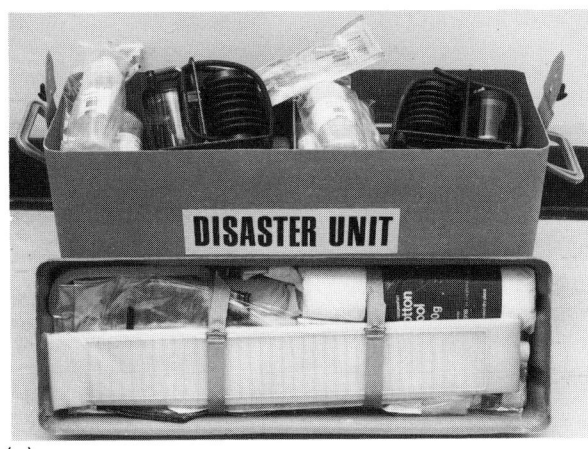

(a)

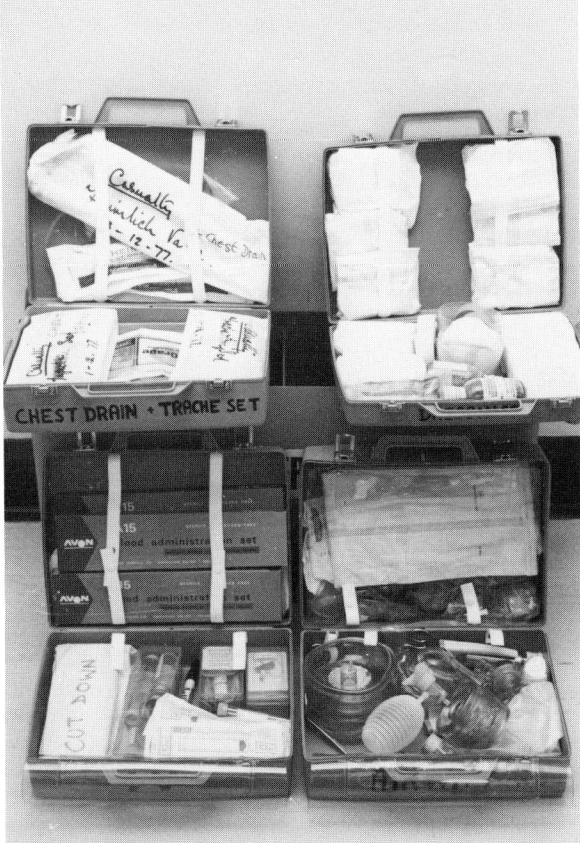

(b)

Fig 44.26 (a) Typical disaster kit. (b) Accompanying containers for specialised equipment.

the provision of basic resuscitation techniques. This is not quite the same as assessing priorities on the basis of severity: some very seriously injured patients may fail to respond to prolonged attempts at resuscitation while others may benefit immediately. It is extremely difficult to evaluate the differing prognoses in such patients, hence the need to place the responsibility for triage on the shoulders of a senior doctor who, incidentally, will be able to withstand criticism if he makes a mistake.

Triage at the scene of the incident

This is most convenient if conducted at the ambulance loading point by the Site Medical Officer. All patients must pass through the triage area, however major or minor their injuries. One important aim is to prevent patients presenting at the hospital unheralded. This will never be completely successful, but because the patients who bypass triage points create many problems, not least for themselves, every attempt should be made to achieve this objective.

Forays into the midst of the disaster scene can hinder rather than help the overall effort. Doctors and others unskilled in the art of search and rescue may well endanger life rather than save it. While the possibility of being injured by a passing vehicle at the scene of a road traffic accident is widely recognised, the risks of falling masonry, radiation, toxic fumes, electrocution, and explosion are often overlooked in industrial disasters.

Triage at the hospital entrance

Patients must enter the hospital by one route only. Despite efforts to regulate their flow at the scene of the disaster, experience shows that many people find their way to hospital independently of the ambulance service. Because it cannot be assumed that such people have received only minor injuries, everyone attending the hospital must pass through a single triage area. However, those with minor injuries should be shielded as far as possible from the seriously ill.

The resuscitation area must be immediately adjacent to the hospital entrance and triage point. In most hospitals this is best accomplished by admitting the patients through the A & E department entrance and using the main treatment rooms of the department and possibly the waiting room as the resuscitation area. Triage at the hospital entrance is the key to the efficient management of a sudden influx of casualties. From the outset it must be conducted by an experienced doctor who can delegate resuscitation and subsequent management to his colleagues.

Triage within the hospital

Triage is a continuous process and to be effective must be applied as long as an imbalance exists between patient demands and medical resources. Bottlenecks are likely to occur, particularly in the operating theatres and the x-ray departments (Rutherford, 1973). Priorities for these facilities can be assessed most effectively when the patients requiring them are in one area where quick comparisons can be made. Thus, all those who may need surgery are put in one ward (Irving, 1976).

A senior surgeon should remain in this ward constantly reassessing priorities for surgery while his colleagues work in the operating theatres. Experienced members of the junior surgical team should carry out most of the straightforward operations under the supervision of the consultants. The more difficult cases are identified and operated on by the consultant staff.

Priorities for x-ray examination are less easy to determine because of the various sources from which requests arise. In general terms, x-ray examinations should be discouraged. They must be forbidden before resuscitation has been initiated. A senior clinician or radiologist should assess all requests for x-ray examinations and permit only those that will help in the immediate management of the patients (Table 15).

A senior doctor must be present in the minor treatment area alert to the possibility that seriously ill patients may have been sent there erroneously. In addition, he advises his juniors how best to manage wounds that could result in long-term disabilities.

All doctors working with the injured must remember that the patients may have other illnesses and be receiving drugs for them. Finally a senior nurse in each area must be given the task of ensuring that all patients have been immunised against tetanus (Table 14).

The assessment of priorities

Triage officers find it helpful to be able to refer to guidelines on the assessment of priorities. These can be drawn up in anticipation of a disaster and can highlight problems that have been shown to be important in previous incidents. However, it is dangerous to develop an extensive algorithm that aims to deal with every possible type of disaster. To encourage adherence to a rigid protocol dampens initiative which is an essential attribute for those involved in disaster management. With this constraint in mind, a classification of priorities is presented as a basic framework to be modified according to local circumstances.

The dead

The importance of confirming and recording death has been mentioned already. In dark, dirty, and noisy environments a defibrillator that picks up an ECG through the paddles is most helpful.

The critically injured

Rarely is the number of patients in this category very high during peacetime. If it is, a distinction must be made between the patients who *may* die and those who *will* die. Major insults to the cardiorespiratory system cause most of the critical injuries. These are detailed in Table 19. These patients must be transferred to the resuscitation area and kept there until stable or transferred to the intensive care area or operating theatre.

Table 19
CRITICAL INJURIES

Airway
  Blocked by mucus, vomit or foreign body
  Distorted by major injury to face, jaw or neck
Circulation
  Hypovolaemic shock
  Cardiogenic shock
Chest
  Tension pneumothorax
  Massive flail chest
  Heart or great vessel injury
  Cardiac tamponade

The seriously injured

Table 20 lists the injuries in the 'serious' group. Patients should pass through the resuscitation area for the rapid placement of intravenous lines and the securing of an adequate airway, then go to the receiving surgical ward – possibly via the x-ray department. In the ward a full clinical assessment is made.

The consultant surgeon on the ward uses this information to determine priorities for surgical intervention.

The slightly injured

These patients are considered not to require urgent medical attention or admission to hospital. They include those with lacerations, contusions and ligament injuries. Depending on the availability of beds, patients with tendon and nerve injuries and embedded foreign bodies may have to be treated on an outpatient basis. Delayed primary closure of contused wounds must be encouraged.

Within the context of a disaster the distinction between serious and slight is based on 'threat to life', but in any other circumstance such a distinction is established after consideration of many other factors including pain, loss of function, and cosmesis. It follows that some patients who are pigeon-holed as 'slightly injured' on the day of the disaster may, in fact, have significant injuries. In recognition of this possibility the records of such patients must be just as good as those whose injuries are more evidently of immediate importance. This makes subsequent management much easier.

The sorrowful

Many people, who do not appear to be physically injured and yet are in need of support, present at the triage point at the scene of a disaster and at the hospital entrance. Such people may be able to support each other, and do this most effectively in a relaxed environment away from the main area of medical activity. Because of this therapeutic isolation, it is important that the group does not contain seriously ill patients whose injuries were not detected at the triage point. Particularly difficult problems can be posed by patients who have sustained head injuries, been influenced by toxic fumes, or become deaf after an explosion.

Coincidental accidents and emergencies

Emergency medical and surgical conditions continue to arise irrespective of the disaster; indeed some cardiovascular emergencies may be provoked by it. While some patients with minor problems decide to seek help elsewhere when they realise that the hospital service is hard-pressed, many attend in the normal way. Provision must be made for their reception and appropriate initial management. This is best done by routing all such patients through the triage point at the hospital entrance.

References

Ayella R.J. ed. (1978). *Radiologic Management of the Massively Traumatised Patient.* p. 297. Baltimore: Williams and Wilkins.

Baker S.P., O'Neill B., Haddon W., Long W.B. (1974). The injury severity score; a method for describing patient with multiple injuries and evaluting emergency care. *J. Trauma*; **14**:187–96.

Bromage C. (1976). Communications. In *Developments in Disaster Management* (Howard J., ed) pp. 33–35. Glasgow: Action for Disaster Committee.

Buchsbaum H.J. (1968). Accidental injury complicating pregnancy. *Amer. J. Obstet. Gynaecol*; **102**:752–69.

Buley R., Lumley J. (1975). Some observations on blood micro-filters. *Ann. Roy. Coll. Surg*; **57(5)**:262–7.

Chandra N., Rudikoff M.T., Weisfeldt M.L. (1980). Simultaneous chest compression and ventilation at high airway pressure during cardiopulmonary resuscitation. Lancet; **i**:175–8.

Clarke S.S., Prudencio R.F. (1972). Lower urinary tract injuries associated with pelvic fractures – diagnosis and management. *Surg. Clin. N.Amer*; **52–1**:183–201.

Don Michael T.A., Lambert E.H., Mehran A. (1968). Mouth to lung airway for cardiac resuscitation. *Lancet*; **ii**:1329.

Easton K.C. (1970). Trauma and the general practitioner. *Proc. Roy. Med*; **63**:1321–3.

Eiseman B., Bond V. (1978). Surgical care of nuclear casualties. *Surg. Gynaecol. Obstet*; **146**:877–83.

Eisenberg R.S. (1980). A new airway for tracheal or oesophageal insertion. *Ann. Emerg. Med*; **9**:270–2.

Gill W., Champion H.R., Long W.B. (1975). Abdominal lavage in blunt trauma. *Brit. J. Surg*; **62(2)**:121–4.

Griffith I.P. (1976). Tracheostomy. *Brit. J. Hosp. Med*; **16(1)**:78–86.

Hanson G.C., Mearns A.J., Light L.H. (1980). Haemodynamic monitoring in the intensive care unit. *Brit. Med. J*; **1**:1448–9.

Harber T., Lucas B.G.B. (1980). An evaluation of some mechanical resuscitators for use in the ambulance service. *Ann. Roy. Coll. Surg. Engl*; **62**:291–4.

Henning R.J., Wiener F., Valdes S., Weilm H. (1979). Measurement of toe temperature for assessing the severity of acute circulatory failure. *Surg. Gynaecol. Obstet*; **149**:1–7.

Hoffman E. (1976). Mortality and morbidity following road accidents. *Ann. Roy. Coll. Surg. Engl*; **58**:233–40.

Horowitz M.S., Schultz C.S., Stinson E.B. *et al.* (1974). Sensitivity and specificity of echocardiographic diagnosis of pericardial effusion. *Circulation*; **50**:239–47.

Irving M.H. (1976). Major disasters: Hospital admission procedures. *Brit. J. Surg*; **63**:731–4.

Irving M.H., Temple J. (1976). Surgical audit: one year's experience in a teaching hospital. *Brit. Med. J*; **2**:746–7.

Jacobs L.M., Ramp J.M., Breay J.M. (1979). An emergency medical system approach to disaster planning. *J. Trauma*; **19**:157–62.

Jennett B., Carlin J. (1978). Preventable mortality and morbidity after head injury. *Injury*; **10**:31–9.

Keen G. (1972). Closed injuries of the thoracic aorta. *Ann. Roy. Coll. Surg. Engl*; **51**:137–56.

Kimbler R.W. (1977). Traumatic rupture of the aortic valve after closed chest injury. *J. Trauma*; **17**:168–70.

Lazarus H.M., Nelson J.A. (1979). A technique for peritoneal lavage without risk or complication. *Surg. Gynaecol. Obstet*; **149**:889–92.

Ledingham I.McA., Mone J.G. (1972). Treatment after exposure to cold. *Lancet*; **i**:534–5.

London P.S. (1979). Abdominal injuries: surgical aspects; a review. *J. Roy. S. Med*; **72**:842–5.

McDowall D.G. (1976). Monitoring the brain. *Anaesthesiology*; **45(2)**:117–34.

Mattox K.L., Pickard L., Allen M.K., Garcia-Rinaldi P. (1978). Suspecting thoracic aortic transection. *J.A.C.E.P*; **7**:12–15.

Milner J. (1976). The fire brigade at Moorgate. In *Developments in Diaster Management* (Howard J., ed) pp. 43–50. Glasgow: Action for Disaster Committee.

Ministry of Health (1954). *Medical Arrangements for Dealing with Major Accidents*. London: HMSO (54) 51.

Moss G.S. (1972). An argument in favour of electrolyte solution for early resuscitation. *Surg. Clin. N.Amer*; **52–1**:3–17.

O'Riordan W.D. (1977). Autotransfusion in the emergency department of a community hospital. *J.A.C.E.P*; **6**:233–7.

Oxer H.F. (1975). Aeromedical evacuation. *Brit. Med. J*; **3**:692–4.

Pardy B.J., Dudley H.A.F. (1977). Pulmonary artery pressure in acute haemorrhage. *Brit. J. Surg*; **64**:1–5.

Parmley L.F., Manlow W.C., Mattingly T.W. (1958). Non penetrating traumatic rupture of the heart. *Circulation*; **18**:371–96.

Pories W.J., Gaudiani V.A. (1975). Cardiac tamponade. *Surg. Clin. N.Amer*; **55–3**:573–89.

Richardson J.W. ed. (1975). *Disaster Planning*. pp. 121. Bristol: Wright.

Ring J., Messmer K. (1977). Incidence and severity of anaphylactoid reactions to colloid substances. *Lancet*; **i**:466–9.

Rose J., Valtonen S., Jennett B. (1977). Avoidable factors contributing death after head injury. *Brit. Med. J*; **2**:615–18.

Rudikoff M.T., Trend P., Weisfeldt M.L. (1977). Mechanisms of blood flow during cardiopulmonary resuscitation. *Circulation*; **56** suppl.111: abstract no.370.

Rudowski W.J. (1980). Evaluation of modern plasma expanders and blood substitutes. *Brit. J. Hosp. Med*; **23**:389–99.

Rutherford W.H. (1973). Experience in the accident and emergency department of the Royal Victoria Hospital with patients from civil disturbances in Belfast 1969–72, with a review of disasters in the United Kingdom 1951–1971. *Injury*; **4**:189–99.

Savage P.E.A. (1975). Documentation. In *Disaster Planning* (Richardson J.W., ed.) pp. 93–97. Bristol: Wright.

Smith J.W.G., Laurance D.R., Evans D.G. (1975). Prevention of tetanus in the wounded. *Brit. Med. J*; **2**:453–5.

Sterling L.C., Zauder H.L., Rogers W. (1975). Intraoperative autotransfusion. *Anaesthesiology*; **43(3)**:337–45.

Stewart R.D. (1977). Training of paramedics. *Brit. J. Anaesth*; **49(7)**:659–71.

Stoner H.B. (1976). Changes in the central nervous system and their role in the metabolic response to injury. In *Metabolism and the Response to Injury* (Wilkinson A.W., Cuthbertson D., ed.) pp. 179–93. London: Pitman Medical.

Teasdale G., Jennett B. (1974). Assessment of coma and impaired consciousness. A practical scale. *Lancet*; **ii**:81–3.

Yates D.W. (1977). Airway patency in fatal accidents. *Brit. Med. J*; **2**:1249–51.

Yates D.W., Little R.A. (1979). Accidental hypothermia. *Resuscitation*; **7**:59–67.

Waddell G. (1975). Movement of patients within hospital. *Brit. Med. J*; **2**:417–19.

Wyler A.R., Reynolds A.F. (1977). An intracranial complication of nasogastric intubation. *J. Neurosurg*; **47**:297–8.

45

Head injury

R.M. KALBAG

The vast majority of head injuries in Britain are managed in the first instance, if not entirely, in general hospitals without direct access to the experience or diagnostic facilities taken for granted in a modern neurosurgical department. This situation is unlikely to change in the foreseeable future. Of all fatal head injuries 21.5% die in accident departments before admission to a ward (Field, 1976). In Sevitt's surveys (1968, 1973) 42% of the deaths occurred within an hour of injury and 69% within 24 h. A feeling of inadequacy and frustration is, therefore, understandable in those working in such conditions. However, almost all the acute fatalities are from overwhelming brain damage; the few avoidable disasters are due to neglect of the simple basic rules of resuscitation and assessment (Jennett and Carlin, 1978), rather than for want of specialist expertise.

The primary brain injury is not amenable to treatment; *the aim of management is to recognise, prevent or correct those secondary complications which might affect the outcome unfavourably:*

1 Anoxia
2 Compression
3 Infection

The degree of sophistication used to achieve these ends will depend on the resources available when the need for action arises, on how urgent that need is and on one's own philosophy.

Advances in medical technology have outstripped the profession's ability to assess their worth. A naive tendency to equate technical feasibility with therapeutic benefit has bedevilled the practice of medicine in the last quarter of a century; this probably reaches its peak in the context of head injury, when decisions about what treatment should be initiated have to be taken quickly, often by inexperienced doctors, mostly trainee surgeons. The very temperament that usually attracts a man of action rather than a thinker to surgery, may drive him to the heroic application of whatever measures are at hand, surgical or otherwise, in a seemingly desperate situation. Moreover, in a moment of crisis to be seen to be doing something is far more comforting to anxious relatives, and a more reliable safeguard against adverse comment later, if there are unfortunate consequences, than inactivity, however rational. The difficulties in establishing the value of some of the methods currently in use in the treatment of head injuries have been reviewed by Jennett *et al.* (1980). While indicating the possible role of ancillary methods in the management of head injuries, the emphasis here will be principally on the underlying concepts and their practical application in the clinical setting.

The primary brain injury

The effects, on the brain, of injury to the head depend on the surface area of the object it strikes, the velocity of impact and whether the head is supported or not. Damage to the scalp or skull is important only as (a) a clue to what might have happened to the brain underneath, and (b) the complications to be suspected.

The blunt acceleration-deceleration injury is the one most often seen in civilian practice: the unsupported head is struck by a moving object or the moving head suddenly comes to rest against a flat unyielding surface such as the road. The resulting rotational forces acting on the easily deformed brain produce widespread stretching, even rupture, of the axons and diffuse neuronal disturbance, with loss of consciousness, the most prominent feature of such injury.

As the brain swirls around within the cranium, it may suffer laceration or contusion against projections into the cavity, notably the lesser wings of the sphenoid. The latter accounts for the damage to the tips of the temporal and under surface of the frontal lobes so frequently seen in fatal cases, as well as for the almost invariable location of acute and subacute haematomas in the anterior temporal region.

Such an injury is closed unless there is also a compound fracture of the skull with laceration of the dura mater, when it is classed as open, and there is the added risk of infection.

In *compression injury*, the head is crushed or trapped between two flat surfaces. The skull base is fractured, with perhaps lower cranial nerve palsies and c.s.f. otorrhoea, but without loss of consciousness. It is a rare injury.

The *penetrating injury*, as the term indicates, is open, and there is always the risk of infection. The effect on the brain depends on the speed of the missile. If the velocity is low, damage is localised and consciousness retained. The point of entry is small and the injury may be missed unless an adequate history is obtained, especially in children. The track in the brain may be little wider than the missile itself.

The energy transferred to the brain varies directly as the square of the missile velocity. A low velocity bullet such as from a hand-gun produces little generalised damage. Modern rifles, however, with a muzzle velocity more than three times that of a hand gun and more than twice the speed of sound, release up to ten times as much energy. This creates an explosive radial force deep to the point of entry, temporary cavitation and a massive increase in intracranial pressure. There is extensive disruption of cerebral tissue with secondary oedema and haemorrhages in the brain, responsible for the rapid, often fatal, deterioration seen in such injuries. Only a high velocity bullet will pass through the skull, where the exit wound is larger than the entry wound (Crockard, 1974).

Anoxia

To an unconscious individual, whatever the cause of that unconsciousness, the greatest immediate threat is anoxia.

At the most elementary level, it may be anoxic anoxia due to airway obstruction from failure to turn the patient into the semi-prone or 'recovery' position, a simple manoeuvre better known to first-aid trainees than many hospital personnel. A 'flail' chest needing tracheal intubation and ventilatory support may call for greater expertise than can be mustered by every doctor faced with the problem; it is one of the situations in which one appreciates the active participation of anaesthetists in resuscitation and intensive care units, so often taken for granted in most general hospitals today. No hospital which cannot provide such an anaesthetic service should have an accident and emergency department.

Shock and massive haemorrhage constitute the twin dangers of stagnant and anaemic anoxia. Their presence should always alert the medical attendant to the probability of damage to other organs. If it is due to a lower limb or pelvic fracture, restoration of blood volume is all that is necessary. Not infrequently, however, an examiner is so bemused by an obvious head injury in an unconscious patient as to overlook injuries to other systems, which may demand immediate attention, such as a haemopneumothorax or a ruptured spleen. Shock is not seen when injury is to the head alone, unless there has been excessive bleeding from a large scalp laceration or in the rare situation of an infant with an intracranial haematoma. A failing circulation interpreted as shock may be seen in the late stage of brain death, when invariably the patient is already apnoeic.

Price and Murray (1972) showed that hypoxia significantly reduces the prospects of recovery from head injury while hypotension prolongs convalescence without necessarily reducing the quality of survival.

A delay in restoring blood pressure can in some cases be lethal in an injured brain that has become ischaemic and lost its capacity for autoregulation, because of which intracranial pressure passively follows the rise in systemic arterial pressure. As a result, there may be a progressive rise in intracranial pressure, mimicking the clinical picture of an intracranial haematoma, namely deterioration in consciousness.

More than 60 years after Haldane's statement that anoxia not only stops the machine, but wrecks the machinery, failure to carry out resuscitation at the earliest opportunity is still too frequent to be dismissed lightly. Of 377 patients referred to a neurosurgical unit in 2 years (Barlett and Neil-Dwyer, 1979) 31 were transferred without adequate attention to the airway, 8 with severe blood loss had not been transfused and 1 patient had arrived with a tension pneumothorax.

There are more subtle forms of hypoxaemia which cannot be corrected merely by ensuring an airway or by tracheal intubation and toilet. Pulmonary insufficiency can occur in severe brain injury as it can in multiple trauma with shock. The effects of the head injury itself on lung functions are not easy to separate from the more direct pulmonary complications such as inhalation of vomit and retention of lung secretions. The result is terminal airway closure with perfusion of blood through the walls of unaerated alveoli, and a functional pulmonary shunt, Frost *et al.* (1979), in a study of 86 patients with severe head injury, were unable to find any cause for increased pulmonary shunting other than the central lesion in 60% of the cases. Perhaps the most dramatic example is the decerebrate patient who is hyperventilating yet hypoxic. Sustained overbreathing produces a high pH and a shift of the O_2 dissociation curve to the left with a consequent reduction in the oxygen available to the tissues. The effect of hyperventilation and decerebrate spasms increases the metabolic rate and aggravates the hypoxia. This is one of the situations in which assisted ventilation is often recommended. The role of such ventilation will be considered in some detail in the section on management.

Hypoxia at a cellular level may result from reduced cerebral perfusion either as one of the consequences of a generalised increase in intracranial pressure or from traumatic arterial spasm.

In the days before CAT scanning, when carotid angiography was the popular investigation in the management of patients with suspected haematomas, the radiological demonstration of traumatic arterial spasm could be anticipated on clinical grounds on rare occasions. Though talking on admission, the patient was restless, confused, uncooperative and even violent; if one could get near enough to examine him, which was generally only feasible after his level of consciousness had declined, he had marked meningism. Deterioration generally occurred over a day or two, and on angiography, the vascular spasm was so intense that the smaller arteries were not demonstrable, circulation was slow, and the patient died in spite of energetic measures to control his intracranial hypertension, and without any intracranial haematoma.

An even more extreme example of the ischaemic brain was seen when, as was almost mandatory in some countries, failure to outline the intracranial vessels on angiography was one of the signs required for the diagnosis of brain death.

Cerebral compression

The principal concern of many doctors faced with an unconscious patient is the possibility of an intracranial haematoma. Autopsy reports do little to allay such fears. About 90% of patients dying from head injury have pathological evidence of raised intracranial pressure, and almost two-thirds have a haematoma, findings which have provided the spur to the increasingly aggressive measures currently fashionable. But *for all practical purposes the single most reliable indication for surgery is a progressive deterioration in consciousness.* Unconsciousness alone or, for that matter, the presence of a neurological deficit, does not signify haematoma, though it may be the consequence of one. Successful outcome after any such surgery will be influenced by the highest level of consciousness, the nature of the lesion responsible for such deterioration, the age of the patient, and, not least, by how deeply unconscious the patient is at the time of operation. The ageing brain reacts adversely to brain injury, so much so that even if there has been an unequivocal decline in responsiveness, operation is futile in the elderly unless the individual has spoken rationally at some stage after injury; even here the quality of survival may leave a lot to be desired. In fact, despite aggressive therapy, good recovery is seen mainly in the young, mostly under the age of 21, few, if any, being over the age of 50.

Intracranial hypertension may result from extradural and intradural haematomas, or brain swelling, which may be focal or generalised. The intradural clot is generally subdural, but is so often associated with laceration and contusion of the adjacent brain, that in the first few days after trauma, it is exceptional to see a purely subdural clot.

Extradural haematoma

The term 'extradural' is to be preferred to 'middle meningeal' haemorrhage in that bleeding is not always from the middle meningeal vessels and even then is not necessarily arterial. Middle meningeal haemorrhage is often thought to be from the artery alone, and that the vascular markings on the inner table of the skull are due to pulsation of the artery. Wood Jones (1912) showed that these grooves contained the middle meningeal veins and the artery took a course entirely outside the groove. This has aetiological significance: veins have thin walls and are more vulnerable than arteries, and the reason why haematomas can follow trivial blows. Nearly a third of the patients in a large series (Gallagher and Browder, 1968) had had such minor injury that they had neither been concussed nor sought medical attention in the first instance (Jamieson, 1970). This also accounts for the frequent failure to find any arterial bleeding point at operation. In some patients, in the course of evolution of the syndrome, there is initially a slow decline in the level of consciousness for a few hours, followed by a sudden, often catastrophic, deterioration. At surgery, one is likely to find arterial bleeding at the anterior meningeal point; the early phase is probably the venous bleeding gradually stripping the dura away from the inner table of the skull; then when the dura gets peeled away at the lateral edge of the lesser wing of the sphenoid, where the anterior branch of the middle meningeal artery may run in a bony canal, the artery is lacerated with second-ary arterial bleeding.

With advancing years, the dura mater becomes increasingly adherent to the calvarium and is difficult to separate from it. Hence the extradural haematoma is essentially an affliction of youth, most of the patients being under the age of 20 and only exceptionally over 50. In the localisation of an extradural haematoma, too much emphasis is laid on the demonstration of a frac-ture crossing vascular markings on skull x-rays. In 1816, Sir Charles Bell showed that when the cadaveric skull was struck with a wooden mallet, the blow caused the dura to become separated from the skull directly beneath the point of impact. Every review on the sub-ject since then has borne out the validity of that observation, and is worth remembering if one is to reduce the mortality and morbidity in what is the most rewarding and simply treated of all the serious acute complications of head injury.

Unfortunately, extradural haematoma is a relatively rare condition, though most of the thousands of 'minor' head injuries admitted for observation into primary surgical wards are there in case they develop one. While a clear lucid interval, in which the patient has spoken after injury, is often present, this may be absent or concealed by alcohol. All that is needed for the diagnosis is unequivocal deterioration in consciousness, without waiting for the classical dilatation of the ipsi-lateral pupil, and for the localisation, the point of exter-nal impact as declared by the scalp bruise, laceration or bogginess. Such an external indication may be absent if the patient was wearing head protection.

A rare, but well recognised, presentation is increas-ing restlessness; it is due to intense headache localised to the site of the haematoma; this patient, even if he cannot talk, virtually points to the clot by rubbing the overlying scalp. Again, rarely, an extradural clot may be the reason for a persistent profuse c.s.f. otorrhoea; obvious deterioration in consciousness only occurs when the haematoma, which is ipsilateral to the c.s.f. fistula expands to occlude the fistula, the escape of c.s.f. through which had till then prevented the intracranial pressure from rising dangerously. The diagnosis need not be considered in severe injuries, where the brain swelling and haemorrhage limit the amount of extradural haematoma necessary to produce compression on its own, and where in any case the prognosis is determined by the extent of the initial brain injury. Who does the operation and whether

ancillary investigations, even a plain x-ray of the skull, are carried out first, depends on how quickly deteriora-tion is occurring. In those parts of the country which are at a distance from a neurosurgical service, the patient's only chance of recovery may be operation by the nearest available surgeon. The operation itself is simple and within the competence of any surgeon worth the name.

In this connection one could do no better than quote Jamieson and Yelland (1968): 'The neurosurgeon who from within his ivory tower writes of the necessity for or desirability of special investigations, radiological or otherwise, instead of emphasising simple clinical appraisal, or who advocates osteoplastic flap cra-niotomy, does a grave disservice to the injured. Not only does he jeopardise the chances of that large num-ber of patients, who cannot benefit directly from his care, but he is also likely to find that his own mortality rate based on such a policy is higher than that desirable or attainable'.

Once a burr hole has been made over the haema-toma, the urgency has eased; the surgeon must resist the temptation to suck away the blood clot, as this will usually set off brisk haemorrhage from the depths of the wound before there is enough exposure to deal with it. If the surgeon feels diffident about cranial surgery, the patient may safely travel to more experienced help, with the wound lightly, but copiously, covered with sterile dressings and a slow intravenous infusion, while brain pulsation slowly delivers the clot on to the dres-sings. On the other hand, he may opt to extend the opening in the skull with bone rongeurs to expose as far as possible the periphery of the haematoma before removing the solid clot and dealing with any bleeding vessels. The resulting skull defect can be repaired in a neurosurgcal department at a later date. Joseph Hill (quoted by Gallagher and Browder, 1968) successfully treated a patient with an extradural haematoma in 1772 in Dumfries; British surgery has little reason to be proud of its achievements otherwise if, more than 200 years later, patients still die while being moved from a district general hospital to a distant neurosurgical department.

Subdural haematoma

Acute subdural haematoma, regrettably, because of the high mortality and morbidity associated with it, is a much commoner complication of head injury than the extradural. It may develop in one of three situations:

1   After high speed deceleration, in which the direc-tion of the force is anteroposterior and the res-training effect of the dural folds is absent, relative movement of brain within the skull results in lac-

eration of the tips of the temporal lobe against the lesser wings of the sphenoid. There may be haematomas on both sides.

2   Where there is a fracture, depressed or not, particularly in infants, in whom the skull is unusually resilient, the bone edges at the time of impact may be driven in sufficiently to injure the cortex beneath it.

3   Bleeding from a tear in a superior cerebral vein may produce a subdural haematoma without brain laceration, notably in the middle-aged and elderly, even after a trivial non-concussional injury. In the acute subdural haematoma such a mechanism is unusual enough to be of no more than anecdotal interest, though it does operate in the chronic subdural.

The effects of the haemorrhage depend on the volume and rate of the bleeding, which itself is related to the severity of the injury. It is customary to classify haematomas as acute, subacute or chronic, depending on the speed of evolution of the clinical picture. The basic pattern is the same in every case, namely, a steady decline in the degree of responsiveness with or without a tendency to recover after the actual injury before deterioration begins. A more logical classification based on Hooper (1969) takes into account the natural history and is of value in any attempts to reconcile controversy about the results of treatment.

1   The 'explosive' or rapidly fatal extravasation usually results from a very violent impact of the type seen in high-speed traffic accidents. The patient is deeply unconscious from the outset, but soon develops the classical signs of tentorial herniation – pupillary dilatation and extensor spasms, leading to apnoea and death within 6–12 h. Active intervention does little more, at best, than prolong the act of dying.

2   Acute subdural haematomas present in the first 24 h, but the course of events is slow enough to allow recognition of an early period of recovery before the deterioration sets in. Mortality is high despite energetic treatment, useful survival rare except in the relatively young. The outlook is best in those who were at least localising pain, if not talking, at some stage after injury.

Haematomas coming to operation within the first three days are generally called acute, but the mortality in those presenting on the second and third days is nearer that of the subacute group, where they are therefore more logically placed from the prognostic point of view.

3   Subacute subdural haematoma. This group consists mostly of patients who do not cause any particular concern at first; then it is noticed that the patient is not

making the expected steady improvement before actual deterioration becomes apparent from the second day onwards to the fourteenth. Surgery here is usually rewarding, though there may be some morbidity in the form of persistent hemiparesis and late post-traumatic epilepsy.

4   The fleeting or fugitive subdural haematoma. Routine angiography or CAT scanning in the assessment of head injured patients with depressed consciousness sometimes shows a subdural haematoma, up to 1 cm in thickness, which is not suspected clinically. If operation is deferred, the patient may make an uninterrupted recovery without showing the expected deterioration, and repeat investigation will show absorption of the clot. On the other hand, if, on the commendable principle of early diagnosis, such patients are submitted to surgery, they would naturally be included in the acute subdural group and help to make the prognosis look better than it actually is.

5   The chronic subdural haematoma is (characteristically) a condition seen in the middle-aged and elderly. A history of head injury often may be lacking and the patient admitted to a medical ward as an atypical stroke. The typical patient is over the age of 50 with a history of fluctuating confusion and drowsiness, and a slow decline; particularly when examined in the semiconscious phase, there is bilateral ptosis, small pupils, neck stiffness without a positive Kernig's sign, generally brisk tendon reflexes without gross hemiparesis, and bilateral extensor plantars. If there is even limited cooperation from the patient in the more lucid phase, conjugate upward gaze is limited. Unlike the acute subdural haematoma which is found low in the anterior temporal region, the chronic lesion is high up over the convexity of the cerebral hemisphere. Generally fluid, burr-hole evacuation may be all that is needed; the prognosis is usually excellent. Disappointing results in the very old are probably due to secondary vascular changes in the brain itself.

A diagnosis of chronic subdural is on occasion proposed when some time after a minor injury, a relatively wide awake elderly patient is seen with a dense hemiplegia. The discrepancy between the level of consciousness and the profound paralysis is that of a stroke; for a surface haematoma to produce a dense contralateral paralysis, the pressure would have to be so high as to render the patient deeply unconscious as well. Nor should a chronic subdural haematoma be attributed to any head injury that occurred more than three months earlier.

Infantile subdural haematoma

This is a good example of a condition in which the frequent absence of a history of trauma, because it is withheld by the parents, leads to wildly incorrect deductions about aetiology, until the presence of bruises, of skull fracture and perhaps of healing fractures of varying ages elsewhere draw attention to the possibility of 'baby battering', euphemistically designated 'non-accidental injury'.

The usual presentation is of an irritable infant, vomiting, feeding poorly and failing to thrive, with seizures and a tense fontanelle. The diagnosis is established by careful needling of the subdural space through the widened coronal suture just lateral to the anterior fontanelle if the latter is not wide or through the outer angles of the fontanelle if it is. If there are retinal haemorrhages, it is evidence of a recent sudden increase in intracranial pressure and, therefore, of recent head injury or severe chest compression.

Acute haematomas large enough to require surgical treatment are rare, probably because such infants do not survive the initial injury. The more chronic lesions are fluid; if small, they may settle down with repeated aspiration, but persistent collections require surgical treatment. Craniotomy and removal of subdural membranes used to be practised widely, but has now been generally replaced by the simple procedure of draining the collection into the pleural or peritoneal cavity; the morbidity is less and the results probably better. The writer's preference is for the simple insertion of a rubber catheter passed subcutaneously from the subdural space into the pleural cavity (Till, 1965). Drainage usually continues for several weeks; no expensive valves are necessary and the catheters can be removed simply after about 3–6 months.

The quality of survival depends upon the damage inflicted by the primary injury, but impaired intelligence and epilepsy are all too common sequelae.

Intracerebral haemorrhage

This is usually from cortical vessels bleeding into softened or contused white matter. Such bleeding is frequently associated with acute subdural bleeding and the two may be clinically indistinguishable; it has been suggested that the two lesions should be placed together under the common heading of intradural haematoma. They are being more readily diagnosed since the advent of CAT scanning, and, again, it is not certain that they invariably need surgical evacuation.

Subdural hygroma

Clear or yellow collections of c.s.f. may be encountered in the subdural space either on exploratory burrholes or as low-density extracerebral collections on computerised tomography in both acute and chronic phases of head injury. They are termed subdural hygromata or hydromata. The acute hygroma probably

occurs as the result of a valvular tear in the arachnoid, analogous to a tension pneumothorax, and sometimes seen in a rapidly deteriorating injury with the escape of clear c.s.f. under high pressure on opening the dura after a burr-hole; and a dramatic improvement in the patient's level of consciousness. The chronic subdural hygroma may be seen in patients who seem not to be making satisfactory progress; their evacuation is said to accelerate recovery. A similar yellow collection is seen in retarded children with an asymmetrical head, produced by localised bulging of the skull over the hygroma. The adjacent brain is atrophic, and the hygroma asymptomatic.

Focal cerebral contusion

Localised areas of brain swelling may occur as a result of contusion. The best known and commonest of such focal lesions is the temporal lobe contusion (McLaurin and Helmer, 1965). The latter is typically seen after a sudden deceleration head injury, often accompanied by an occipital or temporal fracture, in a drowsy restless combative patient who develops a localised progressive hemiparesis maximal about the third day, without pupillary inequality. The diagnosis is made on angiography, and the recommended treatment is temporal lobectomy, but unless the clinical deterioration is steep, careful observation might, in fact, demonstrate the real prospect of spontaneous improvement that is not unusual. McLaurin and Helmer themselves advised that the decision about surgical intervention should rest entirely on the clinical course. This advice tends to be consistently overlooked by those who see areas of focal brain swelling so often present when CAT scanning is used routinely in the assessment of acute head injury.

Generalised brain swelling

This may occur in severe injuries as a complication of anoxia or from the initial deceleration forces. It is particularly in the management of intracranial hypertension that cannot be relieved surgically or persists after the evacuation of offending focal masses that hypertonic solutions, diuretics, corticosteroids and ventilation are used with varying degrees of conviction on the part of the protagonists.

Occult hydrocephalus

Also referred to as normal pressure hydrocephalus, this is a late complication of injury, suspected more often than confirmed or successfully treated. Overt symptoms or signs of raised pressure are lacking, and random measurements of c.s.f. pressure by lumbar puncture are normal. The condition should be considered when a patient fails to recover from a severe head injury after a few weeks and in a patient with a past history of head trauma who develops progressive dementia, gait disturbance and incontinence. Investigation reveals large ventricles and a communicating type of hydrocephalus presumably due to obstruction of c.s.f. channels by organised blood. It is not readily distinguishable from dilatation of the ventricles due to cerebral atrophy, and there is no general agreement on how best to identify the patient who will benefit from one of the shunting procedures used in hydrocephalus (British Medical Journal, 1980). So far the best indication in this respect is the demonstration of high pressure waves during sleep when intracranial pressure is monitored continuously. Because such monitoring shows that the damage is probably caused during the periods of hypertension which are only intermittent, the term occult hydrocephalus is more appropriate to this condition than normal pressure hydrocephalus.

Diagnosis of cerebral compression

Ninety-five percent of patients admitted to hospital after head injury in this country are conscious at the time of admission and deteriorating consciousness heralding cerebral compression should be readily recognised in the occasional patient from this large group who develops a haematoma. In the 5% who reach hospital with altered consciousness, diagnosis will depend on our ability to appreciate the more subtle changes that may occur and to record trends reliably. Terms such as stupor, semicoma and coma are often used in practice, but should be avoided as they mean different things to different people. It is better to denote the state of consciousness as a simple description of the individual's response to speech, and, failing that, to pain. Focal brain damage or measures such as tracheal intubation may make verbal responses difficult to assess. The Glasgow Coma Scale (Teasdale and Jennett, 1974) partly overcomes this problem by adding a third dimension – eye opening – to verbal and motor activity; eye-opening is an index of the state of activity of the arousal mechanisms in the brain stem. The three behavioural responses tested are outlined in Table 1,

the figures in brackets against each level of response denote the score for that particular reaction; as each feature can be scored independently, the total of the three responses serves as an indication of the degree of brain dysfunction, useful in recording data for research purposes.

The response to pain deserves some consideration as it is one of the areas in which mistakes are commonly made, even in some hospital observation charts, where the only question asked or answered is whether the patient responds to pain or not. Such practice ignores the different types of response possible, distinction between which may be crucial in a patient who is localising pain when first seen, and may deteriorate to the stage of decerebrate response to pain without such worsening being seen in the findings recorded. The only normal reaction to pain is localising, where a hand comes up to the site of stimulation. At a lower level, the patient may merely withdraw the arm without localising pain. The movement of the upper limbs is noted, as this is most readily visible in a patient lying partly covered by the bedclothes. Flexion to pain corresponds to the posture conventionally labelled decorticate, and extension to pain as the decerebrate state. The best response between the two sides is taken as reflecting the level of brain function, the lesser being possibly the effect of local damage.

On the Glasgow scale, coma is often defined as the state in which the patient does not open his eyes even to pain, with no better than incomprehensible speech and does not obey simple commands.

Increasing acceptance of the Glasgow Coma Scale has improved communication between peripheral hospital and neurosurgical unit, as well as within the unit itself between various members of staff involved in a patient's care.

What is important in the diagnosis of cerebral compression is to recognise that a patient is deteriorating neurologically whatever the method used to identify such change in consciousness. Lateralising CNS signs like pupillary dilatation or progressive hemiparesis are secondary features that are either late or inconstant. Changes in pulse, blood pressure and respiration are, in practice, more useful as a guide to the extracranial factors that might depress brain function e.g. hypoxia, than as signs of cerebral compression. In fact, if a patient in a coma from the moment of injury deteriorates, it may be more fruitful to look for readily correctable causes of hypoxia by measuring blood gases than for a haematoma.

Once the suspicion of cerebral compression is aroused, whether ancillary investigations are carried out to confirm such suspicions will depend on the circumstances. Even in neurosurgical departments the only hope for a rapidly worsening patient may be immediate surgery on clinical grounds alone.

Table 1
GLASGOW COMA SCALE

Eyes open	Verbal response	Motor response
Spontaneously (4)	Orientated (5)	Obeys commands (6)
To speech (3)	Confused (4)	Localises pain (5)
To pain (2)	Inappropriate (3)	Withdrawal to pain (4)
Not at all (1)	Incomprehensible (2)	Flexion to pain (3)
	None (1)	Extension to pain (2)
		None (1)

The figures in brackets denote the score for each response.

Exploratory burr-holes may be regarded as the most readily available diagnostic tool in a surgeon's armamentarium. The number of negative burr-holes made decreases as the surgeon's experience grows, bearing in mind that the incidence of biologically relevant haematomas is very low. As a working rule, such burr-holes ought to be considered if, when first seen:

1 a patient is deeply unconscious, but known to have spoken after the injury
2 the level of consciousness is declining visibly in the course of examination
3 there is no history available and the patient is decerebrate with one or both pupils widely dilated.

Decerebrate patients with reacting pupils do not harbour clots or raised intracranial pressure.

The differential diagnostic features between extra and intradural haematomas are summarised in Table 2. Even if one ignores this clinical distinction, the localisation of a clot does not as a rule require more than three burr-holes. The first should be at the point of impact, which is seen more clearly after the whole head is shaved, especially if the blow has been to the side or front of the head; if there is no extradural here, and the underlying dura does not look blue to suggest a subdural haemorrhage, the next opening is low in the opposite anterior temporal region just below the temporal crest, and the third, at the corresponding point on the side of impact. Even if the first site reveals an extradural haematoma, it is advisable to make an opening in the opposite temple, unless there was a clear lucid interval or the intracranial pressure low without any measures being taken to lower it, beyond removal of the first clot. If all the burr-holes are negative, and the brain is tense, an additional right frontal hole 2.5 cm

from the mid-line, near the coronal suture, is made and the lateral ventricle correlated; if the ventricle is dilated and large quantities of c.s.f. escape, it is an indication of a clot in the posterior fossa.

Echoencephalography

This is attractive in its simplicity and enjoyed a short-lived popularity in detecting displacement of midline structures, and as a screening test before investigations for more precise localisation of a clot are initiated (Ford and Ambrose, 1963). Its reliability depends on the operator's experience with the equipment; by the time a doctor has acquired such expertise, his clinical sense will have developed sufficiently to make such apparatus superfluous. Recently a computerised echo-encephalograph, the 'midliner', which apparently compensates for the user's lack of familiarity with it, has been introduced in some accident departments. It is said that its routine use would help identify seemingly well patients with midline displacements, who could then be selectively transferred to a neuro-surgical unit for further investigation and eliminate the possibility of fatal delays. The value of such a policy has not been tested.

An echoencephalograph is, perhaps, most useful in the management of multiple injuries requiring ventilatory support, where sedatives obscure the conscious level and makes any deterioration difficult to recognise; bedside serial monitoring of the position of the midline could help identify a developing haematoma.

Computerised axial tomography

This is now the investigation of choice in intracranial disease and has virtually replaced all other diagnostic procedures in the management of head injury. It is relatively quick, completely without risk to the patient and not only localises masses, but can also distinguish between haematoma, oedema and infarction. The principal drawbacks are the cost of the equipment which restricts its availability, and the necessity for the patient to lie still for the 5 min the investigation takes; except for those already deeply unconscious, most head injuries, in whom the desirability of excluding an expanding haematoma is greatest, are restless and uncooperative and, therefore, need a general anaesthetic if the investigation is to be conclusive.

Routine CAT scanning has shown that an intracranial haematoma may be present for some time before clinical signs develop. Many neurosurgeons, therefore, feel that to wait for deteriorating consciousness is delaying action and a consequent increase in avoidable

Table 2
DIFFERENTIAL DIAGNOSIS OF ACUTE HAEMATOMA

	Extradural	Subdural
Incidence	relatively low	much commoner
Age	mostly under 20	extremes of life
Type of accident	often trivial	high speed
Direction of injury	30% not concussed	violent impact
Site of haematoma	lateral	antero posterior,
Prognosis	under point of impact	impact mostly to back of head
	excellent with prompt surgery	low anterior temporal
		poor despite heroic measures

N.B. There are always exceptions. Subdural and intracerebral haemorrhage may be indistinguishable or occur together.

mortality and morbidity (Teasdale *et al.*, 1982) and recommend urgent scanning in:

1 patients not opening eyes to pain, not uttering words and not obeying commands after resuscitation
2 patients with skull fracture who are confused,
   or have neurological symptoms
   or focal neurological signs
   or have had a fit
3 patients with deteriorating consciousness.

Scanning is also advised in patients without skull fracture who are still confused 6–8 h after injury, and in those who have compound or depressed fractures, as a preoperative investigation.

In a patient in whom there is a clear clinical picture of a haematoma, the CAT scan is invaluable, if time and the facilities permit. Precise knowledge of the site and nature of the mass makes a surgeon's task easier than if he had proceeded on clinical considerations alone. Again, a normal scan in a deeply unconscious patient is far more reassuring than negative exploratory burr-holes, which cannot altogether dispel doubts about missing an atypical haematoma. Unfortunately, as shown originally by Ambrose *et al.* (1976), while the introduction of the CAT scan has reduced the number of invasive investigations and exploratory operations, the overall mortality in head injuries has remained unchanged. From the avalanche of papers published since then, one cannot escape the conclusion that, where resources allow routine use of the scan in the initial evaluation of all head injuries, patients are being subjected to surgery for radiological abnormalities without considering their clinical relevance. Such a policy might be justified on the basis of early presymptomatic diagnosis, if past experience with carotid angiography had not already amply demonstrated that indiscriminate investigation will reveal haematomas and contusions that were not suspected clinically and which will mostly resolve without specific treatment. French and Dublin (1977) studied 316 patients who had CAT scans after head injury; 161 (51%) had abnormal scans and in 38% there was more than one abnormality, yet only 91 needed operation. Even among those who were alert and asymptomatic, 13% had abnormalities. A normal scan does not rule out the need for vigilance as 6 patients developed complications later.

Where the sedation required for controlled ventilation makes clinical assessment impossible, there is a natural bias in favour of treating all focal mass lesions seen in the scan surgically. Even in centres with an aggressive approach to head injury, it is being appreciated (Roberson *et al.*, 1979) that on serial scanning no surgically significant lesions are detected in the early post-traumatic period that had not already been signalled by changes in neurological status, intracranial pressure or volume-pressure response (the last two being necessary adjuncts in a ventilated patient). Serial scans and surgical action based on their results become virtually obligatory in such patients, if intracranial pressure is not being monitored.

Practising in a region in which many head injuries are primarily managed in district general hospitals at some distance from the neurosurgical centre, even though there is an efficient on-demand neuroradiological service, one is philosophically committed to the concept that a neurosurgeon should show, by example, that all the worthwhile action necessary within the first few hours after injury can be taken without resort to the diagnostic methods only available in a special department. Autopsies carried out in all fatal cases by a neuropathologist, and discussed at weekly departmental meetings, have shown no reason for a change in this attitude. Such considerations apart, patients submitted for CAT scanning fall into at least one of the following groups:

1 Those with neurological deterioration slow enough not to demand immediate surgery.
2 Those with a stable neurological deficit and not localising pain (this includes patients with decorticate and decerebrate posturing), the morning after admission.
3 Patients requiring ventilation for associated chest trauma, not obeying commands after initial resuscitation are also scanned the morning after admission.
4 Those who were drowsy and confused on admission and have not shown any improvement after 48 h.
5 Patients still obtunded a month after injury, to rule out occult hydrocephalus.

Fresh blood is seen as a dense white image on a CAT scan, diffuse concavo-convex if it is subdural (Fig 45.1) and biconvex if extradural (Fig 45.2). An intracerebral haematoma is roughly rounded with an irregular outline; there is usually surrounding oedema, less dense than normal brain, while contusions have a mottled appearance. At operation, an acute subdural haematoma may be much thicker than the scan appearances suggested. The density of blood decreases with age, and after a few days a subdural haemorrhage may be isodense with the adjacent brain, and may not be recognised other than as a displacement of the midline. A chronic subdural clot has a lower density than brain and if wholly fluid, its outline is biconvex.

Carotid angiography

This has been almost entirely superseded by CAT scanning in the diagnosis of cerebral compression. It

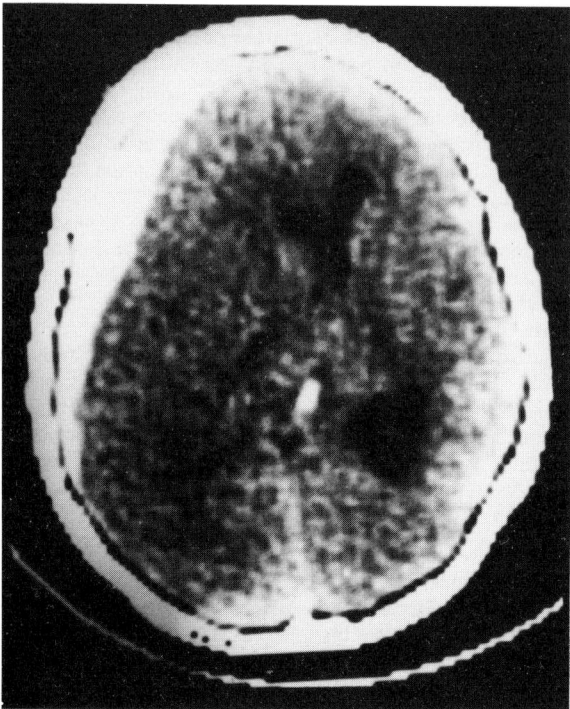

Fig 45.1 CAT scan. Left acute fronto-parietal haematoma.

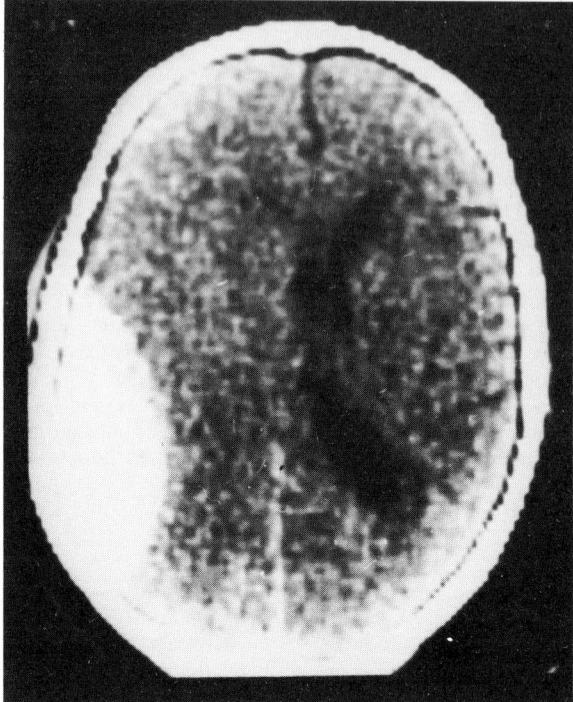

Fig 45.2 CAT scan. Left parietal extradural haematoma.

has a limited application where, in the absence of a midline shift in the scan on an ill patient, symmetrical bilateral isodense subdural haematomas are to be excluded; the author has not come across such a problem. Angiography is still needed in the diagnosis of vascular complications – carotico-cavernous fistula, carotid thrombosis and dural venous sinus thrombosis.

Intracranial pressure monitoring

As experience with monitoring intracranial pressures continuously showed that sustained rises in pressure precede clinical deterioration, the introduction of such monitoring in head injury was a logical development. It serves a dual purpose – the identification of potentially dangerous increases before they are discernible clinically, and the means to judge the success of measures taken to counter such increases. It has added attraction in that there is no clear correlation in a head-injured patient between the conscious level and intracranial pressure, and even more where the treatment of respiratory inadequacy dictates sedation before instituting controlled ventilation.

Price (1980) has reviewed the technical aspects of intracranial pressure monitoring. Lundberg popularised ventricular pressure recording with an in-dwelling catheter connected to an externally placed transducer in 1960; a ventricular catheter not only allows rapid lowering of intracranial pressure where necessary, but also provides a simple means of measuring cerebral compliance by testing the pressure-volume response. The ability of the brain to tolerate increases in the volume of intracranial contents is more relevant to preservation of its functional integrity than the actual pressure itself. Injection into the ventricle or aspiration of 1 ml of fluid should not alter the pressure by more than 3 mmHg if cerebral compliance is normal. Larger changes indicate imminent decompensation. However, in high pressure states, the ventricles are slit-like, and a catheter difficult to place correctly; there is an increased risk of meningitis after long-term monitoring. The extradural space has the lowest risk of infection, but the signal is damped down and less sensitive to changes. The subdural space is more sensitive, but the line is more likely to get blocked.

As with other technical advances, claims that by itself, monitoring has contributed to improved results are questionable, but it is undoubtedly useful in measuring the success or otherwise of measures taken to reduce generalised brain swelling after focal masses have been dealt with or ruled out. Monitoring has helped to demonstrate the futility of gluco-corticoid therapy, often in high dosage, used routinely in severe head injuries (Gudemann *et al.*, 1979).

Infection

Prevention of infection is the third leg of the tripod of head injury management. Infection in a normally closed space like the cranium, in the context of head injury, inevitably means a dural laceration establishing communication between the intradural structures and the outside atmosphere either directly through a compound depressed fracture of the skull vault, or, indirectly through a fracture in the base of the skull opening into the paranasal air sinuses or the middle ear.

Compound depressed fracture of the skull vault

A fracture of the skull vault under a scalp laceration is technically compound, but depression of the fractured fragments and a tear in the dura deep to these are more significant, but can often only be suspected on the basis of the history and the x-ray appearances (Gordon, 1974). More than half such patients will not have lost consciousness, and may, therefore, not be paid the attention they merit in a busy accident department with unfortunate consequences to both patient and doctor.

Ideally all patients with scalp lacerations should have skull x-rays, but this has disadvantages beyond the obvious one of a vast increase in hospital costs and in the work load of the radiology department. Most head injuries arrive outside normal office hours and are assessed by doctors inexperienced in the interpretation of radiographs. The x-rays themselves may not be of adequate diagnostic quality if, as is not unusual, the patient is drunk or uncooperative.

Experienced accident surgeons faced with having to provide a service in far from satisfactory working conditions sometimes advocate a practice, anathema to most neurosurgeons, of probing the wound or, if it is large enough, of palpating the surface of the skull for irregularity, but the scalp laceration may not be directly over the fracture. Despite theoretical objections to such a manoeuvre, instances in which it has caused the patient harm have not been encountered.

What is necessary is to view all scalp lacerations with suspicion, to obtain a clear history of the nature of the object and the velocity at which the wound was produced (especially in children), to shave the hair for at least 5 cm from the edge of the laceration for careful examination under a good light, and, as a last resort, to palpate the wound with the gloved finger for a fracture only if it seems satisfactory x-rays cannot be obtained.

The principles that govern the management of compound fractures elsewhere in the body also apply to the head, i.e. exploration of the wound to remove all contaminated and non-viable tissue and foreign bodies, followed by primary closure. Surgery may be deferred for up to 24 h without increase in morbidity if the wound is cleared immediately and antibiotics given; a delay may even be advisable where the possibility of other complications also requiring operation exists, such as a ruptured spleen.

In some districts in which neurosurgical involvement in the care of trauma is minimal or non-existent, many such fractures are dealt with by no more than cleaning of the wound and a single layer scalp suture with antibiotic cover, a practice which neurosurgeons would deplore. The few disastrous consequences of such a 'primitive' approach seem to be where, because the surrounding hair has not been shaved and the wound inspected carefully, the presence of necrotic brain oozing into the depth of the wound has been missed, and not even antibiotics prescribed. It is doubtful whether a technically compound depressed fracture in which the inner table has split away and the contour of the outer table has been retained or, where the fragments are wedged together so tightly that there is no more than a hairline gap between them and the actual skull, requires further attention than to the scalp wound.

At operation access to the fracture requires either extension of the original laceration, or a separate scalp flap after closing the latter. A burr-hole is made at the edge of the fracture. It may be possible to elevate the fragment by inserting a periosteal elevator underneath. Where this is possible the dura is usually found to be intact. More commonly, especially in the adult, the fragments are impacted, and it may be necessary to use fine bone rongeurs to widen one or more of the fracture lines and carefully remove the pieces of bone taking care not to damage the dura if it is intact, or cause further laceration of the brain if the dura is torn. Damaged brain is sucked away gently and, after meticulous control of bleeding, the dura is repaired with either a patch of pericranium from the intact skull nearby or, for larger defects, fascia lata. The bone fragments are washed in saline and can be replaced safely over the sutured dura to spare the patient a second operation for repair of the skull defect. Topical antibiotics or povidone-iodine are applied to the wound before it is closed, the scalp being sutured in two layers.

In high speed missile wounds, profuse haemorrhage from the scalp and cerebral vessels, and progressive brain swelling, made worse by coughing, vomiting or hypoxia, call for immediate treatment of shock and respiratory inadequacy. This is the one situation in which intermittent positive pressure ventilation is of proven value. Unless uncontrollable haemorrhage demands immediate operation, surgery can wait till the blood volume has been restored and intracranial pressure reduced with ventilation. The devitalised brain tissue usually contains all the in-driven pieces of bone which can be removed without inflicting further injury to the brain, but metallic fragments penetrate more deeply and no special attempt is made to retrieve them. It is particularly important to close the dura where the vitality of the scalp is in doubt. In all cases, full thickness skin cover is essential. Mortality is unfortunately high, being 11% in patients arriving alert in hospital, and 100% in those in coma when first seen (Crockard, 1974).

Compound fracture of the skull base

The heavily buttressed bone at the base of the skull requires considerable force to fracture it. Such force will generally have produced loss of consciousness which should serve to draw attention to the patient, but not necessarily to the internally compound fracture.

C.s.f. otorrhoea is usually profuse and may be obvious when the patient is examined, but not so rhinorrhoea. Unless the fracture line extends into the skull vault or there is air within the cranium, a basal fracture may not be seen on routine skull x-rays. A compound fracture of the anterior cranial fossa should be suspected in patients with a frontal impact who also have fractures of the facial bones or the characteristic black-eye in which the discolouration of the eyelids ends sharply at the bony aperture of the orbit, the so-called 'racoon' or 'eye-shadow' sign and blood in the nostrils. Rhinorrhoea may not develop till the blood clots have dissolved after a few days. Even where there has been a frank meningitis, careful clinical examination may fail to show a rhinorrhoea or x-rays, a fracture.

X-rays films of the quality needed to visualise a basal fracture require the patient's cooperation, and are therefore postponed until consciousness has been fully regained. Films showing the roof of the orbit and the optic foramina are just as likely to reveal fracture lines involving the air-sinuses as tomograms of the anterior cranial fossa. Rhinorrhoea may occur without a fracture in patients in whom the olfactory rootlets have been avulsed from the cribriform plate to produce anosmia.

Where rhinorrhoea or otorrhoea has persisted beyond a week, the necessity for repair of the dural tear is obvious. Fractures of the anterior cranial fossa are usually comminuted and if rhinorrhoea has stopped, it may be due to the defect getting occluded by herniating brain. Therefore, even when rhinorrhoea is transient, exploration is desirable if:

1   the fracture line into a sinus is wide
2   there is a persistent aerocele
3   there has been an attack of meningitis
4   there is bilateral anosmia without fracture.

Operation may be advisable in the absence of a c.s.f. leak in the first three situations mentioned above. The presence of facio-maxillary fractures need not influence the decision; c.s.f. rhinorrhoea at some stage was observed by Leopard (1970) in two-thirds of such patients, but did not require dural repair.

Operation is delayed till all brain swelling has settled, the external sign of which may be taken as disappearance of scalp oedema, usually after the tenth day. Where meningitis has developed, this is treated first. Most dural tears in the anterior cranial fossa are close to the midline and may cross it; a bifrontal craniotomy is, therefore, to be preferred to allow exploration on both sides. In c.s.f. otorrhoea, repair is required less often, but is easier because the defect is usually quite superficial, over the tegmen tympani.

Management

Having considered individually the principal threats to an injured brain, it is now possible to look at the overall management of head injured patients after they have reached the accident department, where medical involvement generally begins.

The few, whose consciousness is depressed when first seen, cause concern, even panic, and correct management calls for a disciplined approach taking into account the order of priorities:

1   Prevention or correction of anoxia
2   A base line assessment with which subsequent progress can be compared
3   History with particular reference to the circumstances and time of the accident and trends in conscious level since.

An adequate examination of the nervous system for practical purposes can be carried out without an ophthalmoscope or tendon hammer, unless there is suspicion of concomitant neurological disease. Apart from care in recording the level of consciousness, only unequivocal features need be considered such as gross hemiparesis, pupillary size and reaction and plantar responses. In the absence of local injury to the neck, neck stiffness may be of diagnostic value. Neck rigidity may result from traumatic subarachnoid haemorrhage, meningitis or herniation of cerebellar tonsils through the foramen magnum. If present from the beginning, it is a sign of blood in the subarachnoid space due to cortical lacerations, which may also lead to the formation of a subdural haematoma; such patients, therefore, deserve more careful observation. If neck stiffness comes on while a patient is being observed, is accompanied by deteriorating consciousness and there is no Kernig's sign, tonsillar herniation demanding urgent relief, has probably occurred. If there is a positive Kernig's sign and, perhaps, pyrexia, meningitis must be ruled out. This is almost the only indication for lumbar puncture after head injury.

Most of the patients admitted to hospital are conscious and rational when first seen. The number of head injuries admitted each year to hospitals in England and Wales has risen steadily over the years, while the mortality rate has remained unchanged. This may suggest improved standards of care, but since the number of severe injuries as judged by the length of in-patient stay haš also been constant, the correct inference probably is that more trivial injuries are being unnecessarily admitted (Field, 1976). The criteria for admission, therefore, merit critical attention in the hope that fewer patients for observation might lead to earlier recognition of serious complications (Strang et al., 1978; Totten and Buxton, 1979). Nothing is lost by sending a patient who has no neurological symptoms, signs or skull fracture, home into the care of a responsible person who is instructed on what symptoms to look for in the unlikely event of complications developing. Costly errors are likely in two situations: when a patient's confusion is thought mistakenly to be due to alcohol, and when a compound fracture of the skull is not recognised. The first can only be avoided by admitting all drunks with any evidence of scalp injury; these may form a substantial group with considerable nuisance value, and are best catered for in a separate small, overnight observation unit attached to the accident and emergency department.

Skull x-rays should ideally be obtained soon after resuscitation and examination, before admission to a ward, so that, should a haematoma develop, knowledge of where a fracture is will help localise it, and help plan treatment if there is a compound fracture. In the conditions that exist in many hospitals, the value of such a practice is questionable in those patients in whom the need for admission is already clear on clinical grounds. Most adult admissions are outside hours when a hospital is fully staffed, and there is invariably a delay in getting such x-rays. If the patient is confused and restless, the radiographs are not of diagnostic quality. An unconscious patient not deep enough to tolerate an endotracheal tube who vomits while flat on his back as the skull is being x-rayed is at risk of inhaling such vomit. Unless there is continual medical or expert nursing supervision with suction facilities in the x-ray department, the danger of anoxic damage or death is too real to be ignored. It is safer to postpone x-rays till the following morning, when most patients will have

regained consciousness and the decision to discharge them may be altered by the demonstration of a compound fracture and more severe head injuries will have become stable. In the rare patient who develops an extradural haematoma, it can be localised just as reliably by reference to the point of external impact, and where time permits, even more accurately by CAT scanning. If treatment of associated injuries, such as chest and spine, demands x-rays, skull films may be obtained at the same time, but such patients are ill enough to deserve the presence of a doctor throughout the procedure.

Over the years there has been no reason to regret this policy, the soundness of which has been reinforced by knowledge of the occasional avoidable death in the x-ray department when such advice has been ignored, and by the findings of Harwood-Nash et al. (1971).

In theory, all asymptomatic patients should have skull x-rays to rule out fracture before a decision not to admit them is made. However, as only 1.3% of such patients, in fact, have a fracture (Strang et al., 1978) there is a case for selection based on the circumstances of the injury, that is, on getting a proper history which is often overlooked.

In-patient care

After admission to hospital, most patients will recover, needing no more than continued observation, maintenance of an airway and general nursing and metabolic care. A close watch on the conscious level being the main purpose of observation, *sedative drugs are avoided*, though confused, restless, even violent patients are not uncommon and pose problems. Exceptions to this policy are when the patient has convulsions or needs controlled ventilation.

Where a patient will tolerate it, an endotracheal tube should be passed; in most cases it is also useful to have a wide bore tube in the stomach for aspiration of contents at first and, if the patient does not recover, for feeding. Most modern endotracheal tubes may be safely left in for up to 7 days or more, by which time some idea of the prognosis is obtained and may determine whether a tracheostomy should be carried out.

Most head injuries occur in previously well hydrated subjects and, if unconscious on admission, are none the worse for being without fluids for up to 24 h by which time they will probably have regained consciousness. Intravenous infusion should, therefore, be unnecessary unless there is shock from associated injuries. If unconsciousness persists, parenteral nutrition may be required till the stomach is able to tolerate nasogastric tube feeding. attention to fluid and electrolyte balance and to sufficient calories in assimilable form is important but elegant expensive solutions to counter the catabolic phase have no proven value in head injury. The aim is to provide 2 l of fluid daily and to work up to a high protein diet providing 2000 calories. The standard hospital diet liquidised and fed through the tube is as good as any proprietary feed (Jones *et al.*, 1980).

Dehydration may still occur if diabetes insipidus develops and is not recognised in an unconscious patient unless electrolytes and urinary output are carefully monitored. In the conscious patient polydipsia and polyuria have no more than a nuisance value. In either case it is readily relieved with Desmopressin which can be given intramuscularly, intravenously or intranasally. Diabetes insipidus after head injury always resolves spontaneously; in any polydipsia persisting beyond a year, compulsive drinking should be excluded. The syndrome of inappropriate secretion of antidiuretic hormone (SIADH) is a rare, but interesting, complication of severe head injury, resulting in deepening coma due to water retention, recognised by the serum electrolyte abnormality and gratifyingly reversed by withholding fluids.

Drugs

Headache is the most frequent symptom and readily relieved by codeine or aspirin. It is most likely to be persistent after traumatic subarachnoid haemorrhage, and if the latter has not been recognised in the acute phase, such continuing headache may be wrongly labelled as part of an accident neurosis.

Prophylactic antibiotics are routinely used in the presence of compound fractures, prolonged coma and dirty scalp lacerations. Penicillin and sulphadimidine are preferred in the first instance despite the widespread occurrence of penicillin-resistant organisms in hospitals.

Post-traumatic epilepsy

Fits occurring in the first week after injury are designated *early post-traumatic epilepsy*. Except in children under the age of 5 in whom it may follow very trivial injury, such epilepsy most commonly occurs in severe injury, particularly with post-traumatic amnesia of more than 24 h, depressed fracture or intracranial haematoma (Jennett, 1975). Its main significance is that 25% of such patients will develop late epilepsy. On its own it does not indicate a haematoma; while a seizure can occur in the course of evolution of a clot, it is never the only sign. Immediate action to control it is only required in status epilepticus; diazepam 10 mg i.v. with another 10 mg i.m. is usually enough, but the dose can be exceeded safely as long as the blood pressure does not drop precipitously and no other drug has been given. Sodium Amylobarbitone in 250 mg doses is equally if not more effective, but not as popular as diazepam. Resistant status is rare if initial treatment is aggressive enough, but occasionally such patients may be better respired mechanically to counteract the respiratory depression that the really large doses of drugs needed may produce.

In any case, routine anticonvulsant treatment to control further attacks and as a prophylaxis against late epilepsy is advisable (Rapport and Penry, 1973) the drug of choice being phenytoin in a dose of 300 mg daily in adults. There is considerable evidence to suggest that regular medication will reduce the incidence of fits even after the drug has been discontinued, but how long such therapy should continue is still undecided (Jennett, 1980). A year is perhaps long enough; unfortunately the personality of most patients who suffer head injuries makes it unlikely that any drug prescribed will be taken regularly if at all.

Even in the absence of early fits, such treatment is also recommended for those at high risk of late epilepsy, namely, depressed fracture, intradural haematoma, prolonged unconsciousness and persistent neurological deficit of cerebral origin.

As an example of how difficult it is to find scientific validation for so many widely accepted practices in medicine, it is worth noting that controlled double-blind trials designed to test the value of prophylactic anticonvulsants have failed to show any difference in the incidence of late post-traumatic epilepsy between treated and placebo groups (Young *et al.*, 1983; McQueen *et al.*, 1983.)

The risk of late epilepsy is 31% after intracranial haematoma, 25% after early epilepsy and 15% with depressed fractures; the last group is weighted by those with prolonged PTA, focal features and dural penetration who have a high incidence of seizures, but where none of these features exists the incidence drops to 3%, and it is, therefore, possible to reassure such patients that the risk of epilepsy is relatively small. *Elevation of a fracture does not reduce the risks*, as is believed by some surgeons.

The time of onset of late epilepsy may have an adverse bearing on the nature of possible employment for a patient who has otherwise made a complete recovery. More than half of those who will develop seizures will have had their first fit within a year, but this may be concealed if a patient is on anticonvulsant drugs during that period; however, 20% may not have their first fit for more than 4 years, and in these the fits are more likely to be frequent and difficult to control. Once late epilepsy has set in, it is safer to assume that it will not remit and the patient will need anticonvulsants in suitable dosage for the rest of his life. An EEG is of little or no value in predicting the prospects of epilepsy in those at risk.

Controlled ventilation

Kramer and Horsley in 1897 thought that, as apnoea precedes cardiac failure in death from head injury, the brain might survive if respiration were maintained. There is certainly a case for controlled ventilation (Frost, 1979) in a situation in which the major problem is hypoxia from respiratory insufficiency, or, at a cellular level, from ischaemia secondary to raised intracranial pressure. Considering that such ventilation has been practised routinely in neurosurgical operations to control brain swelling and reduce intracranial pressure for nearly a quarter of a century, it is surprising that it was not applied earlier to head injuries in which similar problems arose. Since Gordon (1971) introduced routine ventilation early in the management of 'severe' head injury, its popularity has grown steadily. It is around the definitions of severity and, therefore, the clinical criteria for ventilation that arguments revolve. One cannot avoid the impression that the indications expand in direct proportion to the number of ventilators available.

Intermittent positive pressure ventilation is mandatory in the treatment of major *chest trauma* and *fat embolism*. Powers *et al.*, 1972 have suggested that *post-traumatic pulmonary insufficiency*, in multiple injuries, can be prevented by ventilating all patients in shock (defined as a systolic blood pressure of 80 mmHg or less, requiring at least three units of blood transfusion) if their $P\text{AO}_2$ is less than 10 kPa (75 mmHg).

Controlled ventilation is generally recommended, by those with the greatest experience, in patients with:

1   non-specific or no response to pain
2   central neurogenic hyperventilation
3   irregular respiration or hypoventilation
4   intracranial pressure greater than 20 mmHg
5   convulsions
6   and after any procedure under general anaesthesia till at least the preoperative conscious level is regained.

The writer's conservative approach derives partly from the view that, in most cases, respiratory insufficiency is a sign rather than a cause of brain dysfunction, partly from a fear that such ventilation might prevent death without restoring life, and, not least, from a failure to be convinced as yet by the evidence presented by its protagonists. Use of the ventilator is, therefore, limited to:

1   patients with raised intracranial pressure after a haematoma has been ruled out or evacuated
2   patients needing general anaesthesia for investigation or treatment of associated injury such as limb fractures, until the preoperative conscious level has been reached
3   hyperventilating decerebrate or decorticate patients under the age of 21 with intact brain stem reflexes, spastic limbs and a $P\text{AO}_2$ of less than 10 kPa which cannot be raised by increasing the concentration of O_2 inhaled to 40%.

One would also learn from, but hope not to have to apply, the lessons learnt in Belfast (Crockard, 1974) and include mechanical ventilation as part of the resuscitation and treatment of high-velocity missile wounds of the head.

If despite ventilation with a drop of $P\text{aco}_2$ to below 3.3 kPa the intracranial pressure rises to above 50 mmHg and cannot be brought down, the prognosis is poor and ventilation should be discontinued.

Surgery

Of the large numbers admitted to hospital, few will require any surgery beyond the simple suture of scalp lacerations. The more important indications for surgery have been considered already, other than simple depressed fracture and carotico-cavernous fistula.

The only indication for elevation of a *simple depressed fracture* in most patients is cosmetic. Where a focal neurological deficit can be directly related to the point of depression, elevation in the hope of improving the deficit may be rewarding in the rare instance. One sees no logic behind the usual recommendation that all fractures depressed to a greater depth than the thickness of the skull vault should be operated upon, beyond the fact that knowing whether the dura is torn or not will influence the prospect of epilepsy. However, as this cannot materially influence the long-term management in an individual, this slight gain has to be balanced against the patient's personality and attitude.

A *carotico-cavernous fistula* may follow even minor trauma. It may not present for some days, even weeks, after injury, first as a noise in the patient's head, readily confirmed on auscultation, and later by a progressive pulsating exophthalmos.

Spontaneous healing can occur, or the bruit may disappear after angiography. Surgery may be required if the patient finds the noise disturbing, the proptosis unsightly or his vision failing. Simple ligation of the common or internal carotid in the neck is no longer popular as recurrences were frequent. The favoured surgical approach is to trap the fistula with occlusion of the internal carotid above and below and muscle embolisation of the fistula itself before ligating the cervical carotid. However, the same result can be achieved percutaneously during angiography using a catheter with a detachable balloon tip.

Non-operative reduction of intracranial hypertension

Much of the mortality in the very acute head injury is due to raised intracranial pressure, often without any localised haematoma. The logical surgical answer has been to provide room for the swollen brain by removing some of the cranial vault. Limited decompressions with subtemporal craniectomy were found ineffective and led to removal of larger and more, if not all, of the skull vault. But it is now generally acknowledged that such measures are ineffective and those who apparently benefit are probably ones with a good outlook anyway who would have survived without radical surgery.

There are, however, other methods of relieving intracranial pressure, mostly chemical, depending on osmotic dehydration of the brain. Purgatives and diuretics have long been popular, but frusemide in doses of 20 mg i.v. or i.m. is virtually the sole survivor. Of the hypertonic solutions, 20% mannitol is the most popular in a dose of 1–1.5 g/kg given by i.v. infusion over 30 min. The solubility of mannitol is 17.5% and if the supersaturated solution is not to crystallise, it needs to be stored in a warm cabinet. As the solution is often used in an emergency and not inspected for crystals, 15% mannitol is probably safer. Frusemide given at the start of the infusion will help keep the blood volume down and prevent the increase in blood volume which in turn will increase the blood pressure. In patients with extremely high intracranial pressures on the verge of decompensation, when the brain has lost the capacity to regulate its blood flow, intracranial pressure passively follows the systemic arterial pressure, so any rise in the blood pressure could actually make the patient worse. With all hypertonic solutions, there is danger of rebound and after an initial reduction in intracranial pressure, the final level may be higher than at the start. The other disadvantage is that dehydration, by increasing viscosity in blood that already has a tendency to sludge as a result of injury, may be responsible for ischaemic lesions in the brain.

High-dose *corticosteroids*, particularly dexamethasone, have a dramatic action in the lowering of intracranial pressure in patients with tumours and other space occupying lesion. Their value in head injury is controversial and what evidence there is suggests that they are ineffective (Cooper *et al.*, 1979). The only justification for their widespread use is that in a seemingly desperate situation, however slender the support, to give a readily available drug may be better than doing nothing; unfortunately at the dosages often used, the risk of gastrointestinal haemorrhage or perforation cannot be ignored.

The most reliable method of reducing intracranial pressure available in most hospitals is controlled *ven-tilation* with a negative phase, and it is not surprising that ventilation has become the central feature in all dynamic approaches to the care of head injury.

The indiscriminate use of methods to reduce intracranial hypertension is to be deplored. These measures should only be used in two situations; where, because of a clinical deterioration, a haematoma has been ruled out, and when a decision to operate has been made already and one wishes to 'buy' time for the operation. Thoughtless routine administration of any of these methods may mask a developing haematoma, or sometimes even provide room for one.

If one decides to use ventilation, it is only logical to monitor intracranial pressure to test the efficacy of the treatment so that it may be stopped if the pressure still cannot be reduced after 2 h of ventilation.

Hypothermia and *hyperbaric oxygen* have had transient popularity in reducing intracranial pressure and improving cerebral blood flow. However, because of practical problems associated with application, they have been virtually abandoned.

The current fashion is for *barbiturate therapy* (Marshall *et al.*, 1979), used in an attempt to control pressures which have risen about 40 mmHg despite ventilation, lowered Pa_{CO_2}, dexamethasone 20 mg four times a day and mannitol. The mode of action is not clear: although barbiturates slow down metabolism, the assumption that the brain is protected against ischaemia is probably not true. The reduction in intracranial pressure could be due to a constrictive action on cerebral vasculature, and a reduction of cerebral oedema.

Cranial nerve injuries

Cranial nerves, being tethered peripherally, are vulnerable to stretch as the brain moves relative to the skull, or when an exit foramen is involved in a fracture. The first, second, third, sixth and seventh nerves are most often affected.

Anosmia generally follows frontal injury; if really complete, it is accompanied by ageusia and does not recover.

Optic nerve damage is always permanent. It is usually due to indirect injury and there is at least a telltale bruise on the brow above. There may be a fracture line, even a spicule of bone, into the optic foramen; surgical decompression of the nerve has been recommended, but is futile. Any slight recovery that may sometimes occur in a partially blind eye is likely to be seen within a month.

External ocular paresis may be from injury to the sixth or third nerve and is present from the moment of impact. Isolated sixth nerve lesions sometimes develop shortly after relatively minor head injury in children if, otherwise asymptomatic, they have no sinister significance. These palsies recover in 6 to 9 months in most cases.

Facial palsy is usually associated with fracture of the petrous temporal bone, and may not develop till the second to the tenth day after injury. Almost all will recover in under 3 months.

Deafness is more often of the conductive type rather than due to injury to the cochlear nerve itself, and may be seen in patients who also have c.s.f. otorrhoea, facial palsy or postural vertigo.

Postural vertigo

This may be seen after even otherwise trivial injuries, and is commoner than generally appreciated. It is produced by sudden movement of the head. If nystagmus cannot be elicited when the symptom is reproduced by the appropriate movement, the patient may wrongly be diagnosed as suffering from an accident neurosis; electronystagmography will identify the genuine sufferer. Patients with any initiative can adapt to the vertigo by avoiding the specific movement that produces it. Quite early on a definite tendency to recovery can be recognised and vertigo rarely persists longer than a year. Failure to recover, especially apparent deterioration, is due either to a compensation neurosis or reactive depression. In the hope of avoiding the latter, if vertigo seems likely to persist beyond a couple of weeks, drugs such as betahistine or cinnarizine are worth considering, though it is doubtful whether they have any more than a placebo value.

'Best buy' in management

Faced with the claims made for the success of attempts at early diagnosis and aggressive treatment (Becker *et al.*, 1977; Bruce *et al.*, 1978; Marshall *et al.*, 1979), and the frustrations of a shrinking national economy, it helps to recall the words of the neurologist, the late Henry Miller (cited by Jennett *et al.*, 1980): 'As soon as a new, but still unproved, method of treatment is adopted by even a minority of the medical profession, it becomes virtually impossible to conduct the controlled trial that alone can furnish truly reliable evaluation of its efficacy and its hazards.' Such evaluation becomes even more difficult when each treatment schedule contains several components, there is no universally accepted definition of severity, and no single unit admits enough severe head injuries to make a prospective controlled trial feasible. The Glasgow Coma Scale, with its system of scoring, is a worthy attempt to achieve standardisation in the recording of severity and to provide a means of comparing outcome in different

centres (Jennett and Teasdale, 1977). A patient giving no verbal response, not obeying commands and not opening eyes to any stimulus is defined as being in coma; if such coma lasts at least 6 h, immediately following injury or after a lucid interval, the injury is classed as severe. Unfortunately, the most popular new regimens involve intubation and ventilation on arrival in the accident room, using sedation as necessary. Such action artificially lowers the coma score to make the patient seem worse than he actually is, while the duration of coma becomes difficult to assess with any certainty. There is no alternative definition of severity that can overcome this problem.

Nevertheless, the analysis by Jennett *et al.* (1980) of 1000 severe head injuries treated in three different countries deserves attention. There was no significant difference in outcome in the three centres, despite variations in the pattern of admissions and the methods used; corticosteroids had no influence on the results, while the outcome was worse than expected in those who were treated with ventilation. They concluded that the value of treatments proposed for severe head injury needs rigorous scrutiny. Because of the circumstances surrounding acute head injuries, acceptable evidence either way may not be forthcoming for a long time, if ever. Till then each individual has to act on a purely subjective evaluation of the techniques proposed and with the facilities available.

References

Ambrose J., Gooding M.R., Uttley D. (1976). EMI scan in the management of head injuries. *Lancet*; **i**:847–8.

Bartlett J.R., Neil-Dwyer G. (1979). The role of computerised tomography in the care of the injured. *Injury*; **11**:144–7.

Becker D.P., Miller J.D., Ward J.D., Greenberg R.P., Young H.F., Sakalas R. (1977). The outcome from severe head injury with early diagnosis and intensive management. *J. Neurosurg*; **47**:491–502.

British Medical Journal (1980). Cerebral atrophy or hydrocephalus (editorial). *Brit. Med. J*; **1**:348–9.

Bruce D.A., Schut L., Bruno L.A., Wood J.H., Sutton L.N. (1978). Outcome following severe head injuries in children. *J. Neurosurg*; **48**:679–88.

Cooper P.R., Moody S., Clark W.K. *et al.* (1979). Dexamethasone and severe head injury: a prospective double-blind study. *J. Neurosurg*; **51**:307–16.

Crockard H.A. (1974). Bullet injuries of the brain. *Ann. Roy. Coll. Surg. Engl*; **55**:111–23.

Field J.H. (1976). *Epidemiology of Head Injuries in England and Wales*, pp. 28. London: HMSO.

Ford R., Ambrose J. (1963). Echoencephalography. *Brain*; **86**:189–96.

French B.N., Dublin A.B. (1977). The value of computerised tomography in the management of 1000 consecutive head injuries. *Surg. Neurol*; **7**:177–83.

Frost E.A.M. (1979). The physiopathology of respiration in neurosurgical patients. *J. Neurosurg*; **50**:699–714.

Frost E.A.M., Arancibia C.U., Shulman K. (1979). Pulmonary shunt as a prognostic indicator in head injury. *J. Neurosurg*; **50**:768–72.

Gallagher J.P., Browder E.J. (1968). Extradural Haematoma. Experience with 167 patients. *J. Neurosurg*; **29**:1–12.

Gordon D.S. (1974). Depressed fractures and missile wounds of the skull. *Brit. J. Hosp. Med*; **12**:174–92.

Gordon E. (1971). Controlled respiration in the management of patients with traumatic brain injuries. *Acta Anaesthetica Scand*; **15**:193–208.

Gudeman S.K., Miller J.D., Becker D.P. (1979). Failure of high-dosage steroid therapy to influence intra-cranial pressure in patients with severe head injury. *J. Neurosurg*; **51**:301–6.

Harwood-Nash D.C., Hendrick E.B., Hudson A.R. (1971). The significance of skull fracture in children. A study of 1187 patients. *Paediatr. Radiol*; **101**:151–5.

Hooper R. (1969). *Patterns of Acute Head Injury*, pp. 167. London: Edward Arnold.

Jamieson K.G. (1970). Extradural and subdural haematomas, changing patterns and requirements of treatment in Australia. *J. Neurosurg*; **33**:632–5.

Jamieson K.G., Yelland J.D.N. (1968). Extradural haematoma –167 cases. *J. Neurosurg*; **29**:13–23.

Jennett B. (1975). *Epilepsy After Non-missile Head Injuries*, 2nd edn. pp. 179. London: Heinemann Medical.

Jennett B. (1980). Post-traumatic epilepsy: phenytoin prophylaxis (letter). *J. Neurosurg*; **52**:291.

Jennett B., Carlin J. (1978). Preventable mortality and morbidity after head injury. *Injury*; **10**:31–9.

Jennett B., Teasdale G. (1977). Aspects of coma after severe head injury. *Lancet*; **i**:878–1.

Jennett B., Teasdale G., Fry J., Braakman R., Minderhoud J., Heiden J., Kurze T. (1980). Treatment of severe head injury. *J. Neurol., Neurologsurg, Psychiatr*; **43**:289–95.

Jones D.C., Rich A.J., Wright P.D., Johnston I.D.A. (1980). Comparison of proprietary elemental and whole protein diets in unconscious patients with head injury. *Brit. Med. J*; **1**:1493–4.

Leopard P. (1970). Dural tears in maxillo-facial injuries. *Brit. J. Oral Surg*; **8**:222–30.

McLaurin R.L., Helmer F. (1965). The syndrome of temporal lobe contusion. *J. Neurosurg*; **23**:296–303.

McQueen J.K., Blackwood D.H.R., Harris P., Kalbag R.M., Johnson A.L. (1983). Low risk of late post-traumatic seizures following head injury. Implications for clinical trials of prophylaxis. *J. Neurol. Neurosurg. Psychiatr*. (In press).

Marshall L.F., Smith R.W., Shapiro H.M. (1979). The outcome with aggressive treatment in severe head injuries. *J. Neurosurg*; **50**:20–30.

Powers S.R. Jr., Burdge R., Leather R. *et al*. (1972). Studies of pulmonary insufficiency in non-thoracic trauma. *J. Trauma*; **12**:1–14.

Price D.J. (1980). Intracranial pressure monitoring. *Brit. J. Clin. Equip*; **5**:92–8.

Price D.J.E., Murray A. (1972). Influence of hypoxia and hypotension on recovery from head injury. *Injury*; **3**:218–24.

Rapport II. R.L., Penry J.K. (1973). A survey of attitudes towards the prophylaxis of post-traumatic epilepsy. *J. Neurosurg*; **38**:159–66.

Roberson F.C., Kishore P.R.S., Miller J.D., Lipper M.H., Becker D.P. (1979). The value of axial computerised tomography in the management of severe head injury. *Surg. Neurol*; **12**:161–7.

Sevitt S. (1968). Fatal road accidents, injuries, complications and causes of death in 250 subjects. *Brit. J. Surg*; **55**:481–505.

Sevitt S. (1973). Fatal road accidents in Brimingham; times to death and their causes. *Injury*; **4**:281–93.

Strang I., MacMillan R., Jennett B. (1978). Head injuries in accident and emergency departments at Scottish hospitals. *Injury*; **10**:154–9.

Teasdale G., Jennett B. (1974). Assessment of coma and impaired consciousness. A practical scale. *Lancet*; **ii**:81–4.

Teasdale G., Galbraith S., Murray L., Ward P., Gentleman D., McKean M. (1982). Management of intracranial haematoma. *Brit. Med. J*. **285**:1695–7.

Till K. (1965). Subdural haematoma and effusion in infancy. *Brit. Med. J*; **2**:400–2.

Totten J., Buxton R. (1979). Were you knocked out? *Lancet*; **i**:369–70.

Wood Jones F. (1912). The vascular lesion in some cases of middle meningeal haemorrhage. *Lancet*; **ii**:7–12.

Young B., Rapp R.P., Norton J.A., Haak D., Tibbs P.A., Bean J.R. (1983). Failure of prophylactically administered Phenytoin to prevent late post-traumatic seizures. *J. Neurosurg*. **58**:236–41.

Further reading

Braakman R., Schouten H.J.A., Blaauw-van Dishoeck M., Minderhoud I.M. (1983). Megadose steroids in head injury. Results of a prospective double-blind clinical trial. *J. Neurosurg*., **58**:326–30.

46

High velocity missile injuries

W. CAMERON MOFFAT

A missile is any object which is capable of being thrown or projected and, in the broad sense therefore, injuries from missiles may vary from minor superficial abrasions caused by sticks and stones to total annihilation by sophisticated nuclear weapons. In the narrower and commonly understood sense, however, a missile injury arises when the body is struck by a bullet or a fragment of the casing of an explosive device. Wounds so caused have come to be called gunshot wounds (GSW) but it is more informative to describe them as bullet wounds or fragment wounds according to their cause. Throughout this chapter the descriptions refer almost constantly to bullet wounds, but the principles apply equally well to wounds caused by bomb fragments or by secondary missiles such as pieces of masonry, glass, furniture or vehicle parts. If such missiles, even though small, strike the body with sufficient velocity the resultant injury is likely to be much more severe and extensive than expected.

The axiom that correct surgical management is dependent on a knowledge of the cause and mechanisms of disease is no less true in respect of injury and in no form of injury is that truth more apparent than in the treatment of missile wounds. The surgeon who undertakes to treat a high velocity missile wound without understanding their special nature is courting disaster.

The mechanisms of missile injury

Kinetic energy

An everyday common object such as a brick or a bottle, innocent in itself, acquires the potential for injury if it is thrown. The damage it may do will be related to its size and weight and to the speed with which it travels, and this, in turn, will be related to the amount of force used to propel it. This general principle applies to all inert missiles. The kinetic energy (K) created by the propelling force is related to the mass and velocity thus:

$$K = \tfrac{1}{2} mv^2$$

where m is the mass and v the velocity. It must be noted that kinetic energy is much more dependent on velocity than on mass and that whereas doubling the mass will double the available kinetic energy doubling the velocity will quadruple it. This fact has had a powerful influence on the development of military small arms over many years, and in modern times there has been an increasing tendency to produce weapons capable of firing bullets of low mass but at very high muzzle velocities. These high velocity bullets may strike into their targets at speeds of 800 m/s or higher and are capable of inflicting wounds and injury out of all proportion to their size. However not all modern weapons fire high velocity bullets as reference to Table 1 will show.

Table 1

Weapon	Calibre	Missile mass	Muzzle velocity
Pistol	9 mm	11.6 g	170 m/s
Thomson			
Sub-machine gun	11.5 mm	17.2 g	183 m/s
British Army			
FN rifle	7.62 mm	9.3 g	825 m/s
US Army			
Armalite rifle	5.56 mm	3.5 g	975 m/s
Bomb	—	—	1000+ m/s

Many hand guns discharge at speeds of around 200 m/s and whilst bullets from these guns may have a very marked 'knock-down' effect due to their high mass, they do not produce the special effects encountered where the strike velocity achieves or exceeds a figure around 500 m/s. Fragments of bombs or other explosive devices may be travelling at very high velocities close to the point of detonation but lose speed rapidly in flight due to their irregularity.

Stability

The modern bullet, because of its shape, is inherently unstable (Fig 46.1). The centre of mass lies behind the point of air resistance and thus any deviation of the long axis from the line of flight (angle of yaw) will tend to increase until the bullet is induced to tumble end over end. This effect was well seen with the original 'rubber bullets', which were fired from smooth barrelled guns, tumbled in flight, and frequently struck the target side on. Bullet instability is overcome by rifling the weapon barrel, thus causing the bullet to spin round its own long axis, in the same manner as stability is achieved in a spinning top.

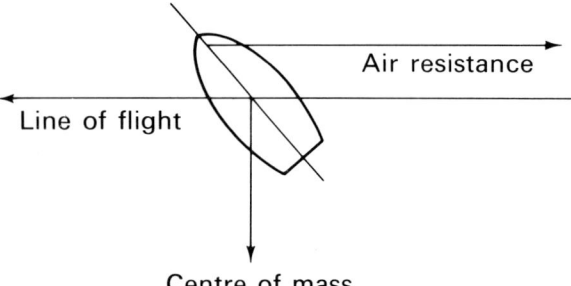

Fig 46.1 Deviation of the long axis of the bullet from the line of flight will eventually induce tumbling.

It should be noted that bullet stability is not fully achieved immediately on discharge, but develops over a distance of some tens of metres depending on the weapon (Fig 46.2). The amount of bullet spin is calculated to achieve nose-on stability in air flight. Once achieved, that stability will be maintained provided the missile remains in air, but should the bullet enter a medium which is denser than air, the spin will be insufficient to maintain stability and it will again exhibit a tendency to yaw and tumble. It is this factor which is of great importance in the production of injury (Fig 46.3).

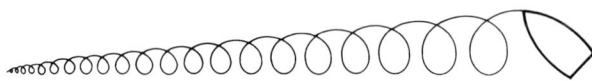

Fig 46.2 Rifling achieves stability gradually.

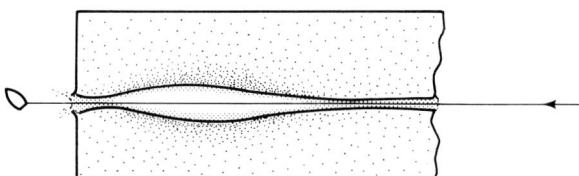

Fig 46.3 Stability is lost in a medium denser than air.

Tissue damage

The high velocity missile inflicts damage in three main ways by:

> Laceration and crushing
> Shock waves
> Cavitation

Laceration and crushing are caused by the physical penetration of the missile and differ little from the effect of penetration by a bayonet or spike. It is the main damaging factor in the case of low velocity missiles striking at speeds below 300 m/s and the effects are serious only in so far as vital organs or major blood vessels may be directly hit.

Shock wave. The effect is interesting and sometimes of importance. When a bomb is detonated a spherical shock wave (blast wave) is set up which travels at the speed of sound in any related medium. Thus in air it travels at around 350 m/s, in water at 1500 m/s and in solid at around 6000 m/s. This shock wave readily reflects from any impeding objects and the reflected waves may be irregular and additive (Fig 46.4). A bul-

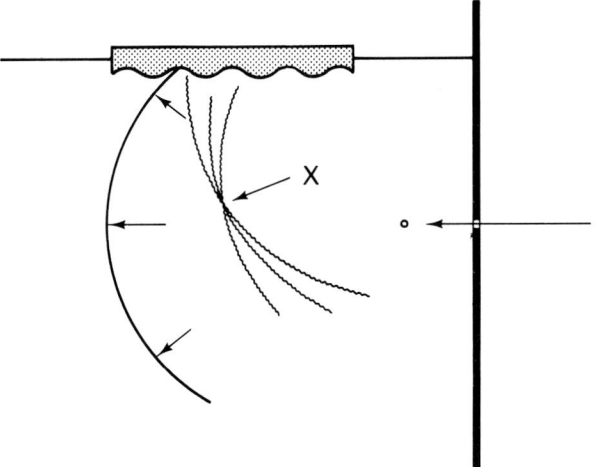

Fig 46.4 Diagram of the shock waves in water set up by a penetrating missile. The reflected waves may be irregular and additive.

let striking a target will set up similar shock waves and if it is a 'mixed medium' target, such as the abdomen, then injury to structures remote from the apparent line of flight may result. Such injury is more likely in thin walled fluid containing structures, such as the bile ducts, or large retroperitoneal veins.

Cavitation. The characteristic features of high velocity bullet wounds depend, however, on the occurrence of cavitation in the target tissues and this special effect requires careful appraisal if the nature of the wound is to be fully understood. The phenomenon can best be studied using ultra high speed cinephotography and by this means observing the passage of bullets through blocks of 20% gelatine, a substance which is lucent and has a density approximately that of muscle. It can be shown that there is little or no cavitational effect where the strike velocity is under 300 m/s. In excess of that speed, however, cavitation does occur and increases in magnitude with rising strike velocity. Figure 46.5 illustrates the effect created by a modern military rifle bullet with a strike velocity around 800 m/s.

The cavitational effect is well seen. It is caused by the violent acceleration of the gelatine away from the missile path and is largely a function of elasticity and inertia. In the moving films it can be seen that cavitation is not a once only phenomenon, but that the cavity is 'pulsatile', forming, collapsing and reforming with decreasing amplitude, during which time the whole block is subject to violent distortion which continues for some time after the cavity has finally settled into a permanent 'wound' track. It will be noted that the cavity is not regular, but greater in the latter part of the

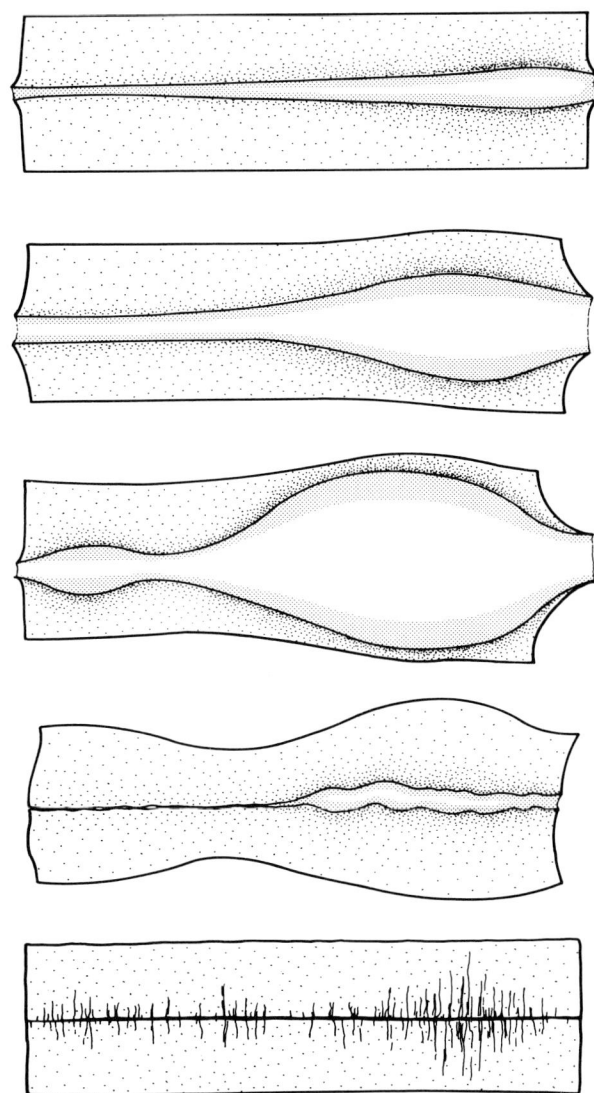

Fig 46.5 The cavitation effect caused by a modern rifle bullet perforating a gelatin block from left to right. Redrawn from high speed cinephotographs.

missile traverse. This is because the bullet has lost stability in the denser medium and has begun to yaw, thus presenting a greater surface area to the target. The bullet is, therefore, more effectively retarded and its kinetic energy consequently more rapidly exchanged.

Retardation and energy exchange

The principle of energy exchange is an important one. A bullet which maintains nose-on stability and perforates a target, emerging with a significant residual velocity, is likely to do less damage than one which penetrates the target, does not emerge and thus exchanges all its kinetic energy. Mathematically if K_E is the energy exchanged then:

$$K_E = \frac{1}{2}\, m(v_1 - v_2)^2$$

where v_1 is the strike velocity and v_2 the emergence velocity. In essence, it is retardation which forces energy exchange and leads to damage, and the more rapid the rate of energy exchange the more intense is the damage likely to be. The factors which affect retardation are considered under two main headings, missile factors and target or tissue factors.

Missile factors:
   Size
   Shape
   Weight
   Velocity
   Material
   Construction

Tissue factors:
   Density
   Elasticity

A missile of relatively high mass and low presenting surface area will be more likely to penetrate or perforate a target than one with relatively low mass and high surface area and this factor has been used in the development of anti-riot missiles, such as the rubber or plastic bullet, where the objective is to deliver a sharp and painful blow and to avoid, as far as possible, internal injury. Missiles made of soft metals are readily deformed and other missiles are so constructed that they break up easily within the target, in each case maximising energy exchange.

Tissues which are highly elastic, such as skin, are able to 'give' under the strain of cavitational forces and are thus able to survive with little permanent damage. Conversely, those which are dense and unyielding will rupture or shatter even though not directly struck by the missile. If bone is struck, not only is the bullet likely to become deformed or fragmented with consequent increase in injury, but the bone will shatter and the fragments will themselves be accelerated within the tissues as secondary missiles and add significantly to the damage.

It is appropriate here also to recognise that missiles do not always travel in straight lines within the target, but are often deflected by fascial planes or bone, often leading to bizarre and unexpected effects. A perforating missile does not always follow a predictable line between entry and exit wounds (Fig 46.6). The human target rarely presents in the anatomical position and this has a profound influence on the possible line of injury (Fig 46.7).

It is important to appreciate the effects of cavitation on muscle, which is sufficiently elastic to allow the

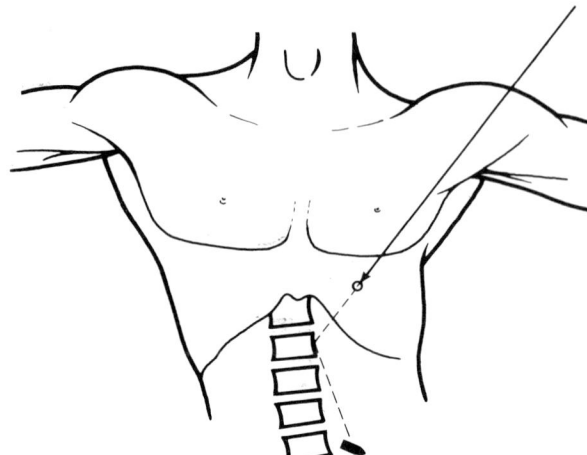

Fig 46.6 A missile does not always follow a predictable line.

formation of a temporary cavity yet sufficiently dense to be damaged in the process. Not only is muscle protein itself directly affected, but the small blood vessels supplying the muscle are damaged and this is highly significant. Muscle which has been subjected to cavitational injury and which lies in relation to the wound tract is not only damaged, but ischaemic.

The effect of cavitation on other tissues is less well defined. Friable tissues such as brain and liver are liable to be shattered and pulped. Gut may be damaged beyond the obvious visible limits. Major blood vessels are remarkably compliant and may escape gross injury, although there is sometimes intimal damage and thrombus in a vessel which appears healthy to the naked eye. Similarly, major nerve trunks may seem undamaged, but suffer neurapraxia or axonotmesis.

Contamination

Figure 46.5 shows that the bullet has entirely perforated the block before the cavity is fully formed and thus entry and exit 'wounds' remain open at the same time. The formation of the cavity creates a near vacuum which is rapidly filled by air from both entry and exit sides. Any contaminants or debris in relation to the entry or exit wounds are likely to be sucked into the temporary cavity and thus the entire wound tract is lined with organisms, dirt, skin scales, hair and possibly clothing fragments. This factor is of especial importance if the wound lies in relation to the buttocks or thighs when the contaminating organisms are likely to be anaerobic clostridia.

Thus high velocity missile wounds are unpredictable,

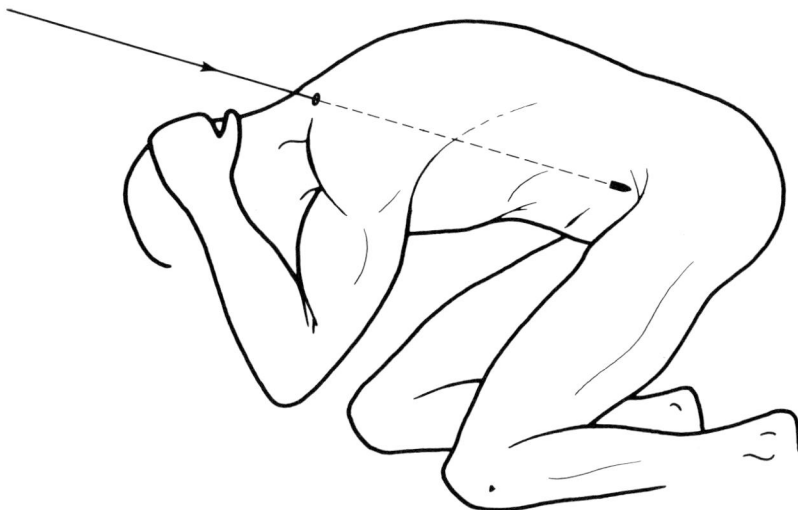

Fig 46.7 The line of injury rarely accords with the anatomical position.

frequently associated with greater damage than is immediately apparent and often contain large amounts of dead muscle. Furthermore, all such wounds arc contaminated from the outset, often with tetanus and gas gangrene, and all of these factors have an important bearing on treatment.

Treatment

The aim of wound treatment is to achieve sound soft tissue healing in the shortest time compatible with safety. The enemies of sound healing are infection and ischaemia and missile wounds should be treated accordingly. Even when it is certain that a wound has been caused by a low velocity weapon, failure to explore the wound is unwise. There is absolutely no doubt that high velocity missile wounds require careful and thorough surgery and that the operation should be a two-stage procedure.

The first operation, *primary wound excision* should be carried out as soon as possible after injury and before contamination in the wound has become established infection. The second operation, *delayed primary closure*, should be done some 4 or 5 days later, provided the wound is healthy at that time. It cannot be too strongly emphasised that a one-stage operation with immediate wound closure, although sometimes successful, is dangerous and unwise.

Naturally an individual patient in peace time presents a different problem to that which pertains in war, be it limited insurrection or full scale conflict. In such circumstances, the problem is not whether or not to oper-ate, but which of many patients should come to operation first. There is a tendency to deal with the most seriously injured first, but this may be unwise for much valuable time and energy may be wasted in an over-ambitious attempt to save a mortally wounded patient while others, less seriously injured, miss the optimum time for surgery.

In such a situation the surgeon in charge must institute some system of casualty sorting or triage (literally = sifting) to ensure that the order in which operations are done is that which is best suited to the needs of the patients overall. Such a system should take account of the fact that a patient's condition is likely to alter during the waiting period and the operating order may need to be changed accordingly (*see* Chapter 44).

General measures

Prior to surgery the patient should receive general and special supportive care as necessary. The quality of first aid particularly with regard to airway management, control of bleeding and application of good splintage and wound dressings may well determine the outcome. The whole patient should be carefully examined, for missile wounds are frequently multiple. Dressings should be disturbed as little as possible since brisk bleeding may recur. Hypovolaemia should be corrected early by infusion of Hartmann's solution prior to whole blood if necessary, and established shock actively managed by blood volume expansion, adequate intravenous analgesia, oxygen, inotropic drugs and possibly vasodilators.

Antibiotics should be administered parenterally. The choice of agent will depend on circumstances, but a mixture of crystalline penicillin and ampicillin is usually satisfactory for wound contaminants. Tetanus toxoid should be given to boost immunity or commence a course. X-rays are frequently helpful in assessment, but are not vital, except in the case of thoracic or abdominal injury, and operation should not be unduly delayed to obtain them. If x-rays are readily available it is often of value to have several oblique views taken in addition to the standard anterior-posterior and lateral.

Primary wound excision

The aims of the operation are:

> To explore the wound thoroughly under direct vision and note carefully all damaged structures
> To remove all dirt, debris, blood clot and other sources of contamination
> To excise all dead and damaged tissues, particularly muscle
> To release tension in muscle groups by wide fasciotomy
> To achieve haemostasis.

In almost all cases the original wound will require generous extension to allow unhindered access throughout its extent. Extending incisions should be made in the long axis of a limb but 'S'-shaped to avoid cutting across a flexure.

Fascia should be widely incised, this is debridement – a word derived from the French *débrider* to unbridle (a horse) or to slit up. It is an important step, for by relieving tension, it may secure the survival of muscle which otherwise might perish from ischaemia or infection or both. As soon as the wound is readily accessible in depth, it should be mopped out using copious quantities of warm saline. This helps to remove debris, foreign bodies and blood clot and to restore normal colour in healthy tissue. It also helps to identify any vessels which are bleeding briskly and these should be ligated using non-absorbable material. Minor bleeding points should not be dealt with at this stage. All dead and damaged muscle must be excised and it is better to err on the side of generous excision and to remove doubtful tissue rather than leave it behind. The best tools for the job are comfortably sprung toothed dissecting forceps and a pair of sharp curved Mayo scissors. Excision should proceed piecemeal and all muscle which does not contract when pinched or bleed when cut should be removed. Muscle which is discoloured or mushy should be sacrificed saving any which is merely bruised. The entire wound should be dealt with under direct vision. There is no place for probing in the surgery of missile wounds. If any fragments of the missile are encountered they are removed, but it is unnecessary to make a prolonged search beyond the wound tract to find the missile. Such action opens up healthy tissue planes to the possibility of infection and increases blood loss.

If the wound is associated with a fracture, the temptation to use metallic fixation should be resisted by all except the most expert in that field, for the price of bone sepsis is high. All viable bone should be preserved, but small loose fragments should be treated as foreign bodies and discarded. Damage to a major blood vessel should be repaired primarily preferably by direct suture, patching or using autogenous vein graft. Synthetic implants are not recommended. In this instance, it is better for the inexperienced to attempt repair if the alternative is amputation. It should be borne in mind that damage to the vessel wall may extend beyond the line of obvious injury. Major nerve trunks should be carefully inspected to ensure that they are intact. If not, no attempt should be made to carry out primary repair, but the divided ends should be marked with a long coloured suture for subsequent identification. Finally all damaged fat, fascia and subcutaneous tissue should be generously excised and the skin margins of the original wound trimmed. Skin is remarkably resistant to missile damage and skin edge excision should be miserly, bearing in mind the intention to obtain closure without tension in a few days' time. If, however, skin has been so damaged or undermined that it is certain to die, then it should be removed.

At the conclusion of excision the wound should again be mopped out with saline and the small bleeding points dealt with by warm packs, diathermy or ligatures cut short to leave as little foreign material as possible. The wound should be left widely open to promote free drainage. The surfaces should be covered with a layer of fine gauze and the cavity lightly filled with fluffed gauze. This should in no way be firm enough to constitute a 'pack'. Paraffin gauze should not be used and additional drains are unnecessary. The dressing should be completed by the application of a generous layer of absorbent wool held in place by wide crepe bandages carefully applied to avoid constriction. Even in the absence of fracture, the final application of a plaster shell is often of benefit for it provides additional splintage and rest for the injured part, but care should be taken to split the plaster to avoid any constrictive effect.

Further general measures

After operation the injured part is elevated, if possible. Many patients are soon fit to move to another centre, although it is unwise to move those with abdominal wounds before bowel function has been reestablished. During the immediate postoperative period antibiotics and general supportive measures are continued. The haemoglobin level is raised to at least 11g/100 ml. Provided the patient's condition remains satisfactory the initial dressings are not disturbed. Should there be general deterioration, or a rise in temperature or pulse rate, or the occurrence of pain in the wound area, infection should be suspected and the patient returned to the operating theatre for wound inspection under anaesthesia.

Delayed primary closure

After a lapse of 4 or 5 days, provided the patient is well, the wound should be ready for closure. On removal of the original dressing, which may be badly stained and smelly, the wound should appear clean and healthy with signs of early granulation. If this is so, the wound is closed using carefully spaced interrupted sutures taking care to obliterate any dead space. Surgeons vary in their choice of skin sutures, but there is some advantage in using monofilament material or stainless steel wire since the stitches should be left in place for at least 14 days and longer if there is an associated fracture which will heal well in a closed plaster. It is important to avoid tension and split skin grafts should be used, if necessary, to cover all or part of the wound or to make good defects left by relieving incisions or flaps. Should the wound be unhealthy, it is further excised or drained and secondary closure done later. After successful closure a less bulky dressing may be applied, although it is still wise to support and rest the injured part by applying appropriate splintage even in the absence of a fracture.

If primary wound excision has been carefully carried out, delayed primary closure will almost always be possible. Early healing of the soft tissues will be achieved and the patient rendered quickly fit for any further specialist procedures.

Exceptions and special cases

Whereas the principles of delayed primary closure are applicable to most missile wounds there are some exceptions. Careful primary wound excision is always required, but in certain sites complete or partial closure should be obtained without delay.

Primary closure is desirable in wounds of the head and face. If the meninges have been penetrated, the dura mater must be carefully repaired prior to accurate skin suturing and it may be necessary to swing a generous scalp flap. The structures of the face are highly vascular so the risks attending primary closure are small, indeed delay allows swelling and distortion making accurate closure difficult.

The chest and abdomen must be closed although it may be wise to leave the outer layers of the wound open. Joint cavities must be closed primarily by synovial suture if possible, but by any available soft tissue if not. Blood vessel repair must be covered by healthy soft tissue.

Further reading

Byrnes D.P., Crockard H.A., Gordon D.S., Gleadhill G.A. (1974). Penetrating cranio cerebral missile injuries in the civil disturbances in Northern Ireland. *Brit. J. Surg.* **61,** 169-76.

Kennedy T.L., Johnston G.W. (1975). Surgery of violence. 1. Civilian bomb injuries. *Brit. Med. J.* **1,** 382–3.

Moffat W.C. (1978). Gunshot wounds of the abdomen. In *Operative Surgery: Accident Surgery* – 3rd edn. (Rob C., Smith R., eds), 242–253. London: Butterworth.

Owen-Smith M.S. (1981). *High Velocity Missile Wounds*. London: Edward Arnold.

Schramek A., Hashmonai M. (1977). Vascular injuries in the extremities in battle casualties. *Brit. J. Surg*; **64,** 644–8.

Stevenson H.M., Wilson W. (1975). Surgery of violence. VII. Gunshot wounds of the trunk. *Brit. Med. J*; **1,** 728–30.

47

Lung blast

D.L. COPPEL and E. McATEER

Blast injuries of the lungs as a result of bomb explosions have been described in the literature following conventional wars (O'Reilly and Gloyne, 1941; Simmons et al., 1969), but in some parts of the world blast injuries are now unfortunately a fairly common emergency in civilian practice (Gray and Coppel, 1973; Caseby and Porter, 1976). Respiratory insufficiency following bomb explosions, however, is relatively rare. Over an 8-year period 714 patients were admitted to the Royal Victoria Hospital, Belfast following bomb explosions and of these 92 required admission to the Respiratory Intensive Care Unit; 21 developed respiratory failure but in only 8 could a confident diagnosis of pure blast injury be made.

Casualties may have multiple injuries but sometimes they are found dead following a bomb explosion without any significant external injury. Characteristically, the only finding might be blood-stained fluid trickling from the nose and mouth (Logan, 1939; Thompson, 1940). Pierre Jans in the eighteenth century suggested that such deaths were caused by 'la grande et prompte dilation d'air' (Hill, 1979). The physiological effects of 'air concussion' were first described in 1920 by Hooker. In a series of animal experiments Zuckerman (1940) showed that the lung damage was caused by direct impact of the pressure wave on the chest wall. Direct exposure of the airway to the blast wave via a tracheostomy did not result in the characteristic lesions of the blast lung syndrome provided the chest wall was adequately protected (Benzinger, 1950).

Characteristics of the blast wave

As a result of a sudden explosive release of energy, a high-pressure shock-wave travels outwards at supersonic speed. The magnitude of this pressure falls off rapidly with distance from the source. At 15 ft from a 125 lb charge a pressure of 200 psi above atmospheric (over-pressure) is reached, but at 50 ft from the same charge the overpressure is only 10 psi. In comparison, a hurricane wind of 120 mph will only exert an overpressure of 0.25 psi. The initial pressure wave is followed by a weaker although longer-lasting negative suction wave, which cannot exceed 15 psi as this corresponds to a perfect vacuum. Clinically, damage to eardrums is possible at overpressure of 5 psi and lung damage may occur at 15 psi (de Candole, 1967).

The damage caused by an explosion is related to:

1 the peak pressure reached
2 the rate at which the pressure rises
3 the duration of the peak pressure.

In clinical practice the likelihood of physical damage is related to the size of the explosion and the proximity of the victim to the source.

The impact of the blast wave causes severe compression of the chest and abdominal wall. As the chest is pushed inwards and the diaphragm elevated, the lungs

are forcibly squeezed. Wedge-shaped areas of haemorrhage are produced and rib markings may be left on the
lung surface. The pressure wave is transmitted through
the chest wall and lung parenchyma faster than through
the airway, so that a large, transient pressure differential is created. Fluid is therefore expelled from the
lungs and pulmonary blood vessels to fill the airways
and alveoli with oedema fluid and blood. Non-uniform
compression of the air and fluid elements within the
lung leads to distortion of the tissues which tear. The
alveolar parenchyma shears away from the vascular
structures and alveolar venous fistulae are created, with
the possibility of air embolisation. Interalveolar septa
become torn so that pockets of emphysema, subpleural
cysts and bullae are formed.

When a blast wave moves through a liquid medium
containing air cavities the energy of the blast is converted into kinetic energy at the liquid-air interface.
Air within the cavity is abruptly compressed – up to a
pressure of 100 000 atmospheres. This causes a violent
disruption of the bubble which implodes after the main
blast has passed thus producing a second detonation
and further local damage.

As the wave passes from high density lung parenchyma to lower density air, a negative reflection occurs
at the interface. Tension is created within the surface of
the first medium which then fragments or spalls (White
and Richmond, 1960).

Spalling and implosion effects cause disruption of cell
morphology and function.

Underwater explosions

Immersion blast injuries were described by Huller
and Bazini (1970). A missile exploded in the water
amongst sailors who had abandoned their ship. The
mechanism of injury to air blast is similar, but the distribution of injury was different; 75% of the sailors said
that they felt the effect of the blast on their bodies.
Severe abdominal pain was the most common complaint in this group. Some describing it as a strong kick
or blow in the abdomen. Although only 18% complained of chest pain, 84% had chest injuries. Apart
from minor skin abrasions probably sustained on the
ship from metallic objects, there was no external sign of
contusion.

At laparatomy tears of bowel wall, peritonitis and
serosal haemorrhage were a common feature. A few
had lacerations of the liver and one a ruptured spleen.
Chest injuries apart from pulmonary oedema included
pneumomediastinum, pneumothoraces, haemothorax,
cystic translucencies and interstitial pulmonary
emphysema. Four of the patients had evidence of
myocardial injury on ECG.

Pathology

At a microscopic level the flat membranous Type I
pneumocytes which normally line the alveoli are destroyed. There is a loss of pulmonary vascular integrity
so that red blood cells and protein-rich fluid leak first
into the interstitial space causing the characteristic pulmonary interstitial oedema, and then into the alveoli.

Widespread infiltration of macrophages and polymorphonuclear cells occurs in response to tissue necrosis. Hyaline membranes are formed from necrotic
epithelial cells, high-protein fluid and fragments of
fibrin.

To compensate for the loss of functional Type I cells,
Type II pneumocytes begin a phase of marked hyperplasia and proliferation. These are large cuboidal cells
with centrally-placed nuclei and they have the ability to
convert to Type I. It is therefore possible to replace the
alveolar lining (Bharucha et al., 1979). The changes in
the lung parenchyma may either resolve or heal with
fibrosis. Recovery of respiratory function depends on:

1 adequate numbers of Type I cells surviving the
   blast injury or
2 rapid conversion of Type II to Type I cells.

Clinical presentation

Patients may be killed outright at the scene of the
explosion or survive long enough to reach hospital.

In the Accident and Emergency Department such
patients are obviously divided into:

1 those with major multiple trauma requiring rapid
   vigorous resuscitation
2 those with minor external injuries who may look
   quite well on admission and initially have no
   respiratory symptoms. The patient may be able to
   describe a sensation of having been struck by a
   blast wave.

The onset of respiratory failure may occur
immediately or be delayed for hours or even days. Both
groups of patients require intensive observation and
supervision in hospital.

The onset of respiratory distress may be quite sudden
and is characterised by:

1 restlessness and confusion
2 progressive dyspnoea
3 dry, irritating cough which may later produce
   frothy sputum or haemoptysis
4 retrosternal pain.

On examination, the patient appears cyanosed and
tachypnoeic. There is often hypotension and usually a
sinus tachycardia. Auscultation of the lungs reveals

diminished air entry in all areas, generalised coarse crepitations, rhonchi and bronchospasm. Chest x-ray shows diffuse lung infiltrations with bilateral pulmonary oedema and haemorrhage, but may be unilateral. There may be pneumothorax, haemothorax or pneumomediastinum. Radiological changes usually occur several hours before clinical symptoms occur and serial chest x-rays are an essential part of early investigations. ECG should be carried out to exclude myocardial injury and continuous monitoring is desirable.

Patients may require emergency surgery shortly after admission, although general anaesthesia is poorly tolerated in the blast lung syndrome (Levinsky *et al.*, 1975). Ideally this should be postponed for 24–28 h, but in practice surgical intervention may be life-saving and the patient must be anaesthetised.

Differential diagnosis

In considering the differential diagnosis of respiratory failure in these circumstances one must exclude penetration of the chest wall by particles energised by the blast (secondary effect) and injuries occurring as a result of the individual being thrown against a solid object (tertiary effect). Other diagnoses include:

1 pneumothorax
2 fluid overload
3 aspiration pneumonitis
4 fat embolism syndrome

and in the next day or two will also include:

5 oxygen toxicity
6 pulmonary embolism
7 septic emboli.

With the onset of respiratory failure there is hypoventilation, decreased lung compliance, and decreased functional residual capacity. Increasing mismatching of ventilation/perfusion occurs as blood is shunted through non-ventilated alveoli and gas exchange is severely impaired.

Treatment

Casualties with associated multiple injuries are often shocked and hypovolaemic on admission. They may require large transfusions of blood and colloid in order to achieve an adequate circulating blood volume. It is almost impossible, in practice, to avoid giving some crystalloid fluids in the initial phase of resuscitation, particularly if a large number of casualties have arrived in a small unit unused to major trauma.

An accurate record of all intravenous fluid replacement must be kept. These patients are very intolerant of clear fluids, especially in the pulmonary capillaries where there is loss of vascular integrity. Fluids rapidly leave the circulation and gross interstitial pulmonary oedema occurs with further impairments of blood-gas exchange.

Central venous measurement (CVP), is a guide to effective circulating volume, but does not detect this leakage of fluid into the pulmonary tissues. It is not necessary to achieve a normal CVP value when estimating the volume to be transfused – but achieving a blood pressure of 80–90 mmHg systolic will allow adequate tissue perfusion.

Urinary output is a helpful guide to the development of fluid overload and if it begins to rise above 3 ml/min, fluid restriction and diuretics should be introduced. Serum and urine osmolality should also be performed. The placement of a Swan Ganz catheter in the pulmonary wedge position will provide additional information in prevention and treatment of fluid overload. The development of pulmonary oedema can be further quantitated to some extent by measuring the alveolar–arterial P_{O_2} difference which will progressively increase.

Adequate oxygenation may be impossible to achieve with 50 to 70% oxygen delivered by a face mask and in these circumstances and especially in the presence of a respiratory acidosis, tracheal intubation and intermittent pressure ventilation (IPV) will be required. Oxygen demand should be reduced where possible by controlling infection, avoiding pyrexia and, if necessary, by cooling the patient. Frequent chest physiotherapy is essential to re-expand areas of atelectasis and allow improved oxygenation. Frequent endobronchial suction is required to remove blood and secretions. Positive End Expiratory Pressure (PEEP) (Coppel, 1979) is invariably required to produce oxygenation compatible with survival. Usually F_IO_2 can be reduced by this technique which thus reduces the risk of pulmonary oxygen toxicity. PEEP increases the intra-alveolar pressure above capillary pressure and helps to control pulmonary oedema. Artificial respiration can be facilitated by using Synchronised Intermittent Mandatory Ventilation (SIMV). This allows evaluation of head and abdominal injuries to be more meaningful than with the use of muscle relaxants or heavy sedation. The adminstration of corticosteroids is somewhat controversial. They are said to act by preserving lysosome integrity, thus decreasing the acute inflammatory response and decreasing capillary permeability. Hydrocortisone 500 mg IV 4-hourly for 10 to 14 days was recommended by McCaughey *et al.* (1973) but they have now modified this to 3 mg/kg Methyl Prednisolone for two or three doses. Prolonged steroid therapy undoubtedly enhances the very real risk of infection. Infusions of albumin are often required to maintain the plasma oncotic pressure. However, if there is a loss in integrity of the pulmonary capillary wall, extravasation of albumin may further increase pulmonary oedema.

Complications of treatment

Pneumothorax

If absent at the onset pneumothoraces may develop with mechanical ventilation. High inflation pressures are often generated in order to produce adequate tidal volumes. This leads to post-traumatic bullae and defects in the pleura. In the past it has been recommended that bilateral chest drainage should be inserted prophylatically, but as this procedure itself is associated with a certain morbidity, it is probably better to monitor the patient closely and institute rapid treatment if a pneumothorax occurs.

Sepsis

This must be treated early and vigorously, but infection is often caused by virulent drug-resistant organisms in a perfect culture media. Pneumonia and septicaemia are frequent causes of death.

Air embolism

There is a theoretical risk that mechanical ventilation, especially with PEEP, may cause embolisation of air through alveolar-venous fistulae. In practice this does not appear to happen, but the possibility should be borne in mind.

Prognosis

Recovery from blast lung damage occurs when:

1 haemorrhage stops and oedema begins to resolve
2 gross repair of parenchymal damage takes place
3 regeneration of Type I pneumocytes occurs, allowing respiratory exchange.

Clinically, less blood and clear fluid are aspirated from the trachea, and the lungs become easier to expand. The inflation pressure required to produce a given tidal volume falls. The lung fields sound clearer on auscultation as coarse crepitations and bronchospasm disappear. The arterial blood gases improve and the F_IO_2 can be steadily reduced to maintain adequate oxygenation.

Chest x-ray. After initial deterioration for 24–48 h, resolution usually begins in 3–5 days.

The outcome of treatment depends on the ability to maintain adequate ventilatory support until the parenchymal damage has resolved and regeneration of Type I pneumocyte is adequate.

Unfortunately, the mortality is high and if recovery is not rapid, infection supervenes which inhibits regeneration of Type I pneumocyte. In the longer term, residual lung damage is said to occur in animals who have survived exposure to blast, but no evidence of permanent lung damage of clinical significance has been found in recent Belfast experiences.

References

Benzinger T. (1950). Physiological effects of blast in air and water. In *US Air Force German Aviation Medicine*, World War II, vol. 2., pp. 1225–59. Washington DC: Department of the Air Force.

Bharucha H., Ferguson D.G., Coppel D.L. (1979). Blast lungs – some histopathological observations. *J. Clin. Path*; **32**:416.

Caseby N.G., Porter M.F. (1976). Blast injuries to the lungs: clinical presentation, management and course. *Injury*; **8,** 1:1–12.

Coppel D.L. (1979). Management of chest injuries. In *Medical Management of the Critically Ill*, Pt 2, pp. 386–97 (Hanson G.C., Wright P.L., eds.). New York: Grune and Stratton.

De Candole C.A. (1967). Blast injury. *Can. Med. Ass. J*; **96**:207–14.

Gray R.C., Coppel D.L. (1973). Blast Injuries of the Lungs. In *Recent Advances in Surgery* (Taylor S., ed) ch. 13. pp. 339–43. Edinburgh: Churchill Livingstone.

Hill J.F. (1979). Blast injury with particular reference to recent terrorist bombing incidents. *Ann. Roy. Coll. Surg. Engl*; **60**:4–11.

Huller T., Bazini Y. (1970). Blast injuries of the chest and abdomen. *Arch. Surg*; **100**:24–30.

Levinsky L., Vidne B., Nudelman I., Saloman J., Kissin L., Levy M.J. (1957). Thoracic injuries in the Yom Kippur War. Experience in a base hospital. *Isr. J. Med. Sci*; **11**:2–3, 275–9.

Logan D.D. (1939). Detonation of high explosives in shell and bombs and its effects. *Brit. Med. J*; **2**:864–6.

McCaughey W., Coppel D.L., Dundee J.W. (1973). Blast injuries to the lungs. A report of two cases. *Anaesthesia*; **28**:2–9.

O'Reilly J.N., Gloyne S.R. (1941). Blast injury of the lungs. *Lancet*; **ii**:423–8.

Simmons R.L., Heisterkamp C.A., Collins J.A., Bredenburg C.A., Martin A.M. (1969). Acute pulmonary edema in battle casualties. *J. Trauma*; **9,9**:760–73.

Thompson F.G. (1940). Notes of penetrating chest wounds. *Brit. Med. J*; **1**:44–6.

White C.S., Richmond D.R. (1960). Blast biology. In *Clinical Cardiopulmonary Physiology*, 2nd edn. (Gordon B.L., ed.) **63**:974–92. New York: Grune and Stratton.

Zuckerman S. (1940). Experimental studies of blast injuries to the lungs. *Lancet*; **ii**:219–24.

48

Microsurgery

ROBERT A. DICKSON

The microscope was first used by Swammerdam and Van der Meer in Holland, but the concept that its powers of magnification could be used for operative surgery took two and a half centuries to be realised. Since the pioneering work of Jacobson and Suarez, who first attempted the anastomosis of vessels less than 3 mm in diameter, it has become routine in microsurgical centres to anastomose vessels whose diameter is less than 1 mm. Thus the last twenty years has seen a revolution in surgery of the musculo-skeletal system and the integument, with the transfer of free skin flaps by microsurgical techniques being an integral part of the work of the musculo-skeletal microsurgeon. Pari-passu with these technical developments, microsurgical centres have appeared and proliferated in many countries.

There is little artistry about the majority of orthopaedic procedures, but the learning of microsurgical techniques develops the dexterity of the surgeon, and this has its rewards when it comes to handling delicate tissue in other operations. Few microsurgeons, however, have sufficient patients requiring their services to maintain the surgical skills that are required, and therefore the microsurgery laboratory is an invaluable adjunct. Here the procedures he will use on patients can be perfected and, at the same time, he can apply himself to many basic scientific questions which have thus far been left unanswered. The author was taught basic microsurgical techniques by Acland in his microsurgery laboratory in Louisville, Kentucky, and was impressed by the small number of simple instru-

ments with which the microsurgical procedures could be performed with practice and patience.

The operating microscope

In the Nuffield Orthopaedic Microsurgery Laboratory there is both a modern fibreoptic illuminated operating microscope (Zeiss Operating Microscope) and another which is 20 years old. The latter is independently illuminated from the side, but it is as good, if not better, optically and is perfectly satisfactory for the great majority of procedures. The type of operating microscope is, therefore, much less important than its proper use.

Microsurgery is nothing more than a battle against unwanted movement and fatigue. In this latter respect the proper use of the operating microscope is most important. There are three vertical heights, which have to be adjusted one to another for optimal microsurgery to be performed with maximum comfort. These are:

1   the surgeon's eyes
2   the operating surface
3   the surgeon's seat.

There is a set routine for this adjustment. The microscope is positioned so that its light shines on the operating surface at a distance of just under 30 cm from the edge of the table. The microscope is then moved on its vertical axis until a test card on the operating surface is in focus. The surgeon's seat is then adjusted so that it is close to the operating surface, and further adjusted on its vertical axis so that a position of comfort is achieved. If it is too low the neck is stretched and this leads to cervical spine discomfort; if it is too high the axial skeleton sags with back discomfort. The eye pieces are then adjusted to suit the interpupillary distance of the surgeon, and this should be noted for future settings. Finally each eye piece, in turn, is focussed individually on the test card at the highest magnification of the microscope. The prescription of the surgeon is thus built into the system, and again this should be noted for future use. Further, when the microscope is accurately focused under the highest magnification it will then be in focus throughout the magnification range of the instrument. It is important to appreciate that high magnification is only required for preparing vessel ends or inserting a microneedle through a delicate piece of tissue and the remainder of the dissection, including tying of knots, is much better performed under a low magnification, thus providing a bigger operative field.

Microsurgical instruments

Those suggested by Acland (1977), can be generally recommended (Fig 48.1). Instruments should have a dull finish to avoid light reflection, and should be not more than 15 cm long for comfortable balance and ease of operation. The inherent spring tension of the instruments should not be excessive lest hand fatigue results.

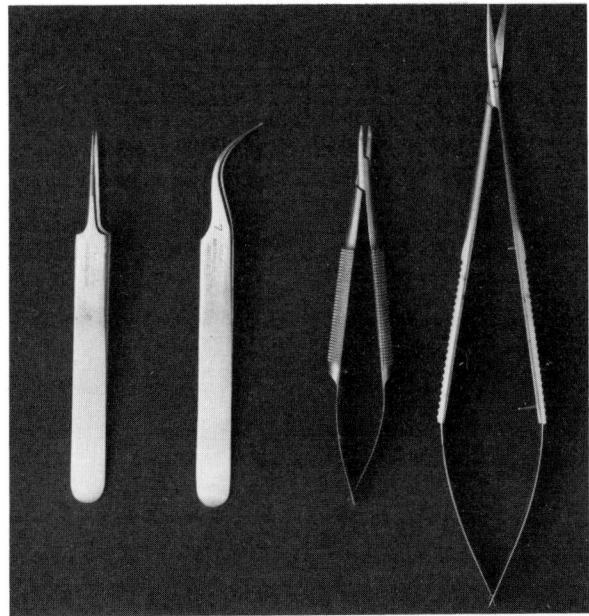

Fig 48.1 The microsurgical instruments required. These are from left to right: (a) straight jeweller's forceps; (b) curved jeweller's forceps; (c) needle holder; (d) scissors.

Steel instruments are the most satisfactory, being cheap and of a comfortable weight, but do have the inconvenience of occasionally becoming magnetic, and therefore an electromagnetic coil is useful to demagnetise instruments when this complication arises. There is no need to purchase titanium instruments, which apart from being expensive are also too light. For the great majority of microsurgical procedures only three instruments are necessary – two pairs of jeweller's forceps and one pair of scissors. The straight No 5 universal pick-up jeweller's forceps are the non-toothed dissecting forceps of microsurgery and are always held in the left hand. A gently curved jeweller's forcep is useful to aid dissection and doubles as a needle-holder, having much more versatility than a conventional microsurgery needle-holder. This is always held in the right hand. A modified straight jeweller's forcep is useful as a vessel dilator. These forceps can be serviced in the microsurgery laboratory with nothing more complicated than jeweller's emery paper and an oil stone. A pair of small sharp-pointed scissors is necessary for fine work, and a larger pair of round-pointed scissors for less exacting work. In order to suture tough tissues a needle-holder becomes necessary.

Microsurgery should be performed in a moist, but bloodless, field and haemostasis is particularly important. Tantalum hemo clips are used for vessels which are greater than 1 mm, while a bipolar coagulator is invaluable for vessels less than 1 mm. Petroleum jelly is useful for the tips of the bipolar coagulator to avoid soft tissue adherence. A 20 ml syringe containing Ringer lactate solution is essential for frequent irrigation of the operating field.

For vessel work a variety of clamps is necessary. Single clamps from 8 mm to 14 mm are useful, but of particular value is the Acland double clamp with approximator so that the vessel ends are held in an apposed position. Microsurgery needles should be of varying sizes and bore up to 150 microns, and 9/0 to 11/0 nylon or polypropylene suture material is recommended.

Maintenance and cleaning of the instruments is particularly important and soaking the instruments singly in a haemolytic enzyme detergent is the recommended method, followed by rinsing with a jet of water from a syringe, and allowing to dry by evaporation. For maximum life microsurgical instruments should be handled with care, never dropped on their points and never handled together with other instruments.

Tying the microsurgical knot

The supinated writing position of the hands is the basic one for holding microsurgical instruments. Unwanted tremor can be abolished by touching the hands together. The technique of picking up the needle is important. It is too small to pick up by hand, and is too fragile to be grasped by more than one instrument. When the thread is unwrapped from the sustaining card and the needle is placed within the microsurgery operative field, the needle will be seen to be lying flat on the operating surface. If the thread at a distance of about 10 cm from the needle is elevated by the left hand forcep, then when it becomes taut the needle will stand up and can be grasped by the curved forcep in the right hand.

The needle must be passed through at 90° to the plane of the material to be sutured, and an equal sized bite should be taken of the two opposing surfaces. Having passed through both surfaces the needle should be drawn through until approximately 1 cm of suture material is left free. The needle will have passed out of the operative field in the process of so doing, but should now be returned to the field and placed in a position where it will be easy to pick up for the next knot. The left hand forcep should now pick up the thread on the side passing to the needle, some 5 cm from the site of the knot. The direction to which the 1 cm short end points should now be noted, and the jaws of the right hand forcep adjusted so that they will be able to close at right angles to the line of the thread. Once the right hand forceps are in this position, the loop can be made with the left hand thread and the forceps in the right hand passed through this to grasp the short end and tie the first half-hitch (Fig 48.2). This procedure is repeated so that a reef knot is obtained. The ends are trimmed with microscissors, and the next knot can now be tied without the eyes being removed from the eye pieces, because the needle was returned to the field after it had been passed through the two apposed surfaces.

Microvascular anastomotic techniques

Artery end-to-end anastomosis

The ease with which this anastomosis is performed depends entirely upon the care taken in preparing the vessel ends (Fig 48.3). Bleeding is irritating and complete haemostasis must be obtained before the repair is carried out. Irrigation with Ringer lactate solution locates the bleeding points exactly. Constant irrigation is also essential to prevent desiccation. Vessel ends should only be handled by the outer adventitia. Too traumatic a dissection leads to spasm, as does the presence of fresh blood on the vessel ends and too low a temperature. Spasm can be relieved by applying 1%

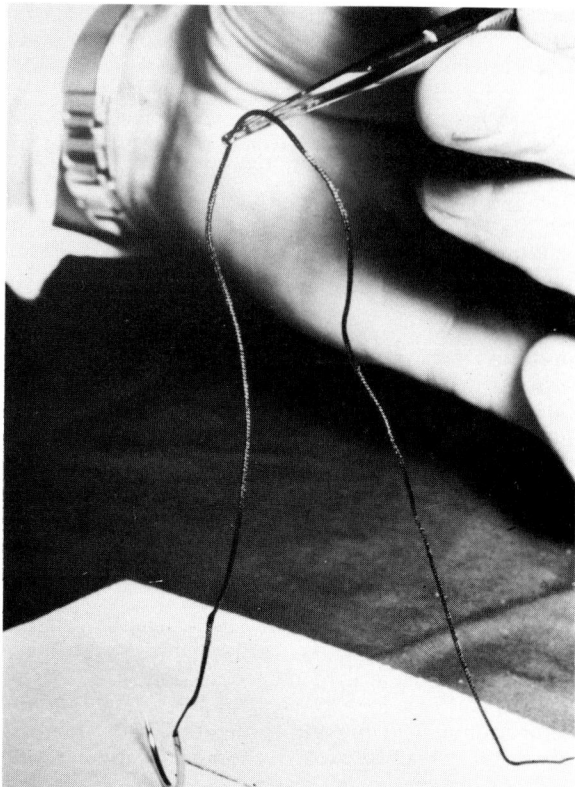

(a)

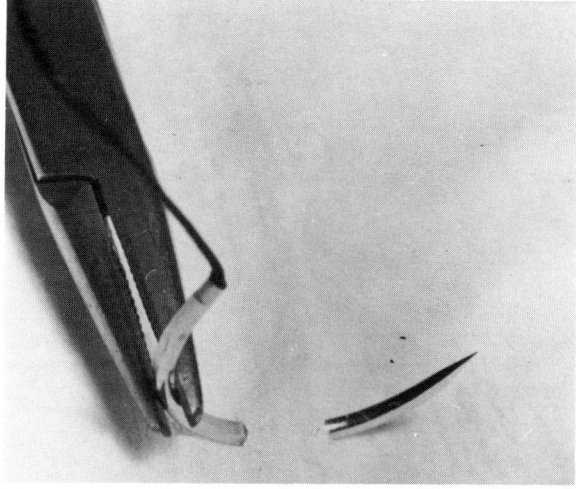

(b)

Fig 48.2 Tying a microsurgical knot. (a) In order to lift the needle from the working surface so that it can be grasped by the needle holder, the thread is lifted until the needle assumes the erect position. (b) The needle is inserted by pushing through approximately half of its length.

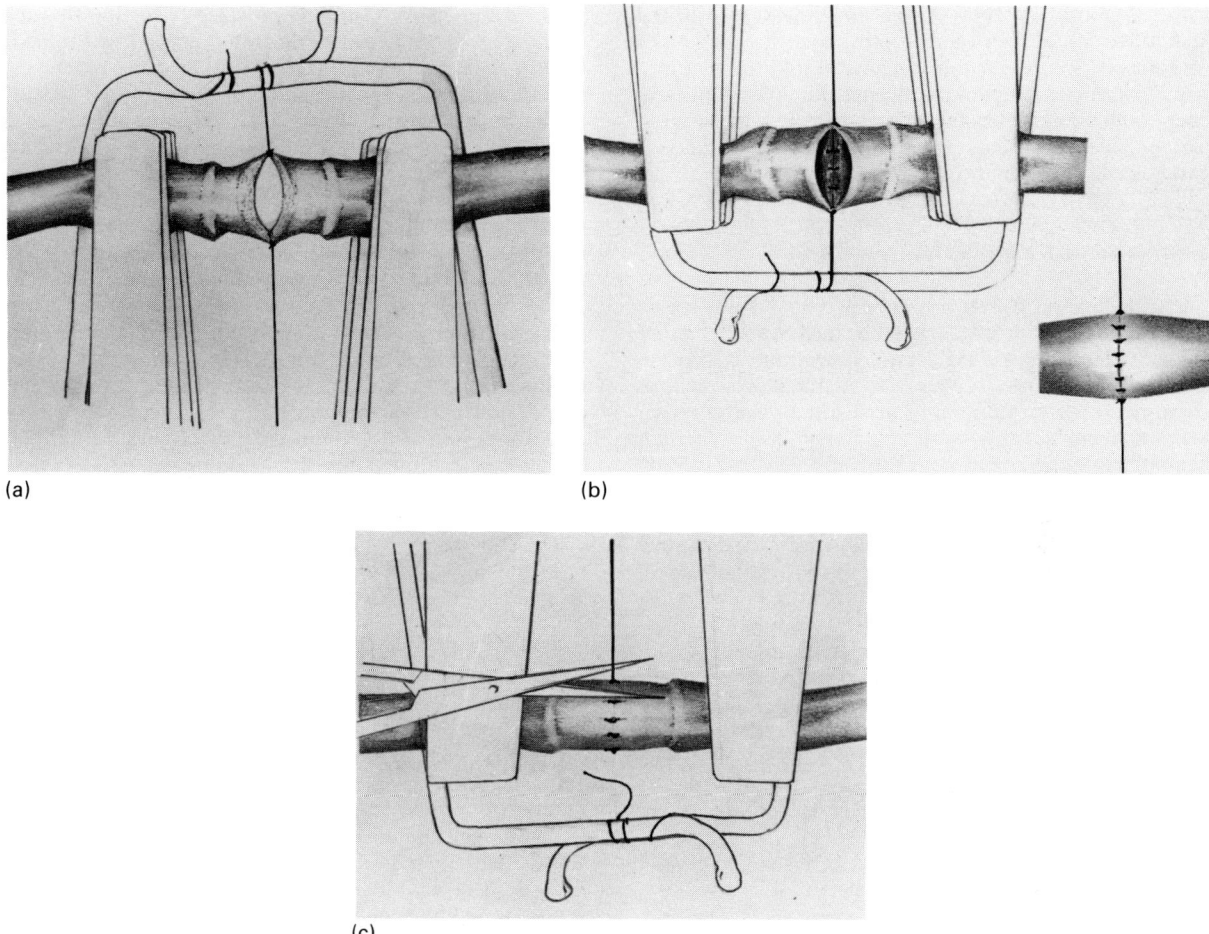

(a)

(b)

(c)

Fig 48.3 Artery end-to-end anastomosis. (a) The microsurgery clamps are applied not more than 3 mm from the vessel ends. The adventitia is removed, and two non-equatorial sutures are inserted and attached under tension to the cleats above and below. (b) The entire clamp is turned over to expose the under surface of the vessel which is now repaired. (c) Finally the stay sutures are cut prior to removal of the clamps.

local anaesthetic to the field. It is important to have a proper diameter vessel out of spasm before the microvascular clamps are applied. Apply the clamps some 2 or 3 mm from the vessel ends. Blood is removed from the vessel ends by gentle compression with a smooth instrument. The adventitia is then removed by pulling this fluffy material in the long axis of the vessel and it easily separates from the media. The vessel ends must now be dilated by stretching the smooth muscle of the vessel wall until the bore is one-and-a-half times its natural size. The clamps are now approximated until there is one vessel's width between the two vessel ends. Two stay sutures are first inserted at positions not equatorial, but approximately two-fifths of the way round the circumference from each other, thus ensur-

ing that, when pulled in opposite directions, the back wall of the vessel sags away, so that there will be no danger of picking up the back wall while suturing the front (Cobbett, 1967). The vessel edge should be everted at both entry and exit points of the needle to ensure a right-angled needle passage. The two stay sutures are attached to the cleats on the Acland clamp. For a 1 mm vessel three sutures should now be inserted between the two stay sutures in the front wall, and then the entire clamp is turned over to expose the back of the vessel. Five or six sutures are required here. The stay sutures are now removed from the clamp and trimmed. Fresh local anaesthetic is applied to the operative field. The clamps are removed 5 min later and any accumulated blood is sucked away. Bleeding stops within 2–3 min. Patency should not be assessed in the first few minutes in order to minimise the danger of thrombosis. Expansile pulsation distal to the anastomosis is a sure sign of patency. Longitudinal pulsation at one point means that the vessel is partially or completely blocked at that point. Milking the vessel as a patency test is traumatic and unnecessary.

Vein anastomosis end-to-end

It is necessary to be more delicate with veins which are thinner than arteries, and the adventitia is more adherent requiring careful sharp dissection rather than teasing for its removal. When the microvascular clamps are applied the terminal apertures collapse, and repair at first may not seem possible. However, copious irrigation facilitates removal of blood and adventitia, and visualisation of the lumen. After insertion of the first two non-equatorial stay sutures the remainder of the anastomosis is straight-forward. For a vein, the sutures can be spaced more widely apart than for an artery of comparable size. The remainder of the repair is as for an artery, and when the clamps are removed the anastomosis should dilate immediately. If this does not occur, then one of the sutures has transfixed both walls of the vein, and should be removed. A gentle milking test has to be used to establish venous patency.

Applied microvascular surgery

Digital replantation

Following the demonstration that small vessels could be anastomosed to salvage an incomplete upper extremity amputation, the first microvascular digital replantation for a complete amputation was performed in 1965 by Komatsu and Tami. Since then experience has not only led to improved results, but also indications and contraindications have become established. Replantation is definitely indicated for thumb loss, digital loss in children, and multiple digit injuries. In the latter situation all digits should be replanted, because relative usefulness cannot be predicted initially, but innervated skin can be rearranged later. The least damaged digit should be transplanted to the most advantageous site. Guillotine or moderate crush injuries have the best prognosis with a survival rate of over 80% in complete amputations and over 90% if the injury is incomplete. Avulsion or diffuse crush injuries have a much lower survival rate, being less than 20% if complete and not more than 70% if incomplete. Amputation occurring through joints and through the area of the fibrous flexor tendon sheath may be associated with poor eventual function. However the thumb, index and middle fingers do not require much active flexion to be usefully functional in the tripod pinch.

Contraindications to replantation are injuries distal to the middle of the middle phalanx, amputation of a single digit especially a border finger, a contaminated wound as from a war or agricultural injury, a double injury to the same digit, the presence of distal damage in the form of local blood extravasation where a vessel has been damaged distally (the red line sign), or if the vessel distal to the injury is tortuous and dilated, indicative of intimal damage (the ribbon sign). If the warm ischaemic time has been greater than 6 h, or if the digit has been improperly treated during transit, then replantation is impractical. A plastic bag around the amputated part surrounded by ice is the best method of transit, and the amputated part should neither be frozen nor perfused, the latter damaging the vessels. Any residual skin bridge attachments should be preserved.

Two microsurgical teams are necessary, one to prepare the replanted digit, and one to prepare the recipient site. Preliminary bone shortening by the order of 1 cm is necessary to avoid tension on repaired soft tissues, and local debridement of dead tissues is another preliminary. All structures should then be repaired commencing with the bone ends, followed by the flexor tendons, extensor tendons, veins, arteries, nerves, soft tissues and finally the skin, in that order (Fig 48.4). The veins and arteries are repaired in precisely the same manner as previously described. Both sets of arteries and veins should be repaired to provide a safety factor. If practical, two to five veins should be repaired for each digit replanted. The skin should be sutured only loosely and there should be no circumferential dress-

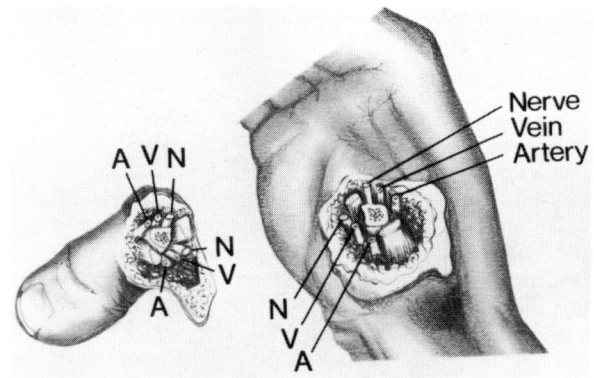

Fig 48.4 Digital replantation. The corresponding nerves, veins, arteries, tendons and bones in the donor and recipient areas must be identified. After ensuring that the ends of all structures are healthy and the bone has been shortened, these corresponding structures are anastomosed.

ings. It is always better to resect vessels until the ends look normal and bridge the gap with a vein graft, than to repair suboptimal vessel ends. Postoperatively heparin, Macrodex and aspirin are given to prevent thrombosis, but are no substitute for proper technique.

The commonest postoperative problem is circulatory obstruction. Arterial insufficiency is the likeliest, giving rise to a bluish mottled digit with a slow capillary return and cool to the touch. Venous blockage is indicated by blueness, turgidity, and a brisk initial capillary return. Local bleeding and infection are the other postoperative problems.

Thumb reconstruction

Primary thumb replantation should always be attempted, but elective thumb reconstruction is necessary if primary replantation was inappropriate, or for thumb hypoplasia or aplasia. Pollicisation (the transposition of a digit for the reconstruction of a new thumb on a neurovascular pedicle) has been performed since 1903 and has been perfected by Buck-Gramcko (1977). The adjacent index finger is used and in his expert hands only one long-term case of vascular insufficiency occurred out of a total of 223. This must be the elective thumb reconstruction procedure of choice. However, since Cobbett first described the elective big toe to thumb transfer in 1969 (Fig 48.5), microsurgery has a role in thumb reconstruction. The first dorsal metatarsal artery (a direct continuation of the dorsalis pedis

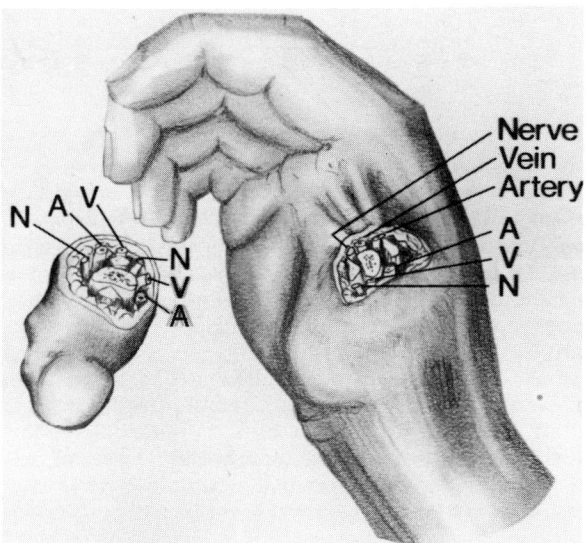

Fig 48.5 Thumb reconstruction. The nerves, veins, arteries, tendons and bones of the great toe are anastomosed to the corresponding structures in the base of the thumb.

artery) is present in almost 90% of individuals and has a calibre of 2–2.5 mm. There are multiple dorsal veins available in the great toe for anastomosis. The medial plantar and common plantar nerves supply the sides of the great toe, and the deep peroneal nerve supplies the dorsum. A good bone fixation of the transplanted digit is assisted by the presence of at least a segment of the first metacarpal. The first dorsal metatarsal artery should be palpated in both feet as either great toe can be transferred and the vascular anatomy may differ.

A skin incision is first planned and marked out on the foot. Through a dorsal S-shaped incision the artery and veins are dissected out. The extensor hallucis longus tendon is located and divided proximally. Through a separate plantar incision the common and medial plantar nerves are identified and through another separate incision just behind the medial malleolus the tendon of flexor hallucis longus is located and divided. Only the vascular supply now connects the toe to the rest of the body and the tourniquet is deflated. Attention is now directed to the hand, and the radial artery and its veni comitantes are located as far proximal as the anatomical snuff-box. The hallux is now attached to bone first, then extensor and flexor tendons, the plantar nerves to the digital nerves and the deep peroneal nerve to the dorsal radial nerve. The veni comitantes are anastomosed and finally the radial artery is joined to the dorsalis pedis artery. The foot incision is closed by swinging the plantar flap over the metatarsal head. The hand is splinted for 2 months postoperatively and then active motion is encouraged.

Free flap transfer

This is the transfer in a single operation of a composite segment of skin and subcutaneous tissue to a distant recipient site by use of microvascular anastomoses (O'Brien *et al.*, 1977). Other tissues such as bone, muscle, and nerve may also be incorporated. Since MacGregor and Jackson's description of the anatomical basis of the groin flap in 1972, this procedure has now become a routine part of the surgical armamentarium of the plastic and reconstructive surgeon with a similar survival rate to the tube pedicle. The first successful microvascular free flap in man was a hair transplantation with a free skin flap based upon the superficial temporal vessels (Harii, 1978). The uses, advantages, disadvantages, preoperative evaluation and techniques have been described by O'Brien *et al.* (1977). This technique is particularly useful in trauma, burns, radical cancer surgery, congenital hypoplasia and aplasia, and thumb contractures. It has the advantages of speeding up the rehabilitation process, being a one stage procedure, and may improve the local vascularity by bringing in new vessels. The donor and recipient sites must be carefully evaluated preoperatively, particularly from the point of view of irradiated vessels. The radiotherapist must, therefore, accurately chart out the extent of the irradiated field, because vessels so damaged are not suitable for anastomosis. The most important aspect of evaluation is palpation of the arterial pulses of the vessels concerned, as arteriography is unreliable, and may cause endothelial damage. The groin flap is the most popular, but the deltopectoral, scalp and forehead flaps are also useful. The first web flap is the most suitable for the hand because of superior sensory endings and lack of hair.

The groin flap is based upon the superficial circumflex iliac artery which was never absent in over 100 cadaver dissections. This vessel is sometimes a branch of the superficial inferior epigastric artery in which case the larger vessel should be selected. The corresponding vein may join the superficial epigastric vein on its way to the long saphenous, in which situation the common trunk is favoured. This flap is centred on the axial vessels with its medial border over the femoral vessels. The delto-pectoral flap is based on the second intercostal vessels, the forehead flap on the anterior branch of the superficial temporal vessels and the scalp flap on the posterior branch of the same vessels. The postauricular flap is based on the vessels of the same name, while neurovascular flaps can be derived from the foot based upon the dorsalis pedis artery or the first dorsal metatarsal artery.

As in all microsurgery transfers, two teams are necessary and the flap is left attached to its feeder vessels until the recipient site is prepared to minimise the ischaemic time. The vessels supplying the flap are then anastomosed by the previously described microvascular techniques to the largest artery and veins in the recipient area. Postoperatively, checks of circulation are necessary and the commonest problem encountered is an arterial block causing vascular insufficiency which will give rise, in addition to the signs of arterial blockage, to a flap which feels empty, whereas a flap suffering from venous blockage feels full. Dependency in the former situation and elevation in the latter are the first aid measures which, if not effective within 2 h, demand re-exploration. O'Brien's experience of 46 groin flaps has provided a total failure of only 16% (O'Brien *et al.*, 1977). Harii (1978) has had a similar experience with 184 skin flaps.

Free vascularised bone grafting

This procedure enjoys its best indication when severe trauma has resulted in an unbridgeable bony defect with amputation as the only alternative means of treatment (Fig 48.6). Animal experiments using vascularised grafts to reconstruct mandibular defects demonstrated

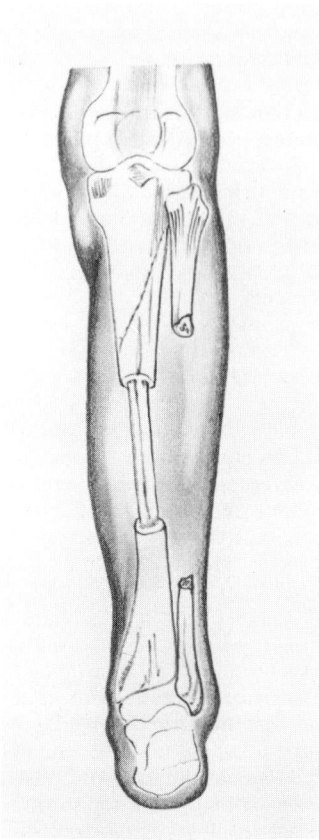

Fig 48.6 Free vascularised bone grafting. The fibula, based on the peroneal vessels, can be used to make good a significant defect in the tibia where amputation is the only alternative.

the feasibility of this procedure and the importance of nutrient vessels which supply the endosteal surface through the attached muscle pedicles. This technique was first introduced into the human situation to bridge a tibial defect and Taylor (1977) has described his clinical experience of this method and stresses the importance of preoperative planning. The optimal donor sites are the fibula, based on the peroneal vessels, of which 23 cm is available in the adult, and ribs based upon posterior intercostal vessels. These provide suitable graft material because they have a predictable endosteal and periosteal blood supply with vessels of sufficient calibre for microvascular anastomosis while leaving an acceptable donor site morbidity. The fibula is ideal in accommodating to the intramedullary diameter of the long bones of the extremities. Furthermore, the veni comitantes follow closely the arterial supply and are applied to the middle two-fourths of the fibula. It is most important to include in the free vascularised bone graft at least 1 cm of surrounding muscle to preserve the important periosteal blood supply. In this particularly challenging type of microsurgery preoperative angiography is essential. The proximal and distal ends of the fibula must be left intact to preclude knee or ankle joint instability.

This procedure is once again performed by two teams of microsurgeons. Through Henry's approach to the fibula posteriorly the popliteal fossa is exposed and the lateral popliteal nerve preserved. The anterior tibial vessels are identified and the lateral head of gastrocnemius and the plantaris are mobilised from the femur taking with them the popliteal vessels and medial popliteal nerve. The soleus muscle is divided in line with the fibula and the posterior tibial vessels traced to the origin of the peroneal vessels which are, in turn, dissected distally preserving the fibular muscular sleeve. After division of the tibialis posterior and flexor hallucis longus the fibula and interosseous membrane are divided leaving the bone graft attached only by its vascular pedicle. The fibular graft is then secured in its new position and, using microvascular techniques the vessels are joined to suitable vessels in the recipient area.

Microneurosurgical techniques

In 1943 Seddon classified nerve injuries into three groups – neuropraxia, axonotmesis and neurotmesis. Neuropraxia is a temporary loss of physiological conduction with no structural damage to the nerve. Axonotmesis implies a loss of axonal continuity but no disruption of the nerve sheath, and recovery is therefore good. Neurotmesis indicates a complete loss of nerve continuity, and it is in this type of injury that nerve repair is indicated.

Surgical anatomy

In 1968 Sunderland established the anatomical substructure of the peripheral nerve. The nerve is surrounded by a connective tissue sheath within which lie bundles of axons, fasciculi, surrounded by a sheath of perineurium. Within each fasciculus each individual axon is surrounded by its own very delicate endoneurial sheath (Fig 48.7). The internal architecture of the peripheral nerve is, however, in a constant state of flux with axonal interchange from one fasciculus to another during the course of the nerve, particularly proximally. This makes identification of corresponding fasciculi difficult if injury has occurred in an area of considerable axonal interchange. Furthermore, the concept that nerve fasciculi are either purely motor or sensory is an

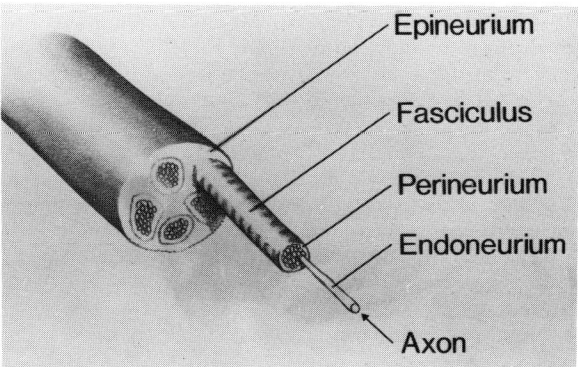

Fig 48.7 The surgical anatomy of the mammalian peripheral nerve. The axons are each surrounded by an endoneurium and then gathered into bundles or fasciculi surrounded by the perineurium. The fasciculi are bound together by the surrounding epineurium.

over simplification. For example, the deep branch of the ulnar nerve, always thought to be motor, is neither purely deep nor purely motor and, in fact, is mostly sensory. Nevertheless, the advent of the operating microscope has improved the results of peripheral nerve repair by enabling fasciculus to be approximated to fasciculus. This is particularly important when one considers the nerve to connective tissue ratio of the cross section of a peripheral nerve may be as low as 1:20. Epineurial coaptation, therefore, if performed with incomplete apposition, malrotation, or buckling may lead to no axonal continuity whatsoever. It must be remembered, however, that while fasciculi can be repaired, the internal substructure of the mammalian peripheral nerve can never be restored to normal and, therefore, there is never a perfect result from surgical reconstruction even with the microscope.

Mechanical properties of mammalian peripheral nerve

The importance of avoiding tension at the site of nerve repair has been stressed. Tension creates fibrous tissue proliferation at the site of repair which considerably diminishes the potential for recovery. This concept is not original and it has been demonstrated that when joints were extended after having been previously flexed to facilitate nerve coaptation, secondary Wallerian degeneration occurred as a result of tension. In addition, it has been shown that the perineurium contains contractile elements being particularly evident when fasciculi are dissected from the surrounding sustaining epineurium. Precisely what tension is required to damage a nerve is not clear, but a small amount of tension is acceptable, because the initial portion of the force-displacement characteristic of the mammalian peripheral nerve is almost horizontal, significant displacement being achieved with minimal or zero force (Kendal *et al.*, 1979). Millesi's (1977) huge experience suggests that if a defect cannot be closed when the nearby joints are in a neutral position then a graft is indicated. This corresponds with a defect in the mammalian peripheral nerve of the order of 0.5 cm.

Interfascicular nerve repair

The debate between the relative advantages of macroneurorrhaphy and microneurorrhaphy continues, but there is little doubt that the improved results obtained by microneurorrhaphy are in all probability due to the improvement in surgical technique which the operating microscope affords. Impeccable technique includes the elimination of tension, the use of an atraumatic technique, proper mapping and aligning of fasciculi, prevention of gaps, avoidance of lengthy nerve mobilisation with its devascularising effect, the use of meticulous intraneural haemostasis, and the minimisation of foreign body reaction. Such technique cannot be employed without the use of the operating microscope.

Interfascicular nerve repair is indicated for cleanly incised fresh nerve injuries with no loss of nerve substance. This is by far the most common nerve injury encountered in civilian practice and the majority occur in the median and ulnar nerves in the forearm.

Using standard hand instruments the wound is explored and excised and the nerve ends identified. Elongation of the incision in an appropriate direction is necessary. A tourniquet is not necessary and its avoidance allows identification of bleeding points and good haemostasis. The ends of the divided nerves should be inspected and the fascicular pattern, both proximally and distally identified. The disposition of the longitudinally running blood vessels aids rotational alignment. Correct fascicular alignment can be achieved in over 90%, but preoperative electrostimulation and the dissection of the distal stump down to its terminal branches, may be necessary.

For interfascicular repair the technique of Millesi (1977) is recommended. The epineurial connective tissue is removed from the proximal and distal stumps, and the perineurium identified by means of its white transverse striations. This is performed under the low magnification of the operating microscope and in peripheral nerve surgery there is only one situation where the high resolution is required and that is for the passage of the microneedle through the perineurium to minimise the amount of axoplasm incorporated in the knot. It has been suggested that a posterior stay suture

in the epineurium is useful initially in bringing the stumps together. If there is no tension only one suture per fasciculus is necessary for perfect coaptation and if this cannot be achieved an interfascicular nerve graft is required (Fig 48.8).

The wound is then closed with standard hand instruments, and after 3 weeks' immobilisation, recovery is monitored by clinical and electrophysiological assessment.

Interfascicular nerve grafting

If there is a loss of nerve tissue substance, a delay between injury and repair, or too great an amount of tension during primary interfascicular repair, then grafting is indicated. When primary nerve repair has failed to produce satisfactory function after 6 months in association with a neuroma-in-continuity, then neuroma excision and interfascicular nerve grafting is similarly indicated.

The nerve is exposed using standard hand surgery instruments, and any redundant fibrous tissue or neuroma is excised until normal nerve tissue is observed proximally and distally. In this respect it is preferable to transect fasciculi at different levels. The wound is now covered with a Ringer lactate-impregnated swab, attention is directed towards the lower extremity, and the lateral sural cutaneous nerve is exposed which is optimal for providing autograft material having a distinct fascicular pattern, no branches in the calf, and a length of 40 cm. In addition the disability after removal of the lateral sural nerve is minimal, with only a small hypo-aesthetic area behind the lateral malleolus. The lateral sural nerve is located alongside the small saphenous vein distally, and by means of up to four horizontal incisions in the lateral side of the calf, the nerve can be delivered up to the popliteal fossa. In the majority of peripheral nerve injuries, one sural nerve will provide all the autograft material necessary, but when reconstructing the brachial plexus the lateral cutaneous nerve of the thigh, the posterior cutaneous nerve of the forearm, and the superficial radial nerve may require to be sacrificed to provide a sufficiency of donor material. The length of autograft removed should be 20% more than that estimated from the defect in order to overcome shrinkage and to allow the graft to be re-routed should the bed of the recipient area be unfavourable.

The autograft is cut into as many pieces as there are fasciculi to be bridged and the graft ends are prepared in the same way as the proximal and distal stumps by removal of the surrounding epineurium. The two anastomoses proximal stump to graft and graft to distal stump are performed exactly as for primary interfascicular nerve repair and the postoperative management is similar (Fig 48.9).

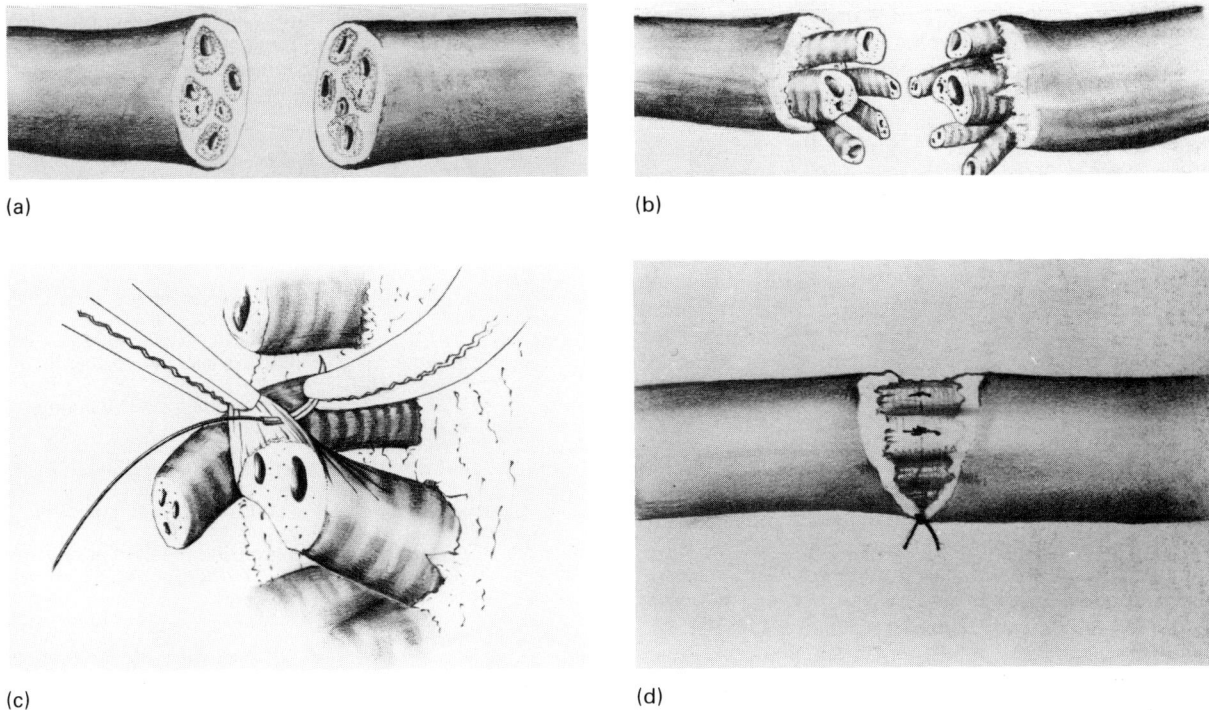

(a)

(b)

(c)

(d)

Fig 48.8 Interfascicular nerve repair. (a) The cut ends of the divided nerve are inspected and the corresponding fasciculi identified. (b) The epineurium is removed from the cut surface thus exposing the intrinsic fasciculi. (c) Corresponding fasciculi are approximated by suturing the perineurium. (d) The anastomosis has been completed. The epineurium can be approximated to reduce tension.

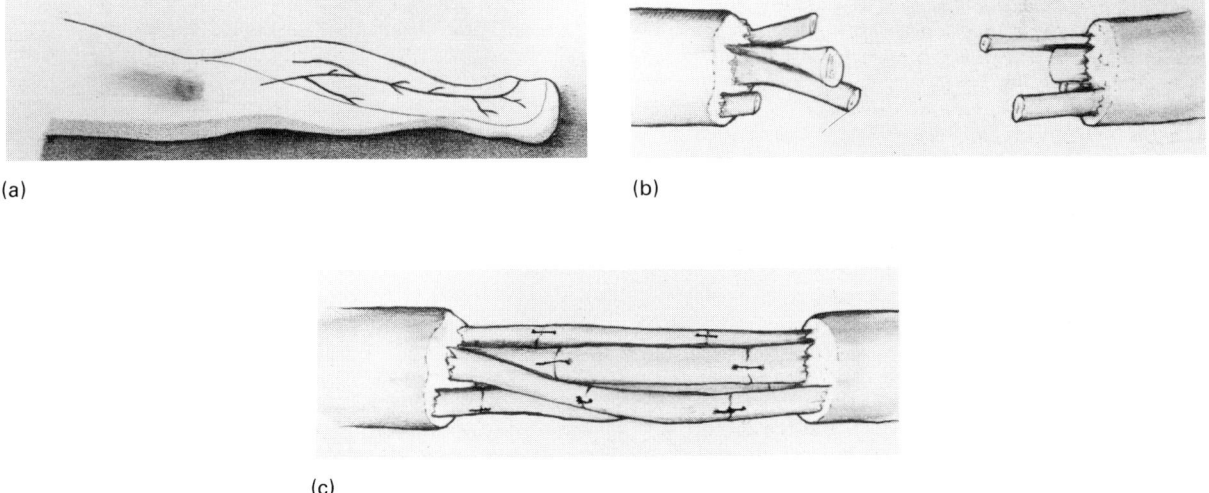

(a)

(b)

(c)

Fig 48.9 Interfascicular nerve grafting. (a) The lateral sural nerve is removed to provide donor material. (b) The fascicular patterns of the nerve ends are identified and the surrounding epineurium trimmed. (c) The gaps between fasciculi are bridged using segments of donor nerve without tension.

An MRC grade of 3 or better motor power can be achieved using interfascicular nerve repair for fresh clean incised injuries of the median and ulnar nerves in the forearm (Millesi, 1977). In 18 radial nerve repairs he achieved an MRC motor power grade of 4 or 5 in over 80% of radial nerve injuries similarly treated. When median nerve injuries are grafted 60% achieve an MRC motor power of grade 4 or 5, and 50% of ulnar nerves.

Brachial plexus injuries are not associated with anywhere near such good results. This is hardly surprising with such proximal injuries in areas of high axonal interchange. Furthermore, the great majority of such injuries are major traction injuries and avulsion of roots from the spinal cord is common. Narakas (1978) with his vast experience of over 10 years of surgical treatment of traction injuries of the brachial plexus has suggested surgical indications and their consequent expectations. One in every three or four traction injuries does not recover spontaneously and these are the ones upon which he seeks to operate at a time of 3–6 weeks after injury. His functional priorities for recovery in order of merit are: (1) elbow control, (2) wrist and finger flexion, (3) shoulder control, (4) wrist and finger extension, and finally (5) intrinsic muscle function. Narakas stresses that a 2-year follow-up period is inadequate for a final assessment and this requires at least 4 or 5 years. He has seen shoulder abduction, elbow flexion, and median nerve sensory recovery occur in 5, 7 and 9 years respectively. In his hands 40% of all patients have a fair result, 20% a good result, and 40% achieve no improvement, with proportionately better results in infraclavicular than supraclavicular injuries.

References

Acland R.D. (1977). Instrumentation for microsurgery. *Orthop. Clin. N. Amer*; **8**:281–94.

Buck-Gramcko D. (1977). Thumb reconstruction by digital transposition. *Orthop. Clin. N. Amer*; **8**:329–42.

Cobbett J.R. (1969). Free digital transfer: report of a case of transfer of a great toe to replace an amputated thumb. *J. Bone, Joint Surg*; **51B**:677–9.

Harii K. (1978). Micro-vascular surgery and its clinical applications. *Clin. Orthop*; **133**:95–105.

Kendall J.P., Stokes I.A.F., O'Hara J.P., Dickson R.A. (1979). Tension and creep phenomena in peripheral nerve. *Acta Orthop. Scand*; **50**:721–25.

MacGregor I.A., Jackson I.T. (1972). The groin flap. *Brit. J. Plast. Surg*; **25**:3–16.

Millesi H. (1977). Interfascicular grafts for repair of peripheral nerves of the upper extremity. *Orthop. Clin. N. Amer*; **8**:387–404.

Narakas A. (1978). Surgical treatment of traction injuries of the brachial plexus. *Clin. Orthop. Relat. Res*; **133**:71–90.

O'Brien B.M., MacLeod A.M., Morrison W.A. (1977). Microvascular free flap transfer. *Orthop. Clin. N. Amer*; **8**:349–66.

Sunderland S. (1968). *Nerve and Nerve Injuries*. London: Livingstone.

Taylor G.I. (1977). Micro-vascular free bone transfer. A clinical technique. *Orthop. Clin. N. Amer*; **8**:425–47.

49

Hand

ROBERT A. DICKSON

Hand function

The thumb, index, and middle fingers form a dynamic tripod of prehension, while the ring and little fingers are responsible for power grip. The position of function of the hand (Fig 49.1) depicts the thumb opposed to both the index and middle fingers with the ring and little fingers flexed towards the palm. The radial three digits are responsible for fine movements while the ulnar two digits are necessary for crude grasp. Although each digit may assume separate responsibilities, the overall function of the hand can be demonstrated by holding a pointer.

The performance of microsurgical operations demonstrates par excellence the position of function of the hand. Support for the hand is achieved by resting the ulnar border of the little finger on the working surface to minimise tremor. The ring finger then rests in contact with the little finger leaving the thumb, index, and middle finger to control the instrument. The instrument rests on the dorsum of the web between thumb and index. The weight-relieving and balancing effect thus leaves the radial three digits to perform only the very fine movements required. Such fine movements are performed by the intrinsic musculature, while the long flexors and extensors of the radial three digits function solely in a synergistic manner to stabilise the articulations of these digits in order that the intrinsic muscles can capitalise upon this added stability.

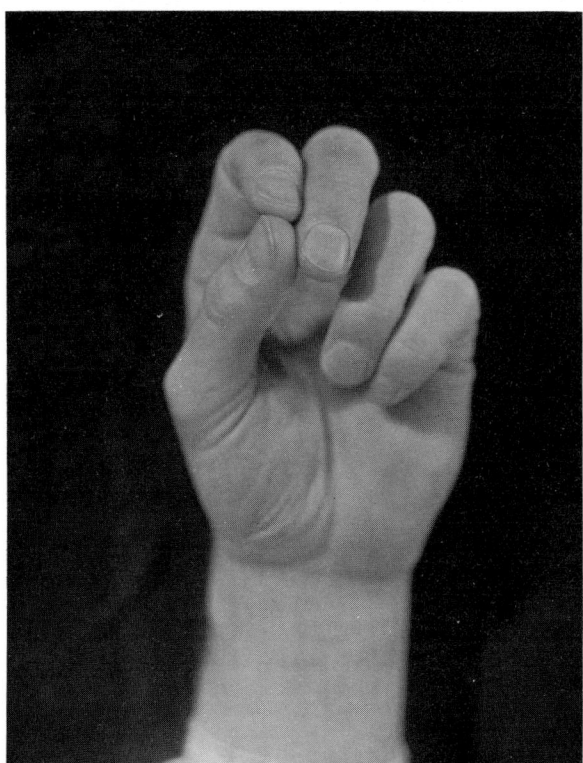

Fig 49.1 The position of function of the hand.

In contradistinction on the ulnar side of the hand, it is the extrinsic musculature which is the more important, the long flexors holding the handle of the pointer or stabilising the hand for fine movement. When all the long flexors of the fingers work together, the finger tips are drawn towards the base of the third metacarpal, Fig 49.2. This is important when treating deformities of the rheumatoid hand and patients with fractures of the hand with malrotation. If an interphalangeal (IP) joint of a rheumatoid finger requires fusion, the position must be that which the joint would normally occupy in

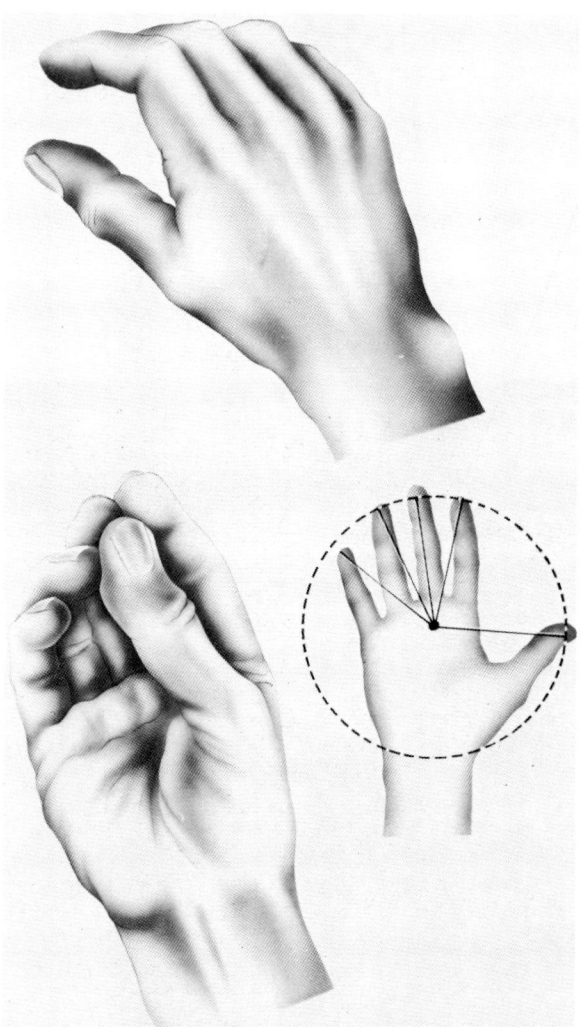

Fig 49.2 All digits flex towards the base of the third metacarpal. In the plane of the palm the thumb nail is perpendicular to the hand. In full opposition the thumb nail is parallel to the hand. (From *Surgery of the Rheumatoid Hand*, 1979, Nicolle F.V., Dickson R.A., eds. London: William Heinemann Medical Books.)

the position of function so that optimal improvement can be realised. Similarly, a finger fracture allowed to heal with malrotation may render the finger progressively less useful the more flexed it is and, eventually, it may completely overlap its neighbour.

Mass flexor action also adducts the fingers and increases the cupping of the palm. The profundus acts mainly at the distal IP joint, the sublimis at the proximal IP joint and the interossei act primarily at the metacarpophalangeal (MP) joints. The long extensors are weaker than their flexor counterparts and abduct the fingers as they extend them. Although providing final extension at the distal IP joint, their primary action is at the MP joint.

The relationship between intrinsic activity and tactile gnosis (stereognosis referable to the hand) is reflected in the considerable proprioceptive nerve supply of the intrinsic muscles. While the dorsal interossei abduct and the palmar interossei adduct the fingers, their main action is in flexion of the MP joints while the lumbricals are important for providing extension of the IP joints.

The thumb is the most important digit in the hand and is responsible for 60% of the hand's function. It has a different arrangement of joints and an extensive intrinsic musculature. The base joint of the thumb is a doubly-concave saddle allowing free range of motion in all directions. Most importantly, it facilitates movement of the thumb from the plane of the palm (when the thumb nail is perpendicular to the palm) to a position of full opposition (when the thumb nail is parallel to the palm). The abductors of the thumb form the first part of this movement, clearing the thumb from the palm. The opponens pollicis rotates the thumb into a position of opposition and then the adductor draws the thumb towards the palm or fingers, thus facilitating pinch or grasp. The distal articulations are hinge joints providing stability in movements of the base of the thumb.

It is important to appreciate the significance of good function in the proximal articulations of the upper extremity – shoulder, elbow, wrist and radioulnar joints – because the hand can only function optimally if it can be readily positioned appropriately. Thus when the hand is examined the status of the other joints should not be overlooked.

The pneumatic tourniquet

Hand surgeons are fortunate in having the opportunity of using the pneumatic tourniquet to provide a dry operative field. Indeed, Bunnell (1948) stated: 'One would no more repair a watch at the bottom of an ink stand, than treat intricate anatomic structures in a bleeding operating area.' However, with the advantages of ischaemia go certain dangers which must be avoided. The tourniquet should be pneumatic and applied to the well-padded upper arm. Furthermore, the surgeon should apply and remove the tourniquet himself, thus avoiding any possibility of leaving the tourniquet on with its disastrous consequences. Before applying the pneumatic tourniquet it is frequently advisable to exsanguinate the upper extremity using an Esmarch bandage, but this should not be performed in the rheumatoid patient or someone with unduly delicate soft tissues. Five minutes of elevation and gentle manual pressure is the favoured method of exsanguination in this situation.

Although much clinical experience and experimental work has accumulated, there is still a wide variation of opinion concerning optimal tourniquet time and pressure. In several hundred operations on the rheumatoid hand no serious side effects were noted with a tourniquet duration of 1.5 h, provided that the pressure did not exceed 300 mm of mercury, and that the tourniquet was well-padded (Nicolle and Dickson, 1979).

However, meticulous technique and peroperative diathermy should be used to minimise the possibility of postoperative haematoma formation. In any situation where much capillary haemorrhage could be anticipated, such as during surgery for Dupuytren's contracture, the tourniquet should be released prior to wound closure.

Skin incisions

It is important to plan out carefully skin incisions preoperatively with particular attention to the possible need for extending the incision. However, the majority of incisions required can be selected from the standard surgical approaches to the front and back of the hand (Fig 49.3; Nicolle and Dickson, 1979). Both the sinusoidal and the volar zig-zag (Bruner, 1967) are standard for approach to the palmar aspect of a finger, and both

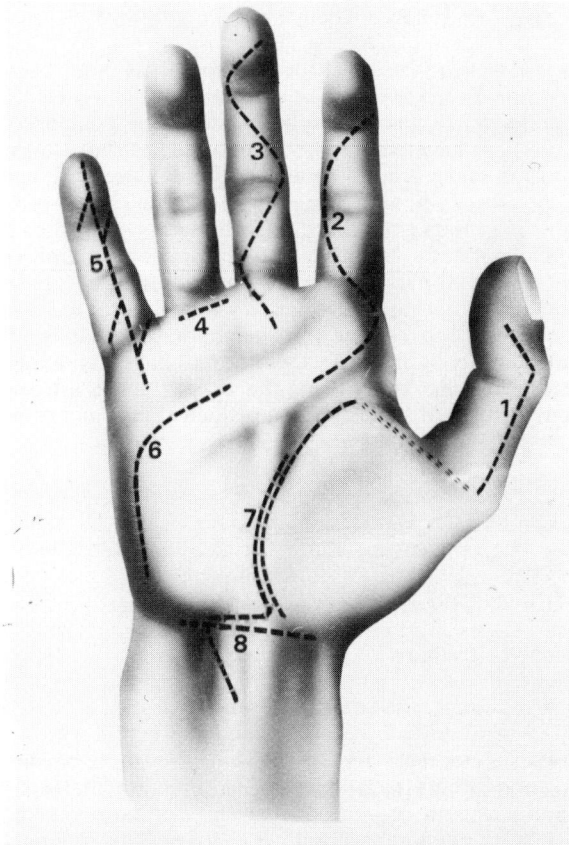

(a)

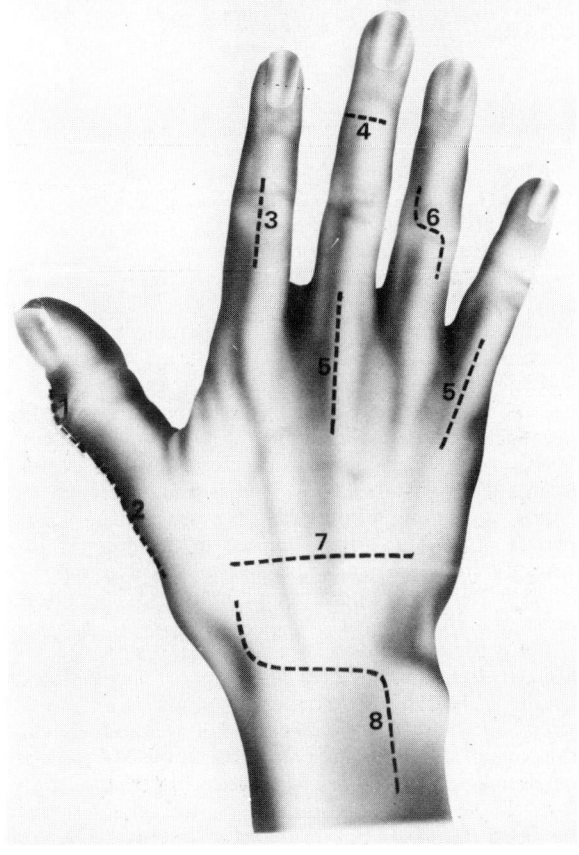

(b)

Fig 49.3 (a) Surgical incisions for exposure of the front of the hand. *(b)* Surgical incisions for exposure of the back of the hand. (From *Surgery of the Rheumatoid Hand*, 1979, Nicolle F.V., Dickson R.A., eds. London: William Heinemann Medical Books.)

have the advantage that they can be readily extended proximally. The volar aspect of the thumb is best exposed using a mid-lateral incision which can then be extended across the first web to join the distal end of the thenar crease. If there is considerable scarring of the palmar aspect of a digit, as is frequently encountered in Dupuytren's contracture, then a straight longitudinal palmar incision with supplementary Z-plasties is preferred. In fashioning the zig-zag incision, it is important to maintain the apices at mid-digital level to avoid contracture, and to curve them to avoid necrosis. The thenar incision can be extended proximally in Z-fashion to expose the structures on the volar aspect of the forearm.

The dorsal aspect of the MP and IP joints of the thumb and fingers is best exposed by individual longitudinal dorsal incisions. They provide excellent exposure of the underlying joint and tendon mechanisms with less retraction than would be required with horizontal incisions and also help to safeguard the integrity of the longitudinally running dorsal veins so important for skin nutrition.

Hand splintage

After minor surgical intervention only the part involved need be dressed or splinted and the hand should always be mobilised at the earliest possible opportunity. However, following operation the entire hand should be carefully dressed and splinted. This not only helps the healing process, but greatly aids patient comfort. A pressure dressing is desirable to maintain haemostasis but should not be excessive. Any dressing which involves the entire hand should extend down to just short of the finger tips thus enabling the pulps to be inspected for neurovascular status. Transverse compression in the region of the MP joints must be avoided as this leads to blockage of the venous drainage and almost certain digital oedema. The use of a supportive plaster of Paris slab incorporated in the dressing provides rigidity. The hand should be elevated for a period of 48 h following operation to minimise haematoma formation and oedema.

When the entire hand is immobilised the proper position of splintage is most important. The collateral ligamentous support of the IP joints is maximally stretched when these joints are fully extended, while the comparable structures referable to the MP joint are maximally stretched in 90° of flexion. In theory, therefore, this should be the optimal position for splintage of the hand, Fig 49.4. However, for physiological reasons the position of rest or function of the hand (*see* Fig 49.1) has also been recommended (Wood-Jones, 1941), because if any degree of stiffness should supervene postoperatively the hand will be in a position very close

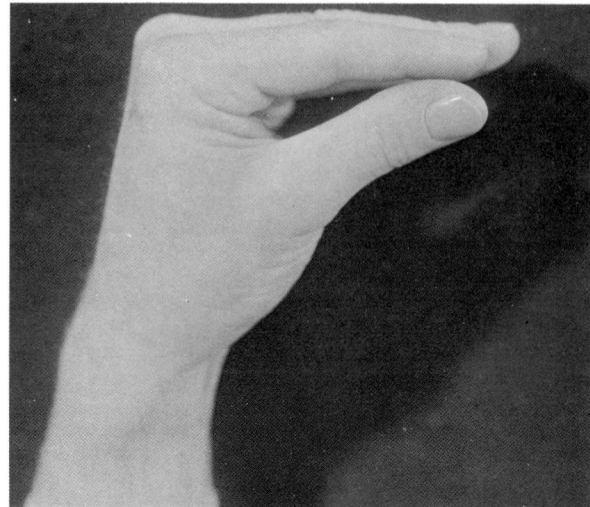

Fig 49.4   The position of safety for hand splintage.

to that which is optimal for function. This latter position is favoured as it may be extremely difficult, or even impossible, to place a swollen hand in the position of safety. No finger should be immobilised in the straight position and no hand should be immobilised for any reason for a period of more than 3 weeks. The position in which a finger should be immobilised is that which it would normally occupy in the position of function of the hand. If the thumb requires immobilisation its position should be one of abduction and opposition. It is useless to strap a finger to its neighbour. This does not satisfactorily immobilise the injured finger and may jeopardise the integrity of the other. These are the golden rules of hand splintage which should never be transgressed.

Fractures of the hand

Metacarpal fractures

Bennett's fracture

This common injury, first described in 1882 is caused by a longitudinal force in a proximal direction with the thumb metacarpal adducted. The dislocation or subluxation occurs in a dorsoradial direction leaving a small fragment of bone on the anterior aspect of the base of the first metacarpal, (Fig 49.5a). This fragment is retained in position by its attachment to the anterior oblique carpometacarpal ligament. If the injury occurs when the thumb is in a markedly adducted position, then the dislocation may occur without leaving any

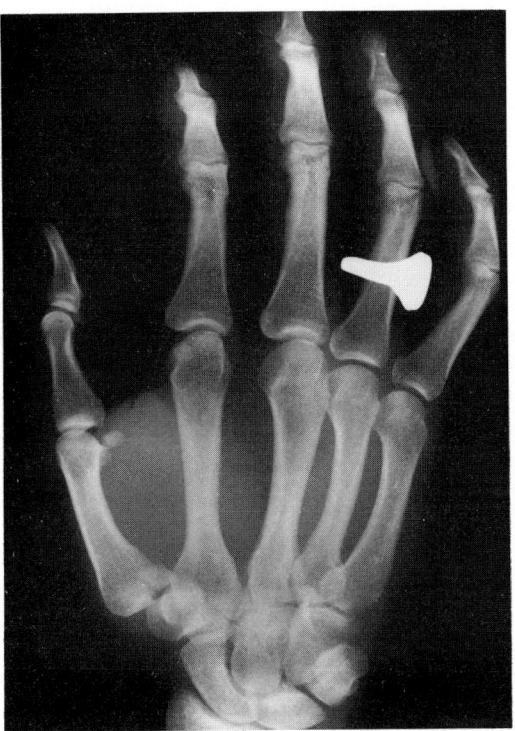

Fig 49.5a Bennett's fracture-dislocation of the first carpo-metacarpal joint.

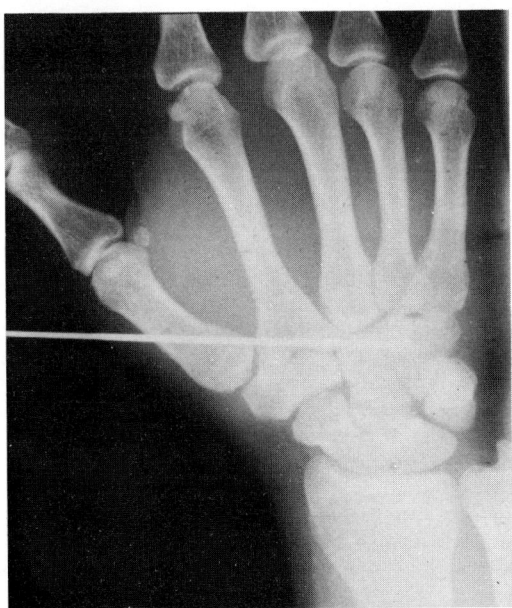

Fig 49.5b Wagner's technique of maintaining the reduction using a Kirschner wire.

bone fragment giving rise to the so-called Bennett's 'fracture without a fracture'.

Treatment. This fracture is readily reduced by longitudinal traction with the thumb fully abducted. By this means the dislocated base of the first metacarpal is brought back into contract with the small anterior fragment left behind. While this position is being secured by means of a plaster of Paris spica, it is convenient to maintain the reduced position by passing a strong Kirschner wire through the shaft of the first metacarpal distal to the injury into the intact second metacarpal (Fig 49.5b).

This is an intra-articular injury and there are many operative treatments described which seek to obtain an anatomical reduction. If the anterior fragment is large enough to sustain a small screw, then, via an anterior approach, the fracture is openly reduced and internally fixed. If the fragment is smaller then a similar position can be achieved using a Kirschner wire. Although anything less than anatomical reduction may give rise to early degenerative osteoarthrosis this is more of theoretical than practical value. In the author's personal experience of over 100 cases of base of thumb arthritis only one has been as a result of a Bennett's fracture, the remainder being associated with primary generalised osteoarthrosis with no previous history of local trauma.

Following 6 weeks immobilisation in a plaster spica union is readily achieved and the patient should commence vigorous active assisted exercises in order to regain a full range of motion.

Metacarpal shaft fractures

The majority of metacarpal shaft fractures are stable, not significantly displaced, and require no specific treatment. However such injuries often result from a severe crush and therefore the soft tissue component of the injury assumes greater importance. There is frequently considerable swelling and contusion, and a period of hospitalisation with the hand elevated in the position of safety forms the basis of treatment. When the oedema has subsided no treatment need be directed towards the underlying fractures and the hand should be mobilised forthwith.

The indications for reduction and immobilisation in metacarpal shaft fractures arise only when there is significant shortening or malrotation. Transverse fractures with malrotation are best reduced by longitudinal traction with the proximal phalanx flexed. The reduction position can be maintained satisfactorily by the retrograde passage of an axial Kirschner wire or small Steinmann pin, (Fig 49.6). Oblique fractures of the metacarpal shafts with shortening are unstable injuries and the technique of Lamb *et al.* (1973) is recommended. After

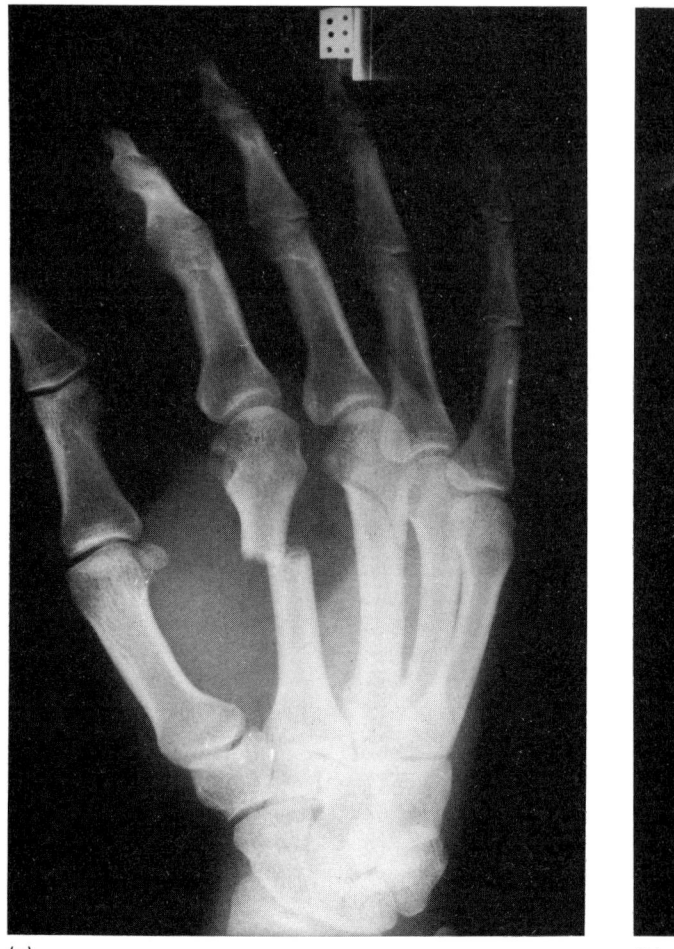 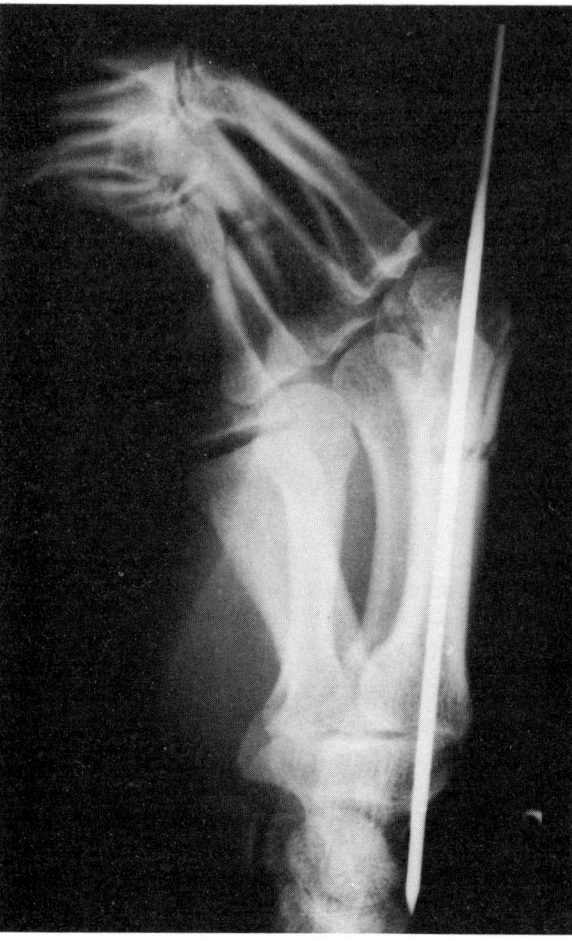

(a)   (b)

Fig 49.6 Displaced transverse metacarpal fractures can be conveniently held reduced by means of an axial Steinman pin or Kirschner wire. (From *The Basis and Practice of Traumatology*, 1983, Hughes S. ed. London: William Heinemann Medical Books.)

reduction by longitudinal traction with the proximal phalanges flexed, two transverse Kirschner wires are passed, one proximal to the fractures and one distal. In order to avoid loss of reduction these wires can be secured on the ulnar side of the hand by means of an external longitudinal Kirschner wire bonded to the two transverse wires using acrylic cement, (Fig 49.7; Dickson, 1975).

Fractures of the metacarpals involving the MP joints

In order to minimise irregularity of the joint surface and to maintain the stability of the collateral ligaments, operative treatment is indicated in these injuries. After open reduction, large fragments can be held in anato-

mical position by means of a small AO cancellous screw whereas smaller fragments are more appropriately secured by a Kirschner wire. On the infrequent occasions when the metacarpal head is severely comminuted it is better to secure alignment and rotation using an axial Kirschner wire followed by the earliest possible mobilisation in an effort to prevent joint stiffness.

If the injury is avulsion of a small piece of bone at the site of attachment of the collateral ligament, open reduction and fixation of this small fragment with a Kirschner wire is indicated.

Although bony injuries of the hand unite in approximately 3 weeks, there is frequently residual pain and swelling lasting many months. Long-term active assisted exercises are therefore essential.

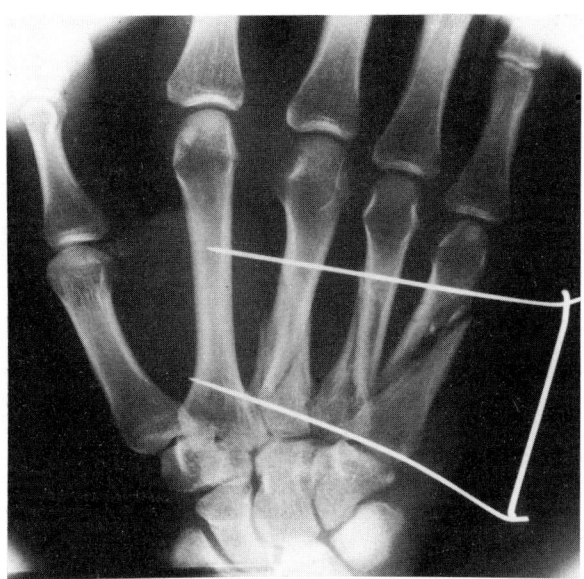

Fig 49.7 Unstable oblique fractures of the metacarpals can be held reduced by two transverse Kirschner wires bonded externally using acrylic cement. (From *The Basis and Practice of Traumatology*, 1983, Hughes S. ed. London: William Heinemann Medical Books.)

Phalangeal injuries

Fractures of the phalanges

The usual mechanism of injury is a direct blow or crushing injury and less commonly the finger is injured as a result of a fall. Approximately one-third of injuries are shaft fractures, one-third are epiphyseal injuries, while joint and finger tip injuries make up 20% each.

As with metacarpal fractures the majority are stable and undisplaced and only symptomatic treatment is indicated. Malrotation or angulation is best treated by closed manipulation followed by immobilisation using a padded aluminium splint. Long unstable fractures of the phalangeal shafts can be secured by AO screws provided the length of the fracture line is at least twice the diameter of the bone (Steel, 1978). Kirschner wires provide a perfectly acceptable alternative. Condylar fragments large enough to sustain an AO screw are best secured in this manner while comminuted articular injuries are best held reduced by Kirschner wires. It is surprising how few patients (60%) obtain a satisfactory result following a phalangeal fracture. They frequently take longer than 3 weeks to unite and fractures of the neck of the bone are notoriously slow.

Fractures of the phalanges in children

Phalangeal fractures are more prevalent in children than adults, but comminution is uncommon. Injuries involving the shaft, joint, epiphysis and finger tip are equally common.

The more common Salter type II epiphyseal injury has a good prognosis due to the degree of remodelling allowed by youth. However, phalangeal neck fractures with displacement in children remain deformed unless corrected because here remodelling does not take place. Although treatment is along the same lines as that for comparable injuries in adults, the proportion of good results is much higher in children except for injuries involving the epiphysis of the base of the distal phalanx.

Boutonnière deformity

This injury is caused by disruption of the central extensor tendon mechanism over the dorsum of the proximal IP joint, Fig 49.8. The site of discontinuity is nearly always in tendon substance itself and only occasionally is a result of avulsion of a small fragment of bone from the base of the proximal phalanx. As a result of this loss of extension the proximal IP joint is held flexed, while the distal IP joint is hyperextended as the lateral extensor bands pass dorsal to the axis of movement of this hinge-joint.

A better prognosis is associated with avulsion of a fragment of bone because this can be replaced using a small Kirschner wire. In contradistinction, repair of the ruptured central slip is disappointing, but should be attempted. It can be reinforced using a distally based flap of extensor mechanism sewn over it (Snow, 1973).

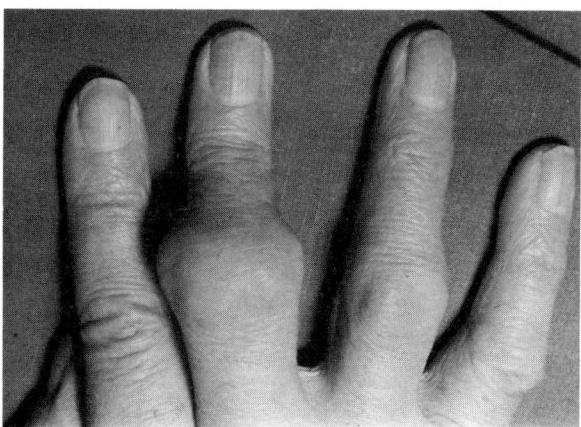

Fig 49.8 Long-standing Boutonnière deformity of the proximal IP joint of the middle finger.

Alternatively, one of the lateral bands of the extensor mechanism can be rerouted over the dorsum of the proximal IP joint.

There are few satisfactory results from this procedure and the outcome for the majority of patients is either a persistent Boutonnière deformity or significant stiffness of the proximal IP joint.

Mallet finger deformity

In this injury the discontinuity in the extensor tendon mechanism occurs over the dorsum of the distal IP joint and is nearly always a closed avulsion injury. An extensor lag, Fig 49.9, develops acutely, often with little or no discomfort. Occasionally a fragment of bone is avulsed from the base of the distal phalanx. In this situation the deformity can be reconstituted by securing the bone fragment in its anatomical position by means of a Kirschner wire. Frequently, however, the damage occurs in tendon substance itself and, even following 4 weeks in a Mallet finger type splint with the distal IP joint extended and the proximal IP joint flexed, the results are disappointing. Fortunately, the functional loss is minimal.

Tendon injuries

Flexor tendon injuries

The palmar aspect of the hand and fingers and distal forearm has been divided arbitrarily into five zones as regards the anatomy, technique and results of flexor tendon repair, (Fig 49.10). Zone 2, extending from the distal palmar crease to the middle of the middle phalanx, is known as 'no man's land'. This is because, until

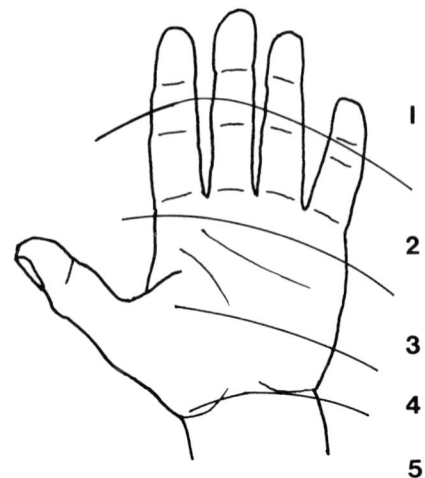

Fig 49.10 The five zones in which flexor tendon injuries can occur. Zone 2 has been referred to as 'no man's land'. (From *The Basis and Practice of Orthopaedics*, 1980, Hughes S.; Sweetnam R., eds. London: William Heinemann Medical Books.).

recently, tendons repaired in this zone became embedded in scar tissue with resultant loss of active motion. If the wound is contaminated, or infected, or there has been delay between injury and presentation, the tendon injury should not be dealt with until there has been sound healing of overlying soft tissue. If there has been loss of tendon substance then repair is preferable, but if excessive then grafting is required. If the superficial tendon alone has been divided, there is no need to proceed with repair as the intact profundus can perform all the functions required of that digit. In Zones 1, 3, 4 and 5 primary repair, if the wound is a clean incised one, is indicated.

Significant recent advances have been made with regard to the management of flexor tendon injuries in 'no man's land'. Because early attempts at restoring continuity yielded such poor results, the pioneers of flexor tendon surgery recommended a free tendon graft in all cases. This was performed 3 weeks after injury when there was sound healing of the integument. Tradition also dictated that if only the profundus was divided the intact sublimis would provide ultimate good function if the distal IP joint was either tenodesed or arthrodesed.

Ten years ago saw results emerging from centres which appeared to employ techniques in direct contravention of traditional principles (Verdan, 1972; Kleinert *et al.*, 1973). They advocated primary repair in 'no man's land' if the profundus tendon alone or both tendons were divided. Their high proportion of good results stimulated much-needed basic work on tendon healing and adhesion formation. It has been shown that

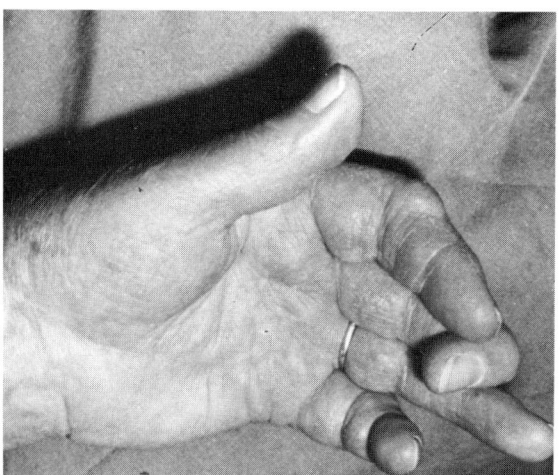

Fig 49.9 Mallet deformity of the distal IP joint.

a significant part of tendon healing comes from the cellular response of the fibrous flexor sheath and the surrounding soft tissues including the synovium. Such adhesions are necessary for the restoration of tendon continuity, but are loose and delicate structures which gradually resorb and do not provide a blockage to active tendon movement. If, however, the site of tendon repair is exposed to unyielding structures such as ligaments, palmar fascia and periosteum, then the tougher and more substantial nature of the adhesions prevents active movement and these mature into fibrous tissue rather than being resorbed.

The principles of flexor tendon repair require a meticulous technique with a minimum of trauma to unyielding structures and careful repair of the fibrous flexor sheath after the tendon anastomosis. The sublimis tendon, if also divided, should never be resected. Its repair not only improves finger strength and dexterity, but also facilitates subsequent gliding of both tendons by limiting adhesion formation.

Clean incised injuries – Zones 2, 3, 4 and 5

When both flexor tendons have been divided, or when the profundus only has been divided, primary repair is indicated. If only the sublimis has been divided, a rare injury, the intact profundus provides nearly full function and no repair is indicated. The technique of repair recommended by Kleinert *et al.* (1973) is favoured, (Fig 49.11). A Bunnell-type interlocking stitch of nylon secures the repair which is gathered neatly by an additional continuous circumferential suture of fine 'Dexon'. The tendon repair is protected for the first 3 weeks by means of a rubber band passed through the tip of the nail and attached to the front of a volar plaster of Paris slab. Movement is permitted immediately postoperatively and at 3 weeks all support is removed and active exercises commenced.

Clean incised injuries – Zone 1

Primary repair is again indicated if the profundus tendon is divided proximal to its last 1.5 cm. However, within 1.5 cm of the distal phalanx, it is preferable to advance the tendon distally and secure it afresh to bone.

Contaminated wounds

Initially, tendon lacerations should be ignored and attention directed towards the skin and soft tissues which should be excised in order to facilitate sound healing. When this has occurred, usually at about 3 weeks, delayed primary repair is carried out.

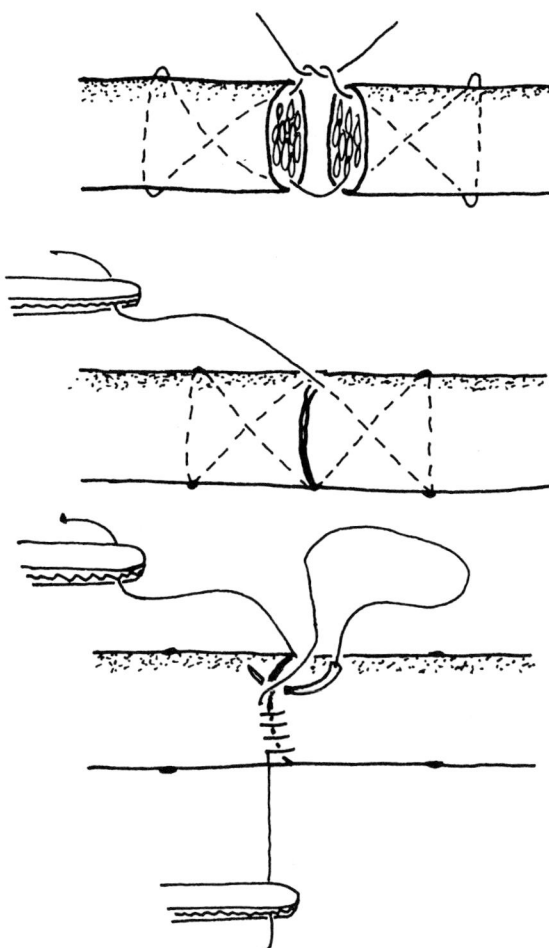

Fig 49.11 Kleinert's technique of repairing a severed flexor tendon. (From *The Basis and Practice of Orthopaedics*, 1980, Hughes S., Sweetnam R., eds. London: William Heinemann Medical Books.)

Other conditions

If there has been a long period of time between injury and repair, or if there has been a significant loss of tendon substance such that the tendon ends cannot be apposed, a free tendon graft is introduced. If the bed in which the tendon graft should lie is unfavourable due to previous infection or crushing, a two-stage tendon graft is preferred using a preliminary silastic rod to generate a new sheath (Hunter, 1965).

Extensor tendon injuries

Extensor tendon injuries have a much better prognosis than their flexor counterparts because of the absence of the fibrous flexor sheath. Extensor tendons are surrounded either by synovium or paratenon, the latter being a condensation of local areolar tissue. For clean incised injuries end-to-end repair should be performed primarily and has a predictably good result. If there has been a significant loss of tendon substance the proximal end can be anastomosed to the side of an adjoining extensor tendon with an equally good result. A contaminated, or otherwise unfavourable, wound should be dealt with by excision, aiming for early healing of the soft tissues and the tendon can be dealt with in a delayed primary fashion some 3 weeks later.

Loss of continuity of the extensor mechanism at the proximal and distal IP joints has a poor prognosis (*vide supra*). When the extensor tendon is divided at the level of the MP joint the latter is inevitably opened. In this situation primary end-to-end repair is the method of choice, but some degree of joint stiffness frequently ensues.

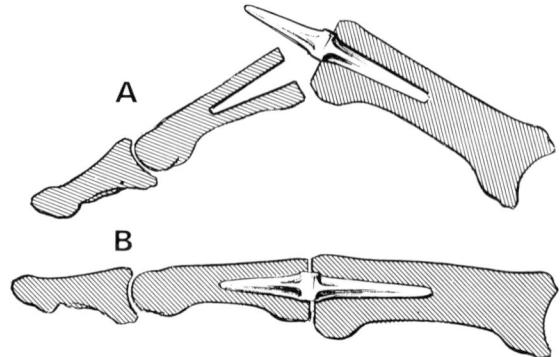

Fig 49.12 Arthrodesis of the MP joint of the thumb is best achieved in the straight position using an intramedullary peg. (From *Surgery of the Rheumatoid Hand*, 1979, Nicolle F.V., Dickson R.A., eds. London: William Heinemann Medical Books.)

Miscellaneous injuries

Poacher's thumb

Poacher's thumb, also known as game-keeper's thumb, is the condition characterised by instability of the MP joint of the thumb. An acute traumatic strain of the ulnar collateral ligament leads to either its rupture or the avulsion of a small fragment of bone at the site of its insertion. Local pain and swelling accompany the injury and when this subsides instability is the main feature.

If the diagnosis is made soon after injury, a good result can be achieved by repair of the ulnar collateral ligament or attachment of the small fragment of bone to its origin by Kirschner wire fixation. All too frequently, however, the patient presents late, by which time the ligamentous structures on the ulnar side of the first MP joint have attenuated and cannot be sutured. In this situation fusion is the treatment of choice. The MP joint of the thumb only moves through a range of hinge motion of 40°–50°; at this articulation stability overrides mobility. A good result is, therefore, achieved by arthrodesis, which is performed in the straight position through a dorsal longitudinal approach (Fig 49.12).

Articular disc tear of the wrist

This troublesome condition, which is also difficult to treat, most frequently affects young adult females. It constitutes a traumatic derangement of the triangular shaped fibrocartilaginous meniscus which joins radius to ulnar styloid just distal to the inferior radioulnar joint. Local pain, tenderness and crepitus are the clinical features which are exacerbated by resisted rotation of the forearm. Coleman (1960) showed arthrographically that radio-opaque dye introduced distally passes proximally beyond the distal radioulnar joint through the torn meniscus.

Surgical removal of the torn disc is frequently disappointing and conservative treatment with local ultrasound, short wave diathermy or anti-inflammatory injection should be persisted with for several months before surgery is contemplated.

The shoulder-hand syndrome

This ill-understood condition tends to affect females in middle age who complain of shoulder pain and limitation of movement in association with pain and swelling of the hand. Steinbrocker *et al.* (1949), when first naming this condition, noted its association with a variety of disorders – e.g. cardiovascular disease, cervical disc disease, frozen shoulder, as well as minor trauma. He considered this to be a reflex neurovascular disturbance similar to Sudek's atrophy.

Examination of shoulder and hand reveal no specific local pathology. The hand is often dark red in colour, with shiny skin and poor capillary return. It is important to recognise this condition and treat it early (Graham and Rosen, 1962). The mainstay of treatment is a short course of oral steroids in association with local ultrasound, short wave diathermy, or heat.

Sudek's atrophy

Although this condition may affect any part of the body, the hand is the most frequently affected. A burning discomfort, swelling, limitation of range of motion, and hyperaemia are the clinical features which are brought on by local trauma which may be so minor as to be undetected by the patient. Hand radiographs frequently demonstrate a remarkable degree of osteoporosis (Fig 49.13).

This condition has a particularly protracted course, but is self-limiting and therefore treatment is symptomatic. In the early acute phase elevation and immobilisation are important while physical therapy is counterproductive. This should be followed by active assisted exercises and wax baths. For the unremitting case an intravenous forearm injection of a long-acting steroid preparation, under tourniquet, is frequently beneficial.

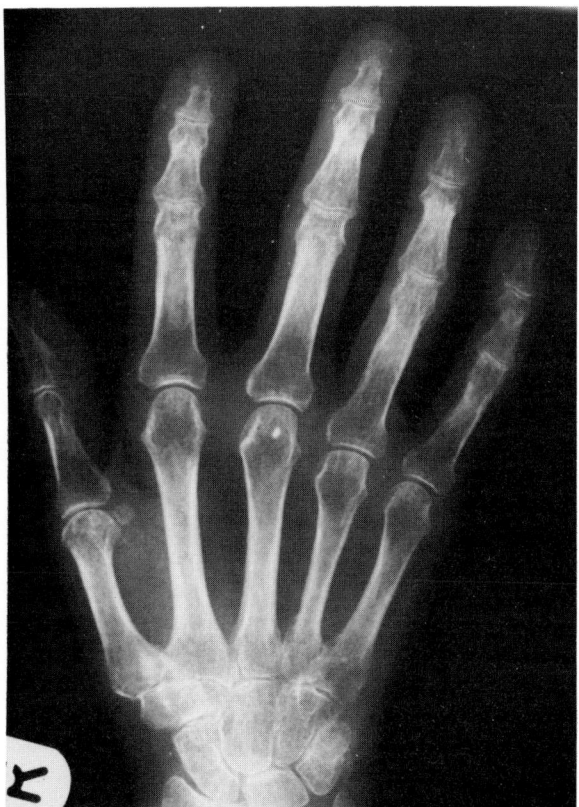

Fig 49.13 Radiograph demonstrating Sudek's atrophy. (From *Mercer's Orthopaedic Surgery*, 1983, 8th edn., Fig 15.24, by courtesy of the editors R.B. Duthie and G. Bentley and the publishers, Edward Arnold.)

Hand infections

Pathogenic organisms may enter the hand by means of a penetrating wound or through a crack in dried skin. The onset is acute with all the cardinal signs of inflammation and the local discomfort is exacerbated if the arm is dependent or local pressure exerted. An anatomical classification of hand infections is fundamental in their understanding (Table 1).

Table 1
ANATOMICAL CLASSIFICATION OF HAND INFECTIONS

ACUTE INFECTIONS

A *Superficial infections* – in one of the layers of the skin
    Subcuticular
    Paronychial
    Subungual
    Furuncular
    Acute spreading infections
    Gangrene

B *Subcutaneous infections*
  (1) Infections of the segment spaces
      distal
      middle
      proximal
  (2) Infections of the synovial sheaths – tenosynovitis
      digital tenosynovitis
      infection of the ulnar bursa
      infection of the radial bursa

C *Infections of the cellular spaces*
    Superficial palmar space
    Deep central palmar space
    Web spaces
    Thenar space
    Hypothenar space
    Dorsal space

D Complications of acute infections
    Septic arthritis
    Osteomyelitis
    Infection of the space of Parona

CHRONIC INFECTIONS

A Tuberculosis
B Syphilis

In-patient treatment is the basis for all serious hand infections. Pathogenic organisms can be isolated in almost 60%, with penicillinase-producing staphylococci being preponderant and the majority of the remainder being Gram-negative organisms or *Escherichia coli*. Cloxacillin is the most useful antibiotic, particularly for those infections which have not yet reached the pus-forming stage or to prevent systemic spread during surgical treatment. Pus should be evacuated at the site of maximum local tenderness although special incisions are frequently necessary to drain the tissue spaces. Elevation and immobilisation of the hand in the position of safety should accompany treatment.

Acute infections

SUPERFICIAL INFECTIONS

Subcuticular

This subepidermal infection of the pulp creates a small superficial abscess which may communicate more deeply by means of a collar-stud extension. This collection should be drained directly over the abscess which is clearly visible and it is important to probe deeply to evacuate subcutaneous extension.

Paronychial

This is the commonest hand infection seen in accident departments and begins on one side of the nail as an infection underneath the eponychium (Fig 49.14). It may extend around the nail folds to the other side of the finger and frequently gives rise to a mass of granulation tissue locally. A longitudinal incision parallel to the lateral side of the nail should be made to evacuate this abscess.

Subungual

A foreign body under the nail, or a penetrating wound of the nail, may give rise to this infection. It also frequently occurs as a local extension of paronychia. The confined space in which this infection occurs gives rise to characteristic severe throbbing pain. The nail is frequently lifted by the underlying collection and removal of this loose nail allows free drainage.

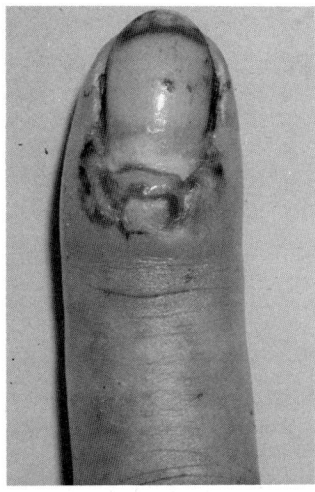

Fig 49.14 A typical paronychia.

Furuncular

The dorsum of the hand and fingers comprises hair-bearing skin and blockage of the follicles gives rise to small superficial boils. Clearance of hair from the infected follicle allows adequate drainage. A carbuncle requires thorough surgical incision.

Acute spreading

The staphylococcus is the commonest organism giving rise to collections of pus, while the haemolytic streptococcus is responsible for spreading infections. If these occur in skin and subcutaneous tissue the term 'cellulitis' is appropriate, whereas the term 'erysipelas' is reserved for cutaneous lymphangitis. These infections spread quickly and give rise to local areas of redness with constitutional upset. The local lymphatics are frequently involved giving rise to red streaks in the skin in a proximal direction. High doses of penicillin combined with local splintage aid rapid resolution.

Gangrene

Any finger infection of severity may block the digital arteries as a result of local pressure (Fig 49.15). Accordingly the signs of inflammation are replaced by temperature reduction, cyanosis, and loss of sensation. Amputation is necessary at the appropriate level.

SUBCUTANEOUS INFECTIONS

Infections of the segment spaces

Distal. The skin of the dorsum of the hand is freely mobile. In contradistinction the skin over the palm of the hand and palmar aspect of the digits is relatively fixed by condensations of fascia running deeply. This is because the palmar aspect of the hand is a working surface and non-extensile skin improves grip.

In the distal pulp space these fascial bands run from the deep surface of the skin to the periosteum of the distal phalanx dividing the pulp into many small compartments containing fat loculi and the terminal ramifications of the digital arteries. Following a minor penetrating wound of the pulp, local signs of inflammation develop. Because this is a closed compartment intensive throbbing pain, particularly at night, is characteristic in association with a tense, red, tender-swelling (Fig 49.16). As the infection subsides the pulp may feel indurated or boggy. Involvement of the underlying distal phalanx is not uncommon in these infections as a consequence of pressure deprivation of blood supply. The bone is then vulnerable to local extension of infection.

In all but the most early infections drainage is essential, not only to evacuate a local collection but to relieve pressure. A lateral incision is recommended in order to avoid a tender scar.

Middle. This corresponds closely with the distal pulp space infection in its clinical features and management, but is less common and less severe. If the penetrating wound causing the infection has also reached the fibrous flexor sheath, then a suppurative tenosynovitis may be a consequence.

Proximal. This is the least common space to be infected and generally occurs in association with a web space infection as the proximal space and web freely communicate. Early incision over the point of maximum tenderness, or over a definitive collection, is recommended.

Infections of the synovial sheaths

Digital tenosynovitis. This disastrous infection has a characteristic clinical picture (Fig 49.17). The finger is held persistently flexed at all joints, tenderness is exquisite and limited to the area of the fibrous flexor sheath, there is a fusiform enlargement of the entire

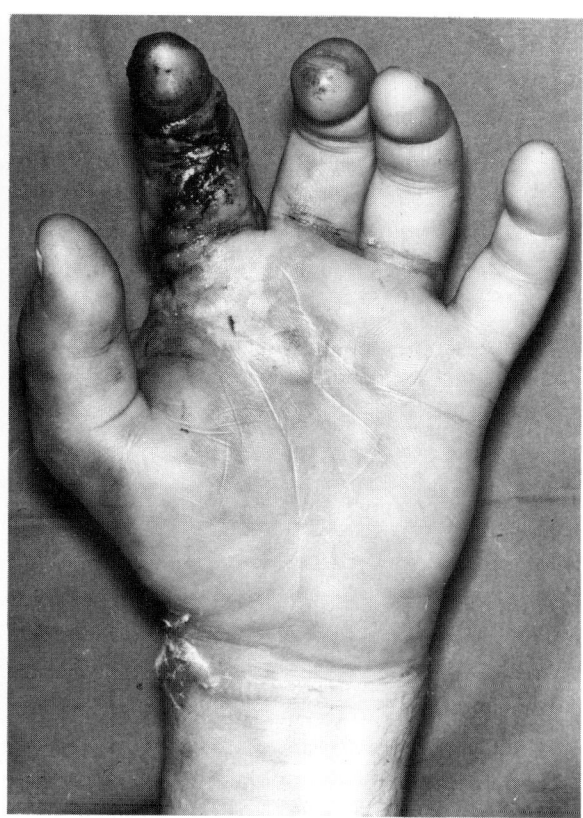

Fig 49.15 Digital infection leading to gangrene.

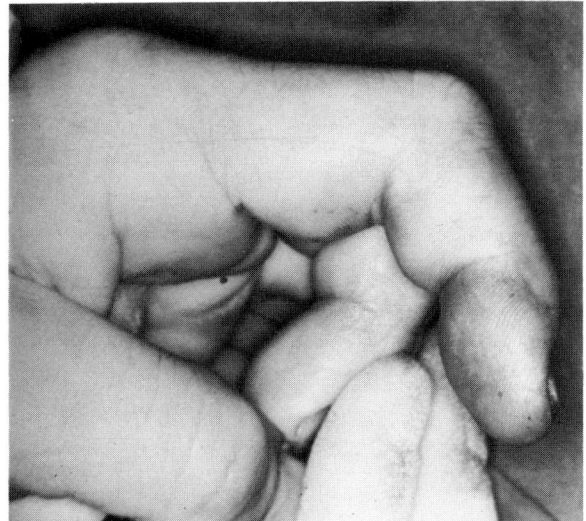

Fig 49.16 Distal segment space infection with a tense, swollen pulp.

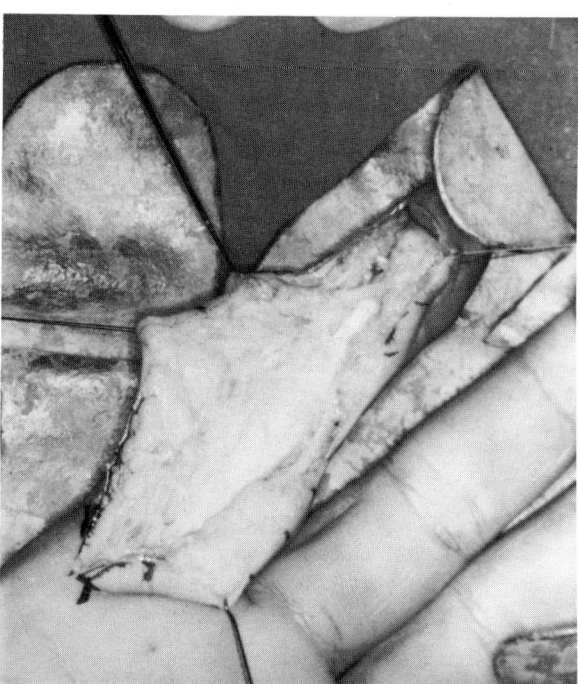

Fig 49.17 Suppurative digital tenosynovitis. The fibrous sheath has been opened and flushed out.

finger, and agonising pain when the finger is straightened. Any penetrating wound of the palmar aspect of the finger can give rise to tenosynovitis and in a quarter of cases, when there is a natural communication with the ulnar bursa, the infection may spread proximally.

Infection of the ulnar bursa. Although this may arise from a wound which penetrates the bursa itself, it more commonly accompanies digital tenosynovitis by proximal extension. As in all severe hand infections the dorsum is particularly swollen, but the diagnostic sign, Kanavel's sign, is maximal tenderness proximal to the distal palmar crease in the line of the fourth web. In addition the little finger is held flexed, 'the hook sign'.

Infection of the radial bursa. Again, although this can be caused by a wound perforating the bursa itself, it more commonly accompanies tenosynovitis of the thumb. In 80% of individuals there is a natural anatomical communication between radial and ulnar bursae and therefore the focus of infection is not well localised and the entire palm may be markedly swollen.

Management of tendon sheath infections. Surgical drainage at the earliest opportunity is the mainstay of treatment combined with appropriate antibiotic administration, elevation and hospitalisation. The radial and ulnar bursae should be opened directly over the point of maximum tenderness. For digital tenosynovitis two incisions are necessary, one at the proximal mouth of the sheath and the other at the level of the distal IP joint crease. This facilitates through-and-through irrigation with a small catheter.

Despite optimal treatment the results are frequently poor with a limited range of active motion resulting from adhesions between tendon and surrounding soft tissue.

INFECTIONS OF THE CELLULAR SPACES

In addition to the thenar space, the hypothenar space and the dorsal space, there are three central spaces first described by Iselin, the superficial palmar space, the deep central palmar space and the web spaces.

The superficial palmar space

This space is situated between the palmar aponeurosis and the long flexor tendons. It is bounded medially by the fourth intermetacarpal space and laterally by the line of the second metacarpal bone. It communicates with the deep central palmar space and the forearm.

The deep central palmar space

Communicating with the forearm and the web spaces via the lumbrical canals, this space is situated beneath the flexor tendons and in front of the interossei. A wound which perforates into this space may give rise to infection, but more commonly the space becomes involved via an infected web or rupture of suppurative tenosynovitis. The entire hand is grossly swollen, as much on the palmar aspect as on the dorsum, (Fig 49.18). There may be a collar-stud link to the superficial space.

Clinically, the hand is held immobile with all fingers flexed. The severity of this infection is evidenced by the degree of constitutional upset. Treatment is surgical and urgent. The point of maximum tenderness is chosen for the site of drainage, but if tenderness is diffuse a transverse midpalmar incision should be used.

The web spaces

These communicate with the palmar spaces proximally and the proximal pulp space distally, and are situated between the slips of the palmar aponeurosis which pass to the four fingers. Each web contains loose fibrofatty tissue through which pass the neurovascular bundles and the tendons of the intrinsic muscles.

The typical clinical picture is separation of the adjacent two fingers with swelling and marked tenderness over the web (Fig 49.19). The collection should be drained through an incision over the point of maximum tenderness on the palmar aspect of the affected web.

The thenar space

This space lies between the thenar fascia and the transverse head of the adductor pollicis, and its medial boundary is the third metacarpal bone. The thenar

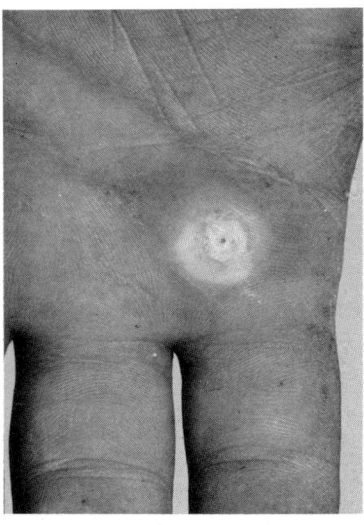

Fig 49.18   Collar-stud extension from deep space.

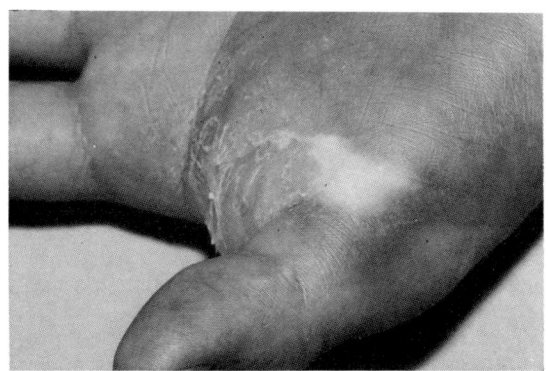

Fig 49.19 Infection of the first web space.

region and radial half of the palm are markedly swollen with exquisite tenderness on local pressure. The thumb is abducted from the index finger. This collection should be drained through an incision on the palmar aspect of the web over the site of maximum tenderness.

The hypothenar space

This is a potential space between the hypothenar muscles and their overlying fascia. There are no natural anatomical communications with this space where local discomfort and tenderness are accurately localised. The space should be drained through a transverse palmar incision over the point of maximum tenderness.

The dorsal space

This space is again a potential one, between the dorsal interosseus muscle fascia and the dorsal skin. This is the space which can become oedematous in any hand infection. A local penetrating wound is the usual cause and there is frequently overlying cellulitis or erysipelas. Because of anatomical boundaries the entire dorsum of the hand is swollen and inflamed.

This space is drained through a transverse incision dorsally over the point of maximum tenderness.

COMPLICATIONS OF ACUTE INFECTIONS OF THE HAND

In addition to the natural communications which exist anatomically through which infections may spread, local bone or joint may be involved in severe or long-standing cases. Furthermore, a severe palmar infection may spread proximally into the forearm between the anterior interosseus muscle fascia and the overlying long flexor tendons – the space of Parona.

Septic arthritis

Signs of inflammation are localised to a joint, usually the proximal IP which is held immobile in the flexed position. This important diagnosis must be made early lest articular damage leads to severe joint destruction.

Osteomyelitis

This usually occurs referable to the distal phalanx consequent upon an untreated distal pulp space infection. Radiographically the bone appears porotic and its tuft eroded. Later frank sequestrum formation may occur. In such cases the bone should be drilled and any necrotic fragments removed.

Infection of the space of Parona

This infection follows untreated sepsis in the radial or ulnar bursae (Fig 49.20). Thus whenever these latter bursae are opened, and pressure over the anterior aspect of the lower forearm causes a further flow of pus, this space is incriminated. The space of Parona should then be opened under a separate incision. Frequently the diagnosis can be made preoperatively when infection of the radial or ulnar bursa is accompanied by symptoms and signs of embarrassment of the median nerve, the most important structure in the space of Parona.

Chronic infections

Tuberculosis may affect the metacarpals and phalanges, particularly in childhood. It is at this age that the vascularity of the short long bones through the nutrient vessel is maximal and liable, therefore, to infection. The medulla is filled with chronic granulation tissue with surrounding endosteal resorption and successive layers of periosteal new bone formation. This gives rise

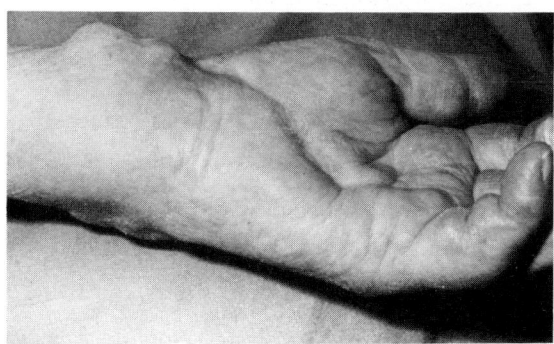

Fig 49.20 Infection of the space of Parona from a severe ulnar bursa abscess.

to a fusiform swelling which is frequently relatively asymptomatic with good preservation of function and minimal local discomfort. If the process is aggressive and untreated there may be extraosseus extension and cold abscess formation.

Tuberculous dactylitis gives rise to a fusiform swelling of the finger with few signs indicative of an underlying infectious process. The differential diagnosis includes syphilitic infection, enchondroma, stress fracture, osteoblastoma and thorn-induced pseudotumour (Dickson and Kemp, 1976; Fig 49.21).

Antituberculous chemotherapy and local splintage are the mainstays of treatment and bring about resolution in the majority. Surgical treatment is sometimes required when there is extensive bone destruction and, therefore, removal of the granulations and cancellous grafting is occasionally necessary.

Congenital abnormalities

At the end of the first two intrauterine months, the upper extremity is a replica of its adult form, growth being the only subsequent change to take place. The insult responsible for producing hand abnormalities, at least half of all musculoskeletal congenital anomalies,

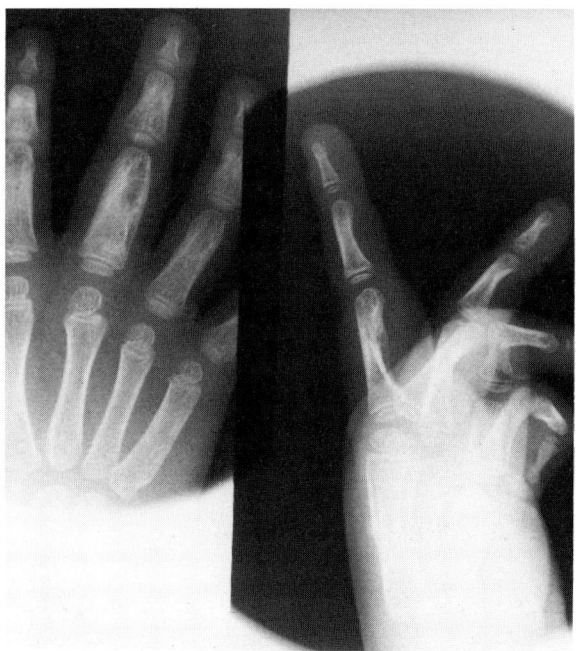

Fig 49.21 Thorn-induced pseudo-tumour in a child's proximal phalanx. (From Dickson R.A., Kemp F.H., 1976, Thorn-induced granulomata of bone, *Hand*; **8**:69–71 by courtesy of the Editor.)

must therefore occur before this. Furthermore, the mesenchymal hand plate appears after 1 month and this therefore limits the time of teratogenic attack to the second intrauterine month, no earlier and no later.

In the management of congenital anomalies of the musculoskeletal system surgical intervention, and the timing thereof, may be very difficult. This is particularly so with reference to the hand in the emotive environment of an otherwise normal growing child. Demands for surgical treatment based upon the cosmetic appearance must be resisted if function may be jeopardised in any way. Function is particularly difficult to assess in the child, who is notoriously good at overcoming the severest deformities with patience and practice.

Congenital malformations of the upper limb have been classified by the American Society for Surgery of the Hand (Entin *et al.*, 1972).

1 Failure of differentiation of parts.
2 Arrest of development of parts.
3 Focal defects.
4 Overgrowth.

Clinical features and treatment of congenital abnormalities

Failure of differentiation of parts

Syndactyly. The most commonly involved digits are the middle and ring fingers joined by skin along their contiguous margins. As in most abnormalities surgical correction before the age of five is inadvisable. The crux of treatment is the careful preoperative planning of the skin incisions so that restoration of existing skin on the radial side of the involved digit is provided, leaving a deficit on the ulnar side which can be covered by a graft.

Camptodactyly and clinodactyly. These are hereditary deformities of a digit in the direction of flexion and lateral deviation respectively (Fig 49.22). The little finger is most commonly involved and consequently function is rarely impaired. With growth the deformity increases and the associated soft tissues provide a component to the contracture. On the rare occasions that surgical treatment is indicated for camptodactyly, when wrist flexion demonstrates passive correctability, a release of flexor digitorum sublimis may prevent a progressive deformity.

Arrest of development of parts

Radial club hand. This deformity occurs in association with radial hypoplasia or aplasia (Fig 49.23). Its

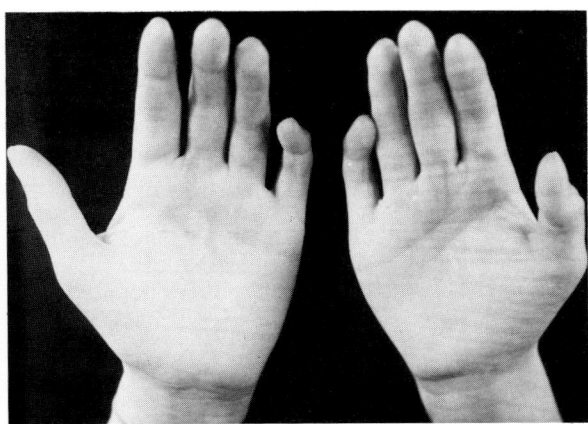

Fig 49.22 Clinodactyly of the little finger with its characteristic lateral deviation deformity.

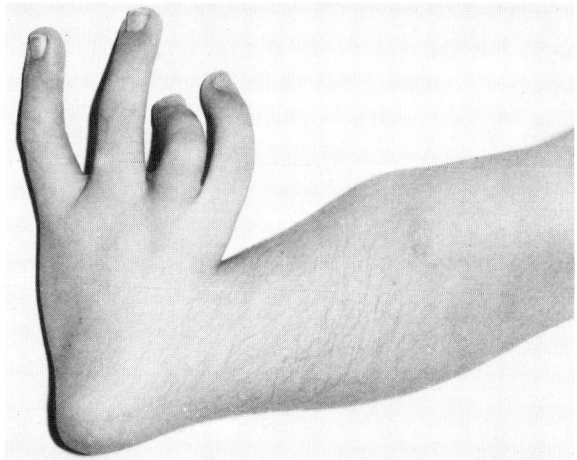

Fig 49.23 Radial club hand in association with radial hypoplasia.

incidence is 1 in 30 000 live births. Treatment is not easy to define but the great experience of Lamb (1977) has yielded the following treatment regime. Conservative treatment in the nature of ratchet splints or night splints is indicated until the child is three to five years of age when operative centralisation of the carpus should be performed in order to correct severe radio-volar displacement.

Lobster claw hand. Most commonly a central deficit separates the rays of the hand, one of which is frequently missing. In the more severe cases there is a single radial and ulnar ray with nothing but a broad cleft between them. Only if the functional capacity of the hand in terms of grip can be improved is operative

treatment indicated which takes the form of closure of the deficit by moving skin from the sides of the cleft. In severe cases this is accompanied by z-elongation of the soft tissues and metacarpal rotation osteotomies.

Focal defects

Congenital constriction rings (Fig 49.24). Surgical treatment is based upon excision of the tight soft tissues making up the groove combined with z-elongation of

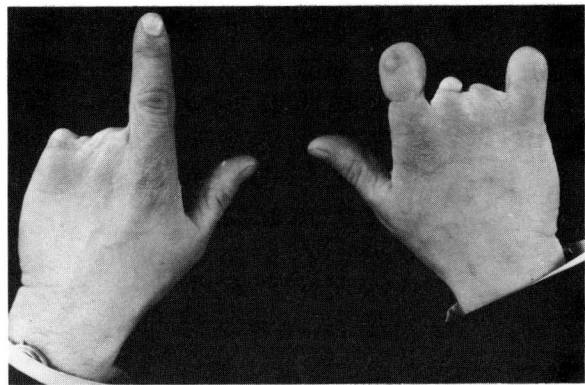

Fig 49.24 Congenital constriction rings. This man drove police cars for many years apparently without any problem.

the skin. In severe cases this is best performed as a multistaged procedure.

Duplications. Supernumerary digits can be unsightly and in this situation surgery is performed for cosmetic considerations. Preoperative radiographic evaluation is mandatory to determine the presence of a residual epiphyseal plate which if not removed may give rise to regrowth.

Overgrowth

Macrodactyly implies a digit bigger in all dimensions than its neighbour for which surgical reduction is seldom indicated.

Rheumatoid disease

A feature of this disease is its predilection for synovial joints and, as it generally commences in the form of a peripheral polyarthropathy, the hands are frequently involved. Unchecked, this progressive disease causes a considerable loss of hand function. Furthermore, a characteristic inflammatory synovitis affects any tissues which have a synovial lining. Thus not only are joints involved but also tendons, ligaments and related soft tissues.

In order to rationalise the treatment of rheumatoid disease affecting the hand in relation to the clinical features, some form of classification based upon staging the disease is essential. That recommended by Barron (1969) is ideal:

Stage 1 – The stage of acute proliferative synovitis
Stage 2 – The stage of soft tissue destruction
Stage 3 – The stage of skeletal collapse.

Stage 1 – *acute proliferative synovitis*

The initial stage of acute synovitis is the province of the rheumatologist using the anti-inflammatory drugs. The hand surgeon, therefore, only becomes involved with a minority of cases of a more aggressive nature. If the phase of acute synovitis remains unchecked then it changes both in its structure and its behaviour. This so-called persistent synovitis is grey, fibrous, adherent and invasive, and damages local tissues in a manner similar to a locally malignant tumour. This is the phase in which surgical treatment has most to offer.

Stage 2 – *soft tissue destruction*

Persistent synovitis

A common site for persistent synovitis is the dorsal synovial bursa which surrounds the extensor tendons (Fig 49.25). The ulnar side of the dorsum of the wrist is first involved and the synovitis does not usually extend to the radial compartment. In the inflammatory phase this gives rise to swelling and local discomfort but if allowed to persist threatens the underlying extensor tendons. The site of rupture of these tendons is in the region of the distal boundary of the extensor retinaculum and is due to pressure and local invasion from synovitis rather than from attrition over roughened bone ends. Persistent synovitis in this area should be removed through a transverse incision over the extensor retinaculum which must be split to liberate the diseased synovium.

Dislocation of the lower end of the ulna

Synovitis in the lower radioulnar joint causes expansion of its capsular support leading to attenuation of the restraining ligaments of the ulnar head. This comes to displace dorsally with swelling and local discomfort particularly on wrist extension and rotational movements of the forearm (Fig 49.26). Synovectomy alone here is impractical and the ulnar head can be removed with no loss of function. This greatly facilitates clearance of diseased synovium and its merit as an operative procedure has been proven over many years. The pronator quadratus muscle is attached down to 1 inch from the ulnar styloid and, therefore, not more than this distance should be removed lest there is subsequent interference with forearm rotation. The overlying extensor tendons should be protected from the cut surface of the ulna by replacing the extensor retinaculum deep to the ulnar extensor tendons.

Extensor tendon rupture

The grey, adherent, invasive dorsal synovitis, if allowed to remain in close proximity to the extensor

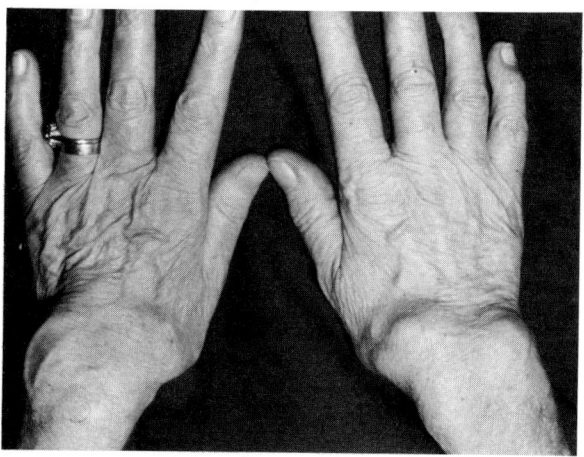

Fig 49.25 Persistent synovitis in the dorsal synovial bursa.

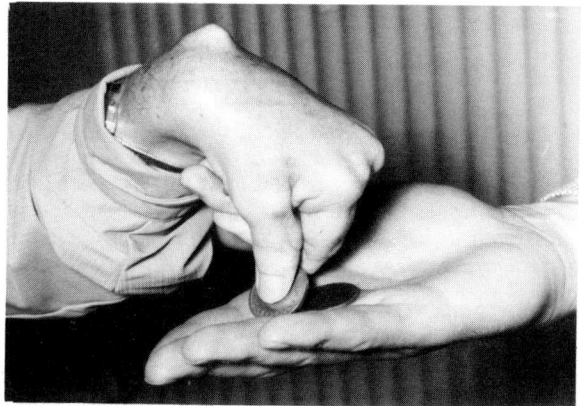

Fig 49.26 Dislocation of the lower end of the ulna in rheumatoid disease.

tendons, attenuates and finally destroys tendon substance. The characteristic painless extensor lag develops indicative of tendon rupture. The ulnar two fingers are commonly affected (Fig 49.27). Surgical treatment should be instituted at once lest more radial

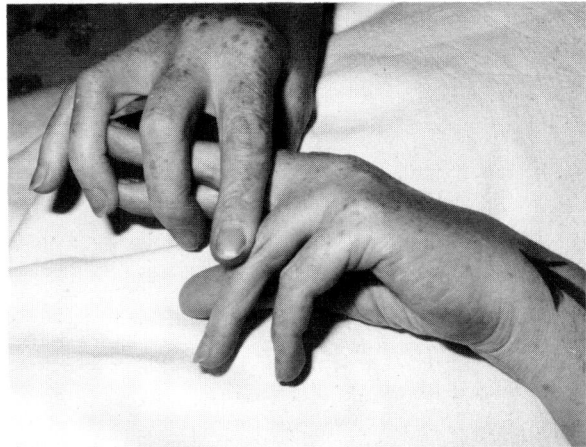

Fig 49.27 The ulnar two long extensor tendons have been ruptured by invasive synovitis.

tendons become similarly involved. The basis of treatment is synovectomy and restoration of tendon continuity. Unfortunately, this cannot be done by end-to-end repair, as in a traumatic rupture, because of the length of tendon substance that has been destroyed. The most effective repair is end-to-side anastomosis to an adjacent intact tendon which is the basis of tendon surgery in the rheumatoid hand.

This form of repair is suitable if only two tendons have been ruptured. Not uncommonly there is loss of continuity of more than two tendons and the single intact tendon cannot take the load applied. In this situation a wrist fusion should be performed which liberates the dorsal extensors of the carpus as motors for the divided tendons (Nicolle and Dickson, 1979).

Rupture of the extensor pollicis longus tendon

This common occurrence should be considered separately from dorsal extensor tendon rupture because in this situation the dorsal synovial bursa may not be enlarged and the local area of synovitis in the region of Lister's tubercle is the incriminating factor. Clinically the patient notices weakness of IP joint extension of the thumb over the preceding few weeks followed by a sudden and painless loss of extension. Because of the length of tendon invaded by diseased synovium, end-to-end repair is not feasible and the optimal method of restoring continuity is by tendon

transfer using the intact extensor indicis proprius. This tendon runs parallel to the extensor digitorum communis tendon to the index finger but lying on the ulnar side where it is conveniently located at the neck of the second metacarpal. It is rerouted through a proximal incision to lie in the line of the divided extensor pollicis longus tendon where it is repaired end-to-side (Fig 49.28).

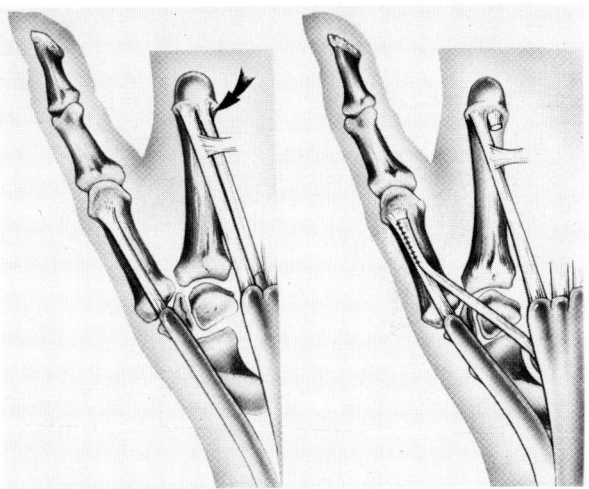

Fig 49.28 The extensor indicis proprius transfer for a ruptured extensor pollicis longus tendon. (From *Surgery of the Rheumatoid Hand*, 1979, Nicolle F.V., Dickson R.A., eds. London: William Heinemann Medical Books.)

Synovitis and rupture of the flexor tendons

This must be considered the most serious soft tissue problem of the rheumatoid hand because of the presence of the fibrous flexor sheath. Even with simple lacerations of flexor tendons in this region, the results are unpredictable, and it can thus be appreciated that if the loss of tendon continuity is a result of invasive synovitis then the potential for adhesion formation subsequently is all the greater. For this reason the palm of the hand and the volar aspect of each digit must be inspected and any fullness, indicative of synovitis treated promptly by synovectomy to protect the flexor tendons.

The site of flexor tendon rupture in the rheumatoid hand is most commonly in the distal palm. The patient complains of a sudden painless lack of active flexion of the IP joints more obvious distally. As with extensor tendon rupture, end-to-end repair is not feasible and the optimal method of restoring tendon continuity is by transfer from an adjacent intact sublimis tendon, (Fig 49.29). If the profundus only has been ruptured then, following synovectomy, a better result is achieved by

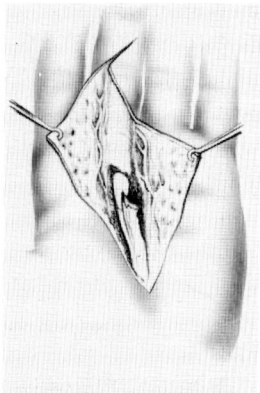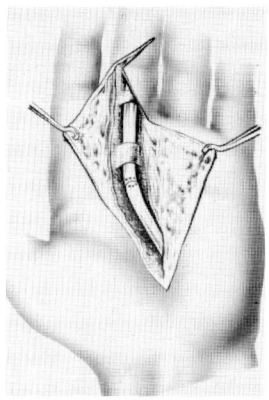

Fig 49.29   The optimal method of restoring flexor tendon continuity is by transfer of an adjacent sublimis tendon. (From *Surgery of the Rheumatoid Hand*, 1979, Nicolle F.V., Dickson R.A., eds. London: William Heinemann Medical Books.)

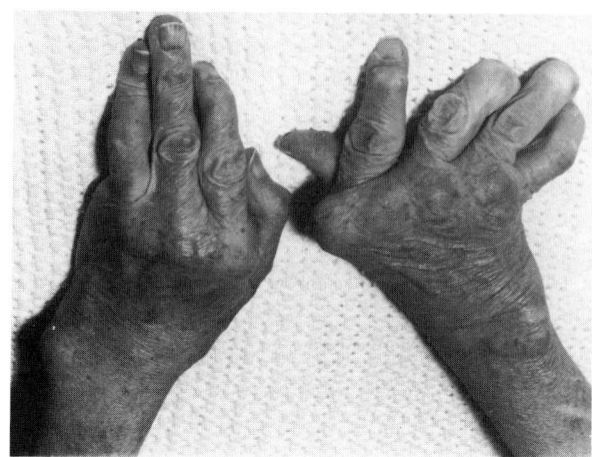

Fig 49.30   Ulnar deviation and volar dislocation.

fusion of the distal IP joint in a position of function. If both tendons have been ruptured and the site of rupture is too distal to be reached by an adjacent sublimis tendon, then a free tendon graft offers the only possible surgical reconstruction, but the results are unsatisfactory because of the potential for adhesion formation in this most unfavourable bed.

Ulnar drift

In the stage of persistent synovitis affecting the MP joint the radial collateral ligament becomes stretched and attenuated. Combined with the natural slope of the metacarpal heads, the fingers drift in an ulnar direction. As a consequence the extensor tendons slip over the metacarpal heads to lie in the gutter between that digit and its ulnar neighbour. Digital realignment by soft tissue reconstructive surgery has been disappointing. Ulnar release followed by imbrication on the radial side of the capsule yields good results, but only in the short term. Harrison (1979) has devised an extensor loop procedure which provides excellent longer term results. By splitting the extensor tendon longitudinally he provides a distally based flap of tendon which he then passes through a drill hole in the base of the proximal phalanx. With the finger now in the corrected position the extensor loop is tightened and stitched back to its source (Fig 49.30). Recurrence is not possible because the extensor tendon is now firmly fixed to bone in the corrected position. This can be performed in association with MP joint arthroplasty when ulnar drift occurs in relation to stage 3 disease.

Swan-neck deformity

With persistent synovitis in the proximal IP joint, the volar soft tissues, the volar plate and the accessory collateral ligaments become attenuated and unable to resist the tendency for the joint to go into hyperextension. This position of hyperextension is then maintained by the intrinsic musculature which, having been stimulated by the pain of local synovitis, contracts secondarily making the deformity uncorrectable passively (Fig 49.31). This 'intrinsic plus deformity' is characterised by inability to flex passively the proximal IP joint with the MP joint fully extended. This is a disabling situation because the fingers can neither flex into the palm on the ulnar side nor oppose the thumb on the radial side for purposes of pinch or fine movement. When the deformity is passively correctable surgical release of the intrinsic inflow yields good results. Only the oblique fibres of the intrinsic tendon as it approaches the dorsal extensor expansion need be divided. In long-standing cases, where the deformity is not correctable passively, IP joint fusion is the procedure of choice. This should be performed in as much flexion as that joint would occupy in the position of function of the hand.

Stage 3 – skeletal collapse

Because the most obvious site of synovitis is in the synovial joints, it would appear that removal of the diseased synovium prior to any joint damage would be of prophylactic benefit. However, unlike the extensor and flexor tendons, this is not so. Synovectomy certainly has benefit in terms of pain relief and improved range of motion, but there is no evidence in favour of preven-

function is considerable, but pain is unusual. Various different types of prostheses have been devised for the rheumatoid hand over the years but the most widely used is the silicone rubber prosthesis devised by Swanson (1972). This acts as a spacer after the eroded articular surfaces have been excised. The success of such prostheses depends largely upon a good range of motion in the more distal articulations. The pattern of disease involvement in the rheumatoid hand favours the surgeon in this respect. The MP joint is four times more frequently the site of severe erosive disease than the proximal IP joint and therefore in the great majority the function of the digit depends very much on the proximal IP joint (Mattingly *et al.*, 1979).

Vainio (1969) believes that prosthetic replacement is an unnecessary adjunct to excision arthroplasty and favours the latter in association with a tendon realigning operation to provide some form of stability for the excised joint. This can be in the form of interosseus transfer, but Harrison (1969) favours his extensor loop procedure in association with excision arthroplasty, thus attempting to provide mobility and correction of ulnar deviation. When the MP joint is to be exposed for either replacement or excision arthroplasty, it is best performed through an individual dorsal longitudinal incision thus protecting the longitudinally orientated veins so important for skin nutrition. The capsule of the joint is excised in the line of the skin incision to expose the eroded bone ends which are then excised prior to insertion of a prosthesis or a tendon realigning procedure (Fig 49.32).

It is important to bear in mind the progressive and widespread nature of the underlying disease process. The lower limb is commonly involved and should a weight-bearing articulation require a replacement or fusion then this should be performed prior to any more delicate surgery on the rheumatoid hand. This is because after surgery on the lower extremity a significant proportion of body weight must be taken through

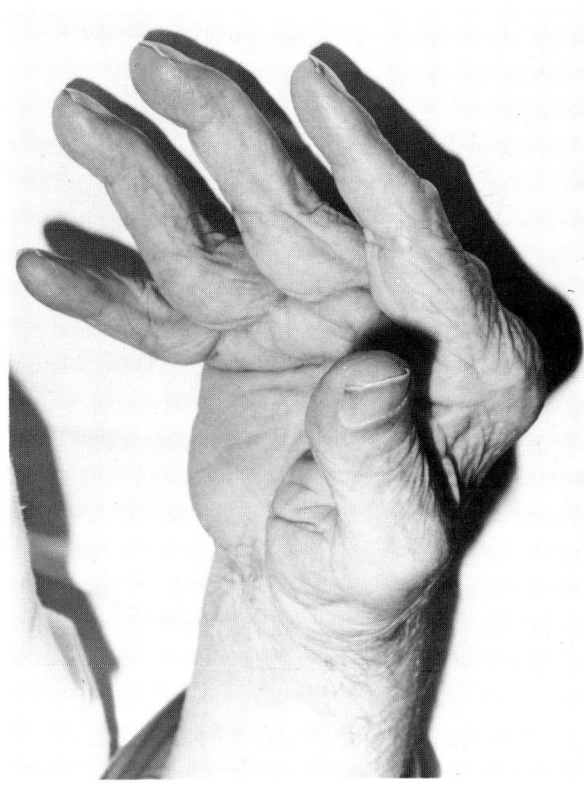

Fig 49.31   The 'intrinsic plus deformity' – the fixed swan-neck deformity.

tion of erosive disease in joints (Arthritis and Rheumatism Council and British Orthopaedic Association, 1976).

There is little therefore that the hand surgeon can do to ward off the long-term effects of destructive synovitis and he therefore finds one of his biggest roles is the reconstruction of joints already severely damaged. The general aims of such surgery must be clearly understood. Whether a joint should be replaced or fused depends largely on its role in hand function. This, in turn, depends upon the need to provide either mobility or stability at a particular articulation (Nicolle, 1973). In each digital ray there is a proximal joint where mobility is of prime importance. In the finger this is the MP joint and in the thumb the carpometacarpal joint. Arthroplasty in these sites is, therefore, the treatment of choice whereas more distal articulations can be fused, stability being more important than mobility.

The metacarpo-phalangeal joint

Unchecked erosive disease of the MP joint leads to dislocation in a volar and ulnar direction. Loss of hand

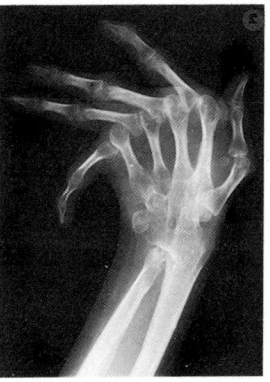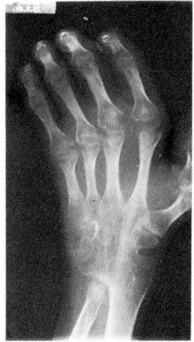

Fig 49.32   Metacarpo-phalangeal joint arthroplasty using silicone rubber prostheses.

the upper extremity via crutches or sticks. Delicate
hand surgery is not designed to withstand such forces
and therefore a properly planned, programme of surgical treatment is fundamental.

The proximal interphalangeal joint

When the proximal IP joint is the site of erosive
rheumatoid disease (Fig 49.33), it frequently takes up a

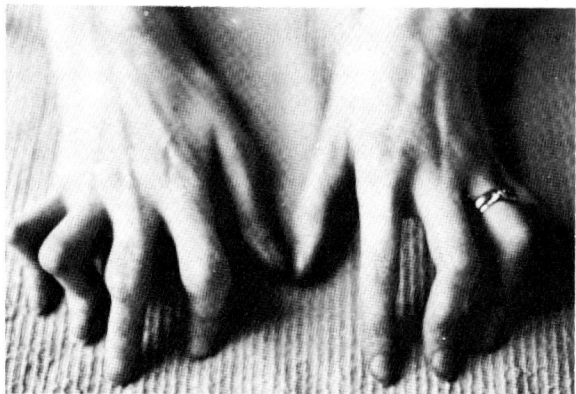

Fig 49.33 Multiple Boutonnière deformities. (From
Surgery of the Rheumatoid Hand, 1979, Nicolle F.V., Dick-
son R.A., eds. London: William Heinemann Medical
Books.)

position of increasing flexion as the dorsal central slip
of the extensor mechanism is attenuated to the point of
rupture. The distal IP joint undergoes compensatory
hyperextension to complete the Boutonnière
deformity. Large objects are difficult to hold particularly on the ulnar side of the hand and function is
markedly impaired. Soft tissue reconstruction of a
Boutonnière deformity in the rheumatoid hand is so
unrewarding as not to be worthwhile and the treatment
of choice is fusion of the joint in the position of function
of the hand. To avoid the cumbersome use of Kirschner
wires, which are non-rigid, an intramedullary peg of
polypropylene is the preferred method of internal
fixation (Harrison and Nicolle, 1974). With such firm
intramedullary support the hand can be mobilised as
soon as the wound has healed. As soon as the joint has
been exposed through a mid-line dorsal incision and the
eroded bone ends resected the appropriate angled peg
can be selected to ensure the correct angle of fusion
(Fig 49.34).

The thumb in rheumatoid disease

Two different types of Z deformity may occur in the
rheumatoid thumb. When the MP joint is flexed and

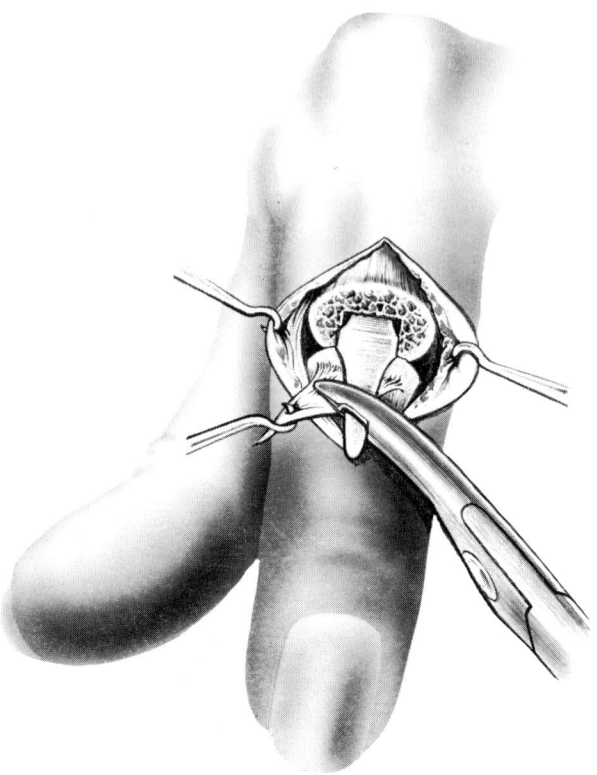

Fig 49.34 Fusion of the proximal IP joint using a rigid
intramedullary peg of polypropylene. (From *Surgery of
the Rheumatoid Hand*, 1979, Nicolle F.V., Dickson R.A.,
eds. London: William Heinemann Medical Books.)

the IP joint extended, this type of Z deformity impli-
cates the MP joint as the site of erosive disease. When
the thumb metacarpal lies adducted and there is compensatory hyperextension at the MP joint with the IP
joint flexed, another Z deformity is produced which
incriminates the carpo-metacarpal joint.

Metacarpo-phalangeal joint disease

The deformity produced here is similar to the
Boutonnière deformity of the proximal IP joint of the
finger. A position of increasing flexion is taken up, but
function is not severely impaired because there is good
preservation of motion at the important base joint of
the thumb. Loss of function therefore usually results
from pain rather than loss of motion. In addition the
MP joint of the thumb does not enjoy as big a range of
motion as is thought, accordingly fusion of this articulation is the method of treatment favoured.

The joint is exposed through a longitudinal incision

and the eroded bone ends resected. An intramedullary peg is again recommended which for this articulation can be straight. The hand can be fully mobilised as soon as the skin has healed.

Carpo-metacarpal joint disease

The nature of this articulation, being a doubly-concave saddle joint, favours movement in all directions. In the early stages of carpo-metacarpal joint disease, local discomfort accompanies all pinching and wringing movements with crepitus palpable on circumduction – the 'axial grind test'. Later, when rigidity supervenes, the thumb comes to lie in the plane of the palm, the first phalanx hyperextends in order to preserve pinch and the IP joint compensatorily flexes (Fig 49.35). This position severely embarrasses hand function and, as capsular and aponeurotic fibrosis supervene, the base of the first metacarpal dislocates in a dorsoradial direction. Finally no movement exists at this articulation and the hand has lost 60% of its function.

Arthroplasty of this joint is the basis of treatment. Simple excision of the trapezium restores mobility but

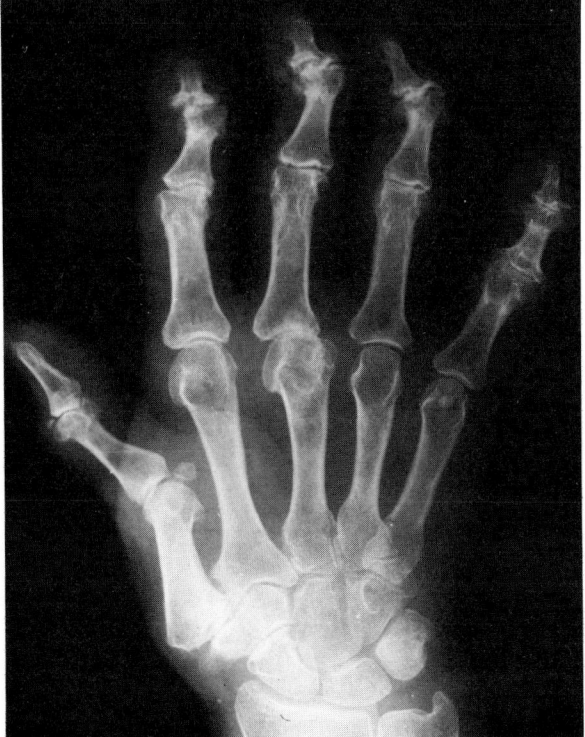

Fig 49.35 The Z-deformity of the thumb associated with carpo-metacarpal joint disease. Note also osteophytes of the distal interphalangeal joints (Heberden's nodes).

leads to instability, and pain is not always relieved. The insertion of a silastic trapezium has an unacceptably high incidence of dislocation. Treatment therefore becomes a compromise, and, following excision of the trapezium, stability is restored by passing a slip of the tendon of flexor carpi radialis through a drill hole in the base of the first metacarpal to act as a soft tissue restraining sling (Eaton and Littler, 1973). If the thumb has been adducted for long, the aponeurosis over the adductor pollicis muscle may have to be divided first to allow passive abduction. For exposure of the carpo-metacarpal joint the anterior thenar crease exposure is favoured. The short muscles of the thumb are erased from their attachment to the radial side of the flexor retinaculum which thereby exposes the front of the joint. After arthroplasty this muscular reattachment provides a firm soft tissue closure anteriorly.

Rheumatoid disease of the wrist joint

This joint is commonly involved with severe erosive rheumatoid disease and the loss of function as a result is very much more severe than would first appear. This is because the hand functions optimally from a painless stable wrist and the effect upon the hand from a painful unstable wrist is considerable. So important is this that once the wrist has been treated function improves to such an extent that hand surgery often becomes unnecessary.

Early in the course of wrist joint disease, when there is joint space narrowing and synovitis, synovectomy would appear appropriate but cannot be performed adequately without causing instability. Accordingly fusion is the treatment for both moderate and severe wrist joint involvement.

The object of fusion is to achieve bony continuity between the radius and the base of the third metacarpal. Both fusion and postoperative comfort are considerably benefited by internal fixation with an axial Steinmann pin. The wrist is exposed through a lazy-S dorsal incision and a trough is created between the base of the third metacarpal and the distal radius. Cancellous bone chips derived from the carpal bones, removed to create this trough, provide a satisfactory fusion mass which can be supplemented by the lower end of the ulna if this has not been previously excised. The Steinmann pin is inserted and the bone chips pressed firmly into place around it (Fig 49.36). It is expedient to repair the extensor retinaculum underneath the extensor tendons thus protecting them from the bone chips. With such firm internal fixation, plaster of Paris support is not necessary and the wrist can be mobilised as soon as the soft tissues have healed.

If an axial Steinmann pin is used, the fusion position must be straight and this is quite satisfactory for the

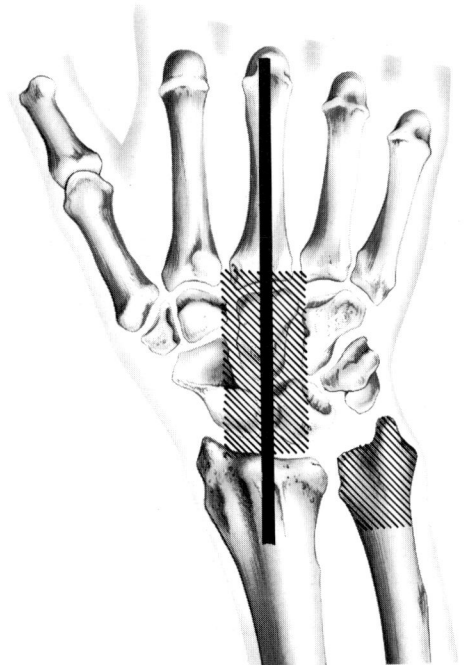

Fig 49.36 Fusion of the rheumatoid wrist. Bone chips are inserted around the axial Steinmann pin. (From *Surgery of the Rheumatoid Hand*, 1979, Nicolle F.V., Dickson R.A., eds. London: William Heinemann Medical Books.)

rheumatoid patient, whether one or both wrists require fusion. It is often said that if both wrists are fused one should be fused in 15° of flexion to retain independent personal hygiene but this can be managed with the straight wrist and our occupational therapist has noted no problems in over 40 wrists fused straight.

Osteoarthrosis

The carpo-metacarpal joint of the thumb

Postmenopausal females are most commonly affected and the clinical course is altogether more insidious than in rheumatoid disease, but the symptoms and signs are similar. Circumduction of the thumb gives rise to painful local crepitus and household activities of the pinching or wringing nature exacerbate symptoms.

Traditionally there have been three methods of treatment for this condition – fusion, trapeziumectomy and arthroplasty. Fusion is an acceptable treatment for a joint involved with osteoarthrosis because it is likely to be the only articulation of that digit involved in this pathological process, unlike rheumatoid disease.

However, while fusion will certainly relieve discomfort, mobility and hand function are sacrificed in this joint of prime mobility. Furthermore, patients do not like the position in which the thumb must be fused for function to be retained, one of abduction and opposition. For these reasons trapeziumectomy is the favoured alternative. However, while mobility is preserved, stability is lost, and after surgery this form of excision arthroplasty is not always painless. Because of the unfortunately high incidence of dorsoradial dislocation of silastic prostheses, some form of soft tissue restraint must be provided for the base of the thumb. Eaton and Littler (1973) favour the use of a sling taken from the flexor carpi radialis tendon.

Such degrees of surgical intervention are certainly indicated when the arthritis at the base of the thumb is severe with an adducted first metacarpal combined with dorsoradial dislocation of the joint. However, in the majority of cases presenting clinically, the joint is only moderately affected radiographically. There is still considerable movement in the form of circumduction available, and there is little or no evidence of subluxation. At this stage a more limited operation would appear to be preferable and silastic interposition arthroplasty fulfils this role (Dickson, 1976). The joint is approached by an anterior thenar crease incision, the short thenar muscles are erased from their retinacular attachment to expose the capsule of the joint. After arthrotomy and a debridement, an appropriate sized disc of silicone rubber sponge is inserted (Fig 49.37). Because of the strong soft tissue cover for this joint when the thenar muscles are reattached, the thumb can be mobilised as soon as the wound has healed.

In the minority of severe cases trapeziumectomy combined with a soft tissue sling from flexor carpi radialis, again performed through an anterior approach, is the treatment of choice.

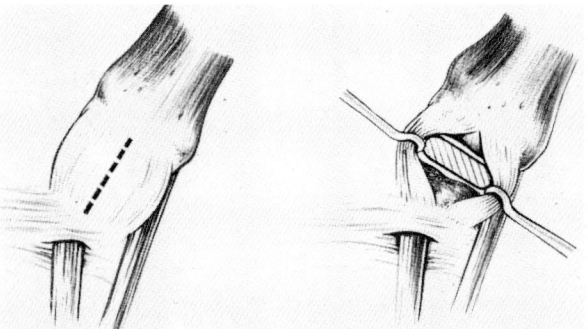

Fig 49.37 Silicone rubber interposition arthroplasty for osteoarthrosis of the base of the thumb. (From *Surgery of the Rheumatoid Hand*, 1979, Nicolle F.V., Dickson R.A., eds. London: William Heinemann Medical Books.)

The distal interphalangeal joint

This is the commonest joint in the body to be involved with degenerative osteoarthrosis and affects particularly postmenopausal females. Osteophyte formation at the base of the distal phalanx gives rise to Heberden's nodes, and destruction of the articular surfaces gives rise to both flexion and lateral deviation deformities. The vast majority of such joints produce few if any symptoms but if associated with degenerative mucous cysts symptoms are common. Simple surgical removal of the cyst gives rise to a high recurrence rate and for symptomatic osteoarthrosis of the distal IP joint, fusion is the treatment of choice. Such destroyed articulations have a very limited range of motion, and restoration of alignment and freedom of discomfort are the surgical aims. An intramedullary peg fusion is the recommended treatment which thereby minimises the duration of fixation and postoperative immobilisation.

Psoriatic arthropathy

Unlike rheumatoid disease men tend to be more frequently affected by psoriatic arthropathy, and the younger the patient the more serious the prognosis. The distal IP joints of the hands are a common site although larger joints can be involved. During the stage of active erosive disease the sedimentation rate is considerably elevated. There is a bad prognosis for joints involved with such aggressive disease and even using high dosages of steroids it is not possible to prevent progression.

The characteristic clinical appearance is a fusiform enlargement of the digit with radiographic osteoporosis and destruction of the distal phalanx (Fig 49.38). While such arthropathy is frequently associated with florid psoriatic skin lesions, sometimes the skin involvement is barely discernible, perhaps just a small patch of psoriasis in the scalp. Treatment is along the same lines as that prescribed for rheumatoid arthropathy and as the distal joints are involved fusion is the procedure of choice.

Gouty arthritis

The proximal IP joints are commonly affected by gouty arthritis. The typical radiographic features are punched out areas of osteolysis with new bone formation around these areas of bone loss. The punched out areas may be replaced by a tophus of urate crystals. Such joints tend to be nodular and hard with periarticular tophi which can be palpated and seen (Fig 49.39).

A severely involved proximal IP joint is best dealt

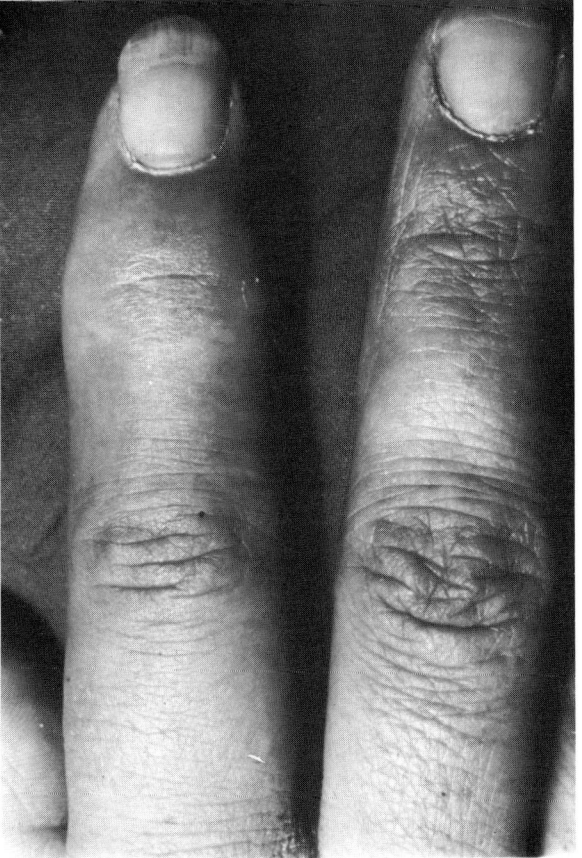

Fig 49.38 Psoriasis of the nail fold with arthroplasty of the distal IP joint. (From *Mercer's Orthopaedic Surgery*, 1983, 8th edn., Fig 15.25, by courtesy of the editors R.B. Duthie and G. Bentley and the publishers, Edward Arnold.)

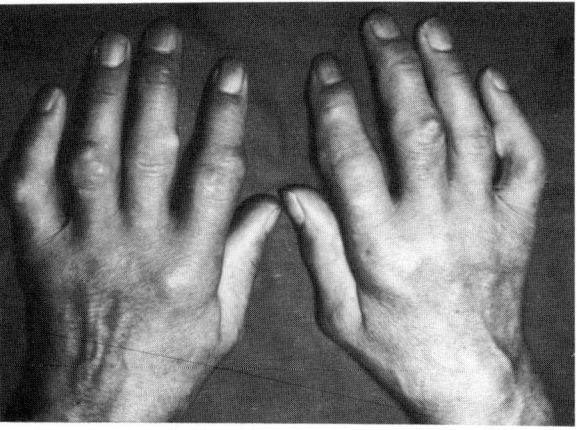

Fig 49.39 Periarticular tophi characterise gouty arthritis.

with by fusion at the angle that that joint would occupy in the *position of function* of the hand. Intramedullary peg fusion is the recommended method of achieving this.

Sarcoidosis

Considered to be a hypersensitivity condition the characteristic lesion is similar to that produced by tuberculosis. Granulomata and large epithelial cells are recognised when striated muscle is biopsied. Although more renowned for its pulmonary lesion, sarcoidosis can present as an arthritis affecting both the hands and feet. The arthropathy produced by sarcoid is seen characteristically on radiographs as large cyst-like spaces in the phalanges. This condition tends to come into the therapeutic range of the rheumatologist or general physician who prescribes steroids when the pulmonary lesions are advanced or when there is impairment of vision, hypercalcaemia or hypersplenism.

Localised swellings of the hand and wrist

Ganglion

The pathological process is cystic degeneration of fibrous tissue in relation to a synovial joint or tendon sheath. They are responsible for half of all local swellings of the hand and wrist and 60% occur on the dorsum of the wrist, 30% on the palmar aspect of the wrist, and 10% in relation to the proximal end of the fibrous flexor sheath in the palm and nowhere else. These cysts are filled with a colourless jelly with a high mucin content. The fibrous walls of the cyst contain nerve fibres which are responsible for the local discomfort experienced when ganglia increase in size (Fig 49.40).

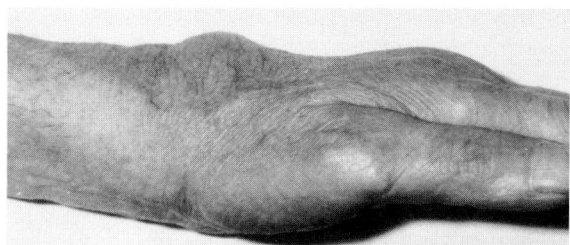

Fig 49.40 A long-standing ganglion. It had recently increased in size with local discomfort. (From *Mercer's Orthopaedic Surgery*, 1983, 8th edn., Fig. 15.14, by courtesy of the editors R.B. Duthie and G. Bentley and the publishers, Edward Arnold.)

Clinical presentation is as a result of the local swelling and discomfort. If the ganglion is in relation to the fibrous flexor sheath on the working surface of the hand, there may be severe local discomfort during hand function. If large enough ganglia will both transilluminate and fluctuate.

Aspiration of the ganglion with injection of an anti-inflammatory agent and surgical excision have a similar success rate. Sometimes the ganglion spontaneously resolves as a result of rupture following a local blow. When approaching wrist ganglia surgically, those on the dorsum are located between the tendons of extensor pollicis longus and extensor digitorum communis, while those on the anterior aspect lie between the tendons of brachio-radialis and flexor carpi radialis. These anatomical relationships are important because unless the attachment of the neck of the ganglion to its parent fibrous tissue structure is located and excised there is a high recurrence rate.

Xanthomas

These are responsible for one-third of all swellings of the hand and wrist and are otherwise called benign synoviomas, foreign body giant cell tumours, or giant cell tumours of tendon sheath. Their characteristic site is on the palmar aspect of the index or middle fingers and they differ histologically from ganglia by having a thicker connective tissue wall with both cellular and myxomatous areas. Giant cells with eosinophilic cytoplasm are also common and keratin and xanthophyl pigments can be detected in the lipid gobule of the contents. Macroscopically they appear grey-yellow with brown streaking.

They present as a result of local swelling and discomfort, sometimes interfering with the action of the long flexor tendons. As a result they may be a cause of trigger finger. Surgical excision is curative in over 90% of cases.

Implantation dermoid cyst

The palmar aspect of the hand and fingers is a working surface and therefore is frequently the site of a minor penetrating injury. During injury epithelial cells are carried into the subdermal layers where the cyst subsequently develops. An overlying scar confirms the diagnosis. As with ganglia and xanthomas, local swelling and discomfort are the cause of clinical presentation. The cyst may appear like a ganglion at surgical removal, but the contents have a high cholesterol content. Less common swellings such as lipoma, fibroma, vascular malformation or neurofibroma may be difficult to differentiate from other hand swellings of the soft tissue variety and can only be diagnosed in hindsight by histological examination.

Enchondroma

This is the commonest bony tumour of the hand and is situated in the centre of a metacarpal or phalanx most commonly in the ulnar two fingers (Fig 49.41). It presents clinically as either a local hard swelling with discomfort or as a pathological fracture. Malignant transformation is negligible except when the tumour is multiple (Ollier's disease).

Noble and Lamb (1974), in reviewing large numbers of these tumours, conclude that there is no difference in outcome whether they are managed conservatively by means of splintage or surgically by means of curettage and bone grafting.

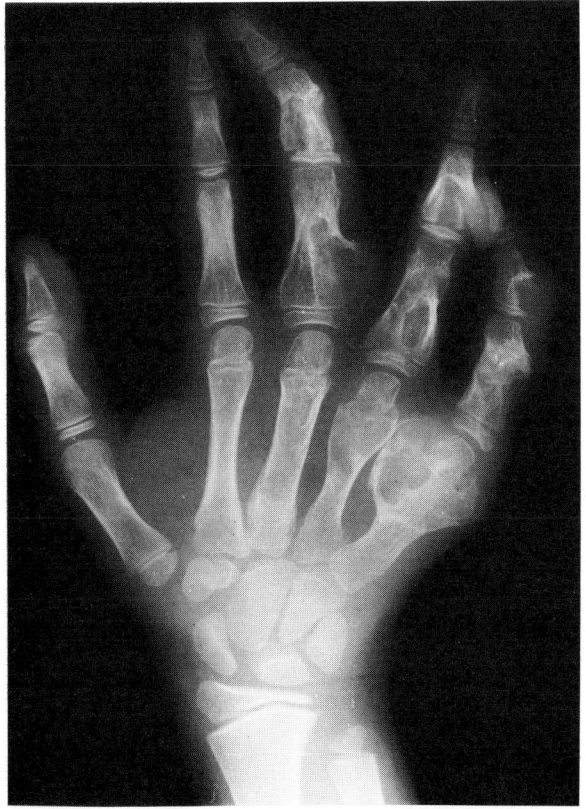

Fig 49.41 Multiple enchondromata.

Lesions of the tendon mechanisms

De Quervain's tendo-vaginitis

In 1895 De Quervain described a fibrosis and narrowing of the sheath surrounding the tendons of abductor pollicis longus and extensor pollicis brevis at the radial syloid. At this point these tendons are enveloped in a condensation of deep fascia for a distance of some 3 cm. Repeated frictional trauma leads to fibrosis and narrowing and, as a consequence, manual workers have a high prevalence. Similar stenotic-type lesions occur in relation to the peroneal tendons and the extensors of the wrist.

Patients, who are more frequently female than male, present as a result of local discomfort which may be sufficient to cause weakness of grasp; the symptoms are exacerbated by extension and ulnar deviation of the wrist. There is tenderness and swelling on palpation of the radial styloid and crepitus can be elicited when the thumb is abducted.

Local ultrasound or anti-inflammatory injection is useful in the short term, but surgical treatment is definitive. The basis of this is to divide the tight stenotic portion of the sheath and knowledge of the surgical anatomy of this condition is important. Variations in these tendons at this site are common. The extensor pollicis longus can run through a separate compartment while the abductor pollicis longus tendon may be in the form of two separate bands. Therefore, at surgery, it is most important to inspect the situation carefully and ensure that the appropriate tunnel has been decompressed.

Trigger finger

This is a stenosing tendo-vaginitis of the long flexor tendons as a result of a discrepancy in size between tendon and its fibrous flexor sheath. The finger can be flexed without difficulty, but the power of extension is insufficient to allow the tendon to extend through its tight sheath and requires passive assistance.

The site of triggering can be detected by palpation where local tenderness and swelling in relation to the mouth of the fibrous flexor sheath can be felt. This swelling is not a nodule attached to the tendon, but is the tendon itself spiralled into a pseudo-nodule. The long flexor tendons are made up of multiple strands which can bunch together to form such a pseudo-nodule which, in turn, makes the tendon too large to re-enter the fibrous flexor sheath with ease on extension.

The condition affects women predominantly and the ring finger is the commonest digit involved. The triggering phenomenon sets up a local synovitis which leads to a further discrepancy in the size of the tendon and its sheath. By the same token rheumatoid synovitis can be a cause of trigger finger.

Ultrasound and injection of an anti-inflammatory drug are effective, but usually only in the short term. A more definitive solution is surgical division longitudinally of the mouth of the fibrous flexor sheath thus allowing the tendon to enjoy its full excursion. The spiralling effect gradually resolves and no pseudo-nodule formation can be detected postoperatively.

Trigger thumb

This is a stenosing tendo-vaginitis affecting the flexor pollicis longus tendon and its fibrous flexor sheath. Unlike trigger finger, this occurs most commonly in infancy and childhood when a flexion deformity is noted in one thumb. This hardly warrants the term trigger thumb because the pathological process is more advanced to the point where the pseudo-nodule is so large that it cannot enter the fibrous flexor sheath even with passive assistance. 'Locked thumb' would be a more appropriate description. Anti-inflammatory analgesic injection and ultrasound are difficult to administer in the young child, and therefore the treatment of choice is surgical division of the mouth of the fibrous flexor sheath.

Dupuytren's contracture

Aetiology

The cause of Dupuytren's contracture is unknown but a recent penetrating wound of the palm is commonly noted in the history. The condition has an autosomal dominant mode of inheritance and there may be an association with long-term epileptic treatment and liver disease, due to alcohol. There is an increased prevalence of knuckle pads, but these are not associated with a necessarily bad prognosis (Fig 49.42).

Hueston (1963) demonstrated two different types of Dupuytren's contracture as regards rapidity of progression. When the condition occurs in young men with a positive family history, the presence of ectopic lesions in the plantar fascia or corpus cavernosum of the penis (Peyronie's disease) it is associated with a particularly bad prognosis, and a high incidence of recurrence after surgical treatment. In contradistinction there is a much more favourable prognosis when the fibrosis is confined to the palm in the older individual.

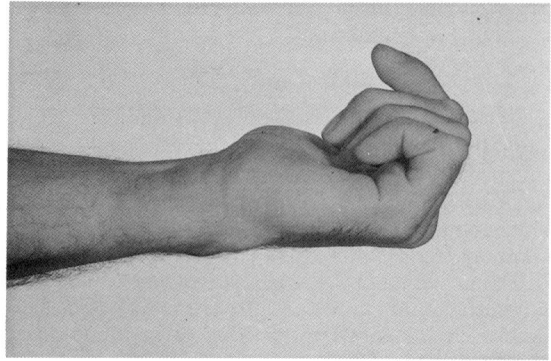

Fig 49.42   Knuckle pads in association with Dupuytren's disease – not a bad prognostic factor.

Pathology

Hueston noted perivascular fibroblastic proliferation in relation to the fibro-fatty tissue of the palm early in the course of Dupuytren's disease. As the fibrotic process continues the skin becomes involved, being attached to the palmar fascia by fibrous septa. Before the stage of contracture, there is isolated nodular thickening usually on the ulnar side of the palm. Gradually the finger is drawn into the palm and the fascial slip to that digit can be palpated as a tight band adherent to the underlying skin (Fig 49.43). So active may this fibroblastic proliferation be that the pathologist may have difficulty in differentiating Dupuytren's contracture from a fibrosarcoma if he did not know the tissue of origin.

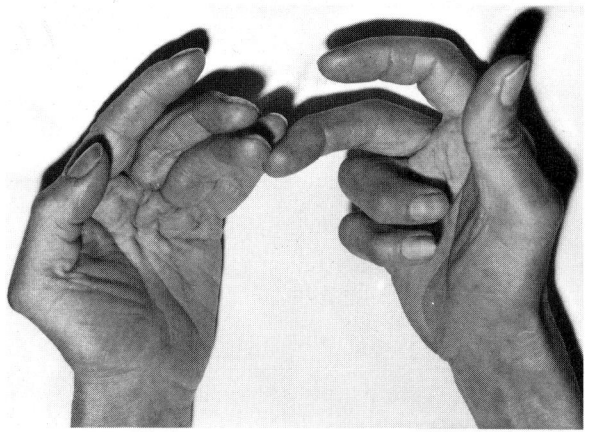

Fig 49.43   Dupuytren's contracture. (From *The Basis and Practice of Orthopaedics*, 1980, Hughes S., Sweetnam R., eds. London: William Heinemann Medical Books.)

Clinical features

Dupuytren's contracture affects 3% of the population, commonly elderly males. Mikkelson (1976) noted that the ring finger is affected in 85% of cases, twice as frequently as the little finger and that the thumb and index finger are never involved alone. The condition is often bilateral and symmetry is common. Pain is not a feature but during an aggressive phase the nodular thickenings of the palm may be tender on palpation. As the slips of the palmar fascia passing down the sides of the involved digit contract, so the finger becomes flexed at either the MP joint, proximal IP joint, or both.

Treatment

Treatment is surgical and is indicated only when a digit is contracted. Nodular thickening of the palmar fascia with no contracture does not require treatment but merits regular observation. Only the contracted fascia to the digit or digits involved should be removed – limited fasciectomy. Radical removal of the entire palmar fascia is now obsolete due to the high incidence of local complications including haematoma formation leading to skin sloughing. Subcutaneous fasciotomy, using a fine tenotome through small skin puncture wounds has been favoured by some although there is almost certain recurrence and a likelihood of damage to the neurovascular bundles by this blind procedure.

The method of removing the tight fascial band depends upon whether the patient is young with a strong diathesis or old with a more simple contracture. In the latter situation the Bruner zig-zag incision is favoured as skin involvement and recurrence are much less common. The zig-zag incision provides excellent exposure to the tight band and when the digital nerves and vessels are exposed on each side throughout the length of the incision, the band can be removed with ease. The operative treatment of those with a strong diathesis is more problematical. Skin involvement is more obvious and recurrence more common. In this situation a straight longitudinal palmar incision is recommended which can be lengthened by z-plasty at the flexion creases in order to provide lengthening of the scar and to place portions of it transversely. Hueston (1963) feels that the surgeon should be even more aggressive. He has noted a higher recurrence rate in those with a strong diathesis even when the palmar skin has been rearranged by z-plasty and consequently suggests that the palmar skin should be replaced by a free full thickness graft at the time of closure. With this addition to his technique he has noted a significantly lower tendency for recurrence.

The postoperative programme is as important as the operative technique. The hand, dressed in a compression bandage, should be elevated for the first 48 h and then the wound inspected so that any local haematoma formation can be evacuated. It should then be rebandaged for a further 10 days until the wound has healed. The sutures can then be removed and an intensive course of physical therapy instituted at once.

The paralytic hand

The paralysed hand represents one of the most challenging problems to the reconstructive hand surgeon. This accounts for the large number of techniques available for its reconstruction.

Clinical features

Whether the paralysis has an associated component of sensory loss depends upon the underlying cause. Conditions of motor loss such as poliomyelitis or progressive muscle atrophy are not associated with sensory impairment, but conditions of the central nervous system such as multiple sclerosis or peripheral nerve compression syndromes give rise to both motor and sensory impairment. Intrinsic paralysis produces the typical claw hand deformity. This has been described by Goldner (1953) as the 'intrinsic minus hand'. A lesion of the median and ulnar nerves at the wrist produces paralysis of the interossei, lumbricals, thenar and hypothenar muscles. There is extension of the MP joints and flexion of the IP joints. The transverse fibres of the extensor hood tighten with MP joint extension thus blocking the action of the long extensor tendons. Paralysis of thumb opposition renders the thumb externally rotated and adducted. With time, the deformities become relatively more fixed as soft tissue contracture, particularly of the collateral ligamentous support of the MP and IP joints supervenes.

Treatment

Treatment of the paralytic hand is mainly by tendon transfer, the prerequisites being a satisfactory range of passive motion of the joints involved and powerful motors.

The thumb

To restore thumb opposition in intrinsic muscle paralysis the flexor digitorum sublimis tendon is used as the motor. It is passed through a pulley on the ulnar side of the wrist across the centre of the abductor pollicis brevis tendon at the level of the MP joint and attached on the lateral side of the IP joint into the extensor pollicis longus tendon. The abductor digiti minimi proprius may be used as an alternative motor.

The fingers

Several different tendon transfer procedures have been described to restore function in the paralysed fingers. The essence of these is to provide flexion of the MP joints by transferring the tendon of an intact muscle into the dorsal expansion of each finger distal to the MP joints with, if necessary, the addition of a free graft. Bunnell (1948) used the flexor sublimis to the middle finger as the motor and divided it into four strands each attached via the lumbrical canal to the radial side of the extensor expansion of each proximal phalanx. Fowler (1947) obtained two strands from the extensor indicis proprius and two from the extensor digiti minimi proprius, whereas Riordan (1959) used the extensor carpi radialis brevis, extensor carpi ulnaris and brachioradialis. These procedures not only prevented MP joint hyperextension, but also provided power for IP joint extension. Brand (1961), in his great experience with the leprosy hand, used a free graft of plantaris tendon with extensor carpi radialis longus as the motor. For severe and long-standing deformity Goldner (1953) recommends IP joint fusion in a functional position and replaces the action of the paralysed first dorsal interosseus with the intact extensor indicis proprius, thus preventing the index finger from drifting ulnarwards during pinch.

Volkmann's ischaemic contracture

This disastrous condition is characterised by ischaemia leading to fibrosis and contracture of the flexor muscles of the forearm. Although it may follow an unreduced supracondylar fracture, it is also unfortunately associated with bandages and casts that are too tight.

Clinical features

The onset is acute with severe forearm and hand pain caused by the ischaemia occurring in a closed fascial compartment. The hand swells and becomes dusky and cyanotic. The fingers are cold to touch and sensation is impaired. The initial acutely painful phase wears off as the forearm flexor musculature is replaced by fibrosis. As a consequence of contracture the fingers adopt the flexed position (Fig 49.44) the finger contracture appearing worse on wrist extension.

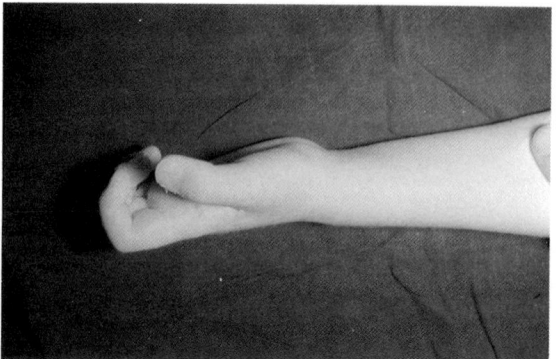

Fig 49.44 Volkmann's ischaemic contracture.

Treatment

This condition is preventable and the management of all supracondylar fractures, or those patients who require a forearm cast or circumferential bandage, must include regular palpation of the radial pulse. If this becomes absent the fracture must at once be remanipulated or opened and a cast or bandage split down to skin. In the acute phase of Volkmann's ischaemia the contracture can be minimised by immediate decompression of the forearm musculature by multiple incisions of its fascial restriction. In the case of the established contracture, surgical lengthening of the forearm flexors by sliding procedures at the musculotendon junction, or sliding of the origin of the forearm flexor muscles from their radial and ulnar attachments distally, form the basis of reconstruction.

References

Arthritis and Rheumatism Council and British Orthopaedic Association (1976). Controlled trial of synovectomy of knee and metacarpo-phalangeal joints in rheumatoid arthritis. *Ann. Rheum. Dis*; **35:**437–42.

Barron J.N. (1969). Assessment of suitability for surgery in general timing of operation. *Ann. Rheum. Dis*; **28:**suppl. 74–6.

Brand P.W. (1961). Tendon grafting – illustrated by a new operation for intrinsic paralysis of the fingers. *J. Bone Jt. Surg*; **43B:**444–53.

Bruner J.M. (1967). The zig-zag volar digital incision for flexor tendon surgery. *Plast. Reconstr. Surg*; **40:**571–4.

Bunnell S. (1948). *Surgery of the Hand*. Philadelphia: JB Lippincott.

Coleman H.M. (1960). Injuries of the articular disc at the wrist. *J. Bone Jt. Surg*; **42B:**522–9.

Dickson R.A. (1975). Rigid fixation of unstable metacarpal fractures using transverse K-wires bonded with acrylic resin. *Hand*; **7:**284–6.

Dickson R.A. (1976). Arthritis of the carpo-metacarpal joint of the thumb. Treatment by silicone interposition arthroplasty. *Hand*; **8:**197–208.

Dickson R.A., Kemp F.H. (1976). Thorn-induced granulomata of bone. *Hand*; **8:**69–71.

Eaton R.G., Littler J.W. (1973). Ligament reconstruction for the painful thumb carpo-metacarpal joint. *J. Bone Jt. Surg*; **55A:**1655–66.

Entin M., Barsky A., Swanson A.B. (1972). Classification of congenital malformations of the hand and upper extremity. *Hand*; **4:**215–9.

Fowler S.B. (1947). Mobilization of the metacarpo-phalangeal joints. *J. Bone Jt. Surg*; **29:**193–202.

Goldner J.L. (1953). Deformities of the hand incidental to pathological changes of the extensor and intrinsic muscle mechanisms. *J. Bone Jt. Surg*; **35A:**115–31.

Graham W., Rosen P. (1962). The shoulder-hand syndrome. *Bull. Rheum. Dis*; **12:**277–8.

Harrison S.H. (1969). Excision arthroplasty of the metacarpo-phalangeal joints. *Hand*; **1:**14–16.

Harrison S.H. (1979). The surgical management of the arthritic hand. *Ann. Roy. Coll. Surg. Engl*; **61:**17–28.

Harrison S.H., Nicolle F.V. (1974). A new intramedullary bone peg for digital arthrodesis. *Brit. J. Plast. Surg*; **27:**240–1.

Hueston J.T. (1963). *Dupuytren's Contracture*. Edinburgh: Churchill Livingstone.

Hunter J. (1965). Artificial tendons. Early development and application. *Amer. J. Surg*; **109:**325–8.

Kleinert H.E., Kutz J.E., Atasoy E., Stormo A. (1973). Primary repair of the flexor tendons. *Orthop. Clin. N.Amer*; **4:**865–76.

Lamb D.W. (1977). Radial club hand. A continuing study of 68 patients with 117 club hands. *J. Bone Jt. Surg*; **59A:**1–13.

Lamb D.W., Abernethy T.A., Raine P.A.M. (1973). Unstable fractures of the metacarpal. A method of treatment by transverse wire fixation to intact metacarpals. *Hand*; **5:**43–8.

Mattingly P.C., Matheson J.A., Dickson R.A. (1979). The distribution of radiological joint damage in the rheumatoid hand. *Rheumatol. Rehabil*; **18:**142–7.

Mikkelsen O.A. (1976). Dupuytren's disease – a study of the pattern of distribution and stage of contracture of the hand. *Hand*; **8:**265–71.

Nicolle F.V. (1973). Recent advances in the management of joint disease in the rheumatoid hand. *Hand*; **5:**91–5.

Nicolle F.V., Dickson R.A. (1979). *Surgery of the Rheumatoid Hand*. London: William Heinemann Medical.

Noble J., Lamb D.W. (1974). Enchondromata of bones of the hand. A review of 40 cases. *Hand*; **6:**275–84.

Riordan D.C. (1959). Surgery of the paralytic hand. *Amer. Acad. Orthopaed. Surg. Inst. C. Lect*; **16:**79–80.

Snow J.W. (1973). Use of a retrograde tendon flap in repairing a severed extensor in the P.I.P. joint area. *Plast. Reconstr. Surg*; **51:**555–8.

Steel W.M. (1978). A.O. small fragment set in hand fractures. *Hand*; **10:**246–53.

Steinbrocker O., Traeger C.H., Batterman R.C. (1949). Therapeutic criteria in rheumatoid arthritis. *J. Amer. Med. Ass*; **140:**659–62.

Swanson A.B. (1972). Flexible implant arthroplasty for arthritic finger joints. *J. Bone Jt. Surg*; **54A:**435–55.

Vainio K. (1969). Secondary operations after joint replacement. *Ann. Rheum. Dis*; **28:**Suppl.89–90.

Verdan C.E. (1972). Half a century of flexor tendon surgery. *J. Bone Jt. Surg*; **54A:**472–91.

Wood Jones F. (1941). *Principles of Anatomy as Seen in the Hand*. London: Balliere Tindall and Cox.

Hernia
NIALL O'HIGGINS

Inguinal hernia

In developmental life the processus vaginalis is an out-pouching of peritoneum which extends downwards anterior to the descending testis. The testis encroaches on the posterior aspect of the processus. The processus, followed by the testis, extends to the scrotum and leads the testis through the inguinal canal into its final intrascrotal position. It becomes obliterated above the testis at the level of the internal ring and loses its connection with the peritoneum. The remnant of the processus vaginalis is the tunica vaginalis which covers the testis anteriorly and on both sides. If the processus becomes obliterated at the superficial inguinal ring rather than at the deep ring, a knuckle of peritoneum extending as far as the external ring forms the basis for indirect inguinal hernia known as a bubonocele. If the peritoneal extension goes down to the scrotal neck, the resulting indirect hernia is known as a funicular hernia. In instances where the processus does not become obliterated there is free communication between the peritoneal cavity and tunica vaginalis. The hernia occurring in these circumstances can enter the scrotum and surround the testis. It is known as a scrotal or complete hernia. A hernia occurring without an obvious predisposing cause is known as a primary ⸳hernia, while a secondary hernia develops as a result of some local or generalised condition. Although most abdominal wall hernias are primary or idiopathic, it is always important to ensure as far as possible that the hernia is not secondary.

Indirect inguinal hernias are twice as common as direct inguinal hernias. An inguinal hernia is about 30 times commoner than a femoral hernia. Recurrences after herniorrhaphy are not uncommon and an average figure of some 10% is reported for both inguinal and femoral hernias. It should be recognised that about one half of the recurrences develop 5 years or more after the repair and that a quarter of recurrences develop more than 10 years after herniorrhaphy. It follows that evaluation of the integrity of a hernia operation is inaccurate unless the patient is followed up for at least 10 years. Indirect inguinal recurrences are extremely rare, most of the recurrences being direct. The incidence of sliding inguinal hernias is about 6% of all inguinal hernias. Sliding hernias are most uncommon in women.

The importance of recognition and treatment of hernia is illustrated by the fact that the operative mortality of uncomplicated hernia approaches zero, whereas when a hernia becomes obstructed, the operative mortality is 10–15%. In the presence of strangulation, where resection of bowel is required, the perioperative mortality is in the region of 30–40%.

Indirect hernia

Indirect inguinal hernia comes through the deep inguinal ring and extends down the inguinal canal as far as the external ring, the neck of the scrotum or even into the scrotum. The internal ring is a rounded defect in the transversalis fascia, which forms the posterior wall of the inguinal canal with the aponeurotic portion of the transversus abdominis muscle. The external ring is a triangular opening in the external oblique aponeurosis, which forms the anterior wall of the inguinal canal. The floor of the canal is formed by the upturned edge of the inguinal ligament. The internal oblique muscle forms an additional part of the anterior wall in the lateral third of the canal. This muscle arches upwards and backwards to form the entire roof of the canal and descends to form an additional posterior boundary on its medial end. It is known here as the conjoined tendon because the fibres join with those of the transversus abdominis muscle and become white and aponeurotic rather than muscular. An indirect inguinal hernia, following the inguinal canal, must take an oblique course to appear at the external ring, which is attached to the margins of the pubic tubercle. An indirect hernia comes through the abdominal wall above and medial to the pubic tubercle.

Direct hernia

A direct inguinal hernia bulges straight forwards through weakened muscular tissue at Hesselbach's triangle. This is an area bounded by the lateral border of the rectus abdominis muscle, the inguinal ligament and the obliquely running inferior epigastric artery. The artery, arising from the external iliac artery lies immediately medial to the internal ring. Direct inguinal hernias usually have a wide neck, are frequently bilateral and are more likely to be secondary to some underlying condition such as chronic bladder neck obstruction than are indirect hernias. In these cases, attention to and treatment of the primary condition takes precedence over the repair of the hernia.

Inguinal hernia in females

Ten per cent of inguinal hernias and hydroceles occur in girls. When they are present, 10% are bilateral and 20% are of the sliding variety, which may contain an ovary or fallopian tube. In adult women, however, sliding hernia is very rare and inguinal hernia is about twenty times less common than in men. Direct inguinal hernias are rare in women, the posterior inguinal wall usually being strong. Indirect inguinal hernias are commoner than are femoral hernias in woman.

High ligation of the sac and excision of the round ligament allows closure of both inguinal rings and obliteration of the inguinal canal to be carried out. A sound repair can almost always be obtained with minimal risk of recurrence.

Clinical features

A hernia in the inguinal region presenting as a swelling is often noticed in children. It is commoner in males than in females and is usually right sided. It appears as a swelling when the child cries or otherwise strains. Such hernias may become irreducible and sometimes require operative treatment if they persist after the second year of life (*see* Chapter 13).

Inspection

In adolescent or adult life an indirect hernia appears as a lump in the groin. It may have followed strenuous exercise during which the patient may feel a sharp or burning sensation in the groin. These hernias, even when reducible, are often uncomfortable or even painful. The pain is experienced over the swelling and along the medial side of the upper thigh below the inguinal ligament, in the area of the skin distribution of the ilioinguinal nerve. The patient can often recognise that the lump comes down in an oblique direction towards the scrotum. A direct inguinal hernia is rarely painful. Thus if an inguinal hernia, although reducible, is painful and if, on questioning about the direction of protrusion, the patient points obliquely downwards with a finger towards the scrotum, the hernia is almost certainly an indirect one. In the physical examination of the patient, it is important in small hernias to ask the patient to stand and strain. This posture and manoeuvre will usually reveal the presence of a hernia if it exists. On coughing, an expansile impulse is seen in the presence of a hernia and if a hernia loses its cough impulse, it is likely to be irreducible and to require prompt surgical treatment. The patient may be able to reduce a hernia himself and should be asked to do so before the examiner attempts reduction. On coughing, the position and direction of the bulge should be sought. If a hernia is below and lateral to the pubic tubercle, it is femoral and, if above and medial to the pubic tubercle, it is inguinal. The obliquity of an inguinal bulge suggests that the hernia is indirect.

Palpation

If there is doubt, a finger should be placed to obliterate the internal ring. If the hernia no longer appears on coughing the diagnosis of an indirect hernia is made. If the inguinal hernia still appears in spite of the occlusion of the internal ring, it is a direct hernia and appears medial to the finger. Some clinicians advise invagination of the scrotum with the little finger so that the finger encounters and encroaches upon the superficial ring. An impulse on coughing, felt at the tip of the examining finger in this position, must come down the inguinal canal and therefore be an indirect hernia. A direct hernia will cause an impulse to be detectable on the volar aspect of the finger tip. This test is usually quite unnecessary, is uncomfortable for the patient and the information yielded by it is often equivocal. Even after meticulous clinical examination it is frequently impossible to be certain whether an inguinal hernia is direct or indirect.

Herniography

The clinical diagnosis of an inguinal hernia may be difficult in infants and children and to improve the diagnostic accuracy, herniography has been developed. It involves the use of radiopaque material (methylglucamine diatrizonte or iothalamate meglumine in a dose of 2 ml/kg body weight) which is injected into the peritoneal cavity below the umbilicus and allowed to flow to the groins by postural adjustment. Radiography of the area then defines the presence or absence of a hernial sac or patent processus vaginalis. It has been used when doubt exists about a hernia, particularly in helping the surgeon to decide whether the contralateral groin needs to be explored at the same operation. The diagnostic accuracy of the procedure is 95%. Nearly half of the children over 2 years of age who have unilateral hernia have patency of the contralateral processus vaginalis and about half of these will develop inguinal hernias (Rowe and Clatworthy, 1971).

Differential diagnosis

Extraperitoneal fat. A collection of extraperitoneal fat may prolapse down the inguinal canal along the spermatic cord and give the appearances of an inguinal hernia. It appears as a painless swelling and is rarely reducible or tender. It is often associated with an impulse on coughing, but rarely enlarges on coughing and does not extend beyond the external ring. A precise diagnosis can only be made at operation.

Femoral hernia. A femoral hernia often coils up from below the inguinal ligament to give the appearance of an inguinal swelling, particularly if it is irreducible. In these circumstances it is worth noting that an inguinal hernia, arising from above the skin fold of the groin, tends to accentuate the groin crease, while a femoral hernia, lying beneath the groin fold tends to obliterate the groin crease.

Incompletely descended testis. This may look and feel like an inguinal hernia, so it is important always to examine the scrotum and confirm the presence of an intrascrotal testis when considering the diagnosis of any groin hernia.

Varicocele. A varicocele, if extensive, can be confused with an inguinal hernia, but the characteristic, soft, irregular and elongated configuration of a varicocele makes its diagnosis easy on clinical grounds.

Inguinal lymphadenopathy, whether primary or secondary, presenting as a swelling in the groin, also enters into the differential diagnosis of hernia in this region. A source of disease or infection in the area drained by the inguinal lymph nodes should be sought and the patient examined for signs of lymphadenopathy elsewhere. Lymph node enlargement in the groin is usually associated with many lumps, either mobile or adherent, and rarely presents as a single discrete swelling. However, an abscess in the area is often difficult to distinguish from an irreducible hernia. The patient may have systemic toxic symptoms or signs, the overlying skin is reddened and the mass is tender and fluctuant. A tuberculous psoas abscess, tracking down behind the inguinal ligament from a focus of tuberculosis in the spine, presents as a lump in the groin. Such a cold abscess has not the typical features of an acute abscess and may not be tender, but fluctuation is detectable in the swelling.

Saphena varix. This presents as a swelling in the groin in the region of the femoral ring and may be mistaken for a femoral hernia. When the patient stands, a varix may be seen as a characteristically smooth, rounded swelling which transmits a slightly bluish hue to the overlying skin. On palpation it is soft and a fluid thrill can be felt when a finger is placed over the swelling and the patient asked to cough. When the patient lies down, the swelling disappears.

Traumatic lesions in the groin, particularly a haematoma of muscle, may be extremely difficult to distinguish from groin hernias. The mechanism of injury is often indirect, the adductor muscle or the straight head of the rectus femoris being torn during violent exercise. This injury occurs typically in young athletes.

Cystic hydrocele of the spermatic cord. A cystic hydrocele of the spermatic cord or the round ligament of the uterus also present as a groin swelling. It is rarely painful or tender and does not usually enlarge on coughing. Definitive diagnosis is made only at operation.

Contents of the inguinal canal

The canal, formed by the track of the processus vaginalis contains the spermatic cord in the male and the round ligament of the uterus in the female. The ilio-inguinal nerve is within the canal. This nerve enters the canal between the internal oblique muscle and the external oblique aponeurosis and is anteriorly placed within the canal. The spermatic cord has three coverings derived as fascial sheaths drawn down into the canal by the passage of the testis towards the scrotum. These layers are extensions of the abdominal wall muscles and fascia. The external oblique is extended downwards over the cord as the external spermatic fascia. Beneath this lies the somewhat thicker cremasteric muscle and fascia derived from the internal oblique and the deepest layer, the internal spermatic fascia, is a downward prolongation of the transversus muscle and tranversalis fascia. The testicular artery, pampiniform venous plexus, lymphatics, nerves and fat, as well as the vas deferens, compose the contents of the spermatic cord.

Hernias which go into the scrotum are nearly always indirect hernias and must be distinguished from primary intrascrotal swellings. If a swelling arises in the scrotum, it is easy to see or feel the upper limit or border and the scrotum with the swelling can be hinged upwards over the lower abdominal wall on the fulcrum of the upper border of the swelling. A scrotal hernia, passing into the scrotum from above cannot be so hinged.

A sliding hernia is one where the peritoneal sac forms part of the wall of the hernia. The bowel component, caecum on the right and sigmoid colon on the left, pushes its way through the neck of the hernia from behind. It is important to bear in mind the possibility of a sliding hernia; otherwise in an attempt to dissect the peritoneal sac completely, the colon may be perforated or a portion of it rendered avascular.

When both a direct and indirect hernia occur simultaneously on the same side, the condition is referred to as a pantaloon hernia.

Littré's hernia is a rarity and consists of a herniation of a Meckel's diverticulum. It has been found in all age groups and occurs in inguinal, femoral and umbilical hernias. The incidence is about 1 in 200 of external groin hernias. As might be expected, intestinal obstruction rarely occurs, but has been described in cases where the ileum may become twisted or kinked about the hernia (Payson *et al.*, 1956).

Principles of repair

The operative treatment of an inguinal hernia (Madden *et al.*, 1971) is determined by two principles:

1   Correct management of the peritoneal sac and the contents of the hernia.

2   Adequate repair of the structure through which the hernia has passed.

In children

If surgical treatment is needed on indirect hernias in children, it is sufficient to identify and isolate the sac, reduce its contents and ligate the sac as high as possible (at the level of or deep to the internal ring). Care must be taken to avoid damage to the delicate structures in the spermatic cord, particularly the testicular blood supply. It is unnecessary to repair the posterior wall, since it is intrinsically sound and will increase in strength with time. As the child grows, the external and internal rings become set obliquely from each other rather than lying directly over each other and this obliquity determines the inguinal canal and seals it off from the peritoneal contents by a shutter mechanism which comes into play when intra-abdominal tension increases (*see* Chapter 13).

In adults

In the adult, a herniorrhaphy must be added to the herniotomy and involves high ligation of the sac and a sound repair of the posterior wall. In a direct inguinal hernia, the neck of the sac is usually wide and bulging and it is not necessary to open the peritoneum. The bladder or ovary may be contained in a direct hernia and may be put at risk if the direct sac is opened. The bulging sac is normally dealt with by imbricating it with non-absorbable material and following this by sound repair of the posterior wall.

Operations for repair of indirect inguinal hernia depend on the size of the hernia and on the strength or laxity of the inguinal tissue. In small indirect hernias, the internal ring is only slightly enlarged. When the hernial sac has been removed and the neck ligated as high as possible, reconstitution of the internal ring on the medial aspect is all that is required. Sutures are placed medial to the cord structures to tighten the internal ring on its medial aspect after the internal ring has been freed completely from the cord structures. When the hernia is larger, a full repair of the posterior wall is required. The entire posterior inguinal wall must be repaired in the presence of a large indirect or a direct inguinal hernia. Many methods have been devised for repair of such hernias with varied success. Whatever method is employed, the layers should be approximated without tension. Relaxing incisions either in the form of a Tanner slide (division of the anterior rectus sheath) or the turning downwards of a flap of rectus sheath, should be used when it is necessary to eliminate tension (Tanner, 1942).

Techniques of repair

Bassini

Through a suprainguinal incision, the superficial and deep fascia are divided along the line of the skin incision to expose the external oblique aponeurosis. This is incised and split along the line of its fibres by sliding partially opened scissors laterally as far as the level of the internal ring and medially to the external ring. The edges of the aponeurosis are held open to expose the ilio-inguinal nerve, the spermatic cord and the hernial sac. The coverings of the sac, external spermatic, cremasteric and internal spermatic fascia are divided and the cord structures protected by passing a tape, rubber sling or ring forceps around them. The edges of the peritoneal sac are identified and cleared as far back as the internal ring. A protrusion of extraperitoneal fat often follows the hernia through the internal ring and should be removed. After the sac has been opened and the contents inspected and replaced, the sac is ligated by a strong transfixion suture.

The transversalis fascia is refashioned throughout the length of the posterior wall and the transversus abdominis and internal oblique are sutured to the upturned edge of the inguinal ligament by interrupted non-absorbable sutures behind the cord as far laterally as the internal ring (Fig 50.1). Particular attention is paid to the medial aspect. The medial two or three sutures

are often placed in the periosteum of the pubic bone in an attempt to make the posterior wall especially strong in this area.

Direct recurrences sometimes follow repair of indirect hernias and the direct bulge is usually at the medial end of the posterior wall. The spermatic cord is replaced on the posterior wall and the inguinal canal reconstituted by suturing the external oblique aponeurosis anterior to the cord. Care must be taken not to tighten the area excessively as sudden straining may cause the tissue to split along the line of the sutures. Proper repair of a hernia depends not on how tightly sutures are placed, but on the restoration of a sound posterior wall sufficiently flexible not to be torn by sudden violent muscular contraction. As a means of overcoming or preventing such tension a Tanner slide manoeuvre is often added. This involves an incision in the anterior rectus sheath 2.5 cm above the hernia repair. The incision is vertical for 2 cm and then almost horizontal and allows the conjoined tendon and internal oblique to fall down without tension on the sutured posterior wall of the inguinal canal (Fig 50.2).

What was described and advocated by Bassini in 1888 was not only, as is commonly thought and practised, the suturing of the conjoined tendon and internal oblique muscle to the inguinal ligament, but also the complete reconstruction of the transversalis fascia including the repair of the internal ring. Bassini's method of repair has been practised throughout the world for almost a century and has been the reference operation against which refinements and developments have been compared.

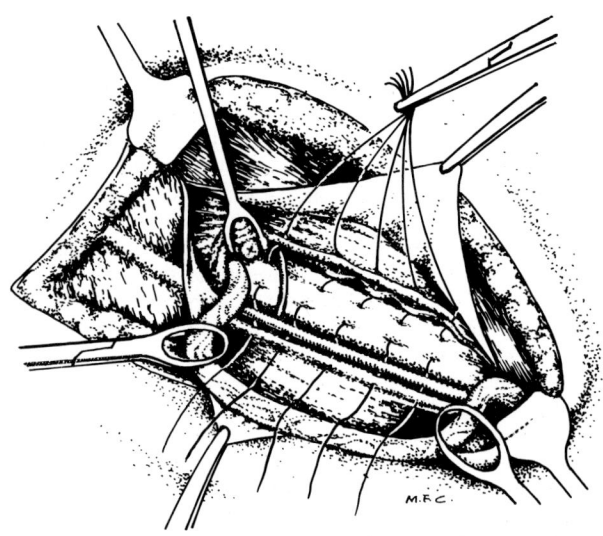

Fig 50.1   Bassini repair of inguinal hernia.

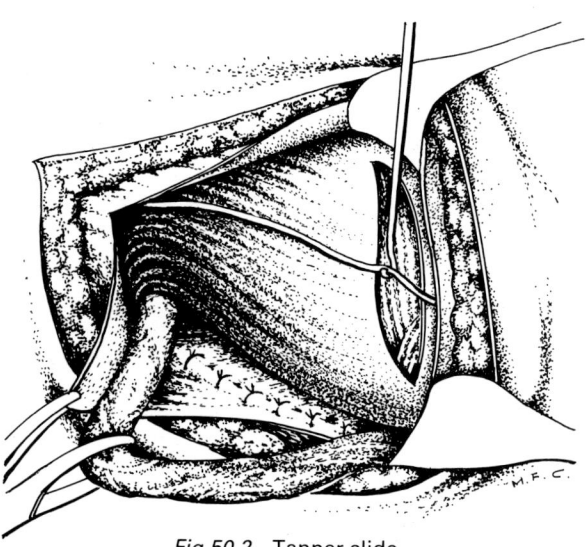

Fig 50.2   Tanner slide.

Halsted

The purpose of the original Halsted repair was to provide an extremely strong posterior wall to the inguinal canal. It is similar to the Bassini repair, but the external oblique aponeurosis is sutured posterior to the cord to reinforce the posterior wall further. The cord now lies subcutaneously. The effect of this operation is to obliterate the inguinal canal completely and the cord comes directly forwards from the internal ring to the subcutaneous space. In effect, there being no inguinal canal, there can be no posterior wall and this operation is now rarely employed.

The repair described above has become known since 1893 as the Halstead I repair to distinguish it from the Halsted II procedure (1903) otherwise known as the Ferguson-Andrews repair, which leaves the cord in its normal position and involves the imbrication of the external oblique aponeurosis. Halsted advised a relaxing incision in the anterior rectus sheath to avoid tension on the herniorrhaphy. The Tanner slide, also in the anterior rectus sheath (Tanner, 1942), describes a relaxing incision vertically in the medial part of the rectus sheath, allowing it and the conjoined tendon to slide laterally. In order to allow accurate placement of sutures and so that the stitches are not tied too tightly, it is advisable that the Tanner slide is carried out before the conjoined tendon is sutured to the inguinal ligament.

Lotheissen-McVay

First described in 1898 for repair of a recurrent inguinal hernia, this repair (Fig 50.3) utilises the pectineal ligament (Cooper's ligament). The operation was popularised and described most clearly by McVay (1966; 1974), who recommended the procedure only when the posterior wall is largely or wholly destroyed by the hernia and not for small to moderate-sized inguinal hernias where the posterior wall is sound. It is, therefore, suitable for large indirect and direct hernias where the posterior inguinal wall is weak. The weakened or destroyed posterior wall is excised leaving a large defect bounded above by the fusion of the transversus abdominis aponeurosis and the transversalis fascia and below by Cooper's ligament medially and the femoral sheath laterally. A relaxing incision in the anterior rectus sheath (Tanner slide) allows the margins of the defect to be apposed. Eight to ten interrupted silk sutures are inserted from medial to lateral, beginning at the pubic tubercle and placed 3 mm apart. The lateral sutures approximate the transversalis fascia above with the anterior femoral sheath below. Care must be taken to avoid compression of the femoral vein at the point where Cooper's ligament merges with the

anterior femoral sheath; a so-called 'transition' suture is inserted while the femoral vein is under direct vision. The external oblique aponeurosis is sutured anterior to the cord.

Mobility of tissues is facilitated in this repair by the use of a relaxing incision. The repair reinforces the posterior inguinal canal, strengthens Hesselbach's triangle and, in effect, obliterates the femoral canal. Direct recurrences are rare with this technique. Difficulty may arise when placing the sutures in Cooper's ligament. It is a rigid and fibrous structure and the utmost care in the placement of sutures is needed to avoid tearing tissue and damaging the femoral vein (Halverson and McVay, 1970).

Andrews

To reinforce the repair of the posterior wall and yet to maintain an oblique inguinal canal, Andrews in 1895 used a Bassini-type repair with additional strengthening of the posterior wall by suture of the upper leaf of the external oblique aponeurosis to the inguinal ligament posterior to the cord structures. The inferior leaf is sutured anterior to the cord to the external oblique aponeurosis at a higher level (Fig 50.4). Imbrication of the external oblique is considered by many to be unnecessary as it adds nothing to the soundness of the posterior wall, and deficiency in the anterior wall is not a problem in inguinal repair.

Shouldice

The Shouldice repair is advised for direct and indirect inguinal hernias and also for recurrent inguinal hernias in both men and women (Glassow 1976; 1978). In the first component of the operation, the cord is freed from the transversalis fascia at the level of the internal inguinal ring. An indirect sac, where present, is freed throughout its extent. Even if no indirect sac is found, the Shouldice repair demands that the small 'knuckle' or protrusion of peritoneum at the level of the internal ring is identified and freed. When a sac is present, it is excised. Freeing of the sac or peritoneum is stressed rather than the 'high ligation' usually advised. The cremaster muscle is excised allowing good visualisation of the entire posterior wall. The second component of the repair is the reconstruction of the transversalis fascia. This structure is routinely and completely identified and divided from the internal ring laterally to the pubic tubercle medially. The upper, medial leaf is then placed in front of the lower, lateral leaf. The free edges of the flaps are fixed by a

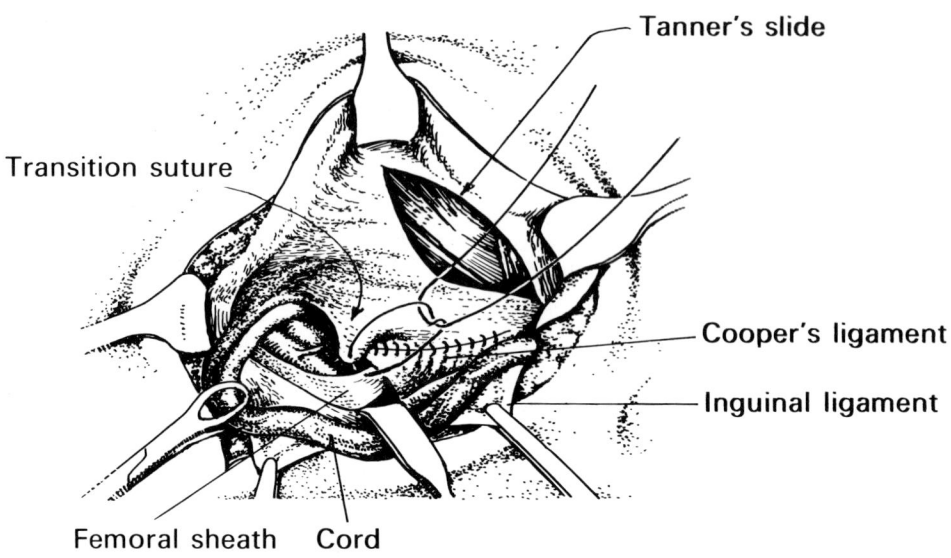

Tanner's slide

Transition suture

Cooper's ligament

Inguinal ligament

Femoral sheath   Cord

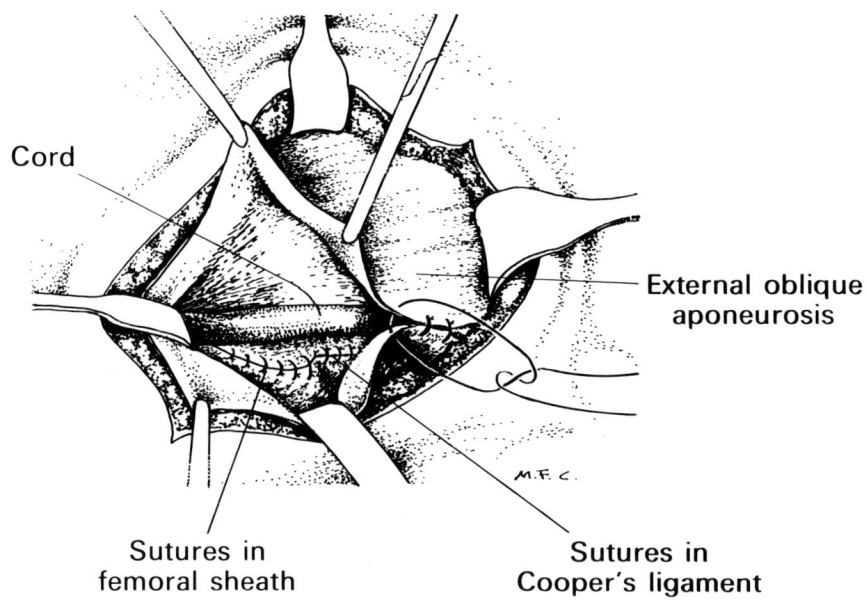

Cord

External oblique
aponeurosis

M.F.C.

Sutures in
femoral sheath

Sutures in
Cooper's ligament

Fig 50.3 Lotheissen-McVay repair.

continuous monofilament stainless steel wire suture of
34 gauge. Anterior to this double-breasted layer, the
internal oblique and transversus abdominis muscles are
joined to the deep surface of the inguinal ligament by a
continuous suture from lateral to medial. This is reinforced by continuing the suture from medial to lateral,
uniting the same sutures at a more superficial level. The

cord is placed on the repaired posterior wall and the
external oblique aponeurosis is reunited anteriorly with
continuous stainless steel wire sutures (Fig 50.5). In the
Shouldice Hospital, 95% of herniorrhaphies are carried
out under local analgesia and the rate of recurrence is
0.6 to 0.8%. The outstanding results with the Shouldice
repair attest to the effectiveness of the procedure. 100

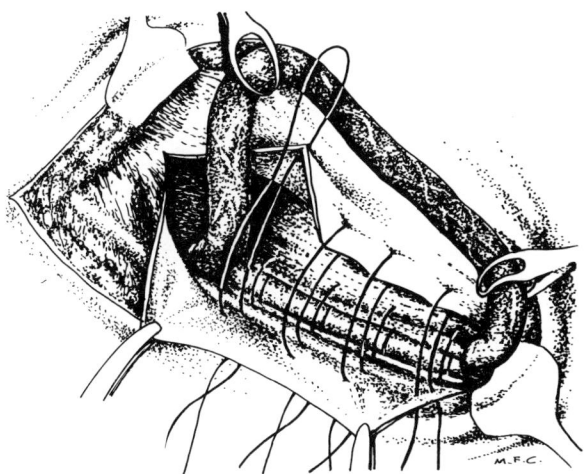

Fig 50.4 Andrews' repair. Upper leaf of external oblique aponeurosis is sutured to the inguinal ligament posterior to the cord. The lower leaf of external oblique is sutured to the external oblique aponeurosis at a higher level anterior to the cord.

to 150 ml of 2% procaine hydrochloride without adrenaline are infiltrated along the entire length of the inguinal canal. The local analgesic is infiltrated subcutaneously at the outset, a second injection is given deep to the aponeurosis once the external oblique has been opened and a third is injected around the internal ring. Monofilament wire is difficult to handle, but other non-absorbable sutures have been used with excellent results. A relaxing incision is not used in this kind of repair.

Preperitoneal approach and iliopubic tract repair

This form of herniorrhaphy (Nyhus and Condon, 1960) is also known as the properitoneal, extraperitoneal or posterior repair. It is a most satisfactory approach for recurrent hernias, since the previous scar tissue is not encountered. It is suitable also for sliding hernias, but requires muscular relaxation of the lower abdominal wall. It is particularly difficult in obese patients and unnecessarily complicated in infants and children where high ligation of the sac without repair is all that is needed. The ilio-pubic tract, first described by Thompson in 1836, is a sheet of fascia, which is attached to the crest of the ilium, covers the psoas muscle and femoral vessels to form part of the anterior

femoral sheath and is attached medially to the superior, pubic ramus and to Cooper's ligament. The lowest fibres are curved backwards to form the medial border of the femoral canal adjacent to the lacunar ligament. The operative approach was first described by Annandale and the technique of repair has been refined and described by Nyhus (1978).

The incision is made 3 cm above the inguinal ligament and must be made above the internal ring. The anterior rectus sheath is incised and the rectus muscle retracted medially. A transverse incision is then made through the musculo-aponeurotic fibres which make up the external oblique aponeurosis, the internal oblique and the transversus abdominis. The transversalis fascia is exposed and incised transversely, care being taken to avoid opening the peritoneum. Retraction of the lower margin of the incision exposes the hernia through the posterior inguinal wall.

If the hernia is *direct*, it is not necessary to excise the peritoneal sac. Inversion of the sac with a purse-string suture may be carried out if the sac bulges excessively. The direct hernia is repaired by uniting the upper and the lower margins with interrupted, non-absorbable sutures. The upper border is made up of the transversalis fascia and transversus abdominis aponeurosis while the lower border consists of the ilio-pubic tract. The medial sutures may incorporate Cooper's ligament as well as the ilio-pubic tract.

With *indirect* hernias, the sac is excised and high ligation carried out. The hernia is then repaired by uniting the anterior crus of the internal ring with the posterior crus of the ilio-pubic tract. For larger hernias, the transversalis fascia is joined to the ilio-pubic tract medial to the cord. Nyhus recommends that an Allis forceps applied to the ilio-pubic tract at the level of the anterior femoral sheath, allows the medial part of the ilio-pubic tract to be defined clearly. Care must be taken to draw the tract forwards when inserting sutures at the level of the femoral vessels so that damage to the vessels may be avoided. Ligation of the inferior epigastric artery and vein is unnecessary. A relaxing incision in the anterior rectus sheath is recommended.

The recurrence rate with preperitoneal approach and repair is much higher with direct than indirect hernias, being about 5% for indirect hernias and about 20% for direct hernias. The recurrence rate for femoral hernia after this operation is about 1%.

Nyhus finds that this approach and repair are suitable for femoral, indirect, inguinal, large sliding and recurrent hernias. It is suitable for irreducible and strangulated hernias. For direct and large indirect hernias, he advises an anterior approach. For small, indirect inguinal hernias, this operation may not be suitable and an anterior approach with high ligation of the sac and repair of the transversalis fascia at the internal ring are preferable.

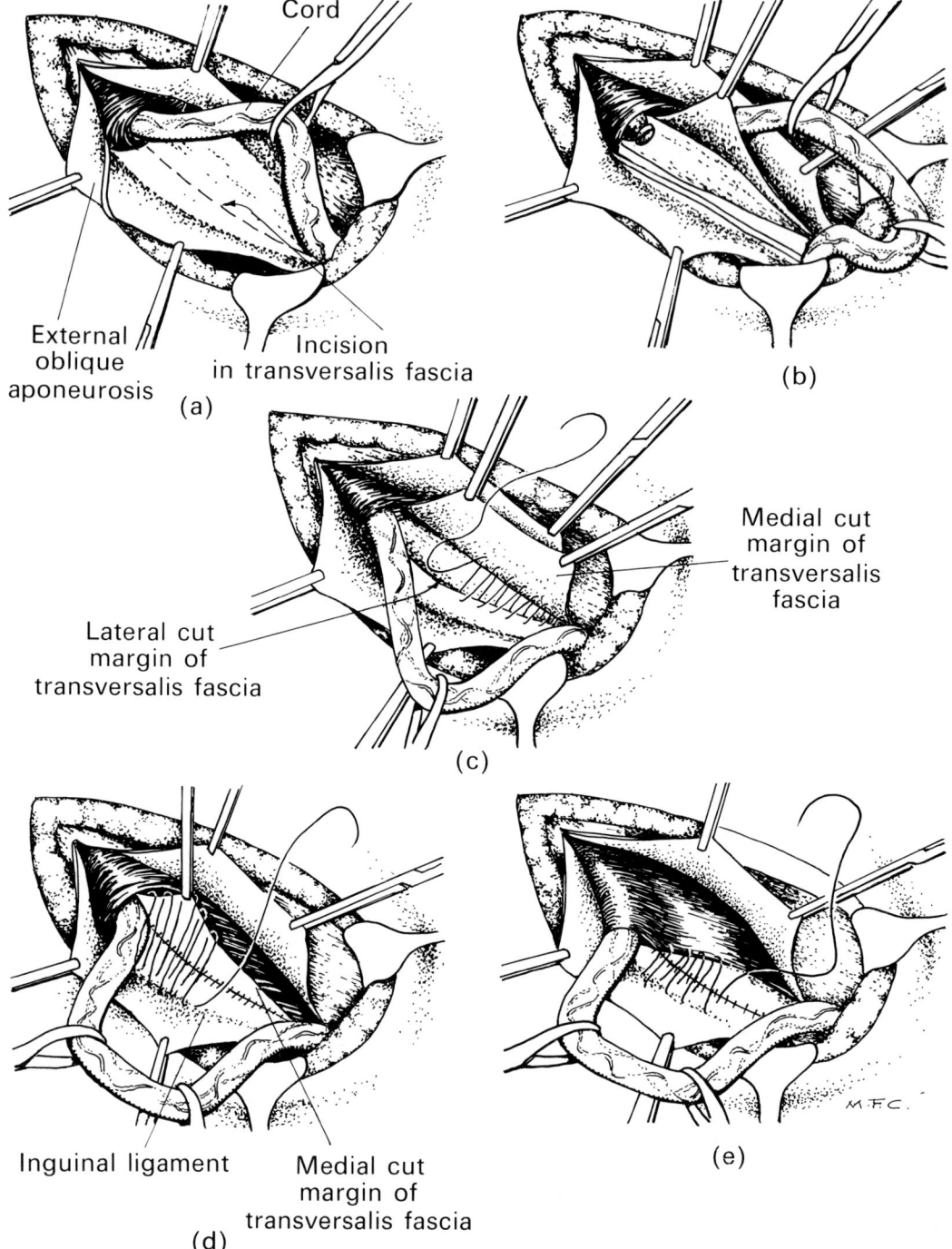

Fig 50.5 Shouldice repair. (c) Lateral cut margin of transversalis fascia sutured to deep surface of lateral flap of transversalis fascia. (d) Medial cut margin of transversalis fascia sutured to inguinal ligament. (e) Internal oblique muscle sutured to under surface of external oblique aponeurosis. (After Shearburn E.W. and Mysers R.N., 1969. *Surgery*; **66**:450.)

Marcy

This type of repair stresses the importance of exposing the transversalis fascia and repairing the basic defect in this layer at the level of the internal ring with sutures which coapt the margins of the defect in the fascia and which include no other structure. Full exposure of the internal ring is aided by removal of the cremaster muscle. When the sac has been dissected free from the cord structures, the internal ring can be clearly identified by forward pressure of the index finger passed from within after the sac has been opened, as advised by Lytle (1945). This allows closure of the peritoneum (high ligation) and repair of the internal ring (transversalis fascia) in two separate layers. Medially, if the transversalis fascia is weakened or attenuated, it may be plicated by suturing it to the ilio-pubic tract or inguinal ligament. This manoeuvre is additional to Marcy's repair of the internal ring as outlined above. If such additional suture is needed, a Tanner slide is used.

The Marcy repair is aimed at preventing indirect recurrences. It is not a repair for direct hernia. For this repair to be conducted properly, it is essential that the margins of the internal ring be defined completely, that the sac and cord structures be dissected from the transversalis fascia and from each other above the internal ring. When the internal ring is small, the transversalis fascia in the immediate vicinity of the ring may be strong enough to accept sutures, but when the ring is large and lax due to stretching by a sizeable hernia, this may not be the case. It then becomes necessary to use the thicker transversalis fascia superiorly (this can be exposed by upward traction on the transversus abdominis muscle) and medially in the area of the inferior epigastric vessels.

Sliding inguinal hernia

Sliding inguinal hernia accounts for about 5% of all inguinal hernias and occurs on the left side four times as commonly as on the right. It is more common in men than in women and its relative incidence increases with age. It is most unusual for such hernias to be irreducible or to strangulate due to the large size of the internal inguinal ring in this kind of patient. Once a sliding hernia has been recognised, it is probably unnecessary to excise the sac. A complete excision of the sac is certainly not required and runs the risk of damage to the colon. Partial excision of the sac with closure by purse-string suture (Zimmerman and Anson, 1967) has been widely used, but the results have not been shown to be superior to freeing of the sac, reduction of the hernia deep to the transversalis fascia and a sound repair of the posterior wall. Excision of a redundant portion of the sac may be needed, but the most important part of

the operative management of this type of hernia is an adequate repair of the defect in the posterior inguinal wall.

Femoral hernia

A femoral hernia, because it usually has a narrow neck and unyielding boundaries, is more likely to become strangulated than an inguinal hernia. A femoral hernia (McVay and Savage, 1961) comes through the femoral canal which lies medial to the femoral vein on the upper and medial aspect of the thigh. The femoral canal is bounded anteriorly by the transversalis fascia and the inguinal ligament, medially by the reflected portion of the ilio-pubic tract and, more superficially, the lacunar ligament and posteriorly by Cooper's ligament. As the hernia enlarges, it extends down the femoral canal through the fossa ovalis, a defect in the fascia lata of the thigh, where the long saphenous vein penetrates to join the femoral vein. Loose fibrous tissue, the cribriform fascia, closes the fossa ovalis.

Repair

Low approach

The low or subinguinal approach to a femoral hernia involves an incision in the skin over the fossa ovalis. The fundus of the hernia is exposed, the sac opened and the contents reduced. A transfixion ligature is placed at the neck of the sac and sutures are placed between the inguinal ligament and the pectineal fascia to close the femoral ring. This procedure rarely effects an adequate repair of the hernia and has the disadvantages that the femoral and external iliac veins cannot be seen along the lateral border of the femoral canal and an accessory obturator artery, coursing along the internal surface of the lacunar ligament, cannot be seen and is prone to injury. The lacunar ligament itself and the reflected ilio-pubic tract can be felt, but not seen, by this approach. Damaged bowel or gangrenous bowel are difficult to deal with through this incision.

In an uncomplicated hernia the low approach is satisfactory, being simple and relatively undisturbing to the patient. It can be carried out under local analgesia. Two or three interrupted non-absorbable sutures on a fish hook needle usually suffice. They should not be pulled tightly in an attempt to approximate Cooper's ligament and the inguinal ligament, but rather tied loosely to form a mesh.

The bladder may be damaged in this approach, especially when the operation is done for irreducible hernia. In these circumstances the hernial contents are retracted and the constricting band at the neck of the sac divided on the medial aspect. A grooved director is passed between the sac and the constricting band. The incision divides Gimbernat's ligament. The contents of the sac can then be drawn downwards gently and inspected for viability. Recurrence rates for femoral herniorraphy using the low approach are around 10% but may be as low as 2.3% (Ponka and Brush, 1971).

Transinguinal

With this incision, the cord structures are lifted from the floor of the inguinal canal which is incised to reveal the femoral hernia after which the hernia is reduced and the sac amputated. The ilio-pubic tract is then sutured to Cooper's ligament. Adjacent blood vessels can be seen throughout the procedure and a sound repair thus effected. The floor of the inguinal canal is closed. The disadvantage of this procedure is that a direct inguinal hernia may occur afterwards.

Lotheissen described the suturing of the conjoint tendon to Cooper's ligament. This combines closure of the femoral hernia with repair of the posterior wall of the inguinal canal which is transgressed during this approach to the femoral hernia.

Properitoneal (posterior)

The properitoneal approach involves an incision in the inguinal region similar to that of repair of an inguinal hernia. After the inguinal canal has been opened and the spermatic cord or round ligament retracted upwards the protruding femoral hernia will be seen beneath the transversalis fascia. Incision of the transversalis fascia will allow the hernial sac to be visible. The hernia is reduced by traction from above. If strangulation is present at the level of the fossa ovalis, a separate vertical incision over the protrusion in the thigh may be needed to free the hernia. The sac is removed and the neck closed with a non-absorbable transfixion ligature. The transversalis fascia is sutured to Cooper's ligament to obliterate the femoral ring. The Moschcowitz repair of a femoral hernia involves suturing the inguinal ligament to Cooper's ligament. A third method is to suture a turned down margin of the external oblique aponeurosis to Cooper's ligament.

Henry

A mid-line lower abdominal incision brought down to the peritoneum which is then reflected from the lower abdominal wall, constitutes the Henry approach to a femoral hernia. This allows bilateral femoral hernias to be dealt with by suturing transversalis fascia to Cooper's ligament, but it does not allow repair of the floor of the inguinal canal and inguinal hernias are, therefore, most difficult to repair by this approach.

McEvedy

The incision described by McEvedy (1950) involves a vertical incision placed above the inner end of the inguinal ligament and extended downwards below the inguinal ligament. The lower part of the anterior rectus sheath is incised 2 cm medial to the lateral border and the rectus muscle is retracted medially. Division of the transversalis fascia exposes the peritoneum and the hernial sac. This exposure allows good access to the femoral hernia and resection of bowel, where necessary, can be carried out conveniently through the approach.

Strangulation

Because of the increased frequency with which elective repair of hernias is carried out, the incidence of strangulation in groin hernias in countries with well developed medical services is declining steadily. In the first half of this century, groin hernias were the commonest cause of intestinal obstruction, accounting for up to 50% of all cases of intestinal obstruction, but now account for about 10%. In many African countries, however, hernia is still responsible for 30–60% of cases of intestinal obstruction. The mortality of this condition depends on whether the irreducible segment of bowel is viable or not. The death rate following operation with resection for gangrenous bowel is declining with better postoperative care, but is still in the region of 35%, while it is about 15% when the intestine is viable. The mortality of strangulated groin hernias increases with age, although it is more closely related to the duration of symptoms than to the age of the patient. The cause of death may be related to local or general peritoneal sepsis or septicaemia and to cardiopulmonary or renal disease (see also Ch. 1).

The diagnosis is rarely difficult, but may not be obvious in obese patients who are unable to give a history of the complaint. It should go without saying that the patient is examined in the erect position if doubt exists. In irreducible inguinal hernia, gentle taxis under sedation may allow the hernia to be reduced, but attempted reduction of an irreducible femoral hernia is unwise, as any damage to the bowel may be aggravated and perforation may be caused. While inguinal hernias are commoner than femoral, the risk of intestinal gangrene from strangulation is higher in femoral hernias. When the pain is constant rather than colicky, when fever or tachycardia develop or when there is any local sign of inflammation in the region of the hernia, strangulation is suspected. While a strangulated hernia is usually tender, it should be noted that the absence of tenderness in a femoral hernia does not rule out strangulation. Intestinal obstruction is usual in patients with strangulation, but Richter's hernia, where only a segment of the circumference of the bowel is incarcerated, is not associated with intestinal obstruction. While Richter's hernia may occur at any hernial site (and indeed was described by Richter in epigastric and ventral hernias), it is commonest in femoral hernias (Rogers, 1959).

Preoperative intraveous fluids are usually required, particularly if there is obstruction of the intestine. In this case, the volume of intravenous fluids required may be considerable. If there is any clinical evidence of major fluid and electrolyte depletion, a central venous pressure line and a urinary catheter should be inserted so that the effect of fluid replacement can be monitored accurately. In addition to sodium, potassium requirements may be high. When gangrene is found and small bowel resection is required, the risk of wound infection and septicaemia is increased and systemic antibiotics effective against Gram-negative and anaerobic organisms are justified. Irrigation of the wound and delayed primary closure of the skin are recommended when heavy contamination exists.

The approach to the strangulated hernia is usually through a suprainguinal incision, although a McEvedy incision allows full exposure if resection of bowel is needed. Another approach is that described by Dennis and Varco (1947) for a strangulated femoral hernia. This involves a vertical incision directly over the swelling for the recognition of gangrene without opening the sac. When gangrene has been recognised, the incision is completed by an incision at right angles to the upper limb of the vertical incision. This T-shaped incision allows exposure of the neck of the sac. By dividing the inguinal ligament, an en-bloc removal of the sac and its contents, including the fibrous neck of the ring, is carried out, the advantage being that no spillage of septic peritoneal fluid occurs.

Preoperative antibiotics, effective against Gram-negative bacilli and bacteroides, should be given and continued after operation. Gentamicin and metronidazole in combination are probably the most effective in these circumstances. The decision to resect the bowel is one of major importance. It is not always easy to decide whether the bowel is viable or not. Absence of pulsation in the arteries, absence of peristaltic activity and the presence of bloody fluid in the sac, if associated with purple or black bowel are important features of gangrene, but are not absolute signs of necrotic bowel. With established gangrene of the bowel, the serosal sheen is lost giving a dull rather than a glistening appearance to this layer. In cases where the bowel is of doubtful viability, the neck of the sac should be released and the damaged bowel covered in warm moist gauze packs for some minutes. If there is still doubt, resection is safer than the alternative of replacing gangrenous bowel. In cases of Richter's hernia,

excision of the gangrenous patch on the wall of the bowel may be possible but in general, it is safer to resect a small length of bowel with end-to-end anastomosis. Otherwise late stenosis may occur due to ischaemic fibrosis and, more serious, perforation of the bowel can occur several days after the operation and result in generalised peritonitis.

Complications of groin herniorrhaphy

Peroperative complications

Bleeding. Vein damage may be a nuisance, but is rarely a problem during hernia surgery in the groin. Damage to the inferior epigastric or circumflex iliac vessels requires that they be isolated and ligated. Unrecognised, this haemorrhage results in localised haematoma formation or in scrotal ecchymosis or haematoma. Damage to the external iliac or femoral vessels is usually identified immediately. It is usually controllable by pressure, but may require careful vascular repair of the involved vessel.

Trauma to the vas deferens. In the repair of recurrent hernia of the inguinal area, deliberate division of the spermatic cord and its structures is sometimes carried out in order to obliterate the deep inguinal ring completely. The incidence of recurrent hernia is lessened by this procedure. Swelling and tenderness of the testis follows this operation in the majority of patients, but the symptoms usually subside gradually.

If the vas has been divided inadvertently, the damage is usually recognised at operation. The cut ends of the vas can be anastomosed by interrupted sutures over an internal splint of monofilament wire which is brought out through the wall of the vas some distance away from the anastomotic site. The splint is removed after the anastomosis has been completed.

Bladder injury. The bladder may be opened in error when the sac of a direct inguinal hernia is opened. The bladder should be repaired with interrupted catgut sutures and an indwelling catheter placed in the bladder and left on free drainage for about 5 days. After closing the bladder, hernial repair can be carried out in the usual fashion.

Interference with blood supply to the testis. A rich anastomotic network of arterioles exists between the testicular artery and branches from the external and internal pudenal vessels as well as the vesical and prostatic vessels. Damage to the main testicular artery may, therefore, not be followed by atrophy to the testis, unless the testis is dissected from the scrotum. These circumstances are especially likely to occur during repair of recurrent hernias.

Intestinal damage. In repairing hernias, great care must be taken not to pick up the bowel in sutures involved in the repair. The bowel is most likely to be damaged during high ligation of the sac. Such an injury may be avoided if the point of the needle is seen at every stage of the pick-up of the suture. The bowel is particularly prone to injury when sliding hernias are encountered, where there is a danger that the wall of the bowel will not be recognised. The bowel may also be damaged by being rendered ischaemic in stripping it away from its blood supply when attempting to identify the sac. If the sac is sought from the anterior aspect, such damage is unlikely.

Damage to the femoral vein. The femoral vein may be compressed by sutures in the region and if the degree of compression is significant, venous thrombosis, swelling of the limb, and pulmonary embolism may occur.

Postoperative complications

In addition to the complications which occur following any procedure, there are relatively specific complications after hernia repair. Pulmonary complications are quite common in patients who have general or spinal anaesthesia, but not with local analgesia.

Retention of urine. The question of any degree of bladder neck obstruction in elderly men ought to be investigated before herniorrhaphy. If there is a doubt about an obstructing prostate, preliminary cystoscopy and, if necessary, prostatectomy should be carried out before the hernia is repaired. Herniorrhaphy can be carried out subsequently or even at the time of prostatectomy. Should the male patient develop retention of urine after herniorrhaphy, reassurance, analgesia and sedation may be all that is required. The patient should have some privacy when attempting to void urine in these circumstances and should not be rushed. In young men, it is very rarely necessary to pass a catheter, but this may be required in elderly male patients who have pre-existing prostatic symptoms which have been overlooked. Once a catheter has been inserted, it is left *in situ* for 1 day and then removed. If the patient develops retention again, the procedure may be repeated on one or two further occasions, but continuing episodes of retention demand investigation and treatment.

Testicular swelling or atrophy. Testicular swelling may occur if there is compression of the venous drainage of the spermatic cord. This condition usually settles after some weeks, but may be uncomfortable or painful during that time. While the testis usually returns to normal size, it may become atrophic. Such atrophy may also occur if the testis is rendered ischaemic by interruption of the arterial supply at operation. Atrophy, if unilateral, does not interfere with fertility, but may cause psychological problems for the patient.

Hydrocele of the cord. This condition may occur if the fundus of the hernial sac has been left *in situ*, particularly if the distal end of the sac has been ligated rather than left open. These conditions are usually quite simple to deal with, aspiration of the straw-coloured fluid being all that is needed. Operation is rarely necessary.

Nerve damage. If the ilio-inguinal nerve is damaged there is a small area of anaesthesia on the medial aspect of the thigh below the inguinal ligament and on the lateral aspect of the scrotum. The ilio-hypogastric nerve may be injured during the operation and gives rise to an area of anaesthesia over the pubis. Trauma to the genital branch of the genitofemoral nerve results in an area of altered sensation to the skin of the penis and scrotum whereas damage to the femoral branch is followed by anaesthesia in the upper part of the later aspect of the thigh. These areas of sensory impairment gradually diminish over a period of some months and generally become unnoticeable within a year.

A more difficult problem related to damage to small nerves in the vicinity of hernial repair is the development of a painful neuroma at the site of nerve section. This condition sometimes causes such pain that re-exploration of the wound is required.

Recurrent hernia. Recurrence of hernia (Thurston Thieme, 1971), has been identified in up to 10% of inguinal and femoral hernias and up to 30% or more in recurrent hernias. While indirect recurrences are uncommon after inguinal herniorrhaphy, direct recurrences are not and femoral hernias may also be encountered. Some of those are undoubtedly missed femoral hernias, but many are due to excessive tension during the primary repair. Recurrences are often asymptomatic and may not be noticed by the patient. When operating on recurrent hernias, it may not be possible to carry out effective repair without tension. In these cases, the use of polypropylene (Marlex) mesh, some 2 cm larger than the defect, should be used. Sutures should be placed from the margins of the defect to the mesh, which is then placed in position over the site of recurrence before the sutures are tied. The utmost care in preventing infection should be taken. With repeated troublesome recurrences the cord structures are sometimes divided and the inguinal canal obliterated completely.

Orchiectomy

In repair of twice or thrice recurrent inguinal hernias, division of the spermatic cord with orchiectomy allows complete closure of the internal and external rings and obliteration of the inguinal canal. The procedure is rarely required. It is usually possible, even in a patient whose hernia has recurred many times, to dissect the cord structures from the surrounding scar tissue and to effect a satisfactory repair, with synthetic material if necessary. In many of these patients, the anatomy of the area has become so deformed and fibrosed that the entire suprainguinal area is weakened in a diffuse fashion. Orchiectomy with transection of the cord has little effect in strengthening the weakened posterior wall or in preventing direct recurrence, which is the more usual type.

Umbilical hernia

In infants

At birth, when the umbilical cord has been ligated, the stump heals by granulation and scarring, leaving a skin-covered cicatrix in the region of the umbilicus. After birth, many infants have a persistent umbilical hernia because of incomplete closure of the defect. This allows protrusion of a knuckle of peritoneum through the umbilicus. At birth about 10% of white children and over 40% of negro infants demonstrate this defect. The reason for this radical difference is not known. In almost all cases, the defect closes spontaneously within 4 years. This fascial defect is particularly common in premature infants. Because there is a tendency to close spontaneously, conservative treatment is the rule, particularly with a small defect of less than 1 cm. No treatment is required with a small defect, but in patients with a hernial neck of more than 1 cm, strapping of the umbilicus is frequently advised in the first 6 months of life. It is doubtful whether this treatment is of benefit and may be harmful because of the risk of skin sepsis associated with it. After the age of 6 months, operation may be required in the rare case in which the hernia becomes irreducible. After the age of 2 years operation is advisable if the hernia persists and enlarges. Strangulation can also occur, although it is a rare event. There is also a risk that the hernia may rupture after injury.

The operation involves a curved incision below the umbilicus. The hernial sac is dissected free of the surrounding linea alba. The neck of the sac is ligated after reduction of the contents and the margins of the defect are coapted with interrupted non-absorbable sutures.

In adults

In the majority of patients a hernia occurring in adult life in the region of the umbilicus is a paraumbilical hernia, which is an acquired condition. It occurs typically in overweight multiparous women. At first there is usually a protrusion of extraperitoneal fat through the linea alba and the peritoneal sac follows the fat pad. The neck of the peritoneal sac remains narrow because of the unyielding nature of the umbilical cicatrix. The sac often protrudes between fibres of the linea alba which becomes attenuated and stretched. This type of hernia is often irreducible and strangulation is likely. Operative treatment should, therefore, be advised. The fundus of the sac becomes adherent to the overlying skin around the umbilicus and frequently contains omentum with protrusions of small and large intestine. The presence of adhesions around the sac and the loculation of the sac through the linea alba are factors which render this type of hernia particularly liable to strangulation. In addition to the risks of complications, this type of hernia usually increases in size and gives rise to a feeling of discomfort and back-ache. Rupture of a paraumbilical hernia, either spontaneously or after trauma, is particularly likely to occur in pregnancy or in patients with ascites. If the ascites is due to cirrhosis of the liver with associated portal hypertension, repair of the umbilical hernia may be followed by haemorrhage from oesophago-gastric varices.

Repair

Unless there is a large protrusion of the umbilicus itself, most surgical repairs can be effected while preserving the umbilicus. Through a subumbilical curved incision, the anterior layer of the rectus sheath is exposed. Removal of fatty tissue around the hernial sac allows the neck of the sac to be delineated. The sac is opened, the hernia reduced and the redundant peritoneum is excised. The sac is then closed with non-absorbable sutures and the repair is carried out. The classical Mayo repair involves the development of a flap of rectus sheath and linea alba above and below the hernia defect. The lower flap is placed under the upper flap and secured by mattress sutures. The free margin of the upper flap is then sutured anteriorly in a 'double-breasted' fashion. More recently, there has been a tendency not to employ a Mayo repair, but merely to coapt the margins of the defect by transverse closure with interrupted sutures. Both methods are satisfactory since recurrence of a paraumbilical hernia is rare. If the margins of the defect are placed widely apart as a result of a large hernia, apposition of the edges may not be possible. In this case a Mersilene mesh may be required. When, as is usual, the patient is fat, a subcutaneous drain is advisable.

Epigastric hernia

Epigastric hernias occur through the linea alba, especially above the umbilicus. The herniation may be of extraperitoneal fat or be a protrusion of peritoneum containing omentum. Many patients have no symptoms from this condition, the incidence of which is about 5% at autopsy. In symptomatic patients, a local pain in the region of the swelling is a common presenting feature. Many patients, however, complain of rather vague upper abdominal discomfort, which is often diffuse in the upper abdomen and not localised to the epigastrium. Typically, the pain worsens when the patient lies down, presumably due to traction on the tissue trapped in the hernia. Sometimes the symptoms are relieved by reclining which allows the hernia to reduce.

In most instances the hernia can be diagnosed by the detection of a small lump in the mid-line or slightly to the left of the mid-line, half way between the xiphisternum and the umbilicus. The swelling may become more obvious if the patient is asked to strain. The swelling is often more difficult to palpate in obese patients. In patients with non-specific symptoms it is advisable to exclude gallbladder and peptic ulcer disease before repair of the epigastric hernia is advised. In symptomatic hernias repair is carried out through a transverse incision. If the hernia consists of fat only, this is removed and the fascial defect closed with interrupted sutures. When a knuckle of peritoneum is protruding, this is reduced and the fascia is repaired in a similar way. Because 20% of these hernias are multiple, a vertical incision is advised by some. This will allow a search to be made for other epigastric hernias and will also allow exploration of the upper abdominal viscera where there is doubt that the symptoms are all due to the epigrastric hernia. The recurrence rate following treatment of epigastric hernia is high, in the region of 15%.

Obturator hernia

An obturator hernia is rare and occurs through the obturator canal which transmits the obturator vessels and nerve. Such hernias are very likely to strangulate because of the firm fibrous and bony edges around the neck of the sac. The condition is much commoner in women than men and generally occurs over the age of 50 years. It is especially likely to occur in patients who have become debilitated or who have lost weight. The patient presents with clinical features of small bowel obstruction or strangulation (Gray *et al.*, 1974).

On examination, there is occasionally a lump to be felt in the upper inner aspect of the thigh and the patient usually holds the affected hip joint in semiflexion. Referred pain to the knee joint along the geniculate branch of the obturator nerve is a common feature. If a groin swelling is present, it may be possible to press on the pubic ramus above the swelling without causing pain and this may help to distinguish the swelling from a femoral hernia. The obturator sign (Howship Romberg) may be positive. In this test the knee and hip are flexed to a right angle and the hip joint internally rotated. This manoeuvre puts the obturator internus muscle on stretch and may cause pain in the presence of an obturator hernia. Rectal and vaginal examination may also reveal the presence of a mass in the side of the pelvis. In most cases of obturator hernia, however, the diagnosis is made at laparotomy when the patient is operated on for intestinal obstruction. In this case, the hernia is reduced by gentle traction. If reduction is difficult, it may be necessary to incise fibres of the obturator membrane, but care must be taken to avoid damage to the obturator vessels. Repair by apposition of the margins of the defect is not possible and a mesh of Marlex or Mersilene may be needed. In cases where the hernia has been diagnosed before operation, a vertical incision extending down from the inguinal ligament on the medial aspect of the femoral vessels allows access to the obturator foramen. In this approach the adductor longus muscle is retracted medially and the fibres of the pectineus muscle are separated or divided along the line of the fibres. The hernia can be reduced from below and repair with a mesh carried out.

Spigelian hernia

A Spigelian hernia is a rare condition and typically occurs at the angle between the lateral border of the rectus abdominus muscle (linea semilunaris) and the linea semicircularis half way between the umbilicus and the pubic symphysis. This type of hernia tends to strangulate and, when irreducible, presents as a swelling about 3 cm above the inguinal ligament. When the hernia is reducible, it may be detectible when the patient is standing and straining. It can be distinguished from an inguinal hernia because of its higher position. Treatment is operative and involves reduction of the hernia, dissection and ligation of the sac and repair of the transversus abdominal muscle around the defect by interrupted non-absorbable sutures (Bertelsen, 1968).

Lumbar hernias

These hernias, occurring in the lumbar region, result from congenital weakness of the muscular wall of the loin or as a result of injury, infection or surgical incisions in the region. Hernias in this region occur in the superior and inferior lumbar triangles. The superior triangle is bounded by the 12th rib, the anterior border of the internal oblique muscle, the lower border of the serratus posterior inferior. The quadratus lumborum muscle is in the floor of the triangle. Herniation through the superior lumbar triangle (triangle of Grynfeltt-Lesshaft) are commoner and larger than hernias through the inferior lumbar triangle (triangle of Petit). The inferior lumbar triangle is bounded by the latissimus dorsi, the external oblique and the iliac crest. Strangulation occurs in about 10% of these hernias and operative repair is advisable. Repair may be difficult because of the weakness of the surrounding muscles and the principle of repair depends on satisfactory closure of the defect in the transversalis fascia. In the presence of a large defect the use of a mesh prosthesis is desirable.

Incisional hernia

Incisional hernias are related to wound infection and to wound dehiscence and, while accurate figures on their frequency are difficult to come by, it can be stated that they occur in about 1% of all laparotomy incisions. Incisional hernia occurs in about one-third of patients who develop a wound dehiscence after operation. Factors predisposing to incisional hernias are the same as those predisposing to wound infection, namely obesity, wound haematoma, steroid therapy, abdominal distension and general conditions associated with delayed healing, such as protein-calorie malnutrition and vitamin and mineral deficiency.

While the neck of the hernial sac is usually large and unlikely to compromise the intestinal lumen or blood supply in incisional hernia, intestinal obstruction does occur. It is related to the presence of fibrous adhesive bands which develop between the serosal intestinal wall and the hernial edge. The presence of an incisional hernia is a constant source of discomfort to the patient, is associated with a heaviness or dragging sensation and, if large, may lead to exaggerated lumbar lordosis, backache and poor posture. While many types of brace, corset and belt have been designed and used to control the protrusion, they are seldom satisfactory. Surgical repair is undoubtedly the best method of dealing with incisional hernias, but the surgeon may be discouraged or dissuaded from advising operation because of the magnitude of the procedure in a patient who often suf-

fers from intercurrent illness, such as marked obesity, hypertension, cardiac or pulmonary disease.

While the operative procedure is the most important aspect of management of a patient with an incisional hernia, a successful outcome can be reached only by assiduous pre- and postoperative care.

Reduction of weight

Patients with incisional hernias are often overweight and a planned reducing diet under the close supervision of a trained dietitian is most important. The handing out of diet sheets with cursory dietary advice is seldom followed by realistic loss of weight. The confidence and total co-operation of the patient in planning his own treatment is mandatory.

Intercurrent disease

Assessment of cardiopulmonary function is essential as control of cardiac failure, treatment of respiratory infection and physiotherapy to the chest are necessary if postoperative cardiopulmonary complications are to be avoided.

Pneumoperitoneum

With massive incisional protrusions, the 'right of domain' may be lost and replacement by reduction of the hernia may not be possible during operation without specific preoperative measures. The technique of pneumoperitoneum, as described by Moreno (1947), allows gradual increase in the intraperitoneal capacity to occur, thus permitting reduction of the hernia in the abdominal cavity without respiratory complications. Before the introduction of this technique, forcible reduction of hernial contents into the abdominal cavity was followed by upward displacement of the diaphragm and the risk of respiratory failure. Gradually increasing amounts of air are injected daily into the peritoneal cavity through a 22-gauge needle and 50 ml syringe. 500 ml of air are injected on the first day and the amount is increased by increments of 200 ml on alternate days until 2500 ml per day are injected on the 21st day. During the course of this progressive pneumoperitoneum, the intra-abdominal capacity increases and allows the hernia to be reduced and repaired with surprising ease. Subcutaneous emphysema and respiratory difficulty may be caused by the procedure. Air may be aspirated if any ventilatory problems arise.

Repair

Operative treatment (Hunter, 1971) of incisional hernia involves a vertical or transverse incision. An ellipse of skin over the hernia is removed and the edges of the fascia are defined by exposing normal tissue about 2 cm lateral to the margins of the fascial defect. The sac is opened, adhesions freed, the hernia reduced and the fascia repaired together with the perintoneum with non-absorbable sutures. Repair of the fascial defect is the most difficult part of the procedure. If the edges of the fascia do not come together without tension, long relaxing fascial incisions are made on each side well away from the margins to be sutured. Alternatively (and preferably, if the defect is large), a mesh of polypropylene (Marlex) is applied external to the peritoneal layer and sutured to the margins of the defect. The mesh may be used as a single layer or in two layers. A modification (Usher, 1970) is to cut strips of Marlex mesh two inches wide, to suture each strip to the margins of the fascial defect, overlap the free margins of the mesh and to suture them together in an overlapping double-breasted fashion. A mesh of polypropylene is more likely to be required in lower abdominal than upper abdominal incisional hernia. Lower abdominal hernias tend to be larger as the recti muscles tend to become more widely spaced. Moreover, the posterior rectus sheath disappears in the lower abdomen tending to separate the margins of the hernia.

Maingot's keel repair is an extraperitoneal procedure involving (i) excision of a wide ellipse of skin around the scar overlying the hernia, (ii) extensive mobilisation of skin and subcutaneous tissue well beyond the margins of the hernial ring and (iii) uniting and inverting the fibro-aponeurotic margins of the hernia with non-absorbable sutures. Longitudinal relaxing incisions along the anterior rectus sheath are made and vacuum drains are placed subcutaneously.

Use of interrupted 'near-and-far' non-absorbable sutures taking alternate large and small bites of tissue from each side of the defect facilitates repair of most incisional hernias. The sutures are not tied until all have been placed. At this stage approximation of the edges of the defect can be carried out by tying the sutures. This can be achieved with surprising ease and lack of tension.

Subcutaneous drains are used during repair of incisional hernias and it is preferable to use a suction drain or one with multiple small side holes.

Parastomal hernias

Paracolostomy or paraileostomy hernias appear as troublesome bulges alongside the stoma and may interfere with the accurate fitting of the appliance. These hernias may cause intestinal obstruction and require operative treatment. The incision should be placed well away from the stoma and if the protrusion is large, an ellipse of skin overlying the hernia is removed. After isolation and excision of the sac, the edge of the defect is sutured to the loop of bowel forming the stoma.

References

Bertelsen S. (1968). The surgical treatment of spigelian hernia. *Surg. Gynaecol. Obstet*; **122**:567–72.

Dennis C., Varco R.L. :1947). Femoral hernia with gangrenous bowel. *Surgery*; **22**:312.

Glassow F. (1976). Inguinal hernia repair. A comparison of the shouldice and Cooper ligament repair of the posterior inguinal wall. *Amer. J. Surg*; **131**:306–11.

Glassow F. (1978). The shouldice repair for inguinal hernia. In *Hernia*, 2nd edn. (Nyhus L.M., Condon R.E., eds.). Philadelphia: Lippincott.

Gray S.W., Skandalakis J.E., Soria R.E., Rowe J.S. Jr. (1974). Strangulated obturator hernia. *Surgery*; **75(1)**:20–7.

Halverson K., McVay C.B. (1970). Inguinal and femoral hernioplasty. A 22-year study of the authors' methods. *Arch. Surg*; **101**:127–35.

Hunter R.R. (1971). Anatomical repair of midline incisional hernia. *Brit. J. Surg*; **5**:888–91.

Lytle W.J. (1945). The internal inguinal ring. *Brit. J. Surg*; **32**:441.

McEvedy P.G. (1950). Femoral hernia. *Ann. R.Coll.Surg. Engl*; **7**:484.

McVay C.B. (1966). Inguinal hernioplasty. Common mistakes and pitfalls. *Surg. Clin. N.Amer*; **46**:1089–1100.

McVay C.B. (1974). The anatomic basis for inguinal and femoral herinoplasty. *Surg. Gynaecol. Obstet*; **139**:931–45.

McVay C.B., Savage L.E. (1961). Etiology of femoral hernia. *Ann. Surg*; **154**:25–32.

Madden J.L., Hakim S., Agorogiannis A.B. (1971). The anatomy and repair of inguinal hernias. *Surg. Clin. N.Amer*; **51**:1269–92.

Maingot R. (1980). Umbilical and incisional hernia. In *Abdominal Operations*, 7th edn., (Maingot R., ed.) p. 1618. New York: Appleton-Century-Crofts.

Moreno I.G. (1947). Chronic eventration and large hernia. Preoperative treatment by progressive pneumoperitoneum. *Surgery*; **22**:945.

Nyhus L.M. (1978). The preperitoneal approach and iliopubic tract repair of inguinal hernia. In *Hernia*, 2nd edn. (Nyhus L.M., Condon R.E., eds.). Philadelphia: Lippincott.

Nyhus L.M., Condon R.E. (1960). Clinical experience with preperitoneal hernial repair for all types of hernia of the groin, with particular reference to the importance of transversalis fascia analogues. *Amer. J. Surg*; **100**:234–44.

Payson B.A., Schneider K.M., Victor M.B. (1956). Strangulation of a Meckel's diverticulum in a femoral hernia (Littre's). *Ann. Surg*; **144**:277.

Ponka J.L., Brush B.E. (1971). Problem of femoral hernia. *Arch. Surg*; **102**:417.

Rogers F.A. (1959). Strangulated femoral hernia: a review of 170 cases. *Ann. Surg*; **149**:9–20.

Rowe M.I., Clatworthy H.W.J. (1971). The other side of the pediatric inguinal hernia. *Surg. Clin. N.Amer*; **51**:1371.

Tanner N.C. (1942). A 'slide' operation for inguinal and femoral hernia. *Brit. J. Surg*; **29**:18.

Thurston Thieme E. (1971). Recurrent inguinal hernia. *Arch. Surg*; **103**:238–41.

Usher F.C. (1970). The repair of incisional and inguinal hernias. *Surg. Gynaecol. Obstet*; **131**:525.

Zimmerman L.M., Anson B.J. (1967). Special forms of hernia. In *Anatomy and Surgery of Hernia*, 2nd edn. Baltimore: Williams and Wilkins.

Patient care

Introduction

From the strategic point of view the opening and the closing pages of any book have a real advantage and it is with this in mind that your editors have grouped together these four subjects at the close of the book.

The subject of fluid and electrolyte balance really came of age during and immediately after the 1939–1945 conflict and now with the introduction of automated equipment for chemical analysis into so many laboratories, it is possible to monitor the patient's progress with considerable accuracy.

Next to the proper maintenance of hydration and electrolyte levels comes nutritional support. Since it is also now possible to give carbohydrate, amino acids and fats entirely by the venous route, the patient's nutrition can be carried on at all times and under any circumstances. It is remarkable how wounds will heal and infection come under control once the body is provided with the normal building blocks of a balanced diet. The use of the term total parenteral nutrition (TPN) is more accurate than hyperalimentation, but the latter was useful in drawing attention to some remarkable salvage operations which were made possible by this method. It must also be remembered that the natural route for feeding a patient is by far the best when it can be used.

Our knowledge of blood replacement also owes much to the impetus it obtained from the stresses and strains of war. However, the later developments which have taken place in this field and the variety of replacements which can now be provided make a peace-time contribution to care in the operating threatre, not only when blood loss is large but also when clotting and bleeding are abnormal.

The final chapter on infection and cross-infection is a veritable storehouse of information. So much of the surgeon's work is created by infection finding its way into the body or by cross-infection from one patient to another. In addition, in recent years anaerobic organisms have provided a new hazard to wound healing, especially following operations in the abdomen. There is little value in a skilful operation well done when the results are marred by the later entry of micro-organisms. Despite all this, antibiotics and chemotherapy have made much possible that could not even be contemplated before their introduction. In their wake, however, these potent substances have brought a host of new problems which are likely to remain with us for a long time to come.

S.T.

Patient care

51

Fluid, electrolyte and nutritional support

RONALD G. CLARK

Technical advances in surgery over the past 50 years have increasingly placed an additional responsibility on the surgeon to develop and apply techniques which can support body function during the critical phases of the patient's illness. About 100 years ago it was appreciated that infective states were associated with abnormalities of protein and carbohydrate metabolism with alterations in body water and salt content. The introduction of blood transfusion about 60 years ago was followed by the development of the intravenous 'drip' in the 1930s and its use uncovered alterations in water and sodium metabolism which were directly attributable to injury and infection. These observations led to the injured state being regarded as one of sodium and water retention. About the same time those features of the metabolic response to surgery which affect protein metabolism were described by Sir David Cuthbertson and form the basis on which modern techniques of nutritional management have developed.

These views of surgical care have developed from the confined one of measuring water balance and blood chemicals to an appreciation of the effects of disease and injury on the composition of the body, of how the mechanism controlling the essential functions of the body are affected and the importance of these effects on morbidity and mortality. The care of the surgical patient should be devoted, first, to the support of the function of the extracellular fluid by administration of water and electrolytes, principally sodium, and secondly to the maintenance of the metabolic processes operating continually within the cells in a concept described as the body cell mass. Although this chapter deals with these two aspects separately their functions are interdependent and this should be reflected in a unified policy of patient management.

Fluid and electrolytes

Not long ago postoperative renal failure, shock, fluid and electrolyte abnormalities and 'biochemical death' were common in routine surgical practice. During the past three decades the incidence of these complications has decreased dramatically because of a better understanding of the importance of maintaining volume and osmotic equilibrium in the body fluids. The physiological background to body function in fluid and electrolyte metabolism is complex and often leads to confusion in the mind of the clinician; yet, paradoxically, the tools which are available for the management of fluid and electrolyte metabolism are limited so that the technique must remain simple. Another factor which leads to confusion is the variety of recommended practices for maintenance of fluid and electrolyte balance, each giving the impression that it alone will succeed. The policy behind fluid and electrolyte maintenance should first of all be based on the philosophy that the patient should be provided with solutions of sufficient volume and content to allow the homeostatic processes to restore and maintain body function.

It is rarely the infusion regimen itself which maintains normality or corrects an abnormality, it is the normal homeostatic processes of the body which achieve this if they are provided with the fluid and substrates of the right type in appropriate quantity.

Management of fluid and electrolyte metabolism is based on an understanding of the following:

1 Properties of the fluids within the various compartments of the body.
2 The mechanisms of homeostasis which maintain the distribution of these fluids.
3 The needs of the patient to maintain function of these fluid spaces.
4 Changes in these mechanisms which can be induced by injury and acute disease.

Properties of the fluid spaces

Body water

Water accounts for 55–60% of the body's weight in the adult male and 40–45% in the adult female, the difference being accounted for by the greater quantity of fat in the female body. This ratio is relatively constant during most of the adult years, starting at 75% of the body weight at birth and decreasing rapidly to adult values in the early years of development and latterly decreasing further with senility. The total amount of water in the body remains remarkably constant for each adult, but should not be regarded as a static pool of fluid within a covering of skin into which fluid is passed at the top and losses leak out at the bottom. Movement of large quantities of fluid and electrolytes takes place within the body which cannot be determined by the measurement of intake and output. There is continuous movement of fluid from the circulation across the capillary membrane and in the lymphatic circulation. Within the alimentary tract in a period of 24 h the movements of fluid amount to 9 l containing 900 mmol of sodium and glomerular filtration accounts for 175 l which contain 20 000 mmol of sodium. In addition there are smaller circulations into the areas which are termed transcellular compartments which include the CSF, synovial fluid and a smaller movement of fluid and electrolytes into the pleural and peritoneal spaces. Changes in any of these internal circulations of fluid can influence significantly the distribution of body fluids.

The water within the body is not a uniform phase and is located in two compartments which are in equilibrium, extracellular and intracellular spaces, each having different functions. The extracellular fluid furnishes the means of transport of materials within the body with, in addition, supportive and environmental functions and is the body compartment the clinician is concerned with most directly in fluid and electrolyte metabolism. The intracellular fluid is the medium in which all metabolic functions take place and is the compartment of the body directly related to nutritional management.

Extracellular fluid (ECF)

The extracellular fluid is composed of the plasma within the blood vessels and the interstitial and transcellular fluid which lie outside the vessel and it is assumed that they are in equilibrium with one another. Approximately 20% of the body weight is accounted for by the ECF which means that in the average adult male the volume is 14–16 l of which 3 l are plasma. The ECF fluid performs a supportive function in the same manner as the skeleton and collagen tissue, providing a medium which engulfs the cells, composed of fluid which permeates a gelatinous ground substance traversed by collagen fibres and applied to the skeleton and tendons. The size of the ECF is related to the skeletal size, but it is capable of a wide range of variation, particularly in diseased states when it is most likely to expand. It behaves not unlike a sponge in which fluid can accumulate without large changes in pressure, the normal pressure being between -8–-4 mmHg. Large volumes of fluid can accumulate in this space before oedema develops which usually occurs when the pressure reaches zero.

The composition of the ECF is maintained by achieving a balance between the concentration of the electrolytes such as the cations, sodium, potassium, calcium and magnesium with their appropriate anions. These maintain osmolality which controls the distribution of fluids within the body. The hydrogen ion content is maintained by groups of substances within the ECF which take part in acid base balance in conjunction with renal and pulmonary mechanisms.

The ECF transports essential substrates and oxygen to the cells and metabolites including carbon dioxide from the cells. The distance between the capillary membrane and the cell membrane is measured in microns and, therefore, transit in the interstitial fluid between the circulation and the cells is relatively rapid.

Composition of ECF. The principal extracellular cation is sodium and there are between 3500 and 4000 mmol of sodium within the body, of which one quarter lies within the bone and is not in rapid equilibrium with the remainder of the body sodium. Therefore, the quantity of sodium which equilibrates with the extracellular space, termed the exchangeable sodium, is between 2400 and 2800 mmol. The concentration of sodium within the extracellular fluid is 140 mmol/l and the extracellular quantity of sodium is between 2000 and 2500 mmol. The sodium content of the body is maintained by a balance between the intake which is normally 100 mmol/day and the losses in the urine of 80–90 mmol with the remaining smaller amount being found in the sweat and faeces. Whereas almost three-quarters of the exchangeable sodium of the body resides in the extracellular space, only 2% of the extracellular potassium is outside the cell at a concentration of 3.6–5.0 mmol/l, the total extracellular potassium being 60 mmol. Calcium is present at a concentration of 2.1–2.6 mmol/l in the plasma of which half is in the unbound ionisable available form, and magnesium is present in the concentration of 1.5 mmol/l. The principal anions in the extracellular fluid are chloride at a concentration of 100 mmol/l and bicarbonate 25 mmol/l, the remainder being much smaller amounts of protein, organic acids e.g. lactate, sulphate and phosphate.

The close relationship between the physical properties of the ECF and its content is exemplified by the fact that sodium and its associated anion are responsible for more than 95% of the osmotic activity and less than 4% is the effect of glucose and urea. The osmolality of plasma is 290 mosmol/kg and changes in sodium concentration are frequently associated with similar alterations in osmolality.

Intracellular fluid (ICF)

Intracellular fluid is contained within the body cell mass, where metabolic processes take place, comprising skeletal and cardiac muscle, the tissues of the gut, liver, kidney, brain, lung and the endocrine and reproductive organs. By its relationship to the body mass the ICF is related less directly to skeletal size than ECF and more directly to heredity, the state of health and nutrition and environmental factors such as employment which determine muscle function. It is, therefore, a component of body composition which is capable of a wide range of variation even in normal health. Intracellular water represents between 25–30% of the body weight in the male and 20–25% of the body weight in the female which means that on average the ICF is in excess of 20 l.

The ICF contains more than 95% of the total potassium in the body and 50% of the magnesium. The major anion is phosphate with a somewhat larger amount of protein and a very small amount of bicarbonate within the cell. Because of its metabolic activity the body cell mass determines a number of related features including the size of the red cell mass, oxygen consumption, cardiac output and resting metabolic expenditure all of which will vary with cell mass. Although convenient to regard the body cell mass as a homogenous compartment, it is divisible into two, one part consisting of those tissues which work ceaselessly to maintain life i.e. the viscera, and the other part comprising tissues which relax between exertions such as skeletal muscle and certain smooth muscles. In severe wasting of the body, the muscle mass diminishes rapidly whereas the size of the viscera does not become less and may be protected until the very late stages of depletion.

On the basis of these differences in function between the extracellular and intracellular space, it is clear why the management of the critically ill, in particular resuscitation, should be devoted first to the restoration of normality in the extracellular space. Control of the intracellular environment cannot be effectively achieved until there is a stable and functionally operative extracellular fluid.

Homeostasis

The body regulates the distribution of water between the various compartments, and the composition of the fluid in these compartments by homeostatic mechanisms. Abnormalities develop in water and sodium metabolism when the controlling influences of these regulators is altered by disease or when their capacity to control the internal environment is exceeded.

The features of the ECF which have the highest priority in homeostasis are volume followed by osmolality. The ECF volume is directly related to the concentration of the osmotic reactive particles within it, 95% of which are the sodium salts; thus water and sodium intake are the items of greatest importance to the clinician. Two hormones, antidiuretic hormone (ADH) and aldosterone, maintain control by their effect on water and sodium balance. An increase in ADH level reduces urine volume by promoting water reabsorption at the distal end of the tubule and a decrease in ADH is followed by a brisk diuresis. The stimulus to ADH activity results from a change in osmolality acting on the osmocentres in the supraoptic and supraventricular nuclei of the hypothalamus. Besides plasma osmolality another effective stimulus for ADH release is a fall in plasma volume irrespective of osmolar status. The sensor areas for this reflex are in the baroceptors in the great vessels and right heart which are sensitive to changes in plasma volume, a decrease inducing an increase in ADH output.

Aldosterone is synthesised in the zona glomerulosa of the adrenal cortex which is sensitive to changes in the plasma concentration of sodium, a reduction inducing an increase in hormone production, but it is likely that a more important stimulus for aldosterone secretion is the renin-angiotensin mechanism. Renin is released from the juxtaglomerular cells around the afferent renal arterioles in response to a drop in circulating volume and it acts on an α_2-globulin to produce angiotensin I which is then converted to angiotensin II, the substance which stimulates aldosterone production.

The renin-angiotensin system may also be activated by renal sympathetic nerves and this may happen irrespective of changes in circulating volume. Thus ADH and aldosterone can each be activated by different physiological stimuli, such as changes in osmolality and sodium concentration, but both can be stimulated by changes in volume or pressure and it is likely that they act in unison *via* all of these mechanisms in their control of the ECF. The roles of other hormones are less clearly defined.

Fluid and electrolyte requirements

The clinician's concern with measurable aspects of fluid and electrolyte metabolism involves the recording of intake and output, but it is unwise to rely solely on the figures on the ward chart and interpretation of their significance must be combined with an understanding of the pathological process and its effects on body spaces and function. In addition, estimation of the concentration of electrolytes in the blood, though done routinely, can be singularly unhelpful in that they may identify an abnormality but rarely identify the cause.

Water and sodium needs are determined by the manner and the rate at which they are lost from the body both by the renal and extrarenal routes. The renal losses in normal circumstances are the means whereby the homeostatic processes regulate the ECF. Extrarenal losses include insensible or invisible losses which occur from the skin by evaporation of sweat, as liquid in the faeces, or as vapour in the lungs and in normal states of health remain constant. Abnormalities of fluid and electrolyte metabolism are most likely to occur when additional extrarenal losses are introduced e.g. nasogastric aspiration, diarrhoea, fistulous drainage, serous drainage or increases in loss from denuded areas of skin such as burns. When this occurs the ability of the homeostatic responses to compensate by their action on the kidney may be overwhelmed or inhibited and the function of the ECF compromised.

Renal losses

The normal daily urine output is 1500 ml with a content of 60–100 mmol sodium. Urine is produced as the end result of a daily glomerular filtrate of 180 l of plasma containing 20 000 mmol of sodium and only very small changes in renal tubular reabsorption are required to produce major changes in the volume and composition of the urine. The minimum urine volume necessary for the excretion of the osmotic load of solutes such as urea is between 600–800 ml/day and failure to achieve this minimum output will lead to accumulation and produce a prerenal uraemia. At the other extreme, large quantities of urine can be pro-duced during a diuresis induced by either pharmacological or endocrine means. The urinary sodium output can be depressed to a few millimole per day during a phase of water and sodium deprivation and can increase to 200–300 mmol/day during a natriuresis. The metabolic processes of the body produce about 600 mosmol daily, comprising urea, hydrogen ion, and potassium and when the urine is maximally concentrated at 1200 mosmol/kg then 600 ml of urine is required for its excretion and, if urine is isotonic to plasma, 2 l of urine would be required illustrating that there is an extensive range of urine output and concentration within which the kidney can play an important part in regulating body fluids.

Extrarenal losses

Insensible losses arise principally by vaporisation of water from the body surfaces and are constant in a normal environment. Provided a patient is lightly clothed or covered, the daily insensible loss from the skin is in the region of 850–1000 ml and from the lungs about 100 ml/day. Heat for vaporisation is generated by the metabolic activity of the patient and will therefore be greater when the metabolic rate is increased in pyrexia, by a change in environment or when insensible water loss is augmented by sweat loss or in burns where the protective function of the skin is lost. Normally the faeces contain 100–200 ml of water but with diarrhoea there is an excess loss of fluid and mucus from the bowel and the volume may increase to 1–2 l/day.

In normal circumstances the sodium content of the insensible losses is low and homeostasis can maintain effective control of the ECF for prolonged periods of time in the presence of a reduced intake, but during a total fast the insensible losses deplete the ECF relentlessly with failure and death after 10–14 days. Abnormal renal losses such as gastrointestinal juices and plasma are outside homeostatic control and isosmolar with plasma containing sodium between 80 and 140 mmol/l depending on the site of loss. Daily replacement of these losses is essential to maintain ECF and it must be by isosmolar solutions, usually saline.

Intake

The normal daily intake of water and sodium is 3.0 l/day and 100 mmol sodium with 60 mmol potassium. The water intake consists of about 1 l of fluid with the remainder contained within the food. Most of the electrolytes are contained within the food, but considerable variation in intake can arise because of taste and style of preparation.

Metabolic response to injury

Following injury or acute disease, the regulators which control the ECF space and the metabolic functions within the body are altered, a reaction called the 'metabolic response to injury'. This reaction, which occurs irrespective of the method of patient management, is related in magnitude to the severity of the physical insult. Although it can be most readily identified following injury, it can be seen in some form following most acute diseases. It is of relatively minor importance in most surgical patients who have an uncomplicated postoperative course and the patient shows little evidence of it apart from some weight loss. It achieves importance in severe illness during intravenous therapy when metabolic problems can arise because of the interaction of therapy and the altered homeostatic responses. At this point in the chapter only those responses affecting the ECF will be discussed.

Injury without replacement therapy

In the untreated state, injury is associated with a reduction in ECF volume. Circulating volume decreases by loss of blood or plasma externally or internally and there may be a relative loss by the effects of anaesthesia on the circulation. In addition, traumatic oedema develops in the injured areas, part of the losses comprising the 'third space', and evaporative losses will increase during the exposure of tissues and viscera. These are all stimuli which one would normally expect to induce a homeostatic response and undoubtedly contribute to the effects of injury on fluid and electrolyte metabolism which would be reversible by replacement of the appropriate fluid lost. However, in addition a stimulus, related to the injury itself, induces an obligatory or inappropriate secretion of those hormones which are involved in the control of the ECF space and which persist for some time, irrespective of management.

The effects of this response are concentrated in the organ which effectively controls ECF, the kidney. Within the first 2–3 days of injury there is an obligatory oliguria when the urine volume is 600–1000 ml with negative free water clearance. The specific gravity of the urine increases and the osmolar excretion is above normal at 800 mosmol/day principally due to the increase in urea output. Sodium excretion decreases rapidly and remains fixed and may almost disappear from the urine within 2–3 days. The potassium excretion is greater than would normally be expected. As long as the volume deficit persists, the phase of antidiuresis and restricted ability of the kidney to excrete sodium will persist so that the urine volume remains low and sodium output is restricted to 1–2 mmol/day. It will be seen from this why the untreated injured patient was at risk of prerenal uraemia and in severe cases to renal tubular necrosis.

Injury with replacement therapy

The patient, who receives replacement therapy during and after his injury, presents the classical description of the metabolic response to injury, namely, water and sodium retention with expansion of the ECF. The obligatory hormonal responses, outlined in the untreated case, remain in operation, but of lesser severity because the deficits incurred by the internal losses of fluids are corrected. There will, therefore, be a phase of antidiuresis and inadequate sodium excretion, particularly in the first 2–3 days when the urine volume will remain in the upper part of the 600–1000 ml range, with negative free water clearance, an increase in specific gravity and increased osmolar and urea excretion. The urinary sodium excretion will be much higher, but not enough to compensate for the sodium intake and the ultimate effect is an expansion of the ECF due to water and sodium retention. The antidiuretic phase may last only 2 or 3 days, whereas the inability to excrete sodium persists for a much longer period. If potassium is infused the urinary excretion is greater than normal.

Mediators

The hormones most directly implicated and about which most is known are ADH and aldosterone, both of whose secretion are increased early in the postoperative period. The responses, though obligatory, are however short lived and do not last as long as their effects. Catecholamines are also increased during this period and could well influence water and sodium metabolism by their action of the renin-angiotensin mechanism *via* the renal sympathetic nerves. Other hormones such as the glucocorticoids may also act. Alterations in renal haemodynamics have some part to play in the immediate postoperative period, but changes in glomerular filtration rate have not been found to persist long enough to be a major factor.

Clinical relevance

In the untreated state the objective of the metabolic response is to conserve the ECF. The changes in renal function are induced more rapidly than would occur were the sole stimulus to be an absence of fluid and electrolytes. The treated state is an example of a homeostatic response without an objective in that the conservation of the ECF continues despite the ability to maintain it by infusion therapy. The ECF will, therefore, expand and the extent will depend on the type of fluid infused. Modern management involves the use of 'balanced salt' solutions such as Hartmann's during the operation and water and sodium infusion until the patient is able to take fluid by mouth. During the first 24–36 h the ECF will expand by 2–3 l and an increase in sodium of 200–300 mmol. When the antidiuresis phase diminishes, sodium retention persists and an infusion of isotonic saline will lead to more sodium retention which stimulates an increase in ADH to retain water and maintain osmolality whereas an administration of 5% dextrose alone will dilute, but not expand, the ECF. Neither of these extremes is acceptable and it is current practice to steer the middle course and give some water and some sodium, but not much of either in a 2.5–3.0 l regimen containing 70–100 mmol of sodium.

Modest expansions of the ECF do not constitute a serious hazard to the average adult postoperative patient, but increased vigilance and monitoring is essential to avoid overloading during intravenous therapy in the young, the elderly and those with cardio-respiratory disease. It is probable that too many patients are given unnecessary intravenous infusion for too long after operation: where there are no extrarenal losses quite small volumes, low in sodium, could be given earlier by mouth with safety. However, where there are extrarenal losses, which are common in gastrointestinal surgery, the need for adequate intravenous replacement of the isosmolar losses is paramount and it is in this group of patients that proper replacement has reduced the incidence of serious abnormalities in fluid and electrolyte metabolism.

Hyponatraemia

A decrease in serum sodium concentration is the most common electrolyte abnormality found in hospital practice. The incidence is highest in surgical patients. Theoretically, hyponatraemia can arise from an increase in ECF, a deficit in sodium or from disproportionate changes in both. In surgical practice, the most common type is a dilutional hyponatraemia arising from an interaction of intravenous therapy and the metabolic response to injury. All infusion regimens are isosmolar on administration but those which contain 5% dextrose rapidly become hypo-osmolar when the dextrose is metabolised and the degree of dilution induced after operation will depend on the quantity of 5% dextrose infused. The usual finding is that of a mild dilution decreasing the serum sodium from 136 to 132 mmol during a four-day infusion; but, if prolonged, the stage is set for severe dilution and eventually water intoxication after some days should the administration of such a regimen be over enthusiastic (*see* Water excess).

Disorders of water metabolism

Dehydration

Pure dehydration is uncommon in clinical practice and is seen rarely in severe prolonged dysphagia, unconscious states, as a consequence of osmotic diuresis e.g. diabetic ketoacidosis and in diabetes insipidus. Dehydration affects both the extra and intracellular water compartment and a loss in excess of 10% of the total body water will produce clinical signs. When severe, the symptoms are those of a reduced ECF volume with hypovolaemia, coma and death after 10–12 days. There is haemoconcentration with a serum sodium of 160–180 mmol/l and osmolality of 340–380 mosmol/l. Severe oliguria and metabolic acidosis develop with an increase in blood urea which also contributes to the increase in serum osmolality. As these patients are unable to drink, rehydration is achieved by infusion of 5% dextrose, but overenthusiasm should be avoided so that the period of rehydration should extend over 48 h in severe cases to allow redistribution of fluid to the intracellular space. If large quantities are infused rapidly into the ECF, there is a risk of internal bleeding particularly in the cerebral circulation, if adequate time has not been allowed for cellular rehydration.

Water excess

An excess of body water is most commonly iatrogenic, following over-administration of water by mouth (as seen in compulsive water and beer drinkers) or by inappropriate intravenous infusion therapy. The latter is seen particularly in postoperative patients who tolerate infusions of pure water or hypotonic fluid badly by virtue of endocrine effects of the metabolic response to injury. It can also arise in cases of Addison's disease or failure of the anterior pituitary gland and in states of inappropriate secretion of ADH such as oatcell carcinoma of the bronchus, acute porphyria, head injury and acute alcoholism. The body sodium content remains normal, but body weight increases as the total body water enlarges and symptoms of lassitude, nausea, headache and coma develop once the total body water increase exceeds 3–4 l. In the advanced stage, the condition is recognised as water intoxication when the serum sodium decreases below 115 mmol/l and the serum osmolality decreases below 250 mosmol/l. Treatment is urgent and demands cessation of water administration until the insensible water losses are sufficient to restore the serum sodium and osmolality to normal. When the condition is acute with the development of coma, a small infusion of hypertonic (5%) saline has been employed in some patients with success, but with the risk of further exaggerating the increase in total water. In other cases, a water diuresis has been induced by the use of mannitol.

Disorders of sodium metabolism

Increased body sodium

An excess of sodium is usually accompanied by an isotonic expansion of the ECF space. The most common cause in surgical practice is the excessive intravenous administration of saline solutions. The other group of patients in which this disorder is commonly seen suffer diseases of the heart, liver and kidney where homeostatic regulation is abnormal; secondary hyperaldosteronism with inappropriate antidiuretic activity may play some part. Increases in body sodium also develop in states of severe hypoalbuminaemia in association with protein-calorie malnutrition, protein-losing states of the bowel and kidney, and in hepatic disease when the plasma colloid osmotic pressure is decreased.

When the expansion of the ECF space is isotonic, the serum sodium and osmolality are normal and only the serum albumin and haematocrit are diminished by dilution. When associated with chronic disease of the heart, liver and kidneys, there is a greater tendency to dilution and development of hyponatraemia and hypoosmolality. The over administration of saline must be stopped. Severe hypoproteinaemia may require the administration of concentrated albumin solution or the appropriate nutritional therapy in association with diuretics but excessive use of diuretics in hypoproteinaemia carries a risk of circulatory collapse. Aldosterone antagonists have a place in the management of chronic liver and renal disease where a secondary hyperaldosteronism is present.

Sodium deficit

Pure losses of sodium from the body are unusual in surgical practice. More commonly salt tends to be lost along with water, usually at a concentration near isotonic. The deficit affects the ECF and when losses exceed 1 l the condition becomes clinically significant. In surgical practice the commonest cause is loss of gastrointestinal fluid from vomiting, fistulae or profuse diarrhoea, less commonly the cause may be renal following a prolonged diuresis. On examination the patient looks drawn and weary complaining of lassitude, faintness and muscle cramps.

While the losses remain isotonic, there is little change in the serum electrolyte pattern and osmolality, but the haematocrit will rise slowly. Later there is dilution especially after intravenous fluids have been given or from cell water which is mobilised to correct the deficit, as a consequence of the catabolic effects of the disease and starvation. Treatment is by the infusion of isotonic solutions to restore the deficit in ECF which

may be many litres. The management of the severely affected case may require the use of central venous pressure (CVP) measurement to monitor therapy. Once repletion is started, potassium depletion may be unmasked which has developed as a consequence of the extrarenal losses, in addition to the loss of intracellular potassium by catabolism.

Disorders of potassium

Deficit of potassium

Potassium resides predominantly within the cells of the body and little indication of its status can be obtained from blood estimation. A reduction in total body potassium need not represent a deficit if the loss occurs with tissue loss, e.g. in protein-calorie restriction. A deficit is a state in which there has been a differential loss of potassium from the cells decreasing the intracellular content or concentration. Potassium depletion can arise from lack of intake which is common in surgical practice or from increased extrarenal losses which is found in many gut conditions such as chronic vomiting, diarrhoea, extensive bowel resection, high small intestinal fistulae and after extensive burns or trauma. Deficits can also arise from increased renal losses of potassium following diuretics such as frusemide and carbonic anhydrase inhibitors and after prolonged exposure to corticosteroids or aldosterone.

The diagnosis of potassium deficiency may not be obvious because it tends to be associated with other clinical states, but it should be suspected when there has been prolonged loss of gastrointestinal secretion and especially where there is severe metabolic alkalosis. Not all cases of hypokalaemia have a potassium deficit but where the serum potassium has been low, particularly in the range of 2–3.5 mmol/l, for some time, the relationship tends to be much more close. The diagnosis is suggested by generalised weakness, anorexia and nausea with fibrillation of skeletal muscle. There is also hypotension and disturbance of GI function such as hypotonia and ileus. ECG changes commonly include a depression of the ST segment, inversion of the T wave and exaggeration of the U wave. The concentrating power of the kidney is diminished and urine of a low specific gravity is produced. Prevention is the best policy: potassium should be given prophylactically, especially to those with extrarenal losses who are most likely to be at risk. Daily infusion of 50 mmol in the form of potassium chloride should be added to most intravenous regimes which are likely to last more than a day or so, and oral supplements should be given where appropriate. In severe depletion the deficit may extend to 400–600 mmol but rapid replacement should not be attempted as it may produce cardiac arrythmias. It is advisable in the treatment of severe states for the patient to have an ECG monitor. It is rarely necessary to replace more than 100–150 mmol of potassium during any 24 h period and it is never essential completely to restore the deficit during intensive management. Potassium depletion is always associated with a deficit of water and sodium which should also be replaced.

Potassium excess

Large increases in body potassium are uncommon and are manifested by the presence of hyperkalaemia with a metabolic acidosis. Renal insufficiency is the common cause – potassium is mobilised from the cell space at a rate faster than the kidneys can excrete it. The rate at which hyperkalaemia develops is dependent on the catabolic stimulus to the cells especially when sepsis and starvation are present. When the serum potassium is increased above 6 mmol/l and ECG changes include the disappearance of P waves and widening of the QRS complex with high peaked T waves, immediate treatment is indicated. When severe hyperkalaemia is present, the intravenous administration of calcium gluconate maintains myocardial stability and the acidosis may require correction by the use of sodium bicarbonate solution. The administration of an insulin/glucose regimen of 300–500 ml 20% glucose + one unit of insulin/3 g glucose will promote transfer of potassium from the extracellular to the intracellular space. Dialysis may be necessary if renal impairment is severe.

Acid-base disturbances

Metabolic acidosis

Metabolic acidosis develops when there is a true or relative increase in the concentration of hydrogen ion in the extracellular space which can arise either by an accumulation of excess acid or by the loss of base from the body. Excess hydrogen ion can arise from lactacidaemia during shock with hypoperfusion of tissues, in ketoacidosis in starvation or diabetes, or where impaired function renders the kidney incapable of excreting hydrogen ion. A relative increase in hydrogen ion develops when fluids of alkaline pH such as pancreatic juice are lost from the body in large quantities, depleting the buffers within the ECF and at the same time creating a deficit in volume which limits the kidneys' capacity to excrete the relative increase in acid. The compensatory mechanism in such cases is the respiratory system and when the acidosis becomes severe the patient develops air hunger. The rapid

respiration rate with deep inspiration reduces the arterial P_{CO_2}.

The arterial blood pH can be reduced to 7.1–7.2 and the P_{CO_2} is less than 33 mmHg and the bicarbonate is reduced from 24 mmol/l to 10 mmol/1. Detection of a metabolic acidosis merely recognises an effect and the major concern should be directed to the underlying cause and administering the specific treatment. Correction of the physical abnormalities in the blood e.g. by the infusion of 4.2% sodium bicarbonate may correct the abnormality in acid base, but it does little to treat the cause. The total amount of alkali to restore normal acid base control can be calculated by estimating the deficit of bicarbonate for each litre of ECF and multiplying this by 20 (the convenient approximation of ECF volume) but it is rarely necessary to titrate completely back to normality. The appropriate treatment of low flow acidosis is the restoration of tissue perfusion by restoring volume. When the acidosis is due to loss of alkaline gastrointestinal juices, the cause is treated by correcting the deficit in ECF volume by infusions of saline or balanced salt solutions to restore renal perfusion and allow the kidney to correct the abnormality. Infusion of hypertonic sodium bicarbonate solution is not recommended for acidosis due to renal insufficiency except where the need is extremely urgent, because of the danger of fluid overload and the development of cardiac failure following the high dosage of sodium in the solution.

Metabolic alkalosis

Metabolic alkalosis describes a state when the blood pH is elevated in association with a loss of hydrogen ion or an absolute increase in the concentration and amount of bicarbonate in the body. It is found most commonly with loss of acid from the stomach, in prolonged vomiting due to pyloric stenosis or prolonged nasogastric suction. The alkalosis is more likely to be severe in duodenal ulceration than in gastric carcinoma. It can also arise after prolonged intakes of alkali by mouth or vein and is seen as a secondary phenomenon in hyperaldosteronism. There is a close link between metabolic alkalosis and the abnormal electrolyte pattern which can be described as hypokalaemic hypochloraemia. The biochemical findings are usually quite clear; the serum sodium may be normal or slightly low, potassium 1.0–2.5 mmol/l, chloride 50–70 mmol/l, pH 7.5–7.56 and bicarbonate 35–45 mmol/l. The patient presents with severe apnoea, dehydration, signs of hypokalaemia and tetany which develop because the ionisable fraction of plasma calcium decreases as the pH increases.

When hydrochloric acid is secreted by the parietal cells of the stomach into the gastric lumen, bicarbonate accumulates temporarily in the ECF and is excreted in the urine as an 'alkaline tide'. In the early stages of vomiting this compensation is maintained. The continual loss of water and sodium induces an aldosterone response which inhibits bicarbonate excretion and promotes even greater urinary loss of potassium than normal which with the persistent loss of potassium in the gastric juice may create a deficit of between 500–600 mmol after 7–10 days. As further potassium is mobilised from the cells, it is replaced by sodium and hydrogen ions which create an intracellular acidosis rendering the renal tubular cells less capable of correcting the alkaline state.

Treatment is devoted to the correction of three major deficits; water, sodium and potassium. Large volumes of saline-containing fluids are essential to restore function of the ECF volume and restore the ability of the kidney to correct some of the metabolic defect. Potassium should also be given in the form of potassium chloride and, although it may take many days before the potassium deficit is fully replenished, the ability of the kidney to correct the alkalosis is restored shortly after the start of the potassium chloride infusion. Where severe alkalotic states have been reported in conditions, such as the Zollinger-Ellison syndrome, dilute hydrochloric acid or ammonium chloride have been employed to replace the hydrogen ion deficit, but their use has been superceded by the H_2 antagonist cimetidine which abolishes gastric acid secretion.

Nutritional care of the surgical patient

A significant proportion of a surgeon's practice involves diseases which can affect the patient's nutrition, particularly so in malignancy, chronic disease of the intestinal tract, after major injury, operation and infection, and in peripheral vascular and cardiac disease. Surgeons have always been conscious of the contributory effect which poor nutrition can have on a patient's response to disease and there is a substantial volume of literature in the 1930s and 1940s commenting upon the problem and describing the methods available at that time. Before the 1960s, correction of nutritional deficit was restricted to manipulation of the oral diet under the guidance of the ward sister or dietitian and in exceptional circumstances various techniques of gastro-intestinal intubation or proctoclysis were used. These techniques were not wholly successful because of poor understanding of the metabolic consequences of disease and also because the preparations used were inadequate.

The first modern advance was the introduction of nutrient solutions for parenteral use in the late 1950s when the early protein solutions were hydrolysates of whole protein containing 70% free amino acids. There were also a variety of fat emulsions based on vegetable oil, the most satisfactory being that derived from soybean. At that time access to the circulation was restricted to peripheral veins and thrombophlebitis, a common complication, tended to limit the period of parenteral nutrition to between 10 and 20 days. This problem was overcome by the introduction of central venous catheterisation enabling safe and long-term access, in some cases permanently. There has been continual improvement and refinement of these solutions which, with the addition of vitamins and minerals, have contributed to the efficacy of the nutritional regimens. A significant recent development has been the increased use of enteral nutrition with the introduction of new techniques and preparations such as the elemental and low residue diets which are readily absorbed from the gastrointestinal tract. These new preparations are soluble in water and can be infused through fine-bore tubes which greatly diminish the complications associated with long-term enteral feeding in the past.

It is now possible to nourish patients efficiently for prolonged periods of time by either the intravenous or enteral route. In the critically ill and severely undernourished this improvement in patient care limits morbidity, improves wound healing and the response to infection and maintains muscle function, particularly cardiac and respiratory. It also allows visceral function within the liver, gut, lung and brain to continue at an optimal level. These benefits are difficult to measure in objective terms, but the newer methods of nutritional assessment are helping identify these effects. Nutritional support is, therefore, routine in modern patient care to maintain the function of the body cell mass and provide optimum conditions for more specific treatment.

In clinical practice the causes of malnutrition are several. Partial or total starvation is often present in association with anorexia, intractable symptoms or obstruction of the GI tract, and this may be combined with excess catabolism with injury or sepsis. In addition the available nutrients may not be used optimally because of dysfunction of the intestine or liver; and when large extrarenal losses are present e.g. in burns or enterocutaneous fistulae, the continuing loss of formed protein may place an additional stress on body protein synthesis.

Factors which affect nutritional status

Starvation

Starvation is the major cause of most clinical nutritional problems and induces a well recognised response by the body to reduce the energy and protein needs of the body. The ultimate effect is a loss in body weight as the body cell mass is depleted, affecting skeletal muscle within the first few weeks, and the viscera later.

There is a gradual reduction in daily urinary excretion of nitrogen from 10 g to 6 g reflecting the reduction in the turnover rate of body protein and decreases in both synthesis and catabolism. The resting energy expenditure also decreases by 30% to reach a plateau by the fourth week of starvation when the rate of depletion in body protein and energy is also less rapid. The source of endogenous energy changes as the patient moves from a state of carbohydrate adaptation to one of fat dependence with utilisation of ketone bodies; during this change-over, amino acids maintain the supply of carbohydrate by gluconeogenesis. Ketonaemia develops gradually during the first week indicating an increased rate of fat mobilisation and then stabilises at the level in the blood of 8–10 times that of a normally nourished individual. The body becomes ketoadapted and capable of utilising ketones as a source of energy, therefore the need to mobilise protein as a source of carbohydrate diminishes. From the early stages the blood glucose diminishes in conjunction with blood insulin levels while free fatty acid levels increase. Throughout this time there is a loss of the intracellular constituents of potassium, calcium, phosphate and sulphate in the urine in a constant proportion to nitrogen excretion indicating that the process is one of dissolution of tissue. There are no differential losses which by themselves would create a metabolic abnormality. This process of adaptation is gradual and the governing factors are the reduction in nutrient substrates, reduction in insulin secretion and increase in hormones responsible for fat mobilisation.

Total starvation is an uncommon finding in clinical practice. Partial starvation where the patient is able to take only a limited amount of nutrition is commoner. This means that the classical picture of starvation which can be expressed in biochemical terms may not always be evident and that the process of adaptation to ketone utilisation may not be complete. However, the ultimate effect on body mass is always one of diminution and the nutritional needs of such patients are, therefore, less than normal. The reintroduction of nutritional care readily reverses the metabolic features of starvation and the condition tends to be relatively easy to manage in clinical practice.

Catabolism

The catabolic process occurs commonly after injury, sepsis or inflammation and develops irrespective of the nutritional intake persisting until the underlying clinical cause resolves. It was first described by Sir David Cuthbertson in the early 1930s who identified the source of increased urinary losses of nitrogen, potassium, sulphate and phosphate after injury as the body cell mass, principally skeletal muscle. The ultimate effect is a loss of cell mass and body protein not unlike starvation, but it differs in that the turnover of proteins is increased and, although both synthesis and catabolism are increased, the balance is in favour of catabolism. There are therefore competing processes between synthesis of new protein for tissue repair, acute phase reactants and antibodies, and catabolism which mobilises intracellular material to provide substrate for these new functions and the conversion of amino acids to carbohydrate. Some indication of the extent of this process can be obtained from measurement of the urinary nitrogen excretion which increases from the normal daily value of 10 g–15 g after an abdominal operation to 18–20 g during severe intra-abdominal sepsis and 20–25 g after moderately severe burns.

Carbohydrate utilisation decreases with hyperglycaemia and a tendency to lactacidaemia and the patient becomes less tolerant to glucose with evidence of insulin resistance. Throughout the period of catabolism the liver is stimulated to produce glucose by gluconeogenesis and appears unresponsive to the normal inhibitory influences of glucose administration. Fat mobilisation is increased and free fatty acids increase in the blood, but ketonaemia may not be evident. There is also an increase in resting energy expenditure which occurs in association with the increase in protein breakdown and also as a result of increased catecholamine activity.

Catabolism is associated with increased circulating levels of glucocorticoids and catecholamines which are considered to be the mediators of the increase in protein metabolism and energy expenditure. The effect of insulin is decreased initially by a reduction in secretion and later by the development of insulin resistance. Glucagon and growth hormone are also increased inducing mobilisation of fat and insulin resistance.

Attempts to achieve nutritional equilibrium during the catabolic state may require intakes far greater than normal while the patient is less tolerant to glucose infusions and may not be able to utilise exogenous amino acids as effectively as the normal individual. In addition, urinary losses of intracellular constituents such as electrolytes and minerals are greatly enhanced in a proportion greater than the loss of body protein so that when prolonged, the catabolic state may set the scene for intracellular deficiencies at later stages. Recent work has shown that depletion of cell mass can be controlled, but any gain by formation of new protein for tissue synthesis must await the passage of the catabolic state.

Nutritional assessment

Clinical assessment of nutritional status is done by the 'eyeball test' from the bottom of the bed and is usually quite sufficient for identifying the seriously undernourished patient when done in conjunction with knowledge of the nutritional intake and an understanding of the pathology.

Objective methods of assessment have been developed recently which may be of value to the clinician who is uncertain of the extent of the problem. The usual procedure is to start with the measurement of the body weight which not only can give an estimate of the quantity of tissue lost, but also of the rate of loss which is equally important. Weight loss of more than 10% should cause the clinician to enquire further and weight losses greater than 20% should remind him of the increased morbidity of severe nutritional depletion. In addition, two anthropometric measurements, the triceps skinfold thickness and arm muscle circumference can give some indication of the loss of body fat and of muscle mass and the triceps skinfold thickness appears to be the more accurate. For routine clinical practice considerable information can be obtained merely by pinching the skin and placing one's fingers around the circumference of the upper arm. Severe undernutrition is frequently associated with hypoalbuminaemia and it is common to find reduced levels of prealbumin, transferrin and folate in the blood. The urinary excretion of urea, nitrogen, creatinine and 3-methyl histidine have all been used as means of assessing the size of the body cell mass or its rate of turnover or for the presence of catabolism. Severe depletion is associated with marked reductions in all of these factors.

The three most commonly employed indicators of nutritional status are serum albumin, triceps skinfold thickness and immune skin tests, but it would be unwise to rely on these alone; they merely augment the clinical impression to employ prophylactic feeding.

Incidence

The incidence of malnutrition is highest in general surgical practice and it is found most frequently in patients with upper GI malignancy, conditions of the lower GI tract such as Crohn's disease and ulcerative colitis, and in complications of GI surgery such as fistulae or extensive intra-abdominal infection. The incidence is relatively low in orthopaedic, neurosurgical and urological patients. Enteral or parenteral feeding is required for about 5%, slightly less than half these patients being malnourished and the remainder having prophylactic nutritional support for enforced starvation.

Methods of administration

Choice of route

Both enteral and parenteral feeding are equally effective and the choice will depend on the clinical circumstances of the patient, the personal preference and the experience of the clinician and local factors such as the number of staff available to supervise. As a general rule the enteral route should be used whenever the GI is intact and there is sufficient available length of small intestine. It is the route of choice in about 60% of patients who require nutritional support, this proportion being somewhat less in surgical practice. Enteral feeding is more physiological, employing the controlling influences of the intestinal mucosa and the liver, but it takes somewhat longer to be fully established and requires the assistance of an interested and dedicated nursing staff. The parenteral route has the advantage of greater accuracy and is more rapidly established, but it is less physiological and has the risk of more serious complications. Intravenous nutrient solutions will always be expensive and the demands placed on nursing staff by parenteral nutrition are equally great in terms of personal supervision and attention to detail. Because of the ease by which a full intake can be established quickly, the parenteral route is more suitable for short-term feeding, especially in the critically ill patient whereas enteral feeding is more applicable to long-term feeding. Often parenteral nutrition is used in the initial phase of acute illness followed by enteral feeding once the nutritional state has been stabilised. However, where the intention of the therapy is total rest to the bowel, or where there is an inadequate length of small intestine, the parenteral route remains the only method of feeding possible.

Dosage and prescription

For nutritional support to be fully effective there must be a balanced intake of fluid, electrolyte, minerals and vitamins with protein and energy as carbohydrate and fat. Fluid and electrolyte metabolism and acid-base balance must be stable and seldom is the indication for feeding so urgent that 24–48 h cannot be spent in achieving equilibrium. Though not a true reflection of body cell mass, body weight can be used to give an approximation of the nutritional needs. For each kilogram of body weight the daily protein requirements are 0.15–0.16 gN and 30–35 kcal* so that a 70 kg semi-ambulant in-patient needs 10–12 gN (60–75 g protein) and 2000–2500 kcal.

---

* 1 kcal = 4.2 kJ.

It is common practice to decide intake first by estimating the protein requirements from the body weight and applying the time honoured ratio of 200 kcal for every 1.0 gN. Accurate titration of the nutritional needs is rarely necessary. In a severely undernourished patient of 35 kg who has lost 40% body weight, the nitrogen loss may be 4–6 gN and the energy expenditure 1100–1300 kcal. As soon as a nutritional intake is established the 'turnover rate' of protein and energy increases and the needs of such patients are best served by a graduated increase to normal intake. In the catabolic patient e.g. in extensive intra-abdominal sepsis the daily 'turnover rate' of protein is increased to 15–20 gN but the energy requiremetns do not increase proportionally and calorie: nitrogen ratio is in the region of 120:1 to 150:1 and, therefore, with the exception of burns, the energy requirements of the catabolic patient rarely exceed 2500–3000 kcal. The catabolic stimulus is of short duration, measured in days rather than weeks, and the need for prolonged administration of supra normal intakes exists for a limited period and may not be technically possible. In such circumstances the objective should be to minimise the losses with an intake which is tolerable to the patient, or in the very acute state give insulin with a high glucose intake to promote additional protein synthesis.

The efficient use of nutritional support requires provision of mineral and vitamin supplements and daily requirements of calcium, iron, magnesium, zinc, copper, manganese and phosphorus are available in additive solutions; additional supplements are usually given in seriously depleted stages. It has not yet been established whether the type of patient who requires nutritional support has vitamin requirements which are greater or less than normal, but there is now a wide range of vitamin preparations for enteral and parenteral use and their inclusion in a nutritional regimen is strongly advised.

Monitoring

Whatever the clinical background, regular monitoring is a wise policy until a state of nutritional equilibrium is established and a standard routine should be designed which is simple, practical and reliable and conforms with the investigative facilities available. Routine screening prior to the start of feeding provides a base-line for later comparison and detects abnormalities. It should include measurement of body weight and height, estimate of renal and extrarenal losses, measurement of haemoglobin level, plasma protein and albumin, electrolytes, osmolality and urea, glucose, calcium, magnesium and phosphate and the routine tests of 'liver function': bilirubin, alkaline phosphatase and aminotransferases. Where possible urinary urea or

nitrogen should be measured to confirm that the estimated protein requirements are realistic.

In the first few days of nutritional support, regular measurement of body weight in conjunction with the estimation in a morning blood sample for urea, electrolytes, glucose and osmolality are routine and the frequency thereafter is dictated by clinical progress. The serum phosphate should be measured daily at the start of parenteral nutrition to detect hypophosphataemia and frequent blood sugar estimations are necessary if insulin and glucose therapy is used. Blood lactate should be measured if sorbitol or fructose are the carbohydrate sources because of the increased incidence of lactacidaemia. Urine volume, urea and osmolality are useful guides to the optimum volume and protein content of the intake. Routine measurements of plasma protein, albumin, calcium, bilirubin and liver function are required less frequently, initially every 2 or 3 days, extending to once weekly and even less frequently for long-term nutritional care. Trace minerals need only be measured monthly.

Clinical assessment of progress is equally important but less easily defined. The general appearance and sense of well-being of the patient, his interest in his surroundings and ability to perform simple physical tasks are useful indices of progress. Rapid changes in weight within the first 2 weeks are likely to represent a change in fluid balance, but thereafter weight increase represents tissue gain which occurs at the average rate of approximately 1 kg every 10 days.

Enteral feeding

There is a steady increase in the number of low residue preparations for enteral nutrition. These are miscible with water and can be infused along enteral tubes of small diameter. Preparations such as blenderised food and supplemental diets still have an important place in clinical nutrition, but they contain too much particulate matter for infusion through anything other than a wide bore tube. They are therefore used principally for 'sip' feeding or 'between meal' supplements. Therefore, one of the factors which determines the choice of diet is the tube bore. Current practice almost universally employs the commercially available 'convenience diets' or low residue diets which are suitably packaged and require little preparation. Palatability remains an important aspect even in tube feeding because of eructation and gastro-oesophageal reflux: the assessment of a patient's response must always include an awareness of unpleasant flavours.

Blenderised and supplemental diets. These are the least expensive form of nutritional support. A blenderised hospital meal produces a thick-coagulable puree somewhat unpalatable and unsuitable for the modern techniques of infusion. It is a hyperosmolar mixture which requires a great deal of additional water to ensure adequate urine output and should be given only where there is an intact stomach and pylorus. It is rarely used nowadays and is about the only preparation which is best given as a bolus and should be given warm. Supplemental diets such as Complan, Casilan, Hycal, Albumaid are whole protein preparations containing carbohydrate and fat which tend to have a high electrolyte content. Generally their use is as an oral supplement.

Low residue enteral feeds. The rapid development of enteral nutrition in hospital practice can be attributed to the development of these preparations. Most are based on whole protein with sufficient carbohydrate and fat and the appropriate range of minerals, vitamins and trace elements. Their osmolality tends to be in the range of 300–500 mosmol/kg, an important property when these diets are infused directly into the small intestine. The protein sources are either milk or vegetable, the carbohydrate in the form of sucrose and the fat is generally of vegetable origin containing medium chain triglycerides. The calorie/nitrogen ratio in these diets ranges between 70:1 to 200:1, the majority being in the lower 100s.

A group of enteral diets which are regarded separately, the 'elemental diets' or 'chemical defined diet' are composed of purified amino acids containing little or no polypeptides, simple carbohydrates which comprise the major part of the energy source and small amounts of fat. The calorie nitrogen ratio is much higher tending to be in excess of 250:1 and their osmolality is therefore, appropriately higher being between 550 and 850 mosmol/l. It has been claimed that the chemically defined diets have the property of reducing faecal bulk to a minimum, but there remains some doubt as to whether this is unique to them.

Routes of administration

Nasogastric intubation. When voluntary oral nutrition is impractical, tube feeding is the alternative and modern practice now uses fine bore tubes of diameter less than 2 mm (Clinifeed, Dobhoff). Tubes of larger diameter have the disadvantage of damaging the throat, lead to bad oral hygiene and induce gastro-oesophageal reflux with the risk of aspiration or oesophagitis with ulceration and stricture. The nasogastric route should always be preferred and the fine-bore tube can be inserted by the use of an introducer wire, by 'piggyback' attached by toffee or gelatin to a larger nasogastric tube which is removed later, inserted directly with a gastro-oesophageal endoscope, or at operation. The position of the tube should always be checked before starting to feed by injecting air and listening over the epigastrium or by x-ray of the upper abdomen.

Gastrostomy. The standard technique for gastrostomy in the past used a wide-bore self-retaining catheter of the Foley or DePezzer type, but gastrostomy has decreased in popularity since the advent of the fine bore nasogastric tube which can be introduced through quite narrow oesophageal strictures.

Jejunostomy. The Witzel type of jejunostomy is no longer necessary. Access can be achieved by the use of a biliary 'T' tube brought out through the greater omentum and abdomen wall or by a needle-catheter jejunostomy using a central venous catheter of 16–18 gauge which is tunnelled through the jejunal wall first subserosally then through the muscle to the submucosal layer where it is tunnelled for a further centimetre before entering the intestinal lumen. Whichever method is used, great care must be taken to ensure that the tube is properly fixed and that the intraperitoneal track of the cannula is protected by omentum. Even with the most meticulous care leakage can occur, but the risk is less with the needle catheter jejunostomy.

Management. The management of enteral feeding is usually fairly simple. All materials used in preparation and in administration must be thoroughly clean. Oral hygiene is of great importance and every facility for mouth-wash and oral toilet must be available. Constant attention to these details is important for co-operation and the patient should be encouraged to move about as much as possible. Enteral solutions should be infused continuously and the rate is adjusted accordingly starting with quarter strength solutions and building up to full strength over 5–6 days to avoid the sudden overloading of a gastrointestinal tract which may have been inactive for some time and undergone villous atrophy. The feed can be placed in a plastic disposable reservoir with drip attachment which reduces the risk of bacterial contamination and a pump used to regulate the rate of administration but the majority of patients appear to be managed quite satisfactorily by a gravity drip feed system.

Complications. Nausea, fullness, regurgitation and vomiting may occur during the first few days, indicating that the volume of administration is excessive. This problem can be solved either by reducing the rate of administration for 2–3 days or when prolonged by giving metaclopropamide (Maxolon). The most frequent complication of enteral feeding is diarrhoea which may be induced by broad spectrum antibiotics, lactase deficiency and the osmolar concentration of the drip feed. Reducing the rate of administration may control diarrhoea but often methyl-cellulose added to the feed or codeine phosphate may be necessary. Milk-based feeds should not be given to patients with lactase deficiency or milk protein allergy.

Parenteral nutrition

Parenteral nutrition remains the term most commonly adopted but others are used, often to the confusion of the uninitiated. 'Complete parenteral nutrition' or 'total parenteral nutrition' (TPN) denotes the intravenous administration of all nutrients including a substantial element of the energy source as fat and 'hyperalimentation', which emanated from the United States, indicates a regimen much in excess of normal requirements of which the predominant energy source is carbohydrate. 'Protein sparing therapy' is a modification of parenteral nutrition which employs amino acid solutions alone and depends on the body's own energy sources for efficient utilisation and is not a technique widely employed. Irrespective of the term used, parenteral nutrition has given the surgeon a valuable tool to manage difficult nutritional problems which in the past often forced him to operate in disadvantageous circumstances. Using this technique the surgeon can buy time and can afford to wait until inflammatory processes resolve allowing better surgical access.

Amino acid solution. Protein synthesis requires a full complement of all 20 amino acids, 8 of which – leucine, isoleucine, valine, methionine, phenyl alanine, tryptophane, lycine and threonine – are essential and must be included in any amino acid solution. The non-essential amino acids can be synthesised, but histidine is considered semi-essential because man's ability to synthesise it is limited and its inclusion is advisable usually in association with most of the other non-essential amino acids which constitute between one half to two-thirds of the total nitrogen source in most amino acid solutions. All modern amino acid solutions are composed of crystalline amino acids in an acceptable balance which avoids antagonism and toxicity. The range of concentration extends from 6.0 gN/l to 17.0 gN/l but the usual choice for routine feeding is in the range of 9–13 gN/l. Some solutions have carbohydrate added, usually of relatively small amount, and most regimens require additional energy in the form of carbohydrate or fat. There appears to be little difference in the nutritional effect of these many amino acid solutions provided the total intake is well balanced.

Carbohydrates. Carbohydrates are essential fuel for the glycolytic tissues such as the central nervous system and red blood cell and have a specific protein sparing effect. They also provide metabolic intermediates for many processes of metabolism. The minimum daily need is 100 g to avoid ketosis, the normal intake being between 200 and 350 g. When the daily intake exceeds 350 g, the osmolar load becomes excessive in the critically ill patient and it has recently been demonstrated that such large carbohydrate loads constitute an additional stress. It is best to limit the intake to the normal range. Glucose should be used wherever possible. It provides 4 cal/g and is available in dextrose solutions ranging in concentration from 5–50% i.e. 200 cal/l–2000 cal/l. It is usual to employ the 15–20% dextrose solution to provide 600–800 cal/l which also acts as a vehicle to provide water as well as energy. Fructose has been used in the past as a substitute for glucose, because it does not cause hyperglycaemia and its rate of disappearance from the circulation is rapid, an action independent of insulin. However, it cannot be used in glycolysis by tissues such as the brain and the red cell and it can potentiate acidotic states by its rapid conversion to lactic acid, thus its use in parenteral feeding is limited. Sorbitol is a polyhydric alcohol and its behaviour is similar to fructose to which it is immediately converted in the body. Ethanol, which has a high calorific value of 7 kcal/g, was used in the early days of parenteral nutrition as an energy source, but it is rarely used in modern practice there being a risk of lacticacidosis and also side effects which can be unpleasant.

Glucose has the advantage of being a carbohydrate freely available to those tissues such as the central nervous system and the red cell which have specific requirements. It also has the additional benefit of stimulating insulin which promotes anabolism.

Fat emulsions. The intravenous fat preparations are emulsions of the vegetable oil, soybean, in water which are stabilised by phospholipids or lecithin, producing fat particles similar to chylomicrons and are metabolised in a manner similar to fat derived from food. They are eliminated from the circulation at a rate of 3–4 g/kg/day, approximately 250 g/day in a 70 kg man. The maximum recommended dosage is 3 g/kg/day which is well above the normal daily infusion which is usually between 50 and 100 g. Fat emulsions are available in 10 and 20% solutions providing 1000 and 2000 kcal/l.

Routes of administration

Access to veins. Almost all parenteral nutrient solutions are hypertonic and should only be infused into the central veins which have a sufficiently large flow to dilute the infusate quickly. The peripheral route must always remain the route of access in the neonate and the small child, but successful therapy requires meticulous care of the catheter site and regular placement of the catheter every 24–48 h. The experience of most centres in this country would indicate that in the adult all peripheral veins tend to become thrombosed within 10–14 days and peripheral veins are, therefore, limited to the use of isotonic solutions.

In the absence of expert assistance it is best for those with only occasional experience in central vein catheterisation to employ a long line catheter inserted through the basilic vein and passed up into the central veins under x-ray control. However, the chance of malposition is much greater by this route and there is also the risk of venous thrombosis due to local trauma to the vein which has tended to limit the use of the long line. In experienced hands the most satisfactory route is by direct percutaneous cannulation of the subclavian vein by the infraclavicular route or alternatively the jugular vein. The subclavian route is more comfortable to the patient and the cannula can also be tunnelled along the chest wall for a few centimetres to minimise the risk of infection tracking along the catheter to the circulation. When cannulation is likely to be prolonged or permanent, a soft silicone catheter e.g. Broviac or Scribner cannula should be formally placed in the central vein and brought out through a long subcutaneous tunnel to the lower chest or upper abdominal wall. The lower siting of this type of catheter makes it easier for the patient to clean and dress without discomfort. Central venous cannulae need not be employed continuously and the cannula can be clamped or capped after loading with a 'heparin lock' so that the patient can mobilise completely on long-term feeding without the encumbrance of a drip feed system. It is not advisable to cannulate *via* the femoral vein because of the high risk of sepsis.

The ideal system for parenteral nutrition is to mix all nutrients in one container. This can be achieved by the adoption of the 'big bag' where all nutrients are prepared in a 3 l plastic container in the pharmacy on prescription. At the moment fat emulsions are only miscible under special conditions and in many centres these continue to be infused separately. The alternative is the multiple bottle system where a succession of bottles is infused either singly or in parallel.

Complications. Infection introduced through the central venous cannula remains the greatest hazard. Patients are frequently undernourished and may already have established sepsis with the risk of self-contamination, or cross infection introduced by the attendant staff. In addition the frequent changing of bottles and drip lines increases the risk of infection. The incidence of sepsis is variable but is currently reported as between 1 and 25%.

The principal cause of sepsis is a breach of aseptic technique contaminating the lumen of the cannula. The adoption of a policy of strict asepsis with careful skin cleansing, the use of antibiotic ointment with regular dressing of the catheter site and a strict aseptic technique while changing bottles or bags, has decreased the incidence of sepsis in this unit from 1 in 40 days of feeding to 1 in 560 days. Positive cultures reveal a variety of organisms ranging from staphylococci and Gram negative organisms to *Candida albicans*. When pyrexia develops during parenteral feeding in the absence of any identifiable cause, it should be assumed that the sepsis is related to the catheter. Blood should be cultured and a short course of broad spectrum antibiotic may be given, but if the pyrexia does not resolve within 48 h the cannula should be withdrawn and the tip cultured.

Metabolic complications are now becoming relatively rare and in the past were probably related to the over enthusiasm of the prescriber. Hyperglycaemia and severe hyperosmolar states were reported regularly some years ago when high carbohydrate infusion loads were popular for administration to critically ill patients intolerant to glucose and with insulin resistance. Should hyperglycaemia occur, the use of exogenous insulin is effective, but the adequacy of the infusion regime should also be reviewed. Severe and sustained hyperglycaemia is uncommon in centres where intravenous fat emulsions are used regularly and the carbohydrate intake is not excessive.

Hypophosphataemia can occur at the beginning of parenteral nutrition, particularly if time has not been spent initially in restoring ECF and electrolyte deficits. The drop in plasma phosphate may first be due to dilution and subsequently to rapid movement of phosphate from the extracellular to the intracellular space as a consequence of the rapid build-up of the metabolic activity within the cells. In severe depletion additional phosphate may be required in the early part of the intravenous regime, but this complication can usually be avoided by a gradual increase in the nutritional intake. Lactacidaemia has also been reported as a complication of parenteral nutrition and is most likely to occur during the infusion of fructose or sorbitol which are rapidly metabolised to lactic acid. If there is already a potential metabolic acidosis, lactacidaemia may follow the infusion of these substances and can produce a dramatic fall in pH. There are usually few complications of fat emulsions if the dosage is maintained within the recommended levels. Excessive administration causes depression of bone marrow, interference with coagulation and reticulo-endothelial function. Conversely, should patients be maintained solely on carbohydrate as an energy source, essential fatty acid deficiency producing dermatitis, diarrhoea, fatty liver and abnormal platelet function can develop after some weeks.

There have been many reports of alterations in liver function during parenteral nutrition. Elevation of the aminotransferase has been noted in several patients during the initial few days of feeding, but this usually resolves after the 10th–14th day, and there are often similar changes in alkaline phosphatase and serum lactic dehydrogenase. It is possible that these changes represent a reaction to high carbohydrate intakes in association with antioxidants in the amino acid solutions such as sodium bisulphate or converted products of some of the amino acids such as tryptophan.

Application of nutritional support

Nutritional support may be required during the convalescence of the most simple disease process e.g. acute appendicitis or an intestinal resection complicated by intestinal fistula while, on the other hand, severely depleted patients can recover without problems from quite extensive surgery. The indications for the use of these techniques, therefore, cannot be specified according to any diagnostic grouping but there are a number of clinical conditions in which nutritional support has a particular role.

Perioperative nutritional support

Preoperative

Some degree of nutritional depletion is evident in one-third to one-half of the patients in a general surgical unit, but serious nutritional change is found only in a small proportion, probably less than 3%. When confronted by a severely depleted patient the surgeon is faced with the choice of operating to restore oral feeding at the earliest opportunity and allow the patient to correct any nutritional deficit later or of delaying operation, to prepare the patient by nutritional support, over 7–10 days. Preoperative nutrition is time-consuming and expensive so that its use even in the severely depleted requires some justification. The Montpellier group have advocated its use in cancer surgery when weight loss exceeds 10% of body weight. They have found that preoperative nutrition increased the resectability rate of cancer of the pancreas and that they were able to operate on patients with cancer of the upper and lower gastrointestinal tract previously considered to be poor risk because of their nutritional status. Other groups have shown that preoperative nutrition in patients with malignant disease of the oesophagus and stomach reduces the incidence of wound infection and improves healing. In severe undernutrition morbidity and mortality were reduced considerably. Preoperative nutrition in cachectic patients has not yet been shown conclusively to reduce morbidity and mortality, but it has been remarked by those conducting such studies that management is improved. The benefit conferred by preoperative feeding is difficult to define exactly. It is unlikely that short periods of 7–10 days achieve any significant increase in muscle mass and any weight gain must be composed of a considerable proportion of water. The most likely benefit is the availability of substrates and a general increase in the turnover of the metabolic processes associated with protein synthesis, which prepares the patient for the increased demands of the postoperative period.

Postoperative

Nutritional support during the immediate postoperative period has a long history, but much of the published work is in normally nourished patients. It is well documented that the catabolic effect of surgery can be modified by nutritional support from the first postoperative day, but as more than 95% of surgical patients have an uncomplicated course with only a temporary interruption of oral feeding there is no reason for adopting a routine policy of postoperative feeding. In those patients where severe nutritional depletion constitutes a risk to surgery, it is unlikely that nutritional support after the event will confer any significant benefit and they are far better nourished in the preoperative period. The best role for postoperative nutrition is a prophylactic one in complex gastrointestinal surgery such as the difficult major gastric or colonic resection with the risk of complications which could delay normal nutrition. Even on this basis for selection, probably only 10–20% of patients will develop a need for nutritional support.

Burns

The catabolic stresses of severe burns are extreme with enormous increases in the demand for fluid and electrolytes, for protein to compensate for the greatly increased nitrogen losses by tissue destruction and by exudation, and for energy to accommodate the hypermetabolic state stimulated by high evaporative losses and increased catecholamine levels. Without additional nutritional support, serious depletion is inevitable within days of severe burning. The oral route is usually available but supplementation with enteral diets or by intravenous infusion may be required. Extensive burns of 40–70% have a substantial mortality but several patients with burns of 75–85% have been treated successfully by parenteral nutrition with weight losses less than 10%. The management of burns is a good example of a clinical situation where nutritional support has contributed to improvement in results. The use of increased ambient temperature, endocrine support employing exogenous insulin with hypertonic glucose and improved care of the burned area have all contributed.

Short bowel syndrome

Almost by definition this is a condition in which parenteral nutrition is the method of choice. Fortunately, this is a rare aftermath of gastrointestinal surgery or disease and tends to be associated most commonly with a vascular catastrophe affecting the superior mesenteric vessels or after extensive inflammatory conditions such as Crohn's disease. Parenteral nutrition should be started as soon as possible after the operation while an assessment is made of the function of the remaining intestine by radiology, measurement of stool volume and content and tests of intestinal absorptive function. Where the remaining length of small intestine appears to be incompatible with normal oral feeding (approximately less than 18–30 cm), the patient on parenteral nutrition should be encouraged to take the optimal oral intake of fluid and a low residue diet. Attempts should be made at regular intervals of 6 weeks to 2 months to increase the intake in the expectation that villous hypertrophy and intestinal hyperplasia will have developed sufficiently to improve absorption. Additional therapeutic manoeuvres include the oral administration of H_2 antagonists to depress gastric secretion, of pancreatic extract and of bile acid absorbants as well as anti-diarrhoea agents such as loperamide and codeine phosphate. There are reports of a return to full oral intake as long as 1 year after operation, indicating that the process of adaptation is gradual and lengthy. Where adaptation is not possible the alternative is permanent home nutrition which is compatible with an active ambulant life in many patients, the longest recorded being in excess of 10 years in Canada.

Entero-cutaneous fistula

Nutritional support has made a major contribution to the dramatic reduction in the mortality of patients with entero-cutaneous fistulae during the past 15 years. The most commonly quoted figure to support this statement is a reduction in mortality from 60–10%, but mortality from entero-cutaneous fistula will obviously vary with the pathology being greater with malignant and high intestinal fistulae. Formerly all cases were treated by parenteral nutrition, but now the greater proportion, especially the low intestinal fistulae, are treated by enteral nutrition using the slow drip infusion of feeds through a fine bore nasogastric tube. Occasionally parenteral and enteral nutrition are employed simultaneously if insufficient nutrient can be given by the enteral route. Nutritional care is only one of a number of factors which contribute to a successful outcome and its effect is greatly enhanced by the eradication of cata-

bolic stimuli such as extensive skin excoriation, by improved stoma care and aggressive management of sepsis, usually intraperitoneal, by appropriate drainage and antibiotic therapy.

Inflammatory bowel disease

Patients with ulcerative colitis and Crohn's disease are often undernourished, especially in the latter condition. The nutritional wellbeing of patients with these conditions can always be improved when there is depletion. During acute episodes of colitis and inflammatory episodes with severe illness, parenteral nutrition greatly facilitates the management by improving nutrition and allowing a period of complete bowel rest which reduces faecal volume and limits the effect on fluid and electrolyte metabolism. Enteral nutrition, often employing fine bore nasogastric feeding when anorexia is intense, is more suitable for the less acute forms of these diseases. Prolonged parenteral nutrition of many months' duration has been advocated as a means of providing bowel rest in patients with Crohn's disease to permit resolution of the secondary inflammatory processes and possibly enable healing to occur. This treatment has been employed in patients who have extensive disease where surgery could result in a short bowel syndrome and in the juvenile with growth failure. The evidence from a number of studies at the moment is conflicting, but it seems that although total resolution with healing is unlikely, resolution of secondary inflammation often permits operation of a lesser extent than was at first envisaged. Excessively prolonged feeding periods may not be necessary and it seems that no further improvement will be gained after 40–60 days of parenteral nutrition.

Nutritional support in liver disease

Impaired nutrition is common in chronic liver disease especially in cirrhosis related to alcoholism and in primary biliary cirrhosis. In uncomplicated states, nutritional management is confined to manipulation of the diet to overcome anorexia, protein intolerance and to avoid imbalances associated with a high alcohol intake. When a patient with chronic liver disease is operated upon, there may be further deterioration in liver function with water and sodium retention. Correction of the hypermetabolic effects of liver disease and the associated water and sodium retention may be achieved by insulin and glucose therapy while protein needs can be met by slow infusion of amino acid solutions, but monitoring may be required because of the danger of encephalopathy. In the presence of coma, amino acid solutions, enriched in the branched-chain amino acids leucine, isoleucine and valine may correct any imbalance in amino acid metabolism.

Nutritional support in the cancer patient

The nutrition of the cancer patient is altered by the effect of disease on the function of the gastrointestinal tract, the nutritional demands of tumour and the metabolic effects of the tumour on the host tissue. In the early stages of malignancy, undernutrition is confined principally to patients who have solid tumours of the upper gastrointestinal tract. It is only in the advanced stage of disease when the tumour mass is large enough to represent any significant catabolic stimulus to the host and has nutritional demands which compete with the host for nutritional intake that undernutrition becomes a signficant feature.

Nutritional support either by the enteral or parenteral route has a role to play in the management of the cancer patient, but it should not be regarded as a therapeutic agent for anything other than nutritional depletion. There is as yet no evidence that improving the nutrition of a cancer patient confers any additional ability to react favourably to the tumour, despite earlier expectations based on studies of immunocompetence that this might be the case. Serious nutritional depletion can be corrected effectively in patients about to undergo major surgery with improvement of the quality of the postoperative management, but there is no evidence to suggest that there is any improvement in the ability of such patients to survive their tumour. In those centres when extensive chemotherapy or radiotherapy is employed in advanced disease, the nutritional complications of therapy can be limited by nutritional support but no strong evidence has yet emerged which demonstrates that the patient is able to tolerate an increase in the dosage of therapy or that survival can be improved by maintaining normal drug metabolism.

Nutritional support is therefore important to the depleted patient with early disease about to undergo surgery, radiotherapy or chemotherapy where reversal of undernutrition improves the quality of life and avoids the deleterious effects of the undernourished state. Intensive support has no place in patients with terminal disease whose nutritional care should be confined to dietetic management.

Further reading

Ballinger W.F., Collins J.A., Drucker W.R., Dudrick S.J., Zeppa R. (1975). *Manual of Surgical Nutrition*. Philadelphia and London: WB Saunders.

Fischer J.E. (1977). Hyperalimentation. In *Advances in Surgery* (Rob C., ed.). Chicago and New York: Year Book Medical.

Goodgame J.T. (1980). A critical assessment of the indications for total parenteral nutrition. *Surg. Gynaecol. Obstet*; **151**:433–41.

Hill G.L. (1981). *Nutrition and the Surgical Patient*. Edinburgh and London: Churchill Livingstone.

Howard A., McLean Baird I. (1981). *Recent Advances in Clinical Nutrition*. London: John Libbey.

Karran S.J., Alberti K.G.M.M. (1980). *Practical Nutritional Support*. Bath: Pitman Medical.

Maxwell M.H., Kleeman C.R. (1972). *Clinical Disorders of Fluid and Electrolyte Metabolism*. New York: McGraw-Hill.

Moore F.D. (1959). *The Metabolic Care of the Surgical Patient*. London: Saunders.

Mullen J.L., Buzby M.D., Mathews D.C., Smale B.F., Rosato E.F. (1980). Reduction of operative morbidity and mortality by combined pre-operative and post-operative support. *Ann. Surg*; **192**:604–13.

Nazari S., Dionigi R., Comodi I., Dionigi P., Campani M. (1982). Preoperative prediction and quantification of septic risk caused by malnutrition. *Surgery*; **117**:266–73.

Richards J.R., Kinney J.M. (1977). *Nutritional Aspects of Care in the Critically Ill*. Edinburgh and London: Churchill Livingstone.

Torosian M.H., Rombeau J.L. (1980). Feeding by tube enterostomy. *Surg. Gynaecol. Obstet*; **150**:918–27.

Wilkinson A.W. (1973). *Body Fluids in Surgery*. Edinburgh and London: Churchill Livingstone.

Yarborough M.F., Curreri P.W. (1981). *Surgical Nutrition*. Edinburgh and London: Churchill Livingstone.

Blood replacement

H.H. GUNSON

Modern transfusion therapy has evolved from the fundamental discoveries of antigenic differences between the red blood cells of individuals, the ability to store blood *in vitro* in a manner which is safe for transfusing from one person to another, and the development of techniques for preparing cellular and plasma components. Blood replacement plays an essential part in many surgical procedures; indeed the ability to perform certain operations has depended on the production of appropriate blood components.

Whilst the primary interest of the surgeon is centred on the rationale for the use of blood products in replacement therapy, a complete understanding of the subject cannot be gained without considering those aspects of blood group serology which are of clinical importance and the associated hazards of transfusion of blood and its products.

Blood groups and blood group antibodies

Antigens

The blood group of a person is an inherited characteristic represented by the presence of antigens on red cells. When the inheritance of one set of antigens is not dependent on another set, the antigens are regarded as belonging to a blood group system, e.g. ABO, Rh, MNSs etc. Several hundred blood group antigens have now been identified and within each blood group system there may be a multiplicity of antigens. Blood group antigens are found in the surface membranes and whilst some are confined to the red cells, others may be present in the cells of other tissues and in a soluble form in certain secretions. It is possible that some antigens serve a function in the maintenance of the integrity of the red cell membrane but for many their purpose, if any, has yet to be defined.

Antibodies

Blood group antibodies are immunoglobulins, a feature which they share with many other antibodies such as those of viral or bacterial origin. Immunoglobulins, whilst they may vary in specificity, possess two different types of polypeptide chains known as the heavy and light chains respectively, and have the ability to combine with a corresponding antigen. Five different types of immunoglobulin are known, viz: IgG, IgM, IgA, IgD and IgE. Blood group antibodies belong principally to the IgG and IgM classes of immunoglobulins or mixtures of the two. However, in some instances IgA immunoglobulins exhibit blood group antibody activity and this may be independent of the other immunoglobulins, particularly in certain instances of acquired haemolytic anaemia, or combined with IgG and IgM.

The presence of an antibody in the serum of a person is normally dependent on stimulation by an antigen. This is a complex process dependent on the interaction of various cell types in the lymphoid system. However, there are certain blood group antibodies for which a clear antigenic stimulation cannot be defined. These are called 'naturally occurring antibodies'. The classical example of such antibodies are those of the ABO blood group system which has considerable importance in transfusion practice and while the exact mechanism of their production is not yet certain, there is a possibility that widespread distribution in animal and vegetable material of substances very similar in nature to group A and B substances may stimulate the production of the antibodies during early life. Many blood group systems have been identified by the discovery of a particular antibody in the serum of a patient which reacts with a proportion of unrelated donor red cells.

Serological tests

It is the ability of an antibody to react with the corresponding antigen on the surface of the red cell which forms the basis of blood group serological tests. The visible result of the antigen-antibody reaction is agglutination or haemolysis of the sensitised red cells.

Agglutination tests

Certain antibodies, often but not exclusively IgM, will agglutinate the appropriate red cells when they are suspended in saline (0.15 M NaCl) at temperatures up to 37°C. Examples of these *saline agglutinins* are anti-A anti-B, some Rh antibodies, anti-Lewis and a variety of cold auto- and allo-agglutinins.

Other antibodies, commonly IgG, are capable of sensitising red cells suspended in saline, but for physico-chemical reasons they will not effect agglutination of the sensitised cells. Examples of such antibodies are many Rh antibodies, anti-Kell, anti-Duffy and anti-Kidd. It is possible to obtain agglutination of the sensitised red cells in one or more ways. Thus:

1 *Suspension in colloid media* e.g. bovine serum albumin.
2 *Pretreatment of the test red cells with certain proteolytic enzymes*, e.g. papain or bromelin, or less satisfactorily for the identification of an antibody, the addition of a solution of proteolytic enzyme to the reacting mixture of antibody and saline-suspended red cells.
3 *Use of antiglobulin serum.* It is possible to raise antibodies in animals to human immunoglobulins

and certain components of complement. After removal of the species-specific antibodies an anti-globulin or 'Coombs' reagent can be obtained. Anti-IgG in this reagent will combine with receptors on IgG antibody immunoglobulin molecules bound to neighbouring red cells and effect agglutination (*see* diagrammatic representation in Fig 52.1). Anti-IgM and anti-IgA can also be present in antiglobulin reagents and may be helpful in antibody detection. With respect to IgM antibodies it is not usually necessary to rely on their interaction with anti-IgM, since many of the antibodies are agglutinins (*see above*) or fix complement and are detected by haemolysis or interaction with anti-complement (anti-C) components in the antiglobulin reagent (*see above*).

Haemolysis

Most IgM and some IgG antibodies have the ability to bind complement. The latter is a complex enzyme cascade of interacting components and if fixation proceeds to completion, damage to the red cell membrane occurs with resultant haemolysis. A few blood group antibodies will haemolyse red cells bearing the corresponding antigens and the commonest are some examples of anti-A and anti-B.

More commonly, complement fixation by blood group antibodies is incomplete with only the first four of the nine components of complement interacting with the immunoglobulin bound to the red cell. Of these four components C3 can be readily detected by the

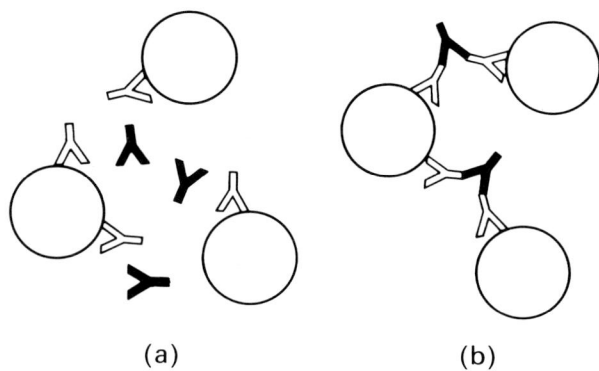

(a)   (b)

Key: ⅄ IgG antibody molecule

Y anti-IgG antibody molecule

Fig 52.1 A diagrammatic representation of the antiglobulin (IgG) reaction with sensitised red cells.

resultant agglutination after interaction of the sensitised cells with anti-C3 present in an antiglobulin reagent. Often, antiglobulin reagents used in routine blood group serology contain a mixture of anti-IgG, anti-IgA and anti-C3.

Compatibility tests

Red cell preparations should be crossmatched prior to transfusion, except in those instances when the transfusion is deemed to be so urgent clinically that no time is available for the tests to be carried out. In these instances group O rhesus negative blood is often used (*see* p. 158), and it is important that the ABO group of such blood is checked prior to issue. Although the compatibility tests are carried out in the laboratory, the procedure commences with the collection of the samples from the patient. It is essential that the patient is clearly identified prior to taking the sample and the specimen tube, containing 5–10 ml clotted blood, is clearly and accurately labelled *before leaving the patient*. The practice of prelabelling several tubes before collecting the samples is dangerous and must be avoided. Multiple number systems are in use at many hospitals and are helpful in avoiding mistakes in identity; one number is placed on a wristband attached to the patient, and the same number is placed on the specimen tube, request card and the units of blood prepared for the patient. Request cards should be fully completed giving proper identification of the patient, the essentials of the diagnosis together with relevant information, e.g. relevant drugs and anticoagulants being administered. If an interval of 2 or 3 days elapses between transfusions, further requests for red cells should be accompanied by a freshly-collected sample from the patient.

In the laboratory the ABO and Rh(D) blood group of the patient is determined and appropriate agglutination and antiglobulin tests are performed. Under normal circumstances compatibility tests between the serum of the patient and donor red cells takes 1–1.5 h to complete. The time can be reduced by using certain modifications, e.g. incorporation of low ionic strength solutions which accelerates binding of the antibody to the red cell.

The blood group systems

Of the many blood group systems which have been defined, two have primary importance with respect to transfusion therapy. A very brief review of these, the ABO and Rh systems, is given below, together with a few comments on other blood group systems which may have some clinical importance.

The ABO blood group system

The ABO blood group system was the first to be discovered and still remains the most important in transfusion practice. The common groups in the ABO system, and their frequencies in the United Kingdom are shown in Table 1, together with the corresponding naturally-occurring antibodies. Anti-A and anti-B react most strongly at temperatures up to 20°C but are still reactive at 37°C and may haemolyse appropriate red cells. They are important antibodies in blood transfusion and fatalities may result if incompatible blood is administered. Anti A_1 is usually a cold-reactive antibody, and apart from an occasional example which reacts strongly at 37°C, can be ignored. The effect of hypothermia during surgical operations will be discussed later. Since group O red cells do not react with anti-A or anti-B, persons of this group can, theoretically, act as donors for persons of other groups. However, the serum of certain group O persons may contain a high titre of anti-A and/or anti-B. If such blood is transfused to patients of group A, B or AB, the transfused antibody may destroy the patient's red cells causing a transfusion reaction. IgG, anti-A and anti-B are most important in this regard and since these most frequently tend to produce haemolysins *in vitro*, i.e. the antibody will lyse the appropriate A or B red cells at 37°C, blood which is haemolysin-free is often made available for transfusions of group O red cells to patients of other ABO groups. However, indiscriminate use of group O blood is to be discouraged and should only be transfused when the clinical condition of the patient is so serious that it is not possible to type the patient before transfusion.

The rhesus blood group system

A vast amount of knowledge on this system has accumulated since its discovery in 1940. It is the most

Table 1
ABO BLOOD GROUPS, THEIR ASSOCIATED ANTIBODIES AND FREQUENCIES IN THE UNITED KINGDOM

Cell group	Serum antibody	Approximate frequency % (UK)
O	anti-A anti-B	47
A_1	anti-B	} 42*
A_2	anti-B (+ anti-A_1)	
B	anti-A	8
A_1B	none	} 3*
A_2B	none (anti-A_1)	

* Approximately 10% of the population is A_2 and 0.7% A_2B.

complex blood group system known in man and it is not possible to include a full description of all the variants of Rh groups. The more common rhesus phenotypes are listed in Table 2, together with frequencies in the United Kingdom. Of the many antigens in the Rhesus blood group system, the D antigen is the most important in blood transfusion. Recipients who are D-antigen negative are commonly referred to as Rh-negative; units of blood for transfusion are not labelled as Rh-negative in the UK unless the red cells are negative also for the C and E antigens (*see* Table 2) although this practice does not apply in all countries. A variant of the D antigen, D^u, occurs occasionally in Caucasians and more commonly in Negroes. Red cells having the D^u characteristic possess either fewer D antigen sites than Rh(D) positive red cells or have reactivity of the D antigen suppressed. Rh negative individuals may develop anti-D from the administration of Rh(D) positive red cells, either as a result of incompatible transfusion or transplacental haemorrhage from a Rh(D) positive fetus. The incidence of anti-D antibodies resulting from pregnancies has diminished following the administration of anti-D immunoglobulin to Rh negative mothers at delivery. The possibility that inadvertent Rh incompatible transfusion to a female may result in the formation of anti-D which cause serious haemolytic disease in future infants should always be borne in mind, and Rh negative blood should be selected when the Rh(D) type of the female patient is uncertain or

unknown. Although the D^u antigen is less likely to stimulate anti-D, such units of blood are usually regarded as Rh(D) positives. The D^u recipient in most instances can safely receive Rh(D) positive blood; however, in a few instances anti-D has been detected in D^u patients receiving Rh(D) positive blood and from a practical point of view it may be preferable to administer Rh negative blood to those patients whose red cells possess weakly reactive D antigens.

Rh(D) positive persons may, on occasions, develop allo-antibodies in the Rhesus system. Anti-E and anti-c are found most commonly. Blood administered should lack the appropriate antigen and it should be noted that with anti-c, Rh negative blood is not suitable (*see* Table 2).

Other blood group systems

From time to time the sera of patients may contain antibodies to one or more of the many blood group systems which have been defined. The clinical importance of such an antibody will depend on its strength and the manner in which it reacts, e.g. at 37°C. The course of action to be taken in patients with an acute clinical condition requiring transfusion of red cells when such antibodies are discovered calls for fine clinical judgement. If the antibody appears to be of clinical significance, then it is to the patient's benefit that an attempt is made to obtain compatible blood. In many instances this can be done by typing units of blood with the appropriate antiserum followed by a compatibility test using the patient's serum.

One blood group system which should be mentioned is Kell. Some 9% of the Caucasians are Kell positive and outside the ABO and rhesus systems, anti-Kell is the commonest immune red cell antibody found. Many hospitals hold a reserve of group O rhesus negative haemolysin-free Kell negative blood to be used for the transfusion of critically ill patients. Use of such blood is justified on the grounds that without knowing the previous transfusion history, or in the case of a female, the obstetric history, the chances of avoiding an incompatible transfusion due to the presence of antibodies in the patient's serum will be reduced to a minimum.

In addition to the antigens of the ABO system, *lymphocytes* and *platelets* possess antigens (HLA) which form a complex polymorphism. Platelets and neutrophils also have specific antigens. Antibodies to the various antigens may be induced as a result of transfusion or pregnancy. Detection of HLA antibodies is conveniently performed by the cytotoxic test; fixation causes the death of the cell which then allows the uptake of a dye, e.g. trypan blue. Leuco-agglutination tests have been described, but the techniques are not easy to carry out with reliability. Platelet antibodies can be detected by complement-fixation tests but antiglobulin radioimmune assay techniques are more sensitive.

Table 2
COMMON RH PHENOTYPES AND THEIR FREQUENCIES IN THE UNITED KINGDOM

	Phenotype	Commonest genotype (CDE notation)	Approximate frequency in UK)
Rh POSITIVE			
	R_1r	CDe/cde	34
	R_2r	cDE/cde	13
	R_1R_2	CDe/cDE	13
	R_1R_1	CDe/CDe	18
	R_2R_2	cDE/cDE	3
	R_0r	cDe/cde	2
Rh NEGATIVE			
	rr	cde/cde	15
	r'r	Cde/cde	1
	r''r	cdE/cde	1

The choice of blood products used for replacement therapy

It is essential that blood transfusion therapy should not be undertaken without a very careful appraisal of the patient's clinical condition. This is important for two reasons. Firstly, there should be clear indications for replacement therapy with blood or its products since each transfusion carries a potential risk. Secondly, it is necessary to determine the nature and type of the blood component required.

Source material for blood components

The source material for most blood components is a donation of whole blood. Transfusion services in most countries have a Code of Practice with respect to the acceptance and rejection of blood donors. Whilst these may vary in detail, in general, healthy adults usually between the ages of 18 and 65 years are used as donors. The decision to take blood from a donor should only be made after considering whether donating will be harmful and whether the blood or blood product derived from the donation will be safe for administration to the patient. Thus, donors would be rejected if suffering from certain illnesses, e.g. anaemia and cardiovascular conditions in which the sudden alteration of the blood volume of the donor or lowering of blood pressure·may cause undesirable side-effects. The most important consideration with respect to the transfusion of the unit of blood is the transmission of diseases such as hepatitis and malaria, and under certain conditions, e.g. cyto-megalovirus.

In certain instances it may be desirable to use specialised blood collection techniques, such as plasmapheresis for the harvesting of large quantities of plasma from donors when the red cells are not required. This is often carried out when specific antibodies are present in the donor's plasma which can be used for the preparation of immunoglobulins. Since the red cells are returned to the donor immediately after the separation of the plasma, the procedure can be performed more frequently than the collection of whole blood donations. Plasmapheresis may be carried out manually using multiple bag systems and also by the use of cell separators. Such machines may also be used for the collection of individual donor platelets and leuco-cytes for transfusion.

The donation of whole blood, anticoagulated with acid citrate dextrose (ACD) or citrate phosphate dextrose (CPD) solutions, can be put to a multiplicity of uses (Fig 52.2). By means of slow-speed centrifugation, the plasma separated from the red cells will be rich in platelets which can be concentrated by further centrifugation. The residual plasma, or that derived from the blood donation following high speed centrifugation, can be used for the preparation of coagulation factors, e.g. factor VIII and factor IX, providing the plasma has been separated from the red cells within 24 h of collection. Other plasma fractions such as fibrinogen and the various specific immunoglobulins can also be prepared. Albumin solutions can be obtained directly from plasma or from the residues remaining after the extraction of other products. Use of each of the above products carries specific indications which will be reviewed in the succeeding sections.

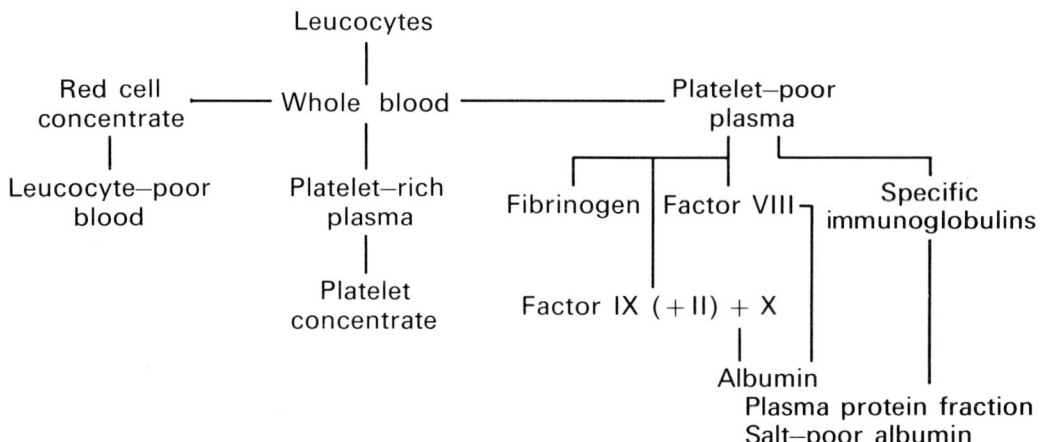

Fig 52.2 Major blood components derived from a donation of whole blood.

The use of red cell preparations

Whole blood and red cell concentrates

The ever increasing need to separate plasma from donations shortly after collection for the preparation of coagulation factors has led to the production of red cell concentrates in large quantities. In England approximately 180–200 ml plasma is removed from a whole blood donation for plasma fractionation. Some of the characteristics of the resulting red cell concentrate are compared with whole blood in Table 3.

Table 3
SOME CHARACTERISTICS OF WHOLE BLOOD AND PLASMA REDUCED BLOOD

Red cell preparation	Residual plasma (ml)	Average PCV %	Total protein (g/unit)
Whole blood	310	38	20
Plasma reduced blood	135	60	9

The term 'plasma reduced blood' is often given to this preparation to distinguish it from more highly concentrated red cells from which additional plasma is removed. It is generally accepted that transfusions of red cell concentrates are of advantage in anaemic states and the smaller volume per gram of haemoglobin transfused may have distinct advantages for an anaemic patient. Indications for transfusion in anaemia, however, should be carefully considered. In patients undergoing elective surgery, there is often sufficient time to correct anaemias by appropriate therapy without having to resort to blood transfusion. When operative procedures are more urgent, or in certain postoperative anaemic states, transfusion of red cell concentrates may be unavoidable.

Because of the availability of red cell concentrates in most Transfusion Centres, considerable efforts have been made to persuade clinicians to consider their use in replacement therapy after acute blood loss. Two objections have been raised against the use of red cell concentrates in such situations:

1   *The rate of flow.* It has been shown that providing the red cells have a PCV of less than 70%, flow through the standard blood filter of 170μ is not impeded, nor is the flow of the undiluted cells through a microaggregate filter (40μ) although additional pressure is required. Plasma reduced blood fulfils this criterion. The use of more concentrated red cells in situations of trauma has distinct disadvantages since they must be prediluted prior to passing through a filter.

2   *Reduction in concentration of plasma proteins.* Providing there is normal cardiac and pulmonary function, the body possesses an extremely efficient compensatory mechanism in the event of haemorrhage. Moderate haemorrhages, up to 20% of the total blood volume, or approximately 1 litre in the average adult, can usually be treated by simply restoring blood volume, and if red cells are given in such circumstances there is no evidence to suggest that whole blood with its higher protein content is more beneficial than red cell concentrates. Haemorrhages up to 30% of the total blood volume can be treated by the use of red cell concentrates, together with crystalloid solutions. It has been proposed that for acute haemorrhage in excess of 2 litres, blood replacement could comprise red cell concentrates with the additional transfusion of fluids containing protein such as modified gelatin. This is not a practice which has gained ready acceptance and most commonly such haemorrhage is treated with whole blood.

A satisfactory guide for the use of whole blood and red cell concentrates can be summarised as follows:

1   Transfusions of red cell concentrates should be used to correct anaemia.
2   For perioperative transfusions, the first two units given to the patient to correct blood loss should be in the form of red cell concentrates. Thereafter, whole blood should be used.
3   Whole blood is used to correct acute massive haemorrhage.

Adoption of the regime outlined above leads, on average, to the use of some 40% of units as whole blood and 60% as red cell concentrates. Red cells are normally stored at $+4°–6°C$ for 21 days after collection, but this time can be extended by the use of certain additives, e.g. adenine will allow up to 35 days storage.

Use of leucocyte poor blood

Febrile, non-haemolytic reactions may be caused by the destruction *in vivo* of transfused leucocytes, probably neutrophils in most instances, but possibly lymphocytes and platelets on other occasions. Such reactions may be so severe that the patient is unable to tolerate transfusions of whole blood or red cell concentrates. It has been known for many years that the removal of approximately 90% of leucocytes from units of blood prevent febrile reactions in a sensitised patient.

It can be seen (Table 4) that differential centrifugation fails to meet this criterion. Even repeated manual washing with 0.15 M sodium chloride solution (saline)

Table 4
AVERAGE REDUCTION OF LEUCOCYTES IN THE VARIOUS METHODS OF PREPARATION OF LEUCOCYTE-POOR BLOOD

Method of preparation	Average removal of leucocytes (%)	Comments
Differential centrifugation	65–85	Unacceptable loss of red cells to achieve high removal of leucocytes
Saline washing manual	80–90	Tedious to perform; loss of red cells
batch	90–95	Requires specialised equipment
frozen-thawed	95–99	Costly; excellent product
Sedimentation dextran	90–95	Requires subsequent saline wash
hydroxy-ethyl starch	90–95	
Filtration scrubbed nylon	60–70	Lymphocytes still present; requires freshly-collected, heparinised blood
cotton wool	90–95	Satisfactory

cannot always achieve satisfactory results without an unacceptable loss of red cells. Over 90% of leucocytes can be removed manually from blood by the use of rouleaux forming agents such as dextran (molecular weight 100–130 000) and hydroxethyl starch, although the antigenicity of dextran necessitates saline washing in addition to the sedimentation. Such manual methods are time consuming when large numbers of units are required and usually have to be performed using multiple entries into the blood pack which are a potential source of contamination, and as a result such products carry a 12-hour shelf life. Automated batch washing procedures can be used to remove in excess of 90% of leucocytes from donations of whole blood. These procedures were developed for the preparation for use of frozen/thawed blood which is virtually leucocyte free. Where frozen blood is available, it is clearly an advantage as starting material. However, the cost of maintaining frozen blood is considerable and is not justified solely on the grounds of producing leucocyte poor blood. Neutrophils can be removed selectively from blood by the use of scrubbed nylon filters. Such preparations have the disadvantage that lymphocytes are still present. Also, such filters require non-refrigerated heparinised, freshly collected blood, a product not readily available in most Transfusion Centres. The recent introduction of a cotton wool filter which will accept blood anticoagulated with citrate solutions have proved useful.

Use of platelet concentrates

Preparation and storage

Platelets can be separated from the red cells in whole blood by means of differential centrifugation and various techniques have been proposed. The principle of each technique involves an initial centrifugation of freshly-collected whole blood at relatively low speed to produce platelet rich plasma. This plasma is separated from the red cell mass taking care to avoid gross contamination with red cells. The platelet rich plasma is recentrifuged to concentrate the platelets. The use of either ACD or CPD as an anticoagulant appears to be equally effective with respect to both the recovery of platelets in the concentrates and *in vivo* survival. Centrifugation of platelets resulting in their close contact causes aggregation, particularly if resuspension is attempted shortly after centrifugation. If the unit of blood is not refrigerated before preparation of the platelet concentrate and centrifugation is carried out at 15–20°C, satisfactory resuspension can be achieved by allowing the concentrate to stand at room temperature for 1–2 h. Careful attention to the technique of platelet preparation is necessary to obtain adequate yield of platelets in the concentrate. On average it should be possible to collected between 5–7 × 10^{10} platelets per single donation of whole blood.

Platelets may be stored at 4°C or 22°C. Whilst those stored at 4°C may be effective haemostatically, their survival *in vivo* is greatly reduced. Such platelets, therefore, are ineffective when used to maintain circulating platelets at a level which prevents haemorrhage. Because of this, it is now common practice to store platelets at 22°C, although it must be recognised that such preparations carry an increased risk of bacterial growth if contaminated. Platelet viability decreases rapidly on storage but a maximum storage period of up to 5 days can now be achieved. Viability can be helped, particularly on storage at 22°C, by maintaining the pH, effected by retaining 50–70 ml residual plasma with the concentrate and subjecting the platelets to continuous agitation during storage. Metabolic activity is much lower at 4°C and such measures are not necessary.

Replacement therapy with platelets

The function of the platelet in haemostatic control will be reviewed in Chapter 53. In this section, however, it is pertinent to comment on the use of platelet concentrates as replacement therapy. The total platelet count has been used as a guide for the administration of platelet concentrates. There is an increasing tendency for spontaneous haemorrhage to occur as the platelet count falls below 100×10^9/l. However, with slowly falling counts, haemorrhage does not occur, usually, until the platelet count falls below 20×10^9/l. In certain patients, particularly those with autoimmune idiopathic thrombocytopenic purpura, platelet counts significantly lower than 20×10^9/l can often be tolerated. Assessment for platelet transfusions must also take into account other factors, e.g. trauma, either surgical or accidental and the presence of infection.

In patients who have congenital or acquired defects of platelet function either due to lack of circulating platelets or qualitative defects in the platelets, surgical procedures may provoke life-threatening haemorrhage, unless adequate replacement therapy is given.

The assessment of the response to the transfused platelet concentrates is often difficult. Increments in the platelet count following transfusion may be helpful under certain circumstances, but there are several conditions such as fever, hypersplenism, the presence of auto- or alloantibodies and haemorrhage which may lead to the sequestration of platelets. Replacement therapy with platelet concentrates in surgical procedures will also depend to some extent on the nature of the underlying cause for the thrombocytopenia. If the patient has the ability to produce normal platelets, e.g. in autoimmune thrombocytopenia, splenectomy is often followed by a rapid rise in the platelet count and haemostasis may be effected without the necessity for platelet transfusion. In patients where hypersplenism is the major causative factor of the thrombocytopenia, removal of the spleen may lead to a rise in the platelet count to levels which will allow haemostasis. Platelet concentrates should be administered to such patients during the operative procedure, but may not be necessary thereafter. When the patient's platelet production is abnormal, either due to primary aplasia of the marrow or secondary following invasive disease or the administration of chemotherapeutic agents, surgical procedures must be accompanied by the transfusion of platelet concentrates. In general, an attempt should be made to maintain the platelet count at $50–70 \times 10^9$/l during the operation and such time afterwards until healing of the wound is established.

It can be seen from the above that it is difficult to give precise recommendations with respect to the dose of platelets required for replacement therapy. If sequestration does not take place, one might expect to find one-third of the number of platelets transfused in the circulation. Laboratory tests such as bleeding time and platelet count may be of some help in assessing the need for transfusion of platelets, but have limited value only. An appraisal of the general clinical state of the patient may be the most reliable guide for the need for transfusion.

It is a commonly held belief that transfusions of freshly collected whole blood are advantageous for treating haemorrhage due to thrombocytopenia. It is difficult to substantiate this form of treatment on a scientific basis and such transfusions have the disadvantage that a large volume of blood may be required to effect haemostasis.

Under certain circumstances, particularly with the presence of alloantibodies, or when surgery is being carried out on a patient with a long-term thrombocytopenia in which prevention of alloimmunisation is important, it may be necessary to use HLA matched platelets. If a patient is a candidate for bone marrow transplanation in the future, then relatives are not suitable as donors. Matched platelets are not required often in surgical practice.

Leucocyte transfusions

Granulocyte transfusions may benefit certain patients suffering from neutropenia in which antibiotics alone will fail to control the infection. Since granulocyte preparations are time consuming and expensive to produce, clinical indications for their use must be carefully assessed. Normally a granulocyte transfusion would only be considered if the patient's granulocyte count was less than 5×10^8 per litre and therapy was available necessary to induce a remission of the primary cause of the neutropenia.

One major factor which has caused delay in the development of granulocyte transfusions is the difficulty of obtaining sufficient quantity of cells. It is generally agreed that to provide clinical effectiveness something in the order of 2×10^{10} granulocytes are required for daily transfusion. Since this represents the yield of granulocytes from approximately ten donations of whole blood, it is usual to harvest granulocytes by either filtration or the use of cell separators. Even with these techniques, particularly the separators, yields of granulocytes from normal blood donors tend to be low because of the trapping of the leucocytes in the red cell mass. Granulocyte yields can be improved by increasing circulating granulocytes with the administration of prednisolone or dexamethasone to the donor, together with a red cell sedimenting agent, such as hydroxyethyl-starch, which induces rouleaux and thus decreases trapping. Patients suffering from chronic granulocytic leukaemia also have been used as a source of mature granulocytes for transfusion. Crossmatching techniques are not yet readily available for neutrophil transfusions. If antibodies are present in the circulation of the patient, troublesome febrile reactions may follow their administration. HLA matching of the leucocytes with those of the patient and leukoaggulutination tests in a specialised laboratory in order to select donors for a recipient may be of assistance in overcoming this problem.

The use of albumin solutions

In general, two preparations of human albumin are available for replacement therapy, (Fig 52.2) i.e. plasma protein fraction which contains more than 90% of the total albumin in the plasma and has a final concentration of 45 g per litre of albumin, and salt poor albumin usually prepared as a 20% solution. Since the concentration of globulin in such preparations is low, it is possible to heat the albumin solutions to 60°C for a period of 10 h so that the products are made virtually free from the risk of transmitting viral hepatitis.

Plasma protein fraction

This is used in the treatment of hypovolaemic shock to restore the circulating blood volume. Considerable controversy exists with respect to the use of albumin instead of infusion of electrolyte solutions such as saline in order to restore the blood volume. There is no doubt that both fluids are effective in restoring blood volume, although if crystalloid solutions are used it is necessary to infuse larger quantities than volume lost (approximately three-fold). Proponents of the use of colloids point out that replacement therapy using crystalloid solutions alone will dilute the plasma proteins, thereby reducing the plasma oncotic pressure. The effect of this could allow the passage of fluid from the intravascular to the interstitial space and thereby favouring development of pulmonary oedema. On the other hand, those who favour the use of crystalloid solutions point out that albumin molecules can enter the pulmonary interstitial compartment relatively freely and are returned to the circulation via the lymphatic system. It has also been argued that the presence of albumin in the infusion fluid also interferes with diuresis, and the resultant increase in plasma volume from decreased excretion will cause increased mobilisation of extravascular water. Such an effect would be detrimental to pulmonary function. However, other experimental work has suggested that there is no significant difference in either the survival rate or the incidence of pulmonary complications whether either crystalloid or colloid solutions are used for replacement in situations of acute trauma requiring laparatomy.

It is important in treating moderate or severe hypovolaemic shock from any cause to institute prompt and rapid transfusion of fluid. It is important also to obtain an assessment of the amount of fluid lost since inadequate replacement may perpetuate shock. A rise in the systolic blood pressure to 100 mmHg is not necessarily an indication for stopping the transfusion. It should be remembered that the underlying defect of haemorrhagic shock is inadequate oxygen transport and with severe blood loss the effectiveness of the compensation which the body is able to make is diminished by the associated depletion of blood volume. Survival from shock, therefore, is dependent on the restoration of oxygen transport and its associated depletion of blood volume and blood flow.

In the face of conflicting observations it is difficult to give clear cut advice with respect to the use of crystalloid or colloid solutions. It appears, however, that for moderate replacement therapy, crystalloid solutions together with the use of red cells as described on p. 855 should be adequate, although for more severe haemorrhages many surgeons will prefer the introduction of colloids as replacement fluid. Whilst prompt and adequate transfusion is essential it is important to avoid overtransfusing.

Salt poor albumin

This is used as a replacement fluid for patients suffering from chronic hypoabluminaemia. There has been considerable doubt regarding the usefulness of albumin in this situation and when the hypoalbuminaemia is due to excretion, it is difficult to justify the use of infused albumin, although it may be that in these conditions and also in ascites, albumin infusions are of value in establishing a diuresis.

Plasma

Plasma contains approximately 30 g per litre of albumin and can be used as a blood volume replacement fluid. Plasma has often taken second place to PPF in recent years because of the dangers of transmission of hepatitis. There is evidence to suggest that in the treatment of adults suffering from severe burns, plasma may be more effective than PPF. Also, plasma frozen within 12–18 h of collection contains most of the major blood coagulation factors and this can be an advantage in the treatment of massive haemorrhages. On the other hand, it has been suggested that vasoactive substances present in freshly-collected plasma may be responsible for its leakage from the circulation, thereby reducing its effectiveness as a volume expander and pooled plasma, stored for 6 months, has been found to be more effective in this regard.

Coagulation factor replacement therapy

Blood coagulation and antiocoagulants are considered in Chapter 53. It is therefore more convenient to consider the use of fresh frozen plasma, factor VII, factor VIII, factor IX preparations and fibrinogen in the replacement thereapy of coagulation factor deficiencies within that section.

Plasma substitutes

Dextran

Dextrans are carbohydrates with various ranges of molecular weight. Molecules with a weight of less than 70000 are rapidly excreted by the kidney, whereas those in excess of 100000 may cause 'sludging' *in vivo* and have an increased tendency to produce rouleaux. Of the available preparations, dextran '70' will provide plasma volume expansion for about 24 h whereas dextran '110' will cause an increase in the plasma volume for a period exceeding 24 h. The latter product, however, has a tendency to produce rouleaux.

It is generally considered that it is best to limit the volume of dextran given over a short period to a patient to 1 litre, since dextran will not replace various plasma constituents such as the blood coagulation factors. It may interfere with haemostasis also, by damaging platelet function. Moreover, many types of dextran are antigenic in man and low levels of dextran antibodies have been found in the sera of certain patients without apparent previous exposure. Such antibodies may cause febrile reactions following the transfusion of dextran and severe anaphylactic reactions have been recorded in a few instances.

Hydroxyethyl-starch (HES)

Although the mean molecular weight of HES preparations is approximately 65000, there is a wide spread in the range of molecular weights in any given preparation and a proportion of molecules remain in the circulation. HES does not appear to be antigenic in man and, although high concentrations have been shown to interfere with blood coagulation, these are rarely achieved in replacement therapy.

Gelatin

Gelatin preparations with molecular size sufficiently large to be retained in the circulation do not remain fluid at normal ambient temperatures and therefore the preparations available tend to contain a large proportion of molecules below 30000 molecular weight. Gelatin has the advantage, however, that it is completely metabolised within the body.

The ill effects of blood transfusion

There are many potential hazards associated with blood transfusion and these are summarised in Table 5. This list is by no means exhaustive and space does not permit more than a brief review of some of the more important aspects.

Table 5
SOME POTENTIAL HAZARDS OF TRANSFUSION

Immunological
  haemolytic transfusion reactions
  allo-immunisation
  leucocyte and platelet incompatibilities
  plasma and urticarial reactions
Bacterial contamination
Transmission of disease
  serum hepatitis B
  non-A, non-B hepatitis
  cytomegalovirus
  E-B virus
  malaria
  syphilis
  brucellosis
Effects of massive transfusion
  altered oxygen transport:reduction of 2,3 DPG
  disseminated intravascular coagulation
  alteration of blood chemistry
  hypothermia
  microemboli

Immunological hazards

Transfusion of incompatible red cells

This may lead to haemolytic transfusion reactions, which are caused by increased red cell destruction. Red cells may be destroyed *intravascularly*, when haemoglobin is liberated into the plasma, or *extravascularly* by removal of damaged red cells by phagocytic cells of the reticulo-endothelial system. Such cells may be removed in either the liver or the spleen.

Whether the red cells are removed intra- or extravascularly, the rate at which they are removed will depend on several factors, e.g. the concentration of antigen, which is dependent on the dose of red cells administered and on the average number of antigen sites per red cell, the concentration of the antibody, the nature of the antibody (IgG or IgM) and the ability of the antibody to fix complement. In general, antibodies which fix complement sufficiently to haemolyse red cells *in vitro* usually cause intravascular lysis with rapid red cell destruction and the most common examples of such antibodies are those in the ABO blood group system, i.e. anti-A and anti-B. Antibodies which have the ability partially to fix complement usually cause extravascular lysis of incompatible red cells.

When intravascular destruction of transfused cells occurs, haemoglobin is liberated into the plasma. Such haemoglobin dissociates to dimers and binds to the haptoglobins. The haemoglobin-haptoglobin complex is removed from the circulation by the liver. Should the amount of haemoglobin exceed that which can be bound to the haptoglobins, unbound haemoglobin will remain in the circulation. This is readily oxidised to methaemoglobin and after dissociation from the globin, the haem binds to haemopexin in the plasma and to albumin to form the methaemalbumin. Haemoglobulinaemia may also occur in certain instances of extravascular red cell destruction and probably arises from the destruction of spherocytes, liberated after phagocytic action on the red cells in the reticulo-endothelial system. Excess haemoglobin in the plasma is excreted by the kidney. The actual presence of haemoglobin in the urine does not in itself appear to be toxic or cause renal damage, but the presence of red cell stroma and other substances released as a result of the antigen-antibody reaction which may interfere with renal blood flow, may lead to renal failure.

Clinically, the rapidity and degree of red cell clearance from the circulation will determine the symptoms in an incompatible transfusion. Initially there is a rise in body temperature and rigors may occurs. With severe intravascular destruction of red cells, other symptoms, such as a varying degree of heat along the length of the vein, skin flushes, constricting pains in the chest and pains in the lumbar region may arise. These are probably secondary to substances liberated as a result of complement fixation. Thromboplastic substances are liberated from lysed red cells and may lead to disseminated intravascular coagulation which in itself can cause haemorrhage and thrombocytopenia (consideration of this condition will be found on p. 878). With extravascular lysis and a slower rate of red cell destruction, jaundice is often the prominent feature, occurring 3 to 6 h after the transfusion. When the red cell destruction is protracted, then the only sign that may be apparent is the failure of the haemoglobin to rise to its expected level following the transfusion.

Transfusion of incompatible plasma

This may result in the destruction of donor red cells if the plasma contains potent antibodies against antigens present on the patient's red cells. Such reactions are usually confined to the transfusion of anti-A and anti-B and the donors have often been referred to as 'dangerous universal donors'. If the concentration and quantity of antibody is high, then there may be serious signs of red cell destruction with haemoglobinuria, although

this occurs relatively infrequently. Jaundice has been reported also in such instances but progressive anaemia is probably the most common finding. In order that the risk of such reactions is minimised, it is recommended that if group O blood has to be administered to patients with other ABO groups then the number of units given are kept to a minimum, that blood known to have a lower than average content of anti-A and anti-B is used (i.e. haemolysin-free) and, where practical, plasma reduced blood is selected.

Delayed haemolytic reactions

These may arise following a massive transfusion of blood to a patient whose serum contains a weak red cell antibody which is absorbed by the high concentration of antigens. Such cells may bind relatively few antibody molecules per cell and may survive for several days before stimulating production of antibody. Increasing concentrations of antibody will allow additional binding and when sufficient antibody molecules per cell are present, destruction of the transfused cells will result. Delayed haemolytic reactions may also be associated with undetected red cell antibodies. This may arise as a result of an error in the compatibility tests, but it is possible for certain immune responses to produce antibody in such a low concentration in the serum that the sensitivity of the serological tests is inadequate to demonstrate the presence of antibody. Common antibodies which contribute to delayed haemolytic reactions of this type are those in the Rhesus and Kidd systems, although involvement of antibodies of other specificities have been reported.

Generally, there are no clinical signs of the destruction of red cells at the time of the transfusion and jaundice is the most common symptom, appearing 4 to 7 days after the transfusion. Occasionally, haemoglobinaemia and haemoglobinuria have been detected. The red cells of the patient may develop a positive direct antiglobulin test and spherocytes are frequently found on blood films.

Decreased red cell survival without detectable antibodies

Uncommonly there may be decreased survival of red cells after transfusion without demonstrable antibody in the serum of the patient. The fact that there is increased cell destruction can be determined by the failure of the haemoglobin to rise and if cell survival studies are done, abnormal curves showing shortened survival are often found. In some instances the removal of the red cells has been so rapid that haemoglobinuria has resulted. The cause of this phenomenon is not known.

Development of blood group alloantibodies

In any transfusion there is a chance that the patient's immune system will respond to antigens present on the surface of the transfused red cells. Theoretically a large number of antigens may cause production of allan-antibodies following transfusion. In practice, however, most transfusions do not lead to immunisation. The production of alloantibodies occurs most frequently in patients who have received multiple transfusions, but it may occur as a result of a single transfusion. This complication should be borne in mind when the transfusion of a single unit of blood to an adult is contemplated; such a transfusion can hardly ever be justified.

If rhesus positive blood is inadvertently transfused to a rhesus negative female patient, the subsequent development of Rh(D) antibodies may be prejudicial to the survival of infants in future pregnancies. It is possible to effect a removal of rhesus positive red cells in such instances by the administration of anti-D immunoglobulin in doses of 25 μg per ml of red cells transfused. Evidence is available to demonstrate that if the transfused cells are removed during a period of 7 days following the transfusion, then the likelihood of Rh(D) antibodies developing is small.

The effects of leucoycte and platelet antibodies

It has been known for many years that leucocyte antibodies can be a cause of febrile reactions. Antibodies to neutrophils are probably responsible for most of such febrile reactions although antibodies to platelets and leucocytes have been implicated. The role of platelets is difficult to assess because suspensions of platelets are almost always contaminated with leucocytes. There is no doubt, however, that platelets can be rapidly removed from the circulation if antibodies are present. Febrile reactions to leucocyte antibodies tend to develop some 30–60 min after the start of the transfusion and may be quite severe.

Plasma and urticarial reactions

Mild allergic reactions manifested by urticaria or other allergic skin manifestations are common in association with blood transfusion. Their exact mechanism has never been fully explained although they are probably immunological in nature. Severe anaphylactic reactions following blood transfusions are rare, the commonest cause of such a reaction is probably the transfusions of a patient whose plasma contains class specific anti-IgA, with normal blood. Such patients, although uncommon, may have serious transfusion problems and only the use of very carefully washed cells may be tolerated.

The effects of bacterial contamination of blood and blood products

Very careful attention has to be paid to the preparation of solutions and containers into which blood or blood products are to be collected so that, as far as possible, bacteria are eliminated from the processes. Many bacteria will produce pyrogens, which consist of bacterial polysaccharide, and are resistant to autoclaving. Severe febrile reaction may result should material containing pryogens be transfused to a patient.

When blood is collected from donors, great care must be taken to avoid contamination. Even with such care it is possible that a certain number of organisms enters the unit of blood, but fortunately in the great majority of instances, such organisms are killed and stored blood is usually sterile. Organisms may gain entry to the blood pack after donation, either through minute pin holes, or as a result of open processes used to prepare certain blood products. It is fortunate now that the use of multiple blood pack systems avoids open treatment of the product in many instances, but certain red cell products, such as washed red cells, cannot be prepared without opening the container. Another factor which helps to diminish bacterial growth in blood is its storage at 4°C. Most organisms will not reproduce at this temperature, but there are certain organisms, particularly in the pseudomonas and coliform groups, which may multiply at 4°C. The presence of such organisms in units of blood can lead to serious transfusion reactions. A unit of blood should not be transfused without a careful inspection to note any signs of deterioration or haemolysis.

Transfusion of heavily contaminated blood to a patient usually results in immediate collapse and often death.

The transmission of disease by blood transfusion

Serum hepatitis

It has been known for many years that there is a possibility of transmission of hepatitis following the transfusion of blood and certain blood products. It was not until the discovery of the hepatitis associated B antigen, formerly known as the Australia or SH antigen and its associated antibody that an effective form of screening routinely for the presence of virus in the blood could be carried out. In the United Kingdom, hepatitis B antigen occurs in only a small proportion of the population, but in other parts of the world it is often a common finding.

Although the testing for the presence of hepatitis B surface antigen has reduced the incidence of post-transfusion hepatitis, it is known that certain instances of jaundice following transfusion are caused by viruses under the collective term, non-A, non-B. Many instances of non-A non-B hepatitis are anicteric and the diagnosis is based on a rise in the transaminase concentration in the patient's serum. At present there is no test for carriers of viruses which cause non-A non-B hepatitis.

Transmission of other viruses

There are several reports of transmission of cytomegalovirus (CMV) following transfusion. These are associated usually with large transfusions to surgical patients often undergoing open heart surgery. The clinical sequela are often referred to as the 'post-transfusion syndrome'. In most instances a mild febrile illness results, but particularly in patients receiving chemotherapy, the illness may be more severe with pulmonary, hepatic or neurological symptoms. CMV infection is commoner after transfusion of fresh blood but it can occur following transfusion of blood which has been stored for several days. Approximately 55% of adults in the UK possess antibodies to CMV. A small proportion of such persons, if used as donors, may transmit CMV infection. It may be beneficial to transfuse blood which is CMV antibody-negative to certain groups of patients, e.g. those undergoing transplantation, neonates, young persons undergoing open cardiac surgery and children suffering from acute lymphoblastic leukaemia.

Infectious mononucleosis may also be transmitted by blood transfusion and several cases have been reported. However, the elimination of transmission of infectious mononucleosis is extremely difficult since most of the adult population possess antibodies to this virus and use of EB virus antibody-negative blood is not practical. However, donors giving a history of infectious mononucleosis are deferred for a period of 2 years after recovery.

Transmission of malaria and other tropical diseases

Malarial parasites can remain viable in stored blood for 7–14 days after collection and may be transmitted to a patient in the red cell mass. With extensive air travel throughout the world, donors must be carefully quesioned to ascertain if they have visited endemic malaria areas.

Transmission of other diseases

At one time *syphilis* was a problem with respect to transfusion. However, since all donations are now screened for the presence of the spirochete and since these organisms do not survive in stored blood longer than 72 h, there is little danger of transmission.

Brucellosis may be transmitted by blood transfusion and donors who give a history of brucellosis because of the chronic nature of this illness are not accepted.

The effects of massive transfusions

It is difficult to define massive transfusion. In general, however, the transfusion of more than 10 units of blood to an adult over a short period can be considered as a massive transfusion. Stored blood has many parameters which differ from blood in the circulation. Thus, platelets are inactive and the concentrations of some of the coagulation factors may be grossly reduced; there is a functional alteration in haemoglobin performance because of depletion of 2,3 diphosphoglycate (2,3-DPG); the presence of the anticoagulant, which is normally based on citrate, will have the effect of removing the ionised calcium from the blood and will also contribute to the acidity of stored blood which is partly due to the citric acid of the anticoagulant and also partly to the lactic acid generated by the metabolism of the red cells during storage. As a result of these changes, administration of large volumes of blood may cause multiple and complex problems for the patient with respect to the haemodynamic function of the blood, alterations in blood chemistry and the effects on haemostasis.

Altered oxygen transport

During storage of red cells the 2,3-DPG level falls almost to undetectable levels at the end of 21 days. 2,3-DPG is one of several factors which controls the affinity of haemoglobin for oxygen. As 2,3-DPG falls, red cells have an increased affinity for oxygen, thus making them less efficient in delivering oxygen to the tissues. It has been difficult to establish clearly whether the transfusion of red cells depleted in 2,3-DPG has the effect of causing cellular injury because of lack of oxygenation. Levels of 2,3-DPG rise fairly rapidly post-transfusion and the patient's levels are usually back to normal in 12–24 h. During the time of the transfusion the effects of poor oxygen released to the tissues can be counteracted to some degree by maintaining a haemoglobin concentration at adequate levels, and the use of CPD blood is clearly advantageous since 2,3-DPG levels do not fall as quickly compared with blood containing ACD. It is advisable with massive transfusions to use the freshest available blood as soon as practical.

Diffuse bleeding

Large transfusions of whole blood may lead to diffuse bleeding. Whilst dilution effects may be contributory, there is evidence to suggest that the lack of platelets and deficiencies in coagulation factors in stored blood are not the only factors involved. Often in such patients there is demonstrable disseminated intravascular coagulation and this in itself will lead to consumption of certain coagulation factors and platelets. A discussion on this aspect of the problem will be found on p. 878.

Altered blood chemistry

Potassium concentration in stored blood increases with the period of storage and can attain levels of 30 mmol/l after 21 days. In most patients receiving massive transfusions, hyperkalaemia is not a complication since with adequate renal function, potassium is eliminated from the circulation rapidly and most patients will have an increased urinary excretion. Complications only arise if more than 100–150 ml/min of blood is exceeded. Problems may occur, however, in anuric patients.

Acidosis. Stored blood has an increased concentration of acid caused partly by the citric and lactic acids. The effect of transfusing the blood with a low pH is very complex. The administration of bicarbonate solution has been recommended, but the use of such solutions may result in complications and should be administered in the critically ill patient only after careful and considered evaluation of biochemical parameters.

Hypocalcaemia. In general, most adults can withstand the infusion of one unit of blood approximately every 5 min without having supplemental injections of calcium. Citrate is removed from the body by metabolism in every nucleated cell and this metabolism is very rapid. It has been noted that there are impaired rates of metabolism of citrate when the patient has hypothermia, diffuse liver disease or is allowed to become hypothermic. The administration of calcium salts to a patient undergoing massive transfusion should be undertaken with very great care since changes in the level of ionised calcium may occur very rapidly and excess calcium is equally dangerous to the patient as low calcium.

Hypothermia

Rapid transfusion of large amounts of blood which have been stored in the refrigerator at 4°C can reduce considerably the body temperature of the patient. Hypothermia may cause several problems, e.g. impairment of citrate metabolism, affinity for oxygen by haemoglobin and the chances of developing hypocalcaemia and acidosis will be increased. It may be an advantage to use warmed blood during massive transfusions, although great care must be taken in procedures for warming blood. Passage of the blood tubing in a thermostatically controlled bath at 37°C may be unsatisfactory for large rapid transfusions and the use of microwave blood warmers has led to haemolysis on certain occasions. It must be stressed that for most transfusions, warming blood is not necessary.

Microemboli

When blood is stored, microaggregates accumulate and these are derived from degraded platelets and white cells together with fibrin. The size of the aggregates is such that most will pass through the normal 170 filters. The significance of the circulation of such particulate matter has not been established with certainty.

Investigation of blood transfusion reactions

It is important that all adverse reactions to the transfusion of blood and blood components are investigated thoroughly. All units of blood should be kept for a reasonable period post-transfusion, so that they are available for investigation should this be required. The following blood samples must be available for tests:

1 The pretransfusion blood sample from the patient.
2 Samples used for crossmatching if they are in addition to the pretransfusion sample.
3 The residue of the donor blood.
4 Samples of blood taken post-transfusion, both clotted and anticoagulated.
5 Any urine passed by the patient.

Although the investigation of a transfusion reaction is largely a matter for the laboratory, the clinical history associated with the transfusion is an important part of this investigation. Records during the transfusion should always be kept meticulously, i.e. the record of the patient's temperature, pulse, the time the transfusion commenced, the volume of blood given and its rate, the time of onset and characteristics of the reaction. Appropriate laboratory tests are carried out to determine whether the ABO group and rhesus group of the patient of post-transfusion samples matches that of the pretransfusion, and the compatibility test is repeated. Investigations for the presence of red cell and leucocyte antibodies are carried out as appropriate. It may be necessary to culture the blood which has been transfused to the patient, and to carry out blood cultures on the patient, although it should be recognised that transfusions of infected blood can occur without evoking septicaemia in the patient.

Blood replacement therapy is important in the treatment of a surgical patient. It can only be managed successfully by a joint approach between the clinician attending the patient and the laboratory staff whose work is concerned with making blood products available. Proper lines of communication must be established and indeed it is a failure of communication that leads to most of the difficulties and complications in transfusion.

It will be noticed that no references have appeared in this chapter. The contents have been obtained from a wide variety of sources and from the personal experience of the author. A list of publications is given which review various aspects of this subject in considerable depth. The reader will, with advantage, be able to extend his or her knowledge of this subject by consulting these texts.

Further reading

Greenwalt T.J., Jamieson G.A. (1978). *The Blood Platelet in Transfusion Therapy*. New York: Liss.
Issit P.D., Issitt C.H. (1976). *Applied Blood Group Serology*. 2nd edn. California: Becton Dickenson.
Mollison P.L. (1979). *Blood Transfusion in Clinical Medicine*. 6th edn. Oxford: Blackwell Scientific Publications.
Race R.R., Sanger R. (1975). *Blood Groups in Man*. 6th edn. Oxford: Blackwell Scientific Publications.

53

Haemostasis and surgery

ALAN SHARP*

The haemostatic mechanism exists to protect the body from trauma and to maintain vascular integrity. In the normal healthy man, there is a delicate balance between this physiological mechanism which is protective to the host and the abnormal overreaction which leads to intravascular thrombosis and tissue damage. This mechanism depends on four main systems (a) the vessel wall, (b) platelets, (c) fibrin formation and (d) fibrinolysis. If this mechanism fails to perform efficiently due to an inherited, acquired or induced defect of any of these four interrelated mechanisms, abnormal bleeding may take place either spontaneously or following trauma or surgical intervention. The converse is intravascular thrombosis. When there is an inherited defect, the haemostatic mechanism of the patient may show evidence of an abnormal tendency to bleed from childhood or even infancy e.g. bleeding from the umbilical cord – Factor XIII deficiency or bleeding after circumcision – Factor VIII deficiency i.e., haemophilia.

By asking the patient specific questions, it is possible to determine whether or not there is likely to be a significant inherited bleeding tendency:

1 *Nose bleeds.* Bleeding that requires the use of towels or a bowl is abnormal.
2 *Tonsils and adenoids.* Removal of these tissues is a significant test of haemostasis. If any patient has had this operation without excessive blood loss, then there is unlikely to be a significant inherited defect. Unfortunately, memories are short lived – length of time in hospital may provide some clue that there were complications.
3 *Tooth extraction.* Again this procedure is a good test of haemostasis. Bleeding for more than 12 h with the presence of blood 'clots' in the mouth is abnormal.
4 *Bruising.* Small spontaneous or minimal trauma bruises are common and normal in the female, but any form of spontaneous bruising in the male should be regarded with suspicion. Any spontaneous bruise that is as large or larger than the palm of the patient's hand is abnormal. Excessive bruising after trauma or surgery is difficult to assess, but should not be ignored.
5 *Menorrhagia.* This is an unreliable guide as too often heavy menstrual loss is regarded as normal by women. If they have had treatment for iron deficiency anaemia, then one should be suspicious that there is excessive menstrual blood loss.
6 *Operations.* Previous successful surgery without excessive bleeding or bruising around the wound would suggest that an inherited defect is unlikely. Yet it is not a 100% exclusive feature as some patients with defects have had successful surgery without bleeding only to bleed excessively following a subsequent operation.

*Dr Sharp died in October, 1983.

7 *Bleeding into deep tissues or joints.* This is a feature of Factor VIII deficiency (Haemophilia) and Factor IX deficiency (Christmas Disease).

8 *Family history.* A carefully taken family history may provide a clue to an autosomal dominant or sex-linked recessive defect. Specific questioning about each 'remembered' member of the family is required, e.g. children, brothers, sisters, cousins, parents, uncles, aunts, grandparents etc. It is striking how little some patients know about their relations; only a positive family history can be considered reliable. If an entirely negative history is obtained, then any abnormal bleeding is likely to be due to an acquired or induced defect.

Often the surgeon or anaesthetist will be confronted with an unconscious patient who is bleeding abnormally following trauma or during surgery and no history will be available. Then, laboratory tests will be the only indicator of abnormality. It must be stressed at this stage that the haematologist requires a fresh sample collected into the correct containers and they should be delivered to the laboratory by the quickest, most reliable route. Postal samples are useless and even between hospital and hospital, transport can be so slow as to cause deterioration of the sample. Further, some tests to be reliable must be collected by special methods at the bed-side. Finally heparin often strays into the circulation and produces abnormal bleeding e.g. via intravenous lines, blood gas estimation.

Analysis of specific defects will be considered in more detail later in this chapter.

Patterns of abnormal bleeding

Post-traumatic

When a specific inherited or acquired defect in the haemostatic mechanism is the cause of abnormal bleeding, the time of onset of the bleeding related to the trauma may provide a rough guide as to which system is involved.

Defects of the vessel wall and platelets characteristically give rise to an immediate excess blood loss. If the mechanism leading to fibrin formation is normal then fibrin will eventually achieve haemostasis especially if pressure can be applied to the bleeding area.

When fibrin formation is delayed or decreased in amount, due to an inherited coagulation factor defect, the characteristic pattern of events is the cessation of bleeding due to the effective vessel/platelet interaction, but the onset of secondary bleeding hours or days later is due to a failure to produce the reinforcing normal fibrin in sufficient amounts or structure. There is some

evidence to suggest that when fibrin formation is slow, due to inadequate thrombin generation, the fibrin so formed is unstable and easily lysed and when this happens granulation tissue may not form normally and so healing will be delayed.

If the fibrinolytic mechanism is activated subsequent to fibrin formation, it is capable of lysing haemostatic fibrin and so causing secondary bleeding up to several days later. As 'local' activation of this mechanism, without detectable changes in the circulating blood is possible, such fibrinolysis may well be a common cause of unexpected secondary, postoperative or traumatic bleeding in normal persons.

Spontaneous bleeding

The pattern of spontaneous bleeding also shows differences. When platelets are deficient in function and number, bleeding from mucosal surfaces is common and deep tissue bleeding is rare. Yet intracerebral haemorrhage is a known cause of death in thrombocytopenic individuals. The pattern of bleeding in the different coagulation deficiencies will be described later, but these do show subtle differences between tissues and the type of bleeding.

Joints (haemarthrosis)	– Haemophilia and Christmas disease
Bleeding into retro-peritoneal space	– Haemophilia, Christmas disease and afibrinogenaemia
Bleeding from veins following venepuncture	– Fibrinogen deficiency
Bleeding from umbilical cord at birth	– Factor XIII deficiency
Haematuria	– Haemophilia, thrombocytopenia
Skin purpura	– Platelet abnormality
Prostate	– Secondary bleeding due to local fibrinolysis
Menorrhagia	– Platelet deficiency, secondary fibrinolysis

Vessel wall

The vessel wall depends on the maintenance of a normal healthy endothelial surface. When the latter is damaged and the subendothelial collagen and microfibrils are exposed, a chain of reactions is initiated which is designed to prevent blood loss.

Within seconds of damage, platelets adhere to the exposed collagen and microfibrils, and platelet aggregates build up around the damaged vessel wall and in the wound tract if there is one – in the first instance this is a reversible reaction. This activation of platelets leads to a further sequence of events:

1   The platelets release their contents and changes take place on their surface.
2   The damaged vessel wall contracts as a consequence of platelet release.
3   The damaged vessel wall becomes permeable and plasma escapes causing a local concentration of red cells in the damaged and contracted vessel.
4   Fibrin forms in and around the platelet aggregates forming a permanent 'plug' in the area of damage by reinforcing the unstable platelet aggregate which is also changed consequent on the thrombin generated to form the fibrin.
5   Fibrinolytic activator released from the damaged vessel wall binds to the fibrin and removes excess fibrin.

Arteries, arterioles, veins and venules all have the ability to contract, but while capillaries do not have any visible contractile mechanism in man, when traumatised they appear to contract. This may be due to emptying caused by contraction of proximal arterioles or may be the result of increased extravascular pressure, consequent on permeability, collapsing these delicate vessels.

Abnormalities in the vessel wall leading to breakdown of haemostasis are rare but are encountered:

1   In scurvy (vitamin C deficiency). The vessel wall becomes fragile due to a defect in collagen synthesis.
2   In Ehlers-Danlos Syndrome, which is inherited as an autosomal dominant trait, abnormal collagen is formed due to a genetic defect.
3   Hereditary telangiectasia (Rendu-Weber Osler Disease) – also inherited as an autosomal dominant defect. This is characterised by multiple foci of abnormal capillaries which are fragile and cannot apparently promote normal haemostasis and contract when damaged. This condition is inherited, but usually does not reveal itself until adult life and often middle age. Thus there is often no history of abnormal bleeding during childhood.

Factors produced by damaged vessel wall

As well as the exposure of subendothelial collagen, damage to endothelium causes certain other changes to take place:

1   Failure of normal prostacyclin (PGI$_2$) production.
2   Release of fibrinolytic activator.

3   Release of increased amounts of parts of the coagulation protein molecule (Factor VIIIR-AG and Factor VIIIR-WF).

Platelets

Platelet formation

Platelets are formed by the megakaryocytes which are unique and easily recognised cells within the marrow. There is controversy as to how the megakaryocytes develop. The conventional theory is that the megakaryocyte nucleus undergoes intracellular division, building up from 2N to 32N by successive stages of intercellular mitoses. When there is a high turnover of platelet production, larger than normal platelets appear in the circulation (metathrombocytes) and it has been shown that these large platelets aggregate more readily than the small ones.

Control of thrombopoiesis

This is apparently regulated by the numbers of circulating platelets in the blood, so when platelet numbers are reduced there is a stimulus to production by the formation of a hormone, thrombocytopoietin. There is some evidence that this hormone is poduced by the kidney-like erythropoietin, but there is no evidence that the two are the same. The relationship to platelet numbers and hormone production suggests that there is a feed-back mechanism.

In situations where platelet numbers are reduced by sequestration in an enlarged spleen, splenectomy is often followed by increased numbers of circulating platelets for a period. It is apparent that the hormone stimulus to platelet production in these situations may not return to normal until some 4 weeks after operation. Occasionally the switch-off mechanism does not occur and the postsplenectomy state is complicated by very high platelet counts.

Blood platelets

Platelets circulate as non-nucleated cytoplasmic fragments in the blood, they vary in diameter between 2 and 4 μm and the numbers are normally between 150 to 300 $\times$ 10^9/l. They survive in the circulation between 7 to 9 days depending on the methods used and appear to have a finite lifespan balanced against random destruction in the circulation, the latter being almost certainly due to maintaining haemostasis in the trauma of everyday life. Platelet survival can be determined by the use of radioactive labels e.g. ^{51}Cr and ^{111}Indium oxide.

The platelet in its undisturbed state is an ellipsoid disc and, considering its small size, it is remarkable the number of materials contained within the cytoplasm and its granules (Table 1).

Table 1

Dense granules	α granules
Serotinin	Platelet factor 4
Calcium	β thromboglobulin
ATP	Growth factor (Mitogenic factor)
ADP	Permeability factor
	Fibrinogen
	? Factor V

In order to maintain normal haemostasis, there must first be normal numbers of platelets. In this connection, there appears to be an excess of circulating platelets in man and $50 \times 10^9/l$ is a sufficient number to achieve normal haemostasis in health. This apparent excess may be a reserve held for the event of excessive trauma, but may be a factor in man's selective tendency to thrombotic disease. Platelets must, however, have normal function as well as number and if any of these are impaired, then they fail to achieve haemostasis despite normal numbers circulating. The two basic functions of platelets which are necessary are the ability to adhere to foreign surfaces and to aggregate. To promote fibrin formation, they must be able to release appropriate materials from their contents.

They also play an important role in the transport of 5 hydroxytryptamine and take up and transport adenine and adenosine for conversion to ATP within the platelet. Platelets have an ill-defined phagocytic function; they engulf virus particles and immune complexes and play a role in locating bacteria in septicaemia prior to neutrophil phagocytosis. The exact mechanism of platelet adhesion is ill-defined, but is almost certainly a specific chemical reaction between the platelet surface and that to which it adheres.

Platelet activation

When platelets adhere to a foreign surface, they become activated and a membrane change takes place with change in platelet shape. Thus the normal discoid platelets put out pseudopod-like structures or dendrites. As well as collagen interaction, other substances, some released by the platelets, promote further activation:

adenosinediphosphate (ADP)	prostaglandins
adrenaline	endotoxin
5 hydroxytryptamine (5HT)	viruses
immune complexes	possible bacterial surfaces
thrombin	

and activation produces aggregation.

The release reaction

Activation and consequent aggregation promote release of materials from the platelet granules (Table 1) and cytosol and unmask the platelet surface phospholipid which promotes blood coagulation. Associated with this activation is the mobilisation of calcium to the cell surface. In addition, platelet Factor 4 and ß thromboglobulin are released and their presence in increased amounts in the circulating blood provide a guide to increased platelet breakdown *in vivo*.

The most exciting discovery in recent years is that when the platelet membrane is damaged, a prostaglandin pathway is activated and the surface lipoprotein is changed by phospholipase to produce arachidonic acid with consequent formation of intermediate endoperoxides PGH_2 and PGG_2, which are platelet aggregating agents. Both these endoperoxides can be converted to thromboxane A2 by the action of thromboxane synthetase. Thromboxane A2 has been found to be the most potent platelet aggregating agent yet discovered and is also an extremely powerful vasoconstrictor, more powerful than angiotension 11. The formation of the endoperoxide PGG_2 and H_2 can be blocked by the use of aspirin which acetylates the cyclooxygenase (Fig 53.1).

While this takes place in the platelets, a similar pathway exists in the vessel wall, especially the endothelium, where the active endoperoxide PGG_2 and H_2 are converted to PGI_2 or prostacyclin which is an inhibitor of platelet aggregation and also a powerful vasodilator. Prostacyclin is produced by arterial endothelium, especially in the pulmonary arterial system. Unlike other prostaglandins, prostacyclin is not metabolised in the lung. Thus prostacyclin produced by normal endothelium prevents platelet adhesion and aggregation while platelet activation by producing thromboxane A2 enhances the tendency to aggregation.

Another effect of platelet release is their inhibitory effect on activator and plasmin and their action on lysis of fibrin. Thus the release of activator from damaged endothelium which usually results in the lysis of unwanted fibrin is inhibited in the proximity of the platelet aggregates, preserving the fibrin in that area.

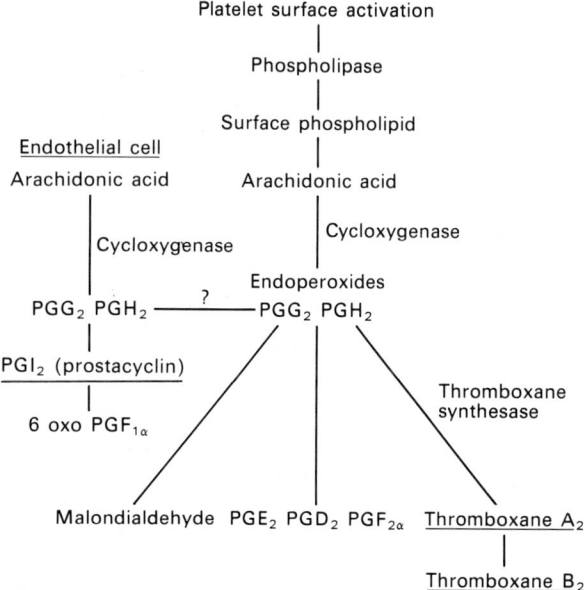

Fig 53.1 Prostaglandin synthesis in the platelet and the vessel wall.

Measurement of platelet function

If platelets fail to function in the normal way in the haemostatic mechanism, then there is a breakdown in primary haemostasis. This failure can be measured by the *bleeding time*. If there is a reduction in numbers or function, the bleeding time is prolonged. *In vitro* tests can be performed to determine platelet adhesion, aggregation and release.

Abnormalities of platelet function

Certain rare abnormalities of platelet function are inherited as recessive traits:

In *thrombasthenia*, there is an abnormality in the glycoprotein of the platelet membrane and these platelets fail to adhere to foreign surfaces or to aggregate when exposed to common inducing agents. The morphology of platelets is normal as is the number of circulating platelets. Other rarer abnormalities of the platelet membrane include the *Bernard Soulier syndrome* in which the platelets are much larger than normal. In some patients with mild bleeding tendencies, there is an abnormality of *the storage pool* within the granules of the platelets.

Acquired abnormalities of platelet function do occur and the effect of certain drugs has been discussed in relation to aspirin and dipyridamole (Persantin). Other drugs such as sulphinpyrazone (Anturan) appear to inhibit the prostaglandin pathway within the platelets, but the effect is far less dramatic than with aspirin, Phenylbutazone and Indomethacin. In other syndromes, namely the myeloproliferative diseases, abnormal platelets are produced in increased numbers. These show an abnormal reaction in two ways. Firstly increased reaction and, therefore, a tendency to thrombosis and secondly, abnormal function with an acquired platelet storage pool defect and apparent hypofunction. Thus one can get the anomaly of a thrombotic tendency and abnormal bleeding in the same patient at the same time.

In *renal failure* platelet abnormalities occur frequently. There is abnormal aggregation and poor lipid availability when the platelets are activated. In the past this has been thought due to high levels of circulating toxins e.g. guanido-succinic acid or magnesium, but recent studies suggest that there are very high levels of prostacyclin in these patients.

In *paraproteinaemias*, due to the presence of large amounts of abnormal globulin, platelet function can be impaired due to coating of its surface with abnormal proteins. Other large molecules e.g. dextran, may have a similar effect. Similarly large highly charged molecules such as heparin, can produce thrombocytopenia.

Thrombocytopenia

The most common acquired disorder is reduction in platelet numbers which below $50 \times 10^9/l$ increases the risk of spontaneous haemorrhage into the skin or internal organs. Yet even when the count is less than $20 \times 10^9/l$ bleeding does not always occur. There is a distinct relationship between numbers and function in thrombocytopaenia. Further, platelets play some role in protection against infection and the presence of infection associated with low numbers of circulating platelets enhances the risk of spontaneous bleeding. The causes of thrombocytopenia are (a) failure of production (b) increased destruction.

Failure of production

This results from marrow damage such as aplasia induced by drugs or by replacement of the normal marrow by foreign cells in leukaemia or carcinomatous myelofibrosis. In megaloblastic anaemia due to deficiency of vitamin B_{12} or folic acid, DNA synthesis in all rapidly dividing cells is impaired and thus platelets as well as white and red cell production is abnormal.

Occasionally congenital thrombocytopenia is encountered and this may be associated with poor production of megakaryocytes. There is a strange association between absence or abnormalities of the radii in the forearm and a lack of megakaryocytes in the marrow.

Increased destruction

Perhaps the most common cause of thrombocytopenia is destruction of circulating platelets produced in the normal marrow.

Immune thrombocytopenia

This may result in the production of antibody by the patient's immune mechanism which either destroys the platelets directly or by reacting with another antigen involves the platelets in the immune complex. When the antibody attacks the platelets, it can cause platelet lysis, activation of the platelet surface or, by coating the platelet, cause it to be removed by the reticulo-endothelial system.

Drug induced thrombocytopenia

Apart from the well-known damage to marrow by certain drugs, e.g. chloramphenicol and phenylbutazone, where megakaryocytes are directly damaged, a drug/platelet link can develop which may produce an antibody specific for that combination. This has been described with sedormid, quinine and quinidine and the antibody can produce dramatic and dangerous thrombocytopenia. It is possible by *in vitro* tests to demonstrate the specificity of such an antibody to the drug. This reaction can occur when only trace amounts of the drug are present e.g. quinine in tonic water. This sensitivity highlights the risks of test dosing such patients with drugs or even skin testing.

Antibodies specific for platelets have also been considered to attack megakaryocytes and endothelial cells, as these have the same antigenic properties. However, recent studies have not confirmed this hypothesis as the turnover of megakaryocytes and platelet production has shown to be increased in immune thrombocytopenic purpura. Vascular lesions consequent on the thrombocytopenia are probably the result of platelet deficiency, platelets being necessary for the maintenance of normal endothelium.

Neonatal thrombocytopenia

A further example of immunothrombocytopenia is its development in the neonate following the transfer of antibody through the placenta from the maternal circulation. This may occur when the mother has or has had immune thrombocytopenia, even if this has been treated by splenectomy.

Alternatively if the baby's platelets carry a different platelet group from the mother, she may become immunised during pregnancy and the antibody passes through the placenta to destroy the infant's normal platelets. In either instance, the thrombocytopenia disappears in 3–5 weeks as the transfer globulin decays in the infant's blood. There is however serious danger of intracerebral haemorrhage due to birth trauma.

Diffuse intravascular coagulation

When explosive intravascular coagulation develops as a sequel to trauma or disease, platelets are involved and thrombocytopenia is usually an early indicator.

Transfusion thrombocytopenia

Patients, whose platelets are PLA1 negative may become sensitised during blood transfusion as the majority of donors have PLA1 positive antigen. This is a rare occurrence, but if a sensitised patient receives a transfusion of PLA1 positive platelets, not only are the positive platelets destroyed, but also the patient's own negative platelets. This is presumably due to the normal platelets becoming involved in the antigen/antibody complex. When this occurs, it is extremely difficult to treat as it is hard to find a suitable negative donor for platelet transfusion.

Apart from this rare immune mechanism, a more frequent cause of thrombocytopenia following transfusion is due to dilution by the use of stored bank blood which does not contain viable platelets. The same can occur following the use of fresh frozen plasma or plasma protein fraction. It is an inevitable consequence if more than 5 l of stored blood is given in a few hours or if more than 2 l of plasma or dextran are transfused in a similar time. When this happens the only solution, if further transfusion is required, is to transfer to as fresh blood as possible or to use a platelet transfusion.

Thrombocythaemia and thrombocytosis

An increase in the platelets count above normal can occur without any obvious harm to the host. In certain forms of myeloproliferative disease, especially chronic myeloid leukaemia, polycythaemia and myelofibrosis, a very large number of platelets may enter the circulation, and the count may rise to greater than a million. This is due to platelets being produced by an abnormal clone of proliferating stem cells. Sometimes this may only affect the megakaryocytes without any increase of red or white cells. Platelets so formed can show the paradoxical association of vascular thrombosis and abnormal bleeding at the same time. Abnormal function is very varied, but there is some evidence that sheer numbers impair the efficiency of platelets. In myeloproliferative syndromes, the platelets often show abnormal morphology being abnormally large with a lack of granules.

In thrombocytosis occurring as a secondary phenomenon, and as a short-lived event in the course of other disease, the platelets often appear abnormally small. The most common cause of such increase in platelets is chronic blood loss with consequently increased levels of erythropoietin and general marrow activity. A similar rise can be seen in acute haemolysis. Where there is no obvious blood loss, thrombocytosis may be an indicator of undiscovered malignant disease e.g. carcinoma of the bronchus. The thrombocytosis following splenectomy for an enlarged spleen or for whatever cause has already been mentioned. Splenic atrophy accompanying malabsorption syndromes may promote a raised, but seldom very high, platelet count as may infection by stimulating white cell production. The vinca-alkaloids, (Vincristine and Vinblastine) used for the treatment of malignant disease can also stimulate platelet production.

Therapy of platelet deficiency states

When deficiencies of platelet numbers or function lead to an abnormal bleeding state, it is essential to treat it, but the discovery of thrombocytopenia without abnormal bleeding is not by itself an indication for treatment. In non-immune thrombocytopenia and in inherited defects, where bleeding is a problem, platelet transfusion (*see* p. 855) should be given. In immune thrombocytopenia, platelet transfusion may be valueless due to the destruction of the platelets by circulating antibody. Steroid therapy has been shown to (a) reduce the tendency to bleed and (b) promote an increase in the platelet count. In children with postviral thrombocytopenia, the platelet count may recover spontaneously, but this may be speeded by steroid therapy for 1–2 weeks. Both parents and doctor sleep better when the platelet count rises quickly!

In adults, the pattern of immune thrombocytopenia differs in that it is often chronic, lasting many years untreated. Steroid therapy may produce a rise in the platelets to normal, but this drops to low and dangerous levels when steroids are withdrawn. In such situations or where there has been no response to steroids, splenectomy should be carried out, preferably after increasing the platelet count once more by steroid therapy. If splenectomy has to be carried out on a severely thrombocytopenic individual, platelet concentrate must be available, but only given after the abdomen has been opened and the splenic pedicle clamped.

If both steroids and splenectomy fail to provide a cure, then some form of immunotherapy may be tried if

spontaneous bleeding is a problem. Yet even if the platelet count does not rise after splenectomy, the patient may have very little trouble with bleeding and immunotherapy should never be given to treat the low platelet count alone. Other surgical intervention in thrombocytopenic states of whatever cause should be avoided if at all possible. There are particular dangers with needle biopsies of internal viscera e.g. liver and kidney, and lumbar puncture should be avoided unless required for therapy (e.g. leukaemia).

Blood coagulation and fibrin formation

Research over the past 20 years has shown that fibrin formation is the result of a complex sequence of enzyme interreactions, some of which are catalysed by other proteins, calcium and lipids. The present concept is based on the cascade defined by Macfarlane in 1965 which has been modified somewhat by subsequent research.

The basis of this cascade (Fig 53.2) is that inactive proteins circulating in the blood are changed becoming active proteolytic enzymes which, in turn, selectively attack the next protein in the sequence converting it into an active enzyme. At each stage there is amplification of the reaction with each enzyme inducing activity

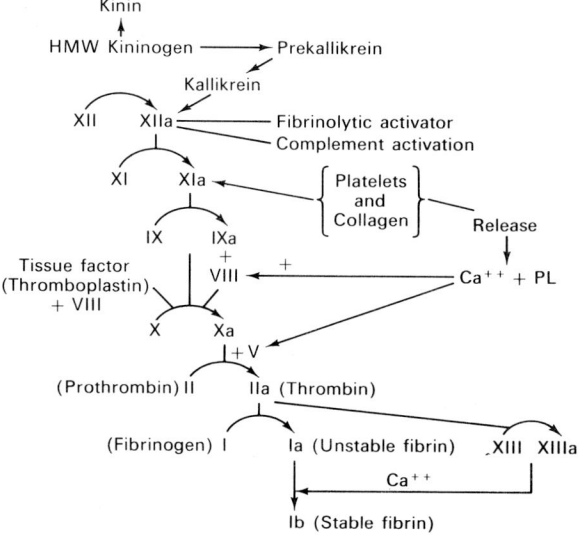

Ca^{++} = Calcium ions
PL   = Phospholipid (tissue or platelet derived)

Fig 53.2 The coagulation 'cascade'.

in many more molecules of the next stage, so that by the time the fibrin is formed a significant amount of fibrin polymer is also formed.

If any factor is absent or deficient due to a genetic abnormality, e.g. Factor VIII in haemophilia or by the action of drugs (anticoagulants), then the cascade fails to function and there is a drastic drop in efficiency. Thus the risk of haemorrhage is increased and in some instances is an inevitable consequence.

Vitamin K dependent proteins

Certain proteins in the cascade are so-called vitamin K dependent, namely Factors IX, X, VII and II. They are manufactured ordinarily in the liver, but absence of vitamin K causes the formation of normal amounts of abnormal proteins which form glutamic acid instead or Y-glutamic acid which is necessary for efficient binding. Oral anticoagulants (warfarin, phenindione) being vitamin K antagonists also impair the formation of Y-glutamic acid. This failure to form Y-glutamic acid does not prevent their activation in the cascade, but slows down the rate of reaction so deterring the amount and rate of thrombin (Factor IIa) formation. Thus, oral anticoagulants when used in therapy only deter fibrin formation and cannot prevent its formation unless used in very large and dangerous doses.

The role of lipids in coagulation

Lipids, including those on the activated platelet surface, attract the same K dependent proteins to their surface by the link of the Y-glutamic acids to Ca^{++} ions by concentrating these inter-reactions. This results in efficient fibrin formation, but at the same time localises the reaction at the site of tissue damage.

The coagulation cascade

Each stage of the intrinsic pathway of the cascade needs to be described in more detail.

Contact phase. Recent studies have revealed that this process by itself is as complex as the total cascade and the theories expressed here are changing rapidly. When blood meets a glass surface in the test tube, it can be shown to have been 'contacted' and the entire cascade moves through to fibrin formation much faster than if the blood is allowed to clot in, say, a plastic tube. The vessel wall in man is not made of glass, but it is now established that when platelet aggregate is formed in its wall by inter-reactions with collagen or microfibrils, or in the wound tract, this complex can activate the coagulation sequence.

Factor XII deficiency. Factor XII deficiency is associated with prolongation of the whole blood clotting time, but the enigma of this situation is that patients with a congenital absence of one or all of these three factors, do not bleed and there is evidence that such patients may have a higher than normal risk of intravascular thrombosis.

Factor XI. Factor XI is activated by XIIa or by the direct action of the platelet-collagen surface to XIa which in turn activates Factor IX. This factor is unstable when freeze-dried, but is present in fresh frozen plasma. Patients with this defect have a higher incidence in Jewish communities.

This tendency to bleed abnormally is mild in the male (nose bleeds and bruising only) but in the female, severe menorrhagia with 'flooding' can be a striking symptom. Mild examples may only show a tendency to excessive blood loss after trauma or surgery.

Treatment is a transfusion of fresh frozen plasma which is effective up to 60 h.

Factor IX (Christmas Factor). This is activated by Factor XIa to form IXa, a serine protease with specificity for Factor X. This is a vitamin K dependent protein. A deficiency of Factor IX (Christmas disease) results in a clinical syndrome identical to that seen in haemophilia (Factor VIII deficiency) and is discussed below.

Factor VIII (Antihaemophiliac globulin). This is a complicated protein complex and may well exist as a loose association of three different molecules, each under separate genetic control.

Factor VII-C (or coagulant fraction) is that part which contributes a catalytic effect to the coagulation cascade enhancing the effect of Factor IXa on Factor X. For maximum efficiency it requires the association of Ca^{++} ions and a lipid surface. It is reduced in amounts to less than 20% of normal in haemophilia. The half-life of this part of the molecule in the circulation is 12 h.

Factor VIIIR-Ag (Factor VIII related antigen). This is closely associated with VIII-C, but is not reduced in amounts in classical haemophilia, but is reduced in association with VIII-C in one form of von Willebrand's syndrome.

Haemophilia and Christmas disease

Impaired synthesis of Factor IX and VII results from sex linked inheritance of a recessive gene defect. The incidence of these defects is 1/1 000 000 for Christmas disease and 1/80 000 approximately for haemophilia. The clinical features vary from severe to mild depending on whether there is 0 activity or higher levels 6–20%. In high grade haemophilia and Christmas disease spontaneous bleeding into joint cavities and deep tissues is frequent with serious damage. Such a tendency shows a curious fluctuation of severity unrelated to the actual levels of Factor VIIIC and IX which tend to remain constant in any one patient or family. Common sites of spontaneous bleeding are:

1 In the joints with consequent acute pain, swelling and the risk of subsequent deformity.
2 In the tongue, with a serious risk of airway obstruction.
3 Into deep tissues – e.g. retroperitoneal space or psoas muscle.

Repeated bleeds into deep tissue or muscle may track along fascial planes and produce pseudo-tumours composed of altered blood. There is only minimal organisation and therefore poor resolution, fortunately such pseudo-tumours are now a rare occurrence. In severe haemophilia and Christmas disease, trivial trauma may result in a life-threatening bleed e.g. into the brain following a head injury. Such bleeds are sometimes diffuse in the brain, but successful treatment without neurological deficit is possible. In mild examples of these syndromes, spontaneous bleeding is rare, but operation or trauma may result in the same excessive bleeding and failure to heal, as is found in patients with severe defects.

Carrier state. As both haemophilia and Christmas disease are inherited as sex linked recessive traits with a defect of the X chromosome, only males are affected. It is frequently necessary to provide genetic counselling to parents of children affected by either syndrome and to affected parents themselves. The affected male will produce carrier daughters, his sons will not be affected (Fig 53.3a). The carrier female can produce normal sons, daughters; affected males and carrier daughters.

Detection of carrier status. Obligate carriers are those who are (a) daughters of a known haemophiliac (b) a female with an affected son.

In those female members of families where haemophilia has occurred who do not fit into any obligate criteria, detection is more complex, but measurement of Factor VIII-C and Factor VIIIR-Ag has increased the ability to detect carriers. By this technique it is possible to detect 70% of possible carriers, but it is impossible to give a guarantee of normality. In the problem case, sex differentiation and the diagnosis of the affected male fetus *in utero* is possible by amniocentesis with an assay level of Factor VIII-C in fetal blood. If it is determined that a suspected carrier has a male fetus with low Factor VIII-C levels, termination of the pregnancy is justified. The occasional female carrier of

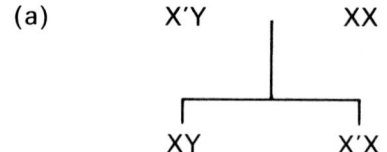

(a)   X'Y   XX

XY   X'X

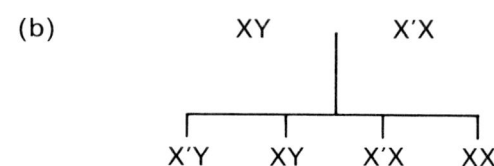

(b)   XY   X'X

X'Y   XY   X'X   XX

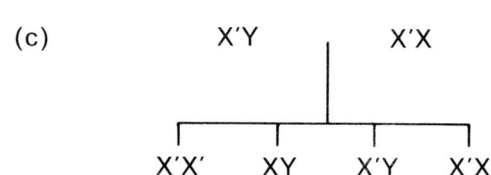

(c)   X'Y   X'X

X'X'   XY   X'Y   X'X

Fig 53.3 The variations of sex linked recessive trait.

haemophilia and Christmas disease with low levels of Factor IX may show a mild tendency to abnormal bleeding.

Treatment

Haemophilia. Having determined the exact defect, treatment is by replacement of the missing factor. All clotting factors are present in fresh frozen plasma (FFP) and this can be used in emergency and in the treatment of mild haemophilia for minor surgery. Enthusiasm for the repeated use of frozen plasma is waning due to the incidence of distressing reactions from antibody produced against IgG subgroups. FFP is not suitable for replacement of Factor IX, but why this is so remains a mystery.

Cryoprecipitate made from fresh plasma contains an increased concentration of Factor VIII-C and fibrinogen and is suitable for the treatment of haemophilia. It is being replaced by the use of freeze-dried Factor VIII concentrate. The content of these concentrates is expressed in units of activity – one unit being equivalent to that in 1 ml of fresh plasma.

Where trauma or surgery have caused bleeding, Factor VIII replacement has to be given which will achieve 50–100% of normal activity in the patient and treatment is continued until healing is complete. As the half-life of Factor VIII-C is 12 h in the circulation, daily infusions are essential.

When there is a need for treatment to abort or prevent spontaneous bleeding (e.g. haemarthrosis), one dose may suffice. The development of home therapy, where the patient or relative gives an infusion, has prevented the scourge of painful haemarthrosis and the crippling deformities that used to follow such recurrent bleeds. Thus the child with haemophilia can lead a relatively normal existence and enjoy uninterrupted education.

Christmas disease. The availability of a concentrate of Factor IX (along with Factor X and II) has revolutionised the treatment of Christmas disease. Again daily infusions are required, but the effective haemostasis level appears to be lower.

Factor X deficiency. Deficiencies of this factor are inherited as an autosomal recessive defect, but are very rare and it is difficult to define the exact pattern of bleeding.

Factor V. Factor V deficiency is inherited as an autosomal factor and appears in the homozygote form. The pattern of bleeding is variable, but usually occurs from mucous membranes and only occasionally do haemarthroses develop. Treatment is straightforward by use of fresh frozen plasma.

Fibrinogen

Thrombin cleaves fibrinogen to form what is known as fibrin monomer. This monomer can circulate as such or form complexes with itself which are sometimes called soluble fibrin monomer complexes (SFMC). Both monomer and the SFMC can polymerise to form the typical fibrin clot, or thrombus to reinforce the haemostatic plug, or in pathological states form an occlusive thrombus.

Abnormal fibrinogen

Congenital hypo- or afibrinogenaemia has been found in some patients although this is a rare deficiency. It can be associated with severe haemorrhage following trauma, but it is not accompanied by a high risk of spontaneous bleeding. Thus patients with this defect have survived for long periods without significant risk to life or organ function, unlike haemophilia or Christmas disease. Acquired hypofibrinogenaemia can occur in severe liver disease and can also be induced by certain forms of anticoagulant therapy, and is a feature of Diffuse Intravascular Coagulation (DIC). Treatment of fibrinogen lack is simple in that

replacement with plasma or fibrinogen concentrate can stop the bleeding very quickly, and the half-life of the transfused fibrinogen is approximately 2–3 days. The necessary haemostatic level for anything other than major trauma is 0.5 g/l and as normal man has a circulating fibrinogen of 2–3 g/l there is an excess in the circulation.

The lack of spontaneous bleeding in the absence of fibrinogen does suggest that the day-to-day maintenance of the vascular system in health depends very largely on the platelets.

Dysfibrinogenaemia

Various types of this have been described where the apparent normal amounts of fibrinogen do not polymerise properly when thrombin is generated. No clinical abnormality is shown in 50%, but defective wound healing, abnormal haemostasis and thrombotic tendencies have been described in association with these rare defects.

Factor XIII

The function of this factor, which is activated by thrombin, is to cross-link the fibrin molecules thus stabilising the polymerised fibrin. Factor XIII deficiency is a rare defect which is inherited as an autosomal recessive trait and only expressed in the homozygous state. It is associated with a mild bleeding tendency after trauma, but bleeding from the umbilical cord at birth is a common feature. Wound healing may be delayed and irregular scar formation is common. Treatment is straightforward with plasma as only 5% of normal levels are required for normal haemostasis and wound healing. One transfusion is often sufficient to deal with post-traumatic or surgical bleeding.

Laboratory diagnosis of specific factor deficiency

When normal spontaneous bleeding following surgery or trauma are encountered it is of vital importance to pinpoint the exact defect (Table 2). Thus the facilities of haematology departments are required, as there is no short cut in establishing such a diagnosis. Once defined and the severity of the defect quantified, therapy is the replacement of the missing factor. Replacement of missing factors does, however, require careful monitoring, especially postoperatively. Daily assays of each deficient factor are necessary as there is considerable variation between individuals as to how they handle the replacement and the transfused protein can vary from batch to batch.

Table 2
LABORATORY TESTS

	Method	Normal range	Prolonged
1. Bleeding time	Ivy method, Template method	3–6 min	Deficiency of platelet numbers or function
2. Whole blood clotting time	Lee and White	3–6 min	Deficiency of Factor XII Severe deficiency of Factor VIII or IX Afibrinogenaemia Heparin therapy
3. Prothrombin time	Quick's one stage thrombo test	Depends on local method	Deficiency of Factors; X, VII, V, II and I
4. Activated partial thromboplastin time	Exact technique depends on local practice	Depends on local method	Deficiency of Factors XII, XI, IX, VIII and a severe deficiency of X, II and I
5. Plasma thrombin clotting time	Variable	10–15 s	Afibrinogenaemia Dysfibrinogenaemia FDP Heparin therapy
6. Fibrinogen level	Fibrinogen titre Claus, Ratmoff and Menzies	1.5–3.0 g/l	Afibrinogenaemia Dysfibrinogenaemia DIC (*see* p. 878)

The combination of tests 3 and 4 allows the defect to be defined in groups. Any abnormality suggesting defect of Factors XII, XI, IX, XIII, X and V requires specific factor assays to determine the exact deficient or missing Factor.

Other tests may be included in the 'screen', e.g. plasma reptilase clotting time, measurement of fibrin fibrinogen degradation products (FDP), tests for fibrinolytic activity.

Anticoagulant therapy

Heparin

Heparin is a useful immediately acting anticoagulant in that it prevents, by linking with anti-thrombin III, the action of Factor Xa and thrombin (IIa). Thus it prevents fibrin formation occurring. However, in its efficiency lies a risk. When used in excess amounts or for prolonged periods of time, spontaneous haemorrhage may occur. When this happens, it will not stop until all the heparin is removed from the circulation by the use of the specific inhibitor, protamine sulphate, (1.0 mg protamine sulphate will neutralise 100 units of heparin). Heparin therapy is not straightforward; the reaction of the patient to any given batch is extremely variable, and the potency of each batch differs. The safest and most effective way of giving heparin is by continuous intravenous drip or using a pump.

Oral anticoagulants

The use of vitamin K antagonists is common practice in medicine for long-term anticoagulant therapy. These, by preventing the formation of normal factors, II, VII, IX and X, deter fibrin formation. It is customary to reduce the overall activity of these factors as measured by the prothrombin time, or a variant of this technique, to between 10–20% of normal level. This is commonly expressed as the ratio of the patient's clotting time to the normal and the therapeutic range is defined as being 2–4 i.e. prolonging the patient's 'prothrombin' time 2–4 times normal. Provided the level of these factors is kept within the therapeutic range, spontaneous bleeding is a rare event, but does occur when careless therapy or the use of another drug potentiates or inhibits the effect of the anticoagulant, e.g. antibiotics, phenylbutazone, aspirin.

When very low levels occur, spontaneous bleeding may take place, and therapy to prevent bleeding or to allow surgery is required. This can be achieved by the use of fresh frozen plasma, or II, IX, X concentrate which will raise the level by some 10–20% of normal. Intravenous vitamin K can also be given, but this may return the prothrombin level to 100% and can, if given in excess amounts, inhibit further use of oral anticoagulants for a time. Although small doses of vitamin K are sometimes recommended, the effect of a dose such as 2 mg is unpredictable and too high a level of II, VII or X may be produced in those who need anticoagulant therapy for life-threatening thrombosis.

Ancrod, defibrase

Certain purified snake venoms have been used as anticoagulants. These two viper venoms contain a coagulant protein which is capable of removing fibrinogen from the circulating blood, thus totally preventing fibrin formation. Their use is not widespread, but they are useful alternatives as anticoagulants to heparin, especially for long-term treatment by intravenous or subcutaneous administration. As well as having an anticoagulant effect, these venoms reduce fibrinogen levels and so lower the viscosity of normal blood, thus improving flow in the microcirculation and damaged vessels. This lowered viscosity, rather than the anticoagulant effect, may be an indication for use. Laboratory control is simple because lowered fibrinogen levels are easy to measure.

Von Willebrand's syndrome (vWS)

In any discussion on haemostasis, perhaps the most perplexing problem in the scientific sense is this complex syndrome. Characteristically it is defined as a syndrome inherited either as an autosomal dominant or as a recessive trait. It expresses in a very variable homozygote form and is found to exist in several diverse heterozygote variants. In the classical form members of such families, both females and males, are affected and several members of each generation. Unlike haemophilia where the defect (mild or severe) remains in any family, in vWS there is variation in any one family, and even in each patient from time to time. Conventionally, this syndrome is characterised by features of both platelet and coagulation deficiency, i.e.:

Normal platelet count
Reduced, but not absent, platelet adhesiveness
Normal platelet aggregation with ADP, noradrenaline, collagen, 5HT and thrombin, but selective absent aggregation with Ristocetin. This latter abnormality is corrected by the addition of normal plasma containing Factor VII-vWF. The prostaglandin pathway and C-AMP levels are normal.

In addition, in the classical form, there are low levels of both Factor VIIIC and Factor VIIIR-AG. The pattern of abnormal bleeding is usually that of a platelet function abnormality with prolonged bleeding time, e.g. there is bleeding from mucous membranes, nose, skin, etc. However, in the more severe examples, when Factor VIIIC and R-AG are below 10% of normal, more serious post-trauma bleeding can develop and haemarthroses and severe gastrointestinal bleeding may occur.

This genetic muddle is more confounded by reports that many variations of this pattern are possible (e.g. normal Factor VIIIC and RAG but absent vW factor). Transfusion of stored or fresh normal plasma results not only in the expected post-transfusion rise of Factor VIIIC and RAG, but there is also evidence of synthesis of both these proteins in that a rise of VIII activity persists for 24 h before decaying at a similar rate to that seen in haemophilia. Further, a similar rise can be induced by plàsma derived from a 'patient with haemophilia', or by stored plasma deficient in Factor VIII. Thus the VIII deficiency in vWS is due to a defective synthesis of the Factor VIII molecule (C, RAG and vWF) and the factor responsible is not carried on the X chromosome.

The problem that this syndrome presents in identification is obvious but, in its severe form treatment is straightforward and simpler than in haemophilia because Factor VIII replacement lasts twice as long. The anomaly is, that in severe forms of this syndrome, it is only necessary to raise the VIIIC levels to approximately 50% to achieve haemostasis and normal healing. It would appear to be unnecessary to return the bleeding time to normal, although this can happen when fresh frozen plasma is used. Although in its fully expressed form this syndrome can cause significant spontaneous and postinjury bleeding, it is not so severe as in haemophilia and wound healing is seldom delayed. Survival into adult life is usual and the defect is widespread in affected families.

Fibrinolytic mechanism (plasminogen/plasmin system)

The fibrinolytic mechanism exists as an important physiological system to limit the formation of excess and, therefore, potentially dangerous fibrin in the vessels. The mechanism, which essentially is much simpler than that of the coagulation sequence, is nevertheless complex.

Basically plasminogen, an inert protein, is cleaved in two stages to form plasmin by the effect of activator, an enzyme defined by its ability to induce the plasminogen to change to plasmin rather than as a chemical entity. Activators may exist in several types:

Vascular endothelial activator. In both veins and arteries, activator can be shown to be secreted from endothelial cells and to be released in greater amount when these are damaged. It is presumed that it also exists as proactivator which can be activated in the damaged cell or excreted into the blood. This activator is probably the most important.

Blood activator. The production of blood activator by the complex 'contact' interaction between Factor XII and the kallikrein system has already been described. This activator, derived from circulating proactivator, is different to vascular activator, but the kinetics of its effect on plasminogen are identical.

Chemically induced activator. A separate activator has been described as being produced by the effect of dextran sulphate, but again this may represent the activation of secreted endothelial proactivator or blood activator.

Tissue activator. Certain tissues appear to be rich in activator, e.g. heart, uterus, endometrium and prostate, but again the amount of activator may be related to the vascular content of the tissue and is probably endothelial activator. The exception to this is the high activity in certain membranes; arachnoid, dura and pleura. The peritoneal serosa does not contain activator.

A further exception is the kidney which secretes a β globulin activator in the urine (Urokinase) which appears to be different from endothelial activator in its action on plasminogen. Tissue culture has shown this is secreted by specific renal cells and its function must be to prevent 'clot' formation in the ureter and bladder.

Leucocyte activator. Leucocytes contain activator of possible importance in the inflammatory process.

Neoplastic activator. Certain types of malignant tumours, e.g. lung, breast, skin, colon, apparently secrete large amounts of a 'Urokinase-like' activator.

Inhibitors of activator

As in the coagulation sequence, inhibitors to neutralise released activator exist (a) α^1 globulin antiactivator, (b) a platelet antiactivator and (c) a Urokinase inhibitor which appears to be specific for that activator and not for blood or endothelial activator.

Plasminogen

Plasminogen circulates in the blood as an active single chain β globulin which exists in two forms with different N-terminal amino acid groups; (a) one with glutamic acid (Plg-Glu) and (b) the other with lysine (Plg-Lys). In man, the majority of the plasminogen exists as Plg-Glu. What is important is that Plg-Lys has a greater affinity to bind to fibrin than Plg-Glu.

Plasmin

Plasmin derived from plasminogen is not readily detectable in plasma as there exists a series of inhibitors which neutralise free plasmin.

One of the mysteries of the fibrinolytic mechanism has been the presence of powerful antiplasmins. Recent studies show that there are three forms:

1 An immediately effective and non-reversible α'-globulin.
2 An immediate but slower acting α^2M macroglobulin.
3 A progressive α' anti-trypsin which destroys formed plasmin slowly.

Anti-thrombin III (especially in association with heparin) has a weak anti-plasmin effect. Plasmin can digest fibrin but can also split the fibrinogen molecule and factors VIII and V.

If formed plasmin is so efficiently neutralised in the blood, the lysis of fibrin appears to be difficult to explain. Two theories have been advanced in the past to explain this puzzle:

1 When fibrin is formed, plasminogen is bound to it and when activator contacts this complex, the generated plasmin is protected from the antiplasmins and digests the fibrin.
2 The reversible plasmin-antiplasmin complex dissociates on contact with fibrin, releasing the plasmin to digest the fibrin.

In recent years several observations suggest that both these theories may be correct.

Once attached to fibrin the plasmin is protected from the various antiplasmins. In addition, the sum of the proteolytic effect of these bound proteins appears to be greater than expected. Thus nature has designed an efficient and effective physiological mechanism for promoting lysis of formed fibrin in both physiological and pathological states.

Thrombolytic therapy. In patients with deep venous thrombosis (DVT) and in pulmonary embolism and in some patients with recent arterial thrombosis or emboli of the limbs, it is possible to enhance normal fibrinolytic activity to remove large amounts of formed fibrin using urokinase, a direct plasminogen activator or by inducing activator formation using Streptokinase (*see* chapter 33).

Action of plasmin on fibrinogen and fibrin

When plasmin acts on fibrinogen or fibrin, the proteolytic activity breaks down these proteins in a predictable way producing fragments of the parent molecule which retain the antigenic properties of fibrinogen, but which also develop neo-antigens for each fragment. The fate of the fragments, always debatable, does not affect treatment.

Acquired haemostatic failure

This may occur in an acute or chronic form in someone who has never had an abnormal tendency to bleed either spontaneously or after trauma. Whenever this occurs it can cause 'clinical' surprise and can be life-threatening e.g. in association with major or minor surgery. Perhaps the commonest cause is deficiency of platelet numbers or function as in renal failure.

Heparin

In modern high technology medicine, a frequent cause of unexpected haemostatic failure is the presence of heparin in the circulating blood at unexpectedly high levels. While this may happen when conventional anticoagulant therapy is being administered, the 'unexpected' episode is usually associated with the use of heparin to maintain patency of intravenous or arterial lines in intensive care. Careless measurement of heparin additions to crystalloid solutions is common in clinical practice and this is not helped by the various multidose ampoules which contain 1000 μ/ml, 5000 μ/ml and 25000 μ/ml of heparin.

When abnormal bleeding is due to heparin and it is essential to reverse the effect, this can be done with protamine sulphate, 1.0 mg neutralises 100 μ heparin. This antidote is effective immediately, but it is important to neutralise all available heparin if bleeding is to be stopped and check this in the laboratory. 'Heparin-rebound' can occur several hours after effective neutralisation due to proteolytic digestion of the protamine with consequent release of the heparin and should be guarded against.

Oral anticoagulants

The action of these has already been described. Although most patients receiving these drugs as therapy are well documented, they can cause unexpected haemostatic failure, e.g. in the unconscious patient after a road accident, in attempted murder or where the doctor has prescribed the wrong drug, e.g. Marevan (warfarin) instead of Mandrax. Occasionally these drugs have been used by unstable persons to cause abnormal bleeding and attract attention, a significant number among members of the nursing profession.

Once the defect is defined, correction can be achieved by vit. K or replacement therapy. A further variant of unexpected haemostatic failure due to anti-coagulants occurs when patients receiving vit. K antagonists are, in addition, given a drug which potentiates them e.g. aspirin, phenylbutazone or broad spectrum antibiotics. The number of substances which potentiate or inhibit the action of anticoagulants increases each year and advice on these inter-reactions should be sought before giving a new drug to a patient receiving warfarin.

Liver failure can result in failure of production of Factors II, VII, X and IX and in severe forms Factor V and Fibrinogen. Such failure can be accompanied by intravascular coagulation with a very confusing resultant picture.

Fibrinolysis can also cause abnormal bleeding. It is exceedingly rare for this to occur in terms of a systemic reaction except in thrombolytic therapy, but occasional cases have been described in patients with carcinoma of the prostate and in cirrhosis of the liver – the latter appears to be more common in alcoholic cirrhosis.

Lysis due to the local release of activator from damaged tissue can cause secondary bleeding e.g. following removal of the prostate, in acute gastric erosion and in association with subdural haemorrhage. When excess lysis is suspected to be the cause of abnormal bleeding, the excess activator can be neutralised by ε-aminocaproic acid (Epsikapron) or tranexamic acid (Cyklokapron). These inhibitors block the binding site for activator and plasminogen on the fibrinogen molecule. Aprotinin (Trasylol) can also be used as this has both an antiplasmin and antiactivator effect *in vitro*, yet its efficiency in reversing excess lysis *in vivo* is less well documented.

Acquired inhibitors of blood coagulation

The appearance of inhibitors with specificity for certain stages of the coagulation sequence are well documented. These are usually IgG antibodies which can totally inhibit one factor or part of the cascade 'sequence'.

Factor VIII inhibitors

Factor VIII inhibitors can develop in high grade haemophiliacs who have received multiple doses of plasma or concentrate. When this happens they are resistant to treatment with Factor VIII replacement. Occasionally, this specific inhibitor can develop in patients with normal levels of Factor VIII e.g. post-pregnancy, in association with malignancy or dissemi-

nated lupus erythematosus (DLE). In both instances, inhibitor has a progressive destruction effect on Factor VIII and treatment is difficult.

A massive transfusion can overcome the antibody effect, but in some instances this cannot be achieved. Recently, the use of partially activated II, X, IX concentrate has been advocated as has exchange plasmapheresis. In the patient with normal Factor VIII levels the autoantibody is often transient and in some can be suppressed by intravenous cyclophosphamide.

Intravascular coagulation and fibrinolysis (ICF) and DIC

When a normal person is exposed to massive trauma e.g. road traffic accident, the whole gamut of platelet activation, fibrin formation and fibrinolysis is 'triggered' off as part of the normal haemostatic reaction to injury and is in this context protective.

In some individuals the stimulus is so great that these reactions result in consumption of platelets, coagulation factors and activation of the fibrinolytic mechanism which can be complicated by bleeding, 'consumption coagulopathy' or clotting due to excess fibrin formation with consequent tissue damage, Diffuse Intravascular Coagulation or DIC. Both these situations can be deleterious and the complication of excess blood loss or tissue damage can increase the mortality.

Opinion and fact relating to this syndrome are varied and controversial, but it is recognised that apart from trauma this sequence of events (Fig 53.4) can occur in a wide variety of situations and is an expression of the body's reaction to injury, infection, malignancy, obstetrical complications, immune complex syndromes and snake bite.

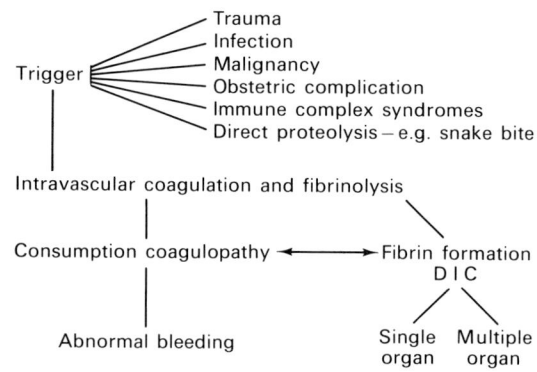

Fig 53.4 The mechanism of diffuse intravascular coagulation.

In only about 10% of those patients with significant changes in the blood does the classic consumption and/or DIC develop. When it does occur it is of prognostic significance. By scoring the clinical and laboratory investigations, it is possible to define four stages of severity.

Clinical features

Tissue damage evident in:

Brain	–	coma
Lung	–	hypoxia
Heart	–	failure
Liver	–	jaundice
Kidney	–	oliguria, anuria
Skin	–	purpura and/or gangrene
Muscle	–	acidosis

Three or more systems involved constitute a 'high' score.

Laboratory tests

Platelet count	– thrombocytopenia
Fibrinogen	– low levels
FDPs	– high levels
Thrombin time	– prolonged
Reptilase time	– prolonged
Ethanol-gel	
Protamine sulphate precipitates	– positive
Prothrombin time	– prolonged
Activated partial thrombo-plastin time	– prolonged
Factor VIII-C, VIII-RAg and Factor V assays	– high or low levels

If 60% of these tests are abnormal it constitutes a high score. (No one test on its own provides a reliable indicator of the existence or severity of this syndrome.)

Prognostic score

Taken together in an analysis of more than 150 patients these scores showed a relationship to mortality (Table 3).

Table 3

Group	Clinical Score	Lab Score	Mortality
1	Low	Low	10%
2	High	Low	11%
3	Low	High	57%
4	High	High	82%

Groups 1 and 2 represent mild examples of ICF and mortality is probably due to the underlying disease. In group 3 the pattern is that of 'consumption coagulopathy' without significant tissue damage. In group 4 there is undoubted DIC with a high consequent mortality due either to the severity of the underlying disease or the DIC tissue damage.

Treatment

Once diagnosed, the treatment of this condition is difficult. Many reports of successful therapy relate to mild examples of ICF which would be expected to recover without treatment. However certain basic guides to treatment can be given:

1   Treat the underlying disease if it is known. In the case of infection this means using the appropriate antibiotic intravenously.
2   Maintain blood volume with plasma or whole blood. Packed cells should not be used as this may result in increased viscosity and tendency to thrombosis. If bleeding is a feature, there is significant depletion of coagulation factors – replacement with fresh frozen plasma or cryoprecipitate is indicated.
3   Anticoagulant therapy. While there is abundant anecdotal evidence of benefit following heparin therapy in individual cases, there is no good aggregate data to justify the use of this therapy in established consumption coagulopathy or DIC. In a few situations heparin therapy may be justified to prevent DIC or coagulopathy e.g. amniotic fluid embolism, incompatible blood transfusion and severe septicaemia.
4   Fibrinolytic therapy. There is experimental evidence, but no data from clinical trials, in man to suggest that induced lytic activity using excess activator in the form of Urokinase or Streptokinase reverses the tissue damage of established DIC.
5   Steroid therapy and fibrinolytic inhibitors. There is no evidence that either form of therapy is of benefit in this syndrome.

Further reading

Bloom A.L., Thomas D.P., eds (1981). *Haemostasis and Thrombosis*. Edinburgh, London, Melbourne and New York: Churchill-Livingstone.
Schmidt R.M., ed (1980). *C.R.C. Handbook Series in Clinical Laboratory Science, Vol. III., Section I. Haematology*. Boca Raton Florida: C.R.C. Press Inc.

Infection in surgery

C.A. BARTZOKAS

'Prevention is better than cure' has always been the microbiologist's most potent dictum. It still is. The main contributions of microbiology to medicine are the introduction of immunisation and the raised consciousness of the principles of hygiene and public health. Despite the development of sensitive, specific and rapid detection techniques and major advances in antimicrobial chemotherapy the problem of infection remains unsolved. Although sophisticated laboratory investigations are now offering additional criteria to 'Koch's Postulates', the efficacy of such results are dependent upon careful and accurate evaluation of an infection.

An understanding of the patient's defences and of the biological and clinical basis of infection is an essential prerequisite for the prevention and elimination of microbial disease. When an infection has occurred, its successful control depends upon an understanding of its epidemiology and the selection of appropriate chemotherapy. The host's resistance to infection, microbial pathogenicity and the hospital environment itself are the main determinants in the pathogenesis of surgical infection. Alterations in any of these factors may result in microbial disease of varied severity.

Host's resistance to infection

Lipids on the skin surface, bacteriocins and other inhibitors control the size of the resident flora: the stratified and cornified epithelium is an efficient mechanical barrier to infection. However, with loss of epithelium the underlying tissues must be protected with sterile dressings or skin homografts. In the respiratory tract the mucociliary flow is a very important clearance mechanism: its impairment results in the infections associated with chronic bronchitis and cystic fibrosis. The flushing action of urine has a similar role in the urinary tract where, again, impairment by diverticulosis, stones or catheterisation facilitates infection.

Humoral and cellular immune defences, acting locally, complement these physical barriers. Food-borne micro-organisms descending the gastrointestinal tract are faced with, among other factors, IgA-type immuno-globulins synthesised locally in the *lamina propia* of the mucous membranes. Whenever the anatomical barriers are breached, a comprehensive second line of defence is normally activated: the invaders are attacked by polymorphonuclear granulocytes and monocytes of the blood and by tissue macrophages. Following engulfment and enzymatic digestion of the target microbes, most of the neutrophils and eosinophils, which have migrated to the injury specifically, die and accumulate, so forming pus. Others are killed by bacterial exotoxins, for example, those produced by staphylococci and streptococci. At the end of this acute inflammatory reaction, the monocytes and macrophages remove the debris of killed host and bacterial cells. Moreover, macrophages form a reservoir of microbial antigen which is slowly released and presented to the T-lymphocytes. A sensitised and activated T-lymphocyte will (a) instruct the circulating B-lymphocytes so that immunoglobulins are produced (humoral immunity) and (b) initiate a classical cell-mediated immune reaction, involving a direct attack upon host cells containing intracellular infectious agents and release of lymphokines. These latter poorly-defined substances stimulate further lymphocyte proliferation and regulate the inflammatory reaction. An intact cell-mediated immunity is essential, therefore, for protection against mainly intracellular infectious agents (e.g. brucellae, mycobacteria, salmonellae). Both neutropenia and a lack of phagocytes or defective phagocytic functions, as in chronic granulomatous disease when the phagocytes are enzymatically deficient, predispose to infection. Similarly, agammaglobulin-aemia or deficiencies in cell-mediated immunity dramatically decrease resistance to infection. The complex armamentarium of proteins, factors and cells which constitutes the immune system is responsible for triggering off the series of reactions against injury known as inflammation. Initially, the release of mediators from damaged mast cells (e.g. histamine, kinins, prostaglandins, serotonin, etc.) leads to vascular changes which promote exudation of polymorpho-nuclear leukocytes. Subsequently, the complement system is activated and later mononuclear cells appear (subacute inflammation). Thus inflammation is intrinsically associated with infection and is intended to eliminate invading microbes and repair tissue injuries.

The terminology of infection

The term 'infection' denotes microbial multiplication in the tissues; 'sepsis' is infection with pyogenic bacteria. Whereas an *infective* disease is one brought about by infection, *infectivity* is a property of the micro-organism, not the disease. Infectivity denotes the capacity of a micro-organism to infect and can be expressed in terms of the numbers of organisms required (infective dose). Inanimate sources are described as 'contaminated' rather than as 'infected'. *Contamination* is not limited to inanimate sources, however. When applied to tissues, this term suggests deposition of organisms without ill effect and without replication. *Colonisation* denotes the continued presence and multiplication of micro-organisms in a specified area. The terms 'pathogenicity' and 'virulence', which describe the relative ability of organisms to cause disease, are increasingly employed interchangeably. Pathogenicity should refer to the overall tendency in behaviour of a defined group of organisms, such as the members of one species, whereas virulence concerns the relative behaviour of individual strains. It is correct,

for example, to speak of BCG as a relatively avirulent strain of the pathogenic *Mycobacterium bovis*. The members of the normal microbial flora of the body surfaces are by tradition termed 'commensals'. When the host's defences are impaired, these same organisms as well as some normally harmless free-living saprophytes, may well take the opportunity to initiate infection; they are then termed 'opportunistic pathogens'.

Disease which has originated from the patient's own normal or altered flora is called *endogenous* (self) infection. Infecting organisms disseminated from the environment or other individuals, are described as *exogenous* (extraneous). When the source of infection is known to be the hospital environment, staff or other in-patients, *hospital* (nosocomial) infection is specified. Infection between patients and/or staff is called *cross-infection*. A postoperative infection of a prosthesis or implant is specified as *xenogenic*.

Factors predisposing to surgical infections

The major determinants of surgical sepsis are the extremes of age, hypertension, cardiovascular disease, immunological deficiences (such as hypo- or agamma-globulinaemia, or arising from immunosuppression with corticosteroids or cytotoxic drugs), haematological disorders, neoplasia, renal diseases, major operations, multiple injuries, disseminated infections and anaesthesia.

Underlying predisposing conditions include nutritional deficiencies, dysproteinaemias, metabolic disorders (e.g. diabetes mellitus), obesity, antibiotic administration, hospitalisation and chronic infections.

Operative circumstances. The traumatisation of tissues and anaesthesia are perhaps the most important factors. The risk in emergency surgery is higher than in elective. Meticulous debridement and irrigation of injuries with copious amounts of saline are definitely superior to local or systemic chemoprophylaxis, although the rapid formation of fibrin may negate the full benefit of irrigation debridement. The nature of the operation and its duration can be crucial. For example, in clean elective operations, particularly those involving areas of poor vascularity, the rate of infection doubles with each hour of the operation. Incisions longer than 15 cm and microdestruction by diathermy increase the opportunities for infection. Devitalised or necrotic tissue being both vulnerable to microbial invasion and offering first class nutritional conditions for bacterial growth, should be debrided drastically. However, even brief interruptions to the vascular flow should be avoided whenever possible, as even temporary ischaemia can alter the oxidation-reduction potential and favour anaerobic proliferation. Paradoxically, inadequate haemostasis, resulting in haematoma provides anaerobic conditions: blood is the optimum bacteriological medium and when clotted the penetration of antimicrobials becomes impossible. Only the gentle manipulation of a dextrous surgeon – as advocated by Paré – can prevent unnecessary tissue necrosis arising from ischaemia, retractor damage or haematoma formation. Foreign bodies (e.g. implants, prostheses, alloplastic grafts, etc.) are obviously deprived from the benefits of both blood flow and defence cells and hence are very susceptible to xenogenic infection. In a septic wound, sutures can act as foreign bodies. The by-pass of anatomic barriers by indwelling catheters and various intravascular manipulations can greatly predispose to colonisation and infection.

Localised surgical sepsis

Surveillance of wound infections

In accidental wounds and burns the nature of the contaminating bacteria reflects the local environment; staphylococci, streptococci, aerobic and anaerobic bacilli, enterobacteria and various other microorganisms are involved. Wound infections are the most frequently encountered form of surgical sepsis and in the UK may account for up to a third of all hospital infections. Although in certain surgical wounds bacterial infection is often predictable, it is nevertheless not always possible to introduce effective prevention. Frequently wounds are contaminated with bacteria without any signs of infection and in such cases local hygiene may be the only treatment necessary.

As various surgical procedures inherently carry different risks of sepsis, it is important to monitor the infection rate separately for each class of operation, particularly when the effect of chemoprophylaxis has to be assessed. The overall incidence of wound infections on a national basis is not known. However, limited surveys of different hospital populations have indicated that the incidence may vary between 4.6% and 14%. The overall wound infection rate, often used for local or national comparisons without the inclusion of data relating to individual classes of operation, can be misleading. In many hospitals all surgical infections are surveyed, classified and computed by the Control of Infection Nurse and the Microbiologist. The following classification for wounds has been proposed by the Committee on Control of Surgical Infection of the American College of Surgeons:

Class I:
(Clean)

Non-traumatic wound in which no inflammation was encountered, no break in

Class I—*contd.*

technique occurred, and respiratory, alimentary and genitourinary tracts were not transected.

Class II:
(Clean-Contaminated)

Non-traumatic wound in which minor break in technique occurred or in which the gastrointestinal, genitourinary, or respiratory tracts were entered without significant spillage.

Class III:
(Contaminated)

A fresh traumatic wound from a relatively clean source or an operative wound in which there is a major break in technique, gross spillage from the gastrointestinal tract, or entrance into the genitourinary or biliary tracts in the presence of infected urine or bile. This includes incisions in which acute, nonpurulent inflammation is encountered.

Class IV:
(Dirty)

Traumatic wound from a dirty source or traumatic wound receiving delayed treatment. Includes operative wounds in which acute bacterial inflammation is encountered or in which clean tissue is transected to gain access to a collection of pus.

The wound infection rate following class I operations is the most sensitive monitor of surgical technique and skill and, theoretically, should be zero %, although in practice it can go up to 5%. The rate of infections in class III operations (without chemoprophylaxis) can be as high as 50%. Detailed wound infection rates should be circulated monthly to the surgeons and members of the Control of Infection Committee. Surprisingly, infection surveillance alone, without any additional precautions or special measures, can appreciably lower the overall infection rate.

Abscesses

Staphylococcal aureus and skin commensals can cause stitch abscesses along the suture line 3–4 days postoperatively. A few days following accidental trauma or surgery, anaerobic streptococci and clostridia and aerobes such as staphylococci and enterobacteria, can be associated with crepitant necrotising cellulitis in soft tissues. This condition should be differentiated from the fulminant *Clostridium perfrigens* gangrene. In the latter, *Clostridium perfrigens*, often in association with other clostridia, may initiate classic gas gangrene. Surgical intervention to excise infected muscle, decompress the facial compartment and introduce hyperbaric oxygen, should be undertaken urgently and the maximum dose of penicillin the patient can tolerate should be administered intravenously. Most clostridia and other anaerobes acting in synergy with the omnipresent *Staphylococcus aureus* can cause deep tissue infections generally known as postoperative gangrene. The pyogenic cocci and enterobacteria can be responsible for the destruction and rapidly spreading necrotising fasciitis (necrotising erysipelas, suppurative fasciitis, acute infective gangrene) associated with heavily contaminated injuries and abdominal surgery. One to two weeks following lower abdominal operations *Staphylococcus aureus* and microaerophilic streptococci, often mixed with coliforms, may cause the rare but synergistic bacterial gangrene (Meleney's, or postoperative synergistic gangrene).

Antibiotics administered for other reasons may delay the presentation of subphrenic, pelvic or paracolic abscesses for several months. The first sign is likely to be unexplained pyrexia. Ultrasound and gallium citrate scanning or computerised tomography have been successfully used for the detection and location of subphrenic abscesses. Administration of an aminoglycoside (e.g. tobramycin) combined with piperacillin or metronidazole during surgical drainage can reduce mortality.

Liver abscesses are uncommon but, when present, are associated with a mortality of up to 80%, particularly when multiple. Ascending cholangitis, chronic cholecystitis and diverticulitis have been identified as sources of bacterial invasion in liver abscesses although the origin of most episodes is not recognised; the organisms usually involved are staphylococci, streptococci and enterobacteria. Elimination of the contributing focus, surgical drainage and parenteral chemotherapy for at least 6 weeks should be undertaken, although percutaneous needle aspiration has been used as a successful alternative to surgery. Blood cultures may reveal the infecting bacteria, but parasitological examination of stool specimens, serological tests and intestinal biopsy are necessary to differentiate amoebic from bacterial abscesses.

Acute cholecystitis in the elderly and obstruction by carcinoma or stones predispose to the formation of biliary tract abscesses by enterobacteria and intestinal anaerobes. Ultrasound or technetium sulphur colloid scanning may be diagnostic. Pre- or peroperative administration of antimicrobials which attain high serum levels are indicated, as antimicrobials excreted in the bile may not penetrate readily into the obstructed gallbladder. Chemoprophylaxis may not reduce the incidence of abscesses in acute pancreatitis.

Surgical progress in implanting devices and foreign materials has provided new territories for bacterial expansion. The absence of blood supply in the prosthesis predisposes to xenogenic infection with skin flora and Gram-negative opportunistic bacteria. Infected vascular grafts can result in thrombosed aneurysms and septicaemia with disseminated septic emboli and metastatic abscesses. Prosthetic hip operations may be followed after 6 to 18 months by osteomyelitis and irreversible joint injury caused by *Staphylococcus aureus* acting alone or in combination with other microorganisms.

Intracerebral abscesses can be formed either by direct extension from chronic ear or sinus infections or haematogenously from a focus usually in the chest or bones. The diagnosis of brain abscesses can be difficult, but fortunately this complication is rare.

Systemic manifestations of surgical sepsis

Fever

Following exposure mainly to endotoxins, but occasionally to exotoxins, the tissue or alveolar macrophages, peripheral polymorphonuclear leukocytes and other defence cells release pyrogens which act by setting the heat-controlling centre in the hypothalmus to a higher temperature. Chills and peripheral vasoconstriction develop while the hypothalamus is adjusting to the new endotoxin-triggered and pyrogen-mediated level.

Septicaemia

When the anatomical barriers to infection have been impaired by accidental or surgical injuries, microorganisms frequently enter the blood-stream. Asymptomatic bacteraemia can originate from minor trauma such as endoscopic manipulations and tooth extraction. During systemic bacterial infection (e.g. meningitis, pneumonia, biliary infection, pyelonephritis) bacteria can also spill over into the blood-stream. Generalised microbial diseases (e.g. leptospirosis, brucellosis, enteric fever) always involve bacteraemia. Low-grade bacteraemia is present in disseminated gonorrhoea and chronic localised infections such as subacute bacterial endocarditis. Rigors should suggest the sudden introduction of organisms into the bloodstream in larger numbers, exogenously (e.g. from contaminated intravenous infusions), endogenously from a focus of infection (e.g. deep seated liver or kidney abscesses, wound sepsis, etc.), or as a result of indwelling catheters through heavily colonised areas. Although neonates, the elderly and immunosuppressed patients may remain afebrile, a raised temperature and pulse, malaise and chills are the classic signs and symptoms of the onset of septicaemia. The terms bacteraemia and septicaemia are often interchanged, but conventionally bacteraemia is a temporary, usually asymptomatic phenomenon and involves small numbers of organisms. Septicaemia, however, is a continuous and indeed progressive life-threatening condition if untreated, accompanied by high temperature and often leading to endotoxic shock.

Since the introduction of antibiotics the incidence of septicaemia caused by *Streptococcus pyogenes* and *Streptococcus pneumoniae* has decreased, while the enterobacteria, including many opportunistic pathogens, are being isolated more frequently. Mortality depends on predisposing factors and can range from 10% in their absence to 90% in cancer patients or leukaemics. Three-quarters of all episodes in surgical patients are hospital acquired. Patients on antibiotics are predisposed to septicaemic infection by strains of *Pseudomonas sp.* or *Klebsiella sp.* often resistant to the antimicrobials concerned. Generally a fifth of all surgical septicaemias originate from the urinary tract, a fifth from the lower intestinal tract and a further fifth from the liver, biliary tract, stomach and upper intestine considered together. Colonised intravenous catheters or shunts and infections of the lungs account for another fifth, while bone, soft tissue and wound infections are responsible for the remaining episodes. Septicaemia originating from the gastrointestinal tract has a special tendency to lead to shock.

The most frequently isolated Gram-positive bacterium from surgical septicaemia is *Staphylococcus aureus*, followed by various streptococcal species, *Staphylococcus albus* and clostridia. *Escherichia coli* is the predominant Gram-negative causative organism, followed by other intestinal organisms such as klebsiellae, bacteroides, pseudomonads and proteus species. Polymicrobial infections in which *Streptococcus faecalis* or *Bacteroides fragilis* are implicated are not uncommon and carry a high mortality. The variety of possible organisms and their unpredictable susceptibility to antimicrobials necessitate urgent laboratory investigation. However, knowledge of the normal flora allows prediction of the organisms likely to be involved in endogenously acquired septicaemias. For instance, both aerobic and anaerobic bacilli are likely to complicate gastrointestinal tract surgery. By monitoring *Staphylococcus aureus* carriage, and the commensal flora generally in immunocompromised patients, predictions can be made for most endogenous infections. In fact, the causative agent in about half of all surgical septicaemias can be anticipated by simply perusing the bacteriological findings in the patient's clinical notes. The therapeutic difficulties that arise are in practice much more likely to be caused by the emergence of resistance in familiar organisms rather than the implication of unusual or uncommon species.

The successful management of septicaemia depends on its early recognition and the identification of the contributing focus. Blood and other relevant specimens (e.g. sputum, urine etc.) must be collected at the earliest suspicion and the causative agent identified and tested for susceptibility to antimicrobials by the most rapid of the newly available techniques. In the last ten years there has been a general increase in both the number of episodes investigated and the rate of laboratory isolation. The improved diagnosis of septicaemia is, in part, due to an increasing awareness among clinicians of the value of laboratory diagnosis which has led to a greater willingness to initiate appropriate tests. As a result, episodes sometimes previously attributed to respiratory failure, pulmonary embolism or myocardial infarctions, are now correctly diagnosed as septicaemia. There has no doubt been a genuine increase in the incidence of septicaemia because of the trend towards major operations and invasive procedures in predisposed patients. In addition, recent advances in microbiological techniques are now being applied to the more rapid detection and identification of the causative organisms. The preparation of more specifically formulated culture media, location of blood culture incubators in the wards and the introduction of a schedule of early subcultures, enable a significant proportion of positive blood cultures to be reported in less than 16 h following collection.

The time taken to report upon blood cultures can be further reduced by radiometry. This automated procedure is based on the detection of $^{14}CO_2$, produced by the microbial metabolism of ^{14}C-labelled substrates which have been incorporated in a specially formulated growth medium. An automated system (BACTEC) can now detect up to 30% of all positive blood cultures within 12 h, 60–70% by 24 h and 80–90% by 48 h. This is a major breakthrough in the rapid diagnosis of septicaemia. However, the benefit of improved laboratory techniques can be negated by the collection of inappropriate specimens. Collection of three 15 ml specimens of blood two-hourly, preferably when the temperature is rising, is sufficient, although when the number of infecting organisms is exceedingly low or they are present intermittently (e.g. endocarditis) more samples may be required. Low standards of aseptic technique during the collection of blood and its inoculation into liquid media can produce misleading contamination of the culture with irrelevant micro-organisms. Antimicrobials which may have been administered up to 3 weeks before the onset of septicaemia may have influenced the susceptibility of the isolate to antimicrobials; if the patient is already on treatment for a concomitant infection, small amounts of antibiotics present in the blood sample may inhibit bacterial growth. On all such occasions relevant data must be relayed to the laboratory so that steps can be taken to inactivate residual antibiotics, and the possibility of altered susceptibilities to antimicrobials can be evaluated. The presumptive focus of infection and provisional diagnosis should also be known to the laboratory. In pyrexia of unknown origin advice should be sought from the microbiologist.

Shock and disseminated intravascular coagulation

Gram-negative bacteria are potent inducers of shock. Over a third of all Gram-negative septicaemias are complicated by ineffective tissue perfusion of which oliguria is a leading clinical expression. The early signs are high temperature, decreased peripheral vascular resistance, raised central venous pressure and increased cardiac output so that, initially, the extremities are warm. Later, as the peripheral vascular resistance is increased and both the central venous pressure and the cardiac output fall, the extremities become cold and the classic manifestations of shock appear. Activation of the coagulation cascade, the release of pro-coagulants and endothelial injury are responsible for disseminated intravascular coagulation (*see* p. 878).

Endogenous infections

From the skin flora

Aerobic micrococci, diphtheroids, Propionibacterium acnes and, in children, *Sarcina sp.* are the predominant commensals of the normal skin flora. These bacteria are resident mainly in the superficial layer of the *stratum corneum* and upper part of the hair follicles. Few can be detected deeper in the follicular canals. Moist and warm areas (e.g. axillae, perineum) may be inhabited by *Alkaligenes sp.*, *Herella sp.*, *Mima sp.* and other Gram-negative organisms. Superficial infections such as eczema, psoriasis, burns, furuncles, cellulitis, fistulae and abscesses greatly increase the microbial burden of the skin and the risks of dispersal and cross-contamination.

Repeated preoperative applications of chlorhexidine or triclosan in alcoholic solution can rapidly and markedly reduce the numbers of superficial resident and transient organisms. Contamination with bacterial spores may be more appropriately dealt with by mechanical cleaning with grease solvents (e.g. Swarfega), followed by treatment with povidone-iodine. It is, of course, preferable to treat skin infections before elective surgery. At least two preoperative baths with added triclosan or chlorhexidine will significantly reduce the number of skin organisms. However, even gentle preoperative shaving may, by traumatising the epidermis, release resident organisms from deep areas. It is better not to shave the skin at all but, if this is considered necessary, then electric hair clippers should be used. If wet shaving is employed, triclosan shaving foam should be used, followed by repeated applications of alcoholic chlorhexidine or triclosan.

From the normal or altered flora of the gastrointestinal tract or body cavities

Normally none but the occasional acid-fast bacterium is found in the stomach. Few micro-organisms ($<10^3$/ ml) are found in the normal jejunum, gallbladder and bile ducts, pancreas, uterus and urinary tract. However, in the presence of obstruction, cancer or inflammation, the numbers increase appreciably. While bile salt, lysosyme and IgA determine those species of bacteria which descend the small intestine, their number is largely controlled by the gastric acid which, in turn, is regulated by the type of diet and frequency of feeding. The microbial community harboured in the normal ileum, appendix and colon is enormous. Microbiologically, the large intestine is simply an efficient continuous culture fermenter using biliary secretions, dietary and intestinal residues to achieve a final concentration of up to 10^{11} organisms per gram of faeces (in English subjects). Factors such as diet, ethnic origin and geographical variation, especially residence in the tropics, can influence the colonic flora in number and species.

Surgery will expose the patient to the risk of infection by his own potentially pathogenic microflora. The longer the preoperative period in hospital, the higher will be the incidence of colonisation with hospital strains, often resistant to antimicrobials. Preparation of the bowel with laxatives, enemata or, better, orthograde lavage (whole-bowel irrigation), supplemented with oral chemoprophylaxis, can appreciably reduce the incidence of postoperative sepsis. Incisions through adhesive plastic drapes cannot prevent parietal contamination and wound sepsis, although it is an advantage to have the surgical towels held in place without the use of metal clips. The value of antiseptic instillation or lavage has not been unequivocally established in comparative, controlled clinical trials, but it would appear that chlorhexidine or povidone-iodine in detergent solution can reduce the bacterial inoculum in accidental trauma. Povidone-iodine was found to be as effective as antibiotics in reducing the incidence of postoperative abdominal sepsis. Peritoneal lavage with noxytiolin or iodophores was also reported to be satisfactory. Intravesicular noxytiolin may reduce infections related to urinary catheterisation. In emergency colonic surgery, 20 min exposure of the bowel flora to iodophor (as an enema) has been shown to reduce the bacterial burden significantly.

Even a small bacterial inoculum may cause local inflammation, but if a suture, incision or anastomosis leaks allowing gross contamination, peritonitis, septicaemia and abscess formation are likely consequences. Spillages of visceral contents should be minimised by careful use of suction and clamps. A heavily contaminated wound may require drainage through separate stab wounds, and systemic chemotherapy. Delayed primary wound closure, as initially practised by Billroth, can prevent deep anaerobic infections, but this benefit has to be balanced against the risk of exogenous contamination of the drains or open dressings. Compared with Penrose drains, wound suction drains are associated with significantly lower infection rates.

Exogenous infections

Peroperatively

A minimum of 10 min surgical scrub with an antiseptic/detergent solution is the single most important factor in preventing peroperative surgeon-induced infection. A 4% chlorhexidine/detergent solution followed by a rinse with alcoholic chlorhexidine will rapidly eliminate transient skin flora, but use of a Triclosan detergent solution may be even more effective since the cumulative bacterial reduction brought about by this antiseptic can maintain protection between handwashings.

Lapses in the proper use of caps, face masks, gloves and gowns are of great importance. Several types of commercially available single-use protective clothing do not meet the intended specifications. For example, a face mask should be an effective barrier, preventing the passage of nasopharyngeal and other organisms in either direction, but many types commercially supplied do not filter bacteria efficiently. All drapes should be

kept dry because when moist, microbial penetration is facilitated. Microbial pollution of the theatre occurs frequently when the occupants sneeze or talk, less frequently when they cough and very rarely during normal breathing. Well's droplet nuclei are bacteria-laden particles which can remain suspended in the air for a considerable time; 1–3 μm residues from dried droplets can remain suspended in the air indefinitely. Generally the number of airborne bacteria-laden particles in the operating theatre is proportional to the number of staff present and general traffic. On many occasions the total number of individuals who come in and out of the operating room may exceed the size of the surgical team by as much as ten-fold.

In comparison with conventional turbulent ventilation systems, unidirectional (laminar) flow and high-efficiency particulate air-filtered (HEPA) systems can reduce airborne bacteria by 100-fold. However, for most operations, conventional, less sophisticated and less expensive precautions are adequate to prevent airborne contamination. Whenever possible class I operations should be programmed first, class III last; a separate theatre should be reserved for class IV procedures (e.g. opening of abscesses). Ultra-violet irradiation is not an effective substitute for mechanical cleaning. The most effective means of reducing the burden of microbial contamination in the operating theatre environment remains simply zeal and attention to detail in manual cleaning of the floor and horizontal surfaces with a quality detergent and hot water, between operations and at the end of each session. Disinfectant mats and plastic overshoes are of limited value.

In the ward

Postoperative exogenous wound infections initiated in the ward are not as significant or as frequent as peroperative infections. However, many infections originate from previous cross-contamination and colonisation of patients with micro-organisms acquired from the hospital milieu. The rate of colonisation with coagulase-positive staphylococci and pseudomonads doubles every week of hospitalisation. Crowded open wards facilitate cross-infection; modern designs, providing separate 4–6 bedded units with adequate toilet facilities and single-bed isolation rooms, are thought to be better.

The wearing of face masks during wound dressings plays only a minor role in preventing contamination. However, domestic cleaning procedures and other activities should be avoided at least 30 min before dressings, as they may increase aerial contamination. Provision of well-equipped sterile dressing packs and training of staff in no-touch aseptic techniques are essential. A well-sutured wound is protected from the ward environment but exudate is a superb medium for bacterial proliferation. Non-drained, clean and dry wounds should not be disturbed; application of antiseptics or antibiotics is not necessary. Drained wounds should be protected by dressings until the drain is removed. Following class III or IV operations or in the management of septic wounds, dressings are essential in preventing cross-infection. Thorough handwashing before and after each aseptic procedure is of paramount importance.

Pathogenic or opportunistic bacteria can be transmitted by direct skin contact or indirectly through instruments, fluids, dressings and bedding, or by airborne droplet nuclei (from the respiratory tract), nebulisers, skin scales and dust. Enterobacteria are transmitted mainly by direct or indirect contact while staphylococcal dissemination is both airborne and by contact. Standard isolation techniques are essential in infectious diseases hospitals, but limited isolation facilities are also a very useful provision in district general hospitals. With the exception of serum hepatitis, surgery in patients with underlying infectious diseases is infrequent. However, isolation of surgical patients can be mandatory for prevention of the dissemination of antibiotic-resistant organisms. Containment (or source) isolation with barrier nursing in a single room under a negative air pressure of not less than 15 air changes per hour is necessary to prevent dissemination of flucloxacillin-resistant staphylococci; barrier nursing is increasingly used to prevent transfer of multiply-resistant enterobacteria between patients. Protective (or reverse) isolation under positive air pressure may prevent the establishment of nosocomial sepsis in transplanted or immunocompromised patients.

Walls, floor and ceiling should be kept domestically clean; the use of disinfectants, unless surfaces become heavily contaminated with body fluids, does not offer special advantages. However, all items which have been in contact with an infectious patient should be sterilised or disinfected after use, and definitely on discharge of the patient. A policy laying down the indications, procedures and frequency of disinfection is invaluable.

Instrumentation in general is the commonest cause of iatrogenic hospital infection. Indwelling urinary catheters, often inserted by inadequately trained staff, account for numerous hospital infections. Urinary catheter-related infections are endogenous from the patient's perineal flora. Bacteria can penetrate through the meatus, through the junction between the distal part and the proximal drainage tube and through reflux from the collection pouch. A closed drainage system, if it remains closed, definitely delays the development of bacteriuria. Antiseptics around the meatus and intravesicular irrigations with noxytiolin can further reduce the incidence of bacteriuria. The insertion of a urinary catheter should be prescribed only when absolutely essential: not infrequently, bladder catheters are inserted merely to measure urinary output! Of the 10–15% of all patients who are subjected to urinary catheterisation, 1 in 5 will suffer infection. More than one catheterised patient in the same ward dramatically increases the cross-infection rate, as unavoidable spillages of urine enrich the environmental bacterial population.

Peripheral and central venous catheters, arterial lines, nasal, oral or endotracheal intubation, parenteral nutrition and other invasive procedures account for three-quarters of all postoperative infections. Thrombophlebitis and septicaemia are major infective complications of intravascular manipulations. Their incidence depends on the location, type and size of catheter, the nature of the infused fluid and duration of the procedure. Sterile intravenous preparations, adequate skin antisepsis and experience in aseptic techniques are essential in preventing iatrogenic infection. In general, applications of antiseptics and antibiotics locally may prevent bacterial invasion, but their value has not been demonstrated unequivocally.

Bacteriology of surgical infections

Aerobic Gram-positive bacteria

Although the high incidence of staphylococcal sepsis experienced in the 1950s and 1960s has declined, *Staphylococcus aureus* is still the predominant pathogen; about half of all Gram-positive infections are due to coagulase-positive staphylococci. One in three of all staphylococcal infections is endogenous. On admission the patients may be carrying penicillin-susceptible strains. However, within two days following admission, most patients will have enriched their flora with hospital strains, usually penicillin-resistant and occasionally flucloxacillin-resistant. The remaining two-thirds of infections are acquired exogenously; most in the operating theatre; some in the wards, mainly by direct contact during dressing procedures. Airborne contamination is important in large exposed wounds or burns, but perhaps more important in replenishing the human reservoir. Isolation of *Staphylococcus aureus* from the anterior nares or perineum of patients or staff indicates carriage, while detection at other body sites may be indicative of no more than a transient presence. Epidemic strains of *Staphylococcus aureus* can be identified by bacteriophage-typing, but the origin and route of infection are variable and not always possible to trace. Treatment and, if necessary, isolation of dispersing patients and/or staff, particularly when colonised or infected with flucloxacillin-resistant strains, are essential for the control of the dissemination of staphylococcal sepsis.

Streptococci in Lancefields groups B, C and G, enterococci, non-haemolytic streptococci and other Gram-positive organisms are sporadically involved in deep infections, particularly when necrotic tissue or foreign bodies are present. Although since the 1940s the incidence of streptococcal sepsis has decreased, sporadic, endemic or epidemic streptococcal or staphylococcal infections can follow dissemination of these organisms from the nasopharynx and body surfaces of carriers, via droplet nuclei or squames.

Aerobic Gram-negative bacteria

Since the early 1960s, the incidence of sepsis due to enterobacteria has increased alarmingly. Three factors may be predisposing to these infections:

1 The invasive procedures of modern surgery (arterial or venous catheters, tracheostomies, parenteral nutrition) create opportunities for microbial colonisation and new routes of microbial penetration into susceptible tissue. Long operations on older and/or immunocompromised patients are major predisposing factors.
2 The predilection of Gram-negative bacilli to establish reservoirs in any humid environment, including antiseptic solutions, has been facilitated by changes in medical care and modern hospital equipment.
3 Indiscriminate chemotherapy enhances the tendency of intestinal bacteria to develop resistance to antimicrobials almost overnight by conjugation and selection.

Gram-negative bacteria are involved in almost any type of surgical sepsis. Initially these are endogenous infections, originating mainly from the patient's colonic flora, but are rapidly transmitted to other patients by direct contamination of the hands, instruments and environment. *Escherichia coli* is the predominant coliform. In many hospitals pseudomonas, proteus and klebsiella infections are endemic.

Anaerobic bacteria

Despite the fact that anaerobes outnumber aerobes in all body cavities, their full pathogenic significance has been recognised widely only in the last decade. The poor record of recovery of anaerobes from conventional clinical specimens can be explained by the two prerequisites for their existence: an oxidation-reduction potential (Eh) as low as -250 mV and absence of oxygen. The high Eh ($+126$ to $+246$ mV) of normal tissue does not allow anaerobiosis. Some anaerobes are more oxygen-labile than others; for example *Clostridium perfrigens* survives at oxygen tensions at which *Clostridium tetani* is killed. The absence of capillary perfusion is the key factor determining the lowered Eh within hollow viscera and the body cavities. When accidental or surgical trauma intrudes upon or occurs in the vicinity of such anaerobic microbial habitats, large numbers of autochthonous flora contaminate tissues in which the Eh has been drastically reduced by ischaemia and interruption of capillary blood flow. The avid consumption of available oxygen by concomitant aerobic organisms further reduces the Eh and thus favours the replication of stricter anaerobes.

Anaerobic growth is commonly associated with abscess formation and such abscesses are prone to rapid extension as the bacterial exotoxins and other poisons produce necrosis in surrounding tissue. The ten exotoxins of *Clostridium perfrigens* are decisive elements in the pathogenesis of clostridial myonecrosis, particularly in predisposed patients (e.g. diabetics, arteriosclerotics, etc.) or in an avascular prosthesis in certain class I operations. Non-clostridial gas-gangrene is a polymicrobial infection with Bacteroides and other intestinal anaerobes. The tetanospasmin and tetanolysin of *Clostridium tetani* can be devastating. Many anaerobes can be involved concomitantly and, occasionally, synergistically in the same infection site.

Anaerobic infections frequently lead to suppurative thrombophlebitis with pulmonary or portal emboli. The resistance to bile of *Bacteroides fragilis* and *Clostridium perfrigens* explains their involvement in biliary tract infections. In lower respiratory infections, *Bacteroides melaninogenicus*, *Peptostreptococcus sp.* or *Veillonella sp.* can be responsible for pneumonitis, extending to necrotising pneumonia or empyema. In the gastrointestinal tract *Bacteroides fragilis* predominates but *Clostridium perfrigens*, *Clostridium septicum* or *Fusobacterium necrophorum* (the spindleform hearse bacterium) can also invade through mucosal ulceration and cause septicaemia and metastatic abscesses. Rupture of the appendix, trauma or a leaking suture will expose the poorly vascularised peritoneum to an enormous inoculum of the colonic polulation. The acute inflammatory response to the aerobic bacilli will predispose to subsequent anaerobic bacterial proliferation and abscess formation: abdominal abscesses being self-sustaining will always require surgical drainage.

Laboratory diagnosis

Microbiological investigations should be instigated without delay upon clinical suspicion of infection in order to:

1 confirm the diagnosis and assess the severity of sepsis;

2 isolate the causative agent(s) and assay their susceptibility to antimicrobials;

3 identify all isolates of a similar biochemical profile for the detection of possible cross-infection, and to establish a detailed knowledge of the distribution, frequency of isolation and antibiotic sensitivity patterns of various infectious agents within the particular hospital concerned.

This is the only basis upon which early, but rational, clinical decisions regarding the treatment and handling of patients can be made subsequently.

Collection of specimens

The collection of specimen material in sufficient quantity from the correct site is essential. Senior surgeons usually delegate this important task to their junior colleagues and juniors to nurses. Of ten specimens received in the laboratory, two will usually have been collected from inappropriate sites. The collection of useful material may be discouraged by the pain and discomfort which sampling may cause to the patient. The importance of thorough preparation of the site before sampling in order to remove contaminants is usually not appreciated; this necessary but time-consuming preliminary step is often omitted. Antiseptic or detergent solutions should be avoided as they can inhibit or kill the significant micro-organisms. Irrigation with saline is satisfactory. If a specimen referred to the laboratory is not representative of the infection and site, or is contaminated with irrelevant micro-organisms, then expensive investigations can only be misleading; three out of ten clinical specimens received at the author's laboratory fall within this category.

The optimum specimen is the actual exudate or tissue taken into a sterile container before blind treatment is commenced. Fluid should be collected into a sterile bottle containing anticoagulant (i.e. sodium citrate) to prevent bacteria being trapped within a clot. Biopsies from lymph nodes or other tissues should be placed into sterile containers with saline to prevent drying. Placing specimens into formalin is of value for histopathological examination only: formaldehyde, at the concentrations used for tissue fixation, will kill all micro-organisms probably within seconds. In special circumstances, quantitative microbiology on tissue biopsy may distinguish contamination from infection: $>10^5$/g bacteria would normally be present in infected tissue. A swab dipped into an exudate is much less satisfactory than collection of the exudate itself in a

sterile bottle. Swabs should be used only when the material available is too limited to be collected by other means; they should be inserted immediately after collection into a non-nutritious transport medium, such as Amies inorganic phosphate base. This system (Transwab) prevents the specimen from drying and preserves delicate organisms and anaerobes during transport. If obligate or facultative anaerobic organisms are suspected, a generous specimen should be placed immediately into a special prereduced and buffered transport medium. The reducing agents present in transport media combine with free oxygen to maintain the anaerobic conditions which are essential for the recovery of these oxygen-labile microbes. Aspirating pus in a syringe and forwarding the filled syringe and attached needle to the laboratory can maintain anaerobes viable for up to 1 h but this practice may contravene Health and Safety regulations. The practice of placing specimens on surgical towels, gauzes or gloves, is not only inefficient – the specimen will dry out – but dangerous: the risk of dissemination of potentially pathogenic micro-organisms to the hospital environment is obvious. Specimens, even when in transport medium, should be transferred to the laboratory and processed immediately. Delay can increase the number of contaminants at the expense of more fastidious organisms.

Microscopic examination

The elementary step of examination of a Gram-stained direct smear can be most informative and must never be omitted. An experienced microbiologist can evaluate a smear within 5 min, whereas the time taken to report on cultures depends on the relatively long period of incubation that bacterial growth requires. Delicate species may not survive the change of environment during collection and transport. However, since the Gram reagents can stain both viable and dead bacteria, such organisms may be detected only on the direct film. Naturally, it is to be expected that macroscopically purulent specimens will contain polymorphonuclear leukocytes in abundance, but the presence of small numbers of such cells in early specimens can provide a valuable clue to the onset of infection. Moreover, a careful analysis of the spatial association between bacteria and pus cells in a film, as for instance in the observation of phagocytosed bacteria, can suggest which of the genera observed are most likely to be of clinical significance in the case under consideration and which, by contrast, are more likely to be 'passengers'. Squames indicate contamination. A list of frequently encountered pathogens with their corresponding Gram reactions and morphologies is presented in Table 1.

Table 1

BACTERIAL MORPHOLOGY AND GRAM REACTION FOR PRESUMPTIVE DIAGNOSIS

	Aerobes and facultative anaerobes	Obligate anaerobes
Gram-positive		
(a) Cocci		
arranged in irregular grape-like clusters	staphylococci	
of uniform size arranged in small groups, or pairs of fours	micrococci	
oval or spherical arranged in chains of varying length	streptococci	peptococci
ovoid or lanceolate arranged in pairs with broad ends opposed	pneumococci	peptostreptococci
(b) Bacilli		
arranged in pairs end-to-end or at an acute angle (V forms)	*Listeria sp.*	
pleomorphic, irregular staining, arranged in palisades, angled pairs or 'chinese lettering'	corynebacteria	
small, branching	*Nocardia sp.*	*Actinomyces sp.*
endospore forming, occurring in chains	*Bacillus sp.*	
endospore bearing, spores often wider than vegetative forms		clostridia
Gram-negative		
(a) Cocci		
oval, arranged in pairs	*Branhamella sp.*	
coccoid	*Acinetobacter sp.*	
minute, occurring in masses		*Veillonella sp.*
(b) Bacilli		
large, single	enterobacteria	
short or pleomorphic; possible bipolar staining	*Moraxella sp.; Pasteurella sp.*	
short or cocci-bacilli arranged singly or in pairs	*Yersinia sp.*	
with rounded ends		*Bacteroides sp.*

Cultures

Direct smear examination must always be supported by culture. Specimens are routinely inoculated on to blood agar and McConkey's agar to be incubated aerobically and on to selective blood agar for anaerobic incubation. Overnight incubation is sufficient for the growth of most pathogens. Aerobic cultures can be reported at 18 h and anaerobic at 36 h, including antibiograms. Fast diagnosis at generic level, plus advice on treatment, can have a decisive role in patient care, whereas a report delayed by several days in order to include the precise bacterial nomenclature will generally have lost most of its practical value.

Full biochemical identification of isolates is normally performed, but for epidemiological rather than clinical reasons.

Rapid diagnostic procedures

There are an increasing number of such sophisticated tests which offer speed and sensitivity without compromising on specificity in any important degree.

Examination of frank pus for obligate anaerobes by gas liquid chromatography takes only 30 min. Immunofluorescence is the classic example of a rapid and specific diagnostic technique. Its specificity depends upon antigen–antibody combination, a reaction detected by conjugating (binding together) purified anti-microbial antibodies with a fluorochrome, which emits visible light when exposed to ultra-violet radiation. In direct immunofluorescence, smears are covered with a fluorescein-conjugated antiserum, specific for the suspected bacterium. The enteropathogenic strains of *Escherichia coli* in faeces, *Streptococcus pneumoniae*, *Neisseria meningitidis* or *Listeria monocytogenes* in cerebrospinal fluid, and *Yersinia pestis*, *Bacillus anthracis*, *Erysipelothrix insidiosa* or the clostridia in exudate or inflamed tissues can be rapidly detected. Application of these tests is limited by the commercial supply of purified reagents, but it is hoped that advances in monoclonal antibody will increase their availability and specificity.

If the patient's defences or current chemotherapy have eliminated viable pathogens from accessible sampling sites, residual bacterial antigen may be specifically detected by counterimmuno-electrophoresis (CIE). Antisera specific to a range of common pathogens are placed into wells cut on an agarose plate and the specimen is put into wells cut opposite; during electrophoresis the negatively charged molecules of the antigen move towards the anode while the antibody molecules move towards the cathode. At the point where these soluble reagents meet and interact specifically, a precipitation line is formed. Thus, *Neisseria meningitidis*, *Streptococcus pneumoniae* and *Haemophilus influenzae* antigens in cerebrospinal, pericardial and pleural fluids, and in sputum, can be detected within 1–4 h. A list of developments in the rapid laboratory diagnosis is presented in Table 2.

Presumptive diagnosis

Given that the nature of the infecting organism is suspected on clinical grounds, or that it has been visualised or provisionally identified, then its antibiotic sensitivity pattern can be predicted. Indeed the susceptibility of certain bacteria to antimicrobials can be so predictable, that *in vitro* sensitivities are not performed (Table 3). For example *Streptococcus pyogenes* and the pneumococcus have retained a high susceptibility to penicillin; the actinomycetes and most clostridia are also fully sensitive to penicillin. Brucellosis, cholera, relapsing fever, the rikettsioses and chlamydial infections respond well to tetracyclines. Lincomycin, metronidazole and erythromycin are active against most important anaerobes. When the presence of anaerobes has been detected, as mentioned previously, by gas liquid chromatography, full identification is not essential since their susceptibility to antimicrobials is still largely predictable.

Susceptibilities to antimicrobials

In vitro the minimum concentration of an antibiotic in mg/l which is inhibitory to the growth of a particular bacterium (MIC) can be determined. Precise quantitative techniques are generally reserved for reference purposes. For routine susceptibilities it is sufficient to place filter paper discs, previously impregnated in a known concentration of the test antimicrobial, on a solid medium inoculated with a standard concentration of the test organism. During incubation the antibiotic diffuses around the disc and, when the required inhibitory concentration is reached, the growth of a sensitive test organism will be inhibited. Interpretation of susceptibilities of micro-organisms to antimicrobials by this simple method has been previously established by extensive studies involving determination of both MIC values and corresponding zone sizes against a large sample of clinical isolates.

In vivo the peak blood level of an antibiotic should exceed the MIC level by two- to four-fold. When the antibiotic is significantly protein-bound or if the infection being treated is of a particularly serious nature, an even higher level is aimed at. The minimum bactericidal concentration (MBC) is a more critical guide than the MIC. The MBC is determined by subculturing a

Table 2

DEVELOPMENTS IN RAPID DETECTION OF BACTERIA IN CLINICAL SPECIMENS

Measurement by	Specimens studied	Time	Agreement with conventional methods
Bioluminescence*	Urine	15 min	89.4%
Chemiluminescence	Urine	NA	NA
Coulter ZBI system	Urine	1–10 min	NA
Counterimmune-electrophoresis*	Various clinical fluids, CSF	1 h	80.0%
Gas liquid chromatography*	Various clinical fluids, blood	30–60 min	NA
Impedance	Various clinical fluids, blood	2.6–3 h	95.8%
Light absorption	Urine Identification of enterobacteria	4–13 h	89.8%
Light scatter	Urine Identification of enterobacteria	5–6 h	89.0%
Limulus amoebocyte lysate pyrogent	Urine, CSF, endotoxin	30 min	poor
Microcalorimetry	Urine	2 h	84.0%
Radiometry of CO_2*	Various clinical fluids, blood	6–24 h	> 90.0%

* This method is applied routinely.

Table 3
CHOICE OF ANTIMICROBIALS FOR PRIMARY SUSCEPTIBILITY TESTING (T) IN SURGICAL SEPSIS

	Staphylo-cocci	Strepto-cocci	Intestinal Gram -ve bacilli	Anae-robes
Penicillin	T	T		T
Flucloxacillin (Clindamycin) (Sodium fusidate)	T			
Clavulanate-potentiated amoxycillin	T	T	T	T
Piperacillin (Azlocillin)			T	
Cefotaxime	T		T	
Latamoxef			T	T
Tobramycin (Amikacin)	T		T	
Erythromycin	T	T		T
Trimethoprim	T	T	T	T
Metronidazole				T

Antimicrobials in parenthesis are reserved for strains insusceptible to the primary choice

minimum inhibited bacterial suspension in order to detect the minimum concentration of antimicrobial which would kill 99.9% of the test organism. In severe infection, i.e. endocarditis, osteomyelitis, meningitis, etc., the concentration of antimicrobial at the site of infection should exceed the MBC rather than the (lower) MIC.

Chemotherapy of surgical infections

Signs of inflammation can vary from a small superficial erythematous area with a little serous discharge, to larger and deeper purulent infections with sinuses, fistulae or cellulitis. Fever, malaise and lymphadenitis, accompanied by peripheral leukocytosis and generalised signs of toxicity, indicate systemic complications. All the characteristics, extent and severity of inflammation should be carefully evaluated. Pain, swelling and a low grade temperature up to 48 h postoperatively, without purulent discharge or signs of severe sepsis, could be attributable to surgical trauma. A rise in temperature following prolonged anaesthesia may be due to pulmonary atelectasis.

Localised, mild or even moderate sepsis without systemic complications in an immunocompetent patient will normally resolve without chemotherapy. Recovery depends much more on the state of the immune system, rather than on chemotherapy. However, intravenous administration of antimicrobials is necessary in severe surgical sepsis in immunocompromised or otherwise predisposed patients and/or in the presence of generalised sepsis. Collection of diagnostic specimens (e.g. wound exudate, pus, urine, sputum, blood) at the onset of a suspected infection, definitely before treatment is initiated, is mandatory.

Empirical chemotherapy

Empirical therapy depends on the evaluation of (a) the anatomic site, signs and degree of inflammation, (b) the nature and class of operation, (c) any predisposing factors, (d) the pattern of previous infections experienced in the patient, and (e) upon a knowledge of the ecology of infecting organisms in the surgical wards of the hospital in question. With these data the most likely organism(s) can be predicted with a high degree of confidence. In septicaemia, determination of the route of entry of micro-organisms into the bloodstream is the key for successful management. A guide to the expected susceptibilities to antimicrobials of hospital pathogens, frequently encountered in surgical sepsis, is presented in Table 4.

Principles of chemotherapy

Rationally prescribed antimicrobials can prevent or treat infections, whether mild or severe. However, their short-term adverse effects are often overestimated while the long-term side-effects are underestimated or ignored. Antimicrobials inappropriately prescribed or administered by a relatively inefficient route can temporarily mask – whilst not eliminating – the primary infection. At the same time the patient is exposed to the risk of occasionally irreversible toxicity and predisposed to superinfection, whilst his acute sepsis may become chronic and the infecting organisms of increased resistance. Even though an individual patient may benefit from a specialist antimicrobial, its use may have been detrimental to the interests of the hospital population at large, because resistant strains emerge. Furthermore, the plethora and variety of antimicrobials available cannot always prevent fatalities from infections due to multiple- or wholly-resistant strains.

A **bactericidal** antibiotic should be preferred whenever chemotherapy is indicated, particularly if the patient's immunity is deficient or when antimicrobials cannot penetrate the focus of infection (e.g. endocarditis). The penicillins, aminoglycosides and cephalosporins are examples of bactericidal classes of antimicrobials. Clindamycin, tetracyclines, suphonamides or other bacteriostatic classes of antimicrobials should not be prescribed on their own as they only inhibit or delay bacterial replication.

A **narrow-spectrum** rather than a wide-spectrum antimicrobial should be preferred when the choice is possible. For example, penicillin in a streptococcal infection is more active, of a narrower spectrum and

Table 4

EXPECTED ANTIBIOGRAMS OF COMMON HOSPITAL PATHOGENS ASSOCIATED WITH SURGICAL SEPSIS

	Pen.[A]	Fluclox.[B]	Clav.-pot.[C] Amoxy.	Piper.[D]	Cefotax.[E]	Latam.[F]	Tobra.[G]	Erythro.[H]	Trimeth.[J]	Metronid.[K]
Staphylococcus aureus (penicillin resistant)	R	$S^{1,2}$	S	R	S	V	S	S	S	R
Streptococcus pyogenes Streptococcus pneumoniae	$S^{1,2}$	S	S	S	S	S	R	S	S	R
Streptococcus faecalis	R	R	$S^{1,2}$	V	R	V	R	R	V	R
Escherichia coli	R	R	S^1	S	S	S	S^2	R	S	R
Klebsiella sp.	R	R	S	V	S	S	$S^{1,2}$	R	S	R
Pseudomonas aeruginosa	R	R	R	S	V	S	$S^{1,2}$	R	R	R
Proteus sp.	R	R	S^1	V	S	S	S^2	R	R	R
Bacteroides sp.	R	R	V	V	R	S	R	R	S	$S^{1,2}$
Other anaerobes including Clostridia	S^1	R	S	S	V	S	R	S	V	S^2

Key:

A = Penicillin
B = Flucloxacillin
C = Clavulanate-potentiated Amoxycillin
D = Piperacillin
E = Cefotaxime
F = Latamoxef
G = Tobramycin/Amikacin
H = Erythromycin
J = Trimethoprim
K = Metronidazole

S = most strains susceptible
R = most strains resistant
V = variable susceptibility
1 = best choice when susceptibility is known
2 = best choice for empirical therapy

less expensive than cephalosporins. Whenever a wide-spectrum drug is administered all the microbial flora, in addition to the infecting organisms, are affected. Commensals, often unrelated to the pathogens, may become insusceptible to the antimicrobial used and this resistance can then be easily transferred *in vivo* to other genera, previously sensitive. Whether wisely or irrationally prescribed, broad-spectrum antimicrobials contribute greatly to the wide-spread problem of antibiotic resistance in the hospital microbial environment and in the community in general.

A **single agent** is preferable, although concomitant administration of antimicrobials can achieve synergy (e.g. penicillin-class + aminoglycoside for *Streptococcus faecalis* or carbenicillin-class + aminoglycoside for *Pseudomonas aeruginosa* infections), prevent inactivation (e.g. clavulanate-potentiated amoxycillin) or the emergence of resistance (e.g. triple regimen in tuberculosis). Combination of two antibiotics may be appropriate when the range of possible agents is wide and unpredictable (e.g. chemoprophylaxis during neutropenia). Combinations of more than two antimicrobials are often a mark of the inexperienced prescriber.

All antimicrobials are either allergenic or toxic or both. The allergenicity of penicillins and cephalosporins, hepatotoxicity of tetracyclines and erythromycin estolate, haematotoxicity of chloramphenicol, high ototoxicity and nephrotoxicity of the early aminoglycosides and the pseudomembranous colitis associated with clindamycin and other wide-spectrum antimicrobials, illustrate some of the risks of chemotherapy. Although in a life-threatening infection sustaining life is more important than, for example, preserving the kidney and hearing functions, the least nephrotoxic and ototoxic antimicrobials should be preferred, if a choice of equally effective drugs is available.

Short-term adverse effects

The toxicity associated with the high dosages of antibiotics which are often unavoidable when treating severe infections, must be balanced against their useful therapeutic effects. Some toxic effects are reversible and most can be prevented by regular assessment of the function of the organs responsible for the drug metabolism and elimination (i.e. liver, kidneys). The serum concentration of potentially toxic antibiotics should always be measured and the dosage adjusted accordingly. It is the duty of the prescriber to warn patients of possible adverse effects: hypersensitivity to penicillins and cephalosporins – mediated by humoral reactions – can range from urticaria to anaphylactic shock: a low grade temperature in the absence of local signs of infection or peripheral leukocytosis, but often accompanied by a mild eosinophilia, may be due to a cellular reaction – delayed hypersensitivity – and simply discontinuing the antibiotic or changing to an alternative can eliminate the symptom.

Long-term adverse effects

Man's evolutionary coexistence with thousands of billions of microbes, conventionally called normal flora, is an expression of Nature's harmony. An advantage to the host, conferred by what is in reality a symbiotic relationship, is an increased resistance to infection supplementing the defence mechanisms. This enormous, but finely balanced, population of bacteria is a functional barrier which can efficiently prevent the establishment of potentially pathogenic micro-organisms. However, if the structure of the microbial community is impaired during antibiotic administration, neoplasms or other debilitating conditions, the host is predisposed to infection. The normal flora, particularly in the respiratory and gastrointestinal tract, when exposed to antimicrobials can be altered, replaced, reduced or eliminated. In the absence of microbial competition and antagonism, minorities of commensals can overgrow and assume pathogenicity. Furthermore, others, not normally constituents of the human flora, can become established. Both these groups can infect, especially when the host's immunity is compromised by an underlying condition. When chemotherapy has selected antibiotic-resistant strains or, even worse, resistance has been transferred between various families of organisms, a subsequent infection will be difficult or impossible to treat. Long courses of wide-spectrum antimicrobials (e.g. ampicillin, cephalosporins) can result in pneumonia, urinary tract infection or wound sepsis with Enterobacteria, often multiply resistant to the antimicrobials in common use. Oral or vaginal moniliasis is a common complication of tetracycline administration.

During or immediately after chemotherapy *Staphylococcus aureus*, *Proteus sp.*, *Pseudomonas sp.* and the Klebsiella-Enterobacter-Serratia group can colonise the bowel with alarming rapidity. Pseudomembranous (entero)colitis is a recently recognised antibiotic-associated intoxication which illustrates the consequences of a disturbance in an ecosystem when exogenous micro-organisms colonise a habitat vacated by the normal residents. Ampicillin, clindamycin, lincomycin and occasionally tetracyclines, but also co-trimoxazole, cephalosporins and metronidazole, can favour the establishment of toxigenic *Clostridium difficile*. Apart from pseudomembranous colitis, the exotoxin of this anaerobe is also suspected of causing antibiotic-associated diarrhoea without pseudomembrane formation and even relapses of some cases of chronic inflammatory bowel disease without history of recent antimicrobial chemotherapy. If diarrhoea complicates antibiotic therapy, specimens of stools should be sent to the laboratory for detection of toxigenic strains and/or toxin. Fortunately this serious opportunistic infection responds well to oral vancomycin.

New antimicrobials

Modifications of established antibiotics in the late 70s led to an explosive increase in the number of compounds available; new antimicrobials are launched at the rate of one per month. For example, over three dozen cephalosporins are available or are in the process of being marketed in the near future. This enormous number of apparently different, but actually very similar, agents, is neither required nor welcome: antagonism among manufacturers, confusion to the surgeon and frustration to the microbiologist are more likely effects than any reduction in the infection rate. Because of the well-defined indications, pharmacokinetics and known toxicity of older and established antimicrobials, only the development of resistance should limit their application. Unless a new antimicrobial has been shown in multi-centre, prospective, randomised, controlled, clinical studies, to be more active, less toxic and perhaps less expensive than their established predecessors, very careful thought should be given to the wisdom of its prescription. Enhanced activity against bacteria which have developed resistance to other antimicrobials is emphasised in the promotion of all new compounds. If they do indeed have a significant advantage, this should be conserved by reserving prescriptions for cases in which full bacteriological investigation has shown that their use is appropriate. Wide-spread use can only hasten the day when the advantage of a new compound is lost through the emergence of resistance.

Although broad-spectrum antimicrobials are invaluable in mixed infections, a general preference for their use must be attributed to a failure to make appropriate microbiological investigations, coupled with a misconception that antibiotics are a panacea. Other factors being equal, a narrow-spectrum antimicrobial is always to be preferred: disturbance of the normal flora, for instance, is then much less of a problem. Generally, narrow-spectrum established antimicrobials cost less than newer wider-spectrum derivatives. The cost of treatment should not be allowed to influence appropriate chemotherapy, but in this competitive field, efficacy and price are not always tied together.

Chemoprophylaxis

A postoperative infection can (a) cause pain and discomfort to the patient, (b) lengthen bed occupancy and hence the cost of treatment, (c) jeopardise fine surgical procedures, and (d) necessitate antibiotic treatment with all the associated adverse effects. Thus, chemoprophylaxis seems logical and desirable. Unfortunately, many poorly designed and badly controlled trials, coupled with a widespread belief in the panacea of antimicrobials, have led to confusion and controversy. Inappropriate chemoprophylaxis will not reduce the incidence of surgical sepsis. Instead the onset of symptoms may be delayed and the associated impairment of the normal flora may predispose to subsequent opportunistic infection. The false security of antimicrobial cover may encourage compromises to be made on wound debridement or irrigation and on aseptic standards generally. The key factors in deciding whether antibiotics should be administered prophylactically are the presence of any local or systemic predisposing factors and the risk of irreversible post-infection sequelae.

Topically applied chemoprophylaxis

In accidental wounds local contamination can be reduced with selected antiseptics. The value of peritoneal lavage with antibiotics is not well established. Antimicrobials will reduce the effective size of the faecal inoculum, but it has not been clearly shown that this is reflected in a reduction in subsequent sepsis. In accidental injuries a combination of neomycin, bacitracin and polymixin, or instillation of cephaloridine has been shown in some, but not all, trials, to reduce the incidence of sepsis in high risk patients, but routine use of these measures will result in resistance. Prospective trials have shown that mechanical bowel preparation, supplemented with oral antibiotics (neomycin combined with metronidazole or erythromycin or tetracyclines) before colorectal surgery can significantly reduce the incidence of sepsis and postoperative complications.

Systemically applied chemoprophylaxis

Although theoretically there should be no sepsis following Class I operations in practice, the rate of infection can be up to 5%. This low level cannot be reduced appreciably by chemoprophylaxis. However, impaired body defences and lowered local resistance due to the presence of prosthetic implants are acknowledged indications for prophylaxis.

Postoperative sepsis in class II operations can be as high as 15%. The record of infections associated with a specific type of operation, the extent and duration of surgery and the immune status of the patient, are the factors to be weighed by the surgeon in determining the risk of infection and necessity for prophylaxis in each individual patient. The infection risk in biliary tract surgery is generally low, but when the common bile duct is opened in circumstances which predispose to infection, for example in the presence of carcinoma or stones, or when there is a history of previous biliary surgery, then chemoprophylaxis may be of value. Chemoprophylaxis in alcohol-related acute pancreatitis cannot reduce the incidence of pancreatic abscesses. In emergency abdominal surgery the rate of postoperative sepsis depends on how long the peritoneum was exposed to bowel flora. At least one in two perforated appendices will result in septic complications, while in the presence of acute inflammation without rupture, the infection rate is much lower. Antimicrobials may be indicated in partial gastrectomy, particularly when cancer or haemorrhage are present. The low concentrations of gastric acid in cancer or gastric ulcers allows the survival of many food-borne bacteria; hence in gastrectomy, chemoprophylaxis may be indicated.

Sepsis in class III operations can be as high as 25% and even 75%; in class IV even higher. In colorectal elective surgery with adequate bowel preparation the rate is about 35–40%. Furthermore, leaking bowel contents (e.g. in anterior resections of the rectum) can increase the infection rate to 70%. Antimicrobials can significantly reduce the infection rate in class III and IV operations, but the numerous published data are beset with deficiencies and inconsistencies so that there is no objective basis upon which to base firm guidelines for chemoprophylaxis. In a superficial, well circumcised abscess, a simple drain is sufficient. At the other extreme, in compound tibia fractures or other extensive injuries, the amputation practised in Lister's time can now be avoided with appropriate chemoprophylaxis.

A knowledge of the most likely infecting organisms and of their usual patterns of susceptibility to antimicrobials is essential in selecting the correct antibiotic. Given adequate infection surveillance data, the identity of the infecting organism can usually be predicted. A narrow-spectrum antimicrobial, specific for the anticipated infecting agent should be preferred, as it is less likely to disturb the normal flora unnecessarily. The route, dose and interval of administration should be carefully determined. The principle of peroperative prophylaxis is to reduce the number (infective dose) or eliminate the bacteria which are likely to be introduced via the operating site during surgery. Consequently, chemotherapy before and after the operation is irrelevant and cannot *per se* decrease surgical sepsis. Parenteral administration is preferable to oral because (a) high concentrations are rapidly and predictably obtained, and (b) exposure of all the intestinal microflora to the antimicrobial before its absorption is avoided, thus minimising problems associated with alterations in the flora and the development of resistance. Doses exceeding the MIC of the likely organisms by four-to six-fold should be administered at such time intervals (preferably twice the antimicrobial's half-life) as to achieve a bacteriocidal concentration in the operation site during the time of surgery.

Conclusions

The patient's immune state and a variety of predisposing factors are the main determinants in the management and prognosis of infections. The initiation of appropriate chemotherapy against anticipated or identified pathogens is not necessarily more important than the contribution of the patient's immune system. Antimicrobials simply allow time for the host to deploy additional defences.

The key to a significant reduction in surgical infections is the attitude and practices of the surgeon himself. When antiseptics were not as refined as today and antibiotics had not yet been discovered, the enormous and almost miraculous advances in surgery were realised by enthusiastic surgical scrub and religious adherence to aseptic no-touch techniques. Handwashing before and after examining patients is still essential in reducing hospital infections; the importance of this principle has changed little since Semmelweis's time. No chemicals can ever substitute the human attention to detail which is the optimum prophylaxis, a point made by Halsted in his advocating of gentle tissue handling. High standards of asepsis complement but do not substitute for gentle surgical technique. Modern antimicrobials are often used in infections which should never have been allowed to occur in the first place. In fact, the surgeon's skill alone remains the single most important determinant of the inception of all surgical infections.

Acknowledgements

I am grateful to Dr C. H. Taylor-Robinson and Mr J. E. Corkill for their pertinent advice and helpful comments during the writing of this chapter.

References

The following references to books, monographs and individual papers cover all the main subjects raised in this chapter and will be found a useful guide to further information.

Altemeier W.A. *et al.* (eds) (1976). *Manual on Control of Infection in Surgical Patients*. Philadelphia: J.B. Lippincott Co.

Altemeier W.A., McDonough J.J., Fullen W.D. (1971). Third-day surgical fever. *Arch. Surg*; **103**:158–66.

Ayliffe G.A.J. (1971). Cross sectional surveys of infection. In *Proceedings of the International Conference on Nosocomial Infections*, pp. 282–84. Chicago: American Hospital Association.

Balows A., Dehaan R., Dowell V.R., Guze L.B. (1974). *Anaerobic Bacteria. Role in Disease*. Springfield Ill: Charles C. Thomas.

Bartlett J.G., Chang T.W., Gurwith M., Gorbach S.L., Onderdonk A.G. (1978). Antibiotic-associated pseudomembranous colitis due to toxin-producing clostridia. *New Engl. J. Med*; **298**:531–34.

Bartlett J.G., Gorbach S.L., Tally F.P., Finegold S.M. (1974). Bacteriology and treatment of primary lung abscess. *Amer. Rev. Resp. Dis*; **109**:510–18.

Benveniste R., Davies J. (1973). Mechanism of antibiotic resistance in bacteria. *Ann. Rev. Biochem*; **42**:471–506.

Berger S.A., Nagar H., Weitzman S. (1978). Prophylactic antibiotics in surgical procedures. *Surg. Gynae. Obstet*; **146**:469–75.

British Medical Journal (1980). Sepsis after bowel surgery. *Brit. Med. J*; **1**:882–3.

Bryant R.G., Hood A.F., Hood C.E. (1971). Factors affecting mortality of Gram-negative bacteraemia. *Arch. Int. Med*; **127**:120–8.

Casewell M.W. (1980). Surveillance of infection in hospitals. *J. Hosp. Infec*; **1**:293–7.

Cherry W.B. (1976). Immunofluorescence tests for bacteria. In *Modern Methods in Medical Microbiology Systems and Trends* (Prier J.E., Bartola J., Friedman H., eds.). Baltimore: University Park Press.

Clarke S.K.R. (1957). Sepsis in surgical wounds with particular reference to *Staphylococcus aureus*. *Brit. J. Surg*; **44**:592–6.

Cohen S. (1977). The role of cell-mediated immunity in the induction of inflammatory responses. *Amer. J. Pathol*; **88**:502–28.

Cruse P.J.E. (1970). Surgical wound sepsis. *Can. Med. Ass. J*; **102**:251–8.

Cruse P.J.E. (1977). Infection surveillance. Identifying the problem and the high risk patient. *S. Med. J*; **70**:(suppl.) 4–8.

Cruse P.J.E., Foord R. (1973). A five-year prospective study of 23 649 surgical wounds. *Arch. Surg*; **107**:206–9.

Daschner F., Borneff J., Jackson G.G., Parker M.T. (1978). Detection, prevention and control of hospital acquired infections. *Infection*; **6**:194–6.

Downes E.M. (1977). Late infection after total hip replacement. *J. Bone Jt. Surg*; **59–B**:42–4.

Eliasson R., Mossberg B., Camner P., Afzelius B.A. (1977). The immotile-cilia syndrome: a congenital ciliary abnormality as an etiologic factor in chronic airway infections and male sterility. *New Engl. J. Med*; **297**:1–6.

England D.M., Rosenblatt J.E. (1977). Anaerobes in human biliary tracts. *J. Clin. Microbiol*; **6**:494–8.

Finch W.T., Sawyers J.L., Schenker S. (1976). A prospective study to determine the efficacy of antibiotics in acute pancreatitis. *Ann. Surg*; **183**:667–71.

Fingold S.M. (1977). *Anaerobic Bacteria in Human Disease*. New York: Academic Press.

Gantz N.M., Gleckman R.A. (1979). *Manual of Clinical Problems in Infectious Disease*. Boston: Little, Brown.

Garrod L.P., Lambert H.P., O'Grady F. (1981). *Antibiotic and Chemotherapy*. Edinburgh: Churchill Livingstone.

Gavan T.L. (1974). *In vitro* antimicrobial susceptibility testing. Clinical implications and limitations. *Med. Clin. N.Amer*; **58**:493–503.

Geddes A.M. (1978). Use of antibiotics. *Brit. Med. J*; **2**:181–4.

Gold R.P., Johnson P.M. (1975). Efficacy of combined liver-lung scintillation imaging. *Radiology*; **117**:105–11.

Goldstone J., Moore W.S. (1974). Infection in vascular prostheses: clinical manifestations and surgical management. *Amer. J. Surg*; **128**:225–33.

Gorbach S.L., Bartlett J.G. (1974). Anaerobic infections. *New Engl. J. Med*; **290**:1177–84, 1237–45, 1289–94.

Gray J.A. (1979). Antibacterial prophylaxis – a clinician's view. *Scott. Med. J*; **?**:141–6.

Green J.W., Wenzel R.P. (1977). Postoperative wound infection: a controlled study of the increased duration of hospital stay and direct cost of hospitalization. *Ann. Surg*; **185**:264–8.

Haley R.W. (1981). C.D.C. guidelines on infection control. *J. Infect*; **2**:117–8.

Hermans P.E. (1977). General principles of antimicrobial therapy. *Mayo Clinic Proc*; **52**:603–10.

Howe C.W. (1954). Postoperative wound infections due to *Staphylococcus aureus*. *New Engl. J. Med*; **251**:411–7.

Howe C.W. (1966). Experimental studies on determinants of wound infection. *Surgery*; **60**:1072–6.

Jepson D.B., Mortensen N. (1980). Prevalence of nosocomial infection and infection control in Denmark. *J. Hosp. Infect*; **I**:237–44.

Karren S. (1980). Septicaemia in surgical patients. In *Controversies in Surgical Sepsis*, pp. 179–90. Eastbourne and New York: Praeger Publishing.

Keighley M.R.B., Drysdale R.B., Quoraishi A.H. (1976). Antibiotics in biliary disease: the relative importance of antibiotic concentrations in the bile and serum. *Gut*: **17**:495–500.

Klimek J., Quintiliani R. (1977). Resistant staphylococci in hospitals. *Lancet*; **i**:255–6.

Krizek T.J., Robson M.C. (1975). Evolution of quantitative bacteriology in wound management. *Amer. J. Surg*; **130**:579–84.

Kucers A., Bennett N. eds. (1979). *The Use of Antibiotics. A Comprehensive Review with Clinical Emphasis*, 3rd edn. London: William Heinemann Medical.

The Lancet (1978). Bowel preparation for surgery. *Lancet*; **ii**:1132–4.

Laufman H. (1978). The control of operating room infection: discipline, defense mechanisms, drugs, design and devices. *Bull. New York Acad. Med*; **54**:465–83.

Lazarchick J., Desouza E., Silva N.A., Nichols D.R. (1973). Pyogenic liver abscess. *Mayo Clin. Proc*; **48**:349.

Levine L., McComb J.A., Dwyer R.C. (1966). Active-passive tetanus immunization. *New Engl. J. Med*; **274**:186–90.

Lidwell O.M. (1980). The ventilation of surgical operating rooms. *J. Hosp. Infect*; **1**:285–7.

Lowbury E.J.L., Ayliffe G.A.J., Geddes A.M., Williams J.D. eds. (1981). *Control of Hospital Infection*. London: Chapman and Hall.

McCabe W.R., Jackson G.G. (1962). Gram-negative bacteremia. I. Etiology and ecology. *Arch. Inter. Med*; **110**:847–55, 856–64.

McLeish A.R., Keighley M.R.B., Bishop H.M. (1977). Selecting patients requiring antibiotics in biliary surgery by immediate gram stains of bile at operation. *Surgery*; **81**:473–7.

Meakins J.L. (1978). Infection control in the surgical intensive care unit. *Can. J. Surg*; **21**:78–81.

Meers P.D. (1980). The organization of infection control in hospitals. *J. Hosp. Infect*; **1**:187–91.

Meers P.D. (1981). Infection in hospitals. *Brit. Med. J*; **282**:1246.

National Health Service (1953). The National Health Service (pay-bed accommodation in hospitals, etc.), No. 420 Regulations, pp. 10–13. London: Her Majesty's Stationary Office.

Polk H.C. Jr., Lopez-Mayor J.F. (1969). Postoperative wound

infection: a prospective study of determinant factors and prevention. *Surgery*; **66**:97–103.

Public Health Laboratory Service (1960). Incidence of surgical wound infection in England and Wales: a report of the Public Health Laboratory Service, Great Britain. *Lancet*: **ii**:659–63.

Raahave D. (1976). Effect of plastic skin and wound drapes on the density of bacteria in operation wounds. *Brit. J. Surg*; **63**:421–6.

Rubin R.H., Swartz M.N., Malt R. (1974). Hepatic abscess: changes in clinical, bacteriologic and therapeutic aspects. *Amer. J. Med*; **57**:601–10.

Rytel M.W. (1975). Counter immunoelectrophoresis in diagnosis of infectious disease. *Hosp Pract*; **10**:75–82.

Saik R.P., Greenburg A.G., Farris J.M. (1975). Spectrum of cholangitis. *Amer. J. Surg*; **130**:143–50.

Saunders R.C. (1970). The changing epidemiology of subphrenic abscess and its clinical and radiological consequences. *Brit. J. Surg*; **57**:449–55.

Sherman N.J., Davis J.R., Jesseph J.E. (1969). Subphrenic abscess: a continuing hazard. *Amer. J. Surg*; **117**:117–23.

Stamm W.E. (1975). Guidelines for prevention of catheter-associated urinary tract infections. *Ann. Int. Med*; **83**:386–9.

Steere A.C., Mallison G.F. (1975). Handwashing practices for the prevention of nosocomial infections. *Ann. Int. Med*; **83**:683–90.

Stone H.H., Hooper C.A., Kolb L.D. (1976). Antibiotic prophylaxis in gastric, biliary and colonic surgery. *Ann. Surg*; **184**:443–52.

Strachan C.J.L., Wise R. (1979). *Surgical Sepsis*. New York: Grune and Stratton.

Swenson R.M., Lorber B., Michaelson T.C. (1974). The bacteriology of intra-abdominal infections. *Arch. Surg*; **109**:398–9.

Wang S.M.S., Wilson S.E. (1977). Subphrenic abscess: the new epidemiology. Arch. Surg; **112**:934–6.

Washington J.A. II (1975). Blood cultures: principles and techniques. *Mayo Clinic. Proc*; **50**:91–8.

Weissman G. (1974). Introduction. In *Mediators of Inflammation* (Weissmann G., ed.). New York: Plenum Publishing.

Wilkinson P.C. (1974). *Chemotaxis and Inflammation*. London: Churchill Livingstone.

Index